THE REQUISITES

Gastrointestinal Imaging

Fourth Edition

Giles W. L. Boland, MD, FACR
Abdominal Imaging and Intervention
Department of Radiology
Massachusetts General Hospital
Professor of Radiology
Harvard Medical School
Boston, Massachusetts

ELSEVIER
SAUNDERS

ELSEVIER
SAUNDERS

1600 John F. Kennedy Blvd.
Ste 1800
Philadelphia, PA 19103-2899

GASTROINTESTINAL IMAGING: THE REQUISITES,
FOURTH EDITION
ISBN: 978-0-323-10199-8

Library of Congress Cataloging-in-Publication Data

Boland, Giles W. L., author.
Gastrointestinal imaging : the requisites / Giles Walter Boland.-- Fourth edition.
p. ; cm.-- (Requisites) (Requisites in radiology)
Preceded by: Gastrointestinal imaging / Robert D. Halpert. 3rd ed. c2006.
Includes bibliographical references and index.
ISBN 978-0-323-10199-8 (hardcover : alk. paper)
I. Halpert, Robert D. (Radiologist) Gastrointestinal imaging. Preceded by (work): II. Title. III. Series: Requisites series. IV. Series: Requisites in radiology.
[DNLM: 1. Digestive System--radiography. 2. Digestive System Diseases--diagnosis. WI 100]
RC804.R6
616.3'07572--dc23

2013029451

Senior Content Strategist: Don Scholz
Content Development Specialist: Lucia Gunzel
Publishing Services Manager: Patricia Tannian
Senior Project Manager: Claire Kramer
Design Direction: Steven Stave

Printed in the United States of America

Last digit is the print number: 9 8 7 6 5

This book is dedicated to my immediate family (Judith, Sam, Holly, Heidi, and Lucy) for their patience in allowing me to spend the many absent hours necessary to complete this work.

–Giles

Preface to the First Edition

In August of 1879, while attending the Annual Meeting of the American Association for the Advancement of Science in Saratoga, New York, the renowned physician Sir William Osler chanced to meet the inventor, Thomas Edison. Edison, having a passing interest in the medical applications of his inventions, suggested to Osler that it might be possible to "illumine the interior of the body by passing a small electric burner into the stomach." Sir William's response is not recorded, but his account of the encounter suggests some degree of amusement at the prospect of passing a tube with a light on the end into the stomach.

Nevertheless, Edison's words were prophetic and 114 years later, endoscopic direct visualization of the mucosal surface has established itself as the standard of gastrointestinal (GI) diagnosis, following several decades of virtual domination of this field by radiologists. However, the expected demise of radiological imaging of the gastrointestinal tract has not occurred. Instead, a collaborative, complementary relationship between endoscopy and radiological imaging of the gut has evolved, spurred on and encouraged by the profound effect of cost constraint and the increasing diagnostic sensitivity and relatively low cost of the radiological procedures.

Barium studies have decreased but not disappeared since the advent of widely available endoscopy. Moreover, the technical refinement of low-cost barium examinations may, in all likelihood, carve out a well-defined niche as a screening examination for many patients.

In addition, the development of other imaging methods has tremendously enhanced the role of imaging in GI diagnosis. Without doubt, the use of helical computer-assisted tomography, real-time ultrasound, and to an increasing extent, magnetic resonance imaging has greatly impacted gastrointestinal imaging. Indeed, modern cross-sectional multiplanar imaging has opened the abdomen for radiological inspection in a way that had been hitherto unattainable. Enhanced liver diagnosis and evaluation of the spleen, pancreas, lymphatics, and the structures surrounding the gut are now possible and signal the beginning of yet a new era in abdominal imaging and diagnosis.

In recent decades, our clinical colleagues have developed what they refer to as the problem-oriented approach to patient care and patient records. This refers to an orderly approach to patient diagnosis and management wherein the problems of greatest concern are appropriately weighted, while diagnoses of lesser importance are not lost sight of or neglected in the process. The goal is to establish a global perspective of patient care. Moreover, it should also facilitate a more readable and organized medical record.

In a similar fashion, we have tried to view the "radiological terrain" through the eyes of a first-year resident, a resident preparing for boards, or possibly a radiologist desiring to acquire a concise and abbreviated review of the specialty of gastrointestinal imaging. It would seem appropriate, from our view, to develop a problem-oriented approach to radiology to best address all of these demands and to attempt to present radiological problem solving (diagnosis) in an organized prioritized fashion.

This is generally referred to in radiology as the pattern approach. However, in keeping with a patient-oriented perspective on the practice of radiology, I would prefer to call these radiological patterns of disease "problems." The irregular thickened gastric fold, from the referring physician's point of view (and especially the patient's perspective) is not a pattern, but a problem! For the attending radiologist, the issue is one of problem solving. Although some may see this as nothing more than hair splitting and semantics (and they may be correct), it is, nevertheless, an accurate reflection of a philosophical perspective on the practice of radiology, no doubt left over from my days as a family practitioner.

The advantage of this approach, as opposed to the disease-oriented method, is to allow a closer paralleling of the real day-to-day world of radiology, and as a result, be of more practical value. The disadvantage is in the complexities of presenting material. In terms of writing a textbook, it is easier to describe a disease and all its radiological presentations, than to start with the radiological problem and work backward toward a reasonable differential diagnosis. The former is the organizational basis of almost all reference texts, while the latter is the daily experience of most radiologists. However, in the problem-oriented clinical management of a patient, problems often overlap, or the same disease may result in several very different problems. In the same way, a disease may have several radiological presentations. Gastric carcinoma, for example, may present as a problem of gastric folds, gastric mass, or ulceration. Hence, the inherent weakness in such a presentation of material.

Accordingly, we have tried to avoid undue redundancy while at the same time overlapping wherever necessary. Usually, the more in depth discussion will be reserved for the most common radiological problem posed by the disease entity.

Robert D. Halpert, MD

Preface

Much has changed in gastrointestinal radiology (and medicine in general) since the last major new edition of this book in 1999, yet in many ways, much has not. Modern imaging tools are now producing images of exquisite anatomical, physiological, and molecular detail, raising the profile of the specialty and increasing the value of our contribution to medicine. Although radiologists (perhaps gastrointestinal radiologists more than most) have an array of modern, sophisticated tools in their arsenal, these may not benefit the patient unless they are used wisely and prudently. The ubiquity of imaging devices has made it too easy sometimes for physicians to recommend imaging to investigate the wide range of clinical presentations and for radiologists to recommend further imaging for the management of the incidentaloma, a common finding for the gastrointestinal radiologist. This larger role that radiologists now enjoy must include taking a commensurately larger responsibility for ensuring that imaging is indicated and will benefit the patient. In short, radiologists and referring physicians should recommend imaging only when the benefits outweigh the costs. The central tenet of the profession—"do no harm"—remains just as important in this era of modern medicine as it ever has been.

This book therefore attempts to discuss not only the range of modalities and the spectrum of imaging findings in gastrointestinal disease, but also the most appropriate imaging for a given clinical context. Furthermore, all available imaging modalities are discussed, not just the most modern. Oral contrast (mostly barium) evaluation of the gut has generally been supplanted by endoscopic or cross-sectional imaging techniques, and it has become difficult for the contemporary resident to become familiar with the art of fluoroscopic contrast gastrointestinal studies. These techniques, however, when performed correctly can still yield exquisite (sometimes unique) detail of gastrointestinal pathology and function and consequently are discussed in some detail alongside the newer, more expensive technologies. It is hoped therefore that the reader will gain a deeper knowledge of how and when best to use a specific imaging modality and technique, as well as appreciate the range of imaging findings in gastrointestinal disease.

I would especially like to thank those who contributed images for this book, Michael Zalis, Francis Scholz, Deborah Hall, Avinash Kambadikone, Dushyant Sahani, Joseph Simeone, Jack Wittenberg, Mukesh Harisinghani, Laura Avery, Michael Gee, Peter Hahn, Susanna Lee, Michael Blake, Sheela Agarwal, Edward Palmer, Damian Dupuy, Koenraad Mortele, Jorge Soto, Chandan Kakkar, Rajagopal Kadavigere, Mitchell Tublin, Kumaresan Sandrasegaran, Christine Menias, Perry Pickhardt, Claudio Cortez, Cheri Canon, Mark Lockhart, and Tracy Jaffe, and many others who offered suggestions for particular cases. A special thank you to Eleni Balasalle for all the help in preparing the figures for this book.

All drawings by Giles Boland.

Giles W. L. Boland

Contents

CHAPTER 1

Esophagus

The esophagus extends from the lower pharynx at the upper esophageal sphincter to the lower esophageal sphincter at the esophageal vestibule, or phrenic ampulla, just above the gastroesophageal (GE) junction. It consists of inner circular and outer longitudinal muscle layers. There is striated (voluntary) muscle for the upper third and smooth muscle for the lower two thirds, and the esophagus has no serosal covering at any point. It is lined by squamous columnar epithelium throughout. The course of the esophagus is normally indented by the aortic arch, left main bronchus, and left atrium.

The esophageal vestibule, or phrenic ampulla, is normally slightly distended (Fig. 1-1). At the upper end of the vestibule is a slight narrowing, or A-ring, caused by smooth muscle (internal esophageal sphincter), which can be normal or may cause slight dysphagia if hypertrophied. The B-ring is at the GE junction itself (at the lower end of the vestibule, also known as phrenic ampulla) and is not seen unless a hiatal hernia is present. The Z line may be seen as a slight narrowing at the lower end of the phrenic ampulla and represents the epithelial junction between the esophagus (squamous) and stomach (columnar) and will not be seen unless a hiatal hernia is present. Dysphagia will not occur unless the B ring in the lower esophagus is less than 12 to 13 mm, when it is known as a Schatzki* ring (see discussion later in chapter).

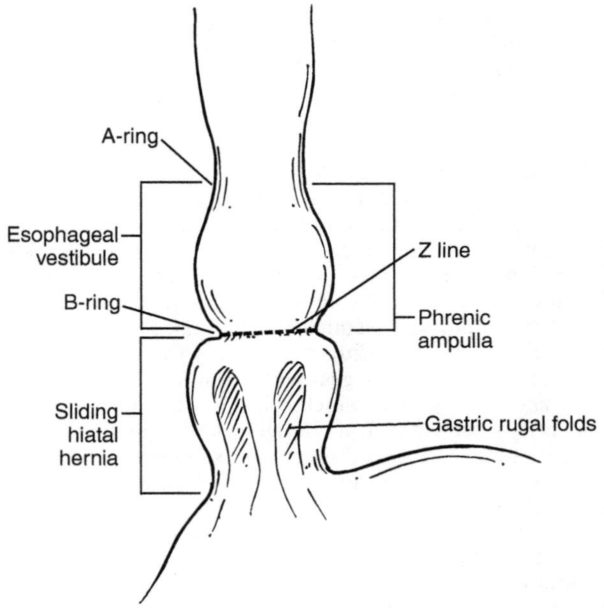

FIGURE 1-1. Schematic representation of lower esophageal anatomy (in the presence of a small hiatal hernia).

TECHNIQUES

Oral Contrast Studies

Although cross-sectional imaging techniques are critical for the evaluation of malignant esophageal disease for staging purposes, most esophageal abnormalities are too small and fine to be accurately evaluated by them. Contrast examination of the esophagus (usually with barium) is an appropriate tool for the evaluation of most esophageal disease, but the radiologist's role has been greatly diminished since the advent and routine use of direct optical endoscopy. However, given that the barium swallow and upper gastrointestinal (UGI) studies can be exquisite tools for the assessment of both morphological (gross appearance of the pharynx, esophagus, GE junction) and functional esophageal abnormalities (pharyngeal function, esophageal dysmotility, gastroesophageal reflux disease [GERD]), radiologists should still be familiar with their use and imaging findings.

A UGI swallow examination is best performed with both single- and double-contrast techniques. Before beginning the examination, the radiologist should further question the patient about his or her symptoms and history. The information gleaned from the patient can offer clues and greater specificity about what the radiologist might expect, and the radiologist might then modify or tailor the examination accordingly. At this point, the radiologist should explain the procedure to the patient because compliance is crucial to obtain an optimal examination. For instance, after the initial ingestion of effervescent gas granules, the patient should try as best as possible to refrain from eructation, which might defeat the purpose of performing a double-contrast examination. Maximal esophageal and gastric distention provides better images and therefore a greater ability to detect subtle disease. In the upright position, the patient then ingests the gas granules, followed by a small sip of water to aid rapid swallowing. The goal is to prevent the granules from "fizzing" in the mouth, which reduces their distensive effect in the esophagus and stomach. The patient then swallows a cup of high-density ("thick") barium, at which point images are taken of the gas-distended esophagus and small mucosal abnormalities can be identified. If any abnormality is identified at this point, multiple tangential views should be taken to allow the radiologist to evaluate the lesion in more detail once the examination is finished. Too often, inadequate oblique and tangential views are taken, resulting in the lesion being visible in a limited plane, which may make formal diagnosis difficult or even impossible. Frequently the examination is performed in conjunction with a UGI series with gastric and duodenal evaluation, and the radiologist will need to then concentrate on these organs while they are maximally distended with air. The radiologist should return later to a final evaluation of the esophagus using a single-contrast examination with low-density ("thin") barium, with the patient typically in the right anterior or prone oblique position. The patient takes several sips of barium, and esophageal motility and distensibility are evaluated as the radiologist observes the stripping waves of esophageal bolus propulsion. The lower esophagus is finally evaluated for hernias and the mucosal B-ring. GERD or a hiatal hernia may not initially be evident, and the patient should be asked to perform a Valsalva* maneuver as a provocative measure to increase intraabdominal

*Richard Schatzki (1901-1992), American radiologist.

*Antonio Maria Valsalva (1666-1723), Italian anatomist.

pressure. This action may elicit either the hiatal hernia or reflux and perhaps be the answer to the patient's symptoms. In this position, the normal longitudinal mucosal relief images are also observed, and this observation may permit variceal visualization. Finally, the stomach and duodenum should be briefly evaluated in case the patient's symptoms are due to disease in these organs.

If the patient's symptom is upper dysphagia, then anteroposterior (AP) and lateral views of the upper esophagus are taken immediately after the ingestion of the effervescent granules. While the patient drinks the barium, the radiologist both observes and performs rapid sequence images (3 to 4 per second) because the barium usually passes through the esophagus too fast for the radiologist to time the exposure correctly. Therefore functional information (i.e., a cricopharyngeus spasm) and morphological disease can be obtained at the same time.

The use of nonionic water-soluble contrast medium, instead of barium, is warranted when there is any risk of aspiration or esophageal leak. Although barium is inert and not toxic if inhaled, it may remain within bronchi for an extended period of time. Ionic contrast medium within the bronchi is hyperosmolar and can cause pulmonary edema and generally should not be used for esophageal examination. Barium is also toxic within the mediastinum and peritoneum, hence the use of nonionic contrast medium if esophageal perforation is suspected. Water-soluble contrast medium, which is less dense than barium, may not identify small leaks. If no initial leak or aspiration is identified, it is then prudent to follow the examination with denser barium, which may identify a small, contained leak. Even if there is some leakage of barium in these circumstances, it will likely be small, given that water-soluble contrast medium failed to identify any leakage.

Contrast studies of the esophagus (including any viscus) are often effective at characterizing the nature of the lesion or abnormality. Extrinsic (extraluminal) masses tend to displace the bowel because of their mass effect and demonstrate shallow, or obtuse, margins on contrast studies (Fig.1-2). Masses that originate in the submucosa (or have an intramural origin) tend to demonstrate sharper, less obtuse margins (Fig. 1-2). Mucosal masses tend to demonstrate acute margins, sometimes pedunculated and sometimes with a stalk. Furthermore, the intraluminal contrast appearances can suggest malignancy or benignity because malignant lesions tend to demonstrate abrupt, sharp margins that are usually irregular (sometimes termed *shouldering*) and are often short (Fig. 1-2). Benign lesions, on the other hand, demonstrate smoother borders with little irregularity, although some larger lesions may ulcerate as they outgrow their vascular supply. These rules of thumb generally apply to the entire gastrointestinal (GI) tract.

Computed Tomography

Computed tomography (CT), although still important in the evaluation of esophageal disease, is not the investigation technique of choice for most diseases unless the patient has esophageal malignancies for which it is used for staging purposes. CT can also be used to evaluate extraluminal or submucosal masses that may impinge on the esophagus because these cannot be observed directly by barium or endoscopic studies. It is also used to evaluate traumatic conditions of perforation, which are iatrogenic, traumatic, or spontaneous. Ideally the patient is asked to drink a cup of contrast material immediately before the CT to delineate the lumen.

Magnetic Resonance Imaging

Magnetic resonance imaging (MRI) has even fewer applications in the esophagus given that respiratory motion artifacts are common when the chest is evaluated with MRI, although it may serve to evaluate mediastinal and paraesophageal abnormalities when CT is not indicated.

Endoscopic Ultrasound

Endoscopic ultrasound has a role in evaluation of submucosal esophageal masses but is rarely performed. Ultrasound has little use otherwise in the esophagus.

Nuclear Medicine

Nuclear medicine still has a role in the functional examination of esophageal motility and reflux disorder, particularly in children. The patient swallows technetium-99m (^{99m}Tc) sulfur colloid, and multiple dynamic views are taken to assess esophageal transit time, particularly in patients with lower esophageal sphincter abnormalities. This test may be used in patients who cannot tolerate manometric endoscopic studies. ^{99m}Tc pertechnetate is also used, particularly in children. After the patient swallows the radiolabelled liquid, multiple dynamic images are obtained for the evaluation of gastroesophageal reflux disease (GERD) or delayed gastric emptying. In an adult, however, the use of positron emission tomography (PET) or PET/CT has become more widespread. The use of PET or PET/CT in the evaluation of the esophagus itself is

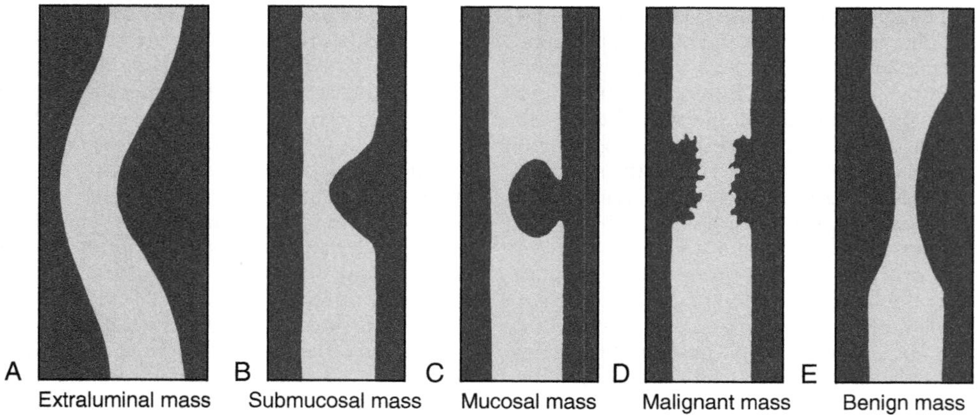

FIGURE 1-2. Schematic representation of extraluminal (**A**), submucosal (**B**), mucosal (**C**), malignant (**D**), and benign (**E**) mass features in contrast imaging of the GI tract.

limited because most primary malignancies can be evaluated directly with endoscopy or by CT. However, PET or PET/CT has proved to be particularly useful in the staging and follow-up assessment of extraesophageal disease, mainly regional lymphadenopathy, which endoscopy cannot see, and CT often cannot determine whether the node is metastatic or benign, particularly if it is small.

DIVERTICULA

Zenker Diverticulum

Zenker* diverticulum is a pulsion diverticulum, usually seen in the elderly, that is due to prolonged intraluminal pressure pushing the esophageal mucosa and submucosa through the medial defect (Killian dehiscence) between the horizontal and oblique fibers of the inferior constrictor muscle at the pharyngoesophageal junction. Patients usually have evidence of esophageal dysmotility and GERD. Patients usually present because of dysphagia, halitosis, and sometimes aspiration pneumonia as fetid food becomes trapped in the diverticulum and steadily enlarges it.

Zenker diverticulum is confirmed at barium swallow as a contrast-filled sac that is posterolateral to the esophagus just above C5-6 and the cricopharyngeus muscle. When it is small, Zenker diverticulum is usually detected best in the true lateral position as a small posterior outpouch, but as it enlarges, it is easy to identify as it extends laterally to avoid the cervical spine (Figs. 1-3 and 1-4). The larger the diverticulum, the greater the compression on the normal esophagus, which can become narrow.

There is an increased incidence of ulceration and carcinoma developing in the diverticulum. Perforation can also occur in patients because of the inadvertent placement of endoscopic instruments or nasogastric tubes.

*Friedrich Albert von Zenker (1825-1898), German pathologist.

Killian-Jamieson Diverticulum

Killian-Jamieson* diverticula are rare; they are observed below the level of the cricopharyngeus muscle, anterolateral to the cervical esophagus. They are also pulsion diverticula through the Killian-Jamieson space (similar to Zenker diverticula) but are much smaller than most Zenker diverticula and therefore produce symptoms and complications less commonly. They are seen as small, rounded, smooth outpouches of the lateral upper esophageal wall (Fig. 1-5). Rarely, they can be large and sometimes confused with Zenker diverticula and can even be observed with CT (Fig. 1-6).

Midesophageal Diverticulum

Midesophageal diverticula are usually anterior, occurring at the level of the carina. They either are due to traction from fibrotic disease in the mediastinum (i.e., healed granulomatous disease), which retracts the whole esophagus toward the fibrotic process, or, more commonly, are due to pulsion from increased intra-esophageal pressure (Figs. 1-7 and 1-8). Traction diverticula in a UGI swallow are usually narrow or triangular with a pointed apex toward the mediastinal disease. Pulsion diverticula typically have a much wider neck, are larger, and fail to empty of barium easily because they have no muscular layer (Fig. 1-9). Most patients with pulsion diverticula have evidence of motility disorders.

Epiphrenic Diverticulum

Epiphrenic diverticula are pulsion diverticula (i.e., the result of increased intraluminal pressure), are found most commonly just cephalad to the GE junction, and are more common in elderly patients with esophageal dysmotility. Most are discovered

*Gustav Killian (1860-1921), German surgeon; Edward Bald Jamieson (1876-1956), Scottish anatomist.

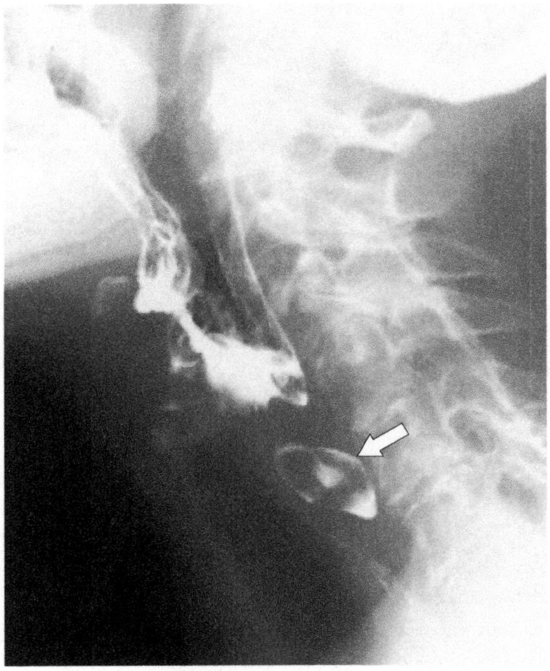

FIGURE 1-3. Lateral UGI swallow in a 76-year-old woman with a small Zenker diverticulum (*arrow*) with a peanut lodged inside.

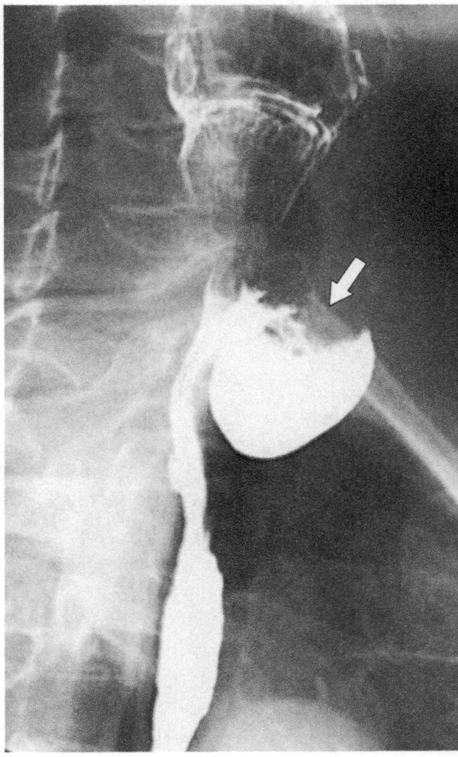

FIGURE 1-4. Left posterior oblique barium swallow in a 69-year-old man with a large outpouching (*arrow*) from the left esophagus due to a Zenker diverticulum.

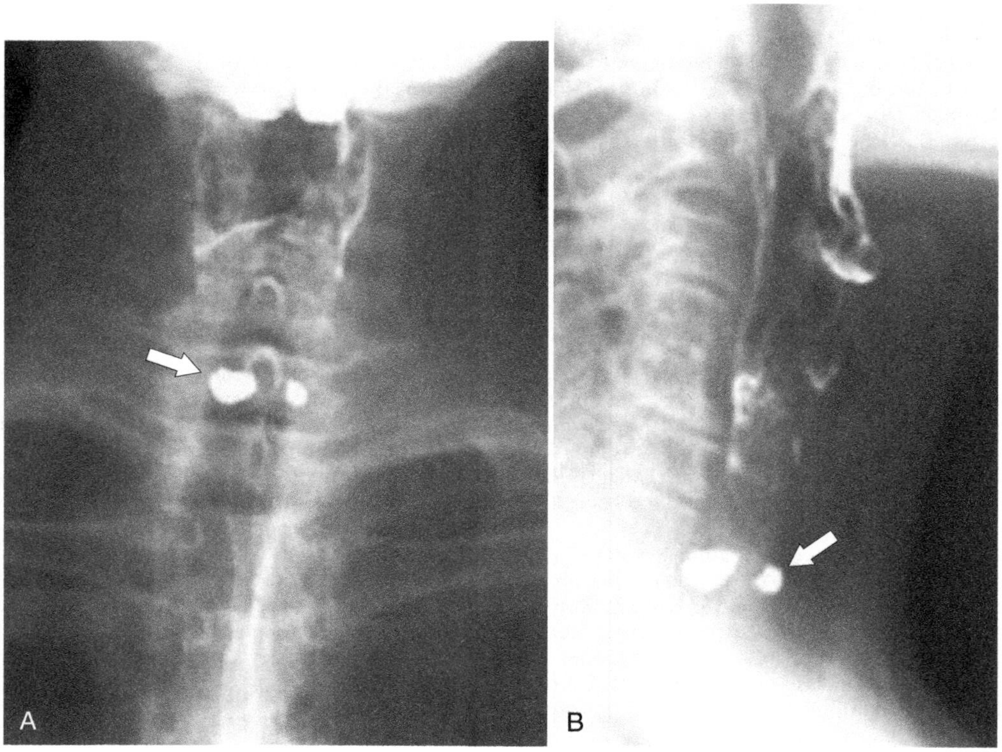

FIGURE 1-5. AP (**A**) and lateral (**B**) barium swallow in a 78-year-old woman with residual contrast on either side of the upper esophagus (*arrows*) due to a Killian-Jamieson diverticula.

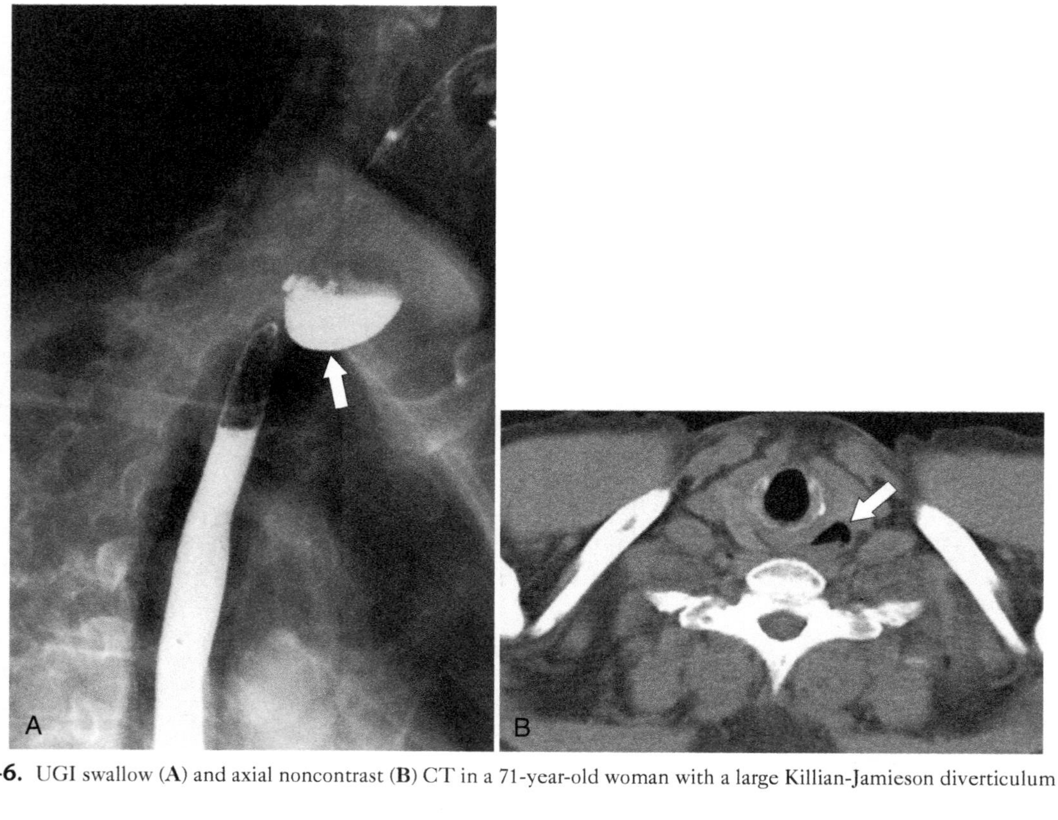

FIGURE 1-6. UGI swallow (**A**) and axial noncontrast (**B**) CT in a 71-year-old woman with a large Killian-Jamieson diverticulum (*arrows*).

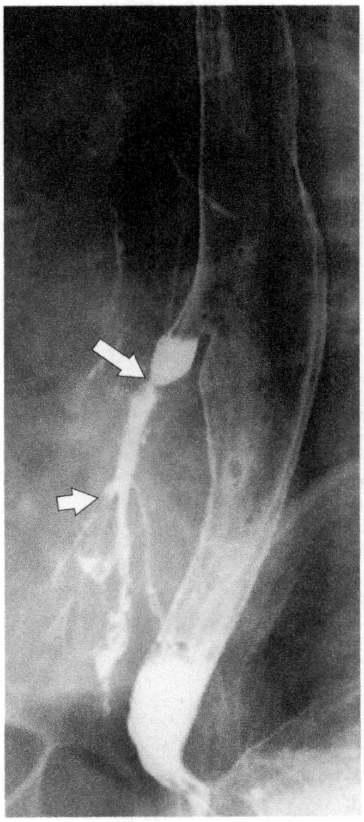

FIGURE 1-7. UGI swallow in a 70-year-old man with a small midesophageal traction diverticulum (*large arrow*) from prior tuberculous mediastinal adenopathy. There is also a tracheoesophageal fistula (*small arrow*).

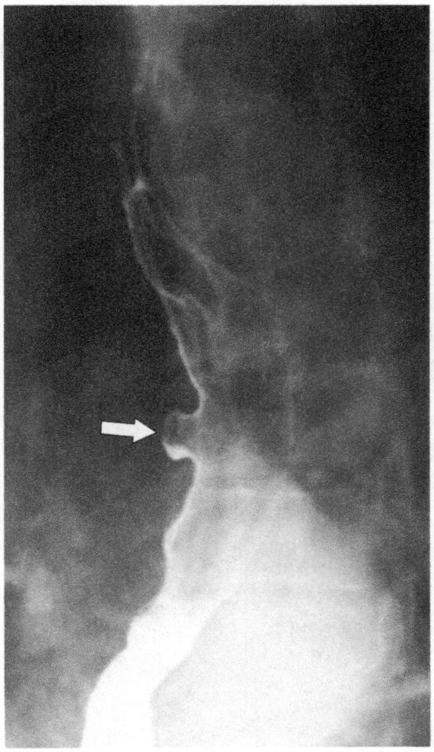

FIGURE 1-8. UGI swallow in a 66-year-old man with a small midesophageal pulsion diverticulum (*arrow*).

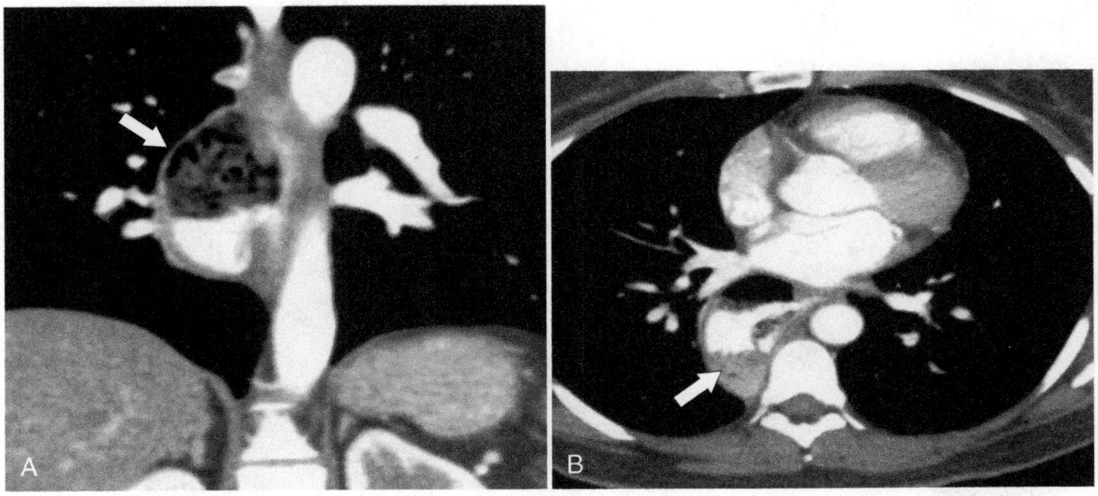

FIGURE 1-9. Coronal (**A**) and axial (**B**) contrast-enhanced CT in a 66-year-old man with a midesophageal pulsion diverticulum (*arrow*). Contrast freely refluxes through the wide-necked orifice (*arrow*).

incidentally, but symptoms include dysphagia, reflux, and aspiration. At a UGI examination, there are obvious wide-necked outpouches in the expected location, and they can be very large (Figs. 1-10 and 1-11).

Intramural Pseudodiverticula

Intramural pseudodiverticula are dilated mucous glands rather than true diverticula. These are seen as single, or more usually multiple, small, flask-like outpouchings from the esophageal lumen. They are associated with GERD and secondary stricture formation. They may be missed at esophagogastroduodenoscopy (EGD) and only observed at a UGI examination as numerous highly characteristic tiny outpouches from the esophageal lumen, typically at right angles (Fig. 1-12). When they are viewed en face, they can be mistaken for ulcer disease, but they are readily classified when viewed in the lateral plane.

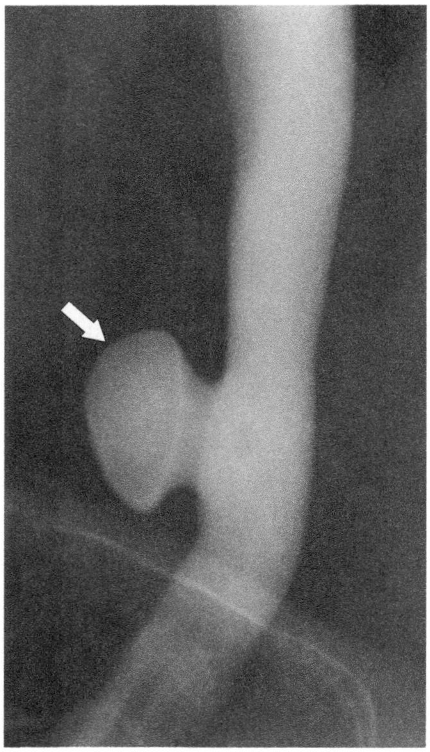

FIGURE 1-10. UGI swallow in a 59-year-old man with an epiphrenic diverticulum (*arrow*).

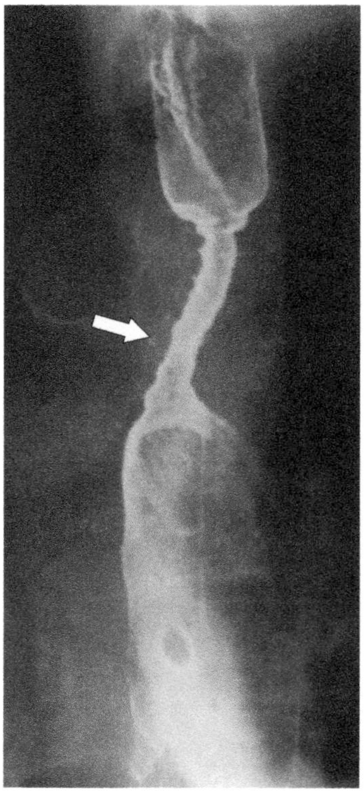

FIGURE 1-12. Esophageal barium swallow study in a 66-year-old man with multiple pseudodiverticula (*arrow*) and stricture due to chronic reflux esophagitis.

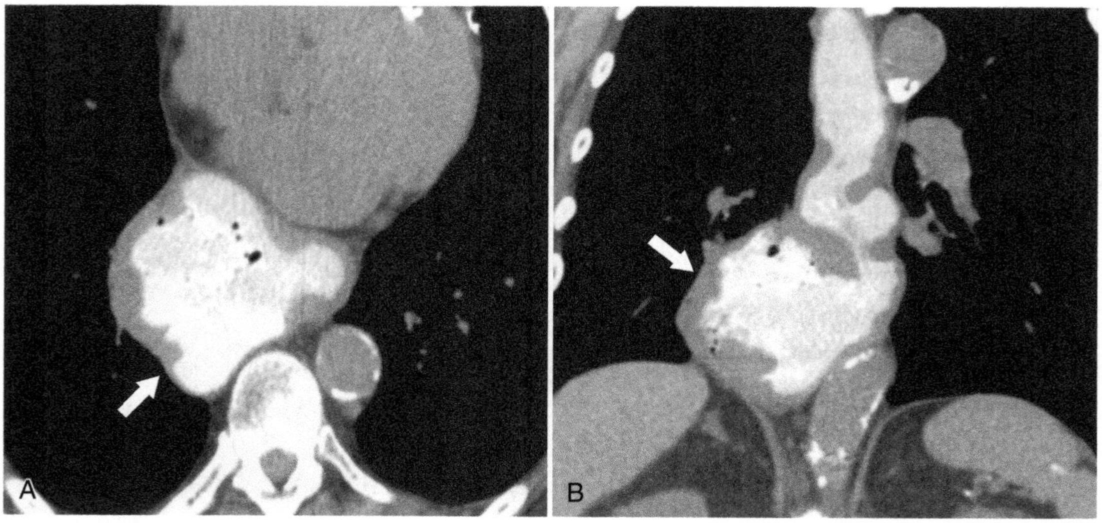

FIGURE 1-11. Axial (**A**) and coronal (**B**) CT in a 77-year-old man with a large, wide-mouthed (*arrow*) epiphrenic diverticulum.

ESOPHAGEAL WEBS AND RINGS

Esophageal webs and rings are usually located in the anterior upper esophagus and result from a variety of causes, which are either idiopathic or secondary to fibrosis from pemphigoid and epidermolysis bullosa, eosinophilic esophagitis, celiac disease, graft-versus-host disease, and Plummer-Vinson* syndrome (Figs. 1-13 and 1-14). The latter is associated with iron deficiency anemia, angular stomatitis, atrophic glossitis, and dysphagia. With lateral views with a UGI examination, these webs are seen as thin (web-like) defects at right angles to the direction of the esophageal lumen, which are usually shelf-like but can be circumferential (Fig. 1-15). Many webs are asymptomatic but can cause dysphagia. Sometimes an anterior web is combined with either posterior osteophyte impression or cricopharyngeal spasm (Fig. 1-16).

Webs can also be identified in the lower esophagus secondary to chronic GERD and are usually due to Schatzki ring. This is a relatively common finding seen in about 10% of the population

*Henry S. Plummer (1874-1936), American physician; Porter P. Vinson (1890-1959), American physician.

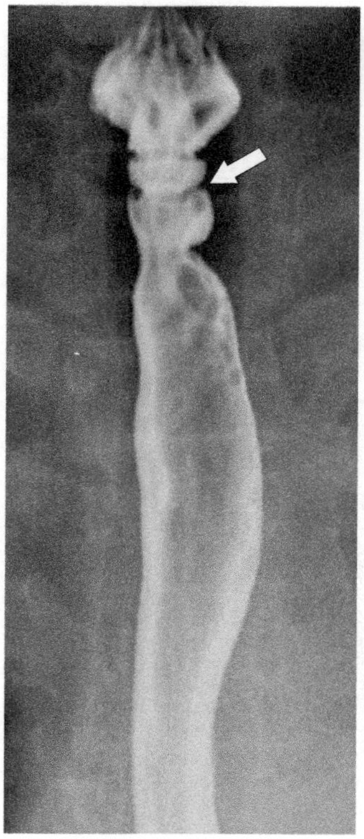

FIGURE 1-13. UGI swallow in a 39-year-old woman with epidermolysis bullosa and several circumferential esophageal webs (*arrow*).

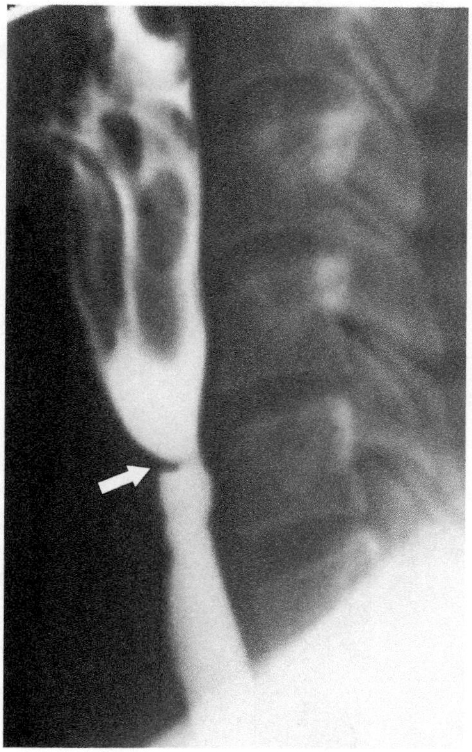

FIGURE 1-14. Barium swallow of the cervical esophagus in a 44-year-old woman demonstrates an anterior esophageal web (*arrow*).

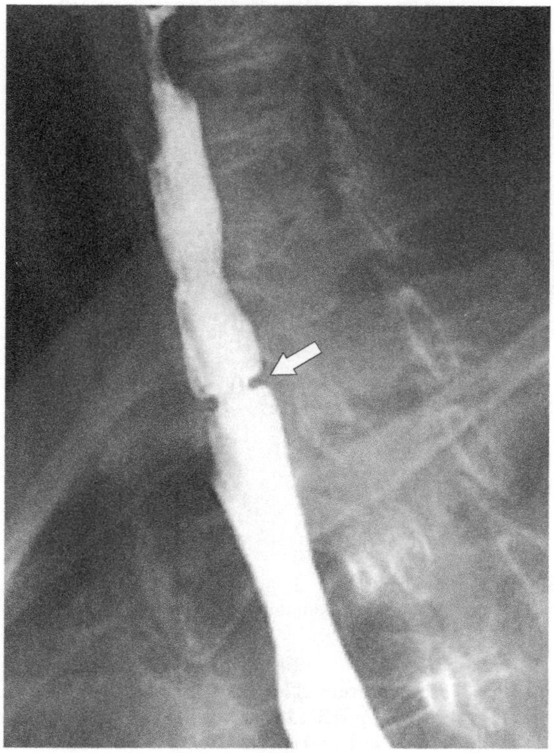

FIGURE 1-15. UGI swallow of the upper esophagus in an 84-year-old woman with a circumferential web (*arrow*).

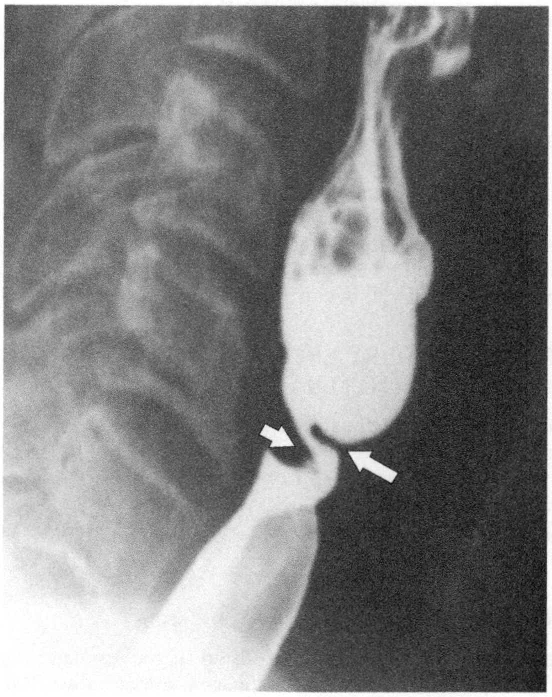

FIGURE 1-16. UGI of the cervical esophagus in a 60-year-old man demonstrating an anterior web (*large arrow*) and posterior impression (*small arrow*) due to cricopharyngeus spasm.

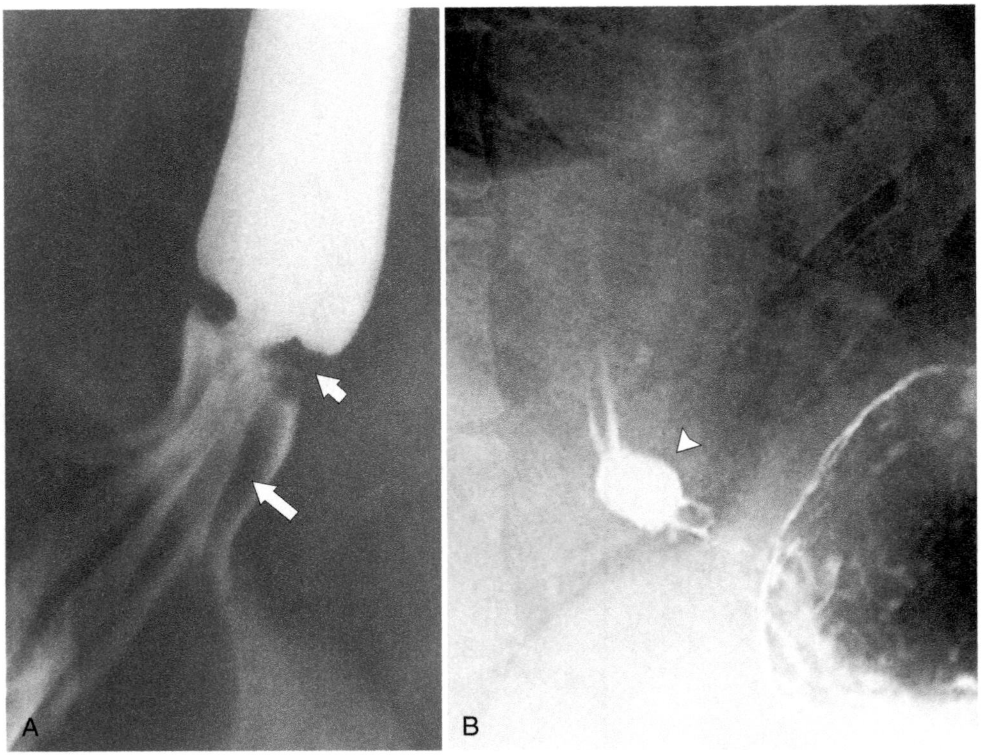

FIGURE 1-17. **A,** Barium swallow in a 64-year-old man with a Schatzki ring (*short arrow*). There is a small hiatal hernia with prominent gastric folds (*long arrow*). **B,** A 13-mm pill (*arrowhead*) failed to pass through the lower esophageal stricture.

and is usually asymptomatic, although about 30% of patients experience dyspeptic symptoms. It is caused by an inflammatory reaction from GERD to the esophageal B-ring, which develops a concentric narrowing resulting in luminal stricture formation, which if 13 mm or less, will likely produce symptoms. Wider rings may or may not be asymptomatic.

The rings are visualized as fixed and smooth associated with a small hiatal hernia below the rings during fluoroscopic observation after the patient swallows thin barium (Fig. 1-17). The rings can be missed on upright swallowing studies and are best elicited with the patient in the prone oblique position, the position most likely to distend the distal esophagus. The diameter of the rings can be confirmed by the patient's swallowing a 13-mm pill in the upright position. Narrowing to 13 mm or less is considered significant, at which point the pill will become stuck at the B-ring (Fig. 1-17).

INFLAMMATORY ESOPHAGOGASTRIC PSEUDOPOLYP OR FOLD

An inflammatory esophagogastric pseudopolyp or fold is an extension of a thickened gastric fold protruding up into the lower esophagus and mimics the appearance of a polyp (it is sometimes termed a *sentinel polyp*) (Fig. 1-18). GERD is usually associated. If the fold is excessively large, a biopsy is recommended to exclude adenocarcinoma at the GE junction.

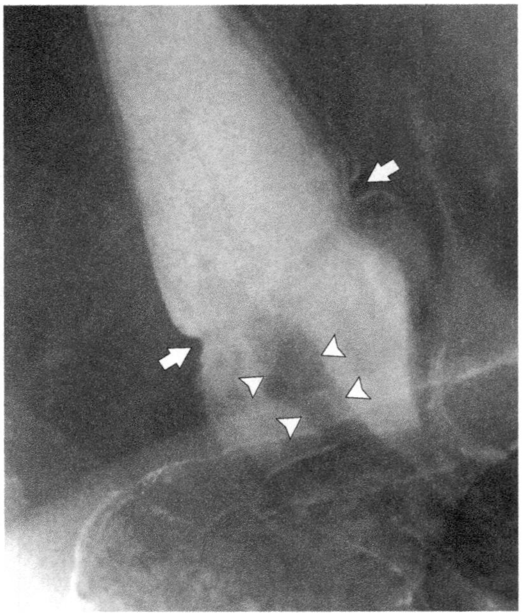

FIGURE 1-18. Barium swallow demonstrating mild B-ring (Schatzki) narrowing (*arrows*) and an inflammatory pseudopolyp (*arrowheads*).

HIATAL HERNIAS

Hiatal hernias are actually an extension of the stomach into the chest as opposed to a primary esophageal abnormality. They are differentiated into sliding (axial) or rolling (paraesophageal) types. In the former, which are far more common (up to 95% of all hiatal hernias), the upper gastric cardia and B-ring (lower esophageal mucosal ring) "slide" up through the diaphragmatic hiatus, typically more than 2 cm. The GE junction therefore lies above the diaphragm in the chest. Most sliding hernias are small and may not be observed at UGI contrast studies unless the patient is examined carefully (usually in the prone oblique position), and many are self-reducible in the erect position. Their significance, even when small, is that patients can have GERD with the resulting symptoms and potential complications. The typical sliding hernia at UGI study demonstrates several cardiac folds passing up into the chest, which may reduce back into the stomach when the patient is upright (Fig. 1-17). There may be a kink in the hiatal hernia because of compression by the adjacent diaphragm. Sliding hiatal hernias can be large with almost the whole stomach being in the chest, but the antrum pylorus remains within the abdomen (Fig. 1-19).

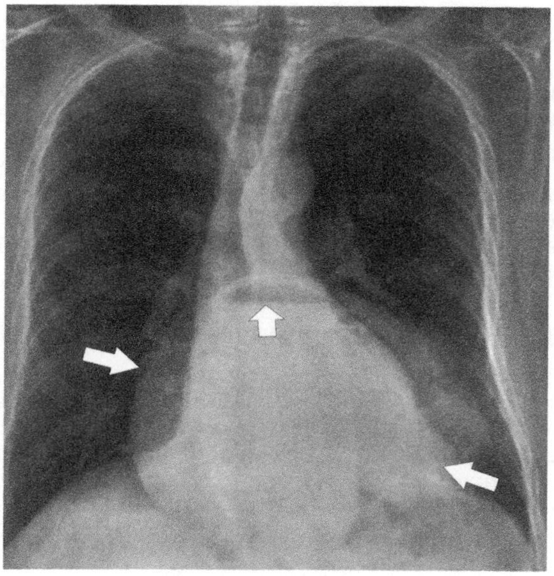

FIGURE 1-19. Chest radiograph in a 56-year-old man with a large hiatal hernia (*large arrows*) and gastric fluid level (*small arrow*). Most of the stomach resides in the chest.

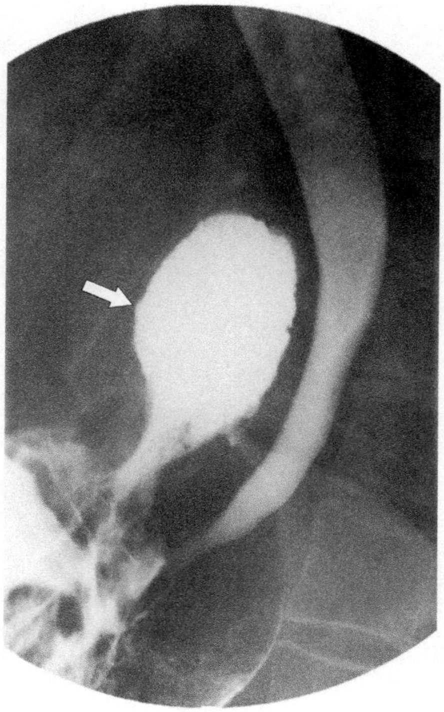

FIGURE 1-20. Barium swallow in a 48-year-old woman with a paraesophageal hernia (*arrow*).

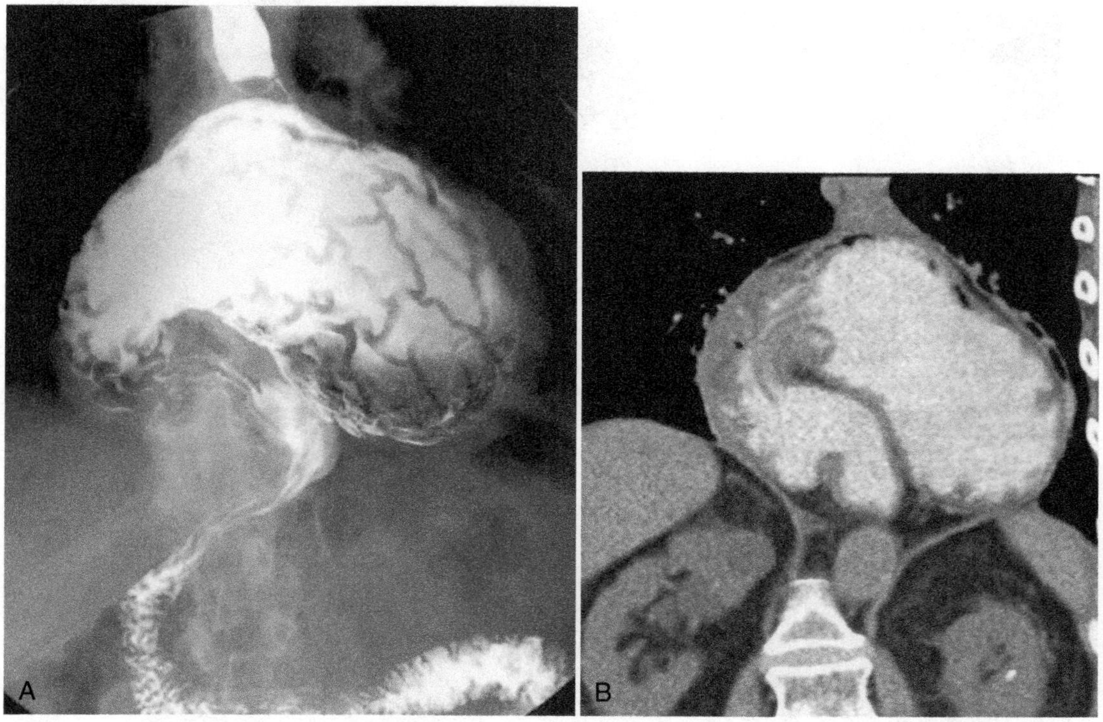

FIGURE 1-21. UGI series (**A**) and coronal noncontrast CT (**B**) in a 52-year-old woman with a nonobstructing organoaxial volvulus resulting in an "upside down" stomach.

Far less common are paraesophageal hernias (rolling hernias) in which the GE junction remains within the abdomen, so reflux is much less likely to occur compared with sliding hiatal hernias. Rather, the gastric fundus passes up into the chest and lies to the left of the lower esophagus (Fig. 1-20). These are generally irreducible but are more likely to be asymptomatic compared with sliding hiatal hernia, due to GERD in the more common sliding hernias. On the other hand, a variant of the paraesophageal hernia occurs when the whole stomach lies "upside down" in the chest because of volvulus, which may be obstructing or nonobstructing (see "Gastric Volvulus" in Chapter 2) and which is at greater risk of strangulation and perforation (Fig. 1-21). This is also the case with the even rarer combination of a sliding hernia and paraesophageal hernia, whereby the GE junction lies in the

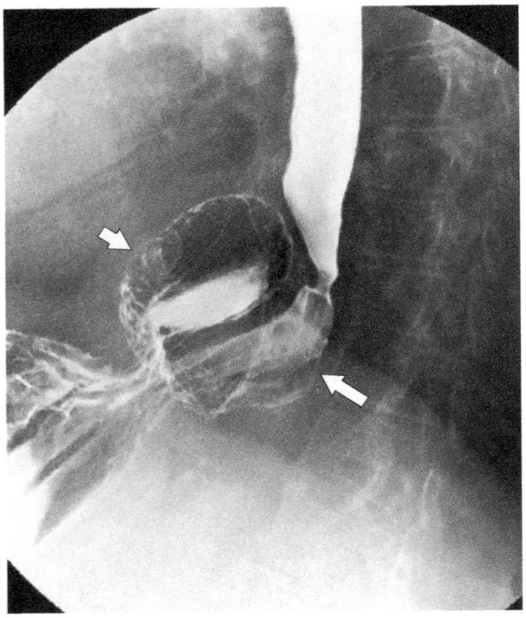

FIGURE 1-22. UGI series in an 86-year-old woman with a sliding hernia with the GE junction in the chest (*large arrow*) and paraesophageal hiatal hernia (*small arrow*).

chest along with the gastric cardia (Fig. 1-22). Therefore, the GE junction lies in the chest with the herniated gastric fundus lying alongside and to the left of the lower esophagus.

Although hernias are best appreciated by UGI series, they are frequently visualized incidentally by CT, which will demonstrate a dilated lower esophagus (actually represents the gastric cardia in the chest) in the lower chest with a variable proportion of mesenteric fat surrounding the herniated stomach (Fig. 1-23). Consequently, there is a slight widening of the diaphragmatic hiatus (>15 mm). A paraesophageal hernia can also be appreciated with the herniated cardia lying alongside the lower esophagus (Fig. 1-24).

EXTRAMURAL ESOPHAGEAL IMPRESSIONS

Extramural esophageal impressions cause smooth and obtuse impressions on the esophagus similar to the extramural masses throughout the GI tract. Most causes are benign (Table 1-1). External malignant masses may ultimately distort the mucosal contour but only after transmural metastatic invasion.

Postcricoid Impression

Also known as postcricoid defect of pharyngeal venous plexus, postcricoid impression is common and not pathological, and it is caused by redundant hypopharyngeal mucosa overlying the central pharyngeal venous plexus positioned approximately at the

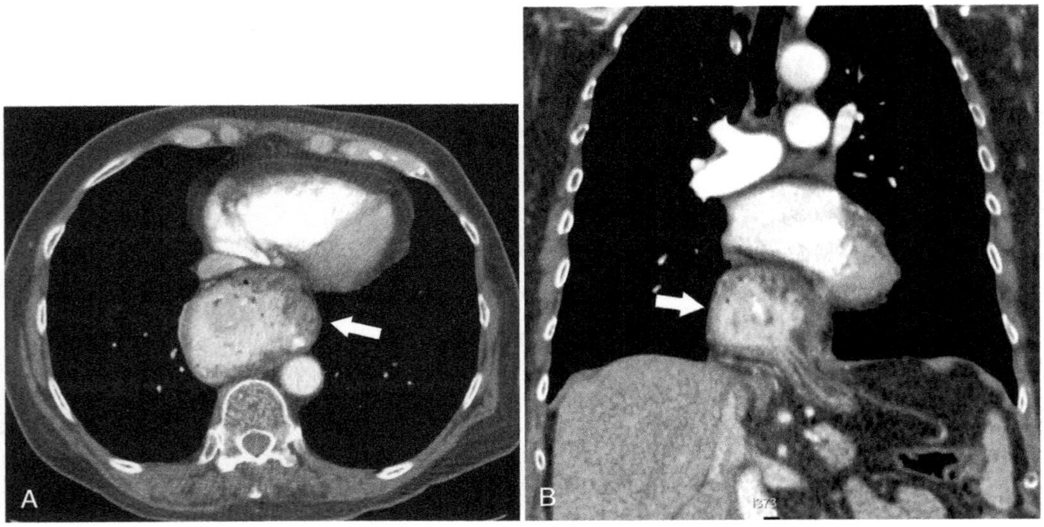

FIGURE 1-23. Axial (**A**) and coronal (**B**) contrast-enhanced CT in a 77-year-old woman with a sliding hiatal hernia (*arrows*).

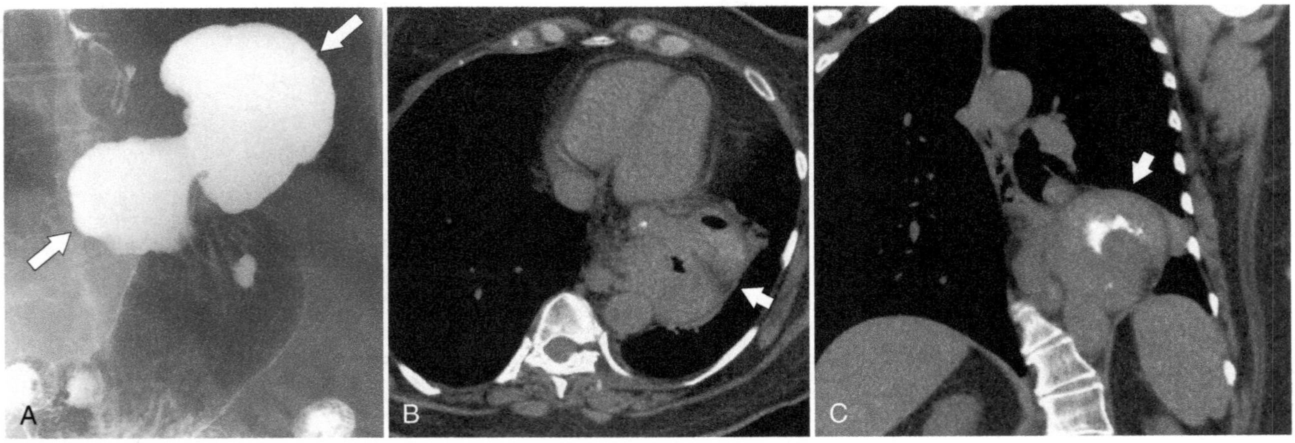

FIGURE 1-24. UGI swallow (**A**) and axial (**B**) and coronal (**C**) noncontrast CT in a 60-year-old woman with a combined sliding and paraesophageal hernia (*arrows*). At CT the GE junction is in the chest.

TABLE 1-1 Extrinsic Esophageal Masses

Benign	Malignant
Postcricoid impression	Mediastinal adenopathy (metastases)
Cricopharyngeal spasm	Lung cancer
Cervical osteophytic disease	Lung metastases
Retropharyngeal masses (e.g., goiter)	
Cardiomegaly	
Vascular anomalies (aberrant vessels, aneurysms, vascular rings)	
Mediastinal adenopathy (e.g., tuberculosis)	

level of C6, just below the cricoid cartilage. It varies in appearance (sometimes smooth, sometimes web-like) and is recognized by its anterior location on the esophagus.

Cricopharyngeal Spasm

This posterior esophageal impression is secondary to hypertrophy and spasm of the cricopharyngeus muscle, the lower portion of the inferior pharyngeal constrictor muscle located posteriorly at the level of C5-6 vertebral body (Figs. 1-16 and 1-25). Normally, after the primary peristaltic wave is initiated, the cricopharyngeus muscle relaxes, allowing the food bolus to pass. Failure to relax due to hypertrophy or spasm is a relatively common cause of dysphagia because the protruding muscle causes localized esophageal dysmotility and relative stricture formation. Usually, symptoms are relatively mild (many patients do not present to their physician) but can result in more marked symptoms depending on the severity of the muscular protrusion. A Zenker diverticulum may ultimately result from the localized increased intraesophageal pressure.

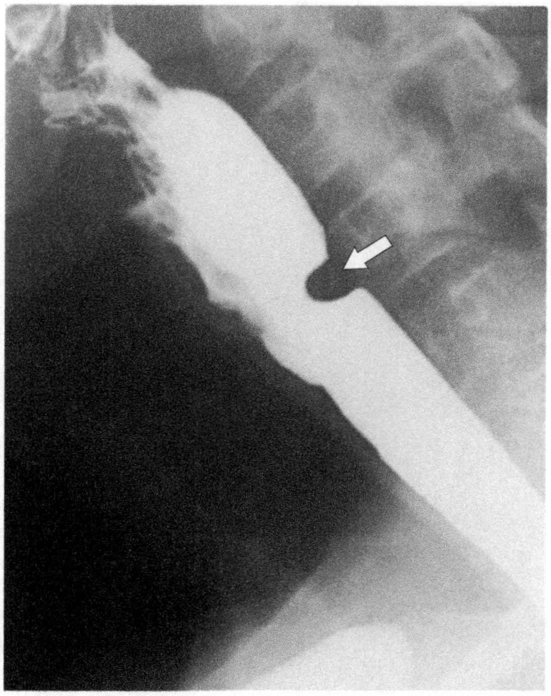

FIGURE 1-25. UGI swallow in a 56-year-old man with cricopharyngeus spasm (*arrow*).

VERTEBRAL OSTEOPHYTIC DISEASE

Anterior vertebral osteophytes or, rarely, anterior cervical disc herniation can cause discrete posterior esophageal indentations, which are usually smooth and sometimes marked (Fig. 1-26).

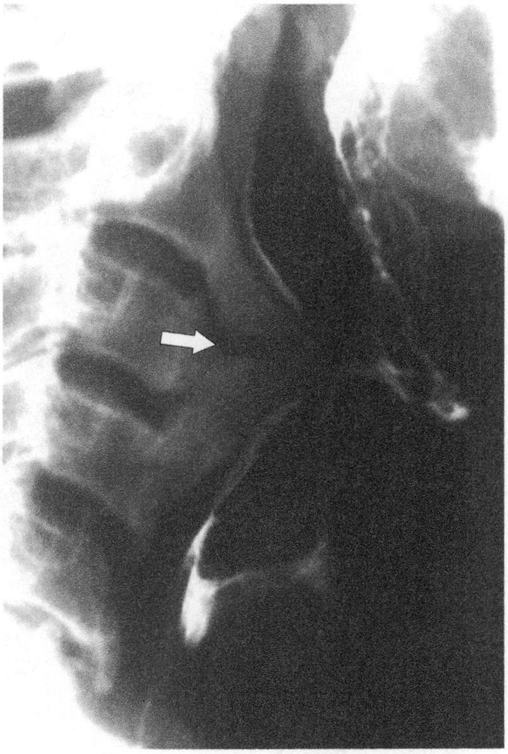

FIGURE 1-26. UGI swallow in a 75-year-old woman with pharyngeal anterior displacement due to vertebral osteophyte disease (*arrow*).

RETROPHARYNGEAL MASSES

The cervical esophagus abuts the vertebral bodies, so pharyngeal disease that extends inferiorly and posterior to the esophagus will produce esophageal deviation. Such retropharyngeal masses include goiter, abscess, hematoma, lymphadenopathy, and parathyroid enlargement (Figs. 1-27 and 1-28).

VASCULAR IMPRESSIONS

Normally the aortic arch and left main bronchus cause smooth external compressions of the esophagus. However, ectatic or aneurysmal dilatation can cause deviation of the esophagus. There are also several congenital vascular anomalies that produce esophageal compressions, which are generally smooth and obliquely angled. Their diagnoses should be suspected by their location either by UGI examination or CT, although contrast-enhanced CT (CECT) (or MRI) will delineate the exact origin and course of the aberrant vessels.

A double aortic arch, the most common form of vascular ring, passes on both sides of the trachea and joins posterior to the esophagus. Barium studies of the esophagus demonstrate bilateral impressions anteriorly and a smooth posterior impression. A right-sided aortic arch, of which there are several types, is recognized by smooth leftward displacement of the barium-filled esophagus in the midthoracic region.

An aberrant right subclavian artery occurs in approximately 1 in 200 individuals and is due to the aberrant origin of the right subclavian artery, usually from a left-sided aortic arch, such that the vessel now has to reach the right axilla by crossing behind the esophagus at an oblique angle. Less commonly, it arises from a right aortic arch. It may be asymptomatic but can cause dysphagia (also known as dysphagia lusoria*). The diagnosis is best made by arterial phase CT where the aberrant vessel is readily observed

---

**lusoria:* Latin for "freak," as in "freak of nature."

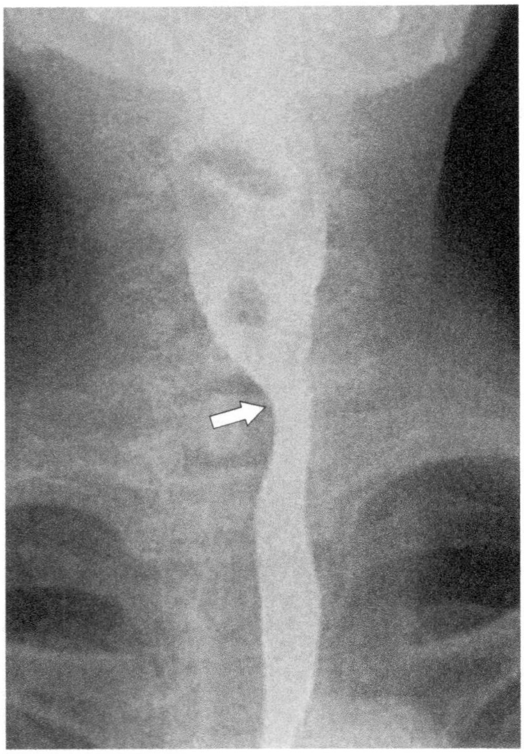

FIGURE 1-27. UGI swallow in a 46-year-old woman with extramural compression of the esophagus (*arrow*) due to a goiter.

crossing behind the esophagus (Fig. 1-29). At UGI examination, there is a classic smooth posterior impression angled upward from the left to the right (Fig. 1-29). An aberrant left subclavian artery is part of a right-sided arch and has similar, but reverse, findings to an aberrant right subclavian artery because it passes from the right and behind the esophagus as it traverses toward the left axilla (Fig. 1-30).

An aberrant left pulmonary artery is an anomaly resulting from the left lung being supplied from the right pulmonary artery, rather than the left pulmonary artery. Because of the location of its origin, this aberrant left pulmonary artery has to cross to the left side of the mediastinum and in doing so causes an anterior extrinsic compression of the thoracic esophagus at the level of the carina, giving the name to the so-called pulmonary sling.

EXTRAMURAL MEDIASTINAL MASSES

Mediastinal lymphadenopathy (benign or malignant) can cause anterior extrinsic impressions on the esophagus, which it may deviate if it is large enough. Other mediastinal masses that cause anterior esophageal impressions include bronchogenic and duplication cysts. Cardiomegaly, particularly left atrial enlargement, causes esophageal deviation if it is significantly dilated. Traction anomalies, including pulmonary fibrotic disease, also cause esophageal deviation (Fig. 1-31).

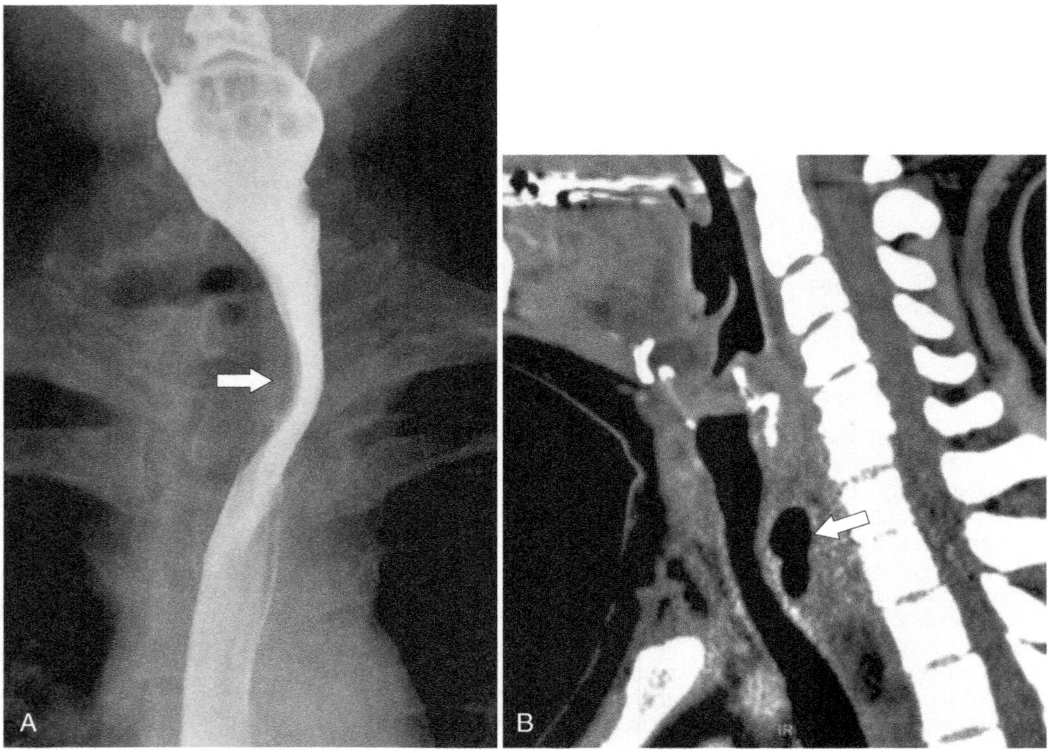

FIGURE 1-28. UGI swallow (**A**) and sagittal noncontrast CT (**B**) in a 54-year-old woman with extramural compression and deviation of the esophagus due to a retropharyngeal abscess that contains gas (*arrows*).

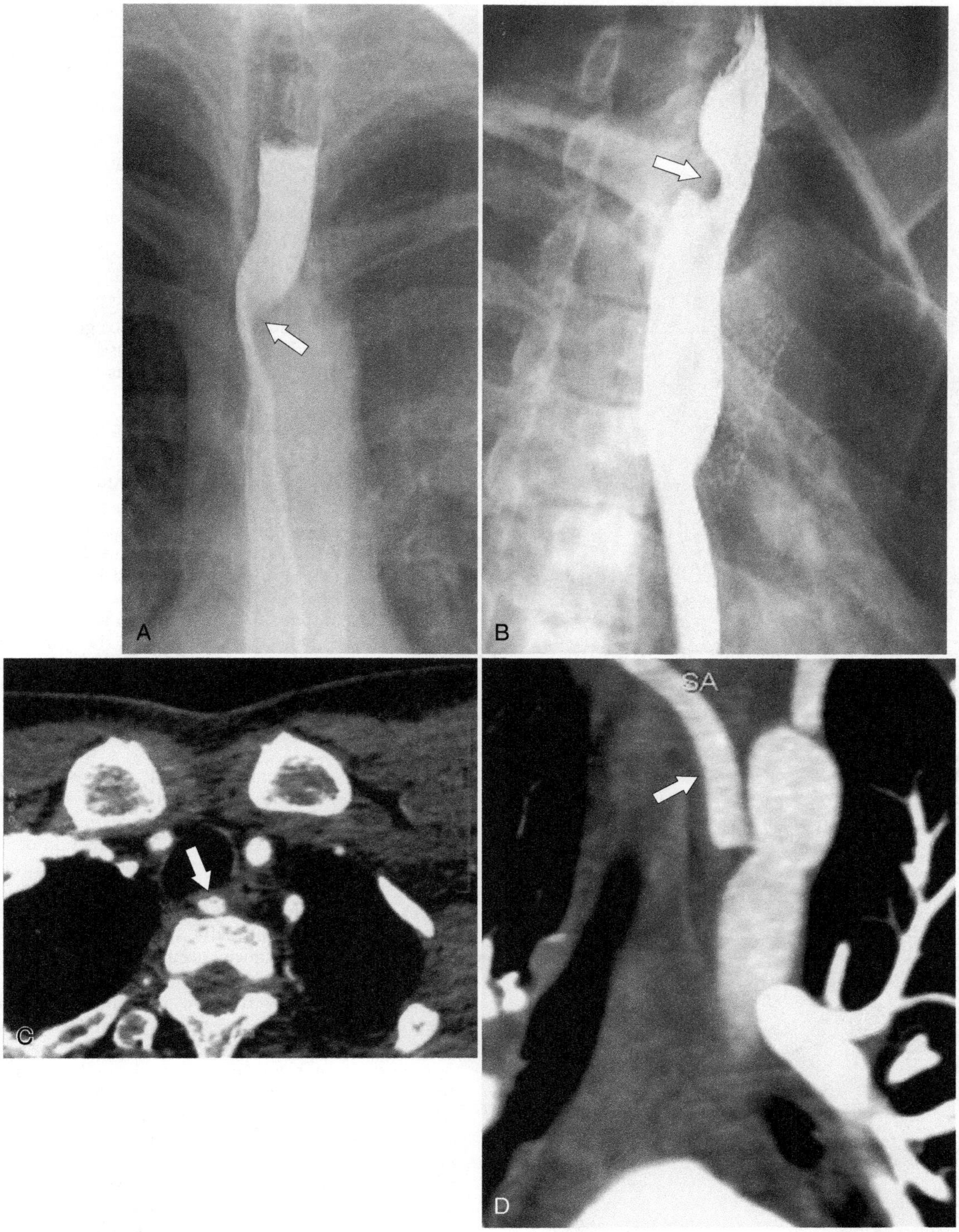

FIGURE 1-29. AP (**A**) and lateral oblique (**B**) UGI swallow and axial (**C**) and coronal (**D**) contrast-enhanced CT in a 35-year-old man. UGI demonstrates a slanting esophageal impression due to an aberrant right subclavian artery (*arrows*, **A** and **B**). CT demonstrates the aberrant vessel passing posterior to the esophagus on the axial view and cephalad to the right on coronal MIP (maximum intensity projection) imaging (*arrows*, **C** and **D**).

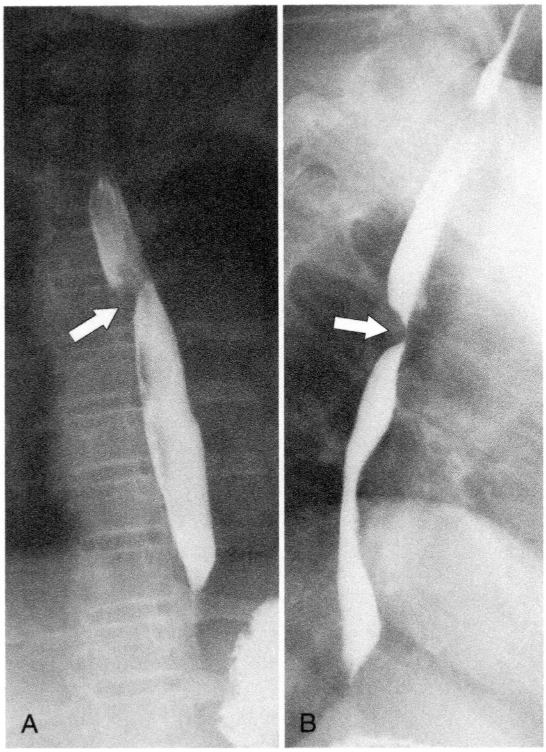

FIGURE 1-30. AP (**A**) and lateral (**B**) barium swallow in a 17-year-old male adolescent with aberrant left subclavian artery. The vessel passes posteriorly and obliquely up and to the left of the esophagus (*arrows*).

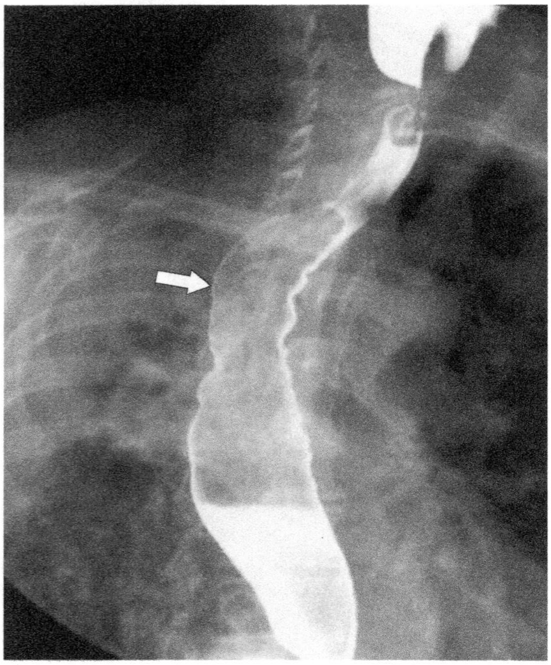

FIGURE 1-31. UGI swallow in a 56-year-old man with right-sided esophageal deviation (*arrow*) due to traction from diffuse right-sided fibrotic pulmonary tuberculosis.

SUBMUCOSAL ESOPHAGEAL MASSES

Esophageal submucosal masses cause smooth esophageal impressions but are less obtuse than extraluminal masses. There are several well-recognized causes, but appearances at UGI series usually cannot be distinguished from one another (Table 1-2).

TABLE 1-2 Esophageal Submucosal Masses

Benign	Malignant
Varices	Metastases
Cyst	Lymphoma
GIST	Kaposi sarcoma
Hemangioma	Malignant GIST
Lipoma	
Neurofibroma	
Fibrovascular polyp	
Granular cell tumor	

GIST, Gastrointestinal stromal tumor.

CT may help, but small, benign masses generally cannot be differentiated, either. However, when masses are malignant or large, some CT features can aid the diagnosis.

Benign Submucosal Masses

Esophageal Varices

Esophageal varices are most commonly secondary to increased portal venous pressure (usually hepatic cirrhosis) with varices in the lower esophagus; these are sometimes termed *uphill varices* because of their caudal to cephalad direction of blood flow. Increased venous pressure is relieved by diverting blood away from the obstruction to the lower pressure of the esophageal venous system, usually the middle to lower third of the esophagus (Fig. 1-32). Venous return from the portal vein is via the coronary vein (left gastric) into the lower esophageal plexus with blood flowing with a cephalad direction and then from esophageal veins into the azygous vein and superior vena cava (SVC). As part of the same venous plexus, it is often associated with gastric fundal varices.

The far less common "downhill" varices form from the upper to middle third of the esophagus and are secondary to superior vena caval obstruction. Blood in "downstream" varices enters the upper esophageal plexus in a caudal direction of flow and reenters the SVC through the azygos in the thoracic esophagus. If the azygos is also obstructed (or the lower SVC), then blood continues in a caudal direction to connect with the coronary vein, then the portal system, and finally the inferior vena cava (IVC). Varices in these circumstances occur along the length of the entire esophagus.

Despite the increased venous pressures that precipitate esophageal variceal formation, esophageal varices are best visualized with the patient horizontal because the venous pressure in the upright position is not sufficient to distend the varicosities. Aside from EGD, they are best visualized when the patient is prone while drinking barium as serpiginous submucosal impressions either in the lower (uphill) or mid to upper (downhill) esophagus. They are also usually well visualized by contrast-enhanced CT or MRI, particularly in the portal venous phase after contrast enhancement as prominent submucosal contrast-filled venous plexuses (Fig. 1-32). Without the use of intravenous (IV) contrast, the esophageal wall will simply appear thickened and therefore difficult to differentiate from other esophageal abnormalities. The findings need to be differentiated from varicoid carcinoma that can also present with serpiginous submucosal fold findings (Fig. 1-33).

Esophageal Cysts

Esophageal cysts represent foregut duplication cysts (congenital) or retention cysts (acquired). The former are usually discovered incidentally, whereas the much rarer retention cysts may be more symptomatic, arising from dilated mucous glands, usually in the distal esophagus.

At UGI, both types appear as submucosal defects, although foregut cysts may calcify and barium may occasionally fill the

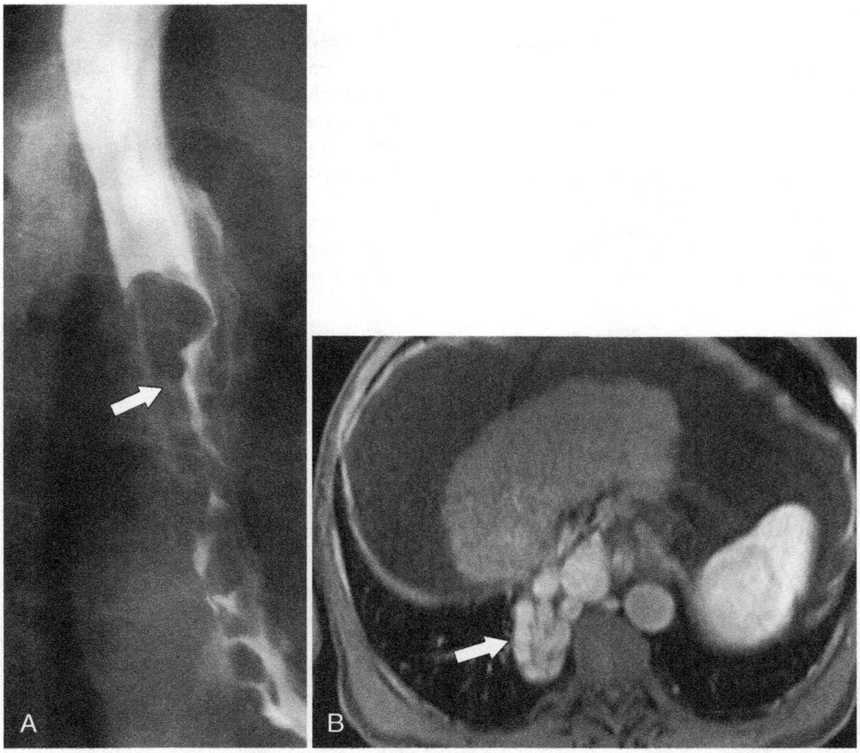

FIGURE 1-32. UGI examination (**A**) and axial contrast-enhanced T1-weighted MRI (**B**) in a 53-year-old man with a serpiginous esophageal filling defect caused by large esophageal varices (*arrows*), a complication of cirrhosis. Note the liver atrophy and diffuse ascites.

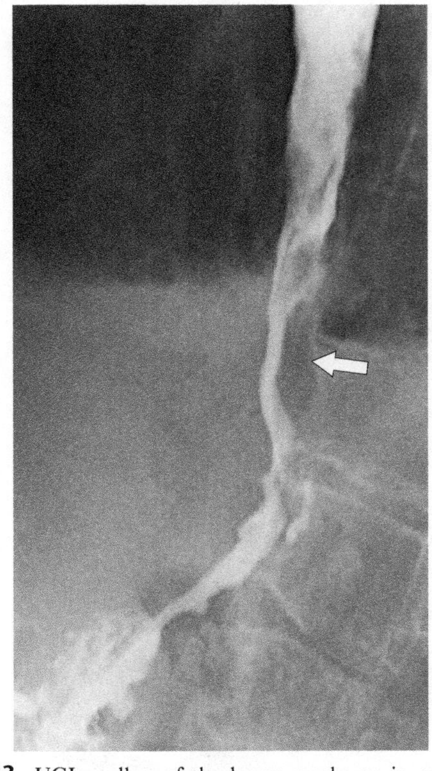

FIGURE 1-33. UGI swallow of the lower esophagus in an 84-year-old man with an infiltrative esophageal adenocarcinoma extending for several centimeters with a varicoid pattern (*arrow*).

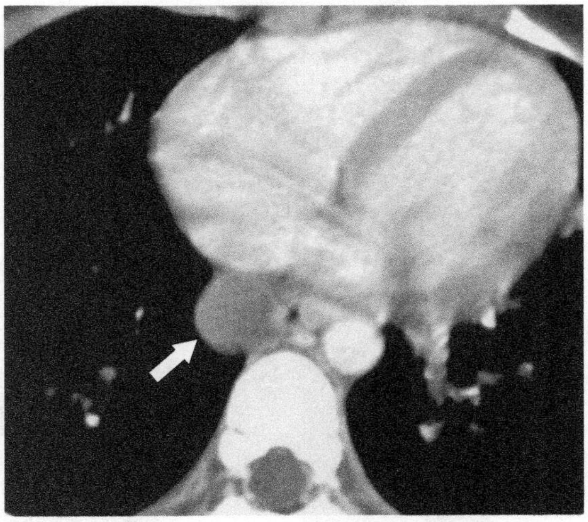

FIGURE 1-34. Axial contrast-enhanced CT in a 10-year-old girl with a hypodense 1.8-cm mass (*arrow*) contiguous with the esophagus due to an esophageal duplication cyst.

retention cyst, giving the appearance of a smooth and rounded mass. They are better visualized at CT as smooth submucosal hypodense lesions (Fig. 1-34).

Esophageal Submucosal Benign Tumors

Common to all these masses is their intramural or submucosal origin (Table 1-3). They therefore cause esophageal narrowing, which at UGI examination is represented by an intraluminal mass with slightly obtuse margins and generally smooth surface. Differentiation between different diagnoses by imaging alone can

TABLE 1-3 Submucosal Benign Esophageal Tumors

Tumor type	Features
GIST	Most common; smaller; may contain amorphous calcification at CT; can be large
Hemangioma	Reddish blue multinodular mass
Lipoma	Fat density on CT
Neurofibroma	May be associated with disease in multiple anatomical sites
Granulosa cell tumor	Broader-based mass
Hamartoma	Contains multiple tissue types (bone, cartilage, fat, muscle)

CT, Computed tomography; *GIST,* gastrointestinal stromal tumor.

be difficult, and the final diagnosis is usually made after surgical resection and histological evaluation (Fig. 1-35). They vary considerably in size with gastrointestinal stromal tumors (GISTs) being the largest (up to 10 cm in diameter) (Fig. 1-36). The masses are generally well outlined by barium en face, and the overlying mucosa may ulcerate (as evidenced by barium pooling in the center of the mass) as they grow.

Fibrovascular Polyp

Fibrovascular polyp is an unusual, benign, submucosal neoplasm of the mid and upper esophagus and consists of fibrovascular and adipose tissue (Fig. 1-37). It may have a long stalk that then elongates in tubular fashion down the length of the esophagus. It sometimes bleeds and can be so long that it can be regurgitated into the pharynx, rarely obstructing the larynx.

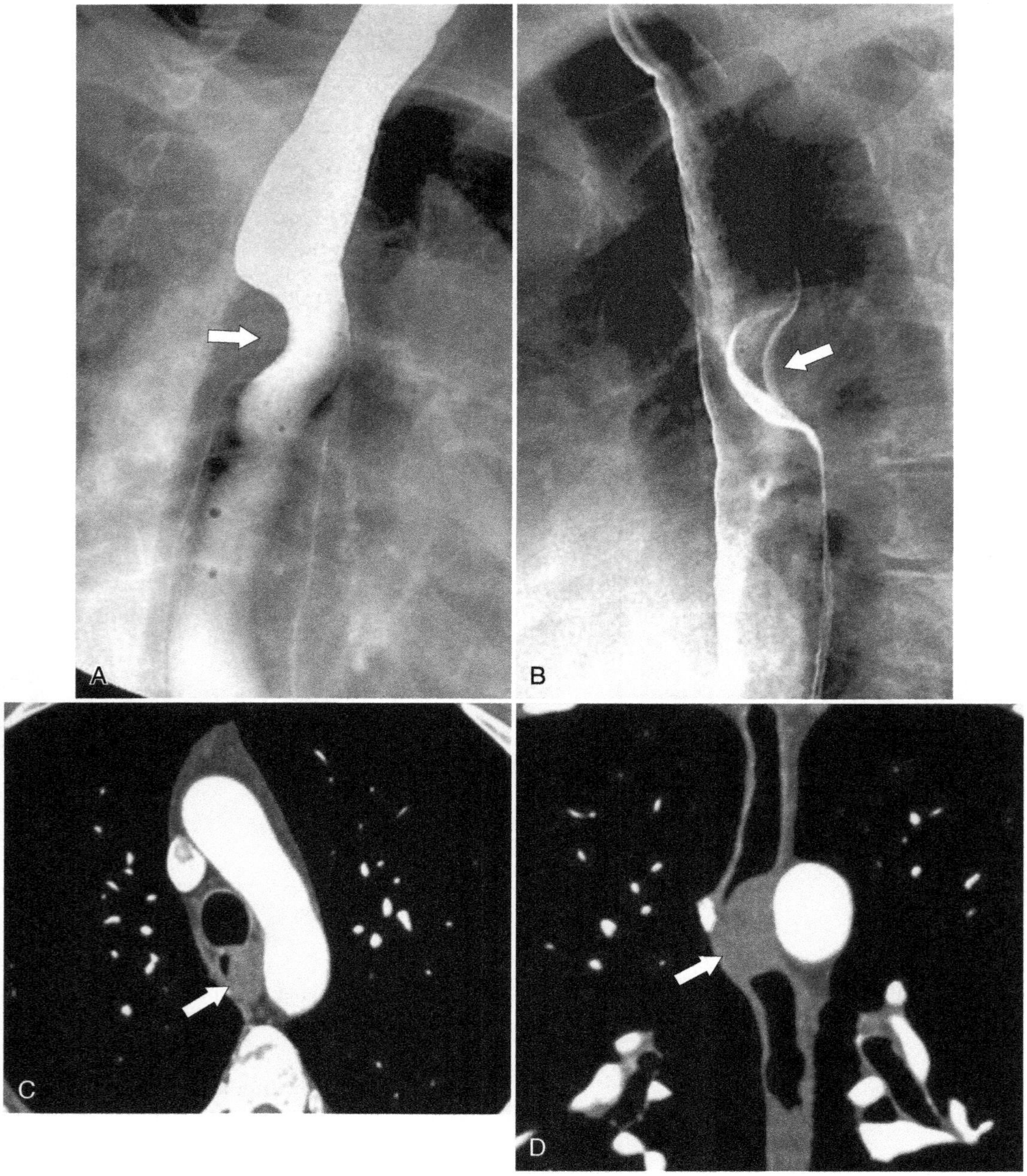

FIGURE 1-35. Single- (**A**) and double-contrast (**B**) UGI series and axial (**C**) and coronal (**D**) contrast-enhanced CT views in a 50-year-old man with a smooth submucosal esophageal impression (*arrows*) due to a GIST.

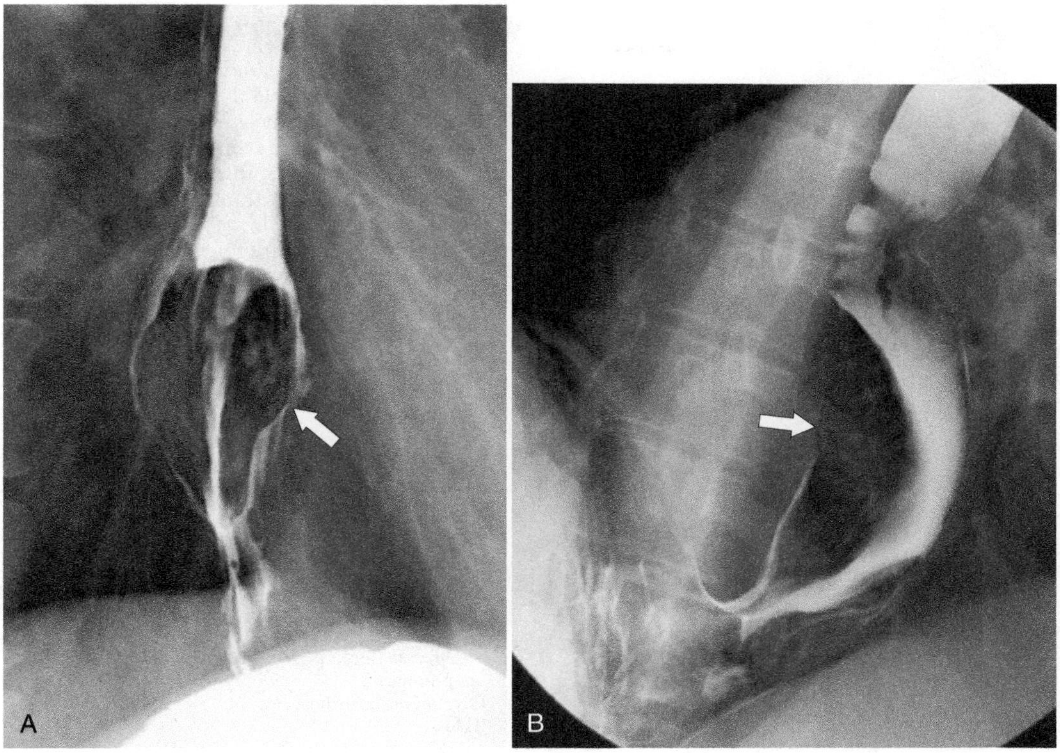

FIGURE 1-36. AP (**A**) and lateral (**B**) UGI swallow in a 31-year-old woman with a large submucosal esophageal impression (*arrows*) due to a GIST.

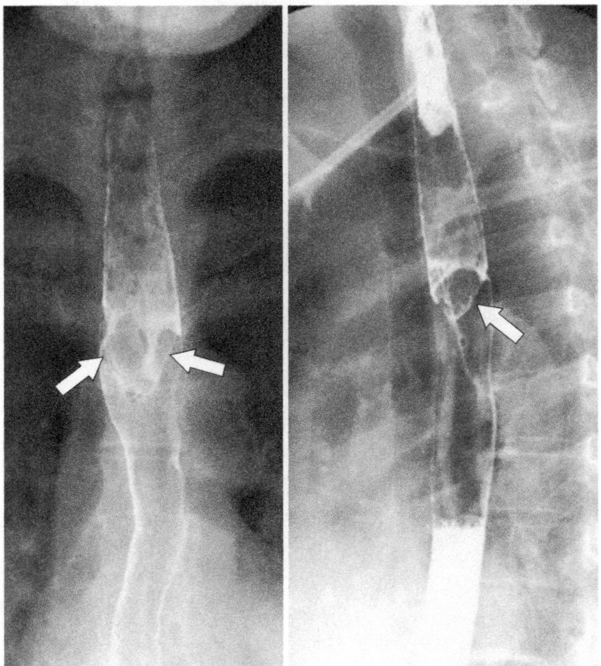

FIGURE 1-37. AP (**A**) and lateral (**B**) UGI swallow in a 50-year-old man with an irregular filling esophageal defect due to a fibrovascular polyp (*arrows*).

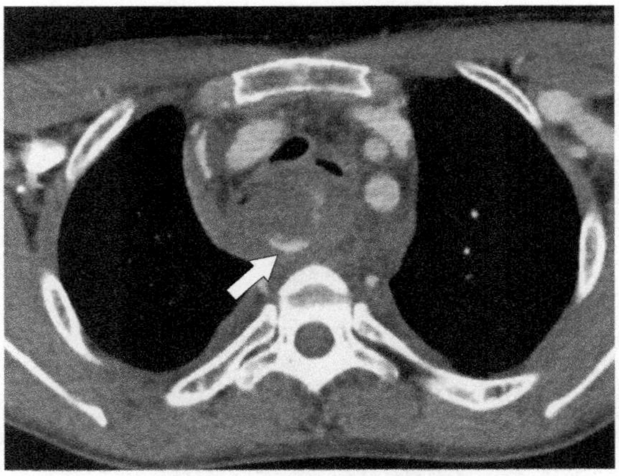

FIGURE 1-38. Axial contrast-enhanced CT in a 66-year-old woman with esophageal hematoma and acute hemorrhage (*arrow*).

Submucosal Hemorrhage

Submucosal hemorrhage is usually iatrogenic from endoscopic procedures or nasogastric tube placement but can be spontaneous in patients with bleeding disorders. The appearances are rarely observed at barium studies but are identified at CT, usually as a circumferential esophageal soft tissue mass, which may be hyperdense if imaged shortly after the acute hemorrhagic event (Fig. 1-38).

Malignant Submucosal Masses

These masses are rare and include metastases (most commonly melanoma, lymphoma, breast) or primary tumors, including sarcomas, mainly Kaposi sarcoma, or malignant GISTs. They often cause mucosal irregularity and ulceration if they invade through the muscularis mucosae and into the mucosa.

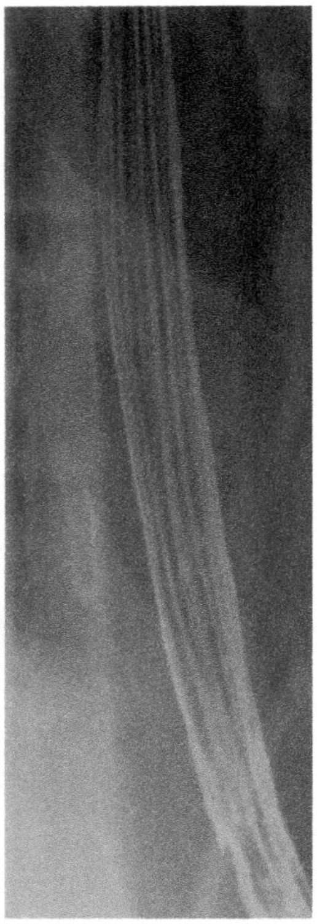

FIGURE 1-39. Barium swallow demonstrating multiple longitudinal esophageal folds.

MUCOSAL ABNORMALITIES

Both benign and malignant mucosal abnormalities are well delineated by good single- and double-contrast technique (Table 1-4). Normal esophageal mucosal folds are mostly longitudinal and extend the length of the esophagus and are best seen on collapsed rather than distended double-contrast views at UGI examination (Fig. 1-39). Conversely, transverse folds, which are also normal, are more difficult to identify and are better seen on double-contrast views. Transverse folds in the esophagus, when observed, are sometimes referred to as a *feline esophagus*, mimicking the normal esophageal folds observed in cats (Fig. 1-40). Thickened edematous benign folds are often seen with esophagitis from any cause, the most common being GERD (Fig. 1-41).

TABLE 1-4 Esophageal Mucosal Abnormalities

Benign	Malignant
Esophagitis (peptic, infectious, caustic, inflammatory, drugs, iatrogenic, radiation, Crohn, Behçet)	Esophageal carcinoma
Ectopic gastric mucosa	Kaposi sarcoma
Neoplastic (leukoplakia, squamous papilloma)	Malignant GIST
Glycogenic acanthosis	Metastases
Tylosis	
Epidermolysis bullosa/pemphigoid	

GIST, Gastrointestinal stromal tumor.

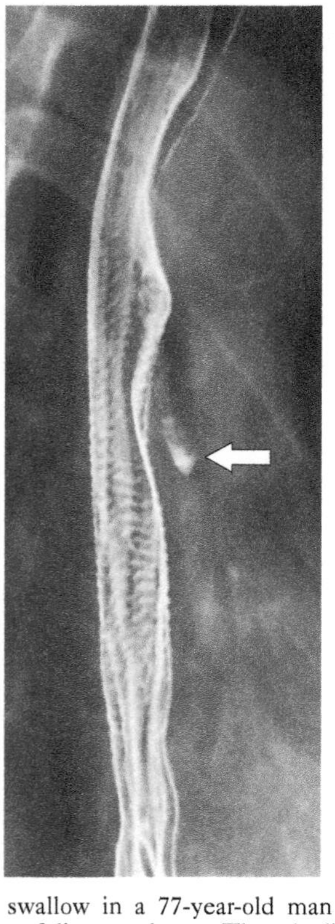

FIGURE 1-40. UGI swallow in a 77-year-old man with multiple fine transverse folds due to a feline esophagus. There is slight aspiration in the trachea and left main bronchus (*arrow*).

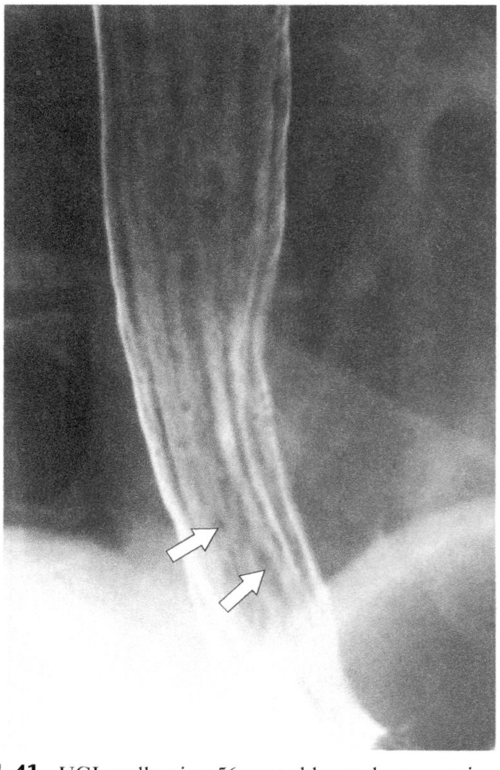

FIGURE 1-41. UGI swallow in a 56-year-old man demonstrating thickening longitudinal esophageal folds and subtle nodular change (*arrows*) due to reflux esophagitis.

BENIGN MUCOSAL DISEASE

Esophagitis

Esophagitis represents the most common mucosal abnormality in clinical practice predominantly because it is due to a wide variety of causes (Table 1-5). Barium studies can be diagnostic and should be performed if endoscopy is contraindicated. Some findings are subtle, and close observation of the whole esophagus is mandatory. Once an abnormality is identified, additional spot views in multiple tangential planes should be taken to maximize the ability of the examination to define the precise cause.

TABLE 1-5 Causes of Esophagitis

Infectious	Herpes *Candida* infection CMV HIV Fungal infection Tuberculosis
Iatrogenic	Radiation therapy Nasogastric tube
Drugs	Tetracycline Nonsteroidal antiinflammatory drug Potassium Iron
Chemical	Reflux esophagitis Corrosives
Inflammatory	Crohn disease Scleroderma Pemphigoid Epidermolysis bullosa

CMV, Cytomegalovirus; *HIV,* human immunodeficiency virus.

Infectious Esophagitis

Infectious esophagitis is most commonly identified in the immunocompromised host (from any cause) and includes herpes simplex, candidiasis, and cytomegalovirus (CMV).

Candida albicans causes the most common infectious esophagitis, which presents with diffuse and painful dysphagia. Most patients are immunosuppressed from either chemotherapy or immune deficiencies, particularly human immunodeficiency virus (HIV), and it is a relatively common manifestation in patients with acquired immune deficiency syndrome (AIDS). The disease may coexist with herpes or CMV esophagitis. Patients with disorders of esophageal motility and the resulting stasis (scleroderma, achalasia, and strictures) are also at risk for *Candida* infection. As its name suggests, the esophageal mucosa is coated with diffuse white (albicans) plaques, which can be present from the tongue (oral thrush) to the lower esophagus. Gastric hyperacidity generally prevents it from spreading below the GE junction.

The imaging findings may lag clinical findings, either with the onset of disease or after treatment (oral antifungal agents are highly effective at treating the disease). When imaging findings are present, they are usually seen from the mid to upper esophagus with multiple and diffuse raised mucosal plaques, sometimes with pseudomembranes and ulcer formation with severe disease (Fig. 1-42). The appearances can sometimes be confused with glycogenic acanthoses, which have randomly deposited mucosal abnormalities, whereas a *Candida* infection tends to have linear mucosal plaques (Figs. 1-42 and 1-43).

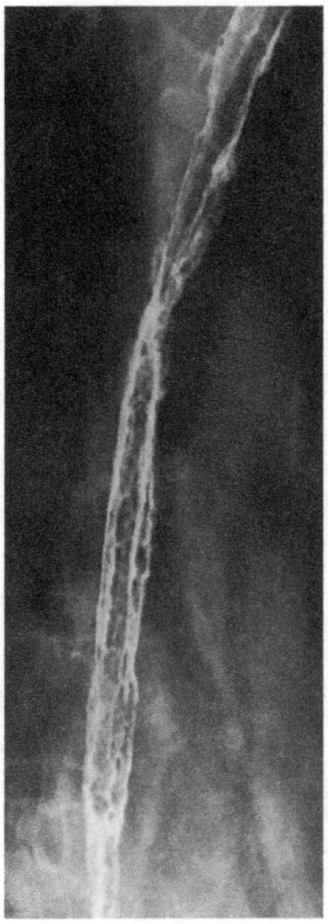

FIGURE 1-42. UGI swallow in 43-year-old woman undergoing chemotherapy for breast cancer and *Candida* esophagitis. There is a "shaggy," plaque-like appearance to the esophageal mucosa.

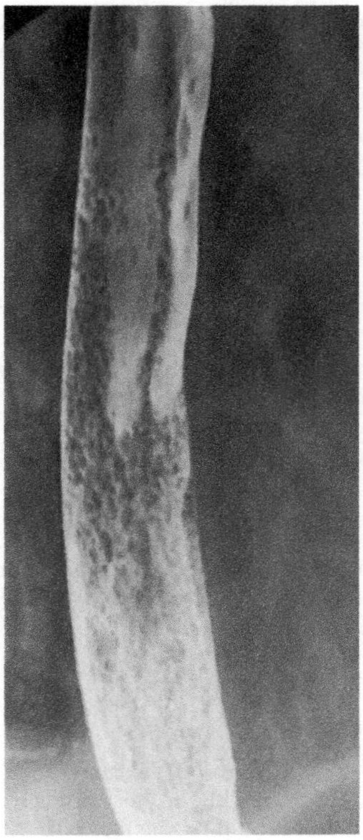

FIGURE 1-43. UGI swallow in a 74-year-old woman with multiple, predominantly rounded or ovoid, randomly distributed mucosal defects due to glycogenic acanthosis.

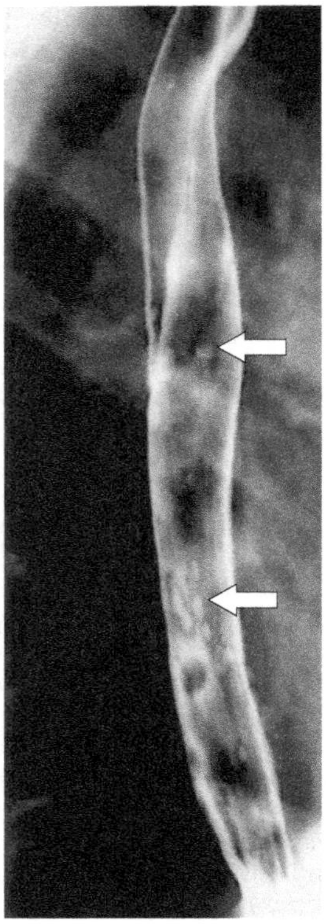

FIGURE 1-44. Barium swallow in a 33-year-old man with immunosuppression showing multiple punctate esophageal ulcers (*arrows*) due to herpes esophagitis.

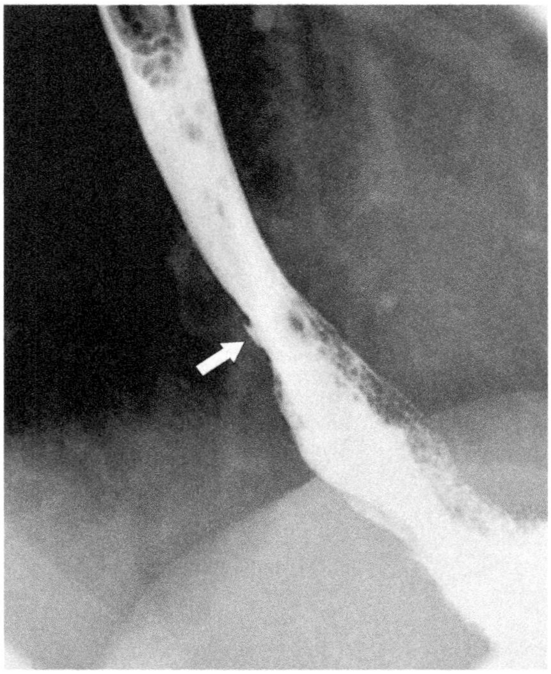

FIGURE 1-45. Barium swallow in a 63-year-old man with subtle esophageal ulcers *(arrow)* caused by reflux esophagitis. There is also a granular appearance to the lower esophagus.

Viral Esophagitis

Herpes, CMV, and HIV esophagitis also typically follow immunocompromised states but can also develop when the esophageal mucosa is damaged from radiation therapy used to treat mediastinal malignancies. With herpes infection, UGI examination will demonstrate multiple small and discrete ulcers separated by normal mucosa, unlike *Candida* infection, in which the mucosa is diffusely involved (Fig. 1-44). CMV and HIV tend to have fewer ulcers, and sometimes there is only a single larger ulcer. Rarely, human papillomavirus and Epstein-Barr* virus can also infect the esophagus.

Fungus

Fungal ulcers result from extension from the mouth and pharynx and demonstrate mucosal, plaque-like disease. The diffusion of barium between these plaques may give the appearance of ulceration; however, this is pseudoulceration.

Tuberculosis

Tuberculosis may result from direct mediastinal extension with ulceration secondary to the extrinsic invasion of the disease, but it can occasionally occur within the esophagus as a result of swallowing infected sputum.

Reflux Esophagitis

Reflux esophagitis is a common disease due to the widespread incidence of GERD; up to 20% of Westerners will have GERD at some time. Any condition that enhances either the production of acid or facilitation of reflux through the GE junction predisposes the patient to lower esophageal ulceration. Therefore, hyperacidity due to Zollinger-Ellison syndrome compounded by GERD can lead to severe esophagitis and ulcer formation. Patients may be asymptomatic, but most will complain of some pain (heartburn) at some time. The disease can be acute and self-limiting or often chronic, requiring adjustment of food intake, antacid medication, and possible histamine (H2) blocker or proton pump inhibitor treatment. The lower esophageal sphincter tone is generally weakened, permitting free retrograde flow of gastric juice. The irritation caused by refluxing gastric acidic juice readily inflames the mucosa and is usually confined to the lower esophagus.

Imaging findings in acute disease include decreased primary peristaltic waves and, sometimes, increased tertiary contractions. There may be an associated esophageal spasm, which tends to give the esophagus a shortened appearance. There is mucosal edema, which can lead to thickened folds, either vertical or transverse, and erosive disease, which is manifested by subtle nodular or granular changes (Fig. 1-41). Further erosive disease can lead to ulceration, seen as subtle, tiny collections of barium with surrounding edematous edges and thickened folds, which may radiate away from the ulcer (Fig. 1-45).

With more chronic disease, a hiatal hernia is almost always present. The mucosa can appear puckered or serrated because of edema and spasm. Pseudodiverticula are classic signs indicative of chronic inflammation (Figs. 1-11 and 1-46). Continued inflammation will ultimately lead to stricture formation, usually of the lower esophagus, represented by a short smooth narrowing typically 1 to 3 cm in length (Fig. 1-47). More severe strictures can develop, with or without ulceration (Fig. 1-48). A benign inflammatory pseudopolyp can also develop, representing a profusely enlarged esophageal fold at the GE junction (see Fig. 1-18).

The greatest risk from GERD is the development of a Barrett* esophagus. This occurs in about 10% of patients with GERD (most also have a hiatal hernia) and chronic esophagitis; therefore it is relatively common in the population. Some patients are

*Michael A. Epstein (1921-2006), British pathologist and virologist; Yvonne M. Barr (1932-), British virologist.

*Norman Barrett (1903-1979), British surgeon.

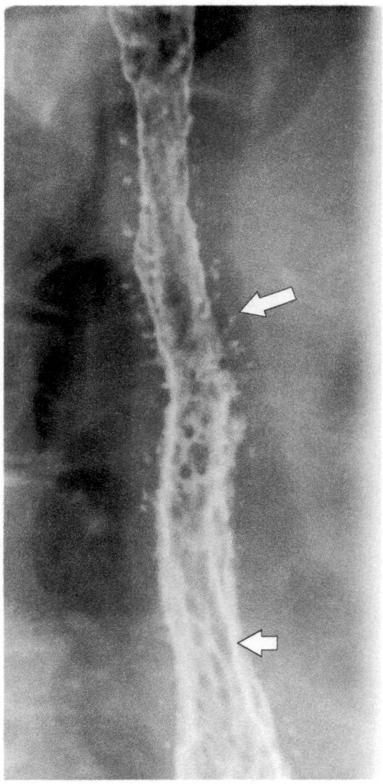

Figure 1-46. Barium swallow in a 43-year-old man with multiple pseudodiverticula (*long arrow*). The patient also has underlying candidiasis (*short arrow*).

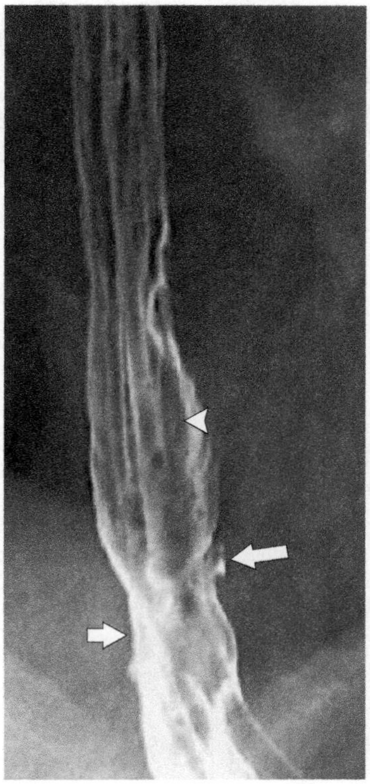

Figure 1-47. UGI swallow in a 57-year-old man with chronic lower esophagitis with a short smooth stricture (*short arrow*), fold thickening (*arrowhead*), and small ulcerations (*long arrow*).

asymptomatic, so the incidence may well be higher. It is more common in males, possibly because it is more commonly associated with centripetal obesity. It requires a histological diagnosis because it represents squamous metaplasia to gastric columnar epithelium, a premalignant condition that can progress to adenocarcinoma in about 0.5% of patients per year. Therefore its detection and follow-up are important. Any patient with symptomatic prolonged GERD should be periodically screened (either with EGD or UGI examination) to determine any presence of the abnormality. Once detected, annual EGD procedures with biopsies of the affected area should be performed to rule out the presence of dysplastic squamous cells.

At UGI examination, Barrett esophagus is recognized by a focal mucosal nodularity, a reticular mucosal pattern, or ulceration and stricture formation in the mid to lower esophagus (Fig. 1-49). Many appear as simple, smooth strictures, but others demonstrate short, narrower strictures, with or without ulceration (Fig. 1-50). Because there is frequent monitoring (usually endoscopy), early esophageal carcinoma can be detected (Fig. 1-51).

Less commonly, biliary reflux can also cause erosions and ulcers of the lower esophagus and is a result of disordered bowel mechanics from partial or complete gastric resections with cholodocho-enteric anastomoses. The alkaline bile refluxes into the lower esophagus, which is as toxic as gastric acid and readily causes edema, erosions, ulceration, and ultimately stricture formation. It is usually best treated by diverting bile away from the stomach remnant and esophagus with a Roux*-en-Y loop of gastroduodenostomy.

Prolonged nasogastric tube insertion interferes with esophageal sphincter closure, and continuous reflux can occur in addition to failure to clear the lower esophagus from refluxed acid due to dysmotility and abnormal peristalsis. Changes of esophagitis mimic those of the more common GERD due to hiatal hernia.

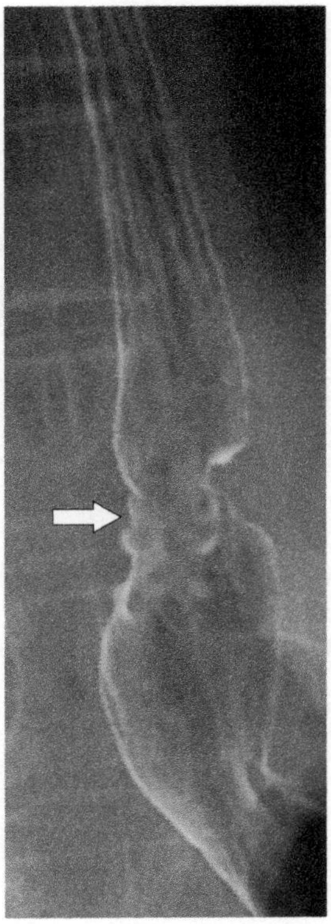

Figure 1-48. Barium swallow in a 59-year-old woman with thickened longitudinal folds due to reflux esophagitis and a lower esophageal irregularity and narrowing (*arrow*) due to a peptic stricture.

---

*César Roux (1857-1934), Swiss surgeon.

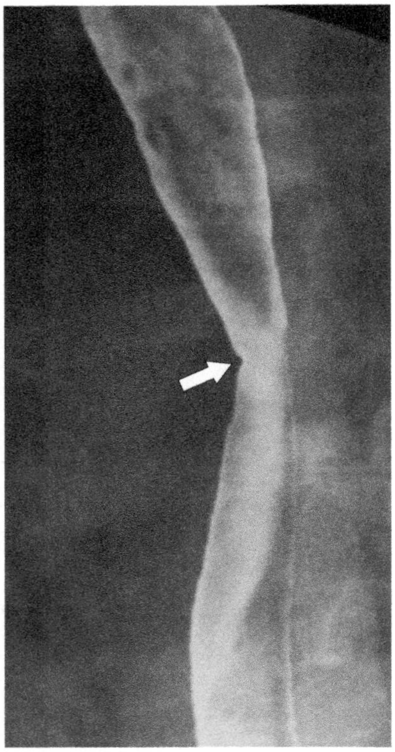

FIGURE 1-49. Barium swallow in a 61-year-old woman with a midesophageal smooth stricture (*arrow*) due to Barrett esophagus.

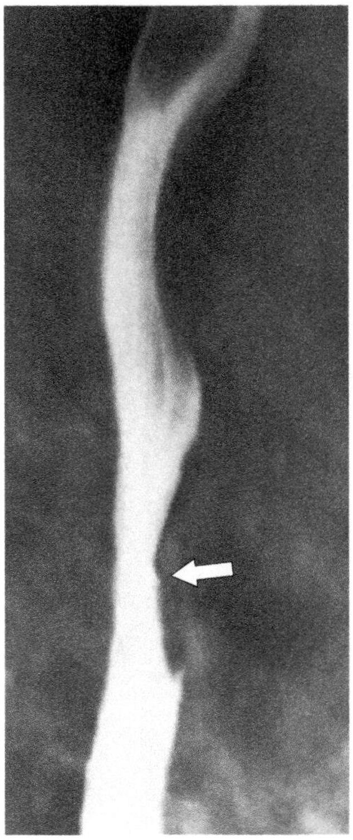

FIGURE 1-51. UGI swallow in a 60-year-old woman with midesophageal stricture due to Barrett esophagus and a plaque-like mucosal defect due to early adenocarcinoma (*arrow*).

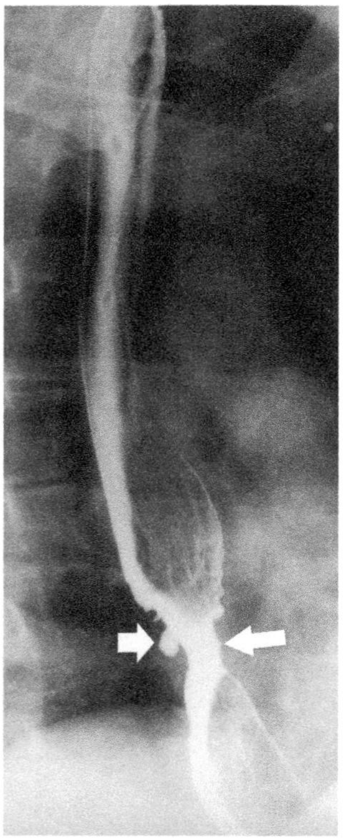

FIGURE 1-50. UGI swallow in a 61-year-old man with a tight, short midesophageal stricture (*long arrow*) and ulcer (*short arrow*) due to Barrett esophagus.

Drug-Induced Esophagitis

Some drugs are caustic to the esophagus if they have prolonged contact with the mucosa because of dysmotility or some other local stricture. Alternatively, if these medications are taken with patients in the supine or prone position before the patients sleep, they can be held up at the level of the aortic arch, left main bronchus, or distal esophagus. These medications include tetracyclines, potassium chloride, quinidine, and nonsteroidal antiinflammatory drugs (NSAIDs). Imaging findings consist of multiple small ulcers that are variable in shape and shallow in depth (Fig. 1-52). Some ulcers are larger and appear more sinister but will ultimately heal by fibrosis and stricture formation (Figs.1-53 and 1-54). Acute alcoholic binges may result in esophageal ulceration, typically of the mid to lower esophagus, although these do not usually lead to stricture formation.

Caustic or Corrosive Esophagitis

Strong liquid alkali or acid ingestion (e.g., lye, a concentrated sodium hydroxide, ammonium chloride, silver nitrate, and other acids) causes a severe erosive and diffuse ulceration of the esophagus, which can be fatal in the acute stage. The stomach and duodenum can be affected if sufficient quantities are swallowed and reach these anatomical regions, but the acute manifestations are most common in the esophagus.

In the acute phase, the esophagus is atonic with extensive ulceration, which may perforate, leading to gas in the mediastinum (Fig. 1-55). It tends to heal by fibrosis and stricture formation (often very narrowed) primarily of the midesophagus, either focally or as a diffusely long stricture (Fig. 1-56). This may retract the stomach partially into the chest because of associated esophageal shortening from the stricture. The ulceration and stricture formation are premalignant for esophageal squamous carcinoma,

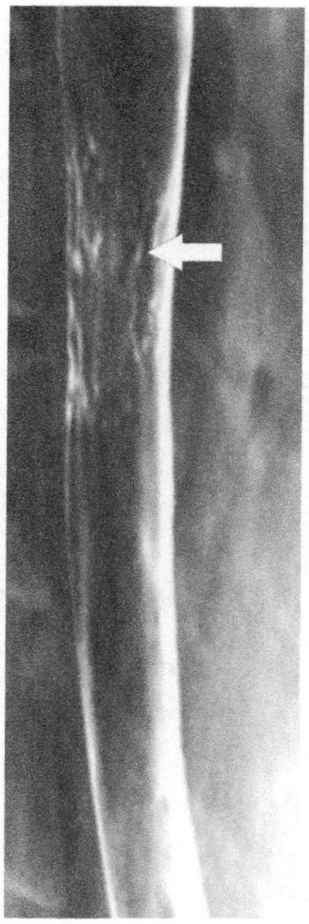

FIGURE 1-52. UGI swallow in a 47-year-old man with midesophageal ulceration (*arrow*) resulting from tetracycline administration.

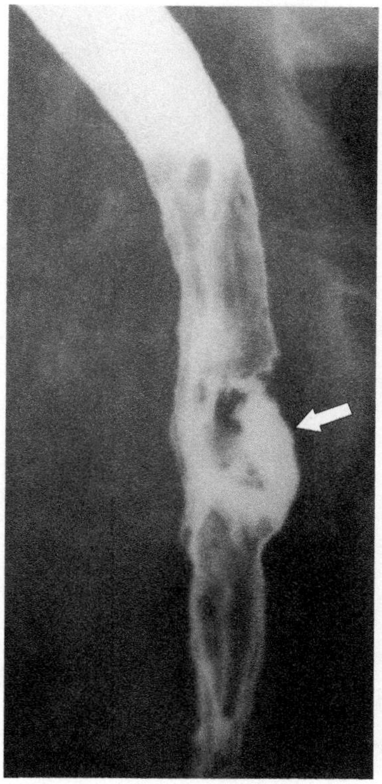

FIGURE 1-53. Barium swallow in a 47-year-old woman with a large midesophageal ulcer (*arrow*) due to ulceration from indomethacin ingestion.

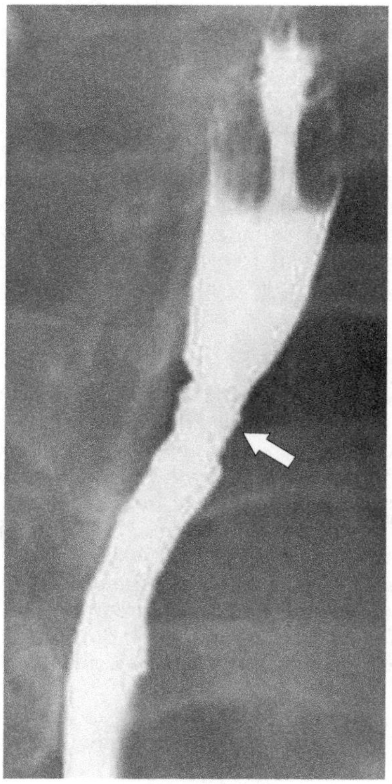

FIGURE 1-54. UGI swallow in a 38-year-old woman with a short narrowing (*arrow*) in the upper esophagus secondary to fibrotic stricture caused by nonsteroidal antiinflammatory drugs.

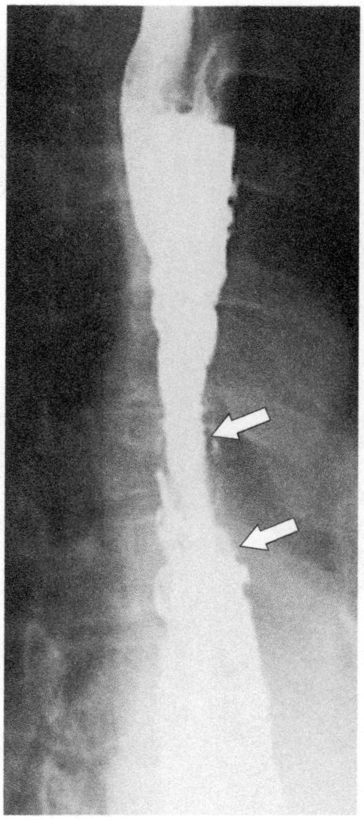

FIGURE 1-55. UGI barium swallow in a 21-year-old woman with recent ingestion of lye demonstrating esophageal narrowing due to edema and ulcers (*arrows*).

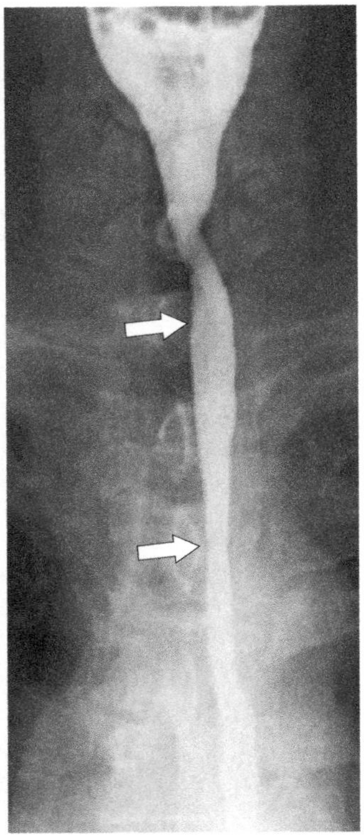

FIGURE 1-56. UGI swallow in a 55-year-old man with a long esophageal stricture (*arrows*) due to previous caustic ingestion.

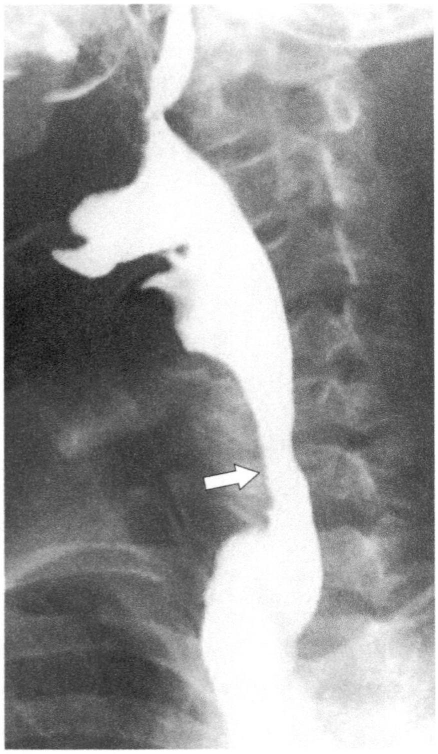

FIGURE 1-57. Barium swallow in a 65-year-old man with prior radiation for thyroid cancer, demonstrating a radiation stricture (*arrow*) in the upper esophagus.

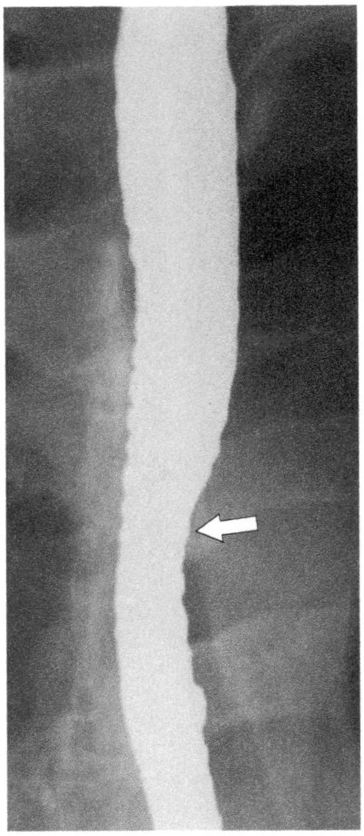

FIGURE 1-58. Barium swallow in a 33-year-old woman with diffuse mild narrowing and nodularity (*arrow*) due to eosinophilic esophagitis.

which may develop 20 years after the ingestion. This would require lifelong repeat endoscopies to exclude malignant transformation in these patients.

Radiation Esophagitis

Radiation esophagitis is less common than in the past because of more recently refined radiation treatment protocols. In the acute phase, there are esophageal edema and a friable esophagus that may cause not only an ulcer, but also a stricture. Fistula formation may then occur between the esophagus and the underlying mediastinal tumor that is being treated or the adjacent normal mediastinum or lung. Healing is by stricture formation, which can be difficult to differentiate from other chronic strictures, although a history of radiation is suggestive (Fig. 1-57).

Eosinophilic Esophagitis

Eosinophilic esophagitis is a poorly understood inflammatory disease that occurs in patients with hyperallergenic conditions with associated hypereosinophilia. Histologically, there is eosinophilic infiltration of all layers of the esophageal wall, and a diagnosis is made at esophageal biopsy. It is associated with other GI eosinophilic conditions (e.g., eosinophilic gastroenteritis). At imaging, there may be diffuse esophageal nodularity, which histologically is filled with eosinophils (Fig. 1-58). More often, however, ulceration and stricture formation are observed (Fig. 1-59). The most specific imaging finding is a "ringed" esophagus due to narrow, fine circumferential focal stricture formation (Fig. 1-60).

Crohn Disease (see Chapter 4)

Only about 3% of patients with Crohn disease have esophageal manifestations, and when present, they are typically concomitant with active small bowel disease. Aphthous ulcerations (discrete

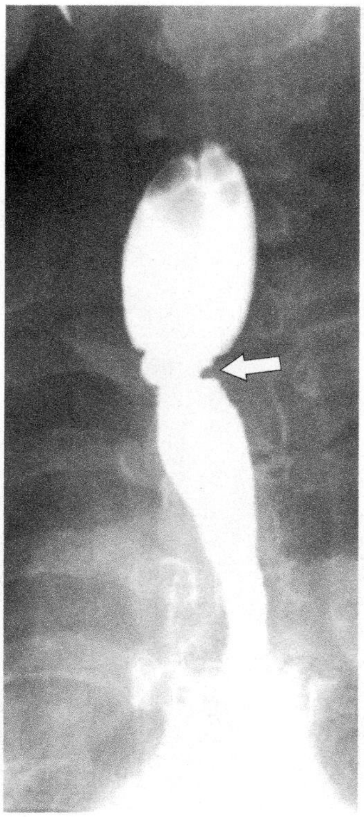

FIGURE 1-59. Barium swallow in a 23-year-old man with an upper esophageal stricture (*arrow*) due to eosinophilic esophagitis.

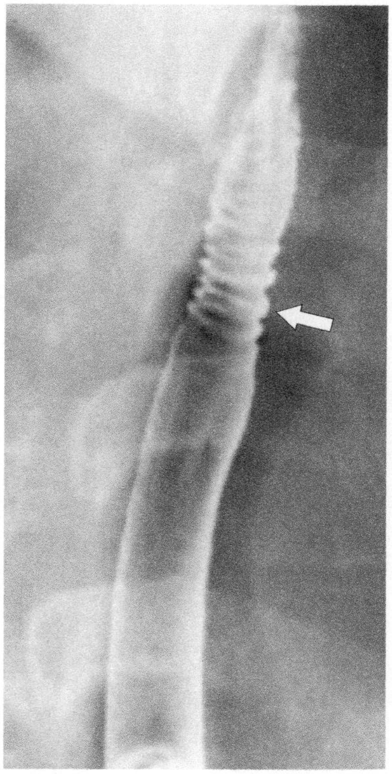

FIGURE 1-60. UGI swallow in a 43-year-old woman with a ring-appearing esophagus (*arrow*) due to eosinophilic esophagitis.

small ulcers with edematous ring) can occur anywhere along the GI tract with Crohn disease, and they appear as a tiny pool of barium surrounded by an edematous halo (see Chapter 2). Other features include small erosions and mucosal polyps, similar to those in the lower small bowel and colon, particularly in its healing phase. Stricture formation and fistula have also been recognized.

Behçet Disease

Behçet* disease is a systemic disease affecting mucous membranes (aphthous ulcers), the skin (erythema nodosum and pyoderma gangrenosum), the eyes (uveitis and optic atrophy), the penis (genital ulcerations), the lungs (pleuritis), the joints (arthritis), the brain (dural sinus thrombosis), and the gut. Its cause is poorly understood, but it is thought to be an immune response to external agents rather than autoimmune, although this is unsubstantiated. It commonly affects the esophagus with findings ranging from esophagitis with or without ulceration and stricture formation.

Pemphigoid

An extension of the epidermal manifestation of this disease can extend to the esophagus with mucosal webs (early in the disease) or bullae (blebs), which are recognized as small nodular mucosal lesions at EGD and UGI examination. These readily ulcerate, and chronic disease can result in esophageal stricture, mostly in the upper esophagus (Fig. 1-61). Some strictures can be very narrow, and a "jet" of barium may be seen below the stricture (Fig. 1-62). There is a risk of malignant degeneration to squamous cell carcinoma.

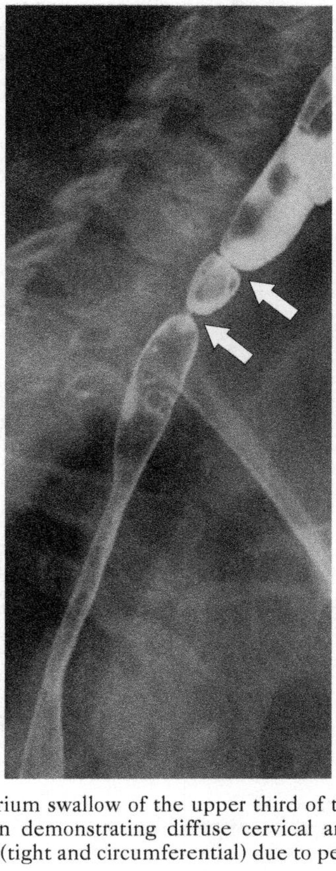

FIGURE 1-61. Barium swallow of the upper third of the esophagus in a 55-year-old woman demonstrating diffuse cervical and upper thoracic strictures (*arrows*) (tight and circumferential) due to pemphigoid.

*Hulusi Behçet (1889-1948), Turkish dermatologist.

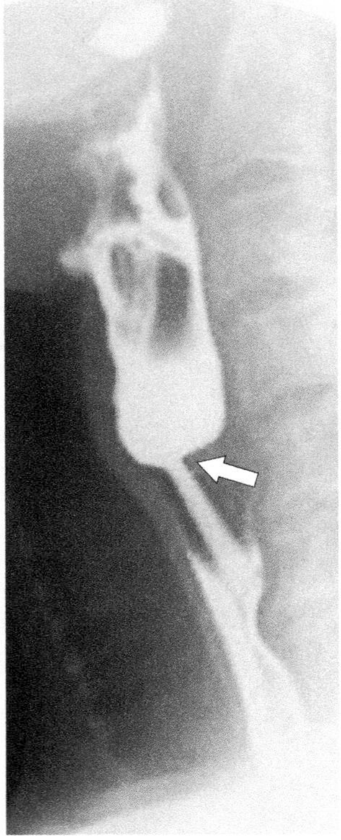

FIGURE 1-62. UGI series in a 49-year-old woman with pemphigoid and a tight stricture (*arrow*) with a barium "jet" caudally.

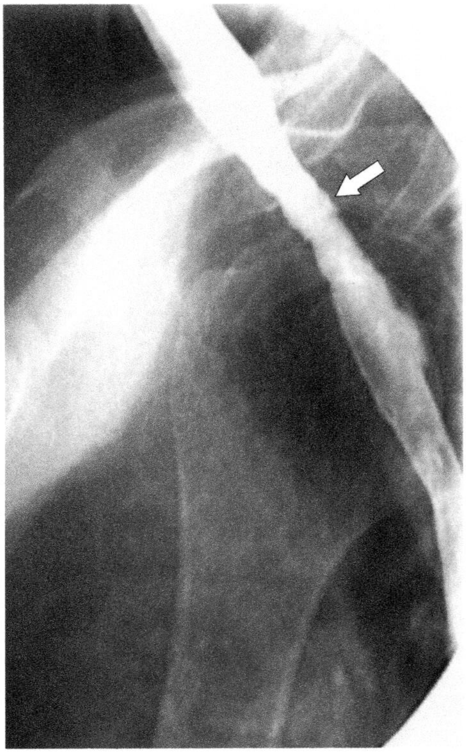

FIGURE 1-64. UGI in a 49-year-old woman with an upper esophageal stricture (*arrow*) due to epidermolysis bullosa.

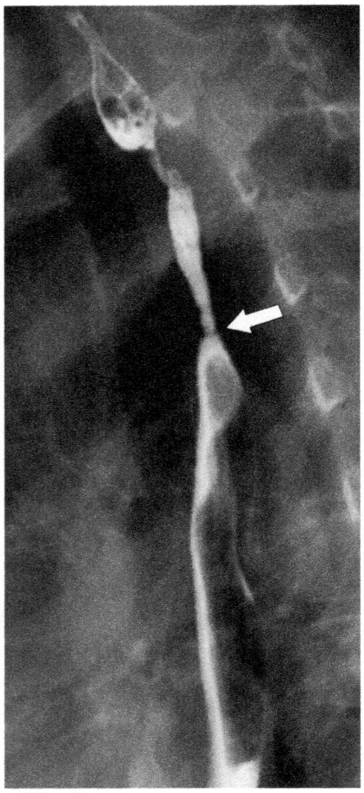

FIGURE 1-63. Oblique UGI swallow of the upper esophagus in a 59-year-old woman with a tight stricture (*arrow*) due to epidermolysis bullosa. The appearance is not dissimilar to pemphigoid.

Epidermolysis Bullosa

Epidermolysis bullosa is similar to pemphigoid with multiple small esophageal bullae that form in the upper esophagus in conjunction with epidermal disease. These ulcerate and result in strictures on healing, with either tight focal strictures or longer tapered strictures (Figs. 1-63 and 1-64). There is a small risk of malignant degeneration.

Tylosis

Tylosis is a rare autosomal dominant disease characterized by hyperkeratinization of the palms of the hands (and sometimes the soles of the feet) with a high risk for squamous esophageal carcinoma (approximately 95% of patients aged 70 years) secondary to esophageal leukoplakia and dysplasia. In the esophagus, focal, small, nonspecific ulcerations can occur along any length of the esophagus, stomach, and small bowel. In the colon, it can produce a colitis similar to ulcerative colitis and is one of the potential causes of a toxic megacolon (see "Thumb-Printing and Toxic Megacolon" in Chapter 5).

Glycogenic Acanthosis

Glycogenic acanthosis is a condition typically seen in the elderly, characterized by small (2 to 10 mm), multiple, disparate, plaque-like mucosal lesions throughout the esophagus, which can be numerous or scattered (Figs. 1-43 and 1-65). These are filled with glycogen deposits, hence their name. Diagnosis is benign, and it is usually detected incidentally and is mostly asymptomatic.

Ectopic Gastric Mucosa

Gastric heterotopia (or ectopic mucosa) in the upper esophagus is present in about 4% of patients and is usually asymptomatic, unlike Barrett esophagus. Ectopic gastric mucosa can produce small, ring-like indentations of the esophagus, usually at the level of the thoracic inlet.

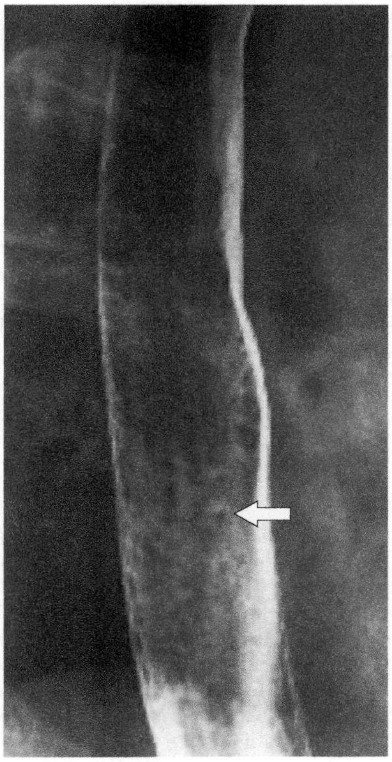

FIGURE 1-65. UGI swallow in an 85-year-old man with multiple small scattered esophageal plaques (*arrow*) due to glycogenic acanthosis.

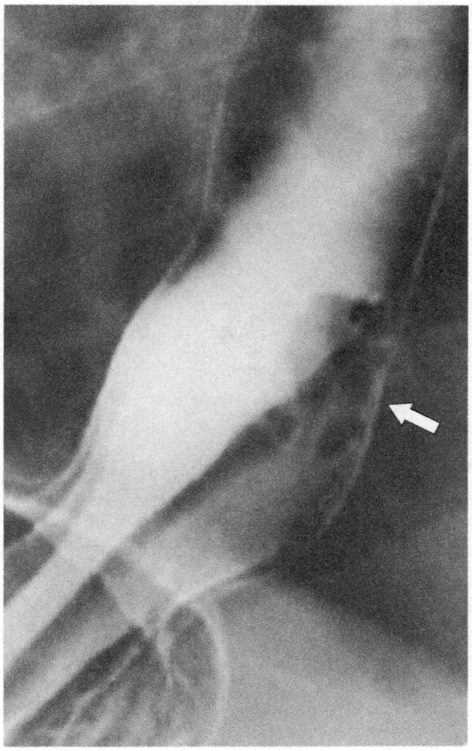

FIGURE 1-66. Barium swallow of the lower esophagus in a 63-year-old woman with an irregular mucosal mass (*arrow*) due to a villous adenoma.

NEOPLASTIC ESOPHAGEAL MUCOSAL ABNORMALITIES

Benign

Squamous Papillomas and Papillomatosis

Squamous papilloma is a rare condition, thought to be mostly benign, but it can be premalignant with the development of squamous carcinoma. A papilloma may be single, but more than one is known as *papillomatosis*. Squamous papillomas are associated with acanthosis nigricans, and at imaging, they appear as single or multiple small polyps.

Villous Adenoma

These adenomas are rarely identified. Like villous adenomatous polyps elsewhere in the GI tract, they appear as frond-like mucosal masses and have premalignant potential (Fig. 1-66).

Hamartoma

Cowden's* disease or multiple hamartoma syndrome, is a rare autosomal dominant-inherited disease that produces widespread hamartomatous disease, particularly of the skin. When it affects the esophagus, multiple small mucosal nodularities can be identified. Similar manifestations can be observed in the colon. These hamartomas are premalignant throughout the body, and frequent patient screening is required.

Leukoplakia

Leukoplakia is due to hyperplastic squamous epithelium that occurs most commonly in the oropharynx because of excessive tobacco use. In the oropharynx it is premalignant, but in the esophagus, where it is less commonly observed, it has debatable malignant potential. When observed, it produces small, whitish, plaque-like mucosal esophageal abnormalities.

*Cowden's syndrome was first mentioned in 1963; Cowden was the first patient seen with the condition.

Box 1-1. Risk Factors for the Development of Esophageal Cancer

- Alcohol
- Tobacco
- Chronic reflux esophagitis/Barrett complex
- HPV infection
- Achalasia
- Caustic ingestion (lye)
- Radiation
- Head and neck cancer
- Plummer-Vinson syndrome
- Celiac disease
- Tylosis (hyperkeratosis)
- Pemphigoid
- Epidermolysis bullosa

HPV, Human papillomavirus.

Malignant

Carcinoma

Carcinoma of the esophagus continues to have high mortality because the development of these tumors is indolent and therefore the tumors present late. Early detection, however, has a 90% 5-year survival. There are multiple predisposing factors (Box 1-1). Males are four times more likely than women to be affected, mostly because of smoking and alcohol habits. Patients present with dysphagia (difficulty swallowing), particularly of solids, and odynophagia (painful swallowing), pain, weight loss, and anorexia.

Most esophageal carcinomas worldwide are squamous (90%), with adenocarcinomas accounting for approximately 5% to 10% (most of which arise from Barrett esophagus) (see "Submucosal Esophageal Masses" earlier in the chapter) (Table 1-6). In

TABLE 1-6 Esophageal Carcinoma

Type	Frequency
Squamous	Worldwide, 90%; Western Europe/ United States, 50%
Adenocarcinoma	Worldwide, 5%-10%; Western Europe/United States, 35%-50%
Spindle cell carcinoma	<1%
Carcinosarcoma	<1%
Primary malignant melanoma	<1%
Oat cell carcinoma	<1%

TABLE 1-7 Staging of Esophageal Carcinoma

Stage	Disease Extension
0	Carcinoma in situ
I	Lamina propria/submucosa
IIA	Transmural but not further extension
IIB	Transmural and regional lymph nodes
III	Regional lymph nodes (or other nodes), invasion of adjacent structures
IVB	Regional or other nodes
IVB	Regional or other nodes and distant metastases

Western Europe and the United States, there has been a marked increase over the last generation in adenocarcinomas so that they now account for nearly 50% of esophageal tumors in some studies. Other tumors are very rare (Table 1-6). Approximately 20% occur in the upper esophagus, 50% in the middle, and 30% in the lower esophagus. The staging is listed in Table 1-7.

The findings at UGI examination depend on the timing of the diagnosis. Early findings may demonstrate small sessile polyps or plaque-like lesions, although with adenocarcinoma, there is usually an associated Barrett esophagus with small plaque-like lesions or more marked irregularity along the Barrett stricture (see Fig. 1-51). Later presentations produce larger lesions, which infiltrate along the length of affected esophagus, with a shelf-like abrupt transition from normal to abnormal esophageal mucosa (not dissimilar to its colonic adenocarcinoma "apple core" counterpart), with resultant luminal stricture formation (Fig. 1-67). The mucosa is distorted, blunted, or destroyed, and nodular masses can arise, which can ulcerate (Fig. 1-68). Other lesions can present as flat ulcers surrounded by an edematous rim. A rarer type is varicoid carcinoma, whereby the neoplasm extends submucosally along a length of esophagus, giving the appearance of varicosities or thickened folds (see Fig. 1-33). The mucosal folds may not be as smooth as those in esophageal varices, and this result gives a clue to the diagnosis. The patient may not have a history of cirrhosis. Some gastric adenocarcinomas invade the lower esophagus and extend a few centimeters above the GE junction (Fig. 1-69). At UGI examination, it can be difficult to know for certain whether these tumors are primarily esophageal extending to the GE junction or vice versa, and the diagnosis may only be made at endoscopy and biopsy.

At CT, the primary tumor can be harder to identify unless it is large, particularly if the esophagus is undistended and empty of oral contrast medium. However, CT is far superior to UGI examination for the identification of any local extension, including regional lymphadenopathy (Fig. 1-70). In stages I and II and early

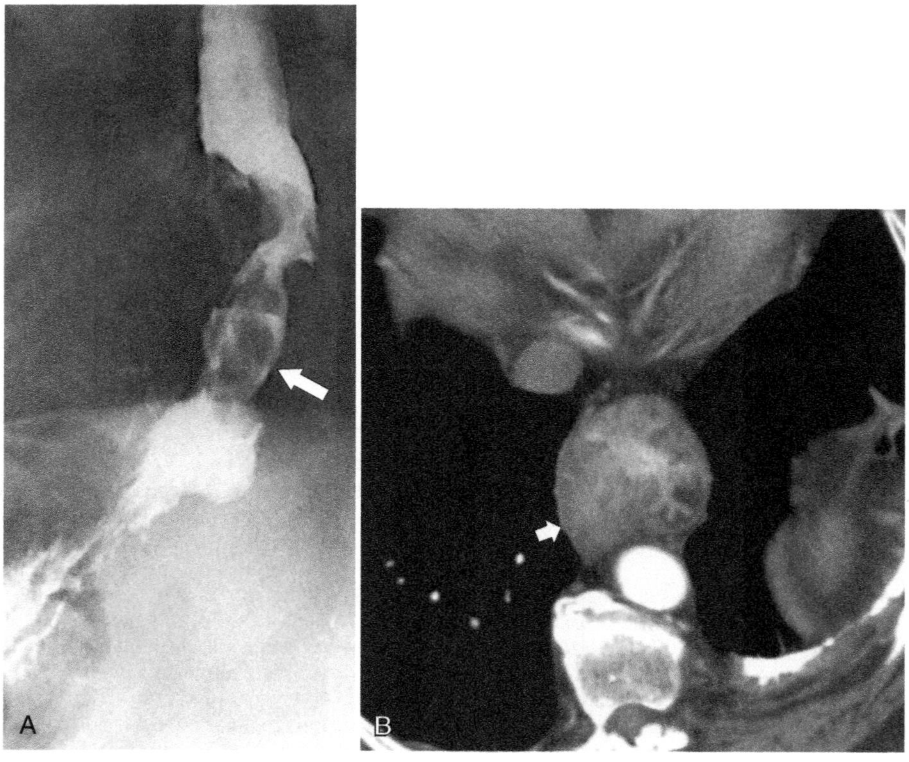

FIGURE 1-67. UGI swallow (**A**) and axial contrast-enhanced CT (**B**) of the lower esophagus in a 68-year-old man with marked mucosal irregularity (**A**; *arrow*) typical of esophageal carcinoma. The lesion is less evident on CT, with eccentric wall thickening (**B**; *arrow*).

stage III, tumors will generally not be identified at CT, although simple esophageal thickening may be present (Table 1-7). Once a tumor develops later in stage III, the mass should be detected by CT as the tumor invades the surrounding mediastinal structures and enlarges regional lymph nodes (Fig. 1-71). Stage IV disease should demonstrate distant dissemination of the disease, particularly to the lungs, liver, and lymph nodes. The detection of these lymph nodes is more readily identifiable by PET/CT, however, which may also aid in detecting more distant disease (particularly lymph nodes) (Fig. 1-71).

Adenocarcinomas look similar to squamous cell carcinomas, even when arising in a Barrett esophagus. By the time the patient is seen, the Barrett stricture has generally been obliterated by the malignant process (Fig. 1-72).

Other carcinomas are rare, and diagnosis will only be made at histological examination. Spindle cell carcinoma is a rare variant of squamous cell carcinoma due to mesenchymal metaplastic transformation. These cells are typically large and polypoid. Oat cell carcinoma, primary esophageal melanoma, and carcinosarcoma are even rarer and present similarly to spindle

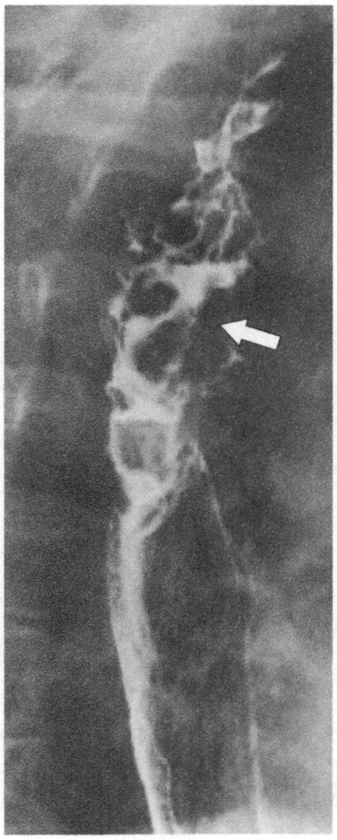

FIGURE 1-68. UGI swallow of the midesophagus in a 54-year-old man with nodular distortion of the mucosal folds (*arrow*) due to esophageal carcinoma.

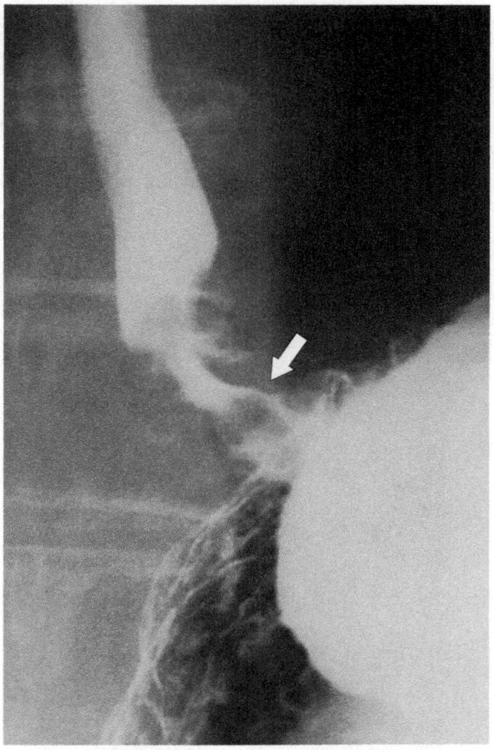

FIGURE 1-69. UGI swallow in a 59-year-old woman with irregular and distorted lower esophageal mucosa due to adenocarcinoma of the gastric cardia infiltrating up into the lower esophagus (*arrow*).

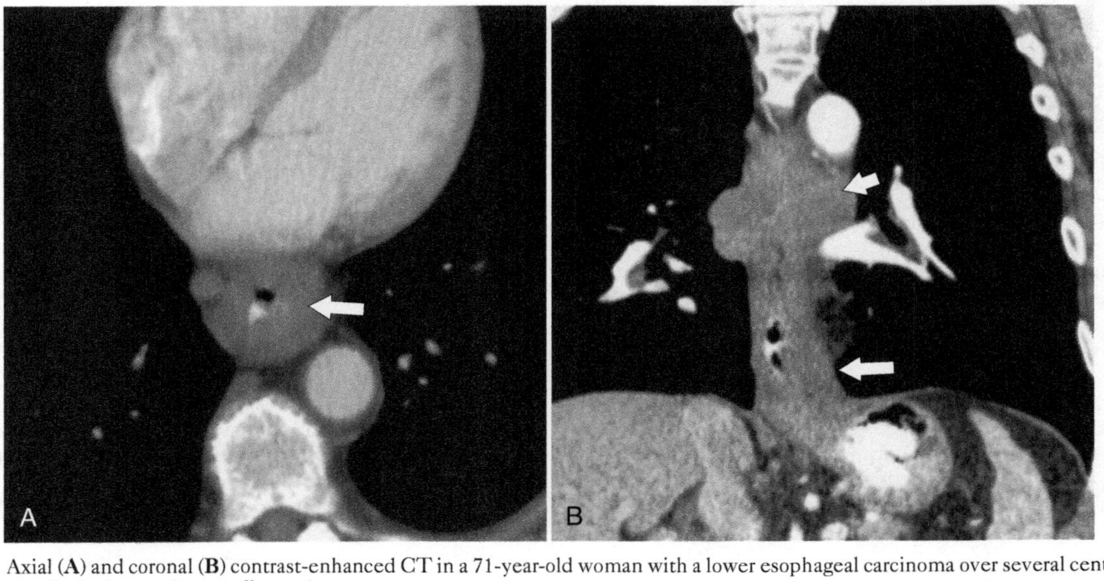

FIGURE 1-70. Axial (**A**) and coronal (**B**) contrast-enhanced CT in a 71-year-old woman with a lower esophageal carcinoma over several centimeters (*large arrow*) with mediastinal adenopathy (*small arrow*).

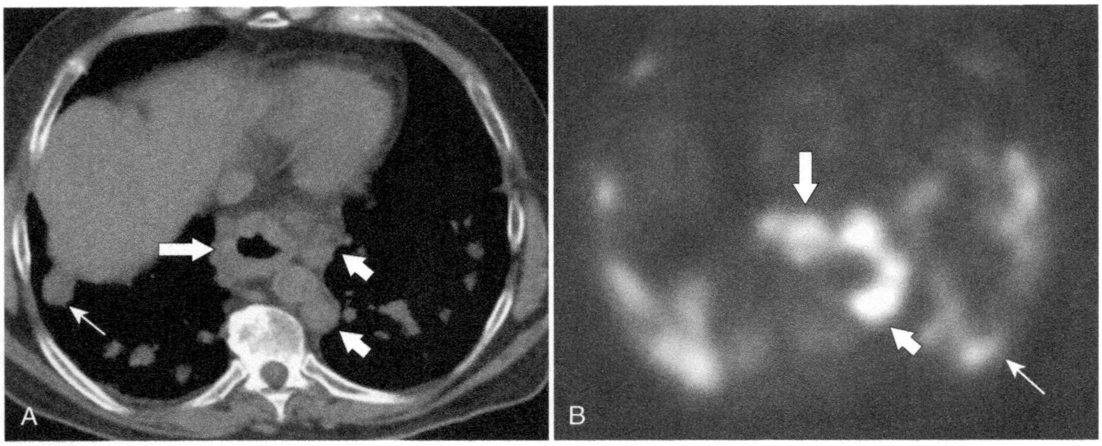

FIGURE 1-71. Axial noncontrast CT (A) and PET (B) in a 70-year-old woman with stage IV esophageal carcinoma (*large arrows*) with multiple paraesophageal lymph nodes (*small arrows*) and lung metastases (*thin arrow*).

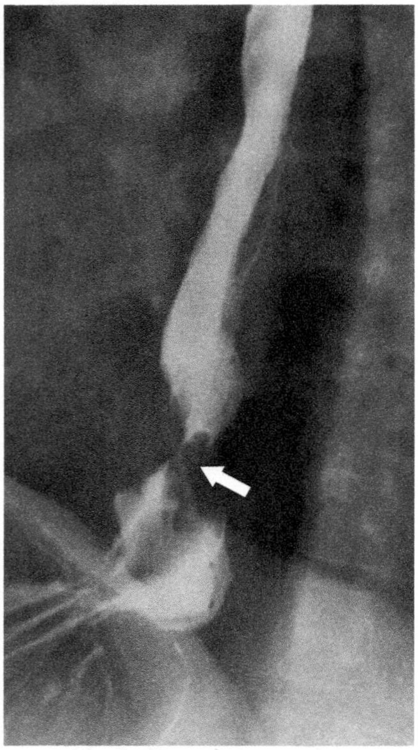

FIGURE 1-72. UGI swallow in a 67-year-old man with a lower esophageal adenocarcinoma (*arrow*) arising in a Barrett esophagus.

cell carcinoma. Superficial spreading carcinoma is a variant of squamous cell carcinoma that is characterized by small mucosal nodules rather than plaque-like or polypoid masses. It has a better prognosis because it is usually confined to the mucosa and submucosa.

Kaposi Sarcoma

Kaposi* sarcoma is caused by a herpes virus and is a systemic disease that typically manifests with purplish skin papular lesions. There are four subtypes, which were originally described in

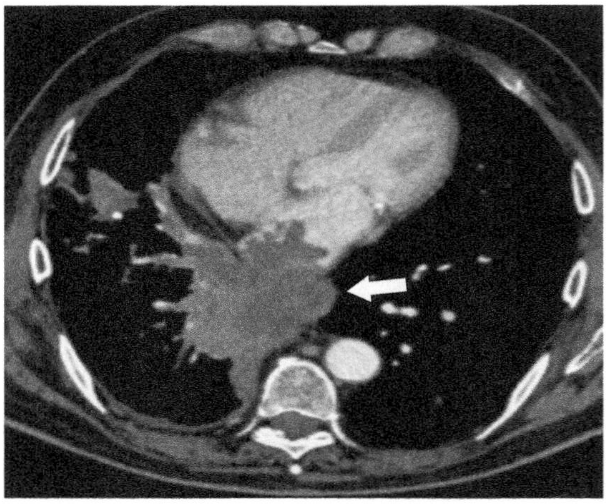

FIGURE 1-73. Axial contrast-enhanced CT in a 66-year-old woman with esophageal invasion (*arrow*) by a large lung cancer.

middle-aged men of Mediterranean and Jewish descent who had vascular cutaneous lesions. This same disease is now observed more commonly in immunocompromised patients, particularly those with AIDS. The former type has a more benign and indolent course, but the type that results from immunosuppression has a more aggressive course. Both the respiratory and GI tracts can be involved, particularly with the immune-suppressed form, with single or multiple submucosal lesions, which often have central ulceration (see Chapter 2).

Metastatic Disease

Metastatic disease results either from local extension (including the larynx, thyroid, and lung), mediastinal nodes (e.g., lymphoma), and gastric extension into the esophagus or rarely from hematogenous spread (breast, melanoma) (Fig. 1-73). In malignancies that directly invade the esophagus from local structures, there may be a smooth extrinsic compression before mucosal nodularity and ulceration are seen, confirming that the malignancy has extended transmurally. As ulceration and necrosis develop, fistula formation can occur, which rarely results from hematogenous metastatic spread (Fig. 1-74). Hematogenous spread from breast cancer typically produces short eccentric strictures, whereas those from melanoma produce submucosal "bull's-eye" ulcerating lesions, as elsewhere in the GI tract. Lymphomatous extension from mediastinal nodes

*Moritz Kaposi (1837-1902), Hungarian dermatologist.

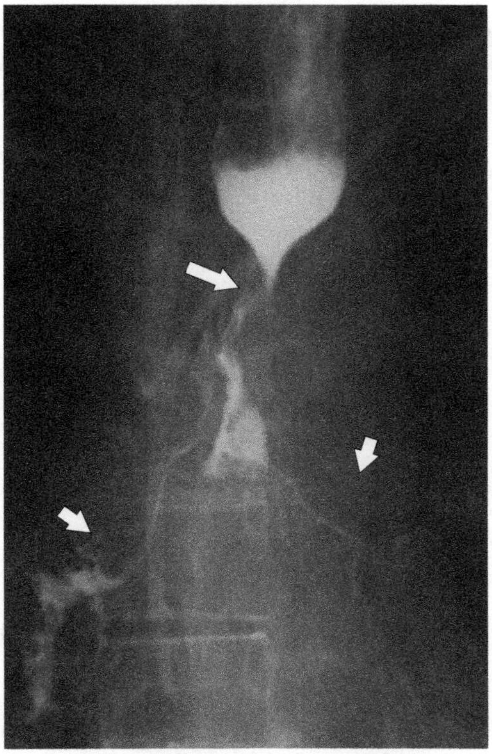

FIGURE 1-74. Nonionic contrast media UGI swallow in a 76-year-old man with metastatic lymphadenopathy to the esophagus, stricture formation (*large arrow*) from lung cancer, and a bronchoesophageal fistula (*small arrows*).

often causes less ulceration; rather, it may produce a more smooth-tapered, achalasia-like appearance.

ESOPHAGEAL MOTILITY DISORDERS

Normal Peristalsis

Peristalsis is a complex neuromuscular and involuntary event involving a primary peristaltic wave that is initiated at the moment of swallowing that propels the food bolus caudally with progressive stripping (or propulsive) waves. This wave is soon followed by the secondary peristaltic wave that results from esophageal distention by the food bolus and is a locally initiated propulsive wave in the area immediately adjacent to the food bolus. Under normal conditions, the result is a smooth, wave-like contraction from upper to lower esophagus. Tertiary contractions are nonpropulsive, random, and disorganized contractions observed more often in the elderly. Dysmotility disorders are caused by disparate causes but are probably most common after stroke, given its frequency in the population (Table 1-8).

Neurogenic Dysmotility

Central or peripheral neuropathies can affect esophageal peristalsis and lead to major dysmotility. It is not uncommon after stroke for the patient to have swallowing difficulties, often with aspiration and its consequent complications. Other causes are listed in Table 1-8. Many of these causes can be sufficiently debilitating that the patient will ultimately require enteral or parenteral feeding; many patients require the placement of gastric or jejunal feeding tubes.

Scleroderma

This autoimmune and chronic systemic disease of uncertain etiology affects the skin, lungs, heart, kidneys, and central nervous system (CNS), and commonly affects the GI tract (second most common manifestation after the skin). It is part of the CREST (calcinosis, Raynaud* phenomenon, esophageal dysmotility, sclerodactyly, and telangiectasia) syndrome. Within the GI tract, the esophagus is most commonly affected (approximately 90% of cases), although small bowel involvement is also common (50%). There is a progressive smooth muscular atrophy secondary to the chronic fibrosing process that affects the lower two thirds of the esophagus (the upper third is striated muscle). The bowel progressively loses function and becomes dilated with the loss of normal peristaltic activity (Fig. 1-75). The resulting fibrosis leads to esophageal widening and distention rather than stricture formation, although GERD is common because the GE junction is typically widely patent. The resulting ulceration can cause stricture formation and even a Barrett esophagus. Dermatomyositis can give similar dysmotility appearances to scleroderma.

TABLE 1-8 Causes of Esophageal Dysmotility

Neurological disease	Brainstem infarction Bulbar palsy Multiple sclerosis Peripheral neuropathies Myasthenia gravis
Local muscular spasm	Cricopharyngeus spasm*
Muscular dysfunction	Dermatomyositis Muscular dystrophy Scleroderma* Achalasia (primary and secondary)* Diffuse esophageal spasm
Inflammatory conditions	Severe esophagitis (e.g., radiation, caustic, GERD)
Systemic disease	Hyperthyroidism, hypothyroidism, amyloidosis, diabetes
Drugs	Anticholinergics (e.g., atropine)

GERD, Gastrointestinal reflux disease.
*See discussion in this chapter.

Achalasia

Achalasia is a smooth muscle motility disorder of the lower esophagus that can be primary or secondary. Primary achalasia is a disease, usually starting in young adulthood, that affects the lower esophagus because of a reduction in myenteric ganglia in Auerbach† (or myenteric) plexus that provide motor function to the lower esophageal sphincter. The lower esophageal sphincter then fails to relax, with the proximal esophagus steadily dilating over months and years as it attempts to propel food through the strictured lower esophagus. Clinically, the resulting stasis can lead to halitosis, aspiration, and secondary infection with candidiasis. It is also a premalignant condition with the risk of secondary squamous carcinoma development, although the diagnosis can be difficult because the patient has a long history of dysphagia and a small tumor can be easily missed for surrounding food debris.

Severe forms can even be recognized on a plain chest radiograph with a posterior mediastinal fluid-filled dilated esophagus, which should be confirmed with UGI examination or ultimately EGD because biopsy of the affected esophageal segment confirms the disease. Esophageal dysmotility at UGI examination varies from mild to almost the complete absence of peristalsis in severe forms. A diffusely dilated esophagus is typically identified as a tight stricture at the GE junction with a "rat-tailed" or "bird-beak"

*Maurice Raynaud (1834-1881), French internal medicine physician.
†Leopold Auerbach (1828-1897), German anatomist.

appearance (Fig. 1-76). Observation under fluoroscopy may not demonstrate the passage of barium into the stomach unless the patient is upright and gravity increases the lower esophageal fluid/barium pressure to overcome the resistance created by the GE junction stricture. However, the passage of barium through the GE sphincter is often slow, if it happens at all. Patients are usually treated with regular endoscopic dilatation where any underlying mucosal malignant change can be observed.

Secondary Achalasia

Secondary achalasia, also known as *pseudoachalasia*, essentially produces the same symptoms and radiological findings as primary achalasia but is caused by invasion of the myenteric plexuses from lower esophageal or GE junction malignancies, particularly carcinoma; lymphoma or even metastatic disease is also recognized (Fig. 1-77). It is therefore seen in older patients and

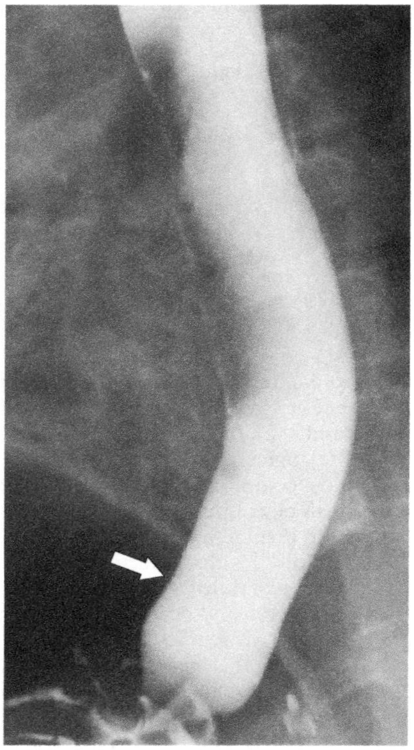

FIGURE 1-75. Barium swallow in a 49-year-old woman with smooth diffuse esophageal dilatation due to scleroderma (*arrow*).

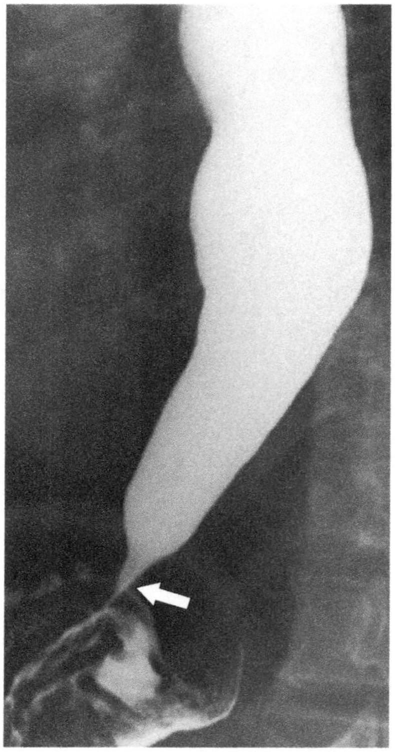

FIGURE 1-76. Barium swallow in a 53-year-old man with achalasia with a diffusely widened esophagus and "rat-tail" stricture at the GE junction (*arrow*).

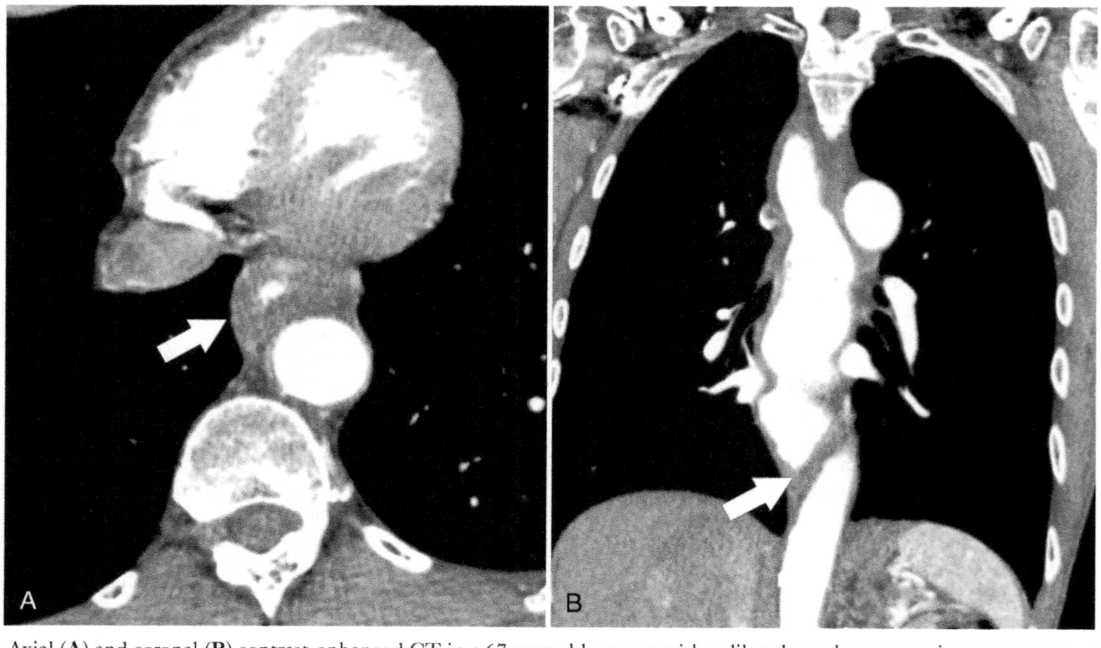

FIGURE 1-77. Axial (**A**) and coronal (**B**) contrast-enhanced CT in a 67-year-old woman with a dilated esophagus tapering to a narrow, smooth stricture at the GE junction (*arrows*) from submucosal esophageal invasion by gastric cancer.

anyone presenting for the first time with symptoms. Radiological findings of achalasia in adults of middle age or in the elderly should raise suspicion of an underlying malignancy. The diagnosis is usually made with EGD and biopsy of the affected segment.

Other causes include scleroderma, severe peptic stricture, surgical postvagotomy, and Chagas* disease. The latter is produced by the trypanosome, *Trypanosoma cruzi*, which is a protozoal infection typically found in poorer living conditions in South America. Infection results from fecal excretion of the protozoa by the reduviid bug subdermally. The resulting complications of infection can take up to 10 years to manifest and affect the esophagus, duodenum, colon, and heart. There is diffuse dilatation of the infected organs secondary to neurotoxic damage of intramural autonomic sympathetic ganglion cells. At imaging, the esophageal abnormalities can appear identical to those of achalasia, although unlike that disease, esophageal contractions can be observed in Chagas disease.

Diffuse Esophageal Spasm

Diffuse esophageal spasm is characterized by repetitive involuntary unexpected esophageal contractions (although hot or cold fluids can trigger the symptoms) that result in intense dysphagia. This spasm can be diagnosed through the observation of these contractions at UGI examination and fluoroscopy with the appearance of a "cork-screw" spasmodic esophagus (Fig. 1-78). The lower esophageal sphincter functions normally.

Presbyesophagus

Presbyesophagus is commonly seen in the elderly in whom there is reduced normal peristaltic activity but increased, haphazard, aperistaltic contractions. The lower esophageal sphincter is usually functioning normally. It is a diagnosis primarily made by fluoroscopic barium examination.

*Carlos Chagas (1879-1934), Brazilian physician.

Trauma

Traumatic disruption to the esophageal mucosa is usually iatrogenic (nasogastric tube insertion, endoscopic perforation, or sclerotherapy for esophageal varices) but can be secondary to ingested fish bones or other sharp foods (e.g., corn chips) (Fig. 1-79). Profuse vomiting with a tear (Mallory-Weiss tear) or frank perforation (Boerhaave syndrome) leads to ulceration and delayed stricture formation in some patients.

Esophageal Foreign Body

There is usually a temporal history of dysphagia related to food ingestion. Typical objects include fish or chicken bones or chunks of meat in adults, but in children, almost anything that can be swallowed has been described (Fig. 1-80). Fish or chicken bones typically become lodged in the upper esophagus just below the cricopharyngeus muscle, whereas meat chunks become stuck above previous strictures (Schatzki ring, peptic or neoplastic lesion). Lateral plain film might identify calcified elements, and UGI examination identifies linear or curved foreign bodies. UGI studies will readily identify larger food boluses, but smaller material can be hard to identify (Fig. 1-81). CT is more likely to identify calcified structures and any related edema, hemorrhage, or abscess (if the foreign body has penetrated the esophageal wall).

Mallory-Weiss Tear

Mallory-Weiss* tear is a rent in the lower esophageal mucosa after prolonged vomiting and retching. Patients usually have hematemesis, melena, or both. This rent is only a mucosal tear

*G. Kenneth Mallory (1900-1986), American pathologist; Soma Weiss (1898-1942), American physician.

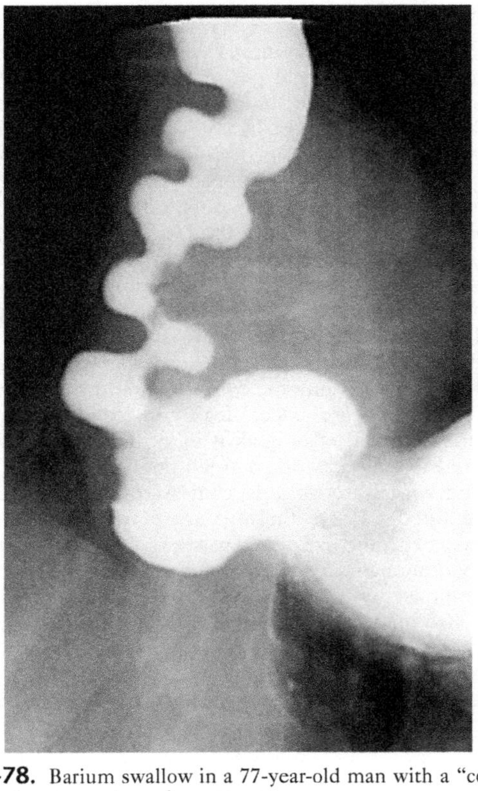

FIGURE 1-78. Barium swallow in a 77-year-old man with a "corkscrew" esophagus due to esophageal spasm.

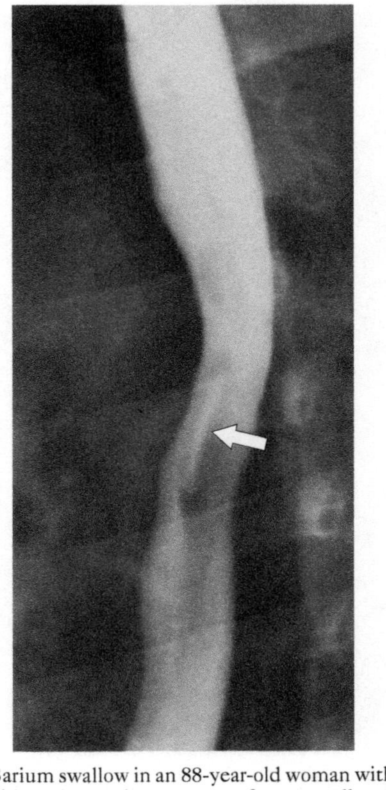

FIGURE 1-79. Barium swallow in an 88-year-old woman with a linear ulcer (*arrow*) in the midesophagus due to trauma from a swallowed toothpick.

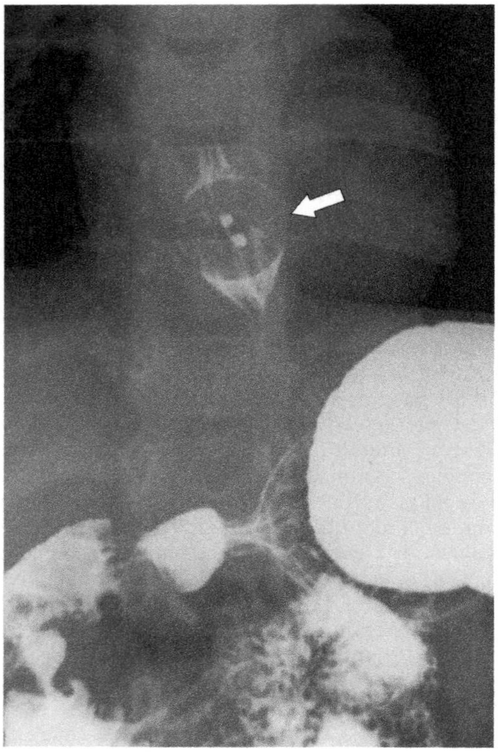

FIGURE 1-80. Barium swallow in a 5-year-old boy with an ingested coat button (*arrow*).

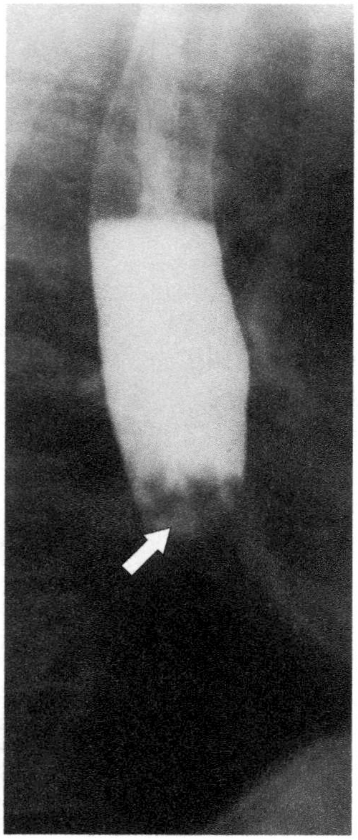

FIGURE 1-81. UGI swallow in a 70-year-old man with a foreign body (steak matter) (*arrow*) completely occluding the esophagus.

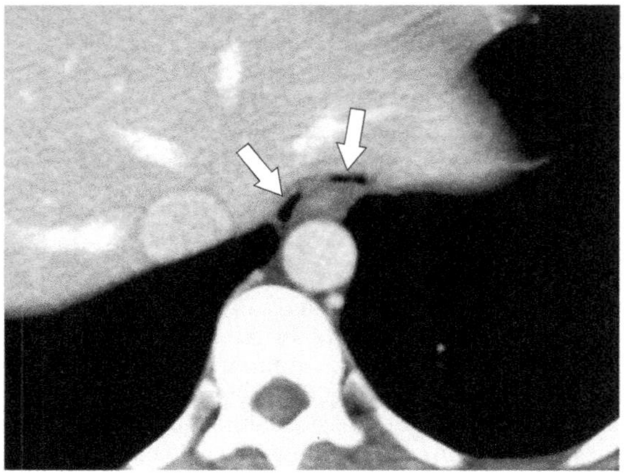

FIGURE 1-82. Axial contrast-enhanced CT in a 48-year-old man with a small ring of submucosal gas (*arrows*) due to a Mallory-Weiss tear.

(rather than full thickness from Boerhaave* syndrome) and is usually self-limiting. The diagnosis can be made by EGD, but a UGI study with water-soluble contrast media may demonstrate a thin, linear collection adjacent to the esophagus. Because the tear is mucosal, though, it is commonly not visualized. If no tear is identified or better visualization is required, then barium can subsequently be used because there is essentially little risk of complete perforation. However, some tears can be more extensive and lead to submucosal hemorrhage, which is recognized as a smooth submucosal mass. At CT, there may be a small linear track of water-soluble contrast medium adjacent to the lower esophagus with or without a small area of gas (Fig. 1-82). This could also identify any submucosal hemorrhage and rule out a complete esophageal wall tear (Boerhaave syndrome).

Boerhaave Syndrome

This is a more severe version of the Mallory-Weiss tear due to a full transmural esophageal perforation also precipitated by a marked sudden increase in esophageal pressure from retching, vomiting, defecation, weight lifting, and seizures. Similar findings can be seen after instrumentation (e.g., perforating EGD, stent placements, or dilatation procedures). There may be mediastinal soft tissue widening and pneumomediastinum by plain radiography due to hemorrhage, fluid, or gas (Fig. 1-83). As the perforation is usually at the left lower esophagus, there may be a left pleural effusion or a left hydropneumothorax (Fig. 1-84). A diagnosis can be made at UGI examination, but barium is initially contraindicated if this condition is suspected because it is highly toxic in the mediastinum and can cause a severe mediastinitis. Rather, water-soluble nonionic contrast should be administered, which may demonstrate a local leak and extravasation of contrast material. Only after no leak is identified should barium be administered to fully exclude a small, localized leak (if no leak is identified with water-soluble contrast medium, then a large leak is excluded). These findings are better demonstrated by CT, however, with the use of oral water-soluble contrast material, which may demonstrate both the site of the leak and mediastinal gas (emphysema) resulting from the perforation (Fig. 1-84). This may also identify mediastinal fluid, including a pericardial effusion, periesophageal fluid, and pleural fluid. Urgent surgical repair is required to prevent severe mediastinitis and possible death; there is a 70% mortality if this rupture is not treated within 24 hours.

*Herman Boerhaave (1668-1738), Dutch physician.

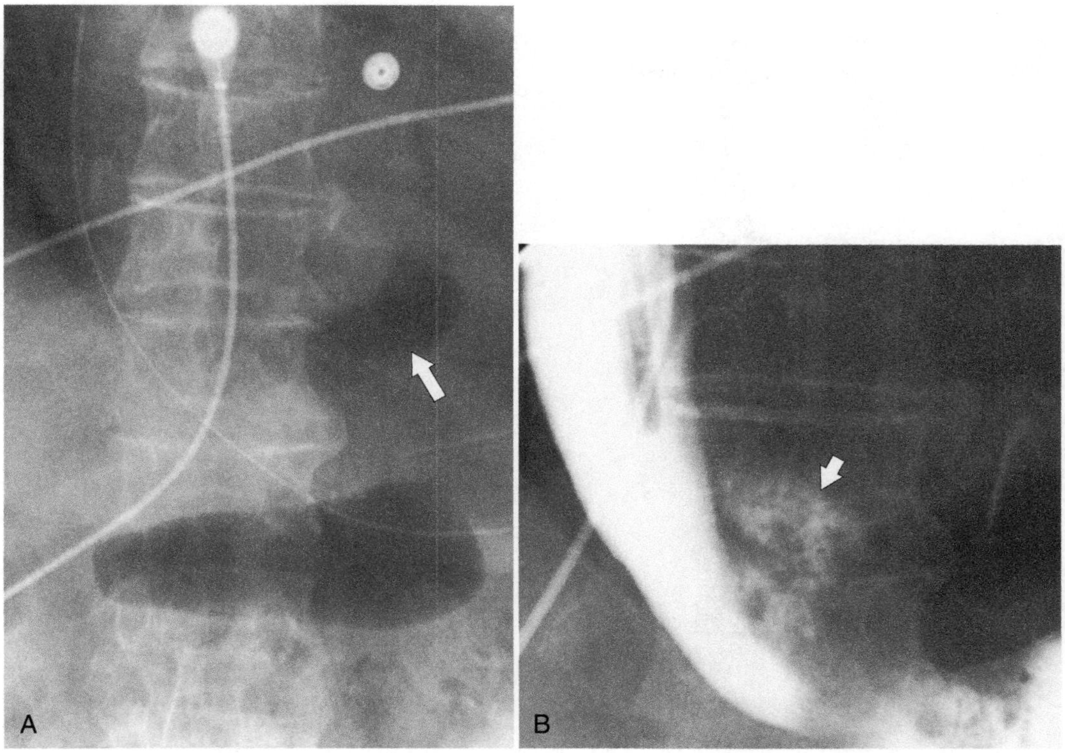

Figure 1-83. Plain radiograph (**A**) and nonionic contrast UGI swallow (**B**) of the lower chest in a 36-year-old man after severe vomiting demonstrating mediastinal gas (*large arrow*). At UGI swallow an esophageal perforation is confirmed with leak of contrast into the mediastinum (*small arrow*) due to a complete (Boerhaave) tear.

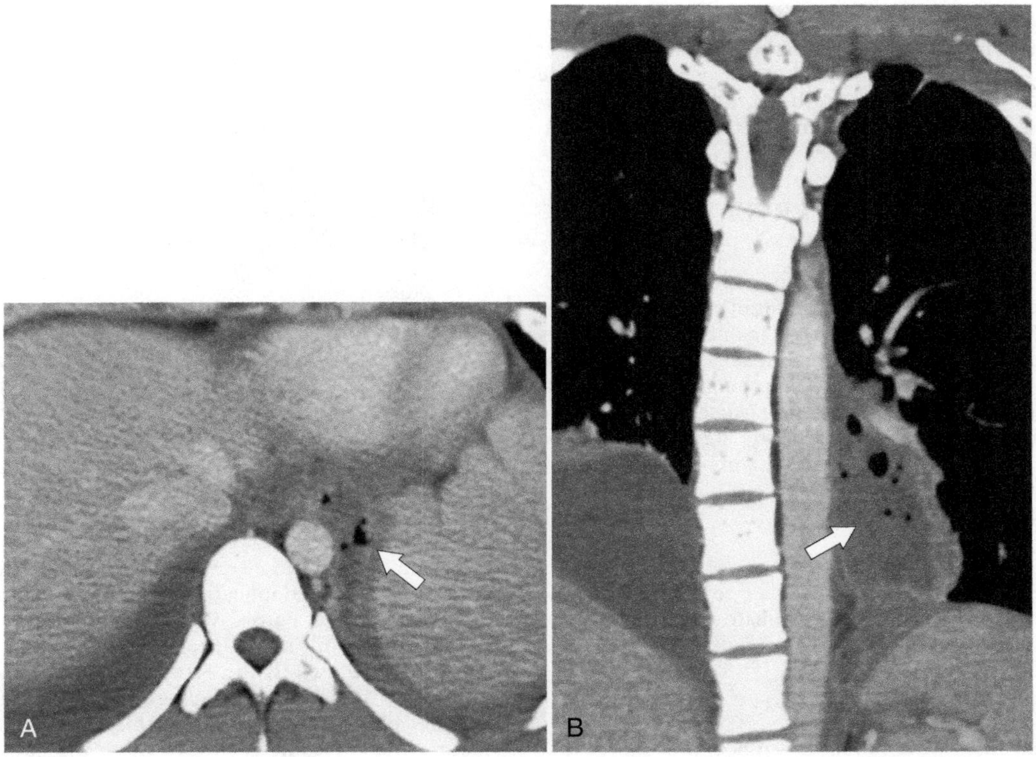

Figure 1-84. Axial (**A**) and coronal (**B**) contrast-enhanced CT in a 44-year-old man with Boerhaave syndrome with mediastinal gas and extraluminal fluid (*arrows*) due to esophageal perforation.

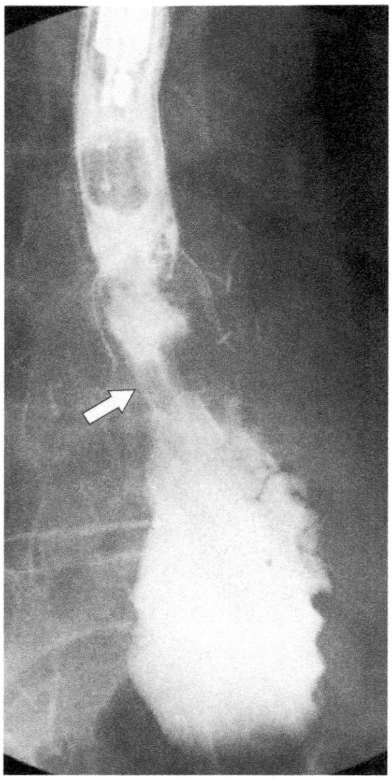

FIGURE 1-85. Barium swallow in a 74-year-old man with recurrent esophageal cancer and stent placement to relieve dysphagia. There is irregularity of the esophageal lumen (*arrow*), but contrast passes through to the stomach.

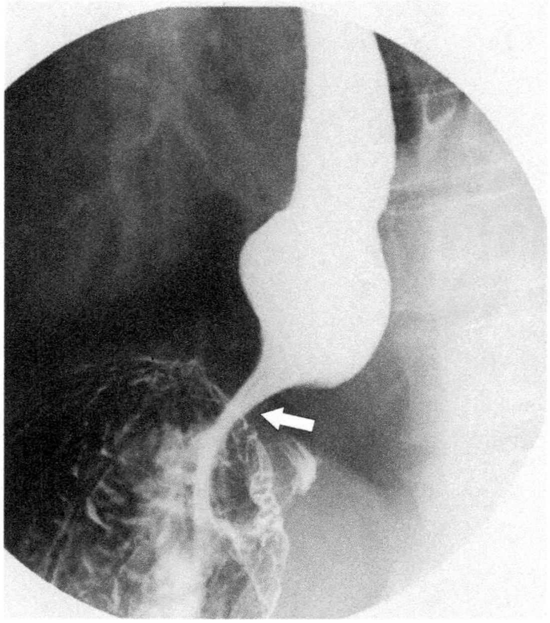

FIGURE 1-86. UGI swallow in a 44-year-old woman with a normal Nissen fundoplication. There is a smooth tapering to the lower esophagus. The "wrap" surrounds the lower esophagus (*arrow*).

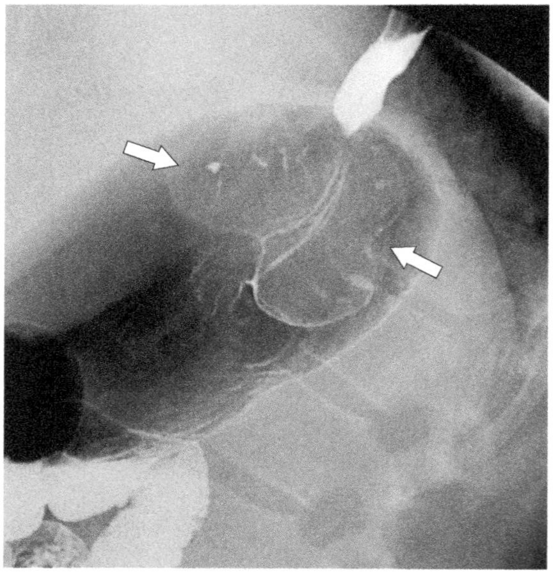

FIGURE 1-87. UGI swallow in a 51-year-old woman with a fundal filling defect (*arrows*) due a normal Nissen fundoplication.

Aortoenteric Fistula

Aortic fistula is secondary to midthoracic invasion of the esophagus from aortic aneurysms, either from atherosclerotic disease or from mycotic or postsurgical complications (e.g, infected aortic grafts). As expected, patients have profuse, bright red hematemesis, and it is often fatal. Contrast-enhanced CT without oral contrast is the investigation of choice.

POSTOPERATIVE AND INTERVENTIONAL PROCEDURES

There are several therapeutic endoscopic esophageal procedures that are performed for either the treatment or relief of benign or malignant esophageal obstruction. These include balloon dilatation for the relief of benign strictures (e.g., achalasia, postcaustic ingestion, drug-induced lesion) and sclerotherapy for the treatment of esophageal varices. Laser therapy is used for debulking malignant disease, and a metallic or plastic stent placement is used to bypass malignant strictures in patients with inoperable esophageal cancer (Fig. 1-85).

Hairy Esophagus

As its name suggests, hairy esophagus is a rare manifestation of skin grafting for pharyngoesophageal reconstructive surgery that presents with hair follicles inside the esophagus.

Fundoplication

Fundoplications constitute a variety of surgical procedures that are aimed at preventing intractable GERD. The fundamental principle is to tighten or compress the lower esophageal sphincter by "wrapping" a portion of the proximal stomach around the lower esophagus, thereby preventing gastric contents from refluxing up into the esophagus. The most common procedure is the Nissen* fundoplication, which is a complete 360-degree wrap (others are partial wraps of approximately 240 to 270 degrees). Complications usually arise because the wrap is too tight or too loose. In the former, there is delayed esophageal emptying, which can be observed at UGI examination, or there can be free reflux and a widened GE junction if the wrap is too loose. Wraps become too loose when the sutures become disrupted and the wrap begins to unfold itself. The wrap can also

*Rudolf Nissen (1896-1981), German surgeon.

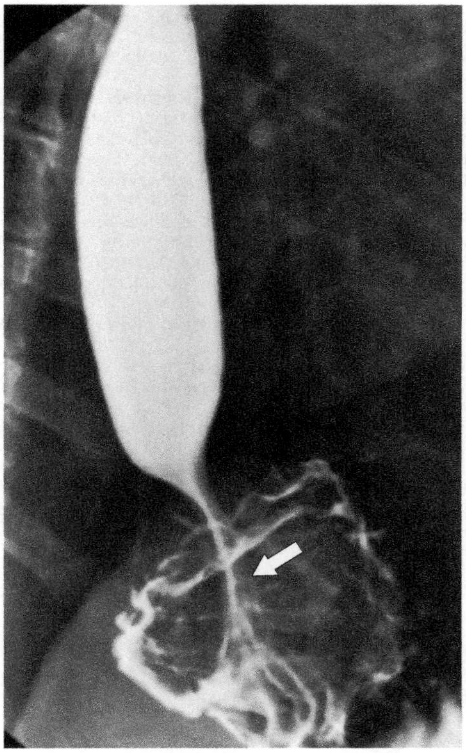

FIGURE 1-88. UGI swallow in a 41-year-old man with a Nissen fundoplication. There is smooth narrowing of the lower esophagus due to the "wrap" being too tight (*arrow*). The esophagus is also dilated.

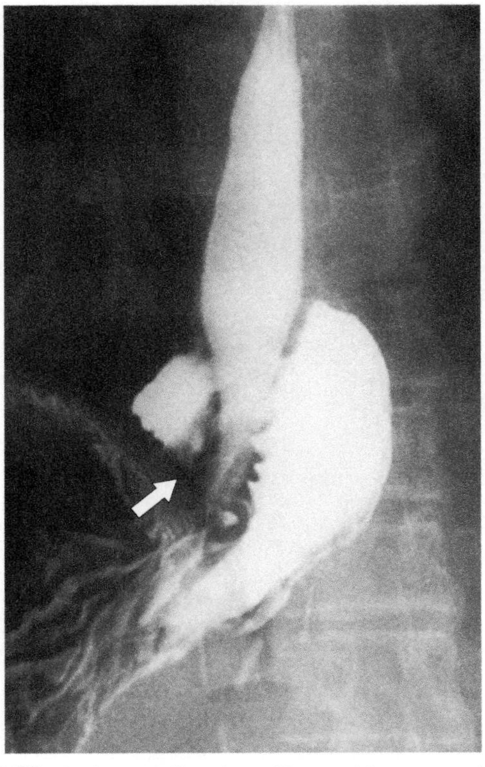

FIGURE 1-89. Barium swallow in a 38-year-old woman with partial unwrapping of the fundoplication (*arrow*).

slide caudally to constrict the middle aspect of the stomach (similar to an hourglass appearance). Conversely, the wrap may herniate into the chest.

The normal appearances with UGI examination demonstrate a smooth tapering of the lower esophagus as it passes through the wrap, which itself may be outlined by barium (Fig. 1-86). Between the esophagus and the wrap is a radiolucent circular band of the constricting gastric wall around the esophagus (Fig. 1-87). At CT, there is a soft tissue mass-like density around the lower esophagus for a few centimeters. Complications, however, are best evaluated by UGI series because CT will generally be unable to determine whether the wrap is too loose or too tight. If the wrap is too tight, the esophagus may be distended, and if it is too loose, the wrap can be seen at barium swallow unfolding and GERD will return (Figs. 1-88 and 1-89). Nonwrap complications are common to most other surgical procedures and include hemorrhage, fluid collections, and abscess in the chest or abdomen due to leaks.

SUGGESTED READINGS

Asrani A et al: Urgent findings on portable chest radiography: what the radiologist should know. AJR Am J Roentgenol 196:S45-S61, 2011.

Bird-Lieberman EL et al: Early diagnosis of oesophageal cancer. Br J Cancer 101(1):1-6, 2009.

Bizekis C et al: Initial experience with minimally invasive Ivor Lewis esophagectomy. Ann Thorac Surg 82(2):402-406, 2006. discussion 406-407.

Bleshman MH et al: The inflammatory esophagogastric polyp and fold. Radiology 128:589-593, 1978.

Buecker A et al: Esophageal perforation: comparison of use of aqueous and barium-containing contrast media. Radiology 202(3):683-686, 1997.

Cheng HT et al: Caustic ingestion in adults: the role of endoscopic classification in predicting outcome. BMC Gastroenterol 8:31, 2008.

De Schipper JP et al: Spontaneous rupture of the oesophagus: Boerhaave's syndrome in 2008. Literature review and treatment algorithm. Dig Surg 26(1):1-6, 2009.

Dibble C et al: Detection of reflux esophagitis on double-contract esophagrams and endoscopy using the histologic findings as the gold standard. Abdom Imaging 29(4):421-425, 2004.

Doo EY et al: Oesophageal strictures caused by the ingestion of corrosive agents: effectiveness of balloon dilatation in children. Clin Radiol 64(3):265-271, 2009.

Ekberg O et al: Dysfunction of the cricopharyngeal muscle: a cineradiographic study of patients with dysphagia. Radiology 143:481-486, 1982.

Freeman RK et al: Esophageal stent placement for the treatment of spontaneous esophageal perforations. Ann Thorac Surg 88(1):194-198, 2009.

Ghahremani GG et al: Glycogenic acanthosis of the esophagus: radiographic and pathologic features. Gastrointest Radiol 9(2):93-98, 1984.

Grant PD et al: Pharyngeal dysphagia: what the radiologist needs to know. Curr Probl Diagn Radiol 38(1):17-32, 2009.

Grishaw EK et al: Functional abnormalities of the esophagus: a prospective analysis of the radiographic findings relative to age and symptoms. AJR Am J Roentgenol 167(3):719-723, 1996.

Gupta S et al: Usefulness of barium strictures of the esophagus. AJR Am J Roentgenol 180(3):737-744, 2003.

Hamilton JM et al: Severe injuries from coin cell battery ingestions: 2 case reports. J Pediatr Surg 44(3):644-647, 2009.

Huang SY et al: Large hiatal hernia with floppy fundus: clinical and radiographic findings. AJR Am J Roentgenol 188(4):960-964, 2007.

Insko EK et al: Benign and malignant lesions of the stomach: evaluation of CT criteria for differentiation. Radiology 228(1):166-171, 2003.

Iyer RB et al: Diagnosis, staging, and follow-up of esophageal cancer. AJR Am J Roentgenol 181(3):785-793, 2003.

Jiang G et al: Thoracoscopic enucleation of esophageal leiomyoma: a retrospective study in 40 cases. Dis Esophagus 22(3):279-283, 2009.

Kang HK et al: Three-dimensional multi-detector row CT portal venography in the evaluation of portosystemic collateral vessels in liver cirrhosis. Radiographics 22(5):1053-1061, 2002.

Kent MS et al: Revisional surgery after esophagectomy: an analysis of 43 patients. Ann Thorac Surg 86(3):975-983, 2008. discussion 967-974.

Kim TJ et al: Multimodality assessment of esophageal cancer: preoperative staging and monitoring of response to therapy. Radiographics 29(2):403-421, 2009.

Kim TJ et al: Postoperative imaging of esophageal cancer: what chest radiologists need to know. Radiographics 27(2):409-429, 2007.

Kim YJ et al: Esophageal varices in cirrhotic patients: evaluation with liver CT. AJR Am J Roentgenol 188(1):139-144, 2007.

Kwee RM: Prediction of tumor response to neoadjuvant therapy in patients with esophageal cancer with use of ^{18}F FDG PET: a systematic review. Radiology 254(3):707-717, 2010.

Lahcene M et al: Esophageal dysmotility in scleroderma: a prospective study of 183 cases. Gastroenterol Clin Biol 33(6-7):466-469, 2009.

Lee SS et al: Superficial esophageal cancer: esophagographic findings correlated with histopathologic findings. Radiology 236(2):535-544, 2005.

Levine MS et al: Diseases of the esophagus: diagnosis with esophagography. Radiology 237(2):414-427, 2005.
Levine MS et al: Esophageal intramural pseudodiverticulosis: a reevaluation. AJR Am J Roentgenol 147:1165-1170, 1986.
Levine MS et al: Double-contrast upper gastrointestinal examination: technique and interpretation. Radiology 168(3):593-602, 1988.
Levine MS et al: Barium studies in modern radiology: do they have a role? Radiology 250(1):18-22, 2009.
Levine MS: Reflux esophagitis and Barrett's esophagus. Semin Roentgenol 29(4):332-340, 1994.
Mahgerefteh SY et al: Radiologic imaging and intervention for gastrointestinal and hepatic complications of hematopoietic stem cell transplantation. Radiology 258(3):660-671, 2011.
Mann NS et al: Barrett's esophagitis in patients with symptomatic reflux esophagitis. Am J Gastroenterol 84(12):1494-1496, 1989.
Mauro MA et al: Epidermolysis bullosa: radiographic findings in 16 cases. AJR Am J Roentgenol 149:925-927, 1987.
Newcomer MK et al: Complications of upper gastrointestinal endoscopy and their management. Gastrointest Endosc Clin N Am 4:551, 1994.
Ntoumazios SK et al: Esophageal involvement in scleroderma: gastroesophageal reflux, the common problem. Semin Arthritis Rheum 36(3):173-181, 2006.
Ott DJ et al: Esophagogastric region and its rings. AJR Am J Roentgenol 142(2):281-287, 1984.
Rantanen TK et al: Gastroesophageal reflux disease as a cause of death is increasing: analysis of fatal cases after medical and surgical treatment. Am J Gastroenterol 102(2):246-253, 2007.
Rubesin S et al: Granular cell tumors of the esophagus. Gastrointest Radiol 10(1):11-15, 1985.
Rubesin SE et al: Killian-Jamieson diverticula: radiographic findings in 16 patients. AJR Am J Roentgenol 177(1):85-89, 2001.
Rubesin SE et al: The tailored double-contrast pharyngogram. Crit Rev Diagn Imaging 28(2):133-179, 1988.
Samadi F et al: Feline esophagus and gastroesophageal reflux. AJR Am J Roentgenol 194(4):972-976, 2010.
Sass DA et al: Portal hypertension and variceal hemorrhage. Med Clin North Am 93(4):837-853, vii-viii, 2009. Savarino E et al: Gastroesophageal reflux and pulmonary fibrosis in scleroderma: a study using pH-impedance monitoring. Am J Respir Crit Care Med 179(5):408-413, 2009.
Schneider JH et al: Transient lower esophageal sphincter relaxation and esophageal motor response. J Surg Res 159(2):714-719, 2010.
Sydow BD et al: Radiographic findings and complications after surgical or endoscopic repair of Zenker's diverticulum in 16 patients. AJR Am J Roentgenol 177(5):1067-1071, 2001. AJR Am J Roentgenol 177(5):1067-1071, 2001 Nov.
Umeoka S et al: Esophageal cancer: evaluation with triple-phase dynamic CT—initial experience. Radiology 239(3):777-783, 2006.
Warshauer DM et al: Imaging manifestations of abdominal sarcoidosis. AJR Am J Roentgenol 182(1):15-28, 2004.
Westerterp M et al: Esophageal cancer: CT, endoscopic US, and FDG PET for assessment of response to neoadjuvant therapy—systematic review. Radiology 236(3):841-851, 2005.
White SB et al: The small-caliber esophagus: radiographic sign of idiopathic eosinophilic esophagitis. Radiology 256(1):127-134, 2010.
Williams VA et al: Achalasia of the esophagus: a surgical disease. J Am Coll Surg 208(1):151-162, 2009.
Yamabe Y et al: Tumor staging of advanced esophageal cancer: combination of double-contrast esophagography and contrast-enhanced CT. AJR Am J Roentgenol 191(3):753-757, 2008.
Yu NC et al: Detection and grading of esophageal varices on liver CT: comparison of standard and thin-section multiplanar reconstructions in diagnostic accuracy. AJR Am J Roentgenol 197(3):643-649, 2011.

Chapter 2

Stomach

NORMAL ANATOMY

The stomach begins at the gastric cardia (the portion that envelops the lower esophagus) and ends after the pylorus. It consists of a fundus, body, lesser and greater curvature, antrum, and pylorus. It has three layers of smooth muscle (outer longitudinal, middle circular, and inner oblique), with gastric rugae (or folds) within. The mucosa is lined by columnar epithelium, within which are numerous mucus- and acid-producing glands. Gastric folds are usually prominent when the stomach is collapsed but are effaced when it is distended. With good double-contrast technique, the normal lower antrum often has a smaller reticulated mucosal appearance, known as areae gastricae (Fig. 2-1).

A contrast (usually barium) examination of the stomach used to be one of the most common imaging examinations before the advent of computed tomography (CT) and endoscopy. It is now rarely performed as a first-line investigation to evaluate for gastric disease. However, knowledge of good upper gastrointestinal (UGI) barium examination technique is still required, particularly because it can detect and characterize most lesions. Small polyps and mucosal lesions are unlikely to be detected by CT, and unless endoscopy is performed, they will be missed.

Barium examination of the stomach usually follows initial examination of the esophagus (see Chapter 1). To promote gastric and duodenal bulb distention, some investigators inject small doses of anticholinergics or glucagon to induce a gastric and duodenal atonic state. Whether or not this is used, the examination of the stomach should not be delayed once the gas granules are swallowed and the initial views of the esophagus with the patient in the upright position have been performed. The patient is immediately placed recumbent to prevent the contrast material from spilling into the duodenum, which usually obscures the stomach, rendering the test inadequate. Once recumbent, the patient is then turned several times to encourage the coating of the mucosa with barium. The sequence of spot radiographs then varies according to institutional preference. Initially, a supine view (to provide an overview of the gastric anatomy) is followed by fundal views, with the patient in the right-side down lateral position (the fundus will be maximally distended with air in this position). After the patient is turned to the supine position (the patient turns to the left), views of the body can be obtained. The patient is then turned to the right anterior oblique position (i.e., the gastric antrum is uppermost) to obtain antral and duodenal bulb views (these regions, being nondependent, will be maximally distended with gas). If there is inadequate coating, the patient is then turned supine again to further coat the antrum and returned to the right anterior oblique position to achieve adequate antral coating and duodenal coating. Further views of the esophagus can now be obtained with low-density (thin) barium with the patient in the prone oblique position, and the patient can be evaluated for hiatal hernia and gastroesophageal reflux disease (GERD). These results may be elicited with the patient in a slight Trendelenburg* position, and gravity is used to provoke the GE junction. The patient is finally turned to the prone position for the evaluation of the antrum and duodenum bulb with compression views. The antral and duodenal bulb anatomy is variable, and the patient may need to be rotated in different obliquities or even lateral positions to view them en face.

*Friedrich Trendelenburg (1844-1924), German surgeon.

CT is not a suitable technique for the examination of mucosal disease, unless there is marked gastritis or mucosal lesions are sufficiently large to be visualized. CT is, however, useful when gastric perforation is suspected. The technique is mostly reserved for evaluating primary and secondary gastric tumors and extragastric inflammatory conditions such as pancreatitis. Magnetic resonance imaging (MRI) has little role in the evaluation of gastric disease.

Positron emission tomography (PET) and PET/CT are increasingly used to evaluate gastric malignancy, particularly for local and distant metastases. Although gastritis can cause increased ^{18}F-fluorodeoxyglucose (FDG) uptake, it is not specific and best evaluated with esophagogastroduodenoscopy (EGD). Gastric emptying studies with technetium-99m (^{99m}Tc) pertechnetate are commonly used to evaluate the pediatric population (see Chapter 1).

GASTRIC DISEASE

Congenital Anomalies

Antral Diaphragm

Antral diaphragm is poorly understood and is likely a result of congenital anomalies in neonates or from fibrotic healing of peptic ulcer disease in adults. There is a mucosal web positioned in the antrum, which, if large enough, can cause gastric outlet obstruction. Antral diaphragm is best recognized by EGD or contrast fluoroscopy, where a thin, well-defined web or diaphragm is seen in the expected location. It may or may not be circumferential.

Pyloric Stenosis

Infantile pyloric stenosis usually presents in males within the first 6 weeks of life, with projectile bilious vomiting due to gastric outlet obstruction from pyloric muscular hypertrophy. Clinically, it may be felt as an olive-shaped mass in the epigastrium. Plain radiograph often demonstrates a distended stomach (Fig. 2-2). Barium examination will confirm gastric distention and outline a bird-beak-like pyloric narrowing (Fig. 2-2). The diagnosis is best made with ultrasound, however, which demonstrates the classic findings of a hypertrophied hypoechoic muscle with

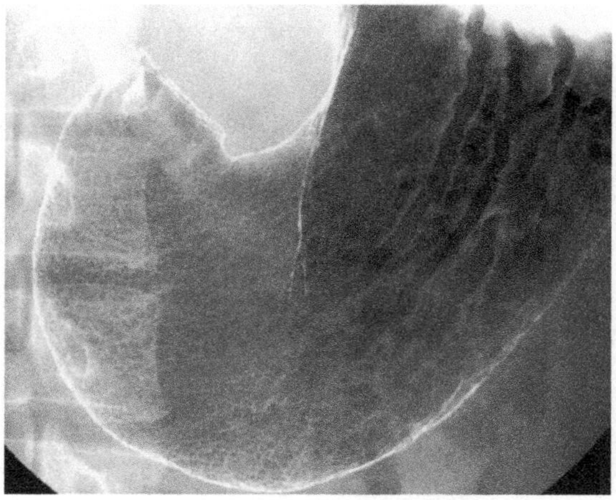

Figure 2-1. Good barium coating at UGI series demonstrates a reticular pattern to the gastric antrum (areae gastricae), which is a normal finding.

measurements that exceed 15 mm longitudinally and 3 mm in diameter of a single wall on transverse images (Fig. 2-3). Treatment is by a pyloromyotomy and is usually curative.

The adult version (hypertrophic pyloric stenosis) is poorly understood and is frequently associated with peptic ulcer disease, which suggests that it is acquired rather than congenital. The findings are similar to those in the neonate with an elongated pyloric channel (up to three times the normal length) and a circumferential mass-like effect within the pylorus, seen by either EGD or contrast studies. Adult pyloric stenosis should be distinguished from prolapsed gastric antral folds that are transient at fluoroscopic evaluation and do not obstruct the gastric outlet.

Gastric Diverticulum

Gastric diverticula can be congenital or acquired, and fundal or antral in location. The fundal diverticulum is usually congenital and the most common of the gastric diverticula. It is positioned posteriorly at the cephalad margin of the lesser curve, close to the inferomedial aspect of the GE junction. It is usually asymptomatic and of no clinical significance, unless it is large whereby stasis and delayed gastric emptying have been recognized. Fundal diverticula can also ulcerate and bleed, and gastric carcinoma has been recognized in the diverticulum.

Gastric diverticula are mostly identified on CT because barium examinations are performed less often. They are readily identifiable, although they are sometimes mistaken for the left adrenal gland on CT, particularly if there is no oral contrast medium within them (Fig. 2-4). Close observation should confirm a connection to the stomach lumen, and a gas/fluid level should clinch the diagnosis (Fig. 2-4). When a UGI series is performed, gas and contrast should outline the diverticulum outside the confines of the normal gastric wall (Fig. 2-5).

Antral diverticula are acquired and are usually small, projecting outward from the antral greater curvature, giving a collar-button appearance; they are sometimes mistaken for a benign gastric ulcer. They may be associated with previous gastric ulcer disease but generally have none of the other features that are usually associated with ulcer disease, including collars and fold thickening. Antral diverticula are also associated with pancreatitis, gastric outlet obstruction, and malignancy.

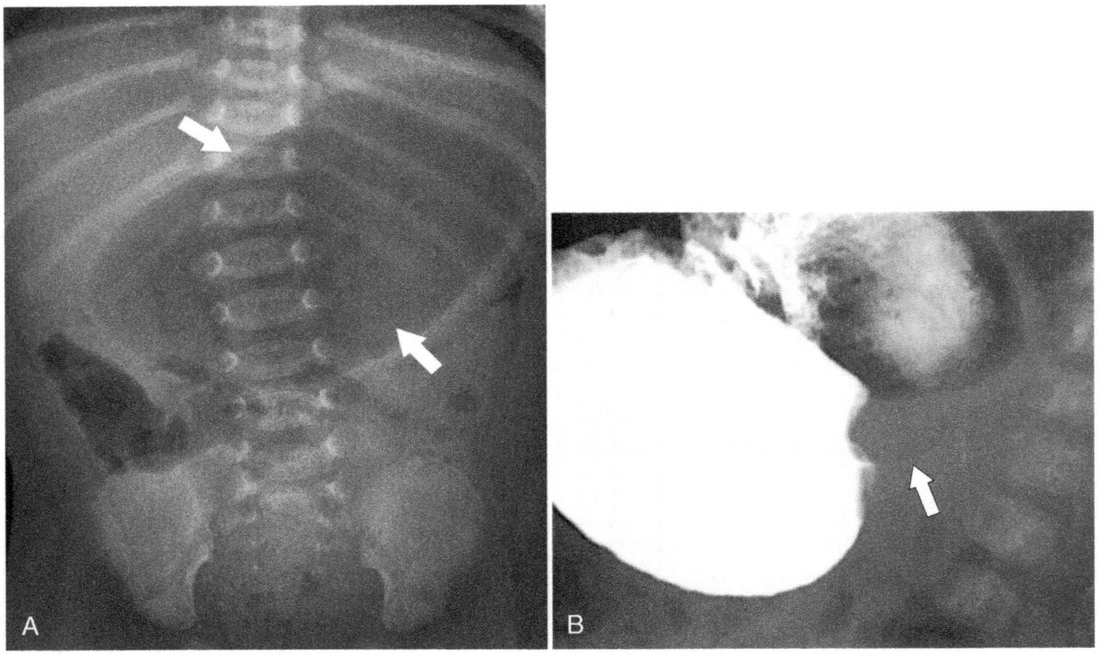

FIGURE 2-2. Abdominal plain radiograph (**A**) and UGI series (**B**) in a 4-week-old boy demonstrating gross gastric dilatation (*arrows*) and a bird-beak appearance to the gastric outlet.

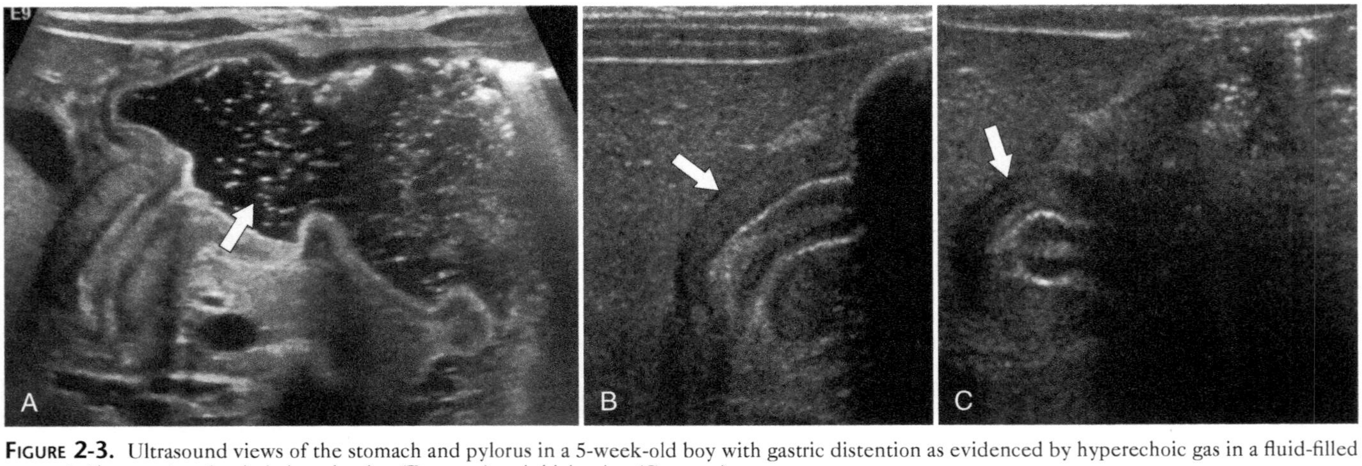

FIGURE 2-3. Ultrasound views of the stomach and pylorus in a 5-week-old boy with gastric distention as evidenced by hyperechoic gas in a fluid-filled stomach (**A**; *arrow*) and pyloric lengthening (**B**; *arrow*) and thickening (**C**; *arrow*).

Hiatal Hernias

Hiatal hernias are classified as either sliding (axial) or rolling (paraesophageal) and are discussed in more detail in Chapter 1. Sliding hernias are far more common and are often visualized on CT (Fig. 2-6). Paraesophageal hernias are uncommon and difficult to identify on CT because they are mostly confused with sliding hernias. Barium studies, however, will identify the gastric fundus within the chest and the GE junction within the abdomen (Fig. 2-7). Even less common are mixed sliding and paraesophageal hernias (Fig. 2-8). Gastroesophageal reflux disease (GERD) is common with sliding hernias, but because the GE junction in paraesophageal hernias lies within the abdomen, reflux is rarely seen. On the other hand, paraesophageal hernias, particularly large ones, are at greater risk for gastric volvulus.

Gastric Volvulus

Gastric volvulus is more common in the elderly, and there are three main types: organoaxial, mesenteroaxial, and mixed organoaxial-mesenteroaxial (Fig. 2-9). Organoaxial occurs when the stomach rotates 180 degrees or more (either anteriorly or posteriorly) around its long axis along a plane from the cardia to the pylorus so that the greater curvature now lies superior to the antrum; it is the so-called upside-down stomach (Fig. 2-10). In organoaxial volvulus, there are two twist points, the esophagogastric junction and the antral-pyloric junction. Contrast medium may not pass through the GE junction, but if it does, it may not then pass through the twisted pylorus. Organoaxial volvulus can be transient and relatively asymptomatic if the twisting is up to, but not more than, 180 degrees. However, when the twisting is complete, it can cause outright obstruction with intense pain, usually little vomiting (because of the obstruction), and difficulty in passing a nasogastric tube. It is usually a surgical emergency that requires the correction of the volvulus to prevent gastric infarction. Organoaxial volvulus is usually a result of large paraesophageal hiatal hernias when a significant proportion or all of the stomach lies in the chest.

Mesenteroaxial volvulus is much less common, and the rotation (to the right or left) is around the mesenteric axis (a perpendicular

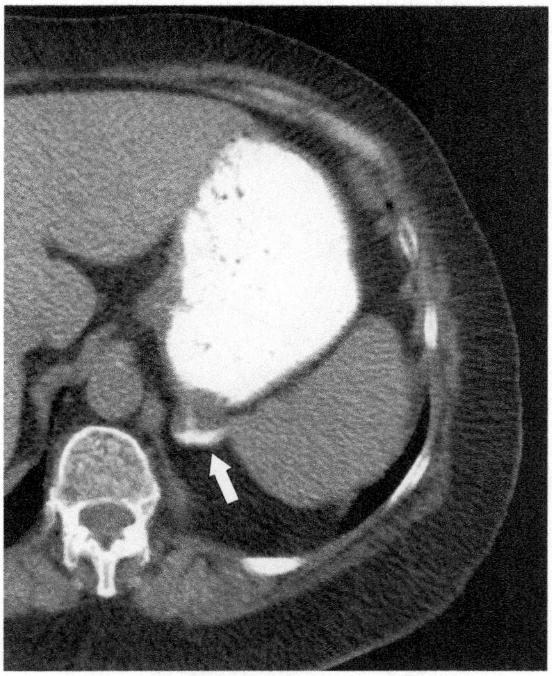

FIGURE 2-4. Axial noncontrast CT in a 51-year-old man with a small gastric fundal diverticulum (*arrow*).

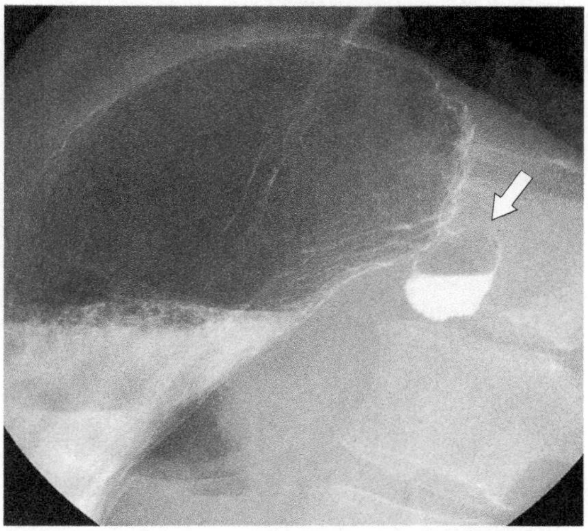

FIGURE 2-5. UGI series in a 40-year-old man with a fundal gastric diverticulum (*arrow*).

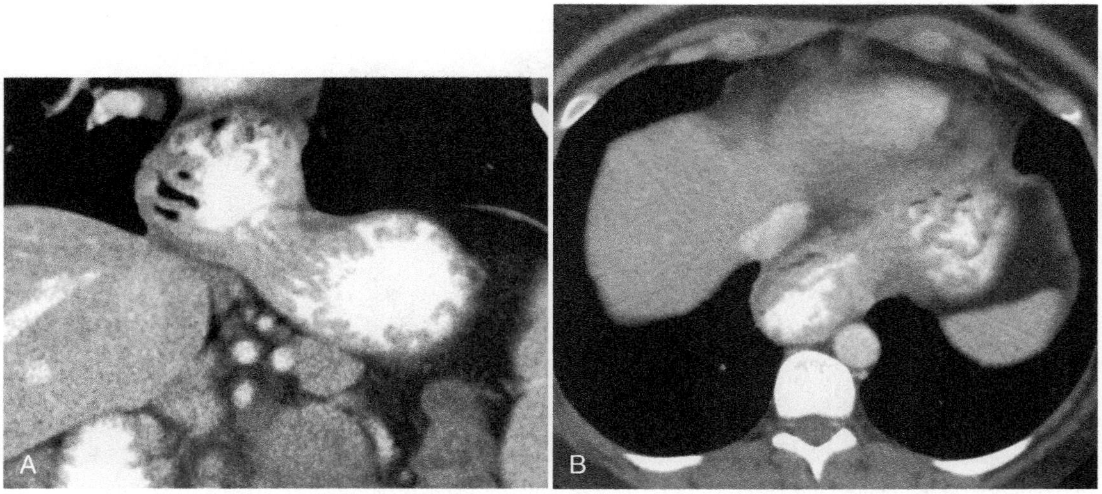

FIGURE 2-6. Coronal (**A**) and axial (**B**) CT in a 47-year-old woman with a sliding hiatal hernia.

line across the stomach from the lesser to the greater curvature) so that fundus comes to lie caudal to the antrum and pylorus (see Fig. 2-9). It is more common in patients with previous diaphragmatic rupture when large portions of the stomach come to lie in the chest. On plain radiograph of the abdomen, there can be a distended viscus in the left upper quadrant with an air-fluid level and collapsed small bowel if the volvulus has caused obstruction. The diagnosis, however, is readily made with UGI examination, which demonstrates the volvulus (Fig. 2-11). On CT, the precise diagnosis can be more difficult, unless multiplanar reformations are made, which should correspond to the UGI coronal series.

Diffuse Gastric Mucosal Thickening

There are many causes of gastric mucosal abnormalities, both benign and malignant (Table 2-1). The most common cause of benign mucosal disease is gastritis, which remains prevalent throughout the world, primarily because of peptic ulcer disease (Table 2-1).

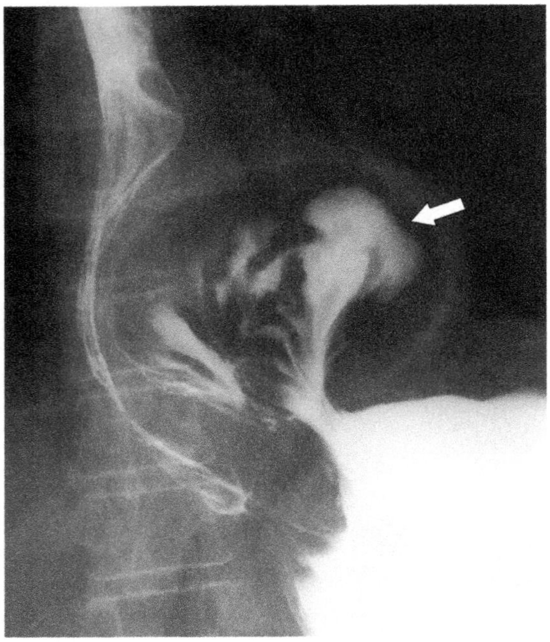

FIGURE 2-7. UGI series in a 72-year-old man with a paraesophageal hernia (*arrow*). The GE junction lies below the diaphragm.

Gastritis

Gastritis is a generic term that refers to gastric mucosa that has become inflamed and edematous; several causes have been isolated (Table 2-2). Many cases (e.g., erosive, antral, *Helicobacter pylori*) completely heal once the offending agent is removed, but others (e.g., granulomatous, caustic, radiation) heal with scarring and luminal narrowing. Imaging with a barium UGI series used to be the investigation of choice for the evaluation of gastritis but has now largely been replaced by direct optical endoscopy and because peptic ulcer disease is now readily treated and cured with antibiotics. However, many of the imaging features of gastritis are characteristic, and contrast evaluation of the gastric mucosa remains a valuable diagnostic tool. In general, however, it is not possible to differentiate the specific cause of gastritis by imaging. Most causes will produce either focal or diffuse gastric wall thickening, which should be readily identified with good single- or double-contrast UGI series (Fig. 2-12). However, because a UGI series is performed less frequently, the imaging findings of gastritis are now usually observed on CT as diffusely thickened folds (Fig. 2-13). Similarly, this is a nonspecific finding, which can sometimes be overdiagnosed in the collapsed stomach. Gastritis, which is mainly an inflammatory condition, may also demonstrate increased FDG uptake, whatever the cause (Figure 2-13). Gastritis commonly may be confined to the antrum, with relative sparing of the body and fundus (Fig. 2-14).

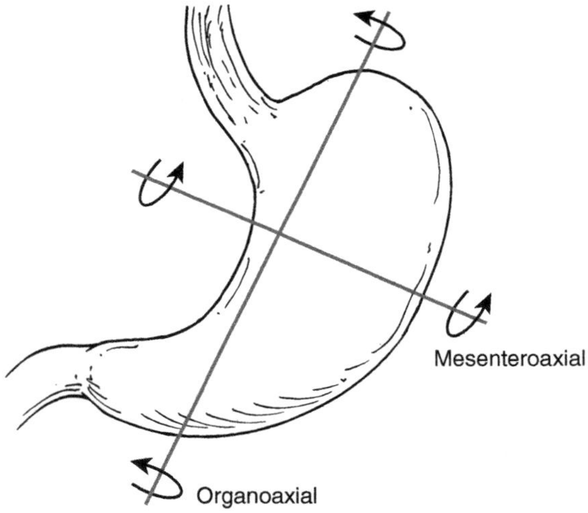

FIGURE 2-9. Schematic representation of organoaxial and mesenteroaxial volvulus.

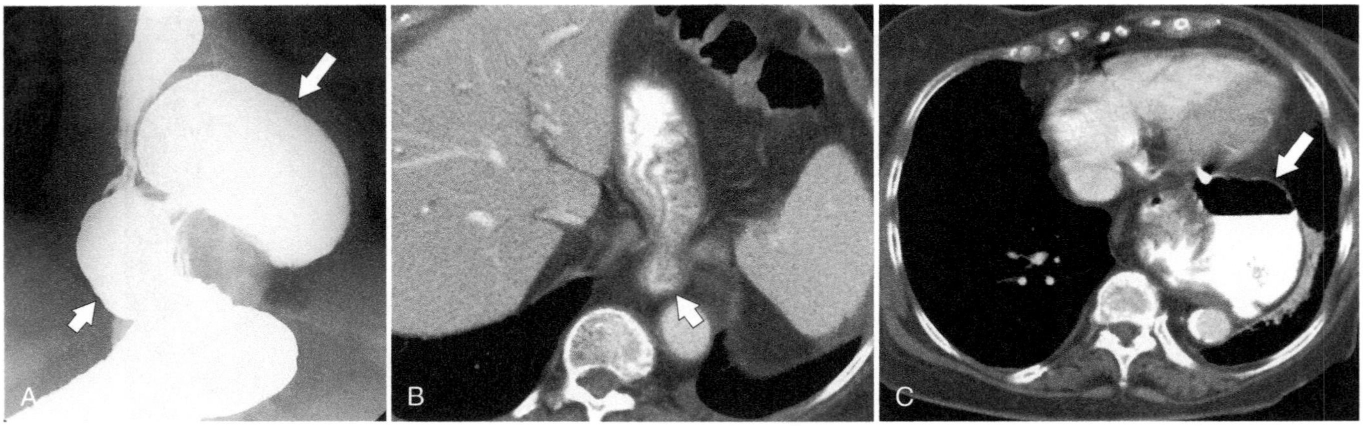

FIGURE 2-8. UGI series and axial contrast-enhanced CT in a 44-year-old woman with both a paraesophageal (*large arrows*) and sliding hiatal hernia (*small arrows*). The GE junction lies below the diaphragm.

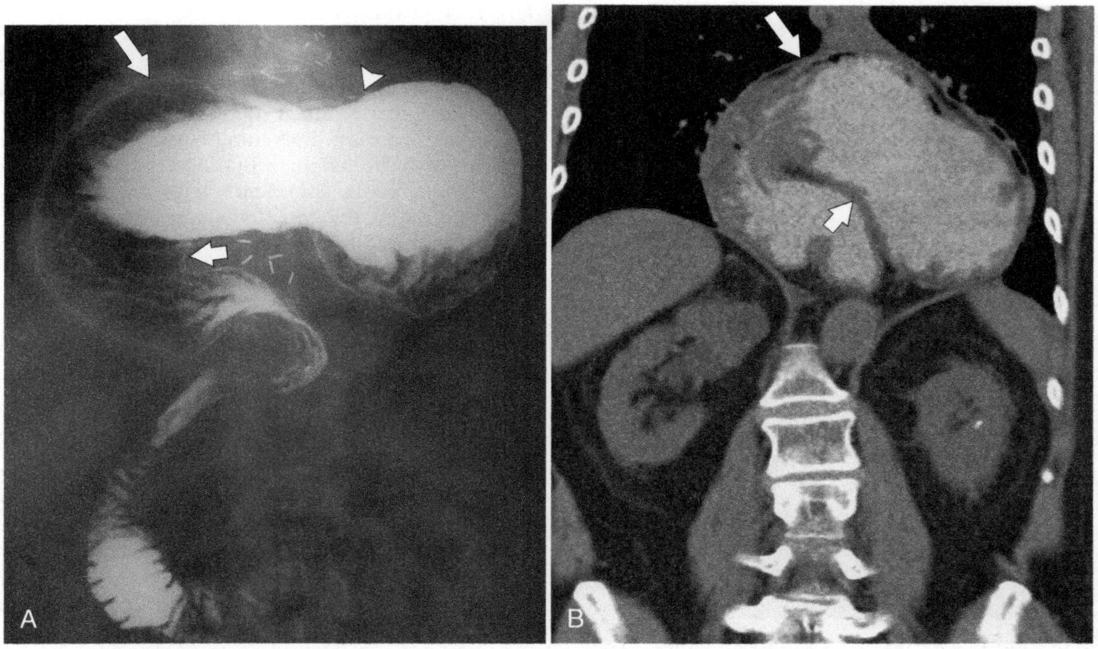

FIGURE 2-10. UGI series (**A**) and coronal CT (**B**) in a 59-year-old woman with an organoaxial volvulus. The greater curvature (*large arrow*) is superior (cephalad) and the lesser curvature inferior (*small arrow*). The GE junction is indicated by the arrowhead.

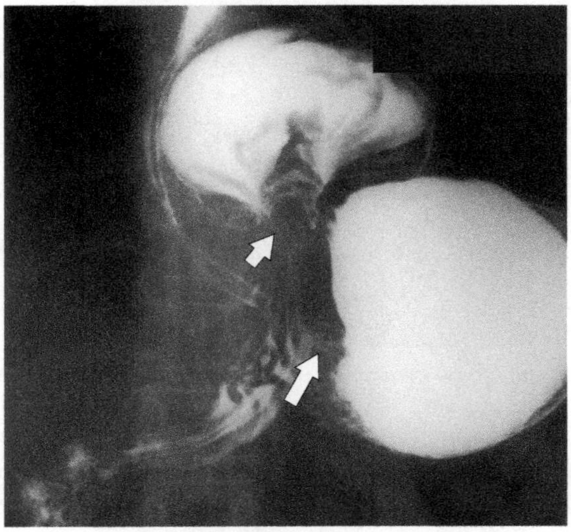

FIGURE 2-11. UGI swallow in a 68-year-old woman with mesenteroaxial volvulus. The GE junction is inferior (*large arrow*) and the pylorus, superior (*small arrow*).

TABLE 2-1 Diffuse Gastric Mucosal Thickening

Benign	Malignant
Gastritis (see Table 2-2)	Carcinoma
Pseudolymphoma	Lymphoma
Varices	Metastases

TABLE 2-2 Causes of Gastritis

Type	Features	Location
H. pylori/peptic	Thick lobulated folds, increased areae gastricae	Antrum and body
Drugs	Often causes erosions when acute	Antrum, body, fundus
Caustic	Thickened folds, ulcers with narrowing when healed	Antrum and body
Radiation	Thickened folds and ulcers and antral narrowing when healed	Antrum, body, fundus
Eosinophilic	Thickened and nodular folds and antral narrowing	Body and antrum
Inflammatory	Aphthous ulcers, thickened folds with larger ulcers in Crohn disease, sarcoid, Behçet syndrome, amyloid	Antrum and body
Infectious	Tuberculosis; syphilis can cause linitis plastica	Antrum and body
Emphysematous	Thickened folds and gas in wall	Antrum and body
Pancreatitis	Thickened folds along greater curvature; gastric narrowing from fluid collections	Body and antrum
Hypertrophic	Large lobulated folds	Body and fundus
Atrophic	Featureless mucosa with decreased folds and narrowed stomach	Antrum, body, fundus

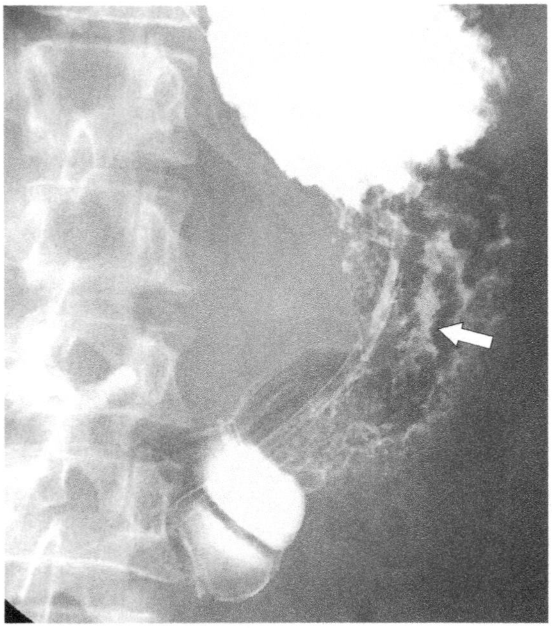

Figure 2-12. UGI series in a 41-year-old woman with diffuse gastric fold thickening (*arrow*) due to profuse gastritis.

Erosive Gastritis

Erosive gastritis evolves from gastritis from several diverse etiologies (Box 2-1). In general, it is not possible to define the precise diagnosis by imaging unless there are other imaging and clinical features that point to the correct disease. They are typified by nodular mucosal thickening (gastritis), predominantly in the antrum, with the hallmark finding at a UGI series of tiny punctate barium pools, sometimes with an edematous radiolucent halo, often along thickened mucosal folds (Fig. 2-15). They must be distinguished from aphthous ulcers and small hematogenous metastases, which can look similar but are usually larger (Figs. 2-16 and 2-17). Good gastric coating is essential because visualization of some gastric erosions can be subtle (Fig. 2-18). Many gastric erosive diseases progress to ulceration, and therefore both are discussed simultaneously.

Peptic Gastritis and Ulcer Disease

Peptic gastritis used to be far more prevalent and was responsible for tens of millions of deaths worldwide. It was widely assumed for centuries to result primarily from "stress" conditions that were presumed to cause gastric hyperacidity and mucosal inflammation, thickening, erosion, and ulcer disease. Over the centuries, many medications were introduced to alleviate the symptoms until a generation ago, when histamine$_2$ (H_2)–receptor antagonists (which block the action of H_2, a powerful gastric acid hormonal promoter) and then proton pump inhibitors (which block hydrochloric acid production) were

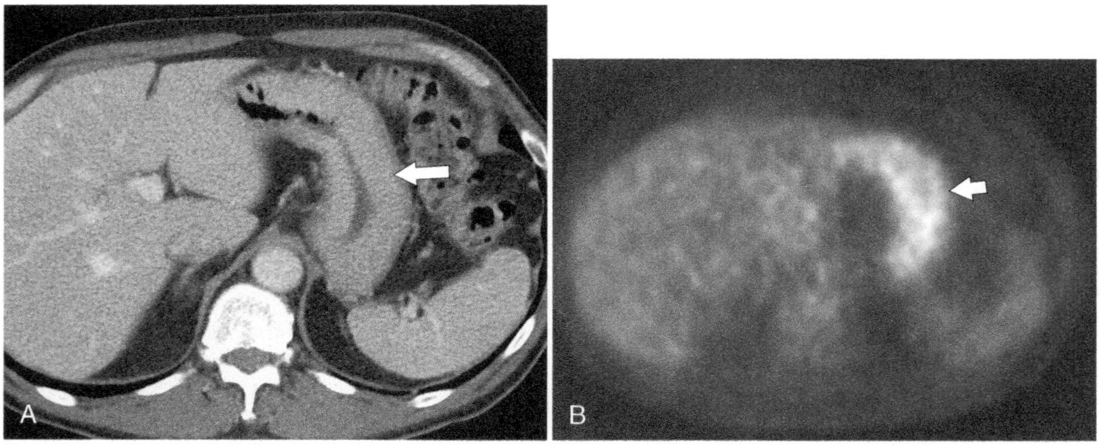

Figure 2-13. Axial contrast-enhanced CT (**A**) and PET (**B**) in a 71-year-old woman with diffuse gastric mucosal thickening (*large arrow*) caused by gastritis; some FDG avidity is also apparent (*small arrow*).

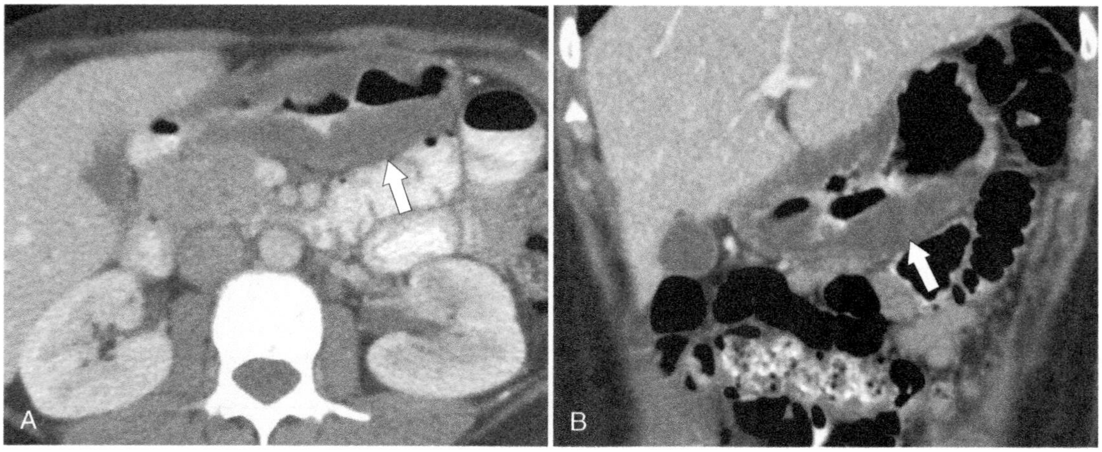

Figure 2-14. Axial (**A**) and coronal (**B**) contrast-enhanced CT in a 56-year-old woman with diffuse gastric mucosal thickening (*arrows*) caused by antral gastritis. The fundus is relatively normal.

introduced. Both drugs have dramatically improved the morbidity and mortality of the disease, but they do not treat the cause. It was not discovered until the early 1980s that almost all peptic ulcer disease was, in fact, due to an infective agent, *H. pylori*, a gram*-negative bacterium present in about 50% of the population. This bacterium causes an excessive production of ammonium, which is toxic to the gastric mucosa. As part of the host's inflammatory response to the bacteria and ammonia production, excessive gastrin is produced that acts on gastric parietal cells to produce more hydrochloric acid (and more parietal cells), setting up an increasing mucosal inflammatory response, predominantly in the gastric antrum (but also throughout the stomach when the infection is severe). Gastric mucosal thickening, erosions, and eventually ulcer disease ensue. The discovery that the disease is primarily infectious and the fact that it is readily treated by antibiotics have completely transformed the outlook for patients with the disease. In practice, almost all erosions and ulcer disease in the stomach and duodenum are related to infection with *H. pylori*, though ulcers can be exacerbated or caused by several drugs and alcohol as listed in Box 2-1. Very rarely, diffuse peptic gastritis and ulcer disease can be caused by Zollinger-Ellison† syndrome.

Ulcers are much more frequent in the duodenum than in the stomach, but erosions are often a precursor to frank ulcer disease and are superficial mucosal defects that have not penetrated the submucosa, as ulcers do. The erosions are a frequent cause of UGI hemorrhage. Of note, some patients suffering from major stress disorders (e.g., burns, septic shock) are also susceptible to superficial gastric erosions known as Curling‡ ulcers. A much smaller proportion (approximately 5%) of gastric ulcers are secondary to malignant disease, primary or secondary.

Patients have epigastric pain, symptoms of GERD, nausea, weight loss, hematemesis, and melena. Gastric ulcer symptoms typically occur during eating a meal, whereas duodenal ulcers occur approximately 2 hours later. Complications of gastric ulcers include blood loss, perforation, gastric outlet obstruction (from the fibrotic healing process), and an increased incidence of adenocarcinoma.

*Hans Christian Joachim Gram (1850-1938), Danish bacteriologist.

†Robert M. Zollinger (1903-1992), American surgeon; Edwin H. Ellison (1918-1970), American surgeon.
‡Thomas Blizard Curling (1811-1888), British surgeon.

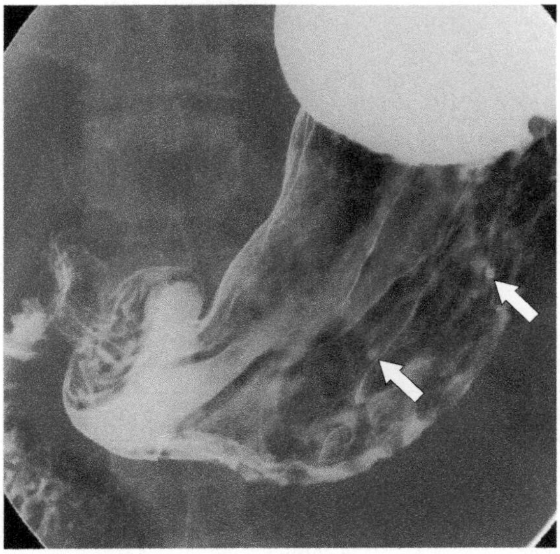

FIGURE 2-15. UGI series in a 52-year-old man with gastric mucosal thickening and multiple small gastric erosions, some of which have punctate pools of barium (*arrows*).

***Box 2-1.* Causes of Gastric Erosions**

- Peptic ulcer disease
- Drugs (aspirin, NSAIDs, steroids, KCl, clopidogrel)
- Alcohol
- Crohn disease
- Infectious (CMV, HSV)
- Behçet syndrome
- Major stress conditions (burns, septic shock)

CMV, Cytomegalovirus; *HSV,* herpes simplex virus; *KCl,* potassium chloride; *NSAIDs,* nonsteroidal antiinflammatory drugs.

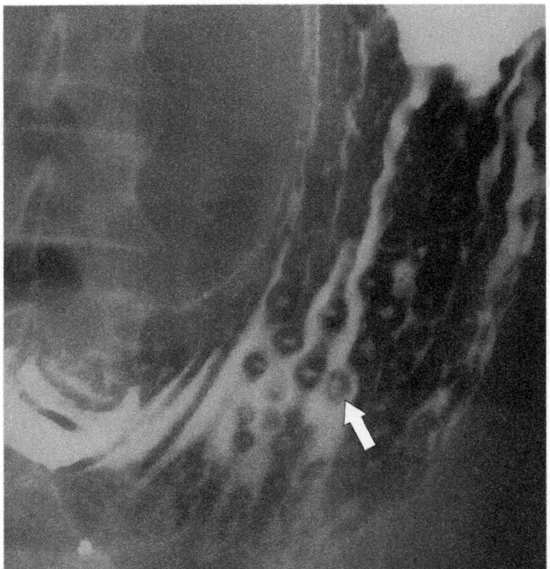

FIGURE 2-16. UGI series in a 60-year-old woman with multiple aphthous ulcers (*arrow*).

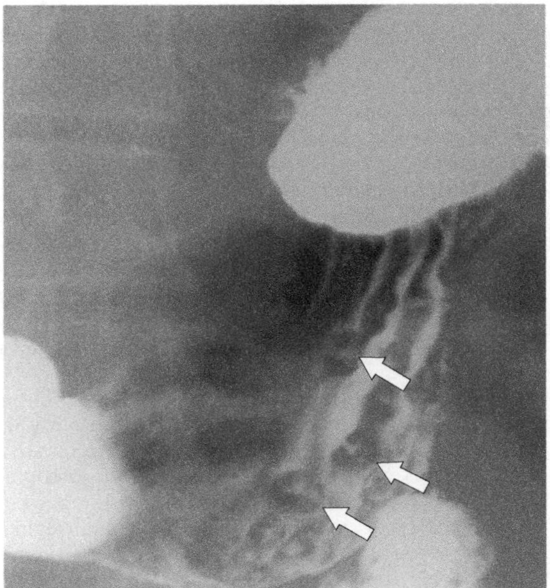

FIGURE 2-17. UGI series in a 54-year-old man with multiple bull's-eye gastric lesions (*arrows*) due to melanoma metastases.

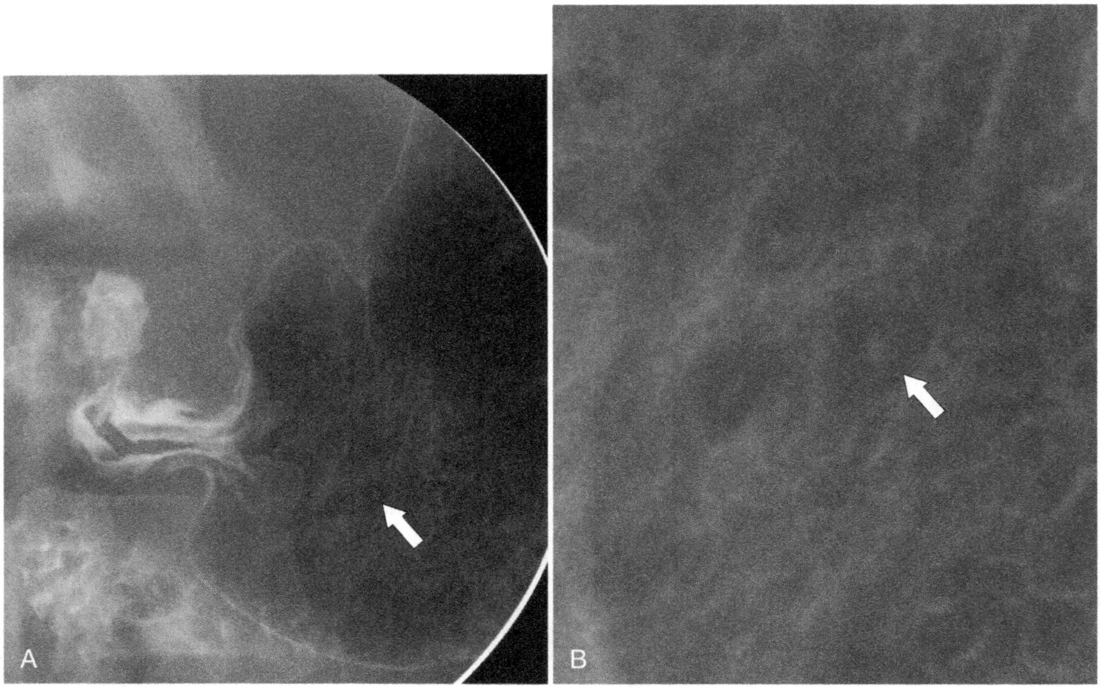

FIGURE 2-18. **A,** UGI in a 54-year-old woman with subtle antral gastric erosions (*arrow*). **B,** A magnified view of the erosions (*arrow*).

The diagnosis is usually made by endoscopy or urea breath test studies. Before the widespread use of EGD to evaluate for gastric ulcer disease, the radiologist should have been able to differentiate most gastric ulcers as benign or malignant, particularly with good double-contrast technique. Single-contrast techniques were useful unless the ulcers were large and florid. However, given the widespread use of EGD to evaluate symptomatic gastric disease and the fact that the disease is less common, it is becoming harder for radiologists to gain sufficient experience with the different imaging presentations of gastric ulcer disease. However, the gastrointestinal (GI) radiologist will still likely identify gastric ulcers from time to time on UGI series, and therefore their detection and differentiation into benign or malignant categories are still required. Certain UGI imaging features should be emphasized (Table 2-3).

Location: Because almost all benign ulcers occur in the antrum, any ulcer identified in the more proximal stomach should be strongly considered as malignant until proved otherwise.

Ulcer position on mound: The inflammatory reaction surrounding a benign ulcer tends to be uniform, and therefore the ulcer tends to be positioned within the center of the surrounding edematous mass (Fig. 2-19). Malignant masses, on the other hand, are often eccentrically placed within the overall mass, dependent on the underlying vascular supply to that part of the tumor (Fig. 2-20).

Ulcer shape: Almost all benign ulcers are uniform and round, even if they are large (Fig. 2-21). However, if they are malignant, there are often other imaging features that will steer the radiologist away from benign disease (see Table 2-3). Most malignant ulcers have irregular ulcer margins (Fig. 2-22).

Ulcer collar: This represents the area of edema around the ulcer and is typically uniform in benign disease; it is also known as a Hampton* line, representing the radiolucent line across the neck of an ulcer (i.e., it separates barium in ulcer from gastric lumen) (Fig. 2-23). Ulcer collars may not be present with malignant disease, but when they are, they are usually thick and irregular.

Ulcer fold convergence: This is a helpful sign for benign disease because folds almost always converge right up to the ulcer margin, whereas this is uncommon in malignant disease where folds, often irregular, fail to meet the ulcer margin (Fig. 2-24).

Mucosal fold shape: Benign folds simply represent edematous changes and are typically smooth and uniform (Fig. 2-24). Malignant folds often contain the malignancy itself as well as

TABLE 2-3 Imaging Differentiation of Benign and Malignant Gastric Ulcer Disease

Features	Benign	Malignant
Age	All adult ages	Elderly
Sex	Equal between males and females	Males more than females
Location	90% antrum (75% lesser curve)	Antrum, but can occur elsewhere
Ulcer position	Central	Eccentric
Ulcer shape	Round	Irregular
Ulcer collar	Uniform (Hampton line)	Irregular
Fold shape	Uniform	Irregular and distorted
Fold convergence	To edge of crater	Does not reach ulcer margins
Projections beyond gastric wall	Yes	No
Multiple	Up to 30%	Uncommon
Associated duodenal ulcer	Frequent	Uncommon
Carman sign	No	Yes
Crescent sign	Yes	No
Response to peptic ulcer treatment	Yes	No

*Aubrey O. Hampton (1900-1955), American radiologist.

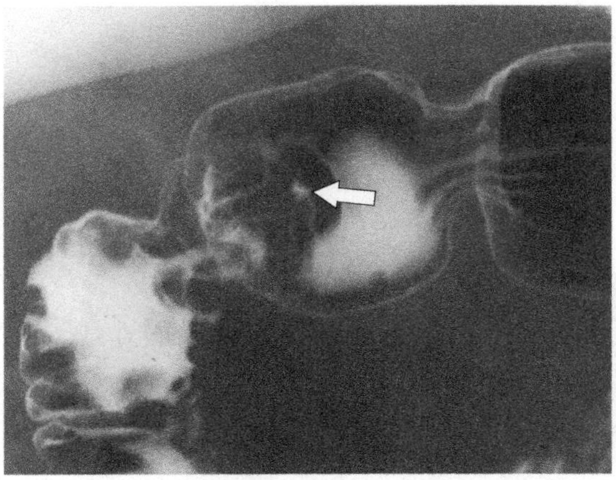

FIGURE 2-19. UGI series in a 44-year-old man with thickened antral folds and a punctate collection of barium at the center (*arrow*) due to an antral ulcer.

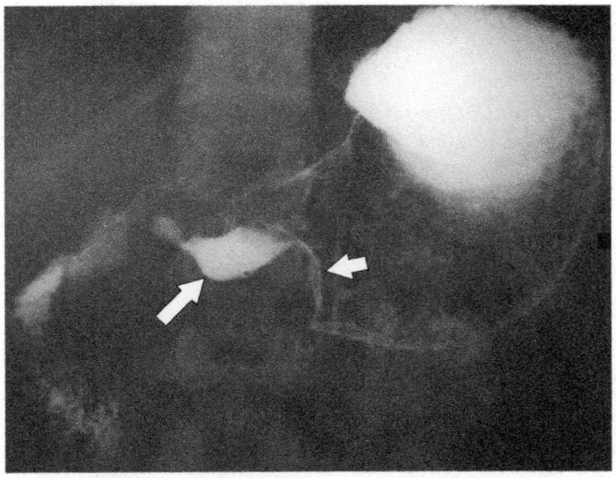

FIGURE 2-20. UGI series in a 60-year-old man with an eccentric gastric ulcer (*large arrow*) within a larger gastric cancer (*small arrow*).

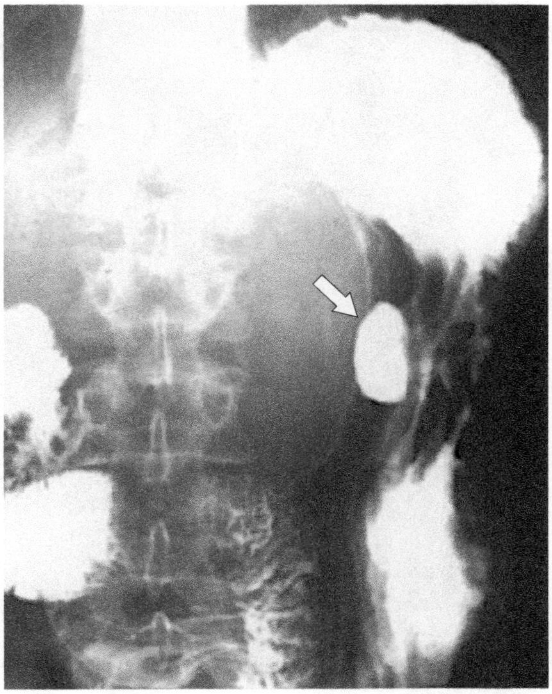

FIGURE 2-21. UGI series in a 76-year-old woman with a larger benign lesser curve ulcer (*arrow*).

edematous changes and so are more typically irregular, amputated, clubbed, or fused (Fig. 2-25).

Visualization of an ulcer within or outside gastric wall: Benign, particularly acute, ulcers often project outside the gastric wall as they erode through the mucosa (see Fig. 2-21). This projection will probably not be appreciated unless visualized tangentially, which underlines the importance of obtaining multiple orthogonal views when any abnormality is identified. Malignant ulcers tend to erode less outside of the stomach wall, but rather, into the gastric lumen as an intraluminal mass (see Fig. 2-22). Occasionally, the position of a chronic benign ulcer can also appear confined within the stomach wall because of the chronic fibrosis, contraction, and distortion of the surrounding gastric wall.

Concurrent duodenal ulcer disease: This is unusual with malignant gastric disease, and its presence strongly suggests benign gastric ulceration.

Carman† *meniscus sign:* This is the radiological representation of a large, flat ulcer with heaped-up edges (Figs. 2-22 and 2-26). There is a radiolucent halo on compression views, which represents the heaped-up edges, with a convex outer shape to the trapped barium in the ulcer crater.

Crescent sign: This represents benignity and is seen in ulcers along the greater curvature of the stomach (usually antrum) where the barium pool protruding outside the mucosa has a concavity away from the gastric lumen and gives the appearance of a crescent.

The complications of benign gastric ulcer disease are potentially fatal. These include hemorrhage after the ulcer erodes into adjacent arterial or venous structures and perforation into either the retroperitoneum or, more commonly, the peritoneum. In most patients, however, the ulcers will heal by fibrosis if left untreated with antibiotics (Fig. 2-27). The fibrosis can be sufficient to cause gastric antral scarring and narrowing, which may be severe enough to cause gastric outlet obstruction (Figs. 2-28 and 2-29). Patients usually have had chronic symptoms of peptic ulcer disease and so generally do not have the short history of symptoms—vomiting, abdominal fullness/mass, and pain—that is associated with gastric outlet obstruction. Should they have such symptoms, however, then other, more sinister causes (e.g., malignancy) should be considered. The obstruction is usually caused by chronic fibrosis and scarring compounded by acute inflammation from recurrent and active ulceration from pyloric channel or duodenal bulb disease. Usually the stomach distends gradually over months and years as luminal distention steadily progresses, and it can be massively distended at the time of presentation. The stomach is usually filled with a mixture of fluid and food residue. Complete obstruction is unusual, and some food, fluid, and gas will pass into the duodenum. The food and fluid are readily identified on plain radiographs (possibly with a fluid level). The site of obstruction can be confirmed with barium studies (presuming no perforation) rather than with water-soluble contrast media because the latter will often be too diluted to yield diagnostic information.

Drug-Induced Gastritis

Alcohol, aspirin, and other nonsteroidal antiinflammatory drugs (NSAIDs) frequently cause focal gastric irritation, particularly with chronic or high-dose use. Erosions and peptic ulcer disease can follow simple gastric mucosal hypertrophy and are the second most-common causes of peptic ulceration, after *H. pylori*–induced peptic disease.

†Russell Daniel Carman (1875-1926), Canadian-born American radiologist.

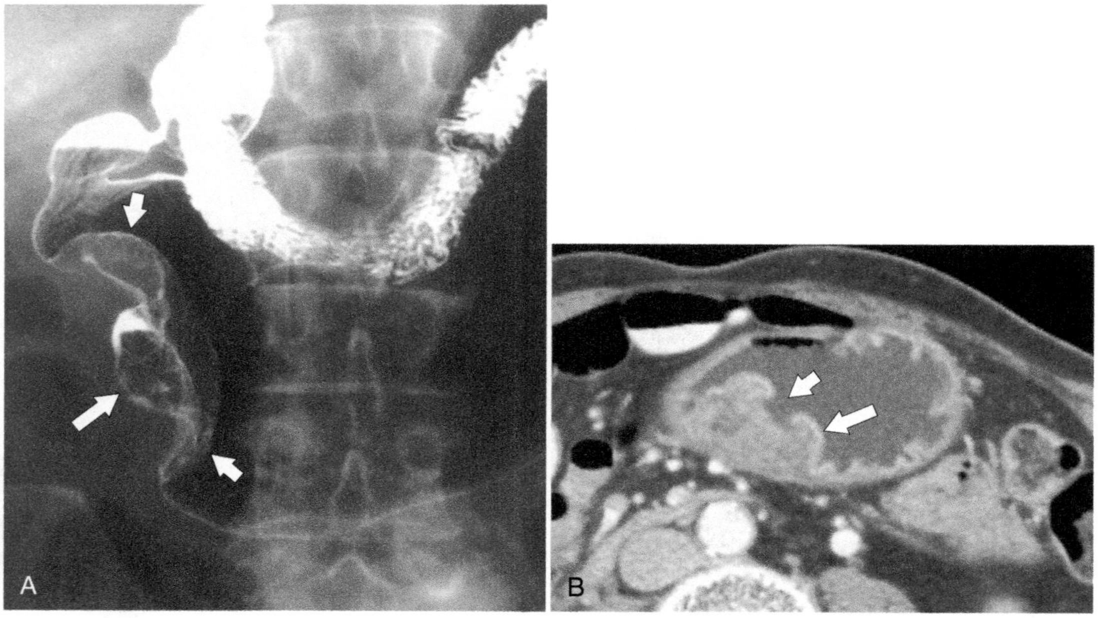

FIGURE 2-22. **A,** UGI in a 71-year-old woman with a large greater curvature malignant ulcer (*large arrow*) with a surrounding irregular mound (*small arrows*) due to infiltrated adenocarcinoma. **B,** Axial contrast-enhanced CT demonstrating a malignant gastric ulcer (*small arrow*), which projects into the gastric lumen surrounded by the malignant mass (*large arrow*).

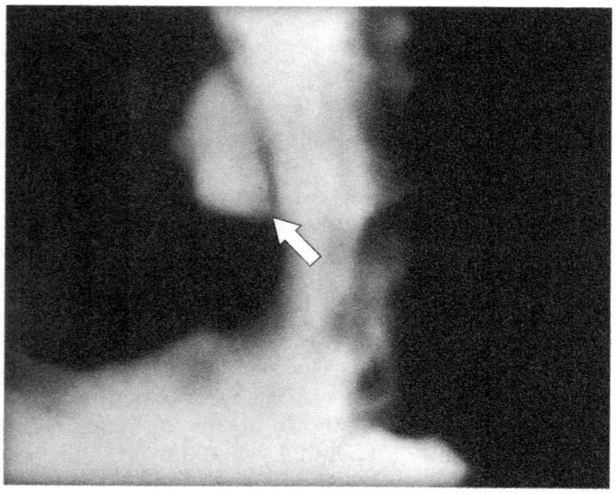

FIGURE 2-23. UGI series in a 61-year-old woman with a benign lesser curve gastric ulcer with a Hampton line (*arrow*) consistent with a benign ulcer.

Corrosive Gastritis

Acute ingestion of alkali or acid will predominantly affect the esophagus, but if enough of the toxin is ingested, it can pass into the stomach (predominantly the antrum if ingested in the upright position) and lead to marked antral mucosal edema and ulceration (Fig. 2-30). A large ingestion of toxin is associated with a poor prognosis because the stomach (or esophagus) can readily perforate in the acute phase (as evidenced at imaging by peritoneal fluid and pneumoperitoneum). If the patient survives, healing usually occurs with antral stricture formation (Fig. 2-31). The appearance can mimic antral narrowing and linitis plastica, common to several other diseases.

Radiation Gastritis

Radiation gastritis is less commonly observed because of the more refined radiation therapy techniques and portals. When observed, it is usually due to the acute radiation effects of nonspecific mucosal thickening, which may ulcerate if the radiation doses were too severe. The healing process occurs by fibrosis with the narrowing of the affected segment.

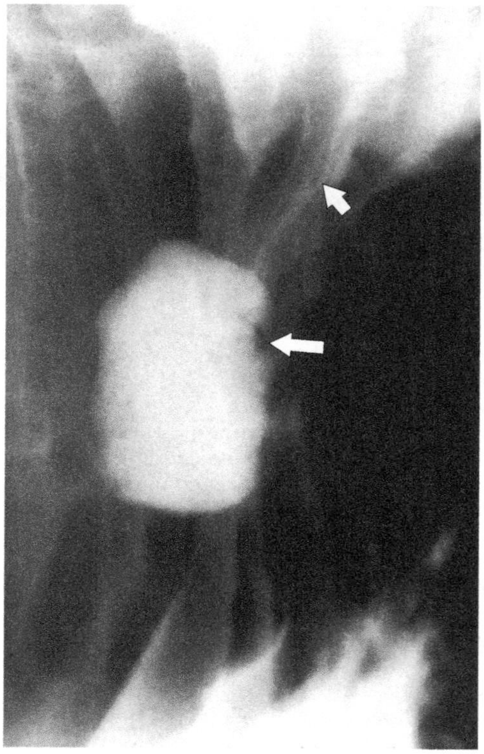

FIGURE 2-24. UGI series in a 69-year-old man with a large benign lesser curve ulcer (*large arrow*) with uniform fold convergence on the ulcer (*small arrow*).

Eosinophilic Gastroenteritis

This rare disease is characterized by diffuse eosinophilic infiltration of the gut, primarily the stomach, but also the esophagus and small and large bowel. It is associated with peripheral eosinophilia, elevated immunoglobulin E (IgE) levels, and food allergies. Patients have nonspecific symptoms of abdominal pain,

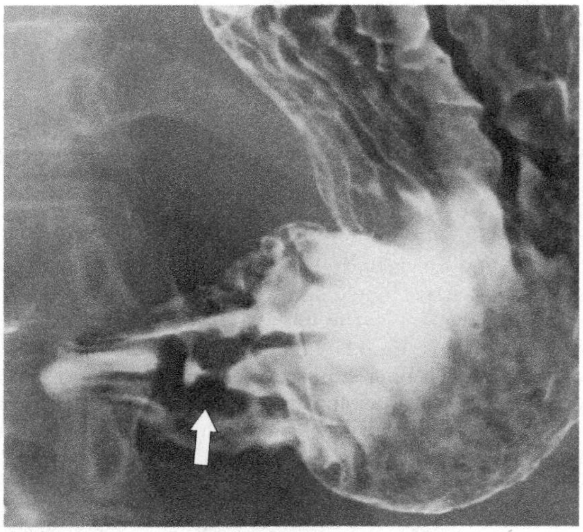

FIGURE 2-25. UGI series of the stomach demonstrating a malignant gastric ulcer. There is a central pooling of barium in the gastric ulcer surrounded by fused and clubbed mucosal folds (*arrow*).

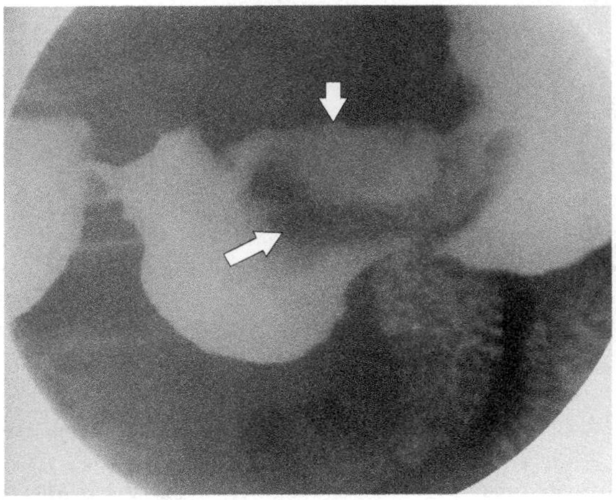

FIGURE 2-26. UGI series in a 70-year-old woman with a radiolucent halo (*large arrow*) due to a Carman meniscus sign that surrounds a central maliginant ulcer crater (*small arrow*).

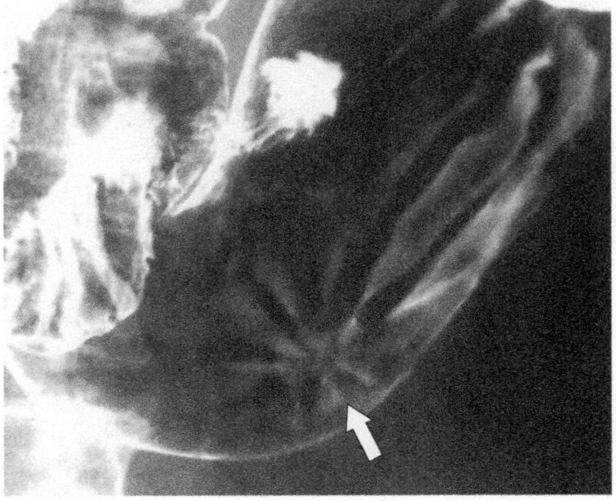

FIGURE 2-27. UGI series in a 72-year-old man with a healing gastric ulcer. Radiating folds (*arrow*) converge on the previous ulcer.

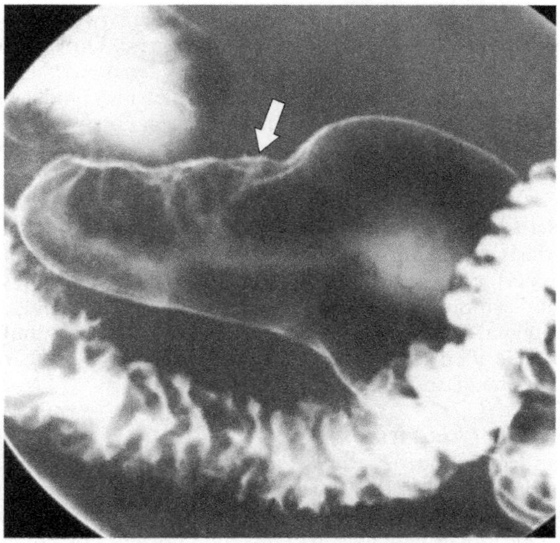

FIGURE 2-28. UGI series in a 59-year-old man with antral deformity (*arrow*) due to chronic scarring from peptic ulcer disease.

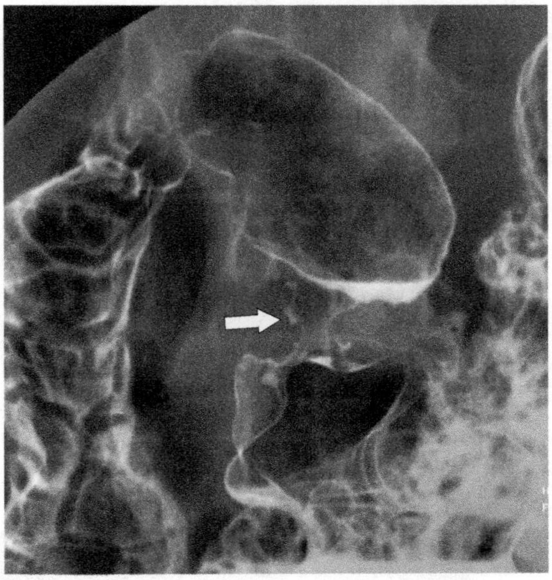

FIGURE 2-29. UGI series in a 48-year-old woman with Zollinger-Ellison syndrome and repetitive antral ulceration with chronic stricture and residual ulcers (*arrow*).

nausea, vomiting, diarrhea, and weight loss. Findings include gastric erosions, ulceration, and diffuse infiltration with mucosal thickening and nodularity, particularly of the distal stomach and proximal small bowel. The latter findings can be difficult to distinguish from other causes of gastric and small bowel thickening, including Crohn disease, Zollinger-Ellison syndrome, and lymphoma. Chronic disease can present with a constricted antral and gastric body, secondary to fibrosis, which is difficult to distinguish from other causes of linitis plastica.

Crohn Disease (see Chapters 4 and 5)

Crohn disease is usually associated with Crohn disease elsewhere in the small bowel and colon and typically demonstrates aphthous ulceration when involving the stomach (see Fig. 2-16). Crohn disease represents a transmural process with submucosal lymphoid follicular proliferation with the ulceration of the overlying mucosa (seen also in the esophagus and small and large bowel). Noncaseating granulomas are characteristic of the disease. On UGI series, there is a small ulcer crater surrounded by an edematous halo or ring (see Fig. 2-16). Healing occurs by fibrosis, which may produce a narrowed antrum with the more proximal stomach mucosa preserved. Occasionally, Crohn disease involves the whole stomach, preventing it from dilatation and giving it a linitis plastica appearance.

Sarcoidosis

Sarcoidosis is rare, although the stomach is the most commonly affected GI organ. Patients have abdominal pain, sometimes diarrhea, and symptoms of GI reflux. Acute disease results in gastritis with mucosal thickening, which can ulcerate. Gastric granulomas can be identified at biopsy. Healing is by fibrosis, which can produce a linitis plastica appearance.

Infectious Gastritis

Phlegmonous gastritis is now rarely observed and results from bacterial infection of the gastric wall (gram-positive streptococci and staphylococci and gram-negative coliforms). It is typically seen in alcoholics who have had repeated episodes of gastritis.

Emphysematous gastritis, which is most commonly seen in elderly patients with poorly controlled diabetes, is similar to patients with emphysematous cholecystitis. It is due to overwhelming mural infection with gas-forming organisms and is fatal if left untreated, so aggressive antibiotic therapy, surgery, or both may be required. The imaging diagnosis is recognized on CT as diffuse gas within the stomach wall and portal venous system, usually in a diabetic patient (Fig. 2-32).

Tuberculosis and syphilis are rare manifestations of gastritis, although tuberculosis is endemic in the developing world, where tuberculous gastritis is more common and may be associated with tuberculosis elsewhere in the body. Acutely, there is nonspecific gastric mucosal thickening, which may progress to ulceration (Fig. 2-33). The chronic fibrosing reaction that both diseases then produce can cause an antral constrictive process, not unlike a linitis plastica finding (Fig. 2-34). Syphilis can produce similar findings (Fig. 2-35).

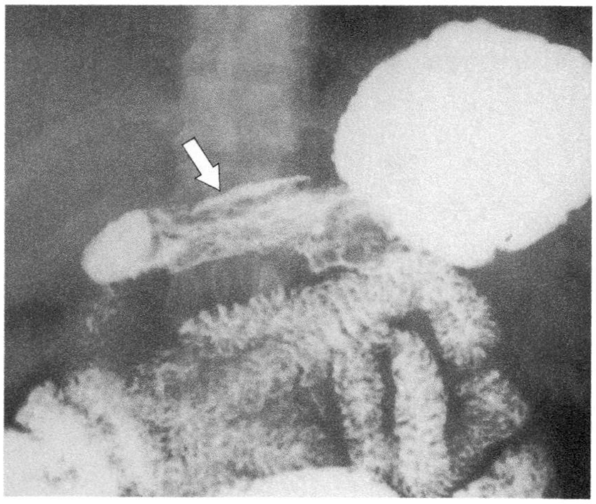

FIGURE 2-30. UGI series in a 39-year-old man with marked gastric wall mucosal thickening and ulceration (*arrow*) after caustic ingestion.

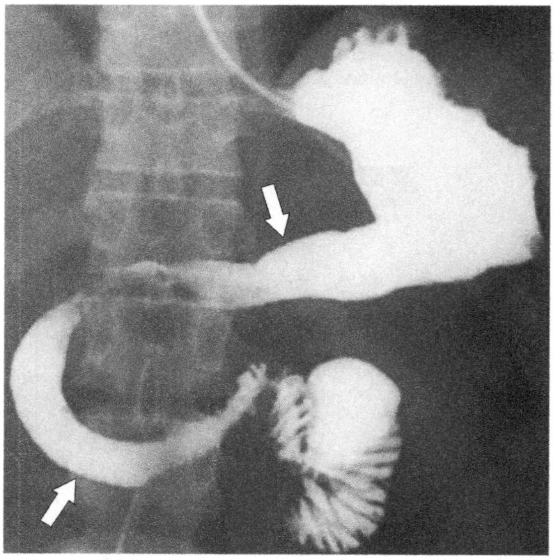

FIGURE 2-31. UGI series and axial contrast-enhanced CT in a 35-year-old man with antral and duodenal fixed strictures (*arrows*) due to prior caustic ingestion.

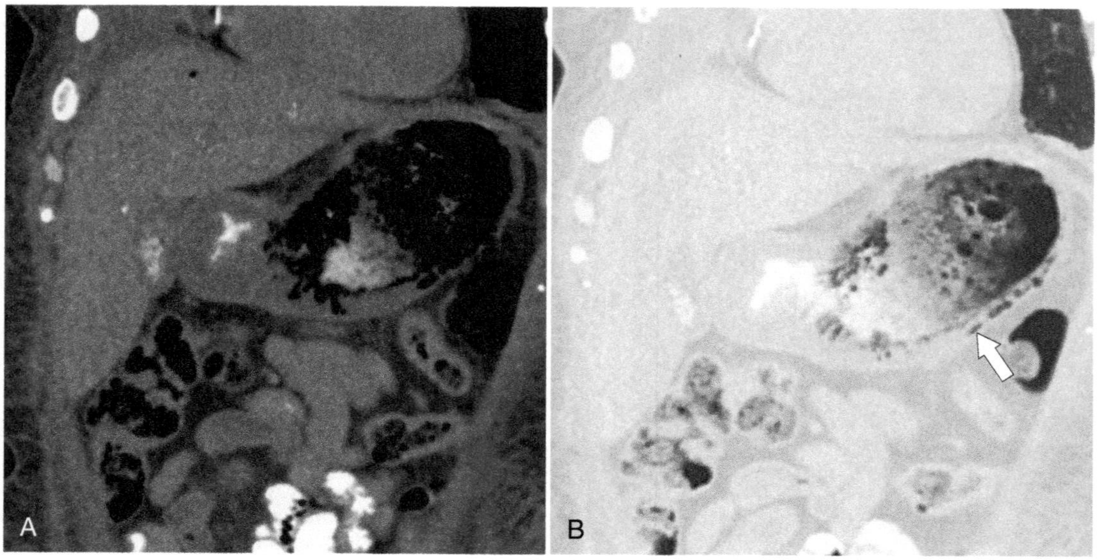

FIGURE 2-32. Coronal CT with soft tissue windows (**A**) and lung window settings (**B**) in a 67-year-old diabetic woman with mural gastric gas (*arrow*) due to emphysematous gastritis.

Candidiasis of the stomach is recognized in the immune-compromised population but is observed less commonly because gastric acid usually neutralizes the yeast organisms. The appearances are similar to those in the esophagus, with multiple small plaque-like filling defects of the gastric lining. They, as with yeast organisms in the esophagus, can bleed if ulceration is severe.

Amyloidosis

Amyloidosis of the stomach, in either its primary or secondary systemic form, is rare and can cause a range of findings, from focal (which may be mass-like) to diffuse mucosal thickening and ulceration. In primary amyloidosis, there is no known underlying predisposing condition, and GI involvement is more common than with the secondary form. One variant of the primary type is focal rather than systemic and can involve only the GI system. In secondary amyloidosis, chronic underlying disease is present, including rheumatoid arthritis, chronic lung disease (tuberculosis/bronchiectasis), and multiple myeloma.

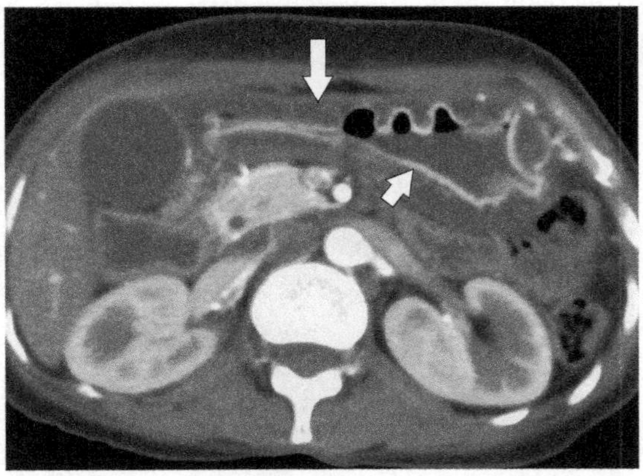

FIGURE 2-33. Axial contrast-enhanced CT in a 35-year-old woman with gastric wall thickening (*large arrow*) and hyperenhancement of the gastric mucosa (*small arrow*) due to tuberculosis.

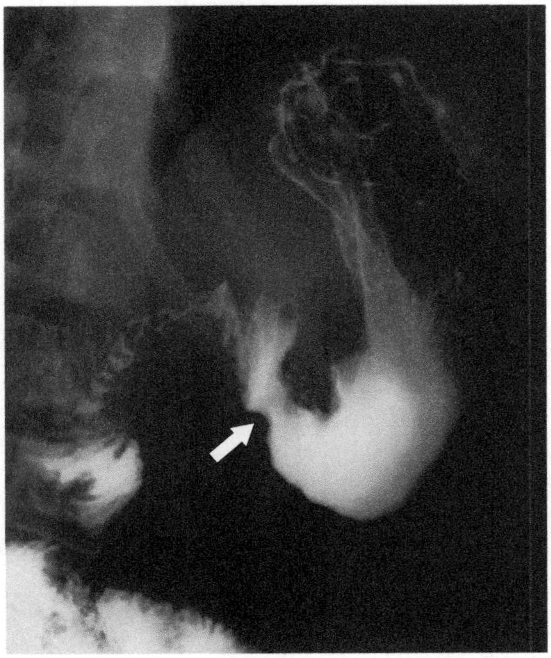

FIGURE 2-34. UGI series in a 70-year-old man with antral narrowing (*arrow*) and a linitis plastica type appearance due to chronic tuberculosis.

Pancreatitis

Severe pancreatitis can cause such diffuse peripancreatic inflammatory change that it can produce gastric wall and mucosal inflammation (Fig. 2-36). The stomach may be narrowed, due to both the inflammatory process and the associated mass effect from peripancreatic acute fluid collections (Fig. 2-37). Once the acute pancreatitis has subsided, the outlet obstruction should subside, although chronic peripancreatic fluid collections (pseudocyst formation) may develop, which can exacerbate any gastric narrowing and cause gastric outlet obstruction (Fig. 2-38).

Ménétrier Disease (Hypertrophic Gastritis)

Ménétrier* disease has an uncertain etiology, is more common in males, and usually follows a viral illness or infection with *H. pylori*. It is characterized by profusely thickened gastric folds throughout the stomach (although it can be focal), with or without ulceration. It is not always associated with hyperacidity, and many patients have reduced gastric acid production (hypochlorhydria) because of parietal cell destruction. There is also secretion of large volumes of mucus, sometimes sufficient to cause hypoalbuminemia. Patients have postprandial epigastric pain, weight loss, and signs of hypoalbuminemia. The diagnosis is

*Pierre E. Ménétrier (1859-1935), French pathologist.

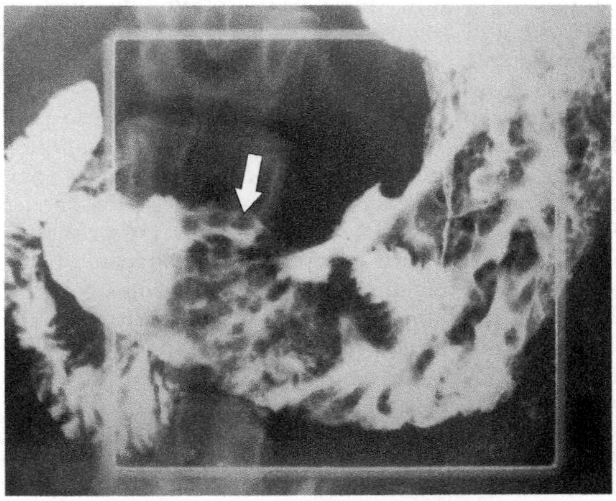

FIGURE 2-35. UGI series in a 39-year-old woman with diffuse gastritis (*arrow*) and ulceration due to syphilis infection.

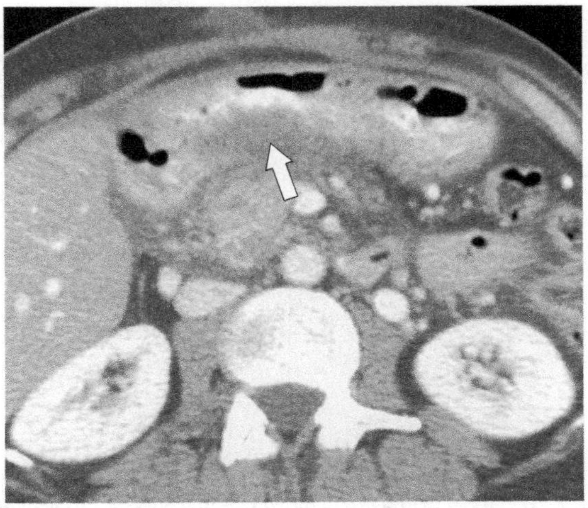

FIGURE 2-36. UGI in a 47-year-old woman with greater curvature inflammation (*arrow*) due to underlying acute pancreatitis.

one of exclusion (i.e., no history of aspirin or excessive alcohol use, negative *H. pylori* test result), although at biopsy, there is characteristic crypt hyperplasia, which is thought to predispose the patient to the development of gastric adenocarcinoma. At imaging, the disease should be suspected if the mucosal folds are grossly thickened, particularly if there are concomitant clinical symptoms (Fig. 2-39). These are usually severe enough to be recognized on CT (Fig. 2-40).

Pseudolymphoma

This uncommon benign disease is due to a lymphoreticular hyperplasia with infiltration of the gastric mucosa. It causes fold thickening that often can ulcerate. The findings can be confused with carcinoma or lymphoma radiologically, especially because anemia is common to both diseases. Pseudolymphoma can also present as a more infiltrative process, again causing confusion between this and other, malignant conditions.

Zollinger-Ellison Syndrome

Zollinger-Ellison* syndrome is the result of a triad of gastric hyperacidity, ulcers, and a gastrin-producing tumor of the pancreas or duodenum. The primary neuroendocrine tumor secretes excessive gastrin, causing parietal cell stimulation and overproduction of gastric acid. This hyperacidity can be profound, leading to massive ulceration of the stomach, particularly the antrum, and proximal small bowel (Figs. 2-29 and 2-41). The hyperacidity in the small bowel also results in excessive small bowel hypersecretion, causing diarrhea and malabsorption. Chronic ulceration can heal with a fibrotic narrowed gastric antrum (Fig. 2-29) and may be sufficiently severe to give a linitis plastica appearance to the stomach.

The primary tumor is hypervascular, but because it is often small, it can be missed, even with a dedicated arterial-phase CT scan through the pancreas and duodenum. It is most commonly found in the duodenal wall (50% to 70%) and pancreas (20% to 40%). A strong clinical suspicion may require the patient to undergo laparotomy and preoperative endoscopic ultrasound or palpation to detect the tumor. Very careful analysis of the pancreas and duodenum is required to identify any arterially enhancing lesions, which may represent the tumor. They are often not identified in the portal venous phase. Liver metastases, when present, are also hypervascular and therefore are best detected with a dedicated arterial-phase CT scan, particularly if they are small.

*Robert M. Zollinger (1903-1992), American surgeon; Edwin H. Ellison (1918-1970), American surgeon.

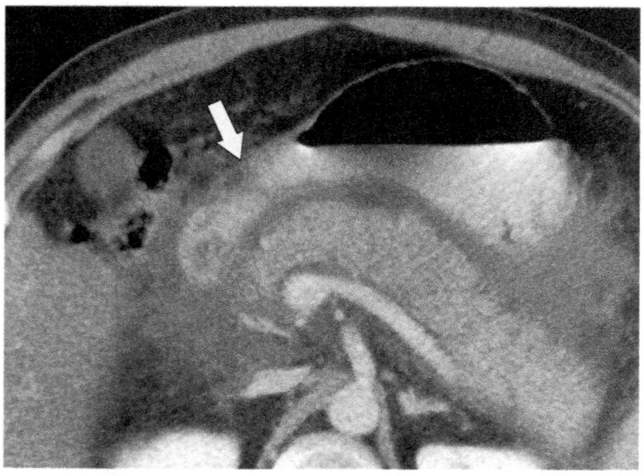

FIGURE 2-37. Axial contrast-enhanced CT in a 64-year-old woman with acute pancreatitis and antral narrowing (*arrow*) due to the acute inflammatory process.

Atrophic Gastritis

In contrast to other forms of gastritis, which are characterized by gastric mucosal thickening, atrophic gastritis results in loss of normal mucosa (Fig. 2-42). It is much less common than other forms of gastritis and is acquired either from a prolonged *H. pylori* infection or from autoimmune causes. The former usually affects the antrum, whereas the latter typically affects the body and fundus. The autoimmune disease is responsible for pernicious anemia. There is antibody destruction of gastric parietal cells, leading to hypochlorhydria and elevated gastrin levels. The ensuing parietal cell loss leads to the loss of protein intrinsic factor (IF) production, which is necessary for normal vitamin B_{12} absorption. Normally, the combined IF-B_{12} molecule is recognized by terminal ileal receptors and transported into the portal circulation. Lack of IF results in vitamin B_{12} malabsorption (as does loss of the normal terminal ileum, e.g., from Crohn disease or surgery). This loss of vitamin B_{12} then results in a megaloblastic-type anemia.

The hypochlorhydria or achlorhydria from parietal cell destruction results in mucosal atrophy, gastritis, and intestinal metaplasia with absent or reduced gastric folds and almost complete loss of the gastric fundus. The stomach demonstrates reduced, but not absent, peristalsis and may demonstrate antral fold thickening

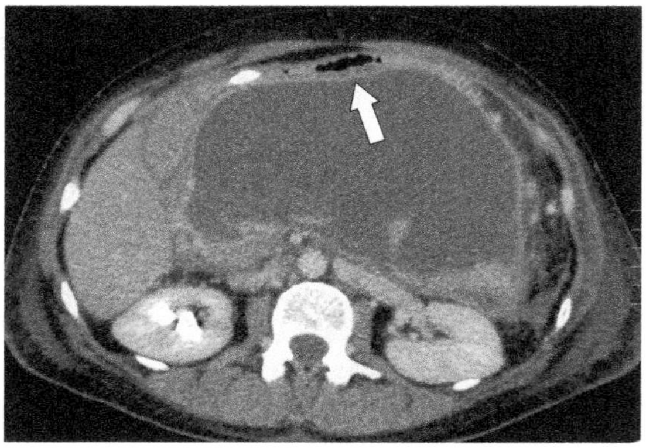

FIGURE 2-38. Axial contrast-enhanced CT in a 47-year-old woman with compression of the stomach (*arrow*) due to a lesser sac pseudocyst from recent pancreatitis (there is the tip of nasogastric tube in the stomach).

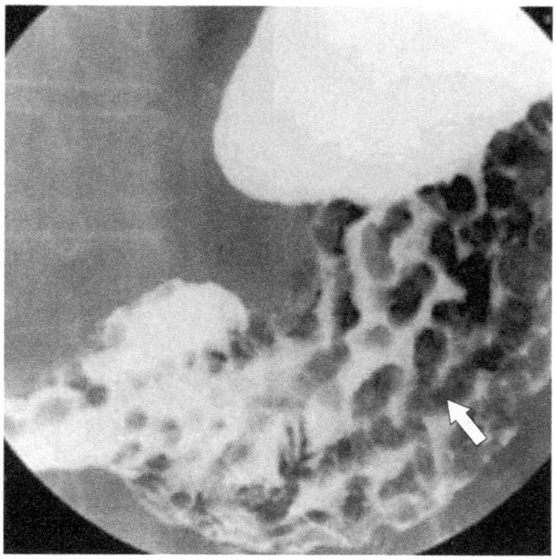

FIGURE 2-39. UGI series in a 55-year-old man with hypertrophic gastritis (*arrow*).

and erosions resulting from a more severe compounding gastritis. Patients with pernicious anemia are at risk of developing carcinoma from the gastric metaplasia.

Solitary Gastric Masses

There are several benign and malignant focal gastric masses, most of which are common to other regions in the GI tract and can be solitary or multiple (Boxes 2-2 and 2-3).

Gastric Polyps

Gastric polyps are mucosal in origin and classified into hyperplastic, adenomatous, and hamartomatous polyps; there is also the rarer inflammatory fibroid polyp.

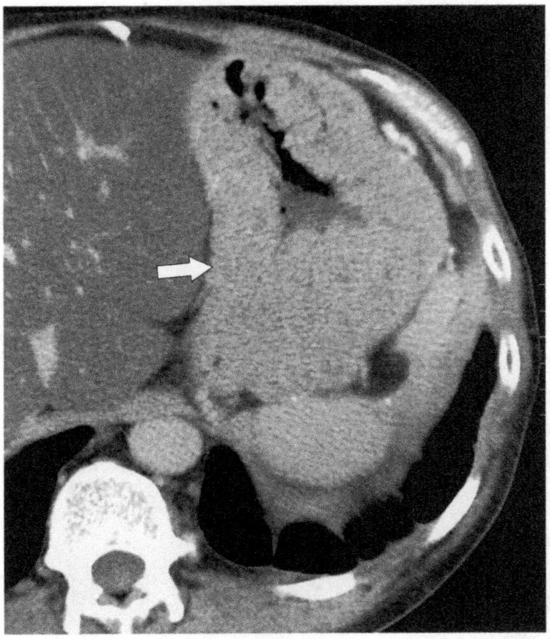

FIGURE 2-40. Axial contrast-enhanced CT in a 52-year-old man with marked gastric mucosal thickening (*arrow*) due to hypertrophic gastritis. There is also marked hepatic steatosis.

Hyperplastic Polyps

Hyperplastic polyps are also known as regenerative or inflammatory polyps because they are thought to result from chronic inflammation. They are the most common benign epithelial tumor in the stomach. They are usually multiple and small (<1 cm), usually in the body or fundus, and are sessile with no stalk (Fig. 2-43). They are difficult to differentiate from other forms of polyps, so their diagnosis is usually made after biopsy. They are not precursors of malignant disease, although there is an increased incidence of gastric carcinoma elsewhere in the stomach.

Adenomatous Polyps

Adenomatous polyps occur more commonly in the distal stomach and are similar to the colonic variety and therefore are predisposed to adenocarcinoma, particularly as they enlarge and therefore require removal. However, unlike the colon, most are sessile, and villous or tubulovillous adenomas are less commonly recognized. They are usually single, but when they are multiple, other polyposis syndromes (familial polyposis coli and Gardner* syndrome) should be considered (Figs. 2-44 and 2-45).

They are best visualized by UGI or EGD as irregular, lobulated surfaces, sometimes cauliflower-like. When larger tubulovillous antral polyps do occur, they often prolapse into the pyloric canal because of peristaltic action and cause gastric outlet obstruction.

Hamartomatous Polyps

Hamartomatous polyps are usually associated with Peutz-Jeghers† or Cronkhite-Canada‡ syndromes (see Chapter 5) and therefore are associated with small bowel (and sometimes large bowel) polyps and mucocutaneous pigmentation. Although there is a slight preponderance for small bowel carcinoma, they only have a very slight association with gastric cancer. They are identified as multiple, small, usually sessile polyps and are diagnosed with the accompanying clinical features (Fig. 2-46). The even rarer

*Eldon J. Gardner (1909-1989), American geneticist.
†Johannes Peutz (1864-1940), Dutch physician; Harold Jeghers (1904-1990), American physician.
‡Leonard W. Cronkhite, Jr., American pediatrician; Wilma J. Canada (1926-), American radiologist.

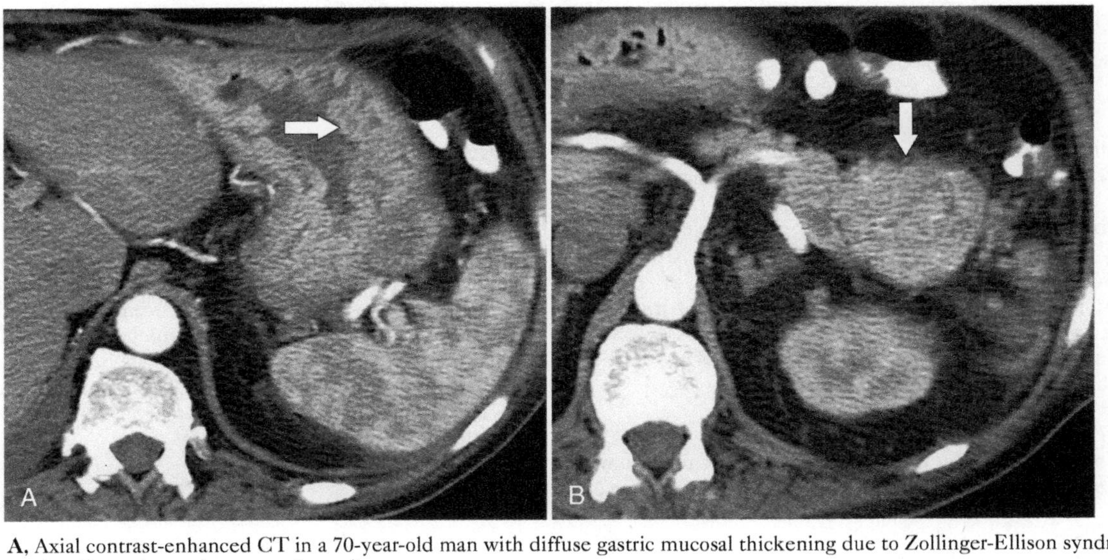

FIGURE 2-41. **A,** Axial contrast-enhanced CT in a 70-year-old man with diffuse gastric mucosal thickening due to Zollinger-Ellison syndrome (*arrow*). **B,** A 4-cm pancreatic tail gastrinoma is present (*arrow*).

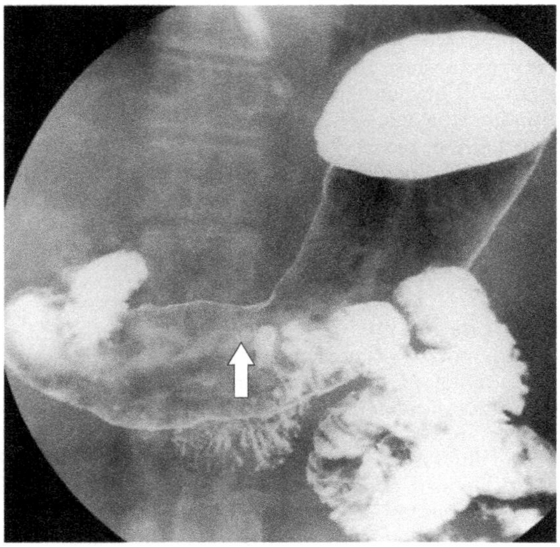

FIGURE 2-42. UGI series in a 60-year-old woman with a featureless stomach due to atrophic gastritis. There is also a small antral polyp (*arrow*).

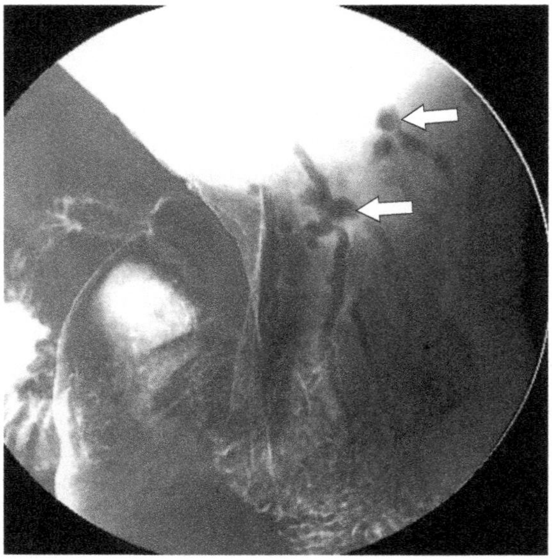

FIGURE 2-43. UGI series in a 47-year-old woman with multiple gastric mucosal lesions (*arrows*) due to hyperplastic polyps.

***Box 2-2.* Benign Gastric Masses**

Polyps (hyperplastic, adenomatous, hamartoma, inflammatory fibroid)
GIST
Hemangioma
Lipoma
Neurofibroma
Paraganglioma
Ectopic pancreas
Carcinoid

GIST, Gastrointestinal stromal tumor.

***Box 2-3.* Malignant Gastric Masses**

Carcinoma
Lymphoma
GIST
Metastases
Kaposi sarcoma

GIST, Gastrointestinal stromal tumor.

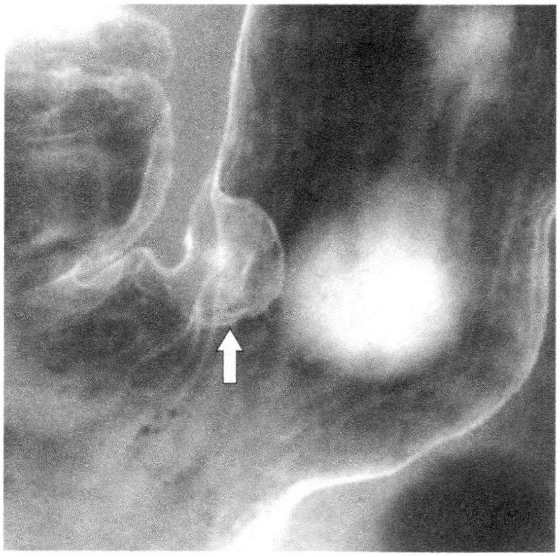

FIGURE 2-44. UGI in a 54-year-old man with a lesser curve smooth mucosal filling defect (*arrow*) due to a gastric adenomatous polyp.

Cowden's* disease (multiple hamartoma syndrome) results in widespread GI hamartomas with thyroid and breast masses.

Inflammatory Fibroid Polyps

Inflammatory fibroid polyps are also known as eosinophilic granulomas because of their histological concentration of eosinophilic cells (not to be confused with eosinophilic gastritis). On imaging they appear as a smooth-walled mucosal mass with or without ulceration, usually in the distal stomach. They are usually asymptomatic.

Benign Intramural Gastric Tumors

Benign intramural gastric tumors include gastrointestinal stromal tumors (GISTs), lipomas, lymphangiomas, hemangiomas, schwannomas, and neurofibromas. A GIST is a nonepithelial sarcoma and the most common submucosal mesenchymal tumor throughout the GI tract, with 70% occurring in the stomach, 20% in the small bowel, and approximately 10% in the esophagus. They usually grow slowly and are mostly benign, but when they are large, they can become malignant and metastasize to distant organs. They are thought to arise from the interstitial cells of Cajal* (responsible for peristaltic regulatory function) and express the c-kit (CD117) receptors, which can be detected by immunohistochemistry. GISTs are part of the Carney† triad of gastric GIST, functioning extraadrenal paraganglioma, and a pulmonary chondroma.

*Cowden's disease. Named after the first described patient.

*Santiago Ramón y Cajal (1852-1934), Spanish pathologist.
†J. Aidan Carney, American pathologist.

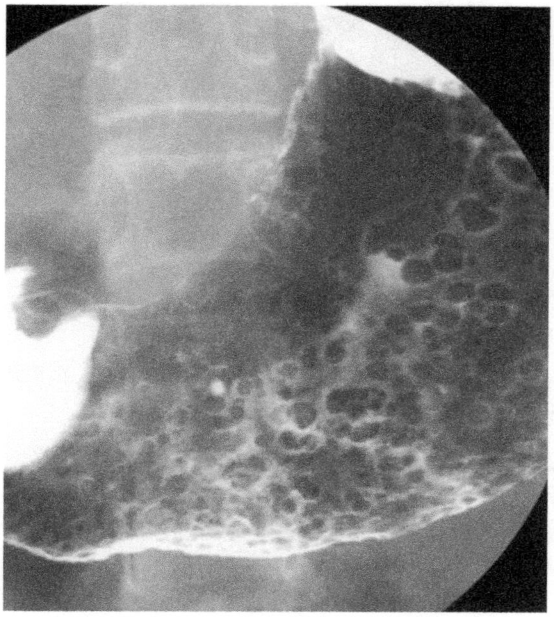

FIGURE 2-45. UGI in a 44-year-old man with Gardner syndrome and multiple gastric adenomatous polyps.

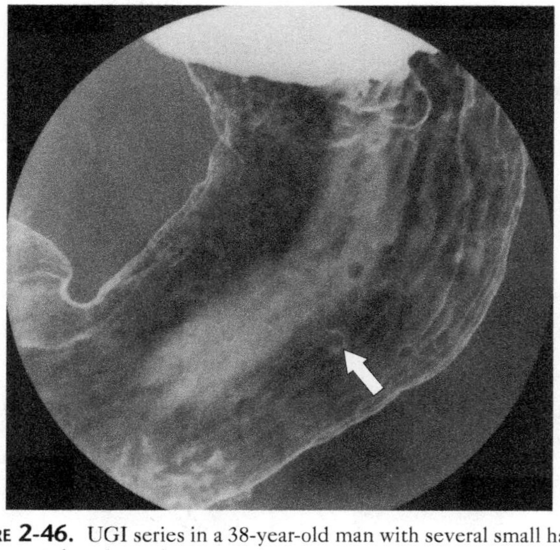

FIGURE 2-46. UGI series in a 38-year-old man with several small hamartomatous polyps (*arrow*).

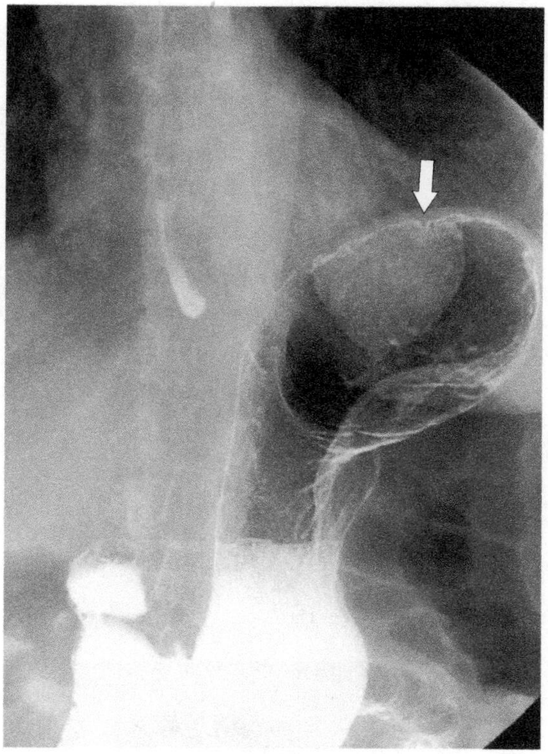

FIGURE 2-47. UGI in a 38-year-old woman demonstrating a smooth, rounded submucosal mass (*arrow*) that proved to be a benign GIST.

Submucosal intramural gastric tumors, including GISTs, all have similar imaging findings at upper GI (Fig. 2-47). They appear with a well-defined border en face, but with a smooth intraluminal projection in profile (side-on), with the characteristic obtuse borders (although this finding is variable depending on the size of the tumor), with similar CT appearances (Figs. 2-27 and 2-48). Some may ulcerate, particularly if larger, which can be seen as a bull's-eye or target lesion (barium pooling in the ulcer crater surrounded by a halo) (Fig. 2-49). If they are larger than 2 cm, they are best evaluated by contrast-enhanced CT, where they demonstrate the features of an intramural mass, which usually extends beyond the confines of the stomach wall. Sometimes, they appear as a predominantly extragastric mass and demonstrate heterogeneous enhancement, with areas of necrosis and ulceration if larger (Fig. 2-50). Calcification is recognized in up to 25% of cases.

Lipomas and lymphangiomas can change shape on compression because of their soft nature (Fig. 2-51). Lipomas typically occur in the gastric antrum and can prolapse into the duodenum. They can be diagnosed by their fatty density on CT (Fig. 2-52). Hemangiomas of the stomach are rare, are usually multiple, and are recognized with associated venous vascular calcification. They are associated with Bean* syndrome (or blue rubber bleb nevus syndrome) and autosomal dominant disease. Patients often have multiple GI hemangiomas, usually in the stomach, that often bleed. Other mesenchymal tumors cannot be differentiated by CT or UGI series and generally require removal for final diagnosis (Fig. 2-53).

Duplication Cysts

Duplication cysts occur anywhere along the GI tract and are rare in the stomach. They are smooth-walled submucosal filling defects, usually along the greater curvature. They may communicate with the stomach and therefore fill with contrast media at fluoroscopy, giving a large diverticulum-like appearance.

Ectopic Pancreas

Ectopic pancreas is usually asymptomatic, although it can bleed occasionally. Some reports state it occurs in up to 10% of patients, but the incidence in clinical practice is likely to be much lower. The submucosa of the gastric antrum or proximal duodenum is the most common site, but its presence in the esophagus to the ileum has been described. Classically, the ectopic pancreas contains small, smooth-filling defects, with a central umbilication that represents a rudimentary pancreatic duct (Fig. 2-54).

Carcinoid

Carcinoids are rare in the stomach and are usually benign. Most probably go undetected, but when they are larger, they may ulcerate and bleed and may therefore be sometimes confused with gastric carcinoma. They are not commonly detected by CT,

*William B. Bean (1909-1989), American physician.

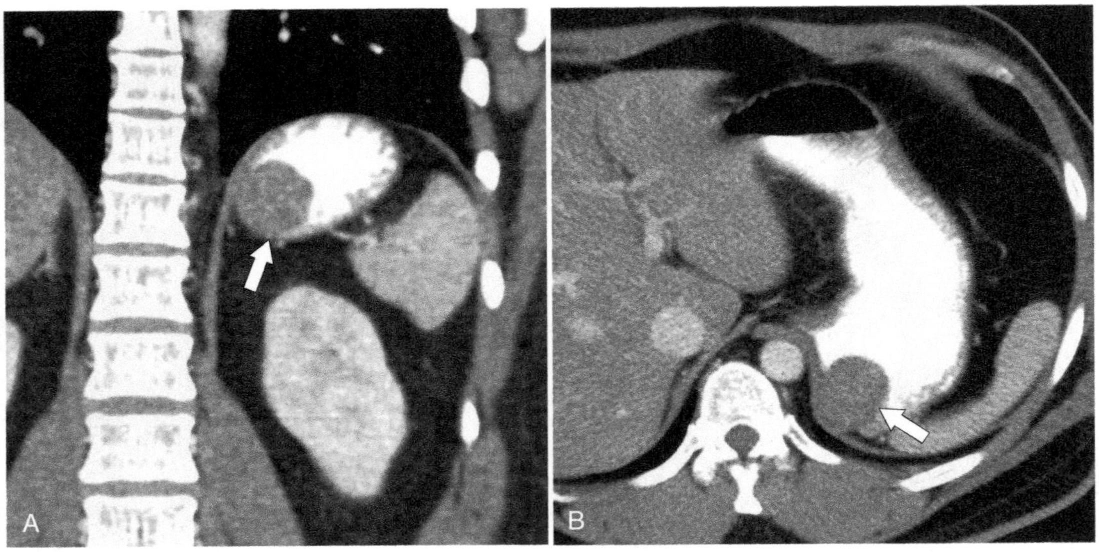

FIGURE 2-48. Axial (**A**) and coronal (**B**) CT in a 44-year-old man with a smooth intraluminal submucosal filling defect at the gastric fundus (*arrows*) due to a GIST.

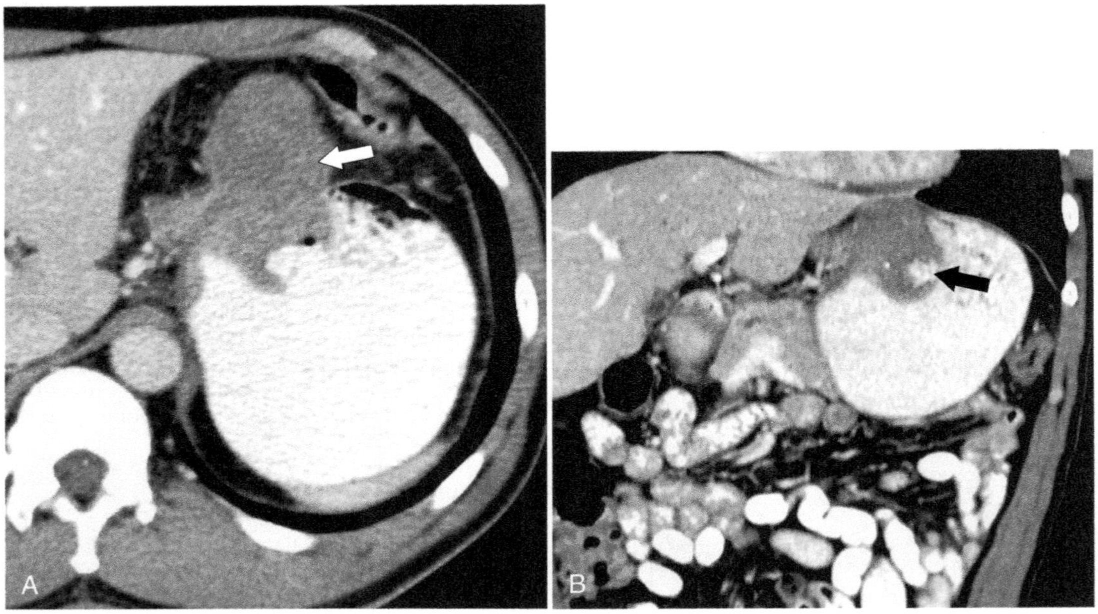

FIGURE 2-49. Axial (**A**) and coronal (**B**) CT in a 55-year-old woman with a transmural gastric mass with ulceration (*arrows*) due to a benign GIST.

but they may appear as generally smooth, rounded hypervascular masses after the administration of intravenous (IV) contrast material (Fig. 2-55).

Gastric Varices

The dilated submucosal gastric vein, like its esophageal equivalent, can cause life-threatening hemorrhage. It can be secondary to portal venous hypertension but is more commonly associated with splenic vein thrombosis (i.e., pancreatic malignancy, pancreatitis, thrombotic disorders).

Diagnosis is usually made by EGD, but on UGI series, there is fold-thickening typically in the fundus because of the dilated submucosal vessels (Fig. 2-56). The diagnosis is usually associated with esophageal varices and may only be visualized with the patient in the prone or supine position that creates enough venous distention to be visible on UGI series. The varices are usually far better visualized by CT than UGI (Fig. 2-57).

Gastric Carcinoma

Gastric carcinoma is the third most common GI malignancy after colonic and pancreatic carcinoma. It arises from the gastric mucosa (it is slightly more common in the gastric fundus), and most gastric carcinomas are adenocarcinomas (95%). It is more common in men, and risk factors include *H. pylori* infection, alcohol, smoking, pernicious anemia, chronic atrophic gastritis, adenomatous polyps, Ménétrier disease, prior gastric surgery (Billroth II), salted and smoked food (especially fish), and foods with high nitrite or nitrate content. Gastric atrophy and carcinoma are associated, but because mild gastric atrophy is common in the elderly, it is not certain whether there is any cause and effect. Therefore it is not unusual for antral and body carcinomas to be associated with gastric atrophy, probably as a simple result of aging. Patients with severe atrophic changes (i.e., those with pernicious anemia), however, are definitely at risk for the development of gastric carcinoma and should be

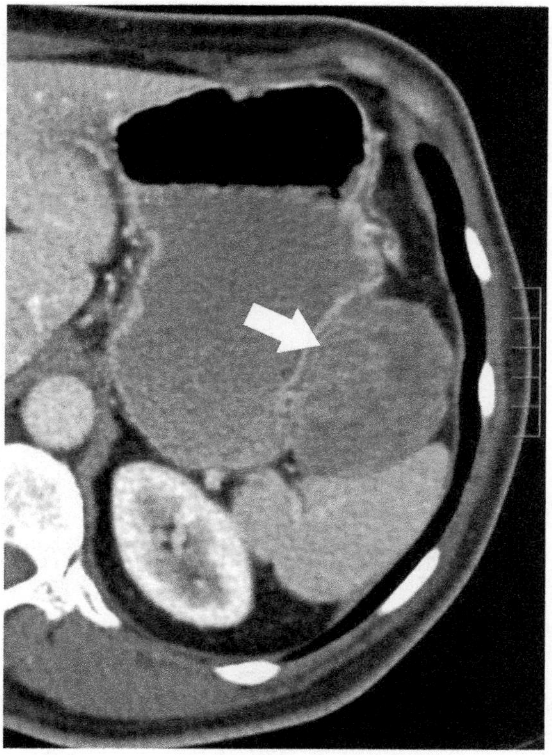

FIGURE 2-50. Axial CT in a 60-year-old woman with a 6-cm predominantly exophytic gastric mass (*arrow*) due to a benign GIST.

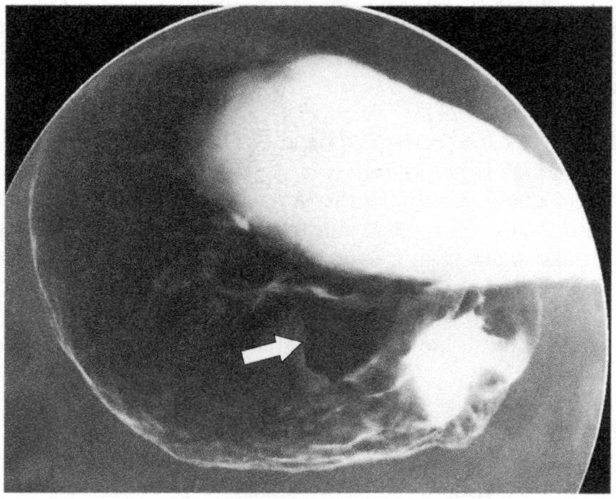

FIGURE 2-51. UGI in a 44-year-old woman with a smooth submucosal mass (*arrow*) due to a lipoma.

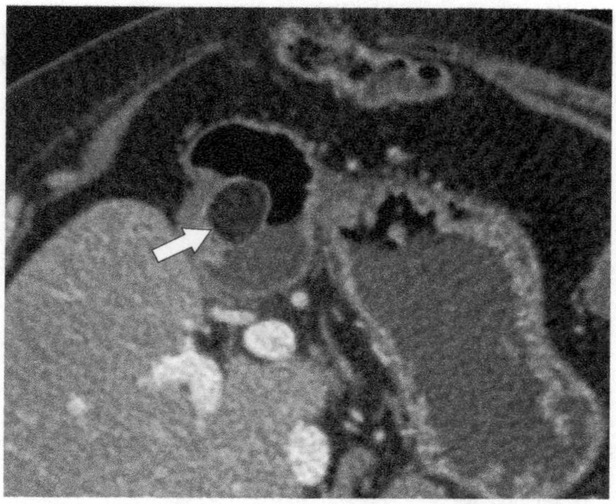

FIGURE 2-52. Axial CT in a 50-year-old woman with a fatty submucosal antral mass (*arrow*) due to an antral gastric lipoma.

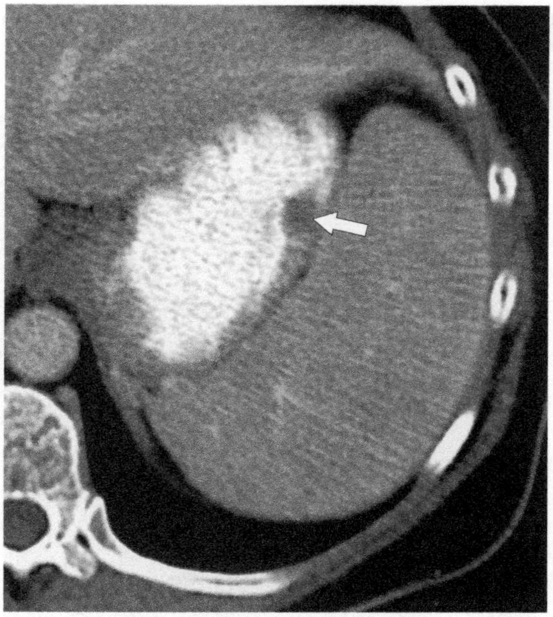

FIGURE 2-53. Axial contrast-enhanced CT in a 33-year-old man with a small submucosal gastric mass (*arrow*) that was proved to be a fibromyxoma at histological examination. This cannot be differentiated from most submucosal masses on CT.

serially monitored (usually by EGD). The staging of gastric cancer follows international TNM staging criteria (Table 2-4).

Patients usually have symptoms of heartburn and a loss of appetite. As the disease progresses, there may be nausea and vomiting from partial gastric outlet obstruction, and many ulcerate and produce hematemesis or melena. Early imaging features on UGI series can vary. These may demonstrate either a small irregular intraluminal polypoid lesion or a raised plaque-like nodular lesion, which may ulcerate. It may also appear like a flat ulcer with edematous walls and radiating irregular or amputated folds that end abruptly (unlike benign ulcers, which demonstrate smooth radiating folds) (Figs. 2-20, 2-22, 2-25, 2-58, and 2-59). As the disease progresses, there is a progressively enlarging irregular polyp or a nodular polyp, often with ulceration as evidenced by an intraluminal filling defect or patches of barium trapped between the polypoid folds (see Fig. 2-59). The tumor margins are shelf-like (acute angled), and the folds converging toward a tumor with or without an ulcer are enlarged, irregular, fused, or nodular (see Fig. 2-25). A classic malignant ulcer feature at UGI series is the Carman meniscus sign (used to differentiate it from benign ulcer disease), whereby an elevated, flattened lesion with a central ulcer crater demonstrates a radiolucent margin or halo on prone compression views because of the raised tumor margins (see Figs. 2-20, 2-22, and 2-25).

Most gastric carcinomas will not be evaluated by UGI series, however, because the diagnosis and initial assessment will be made mostly by EGD. Patients are then referred for a staging CT. The primary tumor, particularly when it is small, can be hard to identify by imaging, and without prior knowledge of an underlying gastric cancer, the radiologist could easily miss it (Fig. 2-60). This problem with identification is compounded by the difficulty of evaluating the nondistended stomach, where gastric wall thickening is often contemplated, but simply represents a normal collapsed stomach. As the tumor increases, however, a discrete mass

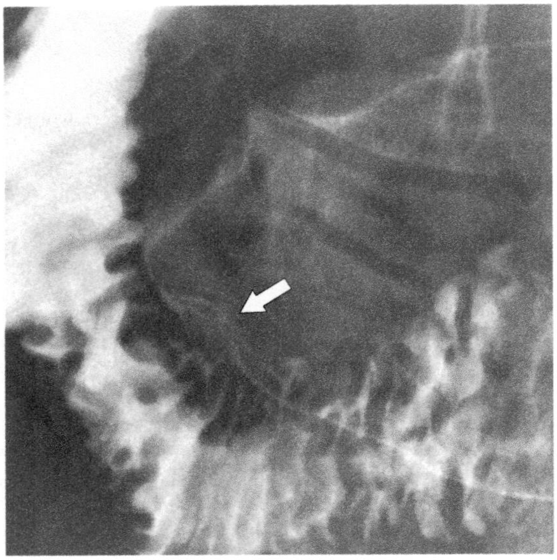

FIGURE 2-54. UGI series in a 40-year-old woman with a small mucosal antral lesion due to ectopic pancreas (*arrow*).

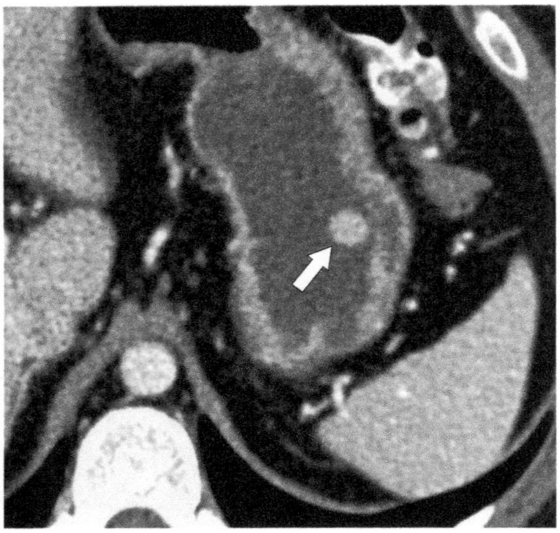

FIGURE 2-55. Axial contrast-enhanced CT in a 49-year-old woman with a 1.5-cm hypervascular intragastric mass (*arrow*) due to gastric carcinoid.

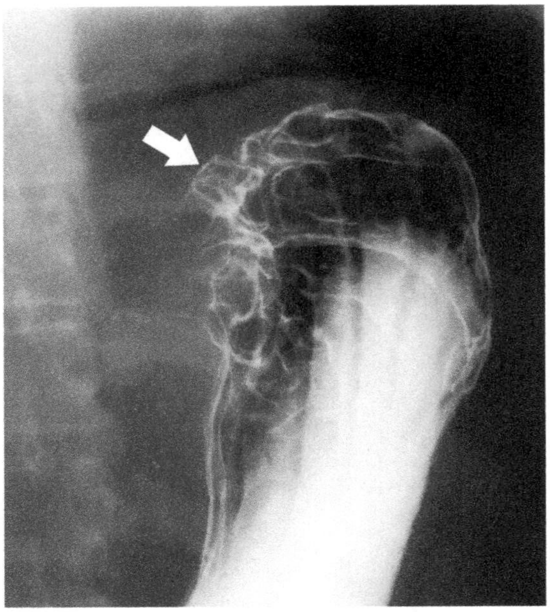

FIGURE 2-56. UGI series in a 64-year-old man with multiple nodular filling defects at the gastric cardia (*arrow*) due to gastric varices.

should be identified, and most tumors will be visualized once they become transmural and stage III and IV cancers develop (Fig. 2-61). Regional lymph nodes may be small and difficult to detect on CT, but their location in relation to the stomach should alert the radiologist to the diagnosis. PET imaging is sometimes used, not as a first-line investigation but rather as a tool for the evaluation of regional and remote metastases, particularly smaller lymphadenopathy (Figs. 2-61 and 2-62). Some tumors appear as if they are lower esophageal tumors, but they represent cardial tumors that invade into the lower esophagus (Fig. 2-62). Others present with the appearance of a leather-bottle stomach (also known as linitis plastica; see later in this chapter), which typically arises in the antrum and infiltrates along the gastric wall, producing a concentric narrow antrum (Figs. 2-63 and 2-64).

A rarer gastric carcinoma, known as scirrhous carcinoma, also typically arises in the antrum and produces a linitis plastica or leather-bottle appearance (Fig. 2-63). This may also extend more proximally to involve the gastric body (Fig. 2-65). Polypoid carcinoma is less common and frequently ulcerates. Such tumors appear as large polypoid and irregular filling defects, usually in the distal stomach, but they can occur elsewhere (see Fig. 2-59).

Gastric carcinoma metastasizes early, to regional lymph nodes, by direct extension, or to a remote area (Figs. 2-62 and 2-66). It has a tendency to metastasize to the ovaries, which is known as Krukenberg* tumor (Fig. 2-67). It can frequently cause peritoneal spread with mesenteric nodular metastases, so-called omental caking (Fig. 2-68).

Malignant Gastrointestinal Stromal Tumors

Malignant GISTs are generally larger than benign GISTs and tend to extend exophytically to the stomach rather than into it (Figs. 2-69 and 2-70). They also infiltrate the gastric wall as a polypoid nodular mass with frequent ulceration (Fig. 2-71). The c-kit (CD117) receptors are effectively targeted by c-kit tyrosine kinase inhibitors (imatinib), which have proved to be highly effective chemotherapeutic agents for malignant GISTs, particularly smaller (< 5 cm) tumors.

Lymphoma

The GI tract is the most common site for extranodal lymphoma (up to 30% of abdominal lymphomas). The stomach is the most common site, followed by the small bowel, and finally the colon. Esophageal involvement is very rare. Although there are many types of lymphoma (the World Health Organization currently lists 43 varieties), the most common lymphomatous GI tract disorders are non-Hodgkin† lymphomas and include those listed in Table 2-5, with diffuse large B cell the most common. The stage is determined by the Ann Arbor classification (Table 2-6).

Primary gastric lymphoma is uncommon (about 2% of all lymphomas), but metastatic lymphoma is much more common, and the stomach is the most common GI site for lymphoma. Most are B-cell, non-Hodgkin lymphomas, ranging from well-differentiated mucosa-associated lymphoid tissue (MALT) type to high-grade large-cell disease. Mantle cell and T-cell lymphomas are rarer recognized types. The latter can be difficult to distinguish from

---

*Friedrich Ernst Krukenberg (1871-1946), German physician.
†Thomas Hodgkin (1798-1866), British physician and pathologist.

Text continued on p. 63

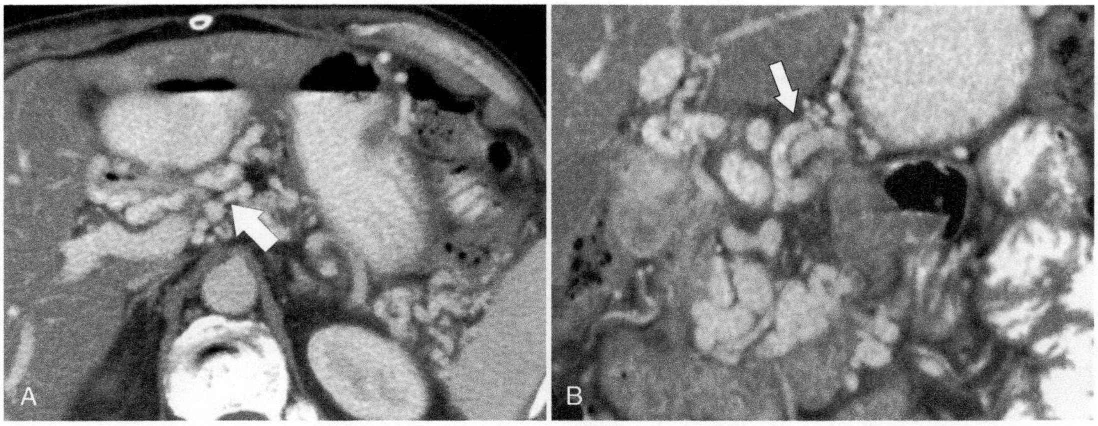

FIGURE 2-57. Axial (**A**) and coronal (**B**) contrast-enhanced CT in a 54-year-old man with chronic pancreatitis and multiple gastric varices (*arrows*).

TABLE 2-4 Staging of Gastric Carcinoma

Stage	Findings
0	Carcinoma in situ; limited to mucosa
1A	Transmucosal (5-year survival 85%)
1B	Transmucosal and up to 6 regional lymph nodes involved or muscularis invaded
II	Transmucosal with 7-15 regional lymph nodes involved or muscularis involvement with 6 regional lymph nodes or serosal involvement without regional lymph nodes
IIIA	Muscularis involvement with 7-15 adjacent nodes; serosal invasion with up to 6 local nodes (5-year survival 50%); local organ invasion but no nodes
IIIB	Serosal involvement with 7-15 regional nodes
IV	Adjacent organs and at least 1 regional lymph node; more than 15 regional nodes; distant metastases

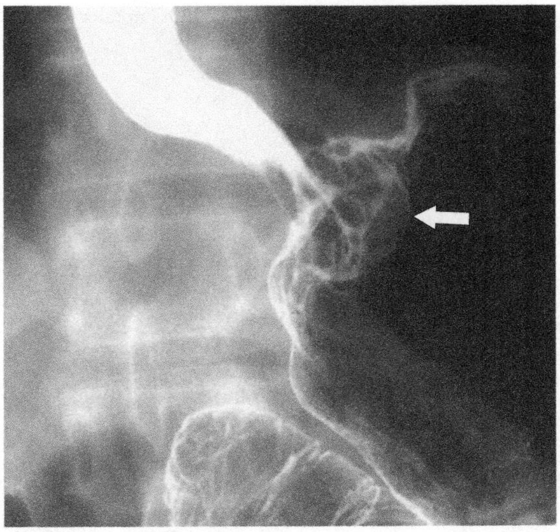

FIGURE 2-59. Barium UGI series in a 44-year-old man with fundal polypoid mass (*arrow*) due to gastric adenocarcinoma.

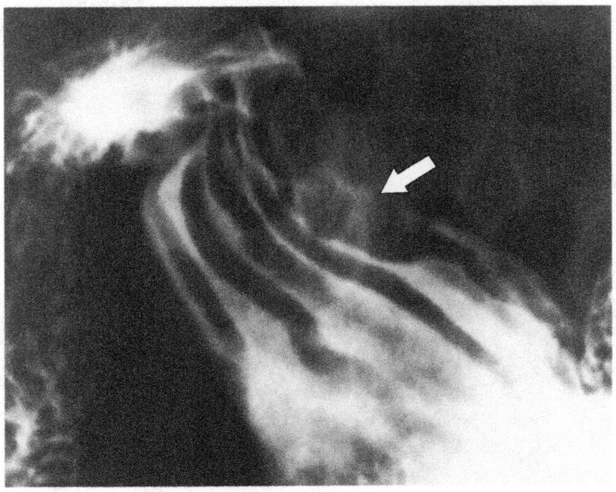

FIGURE 2-58. UGI in a 66-year-old woman with thickened antral folds and a small filling defect (*arrow*) on the distal lesser curve that was proved to be early gastric adenocarcinoma.

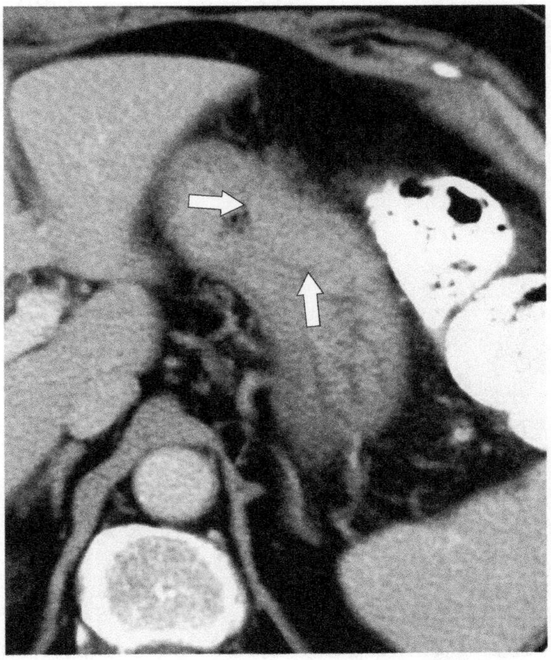

FIGURE 2-60. Axial noncontrast-enhanced CT in a 57-year-old man with a subtle 2-cm gastric mass (*arrows*) that was found to be gastric adenocarcinoma.

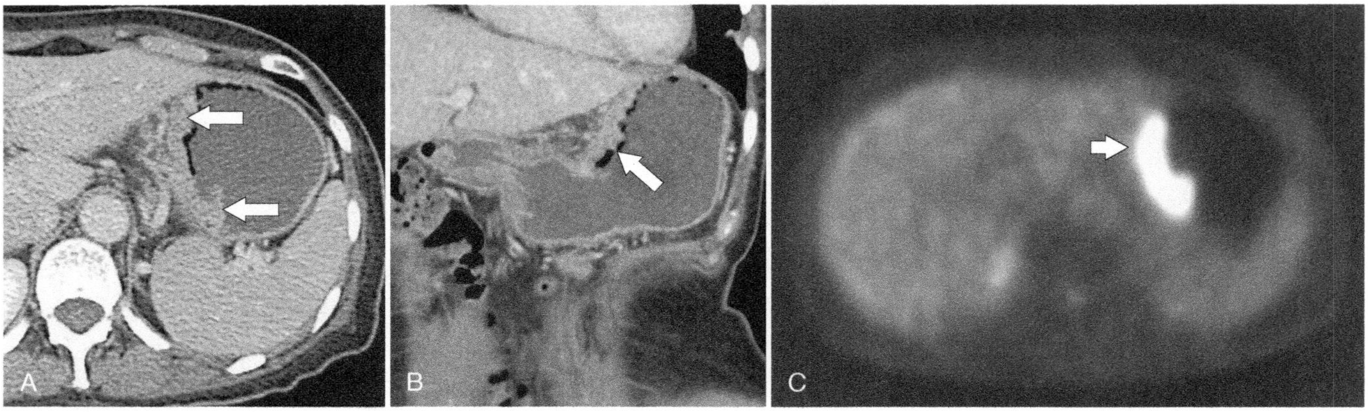

Figure 2-61. Axial contrast-enhanced CT (**A** and **B**) and PET (**C**) in a 62-year-old man with mural thickening of the gastric body (*large arrows*) due to adenocarcinoma, which demonstrates marked FDG uptake (*small arrow*).

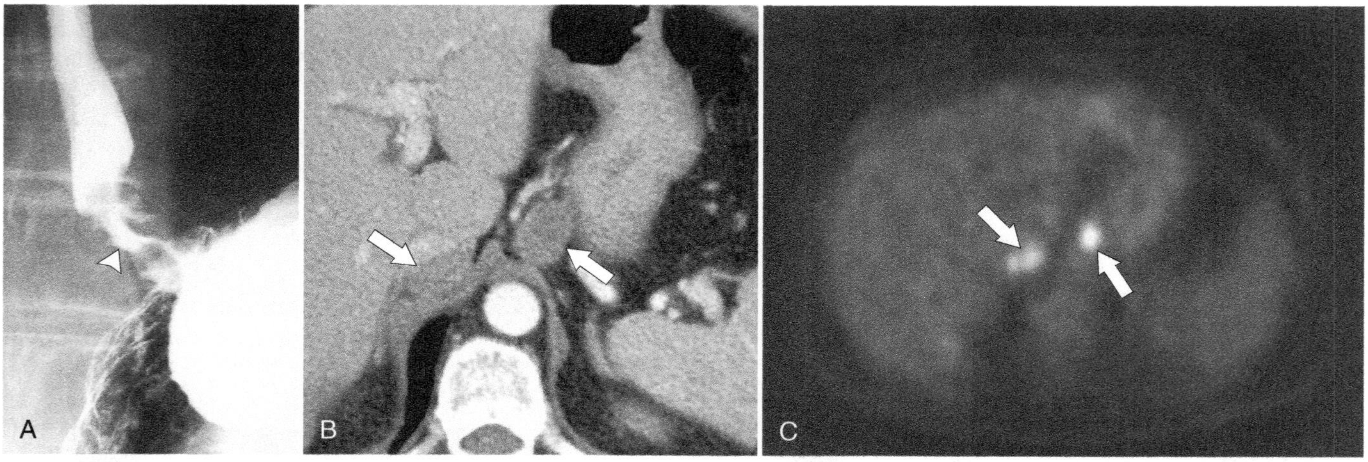

Figure 2-62. Barium swallow, axial contrast-enhanced CT, and PET in a 66-year-old woman with a cardial tumor extending into the lower esophagus (**A**; *arrowhead*) and metastatic lymph nodes (**B**; *arrows*) with uptake on PET (**C**; *arrows*).

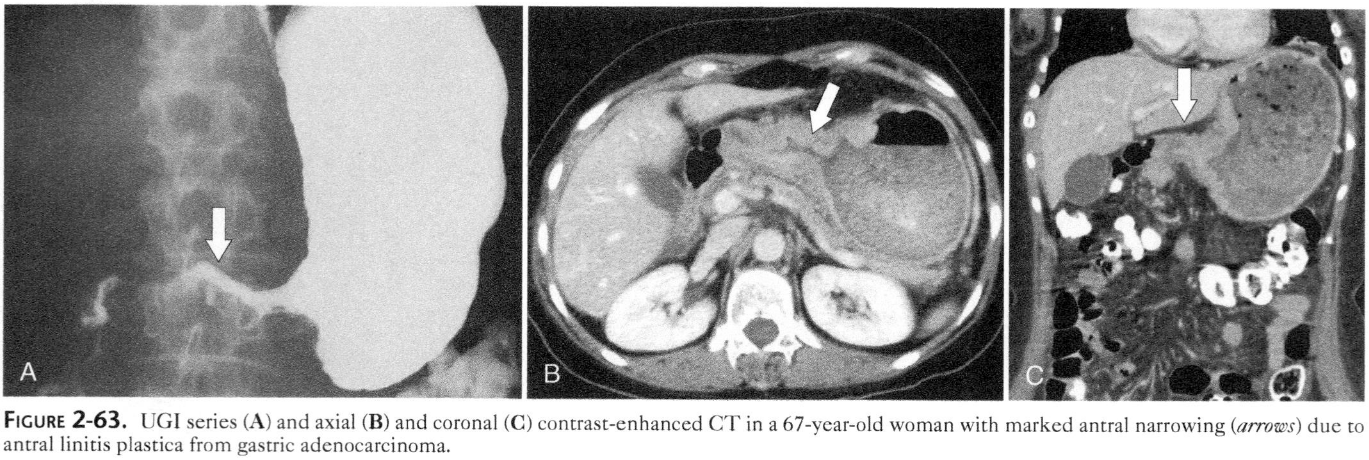

Figure 2-63. UGI series (**A**) and axial (**B**) and coronal (**C**) contrast-enhanced CT in a 67-year-old woman with marked antral narrowing (*arrows*) due to antral linitis plastica from gastric adenocarcinoma.

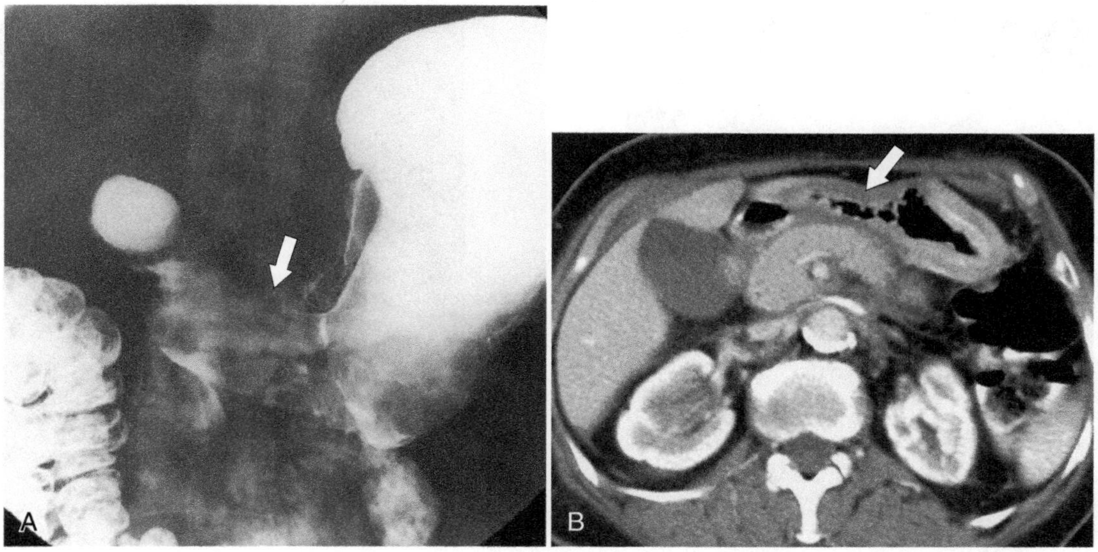

FIGURE 2-64. UGI series (**A**) and axial contrast-enhanced CT (**B**) in a 72-year-old woman with fixed narrowing of the gastric body and antrum (linitis plastica appearance) (*arrows*) due to gastric adenocarcinoma.

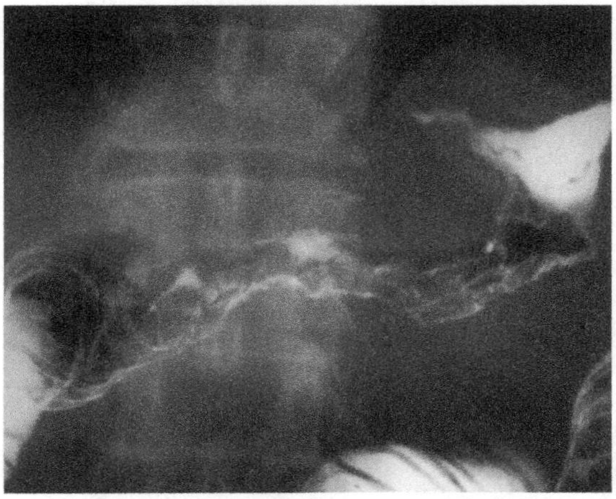

FIGURE 2-65. UGI series in a 66-year-old woman with a linitis plastica–appearing stomach due to scirrhous gastric carcinoma.

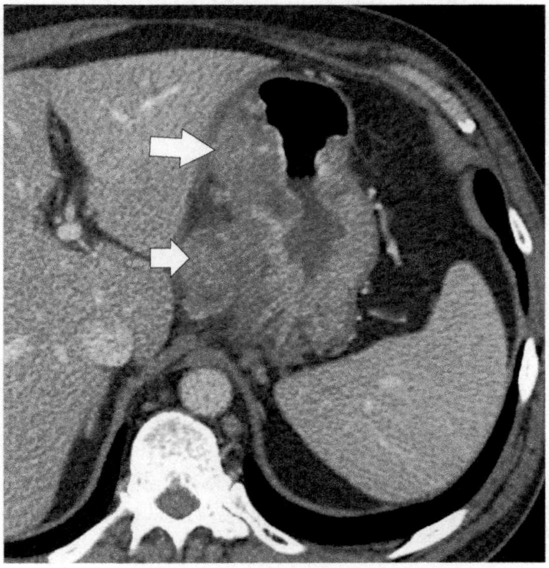

FIGURE 2-66. Axial contrast-enhanced CT in a 70-year-old man with infiltrative mass of the gastric body (*large arrow*) that has spread beyond the confines of the gastric wall (*small arrow*).

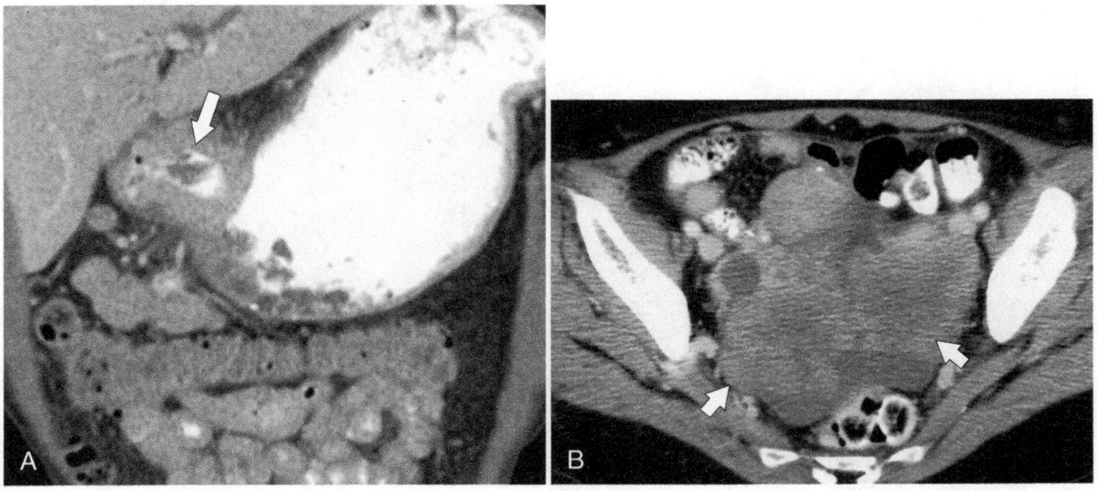

FIGURE 2-67. Coronal and axial-contrast enhanced CT in a 51-year-old woman with an antral gastric carcinoma (**A**; *large arrow*) and bilateral adnexal masses (**B**; *small arrows*) due to Krukenberg metastases.

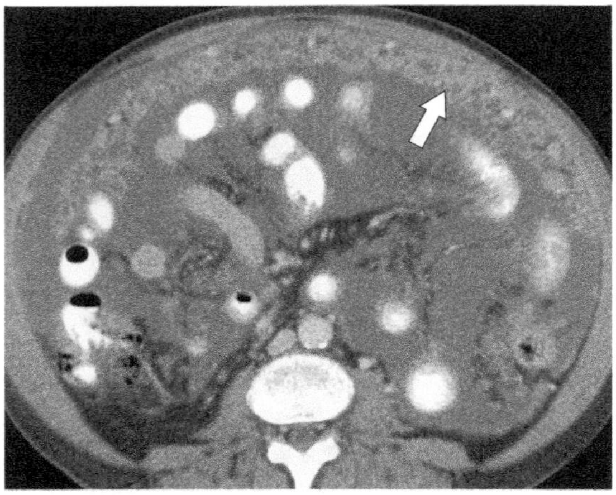

FIGURE 2-68. Axial contrast-enhanced CT in a 50-year-old woman with gastric cancer and peritoneal metastatic disease with ascites and omental cake (*arrow*).

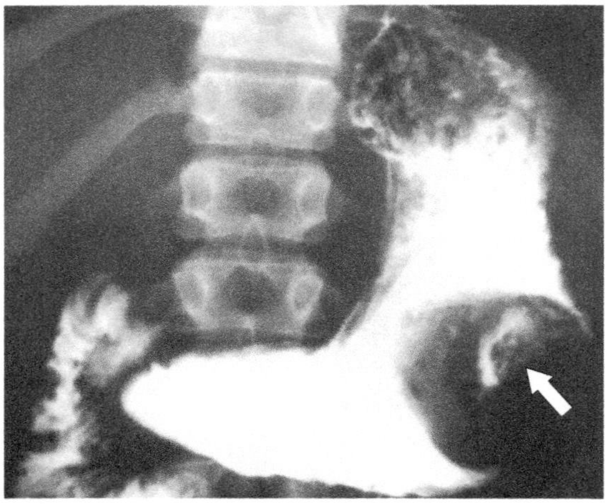

FIGURE 2-69. UGI series in a 47-year-old woman with a large gastric mass with central ulceration (*arrow*) due to a gastric GIST.

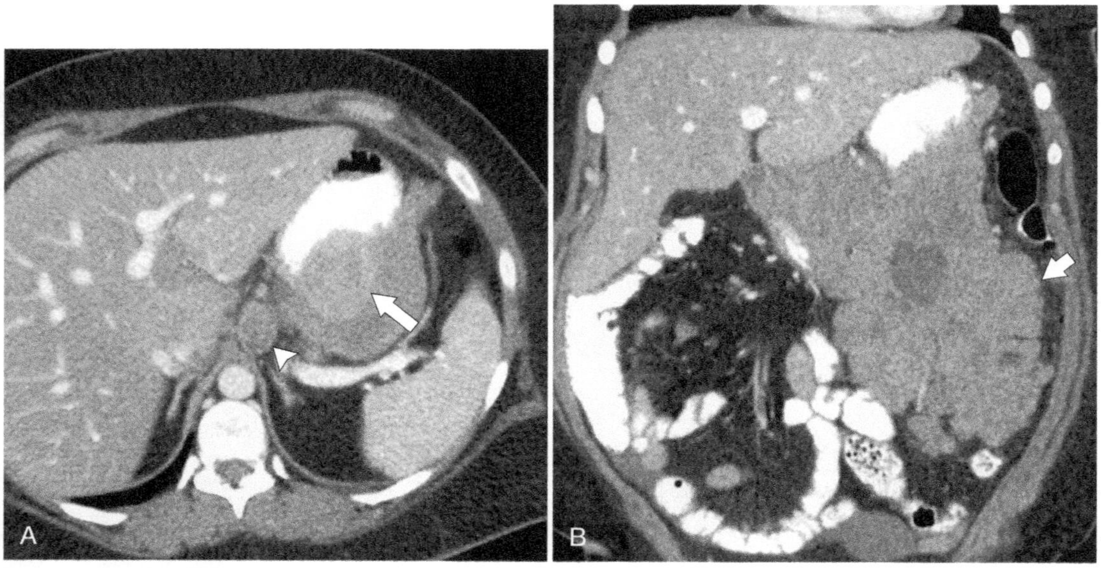

FIGURE 2-70. **A,** Axial and coronal contrast-enhanced CT in a 30-year-old woman with a malignant gastric GIST (*large arrow*). **B,** A large part of the mass (*small arrow*) is exophytic to the stomach. There are perigastric metastatic lymph nodes (*arrowhead*).

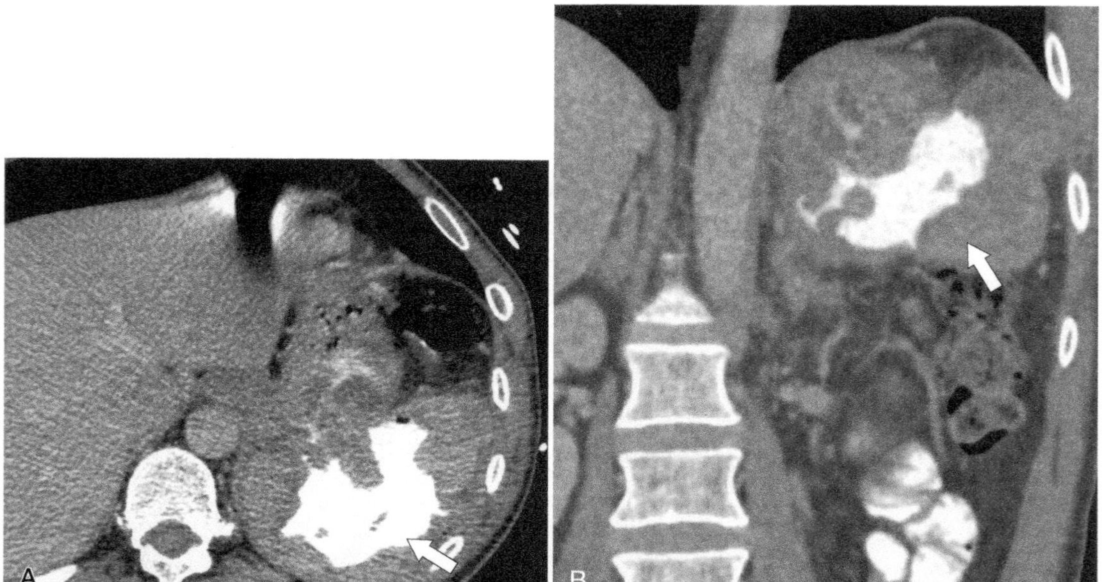

FIGURE 2-71. Axial (**A**) and coronal (**B**) contrast-enhanced CT in a 52-year-old man with diffuse gastric wall thickening (*arrows*) due to a GIST.

TABLE 2-5 Lymphomas Usually Associated with Gastrointestinal Malignancy

B-cell Lymphoma	Grade	Features
Diffuse large B-cell	High grade	Low-grade MALT that has transformed diffuse large B-cell; most common type—anywhere along GI tract
MALT-type	Low grade	*H. pylori* gastritis causative; usually in the stomach, less commonly in the small bowel; low grade in indolent type
Mantle cell	Higher grade	Any area of GI tract; typically polypoid lesions; poorer prognosis
AIDS-related lymphoma	High grade	Second most common malignancy in AIDS patients after Kaposi sarcoma; mainly in the stomach and small bowel; EBV related; aggressive
PTLD	Lower grade	EBV related; GI tract is the most common site
Burkitt lymphoma	High grade	EBV related; 50% curable
T-cell lymphomas	High grade	Subtypes peripheral, anaplastic large cell, angioimmunoblastic and cutaneous
EATL	High grade	Associated with celiac disease; jejunum is mostly involved
Mediterranean	High grade	Spectrum of alpha heavy chain disease and immunoproliferative small intestinal disease

*Denis Burkitt (1911-1993), Irish physician.
AIDS, Acquired immune deficiency syndrome; *EATL*, enteropathy-associated T-cell lymphoma; *EBV*, Epstein-Barr virus; *GI*, gastrointestinal; *MALT*, mucosa-associated lymphoid tissue; *PTLD*, posttransplant lymphoproliferative disorder.

TABLE 2-6 Ann Arbor Staging of Lymphoma

Stage I	Single lymph node region (I); involvement of single extralymphatic organ/site (IA)
Stage II	Two or more lymph node sites on one side of diaphragm (II); involvement of single organ (IIE)
Stage III	Lymph nodes both sides of diaphragm (III); involvement of extralymphatic organ (IIIE); splenic disease (IIIS); both spleen and extralymphatic organ (IIISE)
Stage IV	Diffuse or disseminated involvement of one or more sites; extralymphatic organs

the more common adenocarcinoma. MALT lymphoma most commonly affects the stomach and represents a low-grade B-cell lymphoma. Because of its low grade, it can be difficult to detect with either CT or PET. It is heavily associated with *H. pylori*, which is thought to be causative as a result of the chronic inflammatory reaction induced in the infected stomach. Treatment and eradication of gastric *H. pylori* are often curative.

At imaging, there are various presentations of gastric lymphoma, including a large ulcerating lesion, multiple polypoid lesions (with or without ulceration), or an infiltrating mass that can result in a linitis plastica appearance (Figs. 2-72, 2-73, and 2-74). These features can usually be observed on CT, but differentiation from other malignant diagnoses is sometimes difficult because of similar appearance on imaging. CT will readily demonstrate extragastric extension or remote adenopathy and hepatosplenomegaly.

Posttransplant lymphoproliferative disorder (PTLD) occurs as a complication after prolonged immunosuppression, mostly among transplant recipients. It is due to an uncontrolled proliferation of B cells infected with Epstein-Barr virus (EBV) and the disease; therefore it has similarities with Burkitt lymphoma. The disease can respond to the cessation of the immunosuppressive therapy, although some patients progress to typical non-Hodgkin B-cell lymphoma. Extranodal involvement is much more common than nodal involvement and affects the GI tract most commonly, typically the small bowel, then the colon, stomach, duodenum, and esophagus in descending frequency. Most other abdominal organs can also be involved, including the lung and central nervous system. Implanted allografts can also succumb to disease (e.g., liver, renal, heart/lung).

Imaging features in the bowel are similar to other GI lymphoma, including circumferential wall thickening (sometimes marked) and aneurysmal luminal dilatation. Characteristically, the disease ulcerates and then perforates far more frequently than other types of lymphoma.

Burkitt Lymphoma

This is a B-cell lymphoma first described as an EBV-mediated lymphoma endemic to central Africa. This virally induced tumor (Epstein-Barr*) most often involves the maxilla in younger adults and children, but colonic involvement, particularly of the ascending colon, is well recognized. Other forms of Burkitt lymphoma include the sporadic type, again mediated by EBV, and more commonly produce ileocecal lymphoma. A third variant, termed *immunodeficiency-associated Burkitt lymphoma* (a variant of posttransplant lymphoproliferative disease), occurs in immunosuppressed patients, particularly those with human immunodeficiency virus (HIV) and acquired immune deficiency syndrome (AIDS) but also those taking immunosuppressive drugs.

Metastases

Metastatic disease to the stomach is usually focal and small but can occasionally be larger, particularly with melanoma. These classically result in a bull's-eye mucosal lesion (although simple mucosal masses are also recognized) that appears as a circular metastatic mucosal deposit with a central ulcerated depression (see Fig. 2-17). On UGI examination, contrast will collect in the ulcer crater in the supine position if the lesion is on the posterior wall or conversely on the anterior wall if the patient is in the prone position. These are often multiple and most commonly seen in melanoma, breast cancer, and lung cancer.

Breast cancer and lymphoma can also cause a linitis plastica appearance, infiltrating along the gastric wall rather than producing discrete mucosal masses (Fig. 2-75). Other primary malignancies (e.g., ovarian and pseudomyxoma peritonei) can envelop the stomach with metastatic deposits and give the appearance of linitis plastica (Fig. 2-76). Direct invasion of the stomach from

*Michael A. Epstein (1921-2006), British pathologist and virologist; Yvonne Barr (1932-), British virologist.

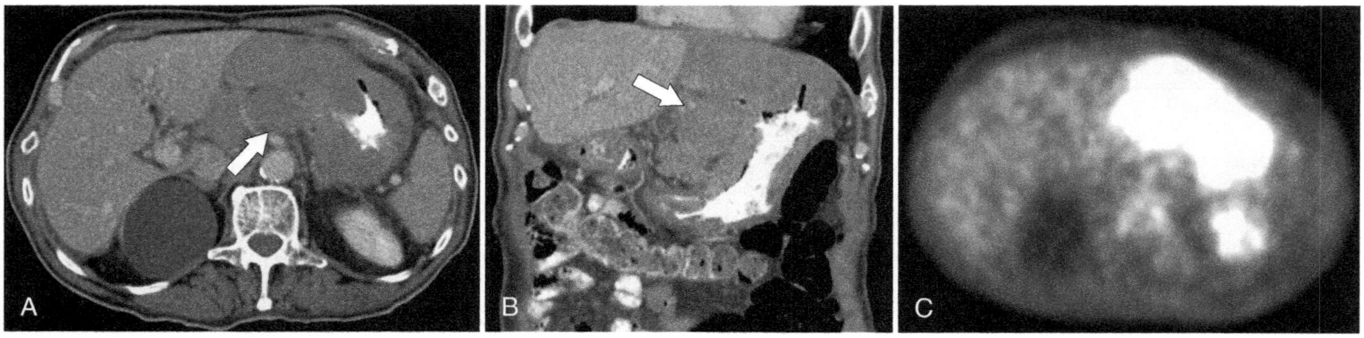

FIGURE 2-72. Axial (**A**) and coronal (**B**) CT and PET (**C**) in a 68-year-old man with a large lobular and polypoid gastric mass (*arrows*) due to gastric lymphoma, which is PET avid.

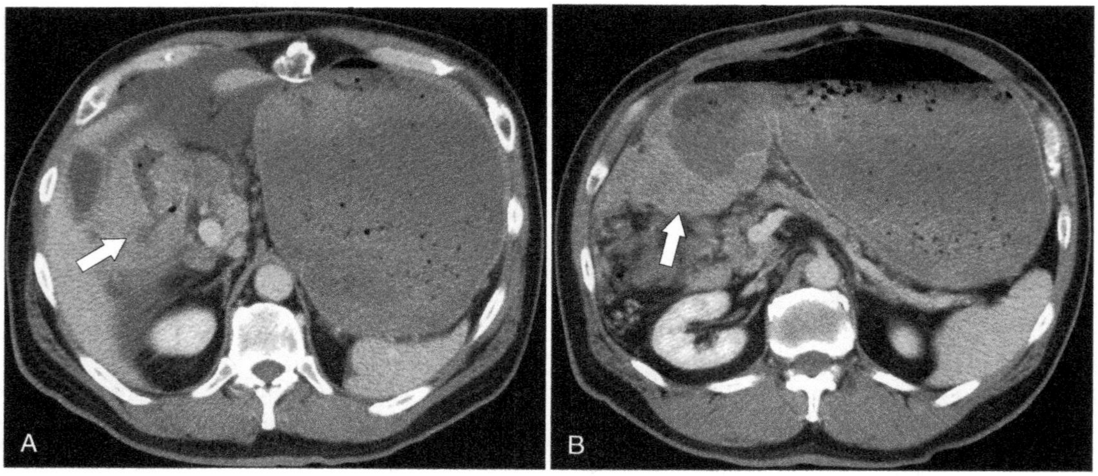

FIGURE 2-73. Axial contrast-enhanced CT in a 56-year-old man with gastric dilatation due to diffuse antral wall circumferential thickening (*arrows*) caused by primary gastric B-cell lymphoma.

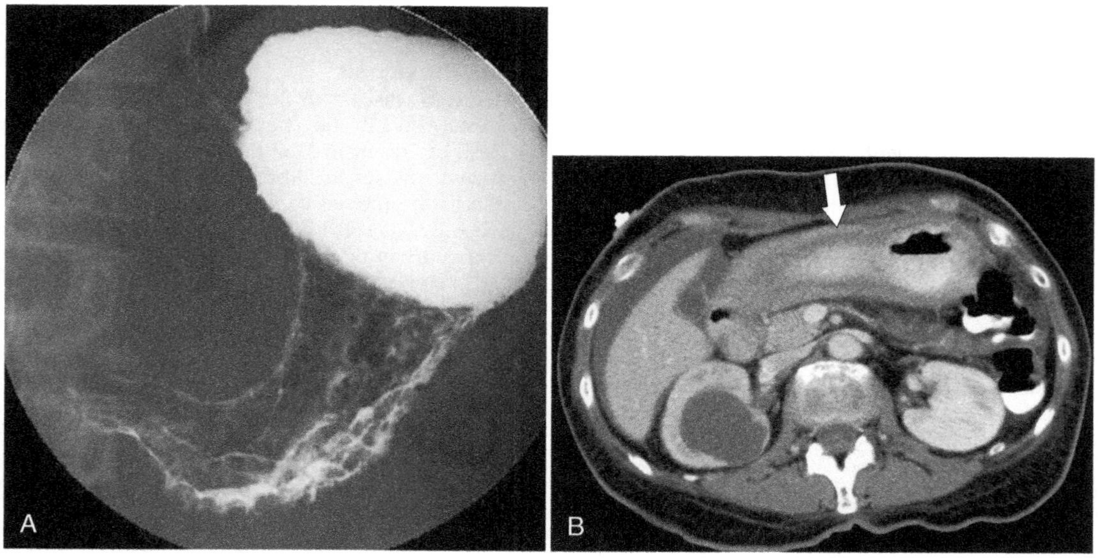

FIGURE 2-74. UGI series (**A**) and axial contrast-enhanced CT (**B**) in a 53-year-old man with fixed diffuse gastric narrowing, mucosal irregularity (*arrow*), and a linitis plastica appearance of the stomach due to gastric lymphoma.

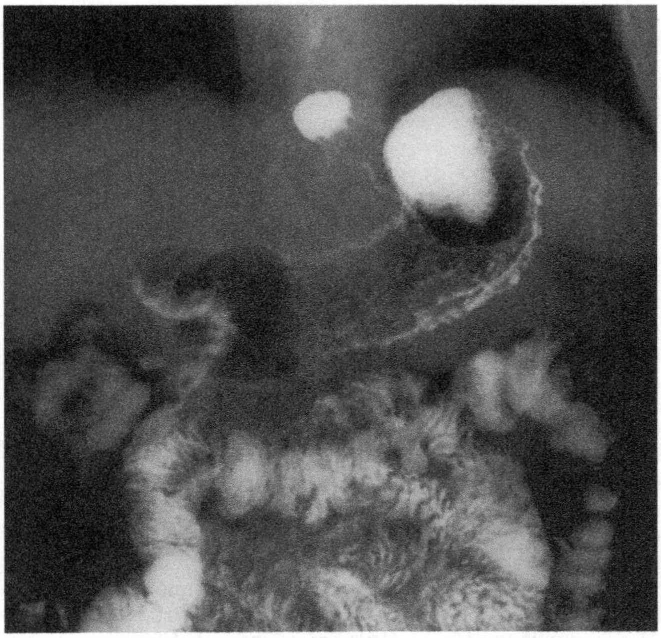

FIGURE 2-75. UGI swallow in a 69-year-old woman with a linitis plastica appearance of the stomach due to breast cancer metastasis. There is incidental sliding hiatal hernia.

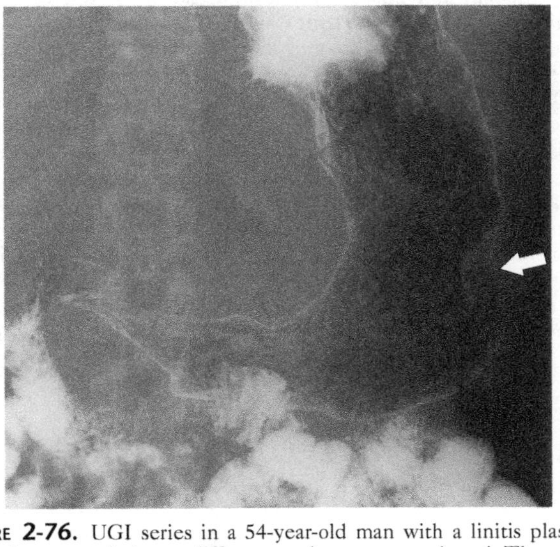

FIGURE 2-76. UGI series in a 54-year-old man with a linitis plastica–appearing stomach due to diffuse pseudomyxoma peritonei. There is an additional submucosal impression on the greater curvature (*arrow*) due to an additional metastatic deposit.

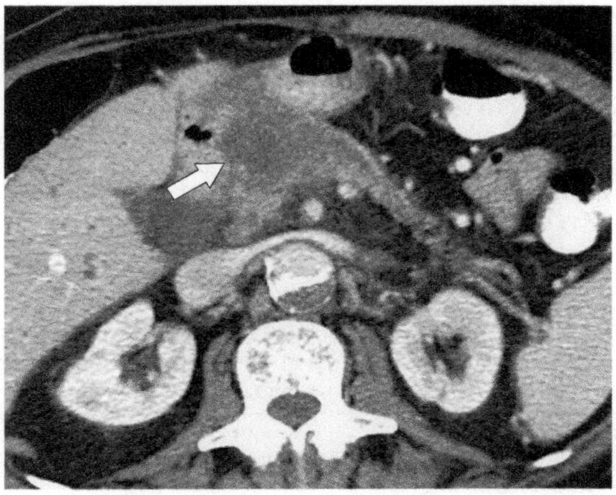

FIGURE 2-77. Axial contrast-enhanced CT in an 83-year-old woman with pancreatic carcinoma that invades the stomach (*arrow*).

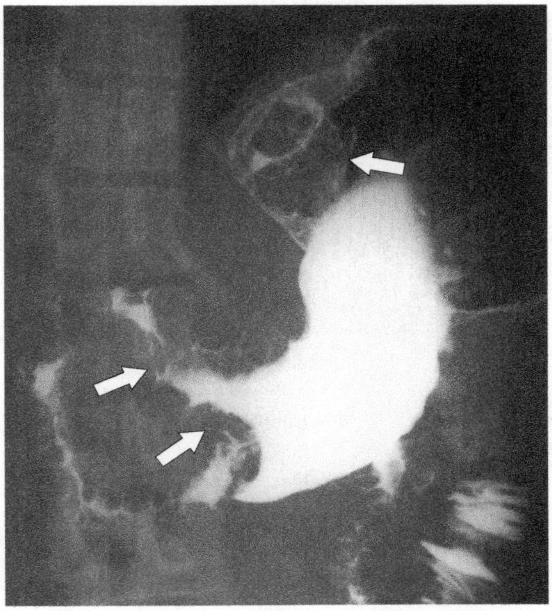

FIGURE 2-78. UGI in a 43-year-old man with a multiple gastric masses (*arrows*) due to Kaposi sarcoma.

adjacent malignancies (e.g., the pancreas) will produce irregular nodular folds and an intraluminal mass if lesions are large (Fig. 2-77). Esophageal cancer can invade the gastric cardia, producing appearances similar to the lower esophageal tumors, with nodular irregular folds and an associated mass.

Kaposi Sarcoma

Kaposi* sarcoma has become more common since the onset of the AIDS epidemic. However, because AIDS can now be effectively treated, this complication is seen less often in developed countries. It is a herpes virus–induced neoplasm that promotes a vascular endothelial tumor, usually of the skin, although involvement of any aspect of the GI tract is relatively common, particularly the esophagus and stomach. Although the lesions are usually asymptomatic, they can ulcerate (particularly when they are large) and cause GI hemorrhage. They are usually multiple and discrete, but they can also be diffuse in nature. They present as large submucosal masses, with or without central ulceration (Fig. 2-78).

Linitis Plastica Stomach

Linitis plastica stomach refers to a constricted, rigid, partial or whole noncontractile stomach thought to resemble the appearance of a leather bottle once used by hikers and travelers. The antrum and body are preferentially affected rather than the gastric fundus. The most common cause is gastric carcinoma, infiltrating diffusely along the gastric wall, rather than causing its more common intraluminal mass. Linitis plastica stomach is more often seen in anaplastic or undifferentiated gastric carcinoma and hence has a very poor prognosis. There are other causes of a linitis plastica stomach, both benign and malignant (Table 2-7).

The diagnosis is readily made by EGD or barium fluoroscopy but should also be recognized at CT. Typically, there is a rigid

*Moritz Kaposi (1837-1902), Hungarian physician and dermatologist.

noncontractile stomach without recognizable mucosal folds, usually starting at the antrum and progressing proximally (see Figs. 2-34, 2-35, 2-64, 2-65, 2-74, and 2-76). In general, it does not extend distally to cross the pylorus. At CT, the stomach lumen is narrowed (particularly in the antrum), with thickened infiltrated tumor in the gastric wall (see Figs. 2-64, 2-73, and 2-74). Associated regional lymphadenopathy and distant metastases are readily observed with the appropriate CT technique.

TABLE 2-7 Causes of Linitis Plastica (Leather-Bottle) Stomach

Malignant	Benign
Gastric carcinoma Lymphoma Metastases (breast, lung)	Eosinophilic gastroenteritis Crohn disease Tuberculosis, syphilis Caustic ingestion Sarcoidosis Zollinger-Ellison syndrome (multiple ulcers)

TABLE 2-8 Causes of Gastric Outlet Obstruction

Congenital	Pyloric stenosis
Mechanical	Bezoar Diaphragmatic hernia Volvulus
Inflammatory	Peptic ulcer disease Pancreatitis Crohn disease
Infection	Tuberculosis Syphilis
Corrosives	Linitis plastica
Malignancy	Carcinoma Lymphoma
Radiation therapy	Radiation stricture

Gastric Outlet Obstruction

There are both benign and malignant causes of gastric outlet obstruction (Table 2-8). Most of the benign gastric causes result in outlet obstruction through fibrosis as a consequence of the healing phases. The most common benign cause is a result of chronic peptic ulcer disease, but as described earlier, this is less prevalent and responds well to antibiotics, so it is now relatively rare.

More common are malignant causes, the most prevalent being gastric cancer (Fig. 2-79) (often scirrhous type) and pancreatic adenocarcinoma (see Fig. 2-63). Both can infiltrate along the gastric wall, causing antral constriction and outlet obstruction. Lymphoma, like that elsewhere in the GI tract or pancreaticobiliary system, tends not to be obstructive but rather mass-like without mechanically constrictive effects. However, if very large, it may ultimately cause outlet obstruction.

Gastric Bezoar

Gastric bezoars are composed of plant and vegetable matter (phytobezoar) or hair (trichobezoar), the first being more common and more likely to cause associated ulcer disease from local abrasion. In general, bezoars do not obstruct unless they are large and act with a ball-valve effect. They are more common after gastric reconstructive surgery when there is a smaller stomach lumen. Trichobezoars tend to be much larger than phytobezoars at presentation, when they are filled with hair and food residue and are typically black in color (Figs. 2-80 and 2-81). Patients often have an underlying psychiatric diagnosis.

The persimmon bezoar is a unique bezoar noted in Native Americans after unripened fruit from the persimmon tree has been eaten. After ingestion, it coagulates with gastric acid into a gelatinous mass, sometimes leading to gastric outlet obstruction.

Other bezoars include lactobezoars, which consist of solidified undigested milk, and pharmacobezoars, which consist of undigested and accumulated multiple medications. Other foreign object bezoars include swallowed drug-filled condoms, typically seen in smugglers, that get lodged in the gastric antrum and pylorus. Rarely, other nondescript foreign objects are swallowed by children or by institutionalized and psychiatric patients.

At imaging, there may be a soft tissue mass noted on plain radiography, but a UGI will readily identify a mottled complex mass

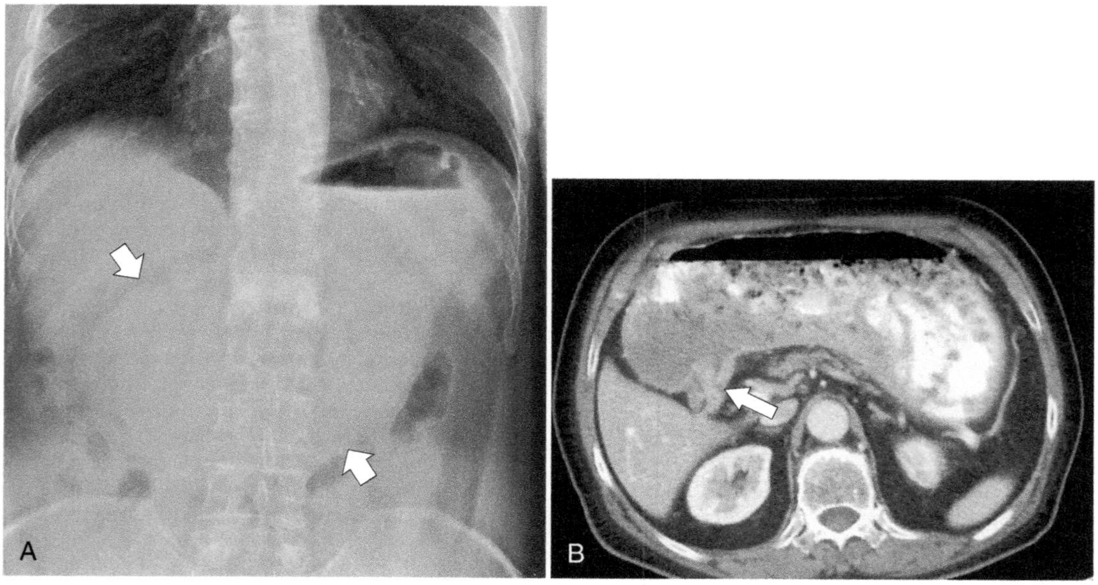

FIGURE 2-79. Plain abdominal radiography (**A**) and axial contrast-enhanced CT (**B**) in a 69-year-old man with gastric outlet obstruction and a distended stomach *(small arrows)* due to an antral gastric cancer (*large arrow*).

with barium interspersed within the bezoar. This tissue can also be identified on CT, which demonstrates a mottled appearance of gas within the bezoar that does not enhance after the administration of IV contrast material.

Functional Obstruction

True atonic conditions that cause gastric distention should be distinguished from chronic air swallowing or ingestions of large quantities of carbonated drinks that simply distend the stomach with gas. The term *gastroparesis* refers to delayed gastric emptying, usually due to atonic conditions rather than to mechanical obstruction. As such, it may be due to autonomic neuropathic causes, most commonly diabetes. As elsewhere in the gut, dehydration and electrolyte disturbance or recent surgery resulting in an ileus can result in temporary loss of gastric contractions. Some acutely ill and terminally ill patients can have agonal atony with an acutely distended, atonic stomach. Many drugs are also responsible for gastroparesis, particularly those with anticholinergic effects; narcotics and antidepressants can cause gastric stasis. At imaging, the dilated stomach is often visualized on plain radiograph, but CT will more likely confirm the nonspecific stomach dilatation (Fig. 2-82).

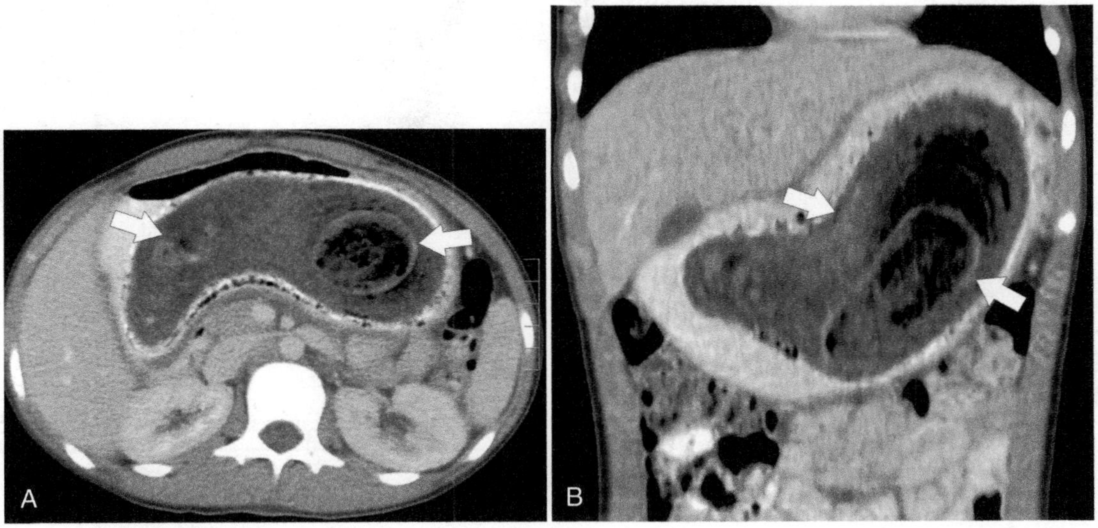

FIGURE 2-80. Axial (**A**) and coronal (**B**) CT in a 16-year-old girl with a large heterogeneous gastric filling defect (*arrows*) due to trichobezoar.

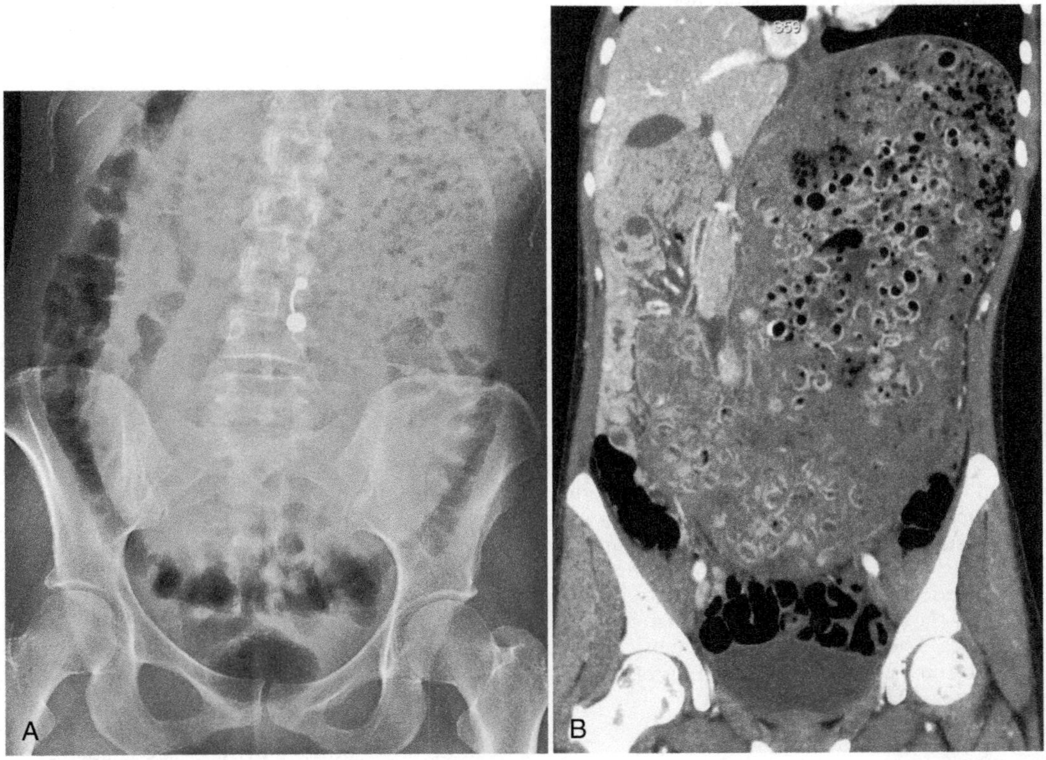

FIGURE 2-81. Abdominal plain radiograph (**A**) and coronal contrast-enhanced CT (**B**) in a 23-year-old woman with gross gastric dilatation and multiple luminal filling defects due to a phytobezoar (overingestion of macaroni).

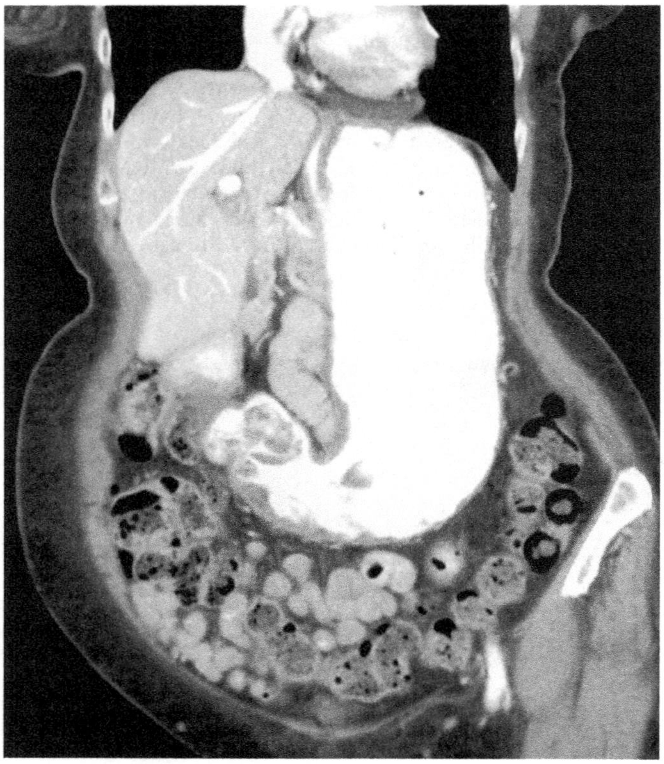

FIGURE 2-82. Coronal conrast-enhanced CT in a 71-year-old woman with gastric atonic dilatation.

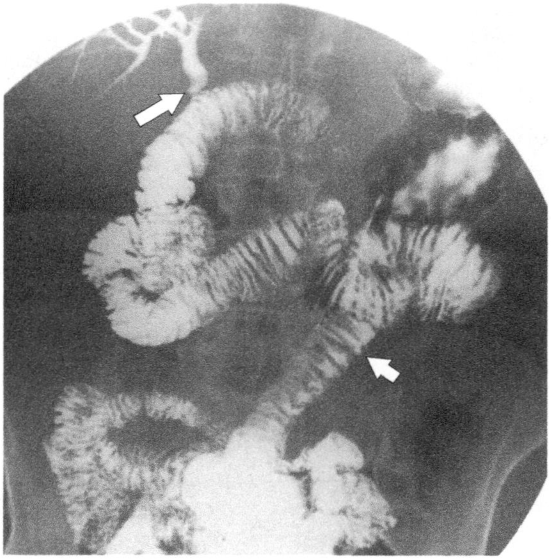

FIGURE 2-83. UGI series in a 56-year-old woman who underwent a normal Roux-en-Y gastric bypass opereation. There is a choledochojejunostomy with the afferent limb (*large arrow*) and normal reflux of contrast into the bile ducts. The efferent limb (*small arrow*) is of normal caliber.

Scleroderma can cause neuromuscular destruction and subsequent atonic stomach, similar to its manifestations elsewhere in the GI tract. Chronic intestinal pseudoobstruction, a very rare entity affecting the neuromuscular plexuses throughout the bowel, can cause an atonic stomach and gastric dilatation. Other neurogenic conditions of central or peripheral neuropathies (syphilis, poliomyelitis, diabetes) can also result in chronic gastric atony.

Postsurgical Stomach

A Billroth* I, or B1, is simply the removal of the pylorus and end-to-end anastomosis of the stomach to the duodenum. A Billroth II, or B2, operation involves antrectomy and a side-to-side anastomosis of the jejunum to the greater curvature of the stomach. The afferent limb consists of the duodenum, which is now a blind ending (with preservation of the normal bile duct anatomy) and a variable length of jejunum. The efferent loop, into which gastric contents should preferentially empty, is the distal component of the side-to-side anastomosis (Fig. 2-83). If stomach contents preferentially empty into the afferent limb, then afferent loop syndrome can develop (see later in chapter).

For the prevention of bile reflux into the stomach, which can cause severe gastritis, a modification of the Billroth II technique involves creation of a Roux†-en-Y anastomosis. In this instance, the afferent duodenal limb is still a blind ending with a normal insertion of the bile duct, but it is inserted into the efferent jejunal limb distal to the gastrojejunal anastomosis. This loop may be brought to the gastric remnant anterior to the transverse mesocolon (antecolic) or posteriorly (retrocolic), with the latter having a shorter loop, which is thought to more closely match normal physiological conditions. The Roux-en-Y anastomosis is also used for hepaticojejunostomy and choledochojejunostomy and is increasingly commonly with gastric bypass surgery.

*Theodor Billroth (1829-1894), German surgeon.
†César Roux (1857-1934), Swiss surgeon.

TABLE 2-9 Complications of Gastric Surgical Procedures

Early	
Leakage	Usually at anastomotic site; fistula may result
Infection	Common to many surgical procedures
Hemorrhage	Common to many surgical procedures
Anastomotic stricture	Usually edema
Esophageal dysmotility	Surgical trauma to esophagus
Ileus	Common in many abdominal surgical procedures.
Late	
Gastroparesis	
Anastomotic stricture	Fibrosis Tumor
Marginal ulcer formation	Gastric acid effect on jejunal mucosa
Gastric cancer	
Obstruction	Gastric outlet obstruction; adhesions; internal hernia intussusception
Malabsorption	Dumping syndrome
Bezoars	
Afferent loop syndrome	

COMPLICATIONS OF GASTRIC SURGICAL PROCEDURES

There are numerous complications to gastric surgery, and they can be divided into early and late (Table 2-9). Some complications (infection and hemorrhage) are common to most surgical procedures.

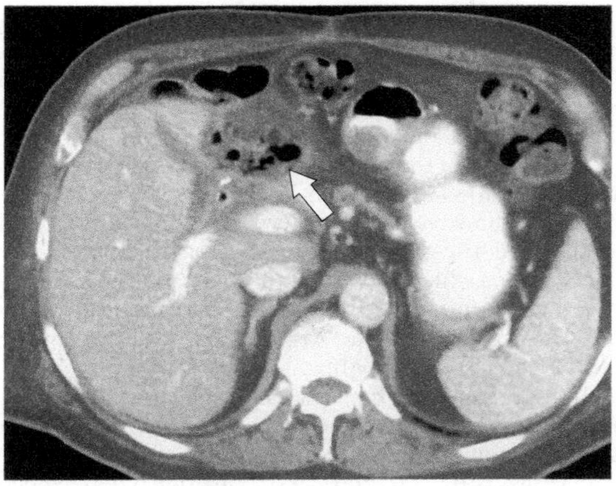

FIGURE 2-84. Axial contrast-enhanced CT in a 67-year-old man who underwent a recent Roux-en-Y procedure and an afferent limb leak with extraluminal gas and fluid (*arrow*).

Leakage

Leakage usually occurs at the anastomotic sites shortly after surgery. Patients are usually imaged with water-soluble contrast media 24 hours after surgery to document any leaks before liquid diets begin. The study is often performed via a nasogastric tube. Leaks will be recognized as collections of contrast, often linear at or near an anastomosis, often in a direction away from or perpendicular to the axis of the organ. It is important to obtain orthogonal views to clearly identify the site, size, and direction of the leak. If no leak is identified, then barium may be administered to better define the anatomy and to determine whether there is any evidence of slow transit time through the stomach or small intestine (both of which are relatively common postsurgically because of ileus and perianastomotic edema). Barium may also identify a small leak missed by water-soluble contrast media. This will likely be of little significance, and the extravasation of barium will likely be minimal, local, and contained. Alternatively, larger leaks will likely be identified on CT, with extraluminal gas, fluid, or contrast material (Fig. 2-84).

Gastroparesis

Delayed gastric emptying with no discernible obstruction is either an early transient (due to an ileus-type picture) or a late and chronic complication of gastric surgery. Either may be due to surgical damage to the vagus nerve. The stomach remains markedly distended with gastric fluid and food, and the patient is often nauseated and vomiting. Bezoars may develop secondary to the gastric stasis.

Marginal Ulcers

Marginal ulcers usually occur in the efferent limb, rather than afferent limb, because of peptic ulceration of the jejunal mucosa, although ischemia secondary to surgical manipulation of the surrounding vasculature can compound the problem (Fig. 2-85). Any predisposing factors (e.g., aspirin, steroid, or alcohol) will also exacerbate the development of an ulcer. These are usually identified by EGD or UGI because they are unlikely to be identified by on CT, unless they are large.

Obstruction

Obstruction may occur early at the gastrojejunal anastomosis because of transitory, self-limiting edema or because of longer-term complications from fibrotic stricture resulting from the surgical procedure or resulting from an anastomotic or marginal ulcer. A more sinister cause results from a gastric carcinoma at the gastrojejunal anastomotic site.

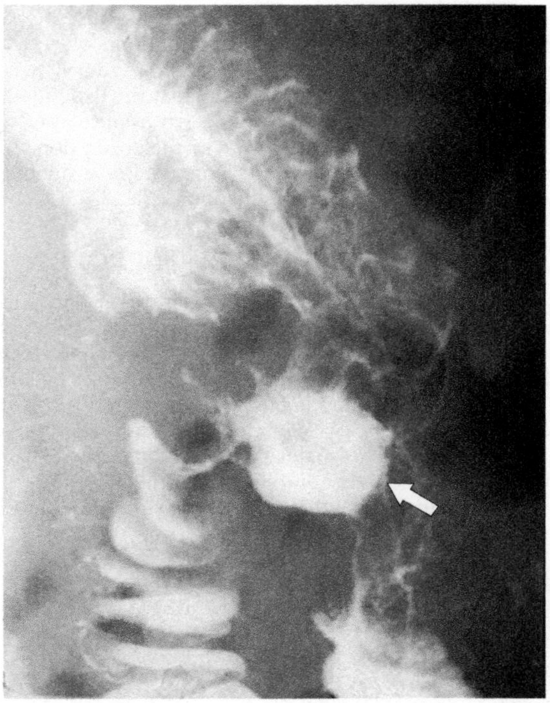

FIGURE 2-85. UGI series in a 67-year-old man after a partial gastrectomy and a Roux-en-Y procedure now with an anastomotic gastrojejunal ulcer (*arrow*).

Internal hernias that develop after gastric surgery occur when a loop of small bowel, usually jejunum, herniates through mesenteric hiatal orifices created at the time of the original operation. Although they are uncommon, the two most common hernias that are associated with gastric surgery involve small bowel herniation through a transmesenteric or transmesocolic peritoneal defect (Figs. 2-86 and 2-87). As the loops become more obstructed because of stricture formation from the narrow hiatal orifice, the patient has increasing abdominal pain, nausea, and vomiting. The loops of small bowel can become strangulated and may undergo volvulus (more commonly identified with transmesenteric hernias).

Obstruction can also occur with intussusception of the jejunum through the gastrojejunal anastomosis. This uncommonly occurs with a jejunojejunal intussusception that progresses retrograde toward the gastrojejunal anastomosis and finally into the anastomosis itself, giving the appearance of an intragastric mass. The mass may have a "coiled-spring" appearance on barium studies, similar to that seen with intussuscepta elsewhere in the small bowel, and if the mass is large enough, it may obstruct the stomach.

Dumping Syndrome

Dumping syndrome is common to all gastric surgical procedures, whereby the rapid delivery of sugars into the small bowel through the gastrojejunal anastomosis creates an osmotic fluid overload in the bowel with diarrhea, palpitations, pallor, sweating, and postural hypotension.

Afferent Loop Syndrome

Afferent loop syndrome is relatively uncommon and is due to the obstruction of the afferent limb (duodenum or jejunum) proximal to the gastrojejunal anastomosis. It results from distention and bacterial overgrowth of the afferent limb. Patients often experience epigastric fullness after eating, and bilious vomiting, sometimes projectile, is a characteristic symptom as the distended loop decompresses abruptly. Bacterial overgrowth from the prolonged stasis of the afferent limb can result in malabsorption. CT is the imaging method of choice and demonstrates a dilated and obstructed loop in the right upper quadrant (Fig. 2-88).

GASTRIC BYPASS (BARIATRIC) SURGERY

There are a variety of surgical procedures designed to promote weight loss in patients with morbid obesity, either for patient preference or for treatment of obesity-associated type II diabetes. The essential surgical goal is to markedly reduce stomach volume to create early satiety after food ingestion, thereby reducing longer-term caloric intake. There two common procedures are Roux-en-Y gastric bypass surgery and laparoscopic adjustable gastric banding (lap band). The former procedure (of which there are several versions) is more common with the creation of a smaller upper gastric remnant (15 to 30 mL) that is directly connected to a loop of jejunum so that food "bypasses" the main larger lower gastric (approximately 400 mL), or excluded, remnant. Because it is still producing gastric secretions, the excluded remnant is still connected to the small bowel with the retained duodenum and proximal jejunum, which is connected to the efferent loop (directly connected to the small upper pouch) via a Roux-en-Y limb (Fig. 2-89).

Increasingly, however, the surgery is being performed laparoscopically, and the separation of the two smaller and larger pouches is often achieved with staples (termed a *sleeve gastrectomy*). This procedure usually results in complete separation (to minimize fistulization into the larger remnant or the connection of the two pouches) (Fig. 2-90).

Complications of the bariatric surgical procedures include infection, hemorrhage, adhesions, intussuscepta, internal hernia formation, anastomotic leakage and fistulization, stricture, and ulceration (Figs. 2-91, 2-92, and 2-93). Nutritional deficiencies can occur, particularly with distal anastomotic procedures. Small leaks are best demonstrated by water-soluble contrast swallow examinations and are seen as contrast material spilling into the peritoneal cavity. This study is routinely performed 24 hours after surgery to check for leaks before more formal liquid feeds start. If no initial leak is seen, barium may be administered to give better depiction of the anatomy and to confirm there is no tiny leak. Larger leaks, which may evolve into abscesses, are best visualized by CT. Internal herniation can be transmesenteric through either the transverse mesocolon or the small bowel mesentery (see Fig. 2-86 and Chapter 4).

An alternative approach to creating the small upper gastric pouch is the laparoscopic adjustable gastric band or lap band. This is an inflatable silicone device, placed approximately 3 cm distal to the GE junction, that effectively mimics the stapling procedure but is less invasive and thought to lead to less morbidity (Figs. 2-94 and 2-95). Unlike the stapling procedure, the larger gastric pouch is not excluded from the digestion process; rather, the band creates a small upper pouch and delays emptying into the larger lower gastric pouch. As the upper pouch fills with food, it also creates early satiety. The ingestion of food therefore stops, and that which was ingested slowly passes into the larger gastric pouch for normal digestion. The band's tightness can be tailored to the patient's weight-loss regimen and can be tightened or loosened accordingly through a small access port under the skin (see Fig. 2-94).

The main complication is that the lap band can "slip" so that the lower larger pouch herniates or prolapses above the band, leaving a larger upper pouch and causing constriction of the stomach at its widest part. This can lead to obstruction or strangulation and

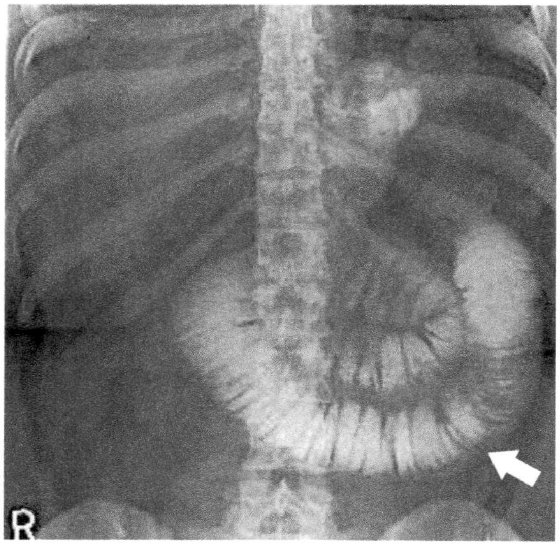

FIGURE 2-86. UGI in a 55-year-old man with prior bariatric surgery now with small bowel obstruction due to a jejunal transmesenteric herniation and volvulus (*arrow*).

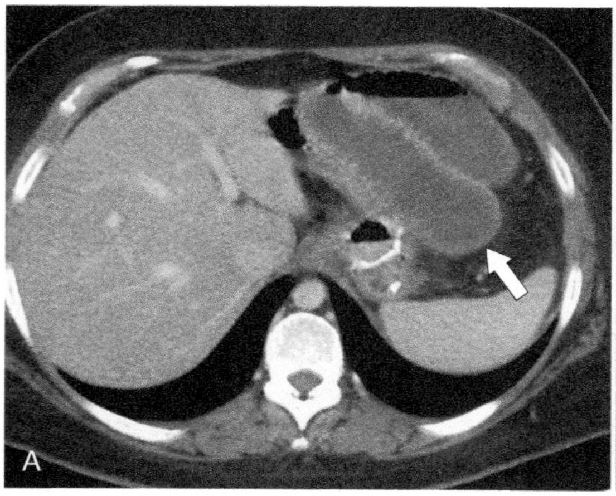

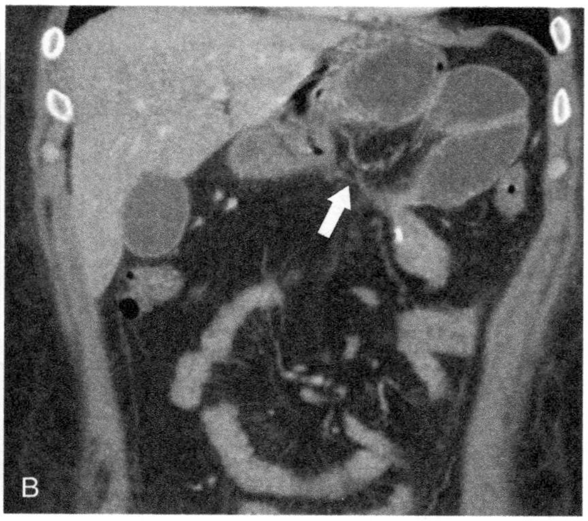

FIGURE 2-87. Axial (**A**) and coronal (**B**) contrast-enhanced CT in a 38-year-old woman after bariatric surgery with jejunal obstruction (*arrows*) due to a closed-loop obstruction.

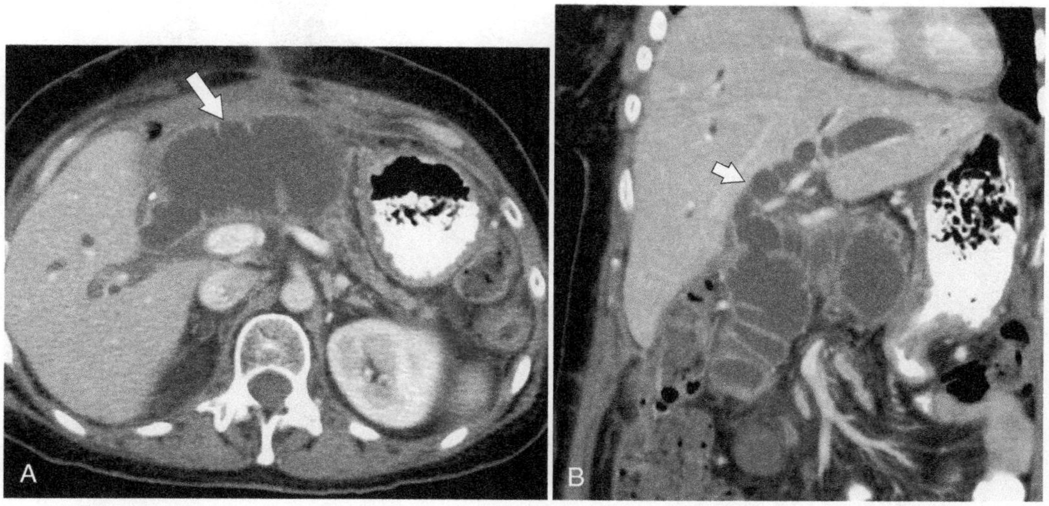

FIGURE 2-88. Axial (A) and coronal (B) contrast-enhanced CT in a 47-year-old woman after a Whipple procedure and an obstructed afferent loop (*large arrow*) with secondary biliary dilatation (*small arrow*).

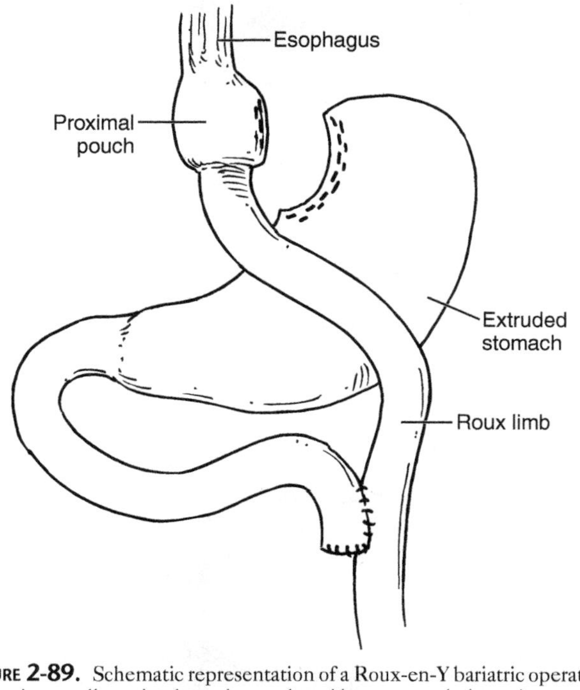

FIGURE 2-89. Schematic representation of a Roux-en-Y bariatric operation. There is a small proximal gastric pouch and larger extruded gastric remnant.

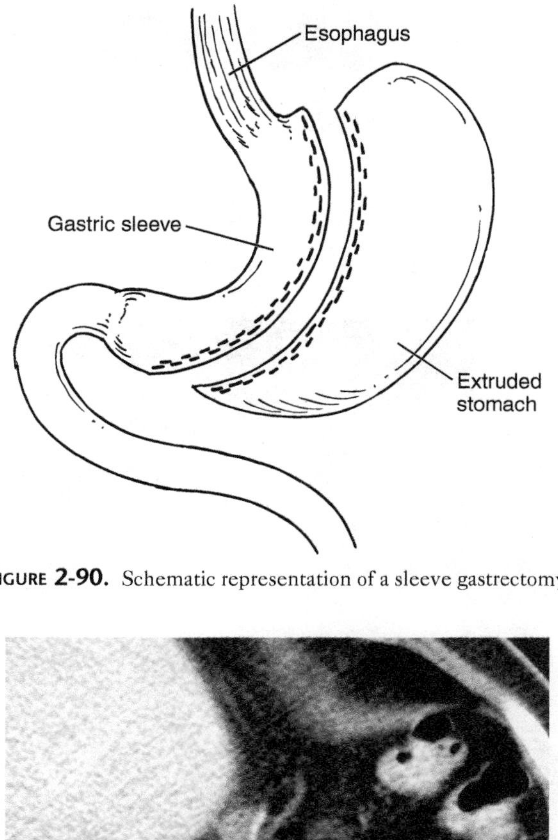

FIGURE 2-90. Schematic representation of a sleeve gastrectomy.

would require urgent surgery (Fig. 2-96). Alternatively, the band can be too "loose" so that the stomach is not constricted and early satiety does not occur. This can be adjusted by tightening the band, assuming it has not slipped distal to its intended position.

Nissen Fundoplication

Nissen* fundoplication is an open or laparoscopic surgical procedure, used to treat GERD, that involves creating a gastric fundal wrap (usually 360 degrees) around the lower esophagus to strengthen the lower esophageal sphincter (see Chapter 1). The procedure is generally effective, although complications of dysphagia, dumping syndrome, achalasia, and a difficulty with belching are recognized. The major complication is loosening of the wrap, with patients having recurrent symptoms of GERD (Fig. 2-97).

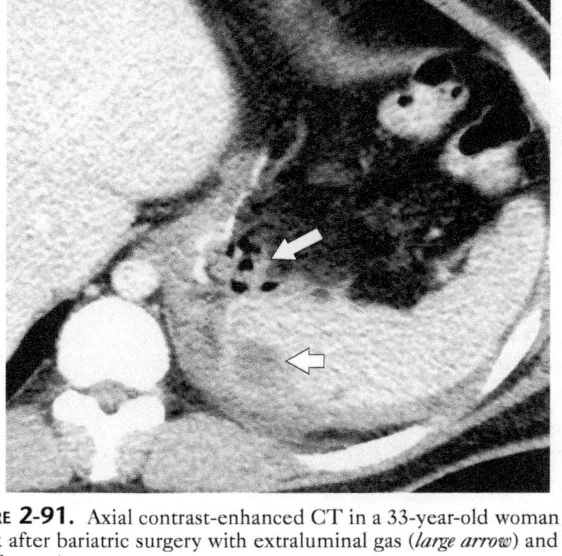

FIGURE 2-91. Axial contrast-enhanced CT in a 33-year-old woman with a leak after bariatric surgery with extraluminal gas (*large arrow*) and fluid (*small arrow*).

*Rudolph Nissen (1896-1981), Swiss surgeon.

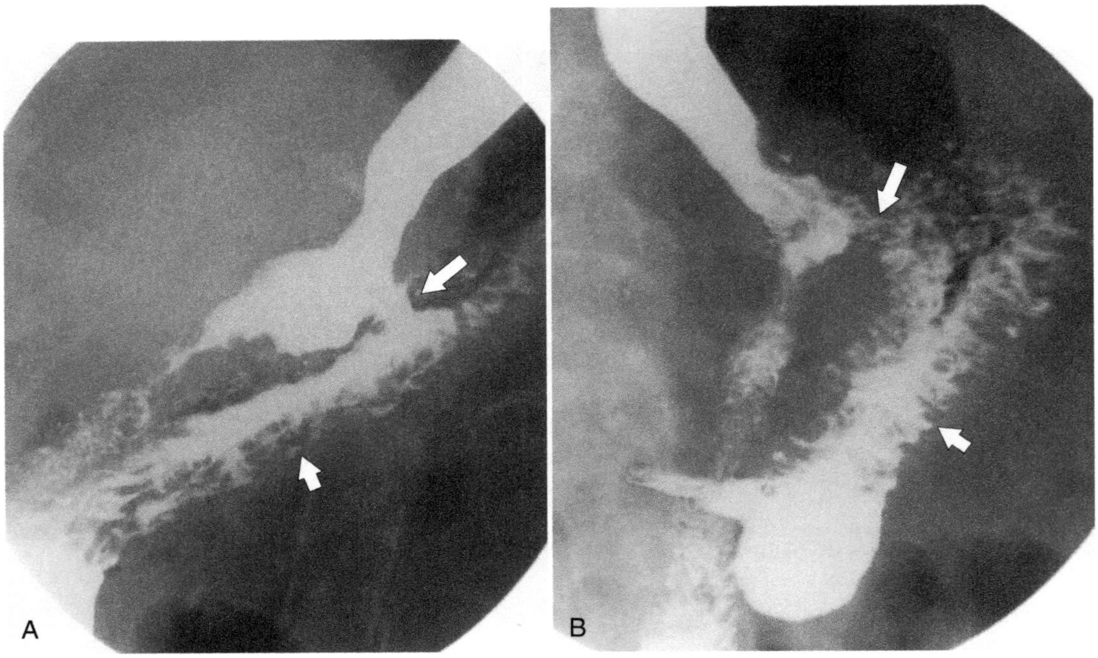

FIGURE 2-92. A and B, UGI swallow in a 36-year-old woman after bariatric surgery with a gastro gastric fistula (*large arrows*). There is contrast in the extruded segment (*small arrows*).

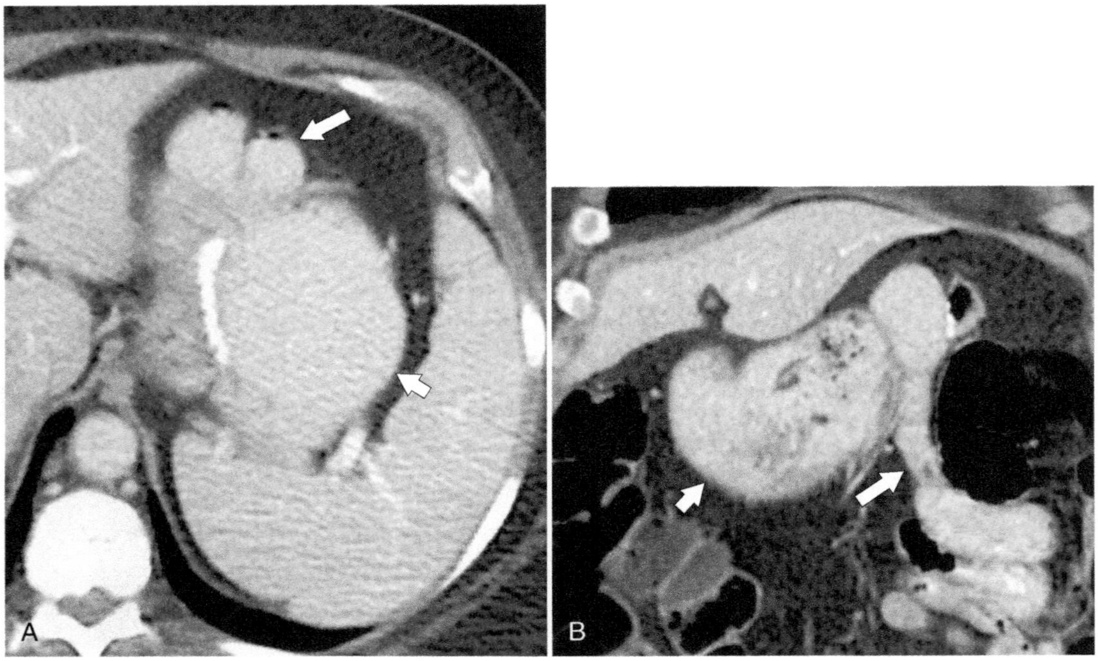

FIGURE 2-93. Axial (A) and coronal (B) CT in a 58-year-old woman with a post-bariatric gastrogastric fistula with contrast present in both the efferent limb (*large arrows*) and extruded stomach (*small arrows*).

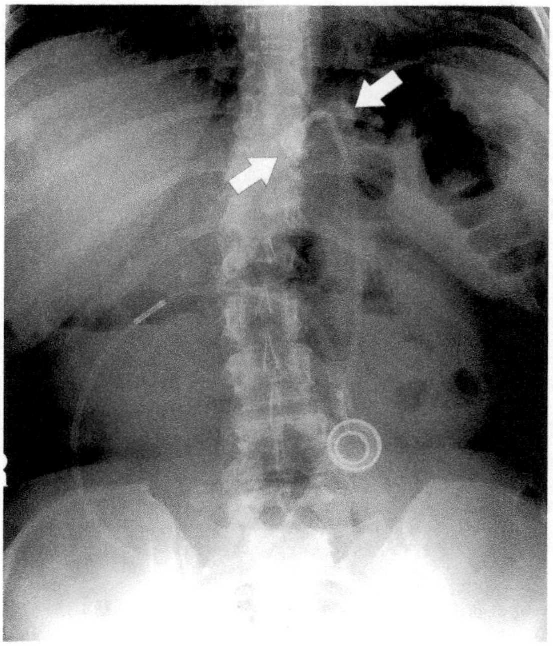

FIGURE 2-94. Abdominal plain radiograph demonstrating a normal lap-band prosthesis (*arrows*).

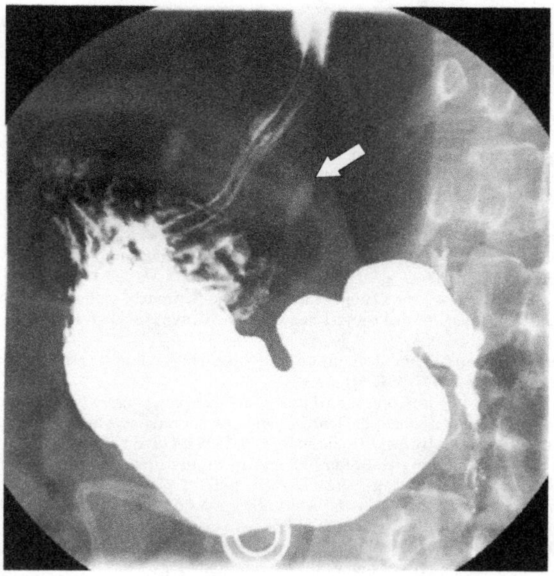

FIGURE 2-96. UGI series in a 39-year-old woman with slipped gastric band. The lap-band has "slipped" cephalad (*arrow*) so there is a very small gastric volume above the ring and the stomach fills normally with barium.

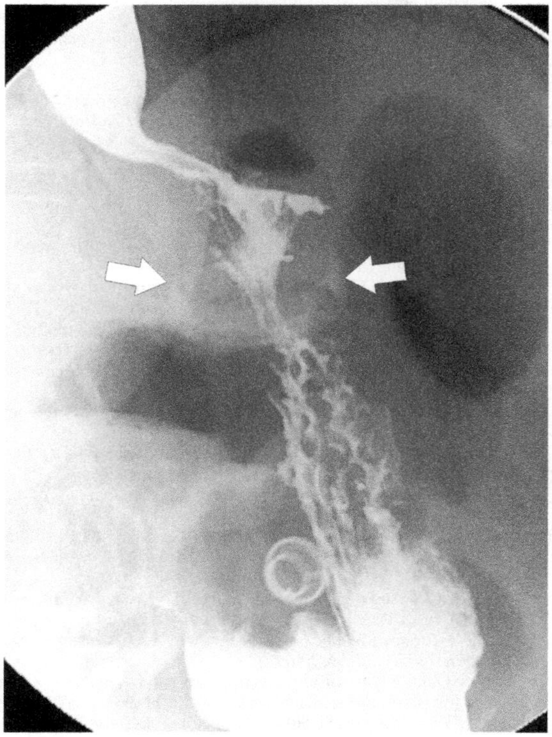

FIGURE 2-95. UGI series in a 33-year-old woman with a normal-appearing lap-band procedure with a small gastric remnant and positioning of the band (*arrows*).

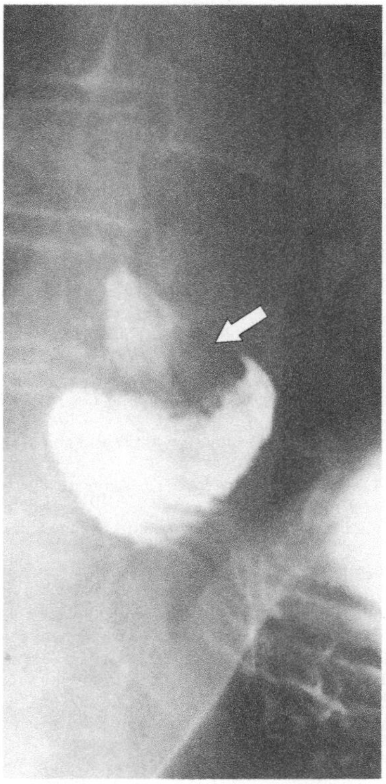

FIGURE 2-97. UGI series in a 51-year-old man with partial unwrapping of the Nissen wrap (*arrow*).

Suggested Readings

Abbara S et al: Intrathoracic stomach revisited. AJR Am J Roentgenol 181(2):403-414, 2003.

Antoch G et al: Comparison of PET, CT, dual-modality PET/CT imaging for monitoring of imatinib (STI571) therapy in patients with gastrointestinal stromal tumors. J Nucl Med 45(3):357-365, 2004.

Asrani AV: The antral pad sign. Radiology 229(2):421-422, 2003.

Balthazar EJ et al: Scirrhous carcinoma of the pyloric channel and distal antrum. AJR Am J Roentgenol 134(4):669-673, 1980.

Ba-Ssalamah A et al: Dedicated multidetector CT of the stomach: spectrum of diseases. Radiographics 23(3):625-644, 2003.

Bawahab M et al: Management of acute paraesophageal hernia. Surg Endosc 23(2):255-259, 2009.

Bechtold RE et al: Cystic changes in hepatic and peritoneal metastases from gastrointestinal stromal tumors treated with Gleevec. Abdom Imaging 28(6):808-814, 2003.

Binstock AJ et al: Carcinoid Tumors of the Stomach: A Clinical and Radiographic Study. AJR 176:947-951, April 2001.

Blachar A et al: Laparoscopic adjustable gastric banding surgery for morbid obesity: imaging of normal anatomic features and postoperative gastrointestinal complications. AJR Am J Roentgenol 188(2):472-479, 2007.

Blaser MJ: Gastric Campylobacter-like organisms, gastritis, and peptic ulcer disease. Gastroenterology 93(2):371-383, 1987.

Blaser MJ: In a world of black and white. *Helicobacter pylori* is gray (editorial). Ann Intern Med 130(8):695-697, 1999.

Burkill GJ: Malignant gastrointestinal stromal tumor: distribution, imaging features, and pattern of metastatic spread. Radiology 226(2):527-532, 2003.

Campbell JB et al: Acute mesentero-axial volvulus of the stomach. Radiology 103(1):53-156, 1972.

Carmack SW et al: The current spectrum of gastric polyps: a 1-year national study of over 120,000 patients. Am J Gastroenterol 104(6):1524-1532, 2009.

Chandler RC et al: Imaging in Bariatric Surgery: A Guide to Postsurgical Anatomy and Common Complications. AJR 190:122-135, January 2008.

Chandler T et al: Gastrointestinal/liver/biliary/pancreas. AJR Am J Roentgenol 196(5):A149-A176, 2011.

Chen CY et al: Differentiation between malignant and benign gastric ulcers: CT virtual gastroscopy versus optical gastroendoscopy. Radiology 252(2):410-417, 2009, doi:10.1148/radiol.2522081249.

Chen CY et al: Gastric cancer: preoperative local staging with 3D multi-detector row CT—correlation with surgical and histopathologic results. Radiology 242(2):472-482, 2007.

Chen CY et al: MDCT for differentiation of category T1 and T2 malignant lesions from benign gastric ulcers. AJR Am J Roentgenol 190(6):1505-1511, 2008.

Chen CY et al: : MDCT of giant gastric folds: differential diagnosis. AJR Am J Roentgenol 195(5):1124-1130, 2010.

Cho JS et al: Heterotopic pancreas in the stomach: CT findings. Radiology 217(1):139-144, 2000.

Choi SH et al: Intussusception in adults: from stomach to rectum. AJR Am J Roentgenol 183(3):691-698, 2004.

Clements JL et al: Antral mucosal diaphragms in adults. AJR Am J Roentgenol 113(6):1105-1111, 1979.

Dickinson RJ et al: Partial gastric diverticula: radiological and endoscopic features in six patients. Gut 27(8):954-957, 1986.

Feczko PJ et al: Gastric polyps: radiological evaluation and clinical significance. Radiology 155(3):581-584, 1985.

Flug J: Gastrointestinal imaging. AJR Am J Roentgenol 198(5):(suppl). E130, 2012.

Friedman J et al: Ménétrier disease. Radiographics 29(1):297-301, 2009. doi:10.1148/rg.291075216.

Gayer G et al: Foreign objects encountered in the abdominal cavity at CT. Radiographics 31(2):409-428, 2011.

Ghanem N et al: Computed tomography in gastrointestinal stromal tumors. Eur Radiol 13(7):1669-1678, 2003.

Gollub MJ: Imaging of gastrointestinal lymphoma. Radiol Clin North Am. 46(2):287-312, 2008, ix.

Gonen C et al: Magnifying endoscopic features of granulomatous gastritis. Dig Dis Sci 54(7):1602-1603, 2009.

Gupta A et al: A prospective study of MR enterography versus capsule endoscopy for the surveillance of adult patients with Peutz-Jeghers syndrome. AJR Am J Roentgenol 195(1):108-116, 2010. doi:10.2214/AJR.09.3174.

Habermann CR et al: Preoperative staging of gastric adenocarcinoma: comparison of helical CT and endoscopic US. Radiology 230(2):465-471, 2004.

Hargunani R et al: Cross-sectional imaging of gastric neoplasia. Clin Radiol 64(4):420-429, 2009.

Hayashi D et al: Mucosa-associated lymphoid tissue lymphoma: multimodality imaging and histopathologic correlation. AJR Am J Roentgenol 195(2): W105-W117, 2010. doi:10.2214/AJR.09.4105.

Ho AS et al: Long-Term Outcome After Chemoembolization and Embolization of Hepatic Metastatic Lesions from Neuroendocrine Tumors. AJR 188:1201-1207, May 2007.

Holdsworth CH et al: CT and PET: early prognostic indicators of response to imatinib mesylate in patients with gastrointestinal stromal tumor. AJR Am J Roentgenol 189(6):W324-W330, 2007.

Horton KM et al: Current role of CT in imaging of the stomach. Radiographics 23(1):75-87, 2003.

Huang SY et al: Large hiatal hernia with floppy fundus: clinical and radiographic findings. AJR Am J Roentgenol 188(4):960-964, 2007.

Hunter TB et al: Medical devices of the abdomen and pelvis. Radiographics 25(2):503-523, 2005.

Hur BY et al: Gastroduodenal glomus tumors: differentiation from other subepithelial lesions based on dynamic contrast-enhanced CT findings. AJR Am J Roentgenol 197(6):1351-1359, 2011. doi:10.2214/AJR.10.6360.

Insko EK et al: Benign and malignant lesions for the stomach: evaluation of CT criteria for differentiation. Radiology 228(1):166-171, 2003.

Johnson PT et al: Hypervascular gastric masses: CT findings and clinical correlates. AJR Am J Roentgenol 195(6):W415-W420, 2010.

Katelaris PH et al: Effect of age. *Helicobacter pylori* infection, and gastritis with atrophy of serum gastrin and gastric acid secretion in healthy men. Gut 34(8):1032-1037, 1993.

Kawamoto S et al: Adjustable laparoscopic gastric banding: demonstrated on multidetector computed tomography with multiplanar reformation and 3-dimensional imaging. J Comput Assist Tomogr 33(2):288-290, 2009.

Kim JY et al: Ectopic pancreas: CT findings with emphasis on differentiation from small gastrointestinal stromal tumor and leiomyoma. Radiology 252(1):92-100, 2009. doi:10.1148/radiol.2521081441.

Kim KA et al: CT Findings in the abdomen and pelvis after gastric carcinoma resection. AJR Am J Roentgenol 179(4):1037-1041, 2002.

Kim T et al: Risk factors for hemorrhage from gastric varices. Hepatology 25(2):307-312, 1997.

Kim YH et al: Staging of T3 and T4 gastric carcinoma with multidetector CT: added value of multiplanar reformations for prediction of adjacent organ invasion. Radiology 250(3):767-775, 2009.

Koplewitz BZ et al: Case 29: Gastric trichobezoar and subphrenic abscess. Radiology 217(3):739-742, 2000.

Kumano S et al: T staging of gastric cancer: role of multi–detector row CT. Radiology 237(3):961-966, 2005.

Lassau N et al: Gastrointestinal stromal tumors treated with imatinib; monitoring response with contrast-enhanced sonography. AJR Am J Roentgenol 187(5):1267-1273, 2006.

Lazarus E et al: CT in the evaluation of nontraumatic abdominal pain in pregnant women. Radiology 244(3):784-790, 2007.

Lee IJ et al: Helical CT evaluation of the preoperative staging of gastric cancer in the remnant stomach. AJR Am J Roentgenol 192(4):902-908, 2009.

Levy AD et al: Duodenal carcinoids: imaging features with clinical-pathologic comparison. Radiology 237(3):967-972, 2005.

Levy AD et al: From the archives of the AFIP: Gastrointestinal carcinoids: imaging features with clinicopathologic comparison. Radiographics 27(1): 237-257, 2007.

Levy AD et al: Gastrointestinal stromal tumors: radiologic features with pathologic correlation. Radiographics 23(2):283-304, 2003, 456; quiz 532.

Liu HT et al: Wandering spleen: an unusual association with gastric volvulus. AJR Am J Roentgenol 188(4):W328-W330, 2007.

Megibow AJ et al: Evaluation of bowel distention and bowel wall appearance by using neutral oral contrast agent for multi-detector row CT. Radiology 238(1):87-95, 2006.

Metz DC et al: Gastrointestinal neuroendocrine tumors: pancreatic endocrine tumors. Gastroenterology 135(5):1469-1492, 2008.

Niraj N et al: Gallium-68-DOTA-NOC PET/CT of patients with gastroenteropancreatic neuroendocrine tumors: a prospective single-center study. AJR Am J Roentgenol 197(5):1221-1228, 2011. doi:10.2214/AJR.11.7298.

Nishie A et al: Comparison of size of proximal gastric pouch and short-term weight loss following routine upper gastrointestinal contrast study after laparoscopic Roux-en-Y gastric bypass. Obes Surg 17(9):1183-1188, 2007.

Okanobu H et al: Giant gastric folds: differential diagnosis at US. Radiology 226(3):686-690, 2003.

Ott DJ et al: Radiographic efficacy in gastric ulcer: comparison of single-contrast and multiphasic examination. AJR Am J Roentgenol 147(4):697-700, 1986.

Park MS et al: Mucinous versus nonmucinous gastric carcinoma: differentiation with helical CT. Radiology 223(2):540-546, 2002.

Pieroni S et al: The "O" sign, a simple and helpful tool in the diagnosis of laparoscopic adjustable gastric band slippage. AJR Am J Roentgenol 195(1):137-141, 2010. doi:10.2214/AJR.09.3933.

Raotma H et al: Clinical and morphological studies of giant hypertrophic gastritis (Ménétrier's disease). Acta Med Scand 195(4):247-252, 1974.

Ripolles T et al: Gastrointestinal bezoars: sonographic and CT characteristics. AJR Am J Roentgenol 177(1):65-69, 2001.

Rubesin SE et al: Double-contrast upper gastrointestinal radiography: a pattern approach for diseases of the stomach. Radiology 246(1):33-48, 2008.

Scheirey CD et al: Radiology of the laparoscopic Roux-en-Y gastric bypass procedure: conceptualization and precise interpretation of results. Radiographics 26(5):1355-1371, 2006.

Shanbhogue AK et al: Spectrum of medication-induced complications in the abdomen: role of cross-sectional imaging. AJR Am J Roentgenol 197(2), W286-W94, 2011. doi:10.2214/AJR.10.5415.

Shinagare AB et al: Pictorial Essay: Hereditary Cancer Syndromes: A Radiologist's Perspective. AJR 197:W1001-W1007, December 2011.

Shivanand G et al: Gastric volvulus: acute and chronic presentation. Clin Imaging 27(4):265-268, 2003.

Sohn J et al: *Helicobacter pylori* gastritis: radiographic findings. Radiology 195(3):763-767, 1995.

Swenson DW et al: Utility of routine barium studies after adjustments of laparoscopically inserted gastric bands. AJR Am J Roentgenol 194(1):129-135, 2010. doi:10.2214/AJR.09.2669.
Timpone VM et al: Abdominal twists and turns: part I, gastrointestinal tract torsions with pathologic correlation. AJR Am J Roentgenol 197(1):86-96, 2011. doi:10.2214/AJR.10.7292.
Torrisi JM et al: CT findings of chemotherapy-induced toxicity: what radiologists need to know about the clinical and radiologic manifestations of chemotherapy toxicity. Radiology 258(1):41-56, 2011. doi:10.1148/radiol.10092129.
Warakaulle DR et al: MDCT appearance of gastrointestinal stromal tumors after therapy with imatinib mesylate. AJR Am J Roentgenol 186(2):510-515, 2006.
Warshauer DM et al: Imaging manifestations of abdominal sarcoidosis. AJR Am J Roentgenol 182(1):15-28, 2004.
Wiesner W et al: Adjustable laparoscopic gastric banding in patients with morbid obesity: radiographic management, results, and postoperative complications. Radiology 216(2):389-394, 2000.
Yoon J et al: GI/liver/biliary/pancreas. AJR Am J Roentgenol 190(4):A111-A128, 2008.

CHAPTER 3

Duodenum

NORMAL ANATOMY

The duodenum is classified into four parts. The first is the duodenal bulb, which is intraperitoneal before it passes posteriorly into the second part, or C-sweep, which is retroperitoneal and fixed. This second part starts at the superior duodenal flexure and ends at the inferior duodenal flexure. The third part, also retroperitoneal, extends transversely from the inferior duodenal flexure to a point where it starts to ascend at the fourth part to its end at the ligament of Treitz.* The duodenum also has four layers: the mucosa, submucosa, inner circular, and outer longitudinal muscle. The mucosa is lined with multiple mucus-secreting Brunner† glands, most of which occur in the proximal duodenum and which can enlarge to cause Brunner gland hypertrophy (see later in chapter). The second part of the duodenum contains two papillae on its medial border, the minor papilla (Santorini‡ or accessory papilla), which is not usually visualized by imaging, and the major papilla (ampulla of Vater§), which can be visualized on upper gastrointestinal (UGI) series (particularly hypotonic duodenography) as a small, rounded filling defect in the midmedial wall of the second part of the duodenum (Fig. 3-1).

IMAGING EVALUATION OF THE DUODENUM

Historically visualization of the duodenum involved UGI contrast studies, but this has now been largely replaced by esophagogastroduodenoscopy (EGD). UGI contrast studies are now usually reserved to evaluate postoperative situations rather than disease de novo. The CT evaluation of the duodenum, though, has become more important. At fluoroscopy and UGI, the duodenal bulb had typically been the area of greatest interest, mainly because of the propensity of duodenal ulcers in the past. These ulcers are now far less common because of effective medications targeting gastric acid production and antibiotic treatment for *Helicobacter pylori* bacteria (see later in chapter). Good single-contrast or double-contrast technique is required to fully evaluate the duodenal bulb. The double-contrast technique, like optimized evaluation of the stomach, is somewhat of an art, and considerable expertise is required to assess patients with the variable anatomy, disease, or both.

The duodenal bulb is typically situated in a posterolateral axis (this can readily be appreciated through observation of its position at axial computed tomography [CT]), knowledge of which is required to fully evaluate bulb disease. The bulb will likely fill adequately with contrast once the patient is positioned in the right side down partial decubitus position. Once filled with barium, the bulb should be brought en face (perpendicular) to the x-ray beam, which usually requires positioning the patient right side up (right anterior oblique). At this point, the bulb should be adequately coated and distended with gas as a double-contrast view. Sometimes the bulb projects directly posteriorly and can be hard to view en face, but rotation of the patient into various positions (e.g., lateral) should bring the bulb en face, sometimes with the patient in a semiprone rather than semisupine position. Other times, the bulb can only be best viewed with the patient standing, which permits the weight of the gastric antrum to "fall away," exposing the relatively fixed duodenal bulb.

Duodenal folds are usually best evaluated in the semisupine (right side up) position, and compression paddles may be required to move the gastric antrum away. In this semisupine position, ulcers may be seen as the pooling of barium on the posterior wall or radiolucent areas on the anterior wall (because the denser barium is now dependent on the posterior wall). Conversely, with the patient in a semiprone position (left side up or left anterior oblique), the barium will pool into ulcers on the anterior wall and not the posterior wall. As with any contrast fluoroscopic technique, any identified disease must be viewed tangentially, and multiple spot views must be taken. Ulcers may not be seen within duodenal folds, unless they are seen tangentially as they protrude outside the duodenal mucosa.

Hypertonic duodenography is a valuable tool for the evaluation of duodenal disease, including the bulb, but is now rarely performed. Hypertonic duodenography is achieved through temporary duodenal spasm after the administration of antispasmodics (glucagon or anticholinergics). Glucagon is relatively contraindicated in diabetics, and patients who are receiving anticholinergic agents should not drive vehicles for up to 4 hours because of the loss of visual accommodation. With appropriate bulb positioning, distortions in the duodenal wall, usually from ulcer disease, should be readily appreciated. If an abnormality is identified, views in multiple planes must be obtained to extract the most diagnostic information from the imaging examination. The second, third, and fourth parts of the duodenum are usually evaluated with single-contrast studies, although hypertonic duodenography should also temporarily distend at least the second part of the duodenum.

CT is not the primary modality for investigating the duodenum but can provide an excellent visualization of gross duodenal disease, including some congenital anomalies, duodenitis, and mural neoplastic lesions, particularly malignant masses. Positron emission tomography/computed tomography (PET/CT) is rarely used unless metastatic spread of duodenal malignancies is being

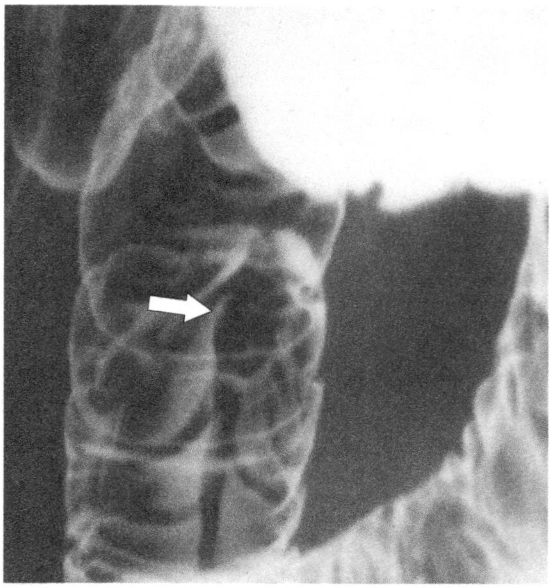

FIGURE 3-1. Normal ampulla of Vater (*arrow*).

*Václav Treitz (1819-1872), Czech pathologist.
†Johann Conrad Brunner (1653-1727), Swiss anatomist.
‡Giovanni Domenico Santorini (1681-1737), Italian anatomist.
§Abraham Vater (1684-1751), German anatomist.

evaluated, in which case it can identify small metastatic nodes that might otherwise be considered indeterminate by CT.

CONGENITAL DUODENAL ANOMALIES

Duodenal Atresia and Web

Duodenal atresia presents very early after birth because of the complete obstruction of the duodenum from the intrauterine failure of duodenal cannulation, which is often associated with Down* syndrome. Patients vomit their feeding, and on plain image, a characteristic "double bubble" is identified representing a gas-filled duodenum proximal to the complete obstruction and an enlarged, gas-filled stomach (Fig. 3-2). Duodenal webs are a form of duodenal atresia, although the duodenal obstruction is not complete; rather there is a diaphragm or membrane or web that causes duodenal stenosis (Fig. 3-3). These may persist into adulthood and present with an intraluminal diverticulum. The thin membrane or web can become stretched and propelled toward the distal duodenal lumen by constant peristalsis, creating the so-called windsock deformity (Fig. 3-4).

Duodenal Duplication

Congenital duplication of the duodenum can be cystic or tubular and may or may not communicate with the lumen. Most are cystic and noncommunicating and located along the medial second part of the duodenum. Patients can have duodenal obstruction, and peptic ulceration or pancreatitis can also occur. At UGI series the affected duodenum is narrowed and displaced in the noncommunicating type, but contrast may fill the cyst when the duplication is communicating. The duplication may be more easily appreciated when it is extraluminal, often identified as a cystic structure medial to the duodenal C-sweep. CT or magnetic resonance imaging (MRI) will usually demonstrate the duplication better (Fig. 3-5). Other diagnoses, including choledochocele, pancreatic pseudocyst, and duodenal diverticulum, may have similar imaging appearances.

*John L. Down (1828-1896), British physician.

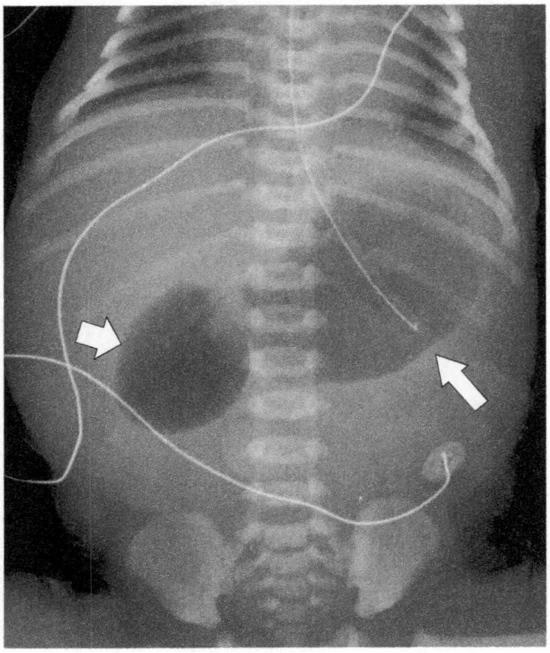

FIGURE 3-2. Plain abdominal film in a neonate with dilatation of the stomach (*large arrow*) and duodenum (*small arrow*) creating the double bubble sign caused by duodenal atresia.

Midgut Malrotation

Midgut malrotation results from malrotation in utero as the duodenum rotates. It is the result of incomplete rotation that is recognized by the ligament of Treitz (represents the junction of the duodenum and jejunum) not migrating to its normal position to the left of the spine. Depending on the degree of malrotation, the ligament of Treitz will be located more inferiorly and to the right. In complete malrotation, it will be located to the right of the spine (Fig. 3-6). The cecal position will vary, usually in the left side of the abdomen with complete malrotation. The intestinal tract is susceptible to volvulus due to abnormal mesenteric anatomy (Fig. 3-7).

Midgut Volvulus

Midgut volvulus is usually diagnosed in childhood and rarely in adulthood. It is an incomplete rotation of the midgut in utero that renders patients susceptible to a volvulus around a congenitally abnormal small bowel mesentery. At UGI series, there is an abrupt tapering of the third part of the duodenum, which is obstructed. Imaging is now usually performed with CT, which

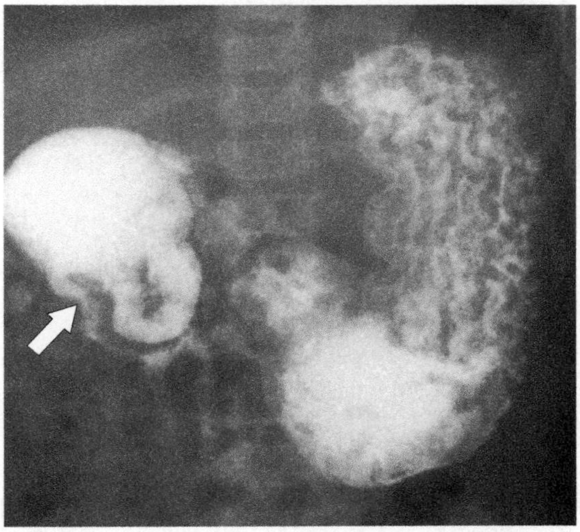

FIGURE 3-3. UGI swallow in a neonate demonstrating a duodenal obstruction (*arrow*) from a congenital duodenal web.

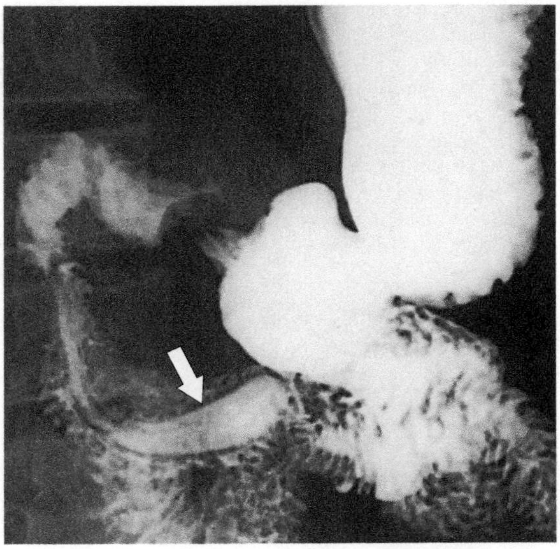

FIGURE 3-4. UGI series demonstrates a tubular filling defect (windsock) in the duodenum due to an intraluminal diverticulum (*arrow*).

identifies a corkscrew or spiral appearance of the mesentery, with the duodenal-jejunal junction positioned inferiorly and to the right of its normal position at the ligament of Treitz (Fig. 3-8). The normal positioning of the superior mesenteric artery (SMA) and superior mesenteric vein (SMV) are frequently reversed (normally the SMA lies to the left of the SMV). UGI series can also demonstrate the corkscrew appearance (Fig. 3-8). An alternative cause of congenital volvulus is a Ladd* band, which is an abnormal fibrous band of tissue at the root of the small bowel mesentery. This abnormality of the mesenteric root also predisposes the patient to malrotation.

*William E. Ladd (1880-1967), American pediatrician.

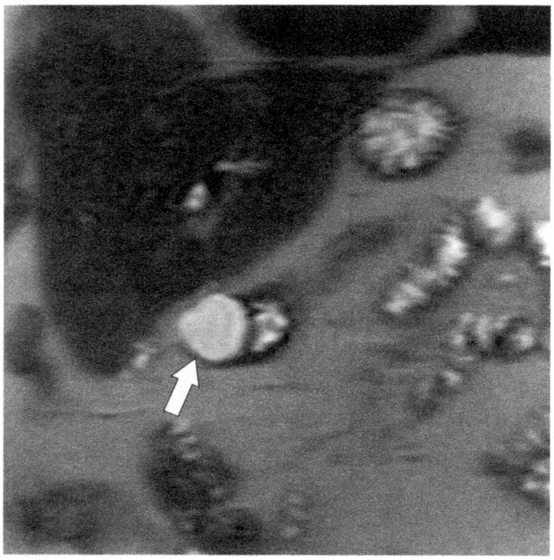

FIGURE 3-5. Coronal T2-weighted MRI in a 34-year-old woman with a hyperintense, smooth, rounded submucosal duodenal mass (*arrow*) due to duodenal duplication.

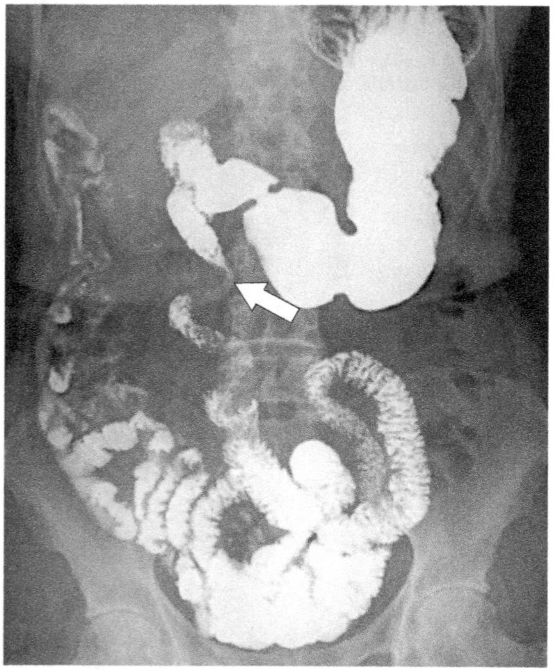

FIGURE 3-6. UGI series and follow-though demonstrating midgut malrotation. The duodenum fails to cross over the midline (*arrow*).

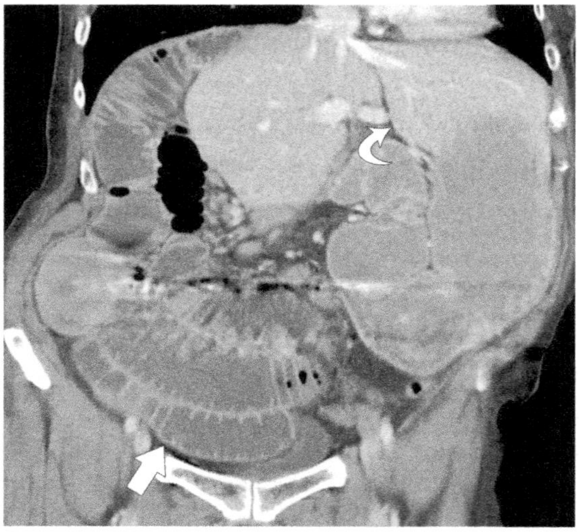

FIGURE 3-7. Coronal contrast-enhanced CT in a 33-year-old man demonstrating a left-sided liver (*curved arrow*) and right-sided bowel (*arrow*). The third and fourth parts of the duodenum do not cross the midline. Volvulus of the small bowel has also occurred, and there is small bowel obstruction.

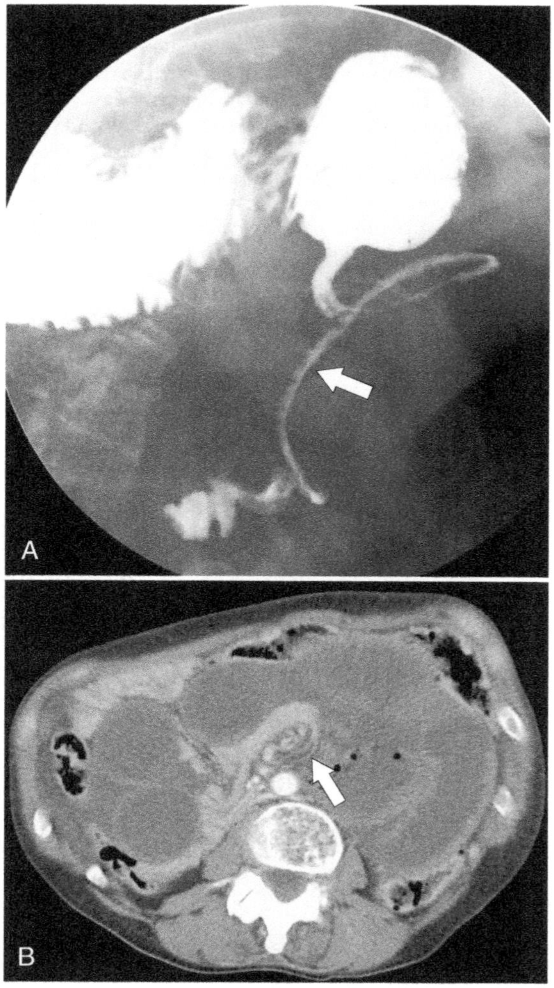

FIGURE 3-8. UGI series (**A**) and axial contrast-enhanced CT (**B**) in a 54-year-old woman with a midgut volvulus (*arrows*) caused by Ladd bands.

Paraduodenal Hernia

Paraduodenal hernias result from congenitally incomplete peritoneal fixation onto the posterior abdominal cavity, creating abnormal peritoneal spaces into which the duodenum and other small bowel can herniate. Therefore the small bowel can be seen in abnormal locations. If it is on the right, the second, third, and fourth parts of the duodenum can be displaced to the right. Left-sided paraduodenal hernias are more common, however, and can sequester large parts of the small bowel into the left upper quadrant, leaving only a small loop of bowel to connect to a normally positioned cecum.

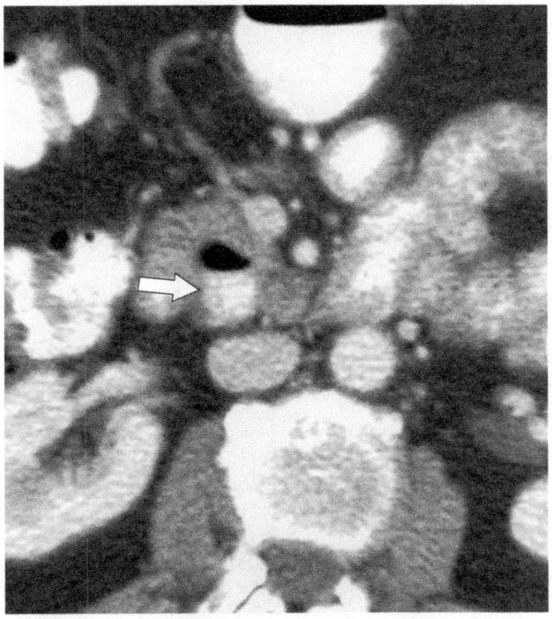

FIGURE 3-9. Axial contrast-enhanced CT in a 61-year-old man with a duodenal diverticulum (*arrow*) with an air/barium fluid level.

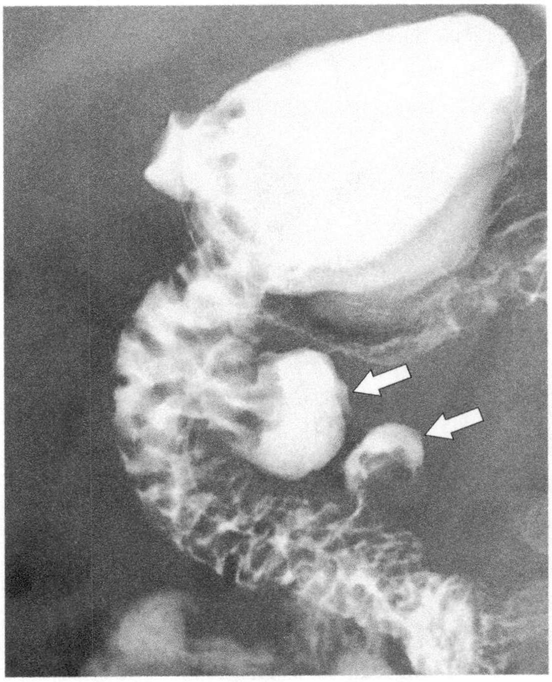

FIGURE 3-10. UGI series in a 38-year-old man with two medial duodenal diverticula (*arrows*).

Duodenal Diverticulum

Extraluminal diverticula are not true diverticula because they represent mucosal herniation through the muscular wall, but they are very common and are frequently identified incidentally at CT or UGI series, occurring mostly on the medial aspect of the second part of the duodenum at or just beyond the periampullary region (Figs. 3-9 and 3-10). Sometimes they can be very large (Fig. 3-11). Less commonly they are in the third and fourth parts of the duodenum (Fig. 3-12). They typically fill with fluid, gas, or both, and knowledge of their frequency, appearance, and location should avoid an erroneous diagnosis of a periduodenal mass or abscess. They are usually insignificant, but there is a risk of inadvertent perforation by endoscopy or feeding-tube placement. Diverticulitis can develop in large diverticula, resulting in fever and upper abdominal pain.

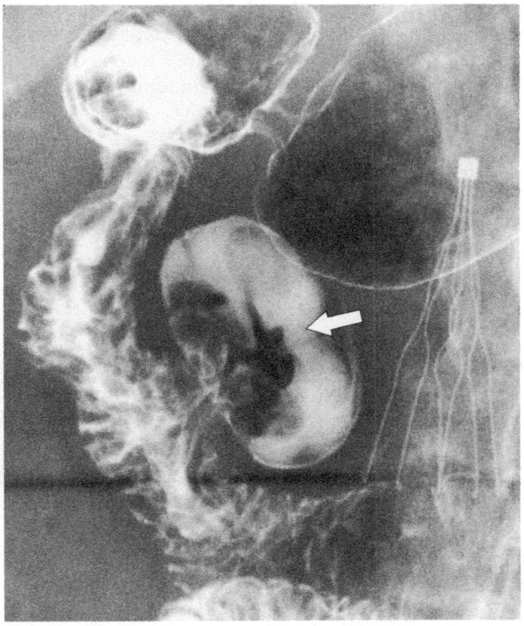

FIGURE 3-11. UGI series in a 65-year-old man with a large medial duodenal diverticulum (*arrow*). Duodenal folds can be seen entering the diverticulum. There is an incidental inferior vena cava filter in situ.

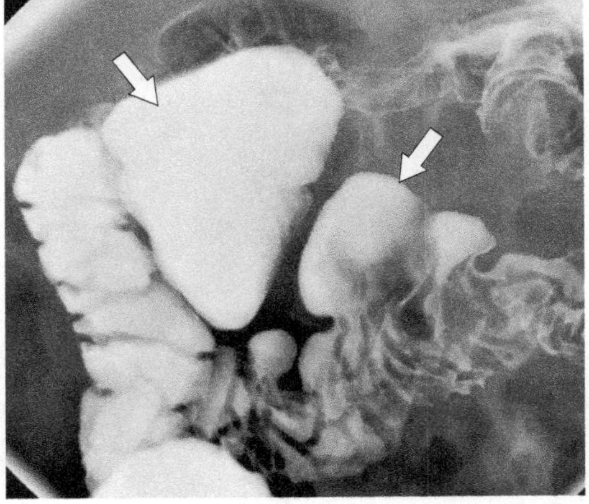

FIGURE 3-12. UGI series in a 61-year-old woman with multiple duodenal diverticula (*arrows*).

Pancreatic Rests

Also known as ectopic pancreas, pancreatic rests are congenital remnants of pancreatic tissue that are most commonly found in the first and second part of the duodenum, although they have also been reported elsewhere in the small bowel and stomach. They are clinically insignificant and usually asymptomatic. They are identified at UGI series or EGD, where they appear as a smooth round or lobulated mucosal filling defect approximately 1 to 2 cm in diameter. A classic central dimple filled with barium, representing the pancreatic ductule remnant, may or may not be present, but it is diagnostic if it is present (Fig. 3-13).

Annular Pancreas

Annular pancreas is an embryological abnormality of pancreatic development that results in the narrowing of the second part of the duodenum because of circumferential constriction by the pancreas. Normal embryological pancreatic development involves a single dorsal and two ventral buds (which fuse early). With normal intestinal rotation at about 7 weeks of gestation, the fused ventral bud rotates behind the duodenum from right to left to fuse with the dorsal bud and forms part of the pancreatic head and the uncinate. Failure of the ventral bud to rotate normally leaves the duodenum encircled by pancreatic tissue. It may remain asymptomatic, particularly with incomplete forms, but complete forms, which may not become symptomatic until adulthood, may require a gastroenterostomy rather than the simple release of the pancreatic annular tissue. At UGI series there is a characteristic narrowed, band-like, and uniform circumferential stricture in the midportion of the second part of the duodenum (Fig. 3-14). CT readily identifies the circumferential pancreatic tissue (Fig. 3-15).

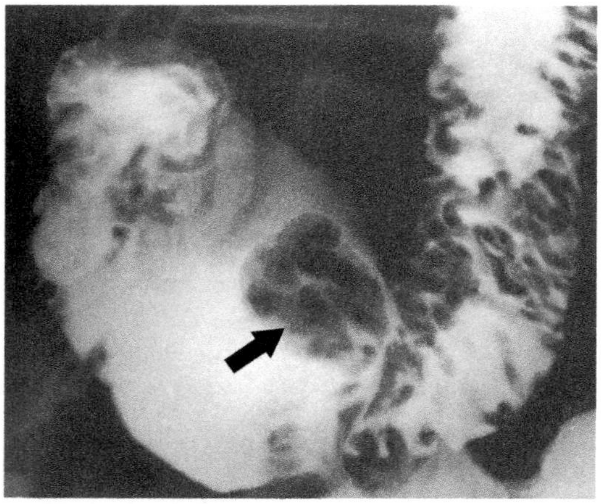

FIGURE 3-13. UGI series demonstrating a small duodenal bulb mass with a central barium collection caused by a pancreatic rest (*arrow*).

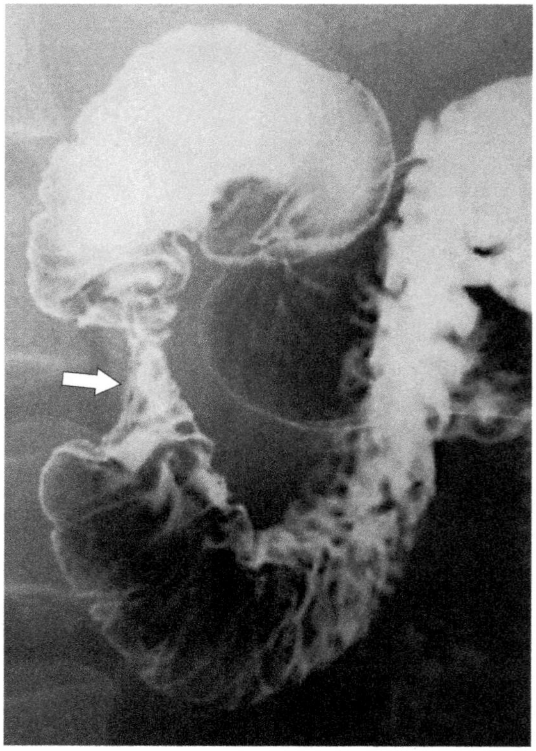

FIGURE 3-14. UGI series in a 45-year-old woman with a stricture of the second part of the duodenum (*arrow*) caused by an annular pancreas.

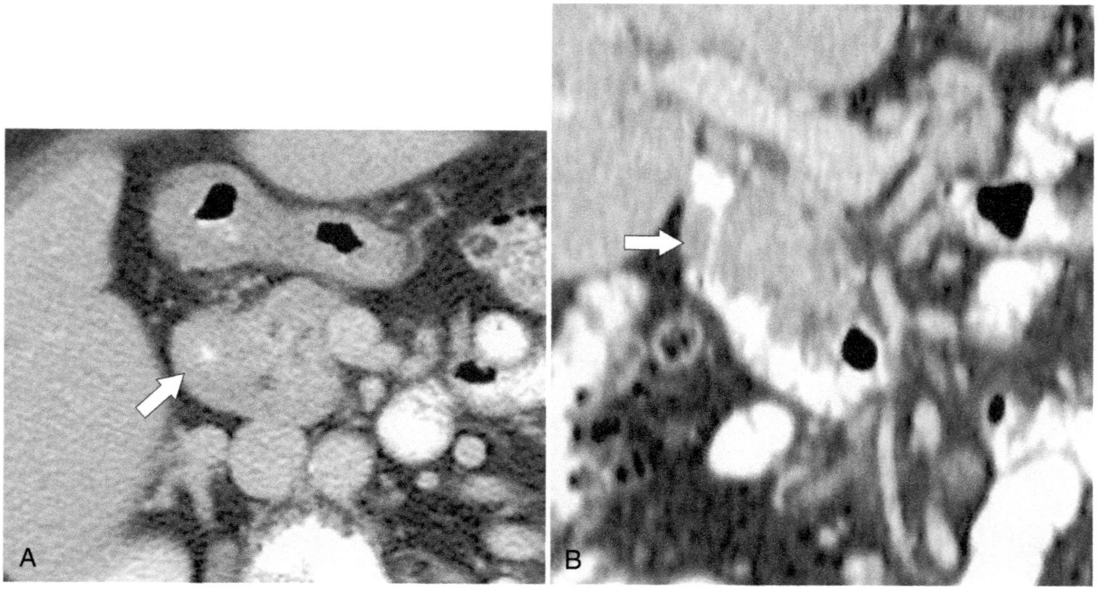

FIGURE 3-15. Axial (**A**) and coronal (**B**) contrast-enhanced CT in a 73-year-old woman with pancreatic annular pancreas (*arrows*) that almost completely occludes the duodenal lumen.

Superior Mesenteric Artery Syndrome

Although SMA syndrome is a congenital abnormality, it usually presents in adulthood, often after significant weight loss from severe acute illness. The theory is that as the retroperitoneal fat is metabolized, the angle between the proximal SMA and aorta becomes more acute, thereby compressing the duodenum that passes left to right immediately beneath this angle. Duodenal and gastric distention then occurs near the obstruction. The diagnosis is made in the correct clinical setting with contrast-enhanced CT demonstrating the features of a dilated duodenum, marked narrowing of the duodenum as it passes behind the SMA, and a relative paucity of retroperitoneal fat (Fig. 3-16). Duodenal narrowing at the level of the SMA, though, can also be a normal finding, and correlation with clinical symptoms is required.

DUODENAL BULB DISEASE

There are a finite number of duodenal bulb diseases, most of which are benign (Box 3-1). Malignant lesions are rare. Normal anatomical structures can impress upon the duodenum (colon and gallbladder), which creates a smooth effacement of the duodenal bulb (Fig. 3-17).

Heterotopic Gastric Mucosa

Heterotopic gastric mucosa represents ectopic gastric mucosa most often situated in the duodenal bulb, although it can occur in the esophagus, jejunum, and even ileum. It can be recognized usually only at double-contrast UGI (or EGD) as small, plaque-like filling defects in a mosaic-like pattern (Fig. 3-18).

Brunner Gland Hyperplasia

Brunner glands secrete alkali, protecting the proximal small intestine from the hyperacidity produced by the gastric mucosa. The cause of their enlargement is uncertain, but multiple Brunner glands can be seen in the duodenal bulb, extending for a short distance into the second part of the duodenum. They are visualized on UGI series, particularly with double-contrast views, which demonstrate multiple small (<5 mm) nodular filling defects (strawberry-like) in the distended duodenal bulb (Fig. 3-19). When there is only one, it is known as Brunner gland adenoma or hamartoma. This can have an appearance similar to flexural pseudotumor if situated at the inferior margin between the duodenal bulb and second part of the duodenum.

Duodenal Flexural Pseudotumor or Pseudopolyp

Duodenal flexural pseudotumor or pseudopolyp is a normal variant in which the angle between the duodenal apex and the descending duodenum is particularly acute, and it is more common in thin, asthenic individuals. The duodenal mucosa on the inner (inferior) aspect of this abrupt angle is sometimes heaped up into the duodenal lumen, giving the spurious appearance of a mass (Fig. 3-20). Repositioning the patient on the fluoroscopy

Box 3-1. Duodenal Bulb Abnormalities

Heterotopic gastric mucosa
Brunner gland hypertrophy and adenoma
Flexural pseudotumor
Peptic erosions and ulcer
Neoplastic (GIST, adenoma, carcinoma, lymphoma)

GIST, Gastrointestinal stromal tumor.

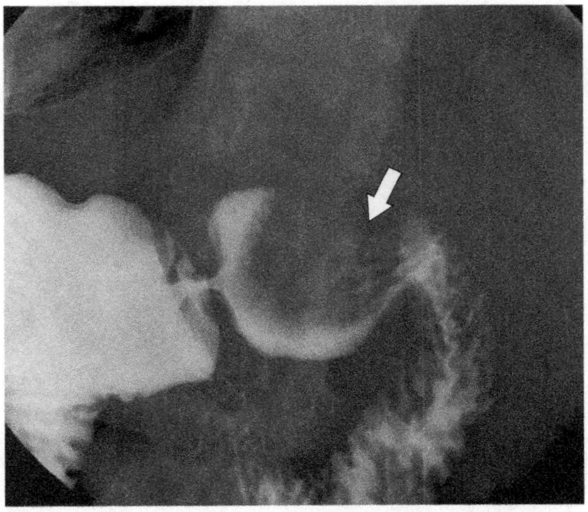

FIGURE 3-17. UGI series in a 39-year-old woman with smooth effacement of the duodenal bulb (*arrow*) caused by duodenal compression by the gallbladder.

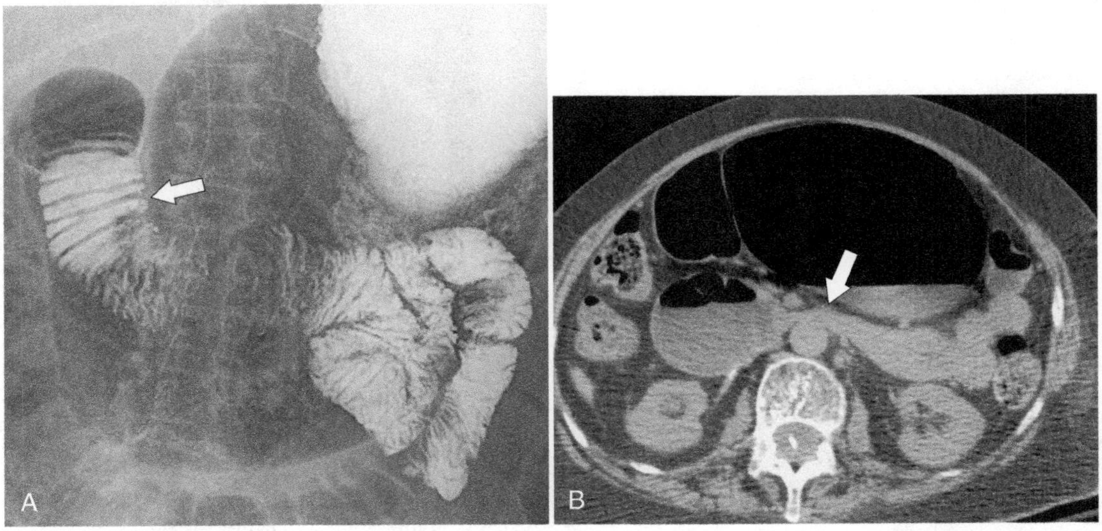

FIGURE 3-16. UGI (**A**) and axial (**B**) contrast-enhanced CT in a 65-year-old woman demonstrating gastric and duodenum dilatation (*arrow* in **A**) and stricture formation (*arrow* in **B**) due to superior mesenteric artery syndrome.

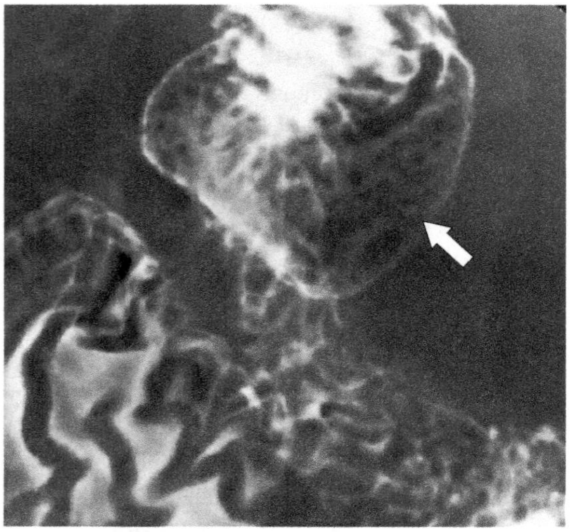

FIGURE 3-18. UGI in a 61-year-old woman with multiple small filling defects in the duodenal bulb (*arrow*) caused by ectopic gastric mucosa.

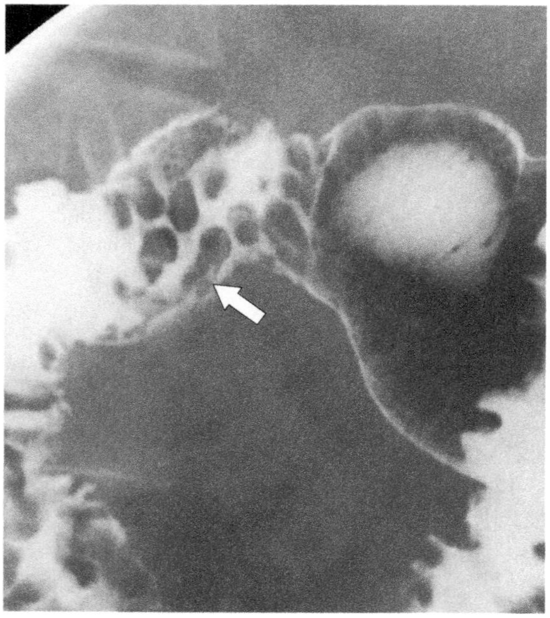

FIGURE 3-19. UGI series in a 55-year-old man with multiple nodular filling defects in the duodenal bulb caused by Brunner gland hypertrophy (*arrow*).

table, though, should diminish the abnormality or make it disappear altogether, which clarifies the diagnosis. At CT, it can appear as a definitive duodenal mass or polyp.

Duodenitis

Most causes of gastritis also cause duodenitis because of the duodenum's proximity to the stomach (see Chapter 2). The imaging features also mimic features of gastritis, including fold thickening and erosions (Fig. 3-21). More severe ulceration can progress to a duodenal ulcer. At CT, there is duodenal wall thickening and thickened folds, but these findings are nonspecific (Fig. 3-22).

Duodenal Ulcer

Although it still an important disease, duodenal ulcer is far less common now that *H. pylori* is known as a causative agent and its treatment is well understood. Furthermore, most patients are now evaluated by EGD, so radiologists will now be unlikely to see many duodenal ulcers in the course of their clinical work.

Duodenal ulcers are two to three times more common than gastric ulcers, but unlike gastric ulcers, almost all duodenal ulcers are benign. Approximately 95% occur in the duodenal bulb, with 5% being postbulbar. Ulcers arise from gastric hyperacidity or other caustic agents such as alcohol or drugs, especially aspirin and nonsteroidal antiinflammatory agents. The disease is frequently associated with the features of peptic disease in the stomach (concomitant gastric fold thickening is common).

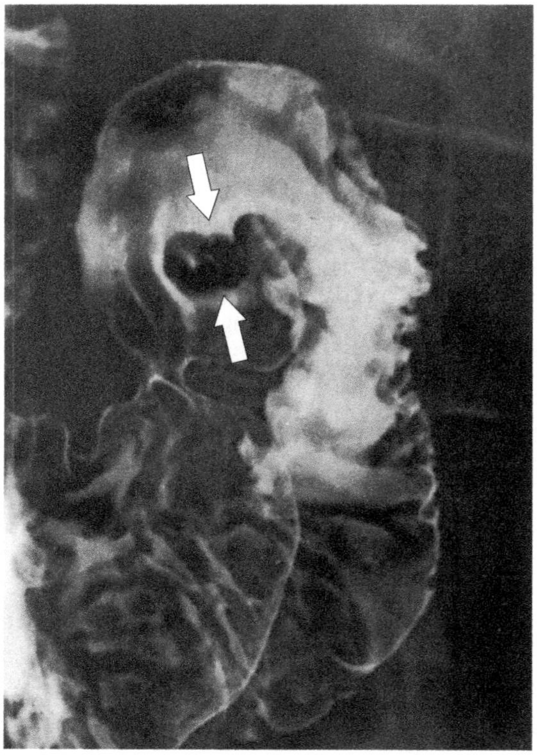

FIGURE 3-20. UGI series demonstrating a smooth duodenal polyp, identified as a duodenal flexural pseudopolyp (*arrows*).

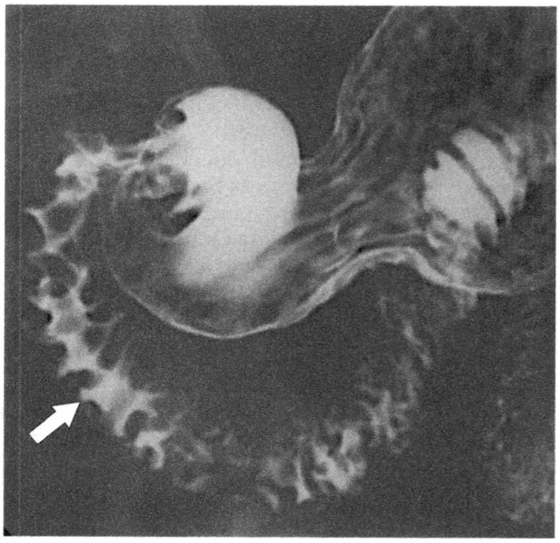

FIGURE 3-21. UGI in a 22-year-old woman with antral and duodenal mucosal thickening caused by gastritis (*arrow*) and secondary duodenitis.

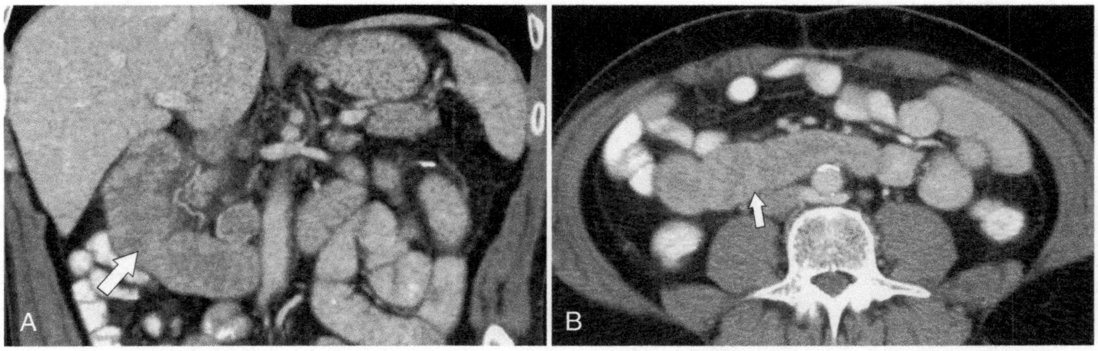

FIGURE 3-22. Coronal (**A**) and axial (**B**) contrast-enhanced CT in a 49-year-old woman with duodenal wall thickening (*arrows*) caused by duodenitis.

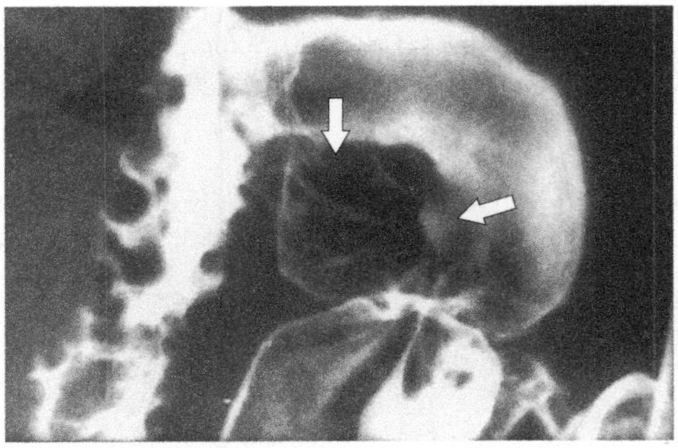

FIGURE 3-23. UGI series in a 44-year-old man with thickened folds (*vertical arrow*) radiating toward an ulcer crater (*horizontal arrow*) from an acute duodenal ulcer.

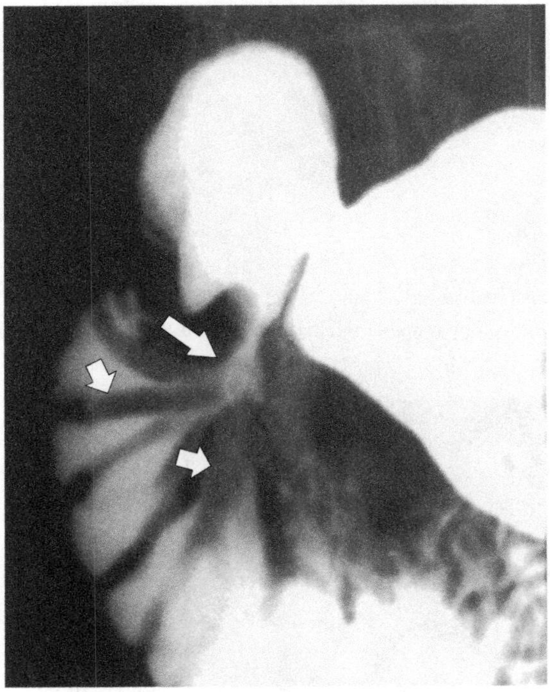

FIGURE 3-24. UGI series in a 61-year-old woman with a postbulbar ulcer (*large arrow*) and radiating thickened duodenal folds (*small arrows*).

Their appearance is best evaluated with single-contrast and double-contrast UGI series, where a persistent pooling of contrast material within the ulcer crater can be observed, especially when the ulcer crater is in the dependent position. There are smooth folds that converge on the acute ulcer (Fig. 3-23). Some ulcers

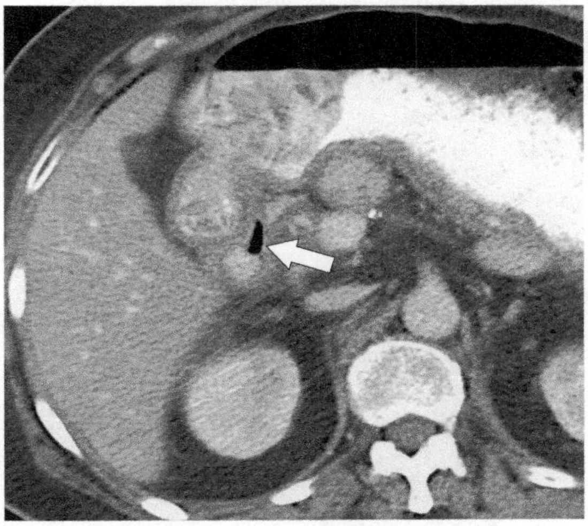

FIGURE 3-25. Axial contrast-enhanced CT in a 46-year-old woman with a perforated duodenal ulcer. There is wall thickening of the proximal duodenal wall, mild surrounding edema, and a sliver of extraluminal gas (*arrow*).

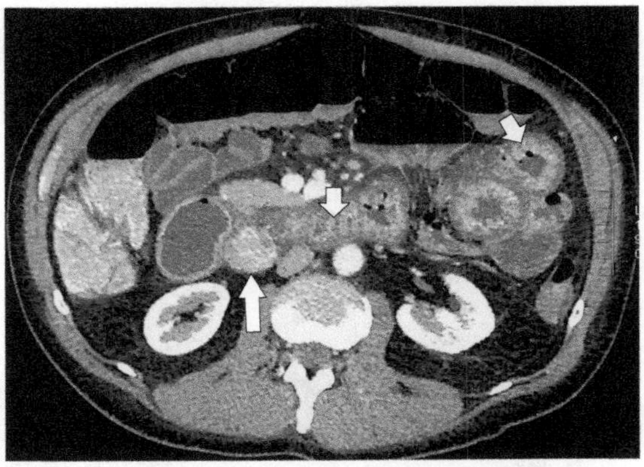

FIGURE 3-26. Axial contrast-enhanced CT in a 36-year-old man with a duodenal gastrinoma (*large arrow*) and Zollinger-Ellison syndrome with marked duodenal and jejunal mucosal thickening (*small arrows*).

form beyond the bulb and are termed *postbulbar ulcers* (Fig. 3-24). Most ulcers cannot be seen with CT, but deep ones are occasionally identified (Fig. 3-25). Postbulbar ulcers are more common in patients with severe gastric hyperacidity such as Zollinger-Ellison syndrome (see Chapter 2). The hyperacidity can be so severe that duodenitis continues into the fourth part of the duodenum and even into the jejunum (Fig. 3-26).

The ulcer typically heals by fibrosis distorting the normal architecture of the duodenal bulb, although both acute ulcers and

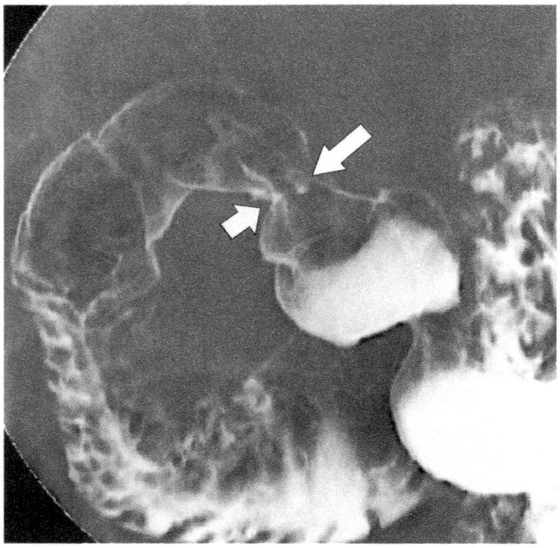

Figure 3-27. UGI series in a 66-year-old woman with proximal duodenal narrowing and distortion (*large arrow*) caused by healing from chronic duodenal ulcer disease. A tiny acute ulcer is also present (*small arrow*).

chronic findings can be seen at the same time (Fig. 3-27). Occasionally the ulcers can be very large, known as *giant duodenal ulcers*, and may mimic the configuration of the bulb itself, potentially leading the radiologist to think that the ulcer is a normal bulb. There should, however, be no duodenal folds within the ulcer itself, and there is persistent pooling of contrast rather than the contrast passing on down the duodenum from the normal peristaltic waves.

The most serious complication is perforation caused by transmural penetration of the ulcer, which mainly occurs into the peritoneum because most (95%) bulbar ulcers are on the anterior wall. Less commonly, retroperitoneal perforation occurs from the rarer posterior wall ulcers. Subtle perforation may require CT analysis with lung "window" contrast settings; otherwise, subtle extraluminal gas may be missed. Perforation can also cause severe hemorrhage with profuse hematemesis or melena. The ulcer itself is often not identified at CT, but the diagnosis is strongly suggested by duodenal mucosal thickening and periduodenal inflammation (stranding), fluid, and gas (Fig. 3-28). Sometimes there is profuse gas that can be both intraperitoneal and extraperitoneal (Fig. 3-29).

Thickened Duodenal Folds

Duodenal mucosal thickening is generally not confined to the bulb unless it is due to peptic ulcer disease. There are several

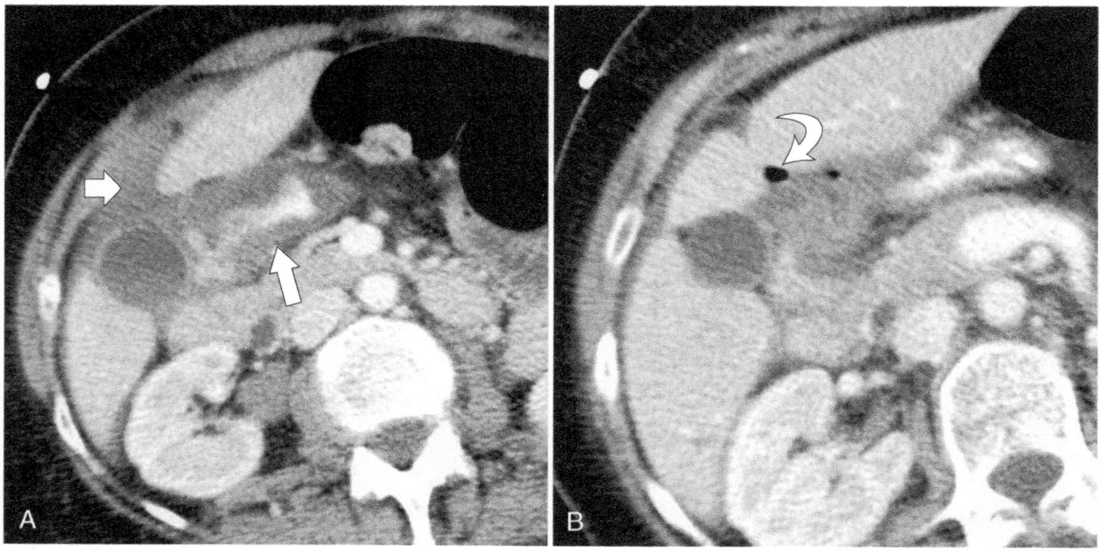

Figure 3-28. Axial CT in a 60-year-old woman with duodenal perforation as evidenced by mucosal thickening (**A**; *arrow*) and periduodenal fluid (**A**; *small arrow*) and pockets of extraluminal gas (**B**; *curved arrow*).

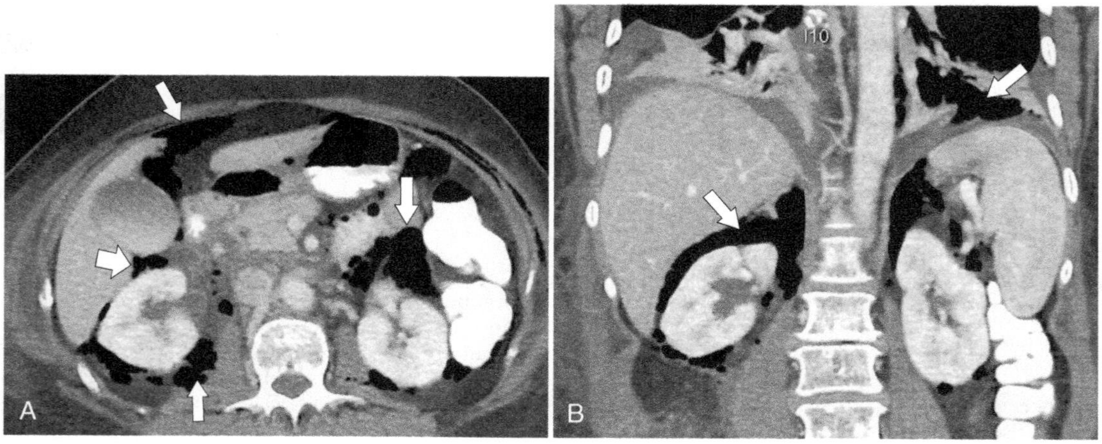

Figure 3-29. Axial (**A**) and coronal (**B**) contrast-enhanced CT in a 62-year-old woman with a perforated duodenal ulcer and diffuse retroperitoneal and peritoneal gas (*arrows*).

BOX 3-2. Thickened Duodenal Folds

Inflammatory: peptic ulcer disease
Pancreatitis, Zollinger-Ellison syndrome
Infectious: parasites, tuberculosis
Caustic ingestion
Crohn disease
Eosinophilic gastroenteritis
Whipple disease
Amyloid
Vascular: varices, hemorrhage
Malignancy: adenocarcinoma, lymphoma

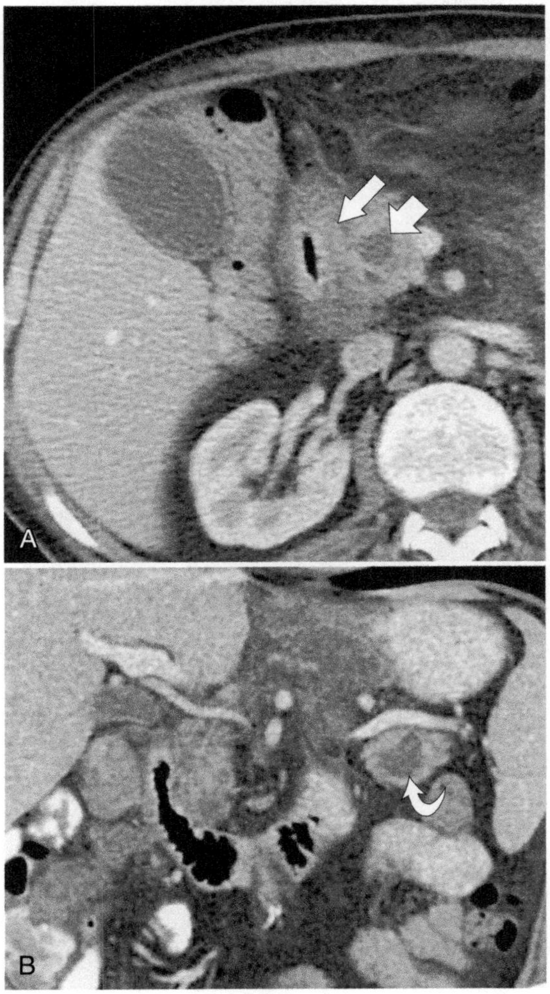

FIGURE 3-30. Axial (**A**) and coronal (**B**) contrast-enhanced CT in a 52-year-old man with duodenal wall thickening (*large arrow*) and luminal narrowing due to acute pancreatitis. There are small fluid collections (*small arrow*) in the pancreatic head and tail (*curved arrow*).

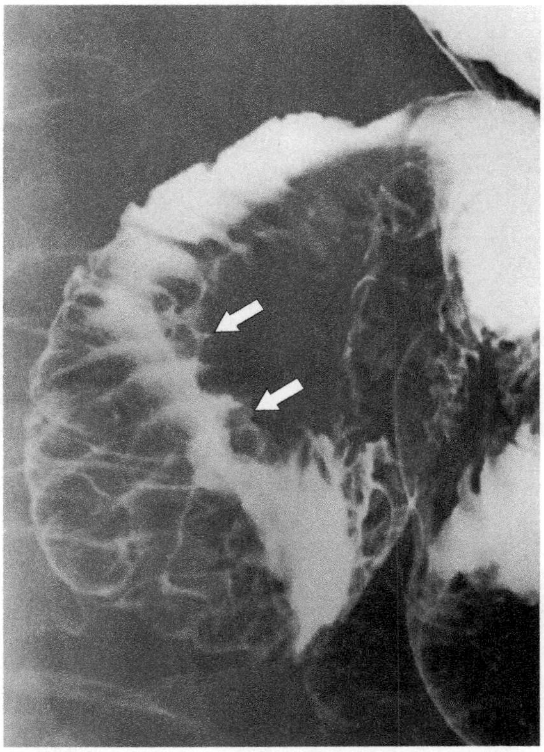

FIGURE 3-31. UGI series demonstrating marked duodenal wall and mucosal thickening caused by acute pancreatitis (*arrows*). There is a "reverse 3" pattern.

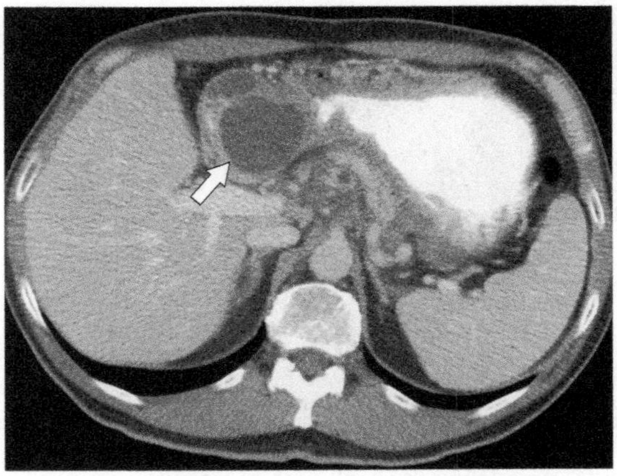

FIGURE 3-32. Axial contrast-enhanced CT in a 52-year-old man with pancreatic pseudocyst (*arrow*) and compression of the second part of the duodenum.

disparate causes, most of which are responsible for mucosal thickening of the gastrointestinal tract elsewhere (Box 3-2). Many intrinsic or extrinsic inflammatory conditions can affect a part of or the entire duodenum. The second part of the duodenum surrounds the pancreatic head, so diseases of the pancreas can have a direct effect on the duodenal wall and mucosa. Pancreatitis frequently causes gastric and duodenal wall inflammation and is usually visualized by CT or UGI series (Figs. 3-30 and 3-31). At UGI series, the medial wall can appear tethered on its medial wall by the inflammatory process, causing medial spiculation that has been described as a "reverse 3" pattern that is also recognized with pancreatic adenocarcinoma. More chronic pancreatic pseudocyst changes can result in duodenal stricture formation (Fig. 3-32). Groove pancreatitis (see Chapter 9), occurring in the duodenal-pancreatic groove, will inevitably cause duodenal thickening (Fig. 3-33). Other adjacent anatomical structures, including the gallbladder (cholecystitis) and colon (diverticulitis), can cause the same effect (Fig. 3-34). Adjacent malignant infiltration may cause nonspecific duodenal thickening early on, but as further duodenal invasion occurs, the duodenal lumen and mucosa will be distorted (Fig. 3-35).

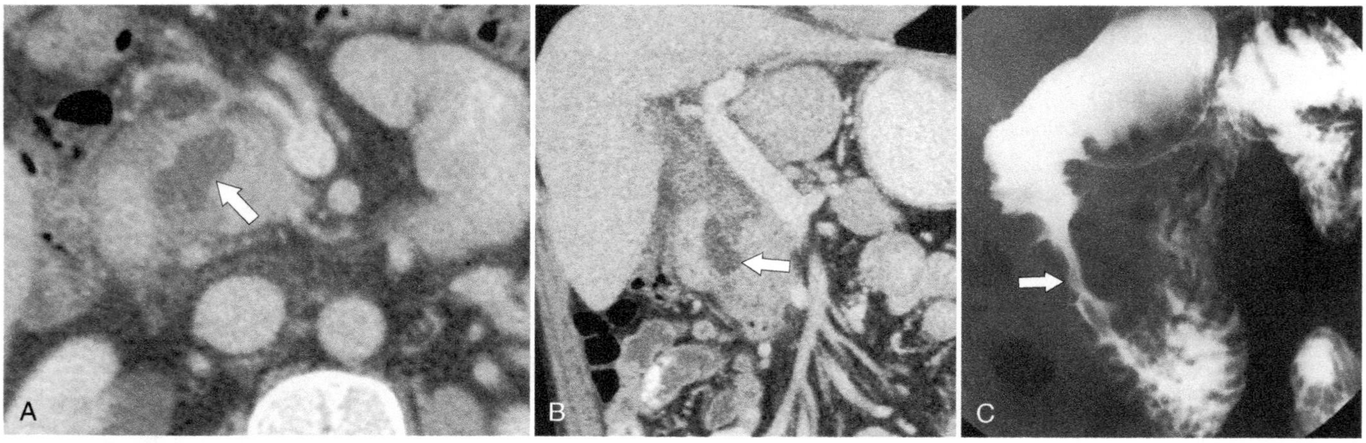

Figure 3-33. Axial (**A**) and coronal (**B**) CT and UGI series (**C**) in a 44-year-old man with inflammation and cystic formation in the pancreatic-duodenal space caused by "groove" pancreatitis (*arrows*).

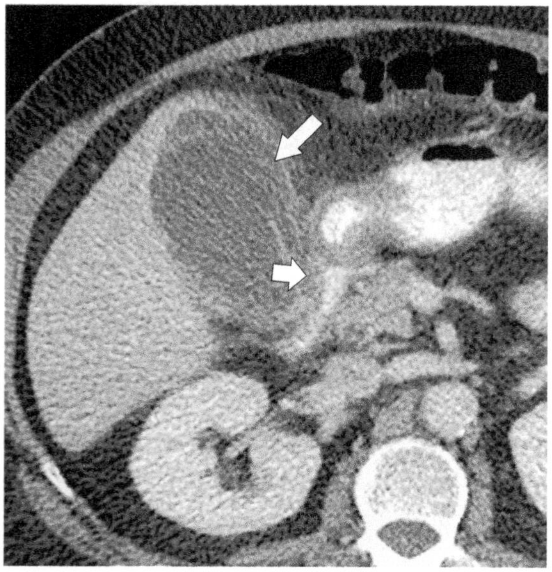

Figure 3-34. Axial contrast-enhanced CT in 79-year-old woman with acute cholecystitis (*large arrow*) with duodenal wall thickening and narrowing (*small arrow*).

INFECTIONS

Tuberculosis (see Chapters 2, 4, and 5), as elsewhere in the GI tract, can produce acute disease with mucosal thickening and ulceration. It also typically heals with fibrosis and stricture formation, leading to proximal duodenal dilatation.

Many parasites can infest the duodenum, in particular, *Strongyloides stercoralis* and *Ancylostoma duodenale* (hookworm) and cause markedly thickened duodenal folds. *Ascaris lumbricoides* more often affects the distal small bowel, but because of its endemic infestation in many developing countries, it is not uncommonly identified in the duodenum. It is also purported to be one of the most common causes worldwide of pancreatitis as a result of the worm tunneling into the pancreatic and/or bile duct and occluding pancreatic secretions from reaching the duodenum. The pancreatitis itself will further contribute to the duodenal fold thickening. The worms are recognized as tubular, elongated filling defects at UGI series or CT (Fig. 3-36).

Giardia lamblia is another common worldwide parasite that infests much of the local population. The protozoan leads to diffuse duodenal and jejunal mucosal thickening, usually with hypersecretion and hypermotility and associated lymphoid hyperplasia (see Chapter 4) (Figs. 3-37 and 3-38).

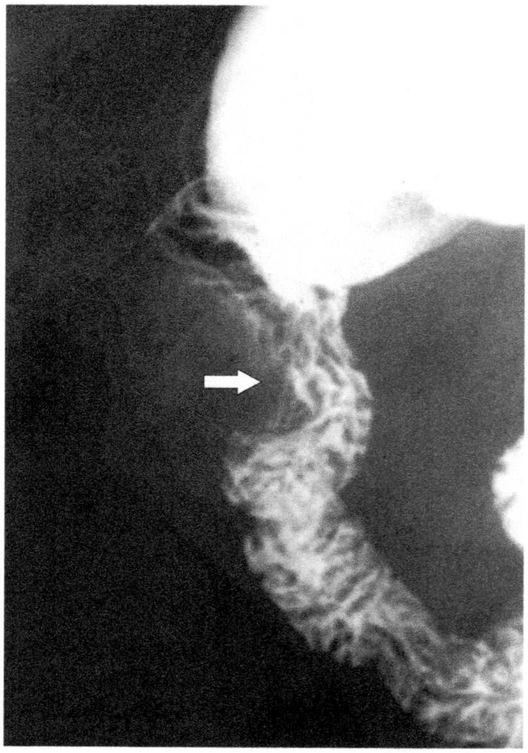

Figure 3-35. UGI series in a 63-year-old man with duodenal distortion (*arrow*) but general preservation of mucosal folds caused by early metastatic invasion by an adjacent hepatic flexure colon cancer.

Caustic Ingestion

Large volumes of caustic ingestion can reach the duodenum and will cause a profound duodenitis. Perforation may occur, but this is usually more proximal in the esophagus or stomach. Fibrotic healing can lead to fixed strictures (see Fig. 3-31).

Crohn Disease (see Chapter 4)

Crohn disease that involves the duodenum usually manifests as thickened folds and ulceration rather than stricture and fistula formation, although these are well-recognized complications (Fig. 3-39). There is usually associated involvement of the terminal ileum, the colon, or both.

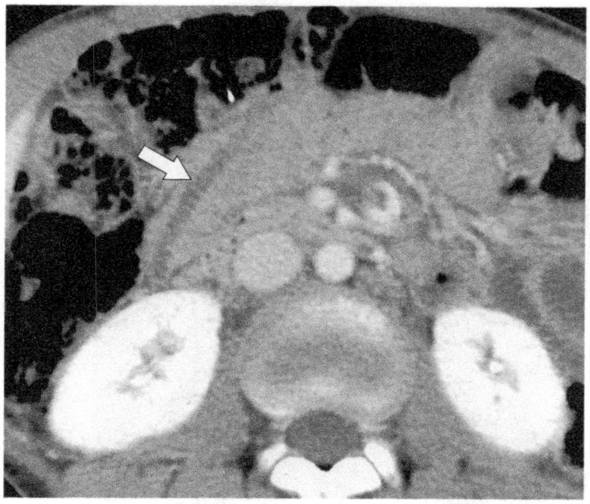

FIGURE 3-36. Axial contrast-enhanced CT in a 12-year-old boy with *Ascaris* worm in the second part of the duodenum (*arrow*).

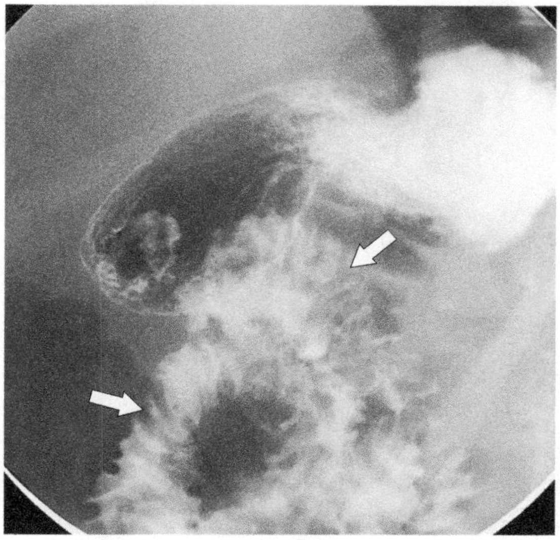

FIGURE 3-37. UGI series in a 10-year-old boy with diffuse duodenal and jejunal thickening (*arrows*) caused by giardiasis.

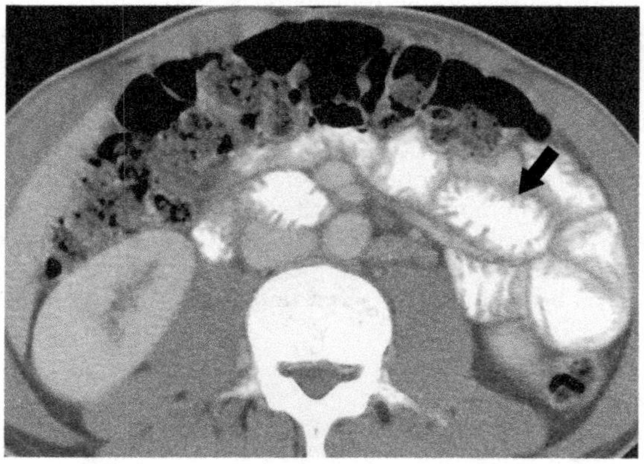

FIGURE 3-38. Axial contrast-enhanced CT in a 29-year-old woman with giardiasis. There is duodenal and jejunal mucosal thickening (*arrow*).

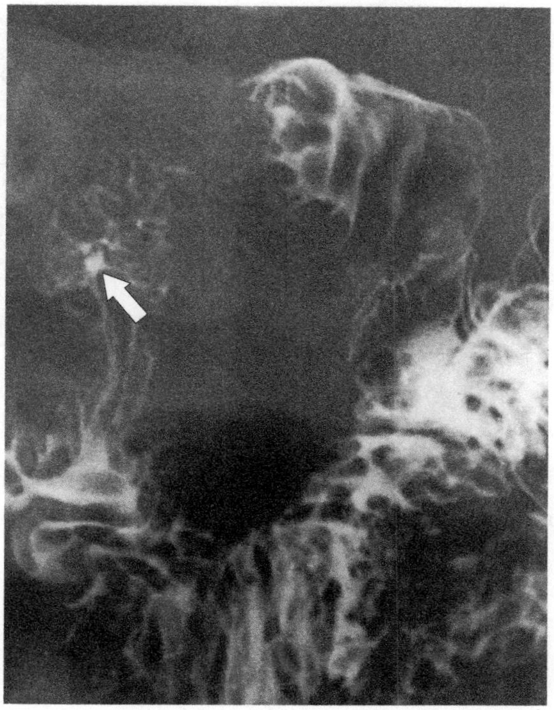

FIGURE 3-39. UGI series in a patient with duodenal Crohn disease demonstrating proximal fold irregularity and ulceration (*arrow*).

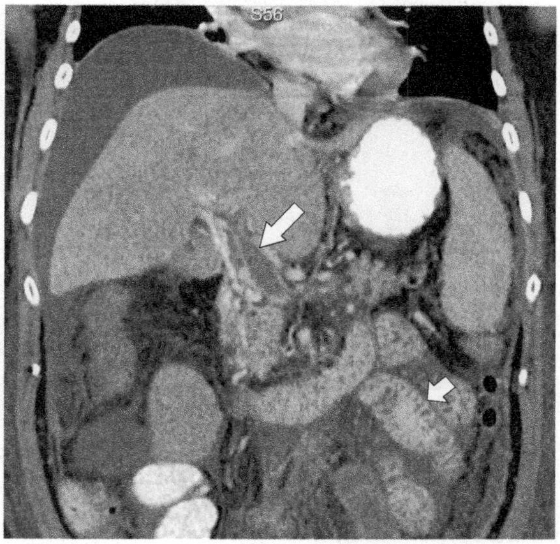

FIGURE 3-40. Coronal contrast-enhanced CT in a 68-year-old woman with a portal vein thrombus (*large arrow*) and diffuse duodenal and jejunal mucosal thickening (*small arrow*). There is associated ascites.

Duodenal Varices

Duodenal varices are rare and result from marked portal hypertension but are a recognized cause of duodenal mucosal thickening, which may be serpiginous in appearance as the dilated veins course through the duodenum.

Portal Hypertension

Any cause of portal hypertension (cirrhosis, portal vein thrombus) can cause duodenal mucosal thickening because of elevated venous pressure (Fig. 3-40).

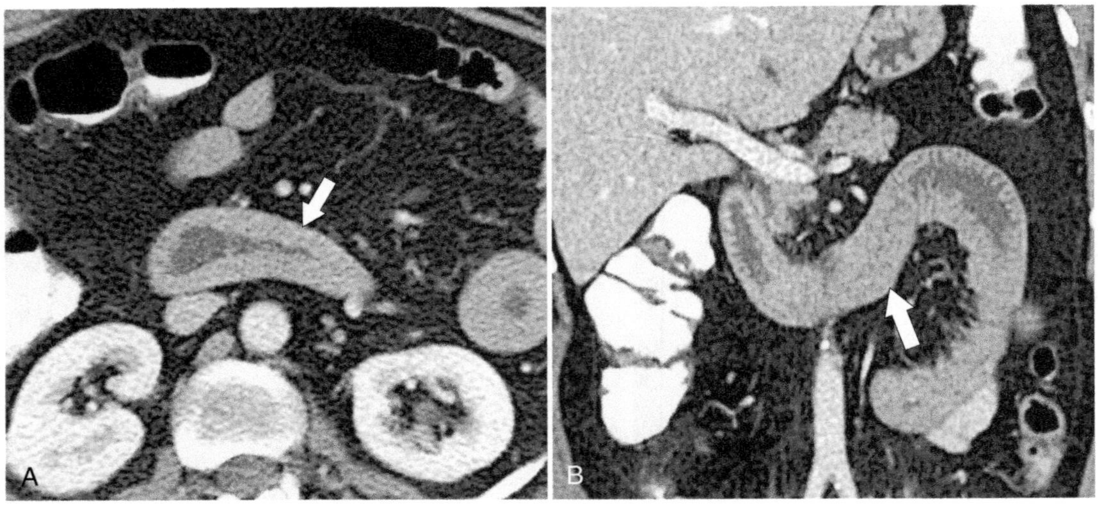

FIGURE 3-41. Axial (**A**) and coronal (**B**) contrast-enhanced CT in a 43-year-old woman with duodenal hemorrhage and diffuse duodenal thickening (*arrows*).

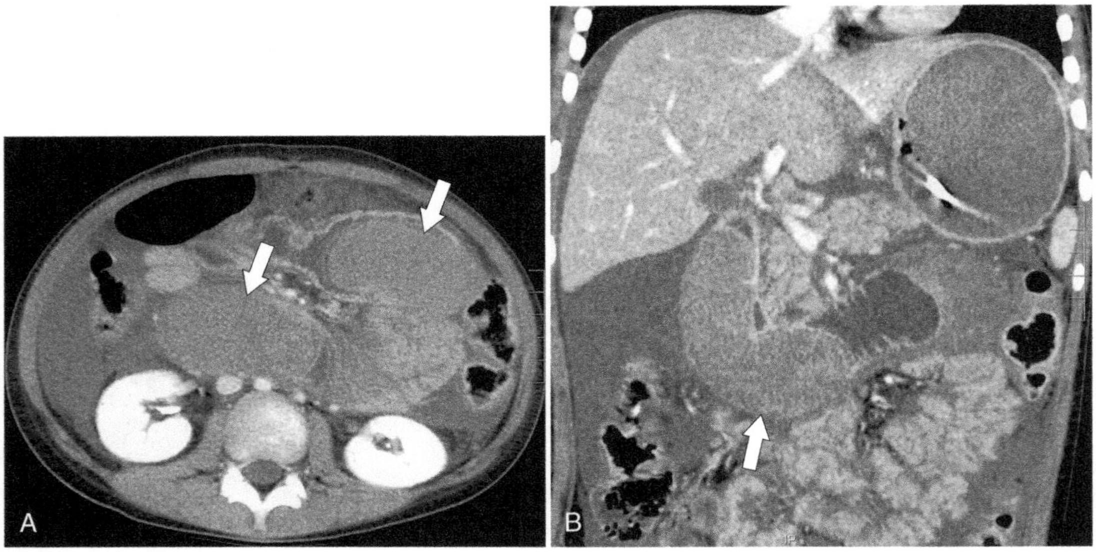

FIGURE 3-42. Axial (**A**) and coronal (**B**) contrast-enhanced CT in a 22-year-old woman after a motor vehicle accident, demonstrating duodenal widening with luminal hemorrhage (*arrows*), mucosal thickening, and ascites.

Lymphoid Hyperplasia

Lymphoid hyperplasia is recognized as multiple tiny filling defects within the duodenum and can be a normal variant in children. When seen in adults, though, it is usually associated with giardiasis and hypogammaglobulinemia.

Duodenal Papillitis

When inflamed, the duodenal papilla can protrude into the duodenal lumen with the appearance of a smooth-walled mass. It is usually a result of an impacted gallstone or pancreatic stone.

Duodenal Hemorrhage

Hemorrhage into the duodenal wall can result spontaneously from trauma, in patients with bleeding diatheses or those taking anticoagulants, and from Henoch-Schönlein purpura (see Chapter 4). The findings can present as either an intramural mass or thickened mucosal folds (Fig. 3-41). Traumatic duodenal injury can result in marked hemorrhage, particularly as the duodenum is relatively fixed in the retroperitoneum and susceptible to acceleration/deceleration forces (Fig. 3-42). At imaging there are thickened and crowded mucosal folds due to the intramural hemorrhage, which at UGI series are thought to resemble a picket fence (see Chapter 4). CT features may even demonstrate a hyperdense duodenal wall, particularly if the patient has been imaged without oral and intravenous contrast material.

Duodenal Masses

Most benign and malignant duodenal masses are common to other lesions elsewhere in the GI tract, although there are some that are unique to the duodenum (Table 3-1).

SUBMUCOSAL MESENCHYMAL DUODENAL TUMORS

Gastrointestinal Stromal Tumor (see Chapter 2)

The duodenum is the second most common site for gastrointestinal stromal tumor (GIST) after the stomach and has similar features to gastric GISTs. These tumors are usually exophytic and eccentric and spare the mucosa, although larger tumors may cause mucosal ulceration. These larger tumors tend to also undergo central necrosis (Fig. 3-43).

Other Benign Submucosal Duodenal Lesions

Duodenal lipomas are relatively common submucosal tumors, and given their malleability, they often appear intraluminal. They are readily characterized at CT because of their fat density (Fig. 3-44). Other rare mesenchymal tumors include hemangioma, lymphangioma, fibroma, and neurofibroma, all of which usually demonstrate features of submucosal lesions (Fig. 3-45).

TABLE 3-1 Duodenal Masses

Congenital	Pancreatic rest Polyposis syndromes
Normal variant	Flexural pseudopolyp Brunner gland hypertrophy
Neoplasia	
Intrinsic	Mesenchymal: GIST, neurofibroma, hemangioma, lipoma Polyps (adenoma, hamartoma) Carcinoid Carcinoma Kaposi sarcoma
Extrinsic	Metastases Lymphoma Pancreatic, gallbladder, colonic, renal, adrenal extension
Inflammatory	Pancreatitis including fluid collections
Extrinsic compression	Gallbladder, hepatic, choledochal cyst, retroperitoneal lymphadenopathy

GIST, Gastrointestinal stromal tumor.

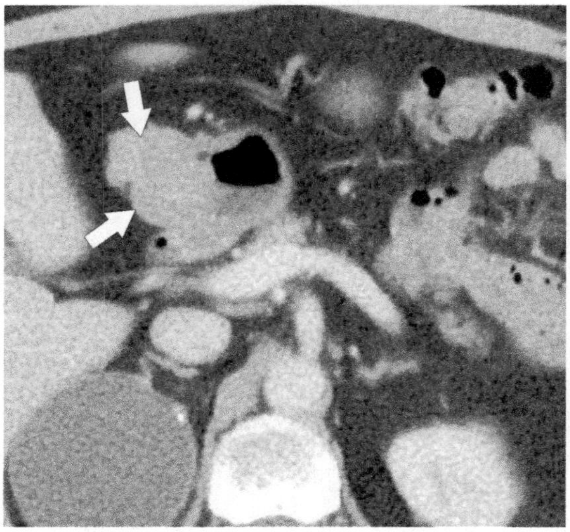

FIGURE 3-43. Axial contrast-enhanced CT in a 56-year-old man with a benign GIST of the first part of the duodenum (*arrows*). The mass is mainly exophytic.

Duodenal Carcinoid

These are submucosal (intramural), usually situated close to the duodenal ampulla, and can range from smooth polyps to irregular invasive masses (Fig. 3-46). In general, they do not arise from enterochromaffin cells, unlike their jejunal and ileal counterparts, and therefore rarely produce serotonin and carcinoid syndrome. Most are gastrin cell (G cell) tumors and therefore some manifest as Zollinger-Ellison syndrome. They are associated with multiple endocrine neoplasia (MEN-1) and neurofibromatosis (NF-1).

Duodenal Polyps

Adenomatous polyps are similar to those elsewhere in the small and large bowel, and these are premalignant, especially if greater

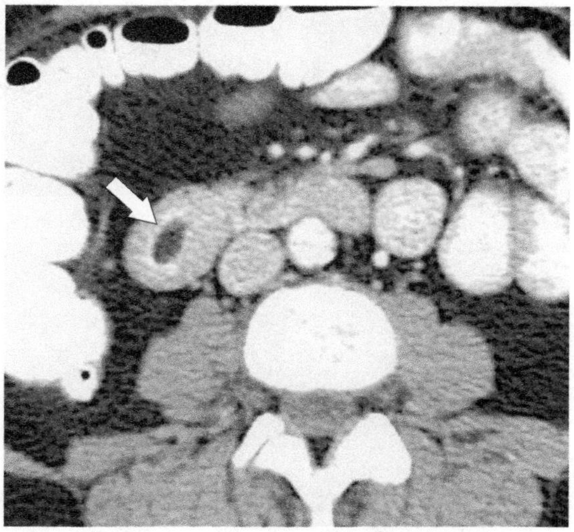

FIGURE 3-44. Axial contrast-enhanced CT in a 44-year-old man with a duodenal lipoma. CT confirms the mass with fat density (*arrow*).

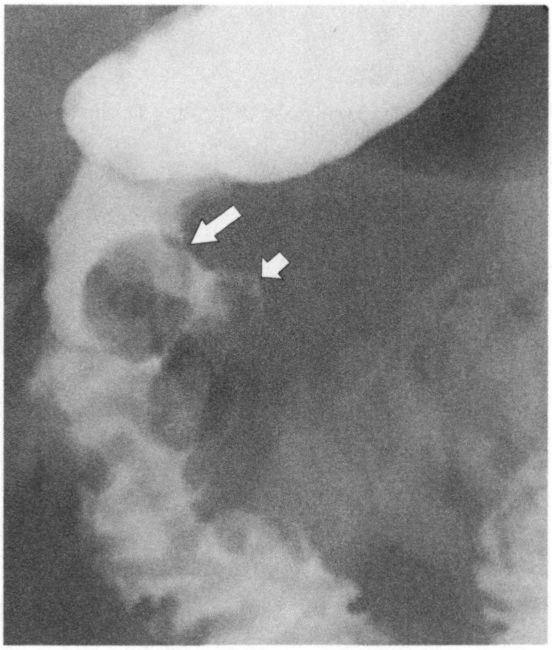

FIGURE 3-45. UGI in a 63-year-old man with a submucosal mass (*large arrow*) caused by a duodenal lymphangioma. There is an associated microperforation (*small arrow*) after recent upper endoscopy and biopsy of the mass.

than 2 cm. Most are tubular with tubulovillous and villous being less common (Fig. 3-47). Patients usually have GI bleeding or obstructive symptoms from intussusception. Adenomatous polyps are more readily recognized at UGI rather than at CT as an irregular polypoid mass, usually close to the duodenal bulb or medial aspect of the second part of the duodenum (Fig. 3-48). Occasionally they appear as a more solid mass (Fig. 3-49).

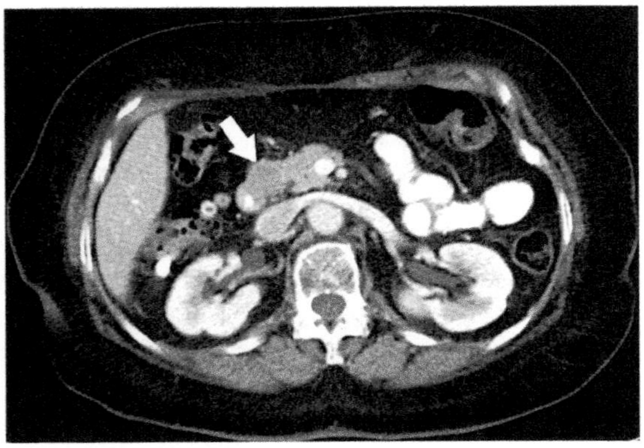

FIGURE 3-46. Axial contrast-enhanced CT in a 42-year-old man with an eccentric 2.5-cm duodenal mass (*arrow*) caused by carcinoid.

Hyperplastic polyps are rare benign epithelial sessile polyps, usually small and multiple within the duodenum. They are far less common than gastric hyperplastic polyps.

Familial polyposis, Peutz-Jeghers syndrome (hamartomatous polyps), Cronkhite-Canada syndrome, and Cowden's disease (see Chapter 5) can all demonstrate duodenal polyposis, although at contrast fluoroscopy, it is not possible to distinguish them. Usually a family history or other manifestations of the disease (e.g., mucocutaneous pigmentation in Peutz-Jeghers syndrome) are a clue to the diagnosis.

Duodenal Carcinoma

Duodenal carcinomas are rare, although they are the most common malignant duodenal tumors. They develop from the adenoma-carcinoma sequence (see Chapter 5), so all duodenal adenomas should be considered premalignant. Other predisposing factors include familial polyposis syndromes, particularly Gardner syndrome. They present with upper abdominal pain, nausea, vomiting, and malignant symptoms of weight loss and anemia. At imaging, they have characteristic features similar to adenocarcinoma elsewhere in the GI tract. Most are in the mid to distal duodenum and present with an irregular intraluminal mass (with or without ulceration) or an apple core appearance, especially if presenting late (Figs. 3-50 and 3-51). Malignancy is confirmed if there is associated regional lymphadenopathy.

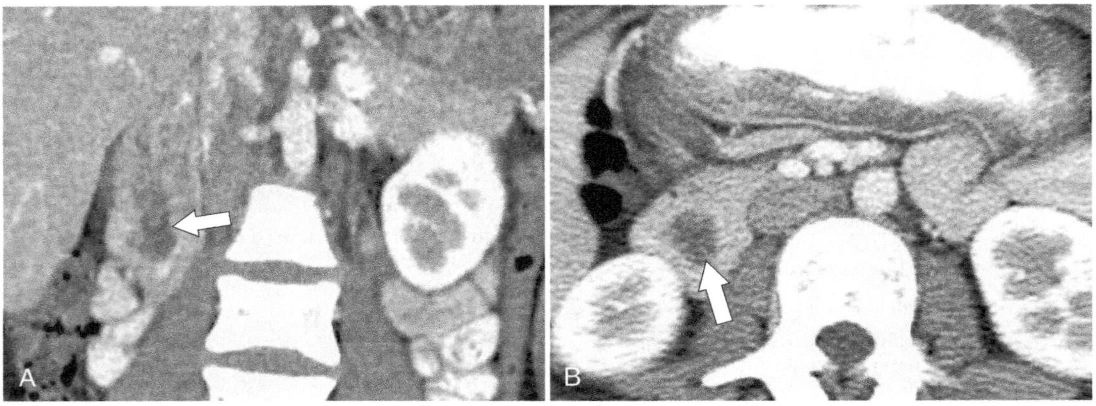

FIGURE 3-47. Coronal (**A**) and axial (**B**) contrast-enhanced CT in a 72-year-old man with a filling defect in the second part of the duodenum (*arrows*) caused by a duodenal villous adenoma.

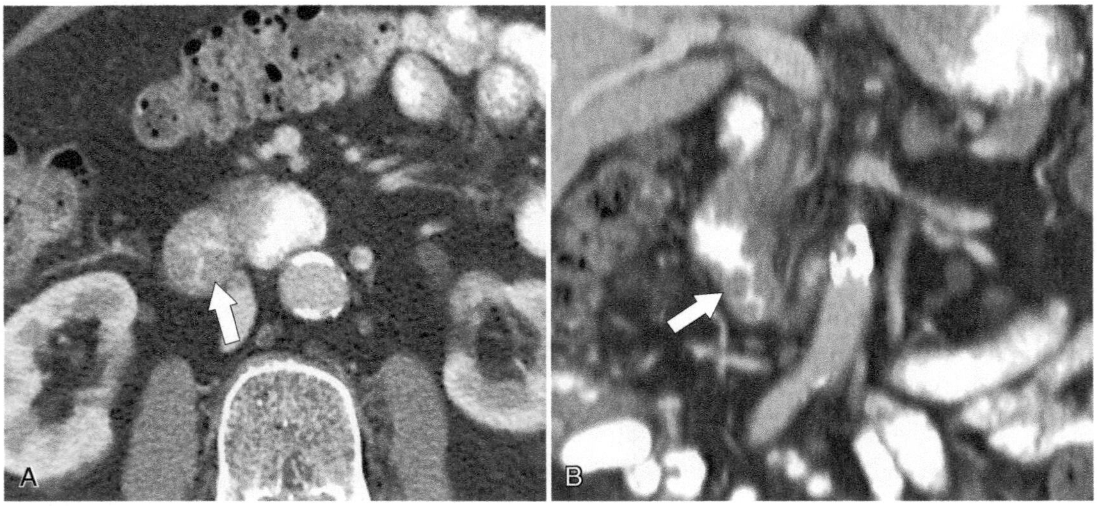

FIGURE 3-48. Axial (**A**) and coronal (**B**) contrast-enhanced CT in a 55-year-old woman with circumferential duodenal wall thickening (*arrows*) due to an adenoma.

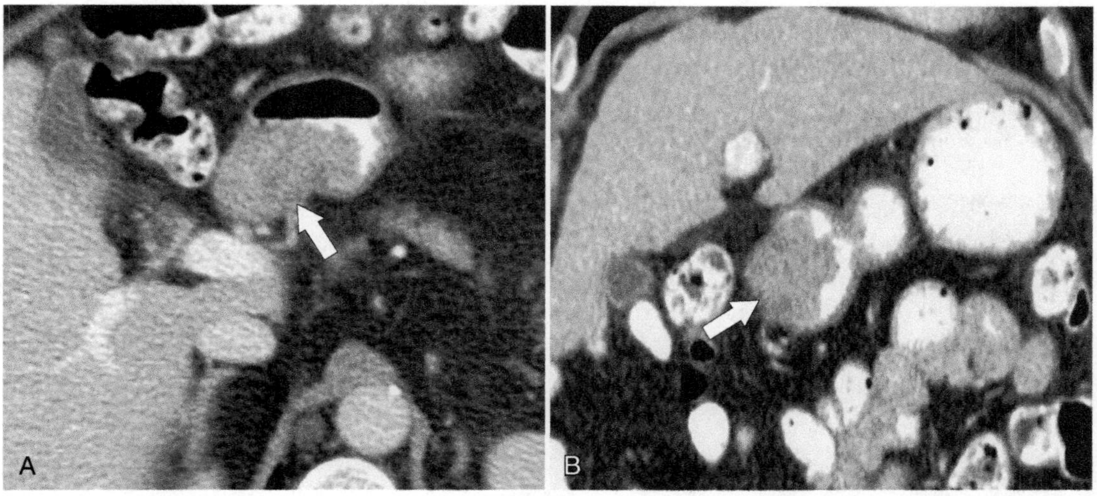

FIGURE 3-49. Axial (**A**) and coronal (**B**) contrast-enhanced CT in a 59-year-old man with an eccentric duodenal mass (*arrows*) due to an adenoma.

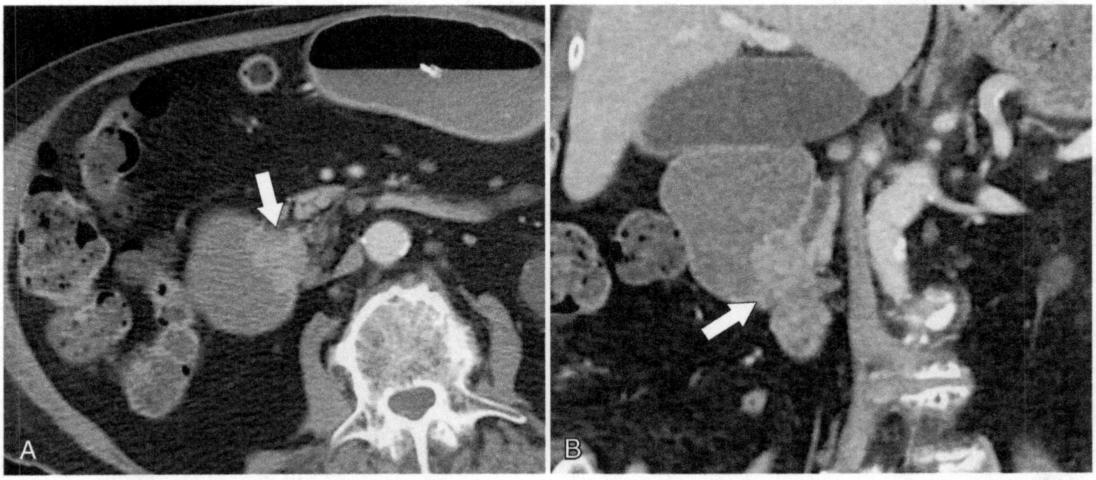

FIGURE 3-50. Axial (**A**) and coronal (**B**) contrast-enhanced CT in a 55-year-old woman with a duodenal malignant stricture (*arrow* in **A**) caused by duodenal adenocarcinoma and resulting in duodenal obstruction. There is also common bile duct dilatation secondary to the mass that involves the ampulla (*arrow* in **B**).

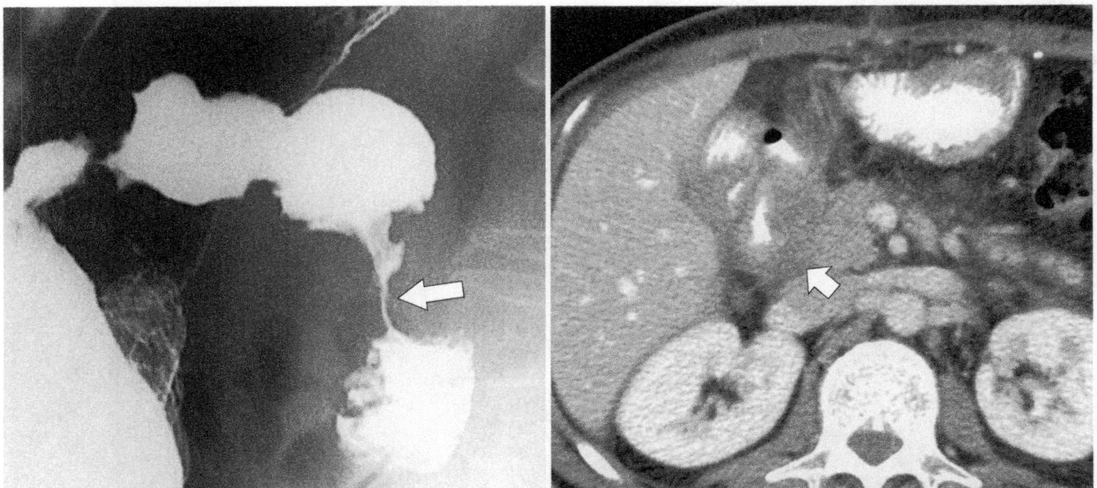

FIGURE 3-51. UGI (**A**) and axial (**B**) contrast-enhanced CT in a 65-year-old woman with duodenal adenocarcinoma and a malignant duodenal stricture, a circumferential duodenal wall mass (*large arrow*) that invades the pancreatic head (*short arrow*).

Malignant Gastrointestinal Stromal Tumor (see Chapter 2)

A malignant GIST, like one elsewhere in the GI tract, presents as a predominantly soft tissue mass that may become necrotic as it enlarges (Fig. 3-52). Some are predominantly eccentric to the affected GI tract. It frequently metastasizes to the liver, often as cystic metastases (see Chapter 6). Surgery to remove the primary tumor is the principal treatment, but c-kit tyrosine kinase inhibitors (i.e., imatinib) can produce dramatic therapeutic responses in patients with metastatic disease, sometimes within days.

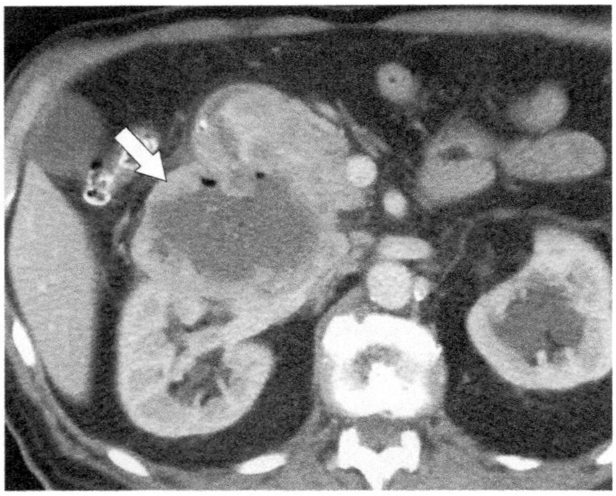

FIGURE 3-52. Contrast-enhanced CT in a 56-year-old man with a 9-cm heterogeneous and partially necrotic mass (*arrow*) caused by a duodenal malignant GIST.

Duodenal Lymphoma

Duodenal lymphoma is usually associated with lymphoma elsewhere and only very rarely involves the duodenum as primary non-Hodgkin disease. Either there is a diffuse polypoid mass, infiltrating mucosal thickening without mass formation, or it appears as an irregular, ill-defined, infiltrating mass (Figs. 3-53, 3-54, and 3-55). As elsewhere in the GI tract, the lymphomatous mass does not usually cause luminal obstruction.

Kaposi Sarcoma

Kaposi sarcoma usually involves the stomach or more distal small bowel, but occasionally the duodenum is involved, demonstrating multiple small rounded polyps, often associated with ulceration. Distinguishing these lesions from other causes of polyps can be difficult by imaging, but a clinical history of acquired immune deficiency syndrome (AIDS) and the presence of cutaneous violaceous lesions are indicators to the diagnosis.

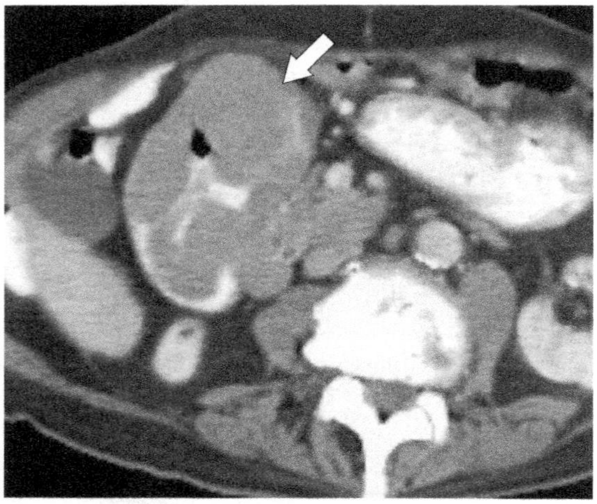

FIGURE 3-53. Axial contrast-enhanced CT in a 77-year-old woman with a circumferential lobulated mass (*arrow*) in the second part of the duodenum caused by duodenal lymphoma.

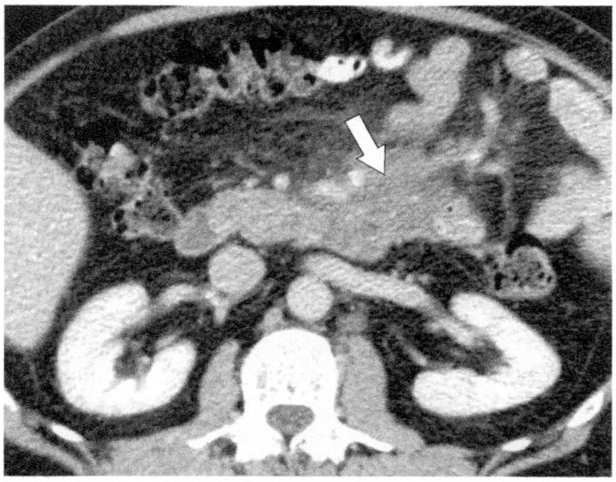

FIGURE 3-55. Axial contrast-enhanced CT in a 55-year-old man with duodenal lymphoma and an ill-defined irregular mass (*arrow*) surrounding the third part of the duodenum.

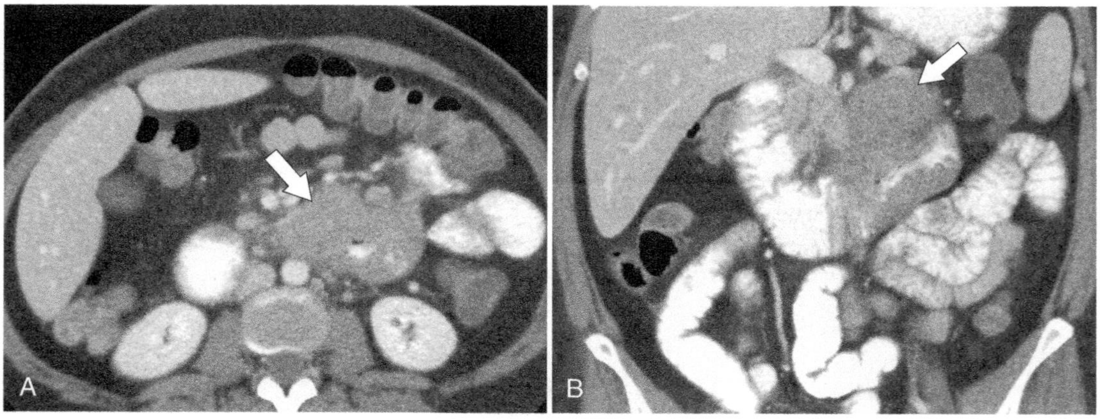

FIGURE 3-54. Axial (**A**) and coronal (**B**) contrast-enhanced CT in a 47-year-old woman with duodenal stricture (*arrows*) (but no obstruction) caused by lymphoma.

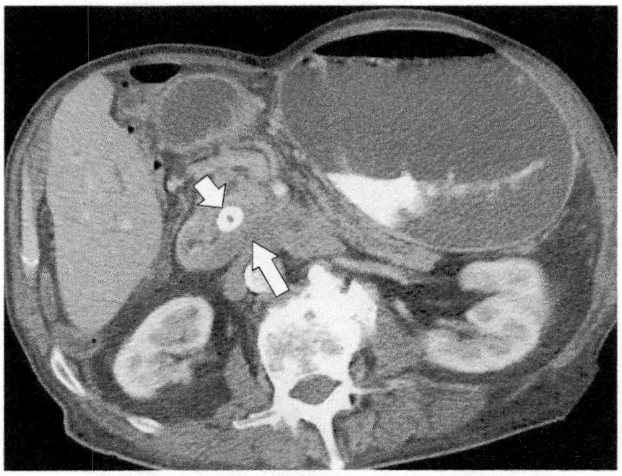

FIGURE 3-56. Axial contrast-enhanced CT in a 74-year-old man with duodenal obstruction (leading to gastric dilatation) from direct duodenal invasion from pancreatic carcinoma (*large arrow*). There is a biliary stent in situ (*small arrow*).

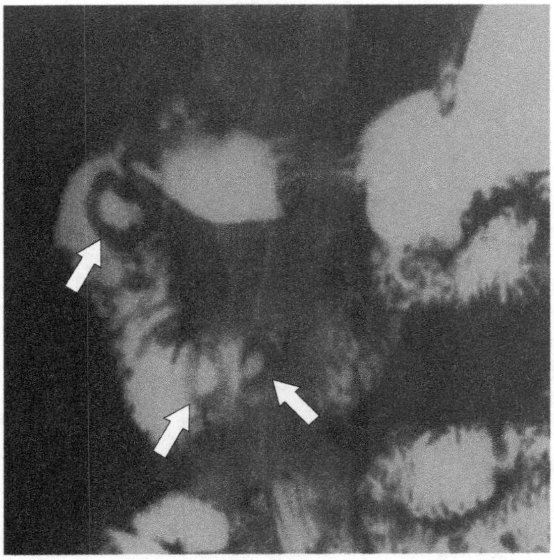

FIGURE 3-57. UGI series in a 47-year-old man with a melanoma metastasis in the second part of the duodenum (*arrows*) with bull's-eye–appearing lesions.

Metastases

Most commonly, metastases are a result of direct extension from adjacent malignancies, particularly pancreatic carcinoma and, less often, colon and gallbladder cancer (Fig. 3-56). Less commonly, metastatic disease is hematogenous (melanoma, breast, lung), producing submucosal masses that may ulcerate and produce a bull's-eye lesion or "target" lesion, similar to those seen in the stomach (Fig. 3-57).

Dilated Duodenum

Similar to the GI tract elsewhere, dilated duodenum can be mechanical or functional (Table 3-2). Functional causes rarely result in absolute obstruction; rather, the duodenum distends and transit time is prolonged (Table 3-3).

TABLE 3-2 Mechanical Duodenal Obstruction

Congenital	Atresia Webs Duplication Diverticulum Annular pancreas Midgut volvulus
Inflammatory	Peptic ulcer disease Crohn disease Pancreatitis Cholecystitis
Infectious	Tuberculosis
Vascular	Hemorrhage (bleeding diatheses, Henoch-Schönlein purpura) Superior mesenteric artery (SMA) syndrome Aorticoduodenal fistula
Neoplastic	Primary (carcinoma, lymphoma) Secondary Local (pancreas, renal, gallbladder, colon) Distant (melanoma, breast)

TABLE 3-3 Functional Duodenal Dilatation

Neuromuscular	Scleroderma, idiopathic intestinal pseudoobstruction, diabetes, Chagas disease
Drugs (anticholinergics)	Narcotic, anticholinergics
Sprue	Dilatation and delayed transit
Severe illness	Burns, shock, trauma
Adynamic ileus	Postsurgical

DUODENAL TRAUMA

Most noniatrogenic duodenal injuries occur in the second or third part of the duodenum because of its fixation by the retroperitoneum. These injuries are either blunt (motor vehicle accidents) or penetrating (stab or gunshot). The investigation of choice is contrast-enhanced CT, which demonstrates intramural duodenal hematoma and extravasation of contrast material from the gastroduodenal artery if the trauma is severe (see Fig. 3-42). There may be duodenal rupture with extraluminal extravasation of oral contrast media (Fig. 3-58). Hepatic, pancreatic, and splenic lacerations are frequently associated.

Traumatic duodenal injuries are a well-recognized complication of EGD and ERCP, particularly in patients with unusual anatomy (e.g., duodenal diverticula, annular pancreas), as this makes the procedure more challenging. Perforation either is blunt by the endoscopic maneuvers or results from biopsy procedures. The injury is usually in the second part of the duodenum, and perforation will therefore be retroperitoneal (Fig. 3-59). Other trauma can result from ingested foreign bodies (Fig. 3-60).

Aorticoduodenal Fistula

This fistula is a life-threatening condition that can present insidiously with relatively minor UGI bleeding or rectal bleeding/

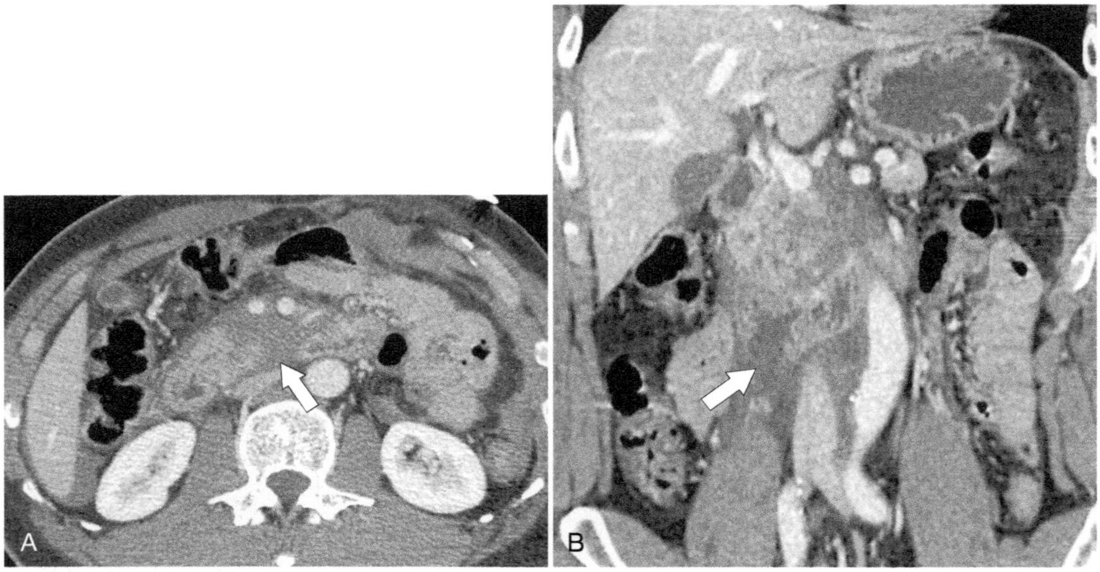

FIGURE 3-58. Axial (**A**) and coronal (**B**) contrast-enhanced CT in a 29-year-old man with duodenal rupture after a motor vehicle accident. There is periduodenal fluid and blood due to duodenal rupture (*arrows*).

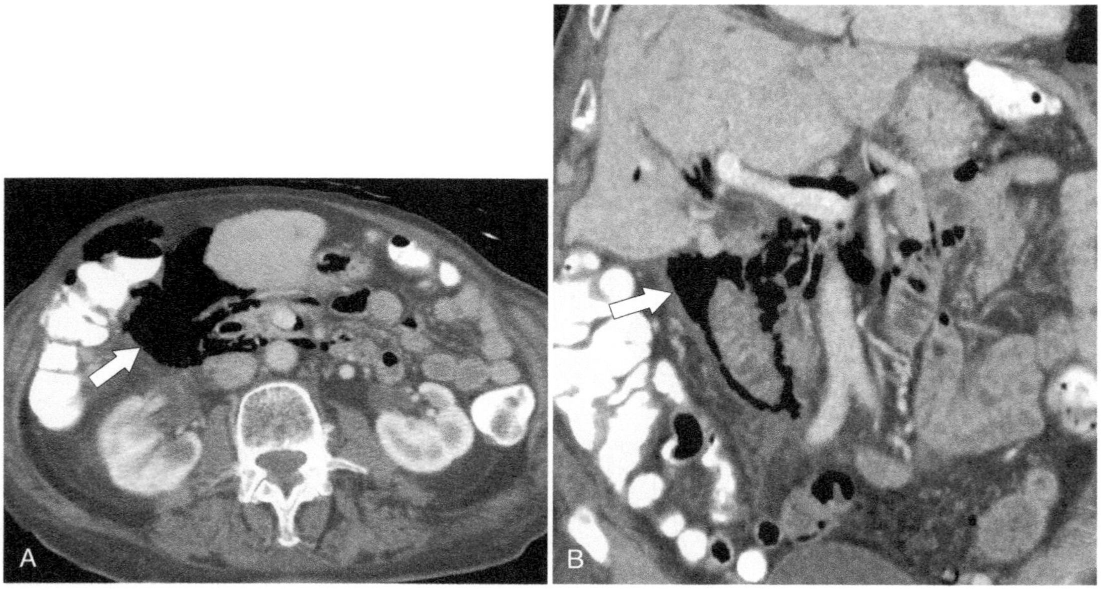

FIGURE 3-59. Axial (**A**) and coronal (**B**) contrast-enhanced CT in a 62-year-old man with duodenal perforation after upper endoscopy. There is retroperitoneal gas surrounding the duodenum (*arrows*).

melena only to be followed some days/weeks later with a massive, often fatal, hemorrhage. It is caused by either aortic (aneurysms, infectious aortitis, postsurgical) or duodenal disease (peptic ulcer, malignancy, radiation change). It is diagnosed by the recognition of gas and inflammatory change between the aorta and duodenum (most often after surgical aneurysmal repair) at CT (Fig. 3-61). Almost all of these fistulas are in the duodenum, but some have been recognized in the jejunum, ileum, stomach, and colon.

POSTOPERATIVE DUODENUM

Most procedures of the duodenum result from gastric procedures that create duodenal afferent loops and are discussed in Chapter 2, in conjunction with the postoperative stomach. Nonsurgical palliation of duodenal obstruction (e.g., from pancreatic adenocarcinoma) can be achieved by endoscopic or fluoroscopic placement of metallic stents to bypass the stricture. These are often temporary, though, and are prone, ultimately, to obstruction due to continued invasion and overgrowth by the primary tumor (Fig. 3-62).

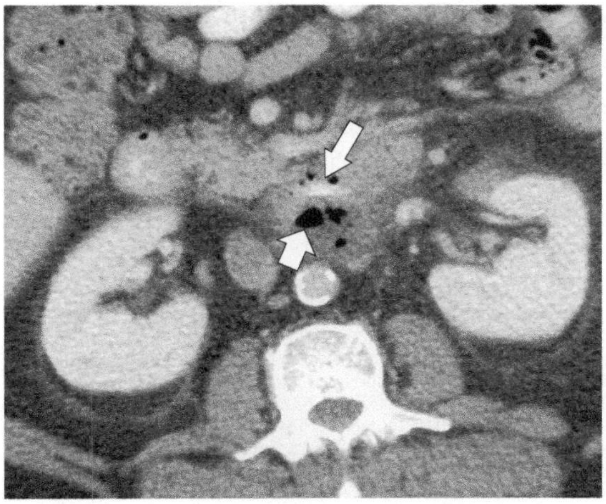

FIGURE 3-60. Axial contrast-enhanced CT in a 58-year-old man with duodenal perforation caused by a chicken bone (*large arrow*). There is an extraluminal collection of fluid and gas (*small arrow*).

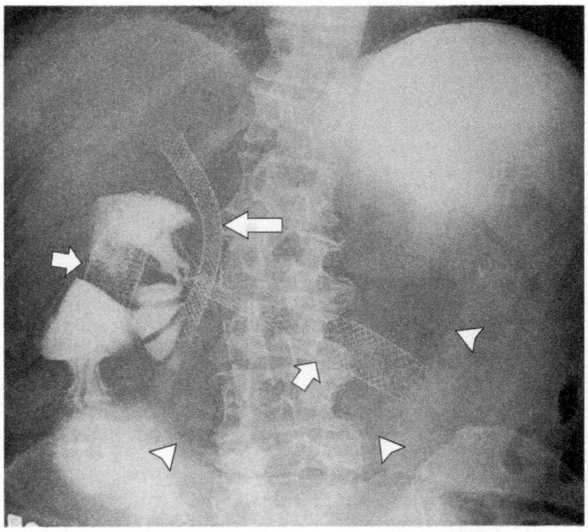

FIGURE 3-62. UGI series with water-soluble contrast media in a 69-year-old woman with biliary (*large arrow*) and duodenal (*small arrows*) metallic stents. There is gross gastric distention (*arrowheads*) caused by an obstructed duodenal stent.

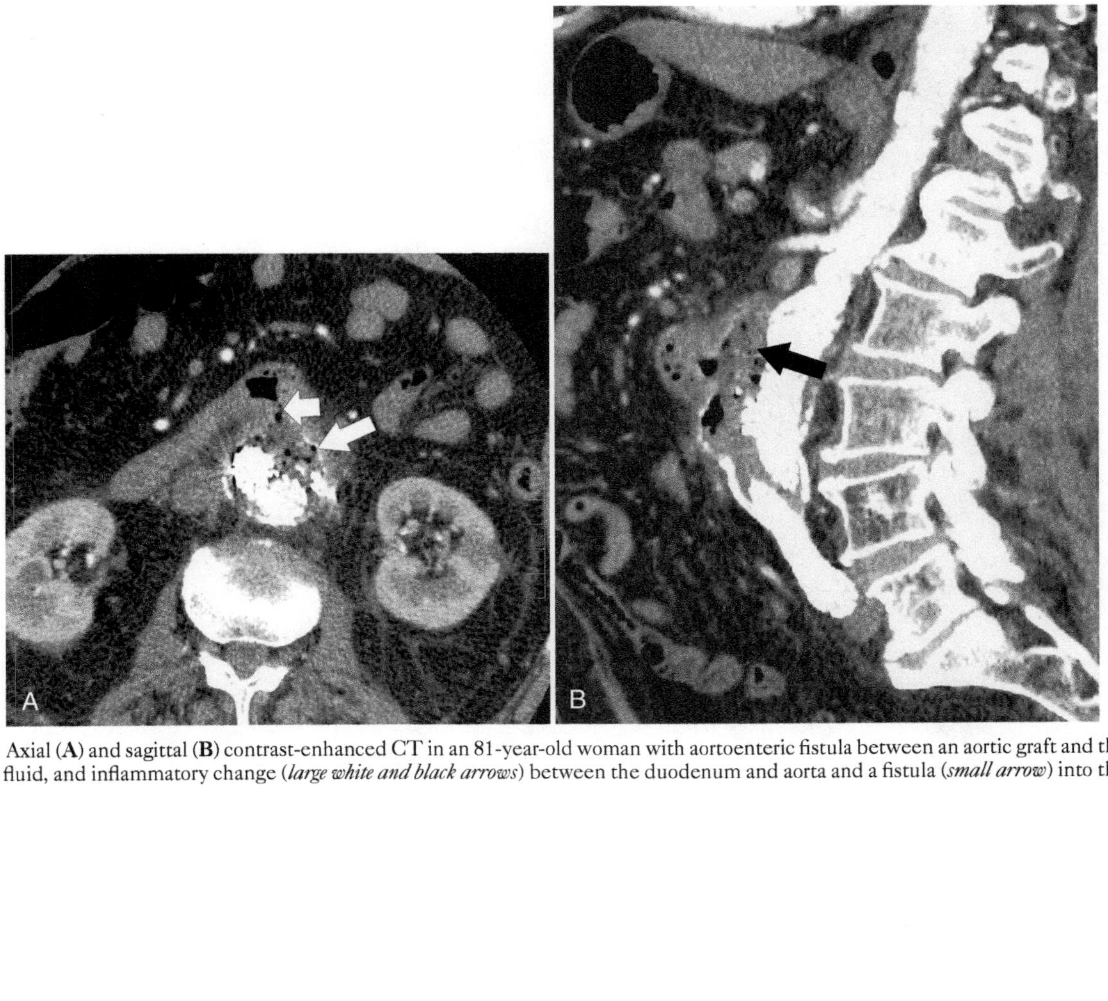

FIGURE 3-61. Axial (A) and sagittal (B) contrast-enhanced CT in an 81-year-old woman with aortoenteric fistula between an aortic graft and the duodenum. There are gas, fluid, and inflammatory change (*large white and black arrows*) between the duodenum and aorta and a fistula (*small arrow*) into the duodenum.

Suggested Readings

Agarwal GA et al: Multidetector row CT of superior mesenteric artery syndrome. J Clin Gastroenterol 41(1):62-65, 2007.

Baichi MM et al: Small-bowel masses found and missed on capsule endoscopy for obscure bleeding. Scand J Gastroenterol 42(9):1127-1132, 2007.

Bradford D et al: Early duodenal cancer: detection on double-contrast upper gastrointestinal radiography. AJR 174:1564-1566, 2000.

Cronin CG et al: Duodenal abnormalities at MR small-bowel follow-through. AJR 191:1082-1092, 2008.

Cronin CG et al: Hypotonic MR duodenography with water ingestion alone: feasibility and technique. Eur Radiol 19(7):1731-1735, 2009.

Gelfand DW et al: Radiologic evaluation of gastritis and duodenitis. AJR 173:357-361, 1999.

Geraci G et al: Secondary aortoduodenal fistula. World J Gastroenterol 14(3):484-486, 2008.

GI/liver/biliary/pancreas. AJR 188(5):A125-A140, 2007.

Izgur V et al: Best cases from the AFIP: villous duodenal adenoma. Radiographics 30(1):295-299, 2010.

Jayaraman MV et al: CT of the duodenum: an overlooked segment gets its due. Radiographics 21:S147-S160, 2001. Spec No.

Kim HC et al: Gastrointestinal stromal tumors of the duodenum: CT and barium study findings. AJR AM J Roentgenol 183(2):415-419, 2004.

Levy AD et al: Duodenal carcinoids: imaging features with clinical-pathologic comparison. Radiology 237(3):967-972, 2005.

Linsenmaier U: Diagnosis and classification of pancreatic and duodenal injuries in emergency radiology. Radiographics 28(6):1591-1602, 2008.

Materne R: The duodenal wind sock sign. Radiology 218(3):749-750, 2001.

Mylona S et al: Aorto-enteric fistula: CT findings. Abdom Imaging 32(3):339-337. 2007.

Newton EB et al: Giant duodenal ulcers. World J Gastroenterol 14(32):4995-4999, 2008.

Oguro S et al: 64-Slice multidetector computed tomography evaluation of gastrointestinal tract perforation site: detectability of direct findings in upper and lower GI tract. Eur Radiol 20(6):1396-1403, 2010.

Patel ND et al: Brunner's gland hyperplasia and hamartoma: imaging features with clinicopathologic correlation. AJR Am J Roentgenol 187(3):715-722, 2006.

Pearl MS et al: CT findings in duodenal diverticulitis. AJR 187:W392-W395, 2006.

Scholz FJ et al: Intramural fat in the duodenum and proximal small intestine in patients with celiac disease, AJR 189:786-790, 2007.

Sol YL et al: Early infectious complications of percutaneous metallic stent insertion for malignant biliary obstruction. AJR 194:261-265, 2010.

Struck A et al: Non-ampullary duodenal adenocarcinoma: factors important for relapse and survival. J Surg Oncol 100(2):144-148, 2009.

Sugita R et al: Periampullary tumors: high-spatial-resolution MR imaging and histopathologic findings in ampullary region specimens. Radiology 231(3): 767-774, 2004.

Triantopoulou C et al: Groove pancreatitis: a diagnostic challenge. Eur Radiol 19(7):1736-1743, 2009.

Yagan N et al: Extension of air into the right perirenal space after duodenal perforation: CT findings. Radiology 250(3):740-748, 2009.

Chapter 4

Small Bowel

ANATOMY

The embryological development of the small bowel (midgut) is complicated, involving herniation into the umbilical cord and a 270-degree counterclockwise rotation before returning to the abdominal cavity. As a result, it is not surprising that there are several congenital rotation anomalies that can result in malrotation and volvulus and that emerge in the neonatal period, infancy, or even adulthood.

The small bowel is defined by the duodenum, jejunum, and ileum, but most radiologists refer to the small bowel as beginning at the ligament of Treitz (duodenojejunal flexure), which therefore consists of just the jejunum and ileum, ending at the ileocecal valve. The jejunum lies predominantly in the left side of the abdomen, whereas the ileum lies predominantly in the lower and right side of the abdomen. Other differences between the two include a thicker jejunal wall, and the valvulae conniventes are more compact in the jejunum. There is a richer vascular supply to jejunum via the small bowel mesentery that traverses the posterior abdominal wall in a direction from lower right to upper left. The ileum contains more lymphoid tissue, known as Peyer* patches. Arterial supply is via the superior mesenteric artery, and venous return is via the superior mesenteric and portal vein to the liver.

EXAMINATION TECHNIQUES

Plain radiography is still a relatively common imaging procedure despite the advent of cross-sectional imaging, because gross anatomical and functional abnormalities can be generally identified.

The standard view is the supine anteroposterior (AP) kidneys-ureter-bladder (KUB), which can be supplemented with an AP upright plain radiograph in patients who are suspected to have bowel obstruction. Supine images readily identify any abnormal air-filled loops, although a bowel distended by only fluid (no gas) may be difficult to identify. Air-fluid levels are identified on the upright plain radiograph with nondependent air situated above the denser dependent fluid.

Fluoroscopic contrast studies include the small bowel follow-through (SBFT), which is a follow-up examination of the stomach and esophagus or is sometimes performed as a small bowel series only when the stomach and esophagus are not formally evaluated. Barium (40% weight/volume suspension) should be used (unless a perforation is suspected) because the denser material better outlines the small bowel lumen and is more likely to identify a fistula formation. Sometimes the radiologist is asked to perform a water-soluble contrast small bowel series by the referring physician out of concern that there may be an underlying perforation. In many instances, this contrast is likely to be of little benefit unless the abnormality is in the proximal small bowel because the contrast will be readily diluted with small bowel fluid, making the identification of subtle abnormalities almost impossible. Furthermore, hypertonic water-soluble contrast medium is further diluted once fluid is absorbed into the small bowel lumen by osmosis. Water-soluble contrast material is reserved to check the positions of tube placements (gastric, jejunal, or abscess tubes). On the other hand, if there is any suggestion of bowel perforation, barium is contraindicated because it can potentially cause a lethal peritonitis.

Alternatively, for better definition of the small bowel, the intubation and direct administration of contrast medium into the jejunum are often required, a process called *small bowel enteroclysis* or *enema*. However, this technique can be difficult to perform for the inexperienced practitioner and can be uncomfortable for the patient. A small bowel enema tube (12-14 French*) is passed fluoroscopically into the proximal jejunum, just beyond the ligament of Treitz.† The technique requires familiarity with the anatomy, especially when passing the tube through the pylorus and around the duodenal C loop. Barium is used either alone (40% weight/volume) or with air or methylcellulose to produce a double-contrast enema (with barium 50% to 80% weight/volume).

Whichever technique is used (SBFT or enteroclysis), the radiologist should periodically palpate the small bowel while the patient is still on the fluoroscopic table to displace loops of small bowel away from each other to identify any disease. Otherwise, abnormalities may remain hidden by the overlapping loops filled with dense barium. Any abnormality should be recorded with spot images and in orthogonal planes. An abnormality in one plane may be better appreciated in another.

A peroral pneumocolon is almost never performed today as the region can usually be evaluated by optical endoscopy. This technique involves insufflating the colon with air once the barium has reached the terminal ileum or colon in an effort to obtain a double-contrast view of the terminal ileum. The passage of air into the terminal ileum is encouraged with the administration of intravenous glucagon. Alternatively, barium can be refluxed into the terminal ileum from a double-contrast barium enema examination.

Computed tomographic (CT) evaluation of the small bowel, while nonspecific, is commonly used to evaluate for small bowel wall and/or mucosal thickening. It is the investigation of choice for evaluation of the acute abdomen. This is best performed with the use of intravenous contrast medium after the use of oral contrast agents (barium- or iodine-based products). For the specific evaluation of the small bowel mucosa, water-based agents may be preferable because these can better delineate finer mucosal details. An extension of the fluoroscopic small bowel enema (enteroclysis) can be used, providing even better small bowel distention and the delineation of small bowel folds. This also requires positioning a catheter in the proximal jejunum and instilling neutral contrast agents into the small bowel. These techniques have now been largely superseded by double balloon endoscopy and capsule endoscopy, which permit direct small bowel mucosal visualization.

Magnetic resonance enteroclysis has gained acceptance recently as a method for the evaluation of small bowel disease, particularly for those patients with chronic Crohn disease; this method avoids the radiation dose from multiple CT procedures. Isosmotic water is ingested, and coronal T2 and post-contrast T1-weighted images are obtained. These outline mural and mucosal abnormalities, including the presence of fistulas or abscesses. Contrast-enhanced magnetic resonance imaging (MRI) can also demonstrate features of mesenteric and mucosal hyperemia, wall thickening, and many of the complications of Crohn disease.

Ultrasound has little use in the small bowel, particularly for adults, but it can demonstrate wall thickening in infants and children, particularly when it is due to hemorrhage. It is also a useful technique for the evaluation of intussusception in children.

---

*Johann Conrad Peyer (1653-1712), Swiss anatomist.

*Joseph-Frédéric-Benoît Charrière (1803-1878), French surgical appliance maker (in the French language the abbreviation is Ch or CH after the inventor, but in English it is Fr, short for French).

†Václav Treitz (1819-1872), Czech pathologist.

Angiography is used to evaluate and treat small bowel bleeding disorders, which are sometimes fatal if left untreated. Nuclear medicine techniques are reserved for specific circumstances, which include evaluating for ectopic gastric mucosa with technetium-99m (^{99m}Tc) pertechnetate, as in a Meckel* diverticulum.

CONGENITAL ABNORMALITIES

Duplication Cyst

Duplication cyst is also termed *enteric duplication cyst* and occurs anywhere along the gastrointestinal (GI) tract, although it is most common in the small intestine. Duplication cysts represent embryological abnormalities that are lined by intestinal mucosa and are contiguous with the small intestine wall. They generally do not communicate with the small bowel lumen but occasionally do. They are recognized as smooth, homogeneous, rounded masses in the small bowel mesentery contiguous with a loop of intestine. Their density varies from simple water density to proteinaceous, denser material (Fig. 4-1).

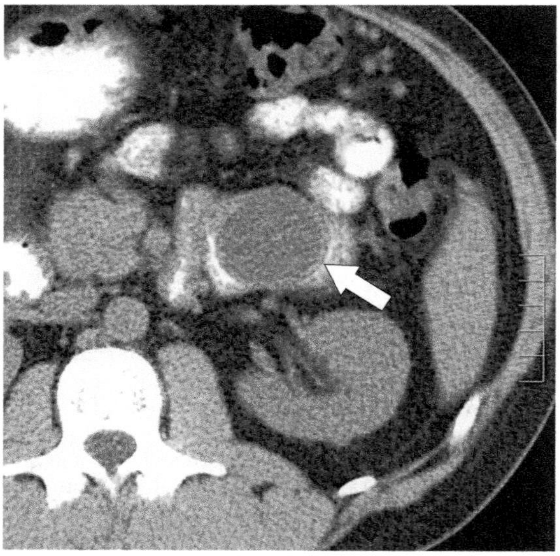

FIGURE 4-1. Axial noncontrast CT in a 42-year-old woman with a 3-cm hypodense rounded mass (*arrow*) due to a jejenual duplication cyst.

Congenital Malrotation

The bowel originally develops in an extraabdominal position before rotating counterclockwise 270 degrees centered around the superior mesenteric artery before entering the abdomen, ending up with the jejunum in the left upper quadrant and the cecum and terminal ileum in the right lower quadrant. Disruption to this normal rotation leads to malrotation, of which there are numerous variants depending on the degree of rotation short of 270 degrees. Sometimes there is no rotation at all, or complete malrotation with the entire small bowel on the right side of the patient and colon on the left (Fig. 4-2). Partial malrotation is sometimes difficult to appreciate or diagnose. The cardinal finding is that the duodenum, usually identified by upper gastrointestinal (UGI) series or SBFT, fails to fully cross the midline from the right to the left and that the ligament of Treitz is to the right of the midline (see Chapter 3). Some of these malrotations are prone to volvulus (twisting of the bowel around its mesentery). It is more common in children, mostly because of a midgut volvulus (Fig. 4-3). The presence of a volvulus usually partially or completely constricts the vascular supply, rendering it a surgical emergency to prevent bowel infarction. The investigation of choice is CT, which will demonstrate the multiple loops of dilated small bowel converging to a narrowing and constriction often to a circular loop (see later this chapter).

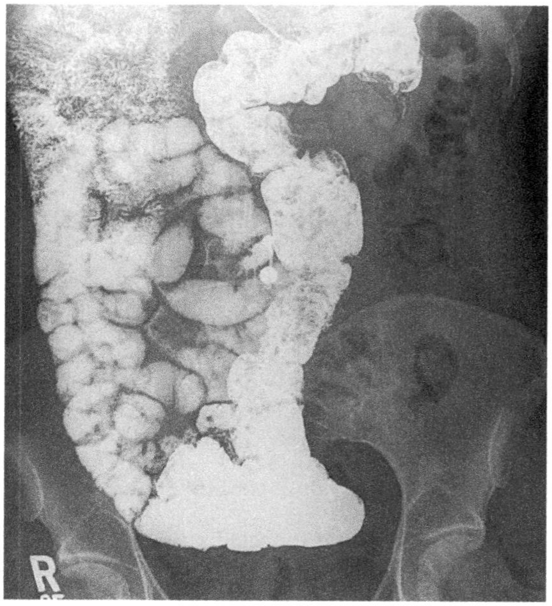

FIGURE 4-2. SBFT in a 36-year-old woman with malrotation with small bowel on the right and colon on the left.

Meckel Diverticulum

Meckel diverticulum is the most common congenital malformation of the small bowel and is due to a remnant of the omphalomesenteric or vitelline duct (connection from the yolk sac to the bowel). It is a small, blind ending pouch containing all layers of the bowel wall, about 3 to 5 cm long on the antimesenteric ileal border and approximately 60 to 100 cm from the ileocecal valve. It is noted for the "rule of 2's": it is located 2 feet from the ileocecal valve, present in 2% of the population, and usually present before the age of 2. Most patients are asymptomatic, however, but those who do show symptoms usually do so before the age of 2, mostly with hemorrhage and melena due to peptic ulceration from ectopic gastric mucosa (present in 50% of patients). Adults can also have rectal bleeding but more commonly complain of obstructive symptoms. These occur when there is Meckel inversion (prolapse into small bowel), intussusception or volvulus from inflammatory diverticulitis (enterolith formation may be the precipitating cause of inflammatory change), and possible perforation. Very rarely, malignant transformation can also occur. The diagnosis is usually

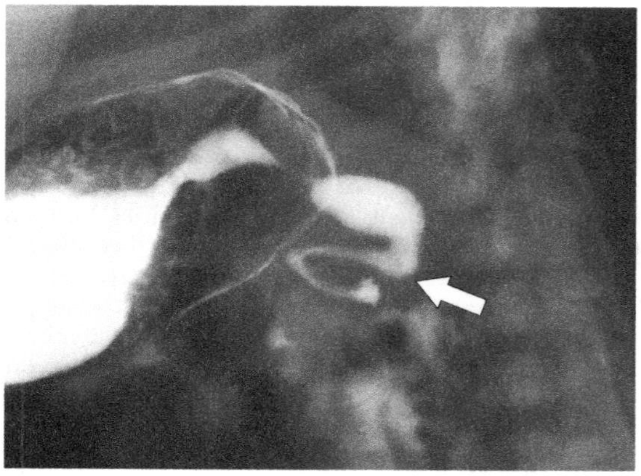

FIGURE 4-3. SBFT in an infant boy with midgut volvulus and a corkscrew abnormality (*arrow*).

*Johann Freidrich Meckel (1781-1833), German anatomist.

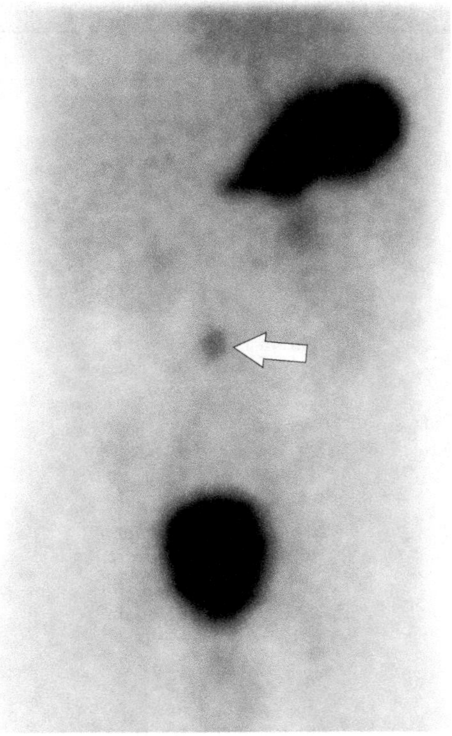

FIGURE 4-4. ^{99m}Tc scan in a 14-year-old boy with a focus on uptake in the midabdomen (*arrow*) due to a Meckel diverticulum.

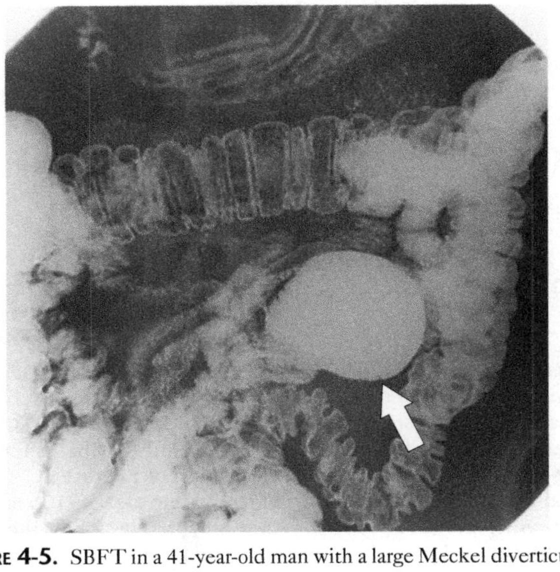

FIGURE 4-5. SBFT in a 41-year-old man with a large Meckel diverticulum (*arrow*).

made with ^{99m}Tc imaging, which has a 95% accuracy for detecting ectopic gastric mucosa (Fig. 4-4). Fluoroscopy may demonstrate the narrowed neck blind-ending sac on the antimesenteric border. Some diverticula can be large but may be difficult to differentiate from smaller enteric duplication cysts (Fig. 4-5). Smaller diverticula will be harder to identify both by SBFT (because of overlying barium-filled small bowel loops) and CT, although with good oral contrast technique, the diverticulum may be identified, sometimes opacified by oral contrast media (Fig. 4-6). Occasionally the diverticulum can become inverted as seen within the ileal lumen with or without intussusception (Fig. 4-7).

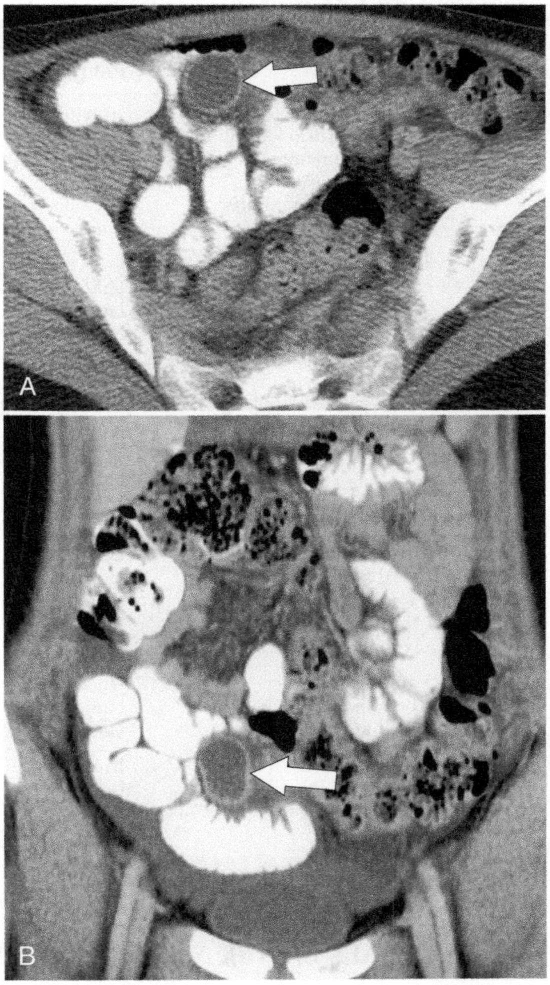

FIGURE 4-6. Axial (**A**) and coronal (**B**) contrast-enhanced CT in a 26-year-old woman with a 2.5-cm cystic mass (*arrows*) continguous to the terminal ileum due to a Meckel diverticulum.

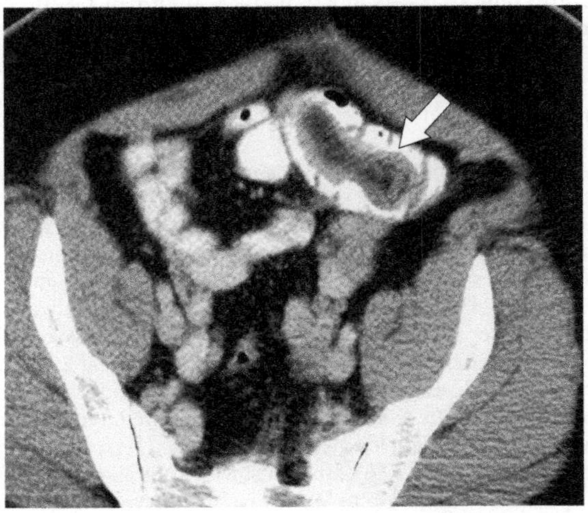

FIGURE 4-7. Axial CT in a 34-year-old woman with a tubular filling defect in the distal ileum (*arrow*) due to an inverted Meckel diverticulum.

TABLE 4-1 Small Bowel Fold Thickening

Type	Disease	Fold Thickening
Inflammatory	Crohn disease	Irregular
	Zollinger-Ellison syndrome	Irregular
	Adjacent inflammatory disease	Regular/irregular
	Behçet disease	Irregular
	Ulcerative ileojejunitis	Irregular
	Vasculitis	Uniform
Autoimmune	Lactose intolerance	Uniform
	Celiac disease	Uniform
	Tropical sprue	Uniform
	Eosinophilic enteritis	Irregular/uniform
	Graft-versus-host disease	Irregular
	Mastocytosis	Uniform/irregular
	Angioneurotic edema	Uniform/irregular
	Waldenström	Uniform
	macroglobulinemia	Uniform
Vascular	Intramural hemorrhage	Uniform
	Ischemia	Uniform/irregular
	Radiation	Uniform
	Shock bowel	Uniform
	Portal hypertension	Uniform
	Vascular infarction	Uniform
	Congestive heart failure	Uniform
	Hypoproteinemia	Uniform
Congenital	Lymphangiectasia	Uniform
	Abetalipoproteinemia	Uniform
	Angioneurotic edema	Uniform
Infection	Whipple disease	Irregular
	Bacterial, viral, fungal protozoal, parasitic infections	Irregular
Neoplastic	Lymphoma	Irregular
	Endometriosis	Irregular

MUCOSAL SMALL BOWEL ABNORMALITIES

Small bowel mucosal or fold thickening has numerous causes, and even the most experienced GI radiologist will probably struggle to remember them all when challenged (Table 4-1). This is compounded by the fact that many of the causes are rare and that the mucosal fold thickening can be further subdivided into uniform versus irregular (or nodular) thickening. Furthermore, these different types of mucosal thickening can be difficult to differentiate from one another, and sometimes a single diagnosis can manifest with both regular and irregular fold thickening.

Crohn Disease

Crohn* disease is also known as *regional* or *terminal ileitis*. It is thought to be an autoimmune disease, although so far there is no known definitive causative agent. It has widespread manifestations, mainly of the GI tract, resulting in inflammatory changes from the mouth to the anus, but most commonly in the small intestine, particularly the terminal ileum. Hence, it is known as an inflammatory bowel disease (along with ulcerative colitis) and is a transmural process and characterized by noncaseating granulomas during histological examination. It is primarily a disease of the West and has a bimodal presentation, either in the early 20s or in the 50s. Symptoms are mainly abdominal pain and diarrhea, weight loss, fever, and melena. Typically the disease is intermittent in up to 80% of patients, with approximately 20% having only a single attack. Up to 50% of patients have recurrent disease even after surgery, usually in the proximal portion of small bowel that remains. Patients are also at increased risk of adenocarcinoma developing in the inflamed areas, in both the small bowel and colon, and therefore regular endoscopic screening is recommended in patients with Crohn disease. Crohn disease is associated with systemic clinical

*Burrill B. Crohn (1884-1983), American gastroenterologist.

TABLE 4-2 Small Bowel Imaging Findings of Crohn Disease

Imaging Finding	Mechanism and Terminology	Figure
Mesenteric hyperemia	Vasa recta hyperemia (comb sign)	4-8
Mucosal and muscularis enhancement	Hyperemic response	4-9 to 4-11
Mural thickening	Transmural inflammatory change Mural stratification—target sign	4-12 to 4-15
Ulcers	Aphthous (target lesions) Cobblestoning (longitudinal and transverse)	4-16 and 4-17
Sinus, fistula, and fissure formation	Deep inflammatory response, ulceration and penetration through wall; trefoil appearance with fistula	4-18 to 4-20
Abscess	Secondary infection from deep penetrating ulceration	4-21
Lymphoid hyperplasia	Small (up to 3 mm) nodular mucosal lesions; immune response	4-22
Lymphadenopathy	Mesenteric adenopathy	4-23
Stricture	String sign—edema, ulceration, or fibrosis	4-24 and 4-25
Segmental narrowing	Skip lesions from fibrosis	4-26
Pseudopolyps	Postinflammatory filiform; islands of normal mucosa surrounded by ulcerations	4-27
Sacculations	Antimesenteric border (increased intraluminal pressure)	4-28
Fat-halo sign on CT	Submucosal fat surrounded by soft tissue, mucosa, serosa, muscularis propria	4-29
Malignant transformation	Mural enhancement, wall thickening	4-30

CT, Computed tomography.

disease of uveitis, episcleritis, seronegative spondyloarthropathy, erythema nodosum, pyoderma gangrenosum, and gallstone formation (because of poor absorption of bile salt from terminal ileal disease).

Patients are typically between ages 15 and 25 when they have their first clinical attack. In the acute phase of the disease, there is mural thickening with mucosal edema and fine ulceration, leading to spasm and luminal narrowing. As the acute phase worsens, the ulcers may deepen and create fistulas with the adjacent small or large bowel. Further disease progression yields fibrotic changes and small bowel stricture formation. Specific signs of Crohn disease are "skip lesions," representing alternating areas of normal bowel (small or large) and affected segments, and "cobblestoning," representing areas of mucosal ulceration separated by regions of more normal mucosa.

The diagnosis can be made by capsule endoscopy or colonoscopy by passing the scope through the ileocecal valve into the terminal ileum and recognizing inflammatory ulcerative changes that will strongly suggest the diagnosis, which can be confirmed with ileal biopsy. Imaging, however, plays a key role in the diagnosis because the disease usually demonstrates highly characteristic imaging features, particularly in the small bowel (Table 4-2). It is one of the few remaining major indications for SBFT, which should identify either the acute or more chronic changes of the disease. CT is also highly informative and often diagnostic and

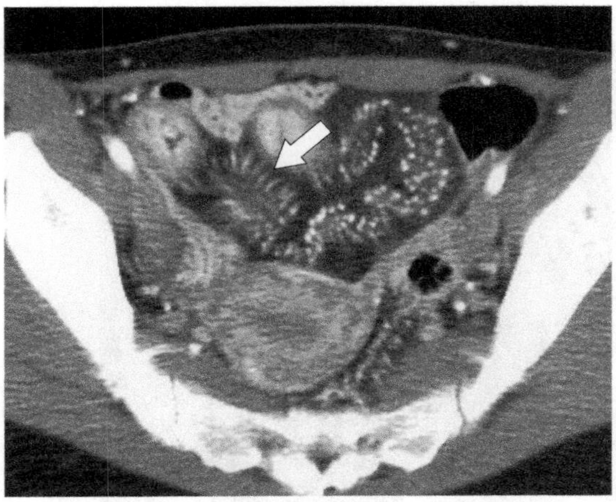

Figure 4-8. Axial contrast-enhanced CT in a 39-year-old woman with mesenteric hyperemia and a “comb sign” (*arrow*).

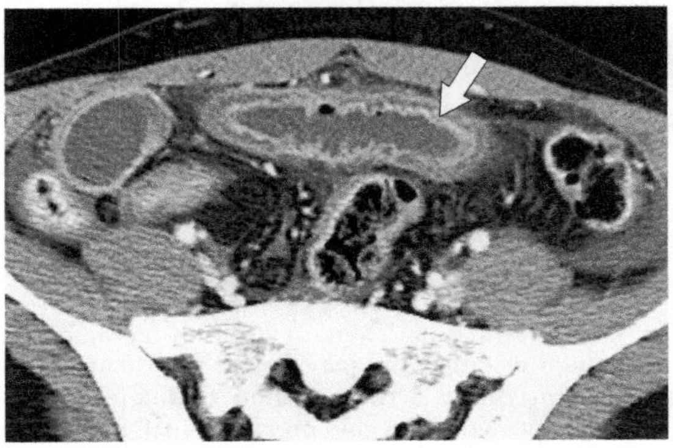

Figure 4-9. Axial contrast-enhanced CT in a 37-year-old woman with mucosal hyperemia (*arrow*) and wall thickening.

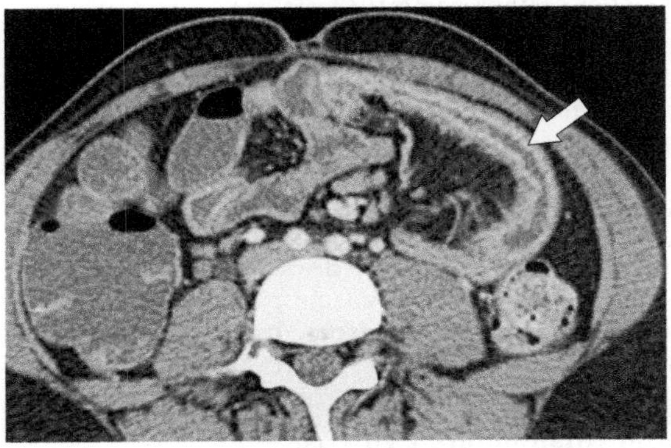

Figure 4-10. CT enteroclysis in a 35-year-old man with a long segment of ileal wall thickening, mucosal hyperemia, and stricture (*arrow*).

is now the investigative tool of choice. However, given that the disease presents in early adulthood and is often chronic, there are natural concerns about cumulative lifetime radiation doses from repetitive CT examinations. MRI has therefore proved useful, particularly for the evaluation of acute or subacute disease and extraluminal complications. Magnetic resonance enterography uses fast T1-weighted and T2-weighted pulse sequences to avoid bowel wall motion distortion, and the use of intravenous gadolinium demonstrates mucosal inflammatory hyperemia, which can be confirmed by diffusion-weighted imaging with increased signal. Furthermore, multiplanar imaging is performed, allowing a better appreciation of the extent of disease.

In the acute phase, there is mesenteric and mucosal hyperemia, which can persist despite symptom improvement (Figs. 4-8 to 4-11). Depending on the severity of the acute attack, there will be a variable amount of small bowel wall thickening, which can be quite marked. Mural stratification or a “target” or “double halo” sign (on the cross section of small bowel) represents inner (mucosal) and outer (muscularis and serosa) hyperemic and enhancing layers because of the acute inflammatory process, separated by an edematous, lower density, submucosal layer (Figs. 4-12 to 4-15). Ulceration frequently occurs, including characteristic aphthous ulcers, which will be difficult to detect by CT but can be visualized by high-quality SBFT (Figs. 4-16 and 4-17). The ulceration may be associated with fissure (small sinus tracts) and fistula formation (Figs. 4-18 and 4-19). Fistula formation is one of the hallmarks of Crohn disease because it is a transmural process. Fistulas can be enteroenteric, enterocolic, and enterocutaneous (Fig. 4-20). Uncommonly, enterocystic (bladder) fistulas may develop, which will be evidenced by gas within the bladder associated with an inflamed small bowel mass. Abscess formation due to small bowel perforation is relatively common with the acute attack (Fig. 4-21). The disease is associated with pronounced lymphatic reaction with lymphoid hyperplasia and regional adenopathy (Figs. 4-22 and 4-23). Stricturing can occur during the acute edematous inflammatory stage or after chronic fibrotic changes. The string sign refers to marked luminal narrowing, often in the terminal ileum, which was originally described as part of the acute ulcerative and inflammatory stage but now also can refer to a long stricture from chronic disease (Figs. 4-24 and 4-25). One of the classic Crohn findings is “skip” lesions, which differentiates the disease from almost every other. All these described acute findings can occur in one or more small bowel segments at the same time, or elsewhere in the GI tract, including the stomach, duodenum, colon, and esophagus. Skip lesions are also observed in chronic disease (Fig. 4-26). Pseudopolyp or filiform polyp formation is a rarer chronic manifestation of Crohn disease, more often observed in the colon, where it can also be secondary to ulcerative colitis. It likely represents the reparative proliferative mucosal process that occurs between areas of previous ulcer formation (Fig. 4-27). Fibrotic changes are also responsible for

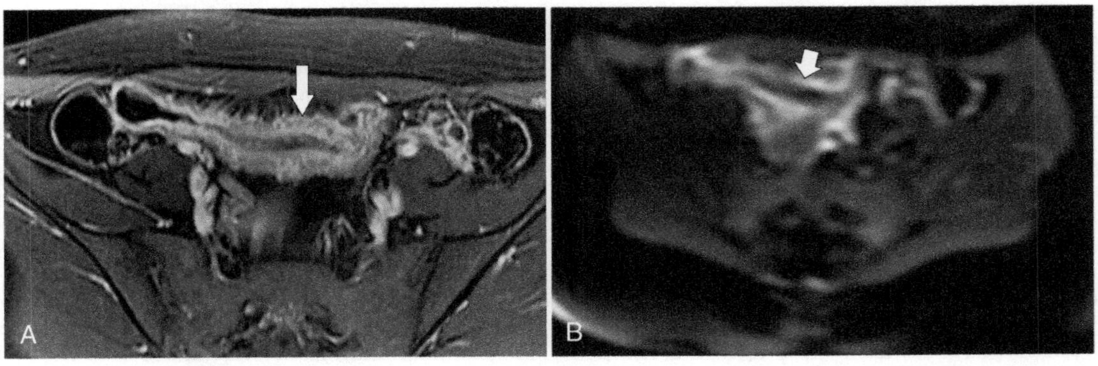

Figure 4-11. Axial contrast-enhanced (**A**) and diffusion-weighted MRI (**B**) in a 31-year-old man demonstrating mucosal hyperemia, wall thickening (*arrow* in **A**), and increased signal at diffusion-weighted imaging (DWI) (*arrow* in **B**) due to Crohn disease of the terminal ileum.

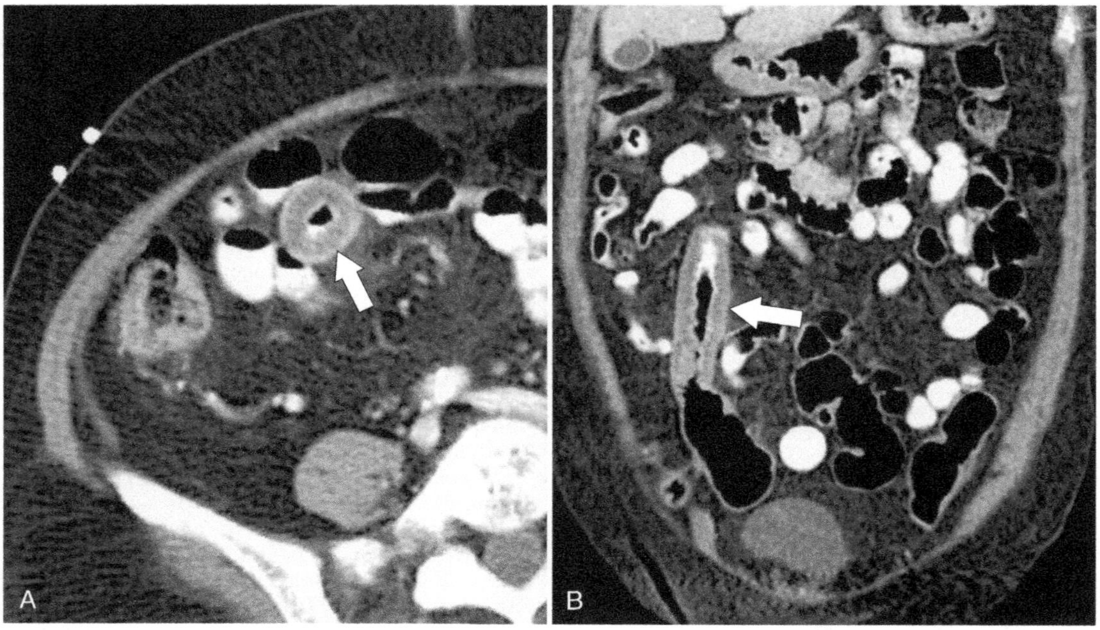

FIGURE 4-12. Axial (A) and coronal (B) contrast-enhanced CT in a 44-year-old woman with terminal ileal thickening and mural stratification (*arrows*).

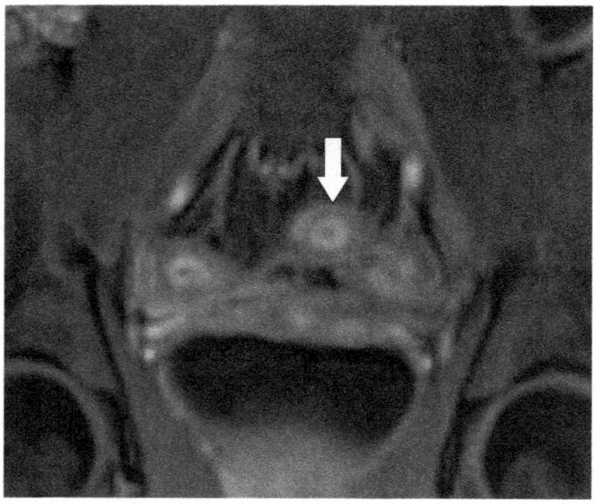

FIGURE 4-13. Coronal T1-weighted postcontrast fat-saturated MRI in a 39-year-old woman with terminal ileal thickening and mural stratification (*arrow*) due to acute Crohn disease.

pseudosacculation formation, in which eccentric small bowel dilatation or sacculation occurs on the antimesenteric border, reflecting the asymmetrical granulomatous involvement on the mesenteric side of the intestine. The mesenteric side becomes fibrotic with more normal, distensible small bowel on the antimesenteric side (Fig. 4-28). The fat-halo sign recognized at CT, which can also be seen in the colon with both Crohn disease and ulcerative colitis, represents an inner mucosal and outer serosal/muscularis layer of soft tissue attenuation, separated by low-density submucosa and muscularis due to the chronic fatty submucosal fatty infiltration (Fig. 4-29). Finally, patients with Crohn disease are susceptible to malignant adenocarcinoma degeneration of the chronically inflamed bowel wall. This may present either as a mass lesion or rarely as a subtle infiltrative form, which is hard to distinguish by imaging techniques (Fig. 4-30).

Zollinger-Ellison Syndrome (see Chapter 3)

Zollinger-Ellison syndrome is due to a gastrin-producing neuroendocrine tumor of either the pancreas or the duodenum. The excessive gastrin causes hypersecretion of hydrochloric acid, with diffuse gastric, duodenal, and proximal small bowel mucosal thickening and ulceration (Fig. 4-31).

Behçet Disease (see Chapter 5)

This multisystemic, primarily vasculitic, disorder usually results in mucocutaneous and genital ulceration and ocular uveitis but can also produce Crohn-like aphthoid and/or linear ulceration throughout the GI tract, most often in the ileocecal region.

Ulcerative Ileojejunitis

Ulcerative ileojejunitis is a rare disease of unknown cause with jejunal and ileal ulceration, causing pain, bleeding, malabsorption, and perforation when severe. It may be associated with lymphoma.

Adjacent Inflammatory Disease

Any adjacent or contiguous mesenteric inflammatory disease (e.g., appendicitis, cholecystitis, colitis) can cause focal small bowel luminal thickening and mucosal disease. For instance, endometrial tissue can deposit throughout the mesentery and sometimes onto the serosal surface of the distal ileum. It typically causes submucosal hemorrhage and pain during menstruation. If SBFT is performed, there may be a focal small mass with distorted bowel lumen and irregular folds. Many of these are small and hard to identify, even by CT (Fig. 4-32). The best imaging method is small bowel CT enterography, imaging directly with endoscopic capsule visualization, or both. Complications of endometrioma include hemorrhage, intussusception, and obstruction.

Drugs

Nonsteroidal antiinflammatory drugs (NSAIDs) of all types, especially enteric and slow-release formulations, can cause not

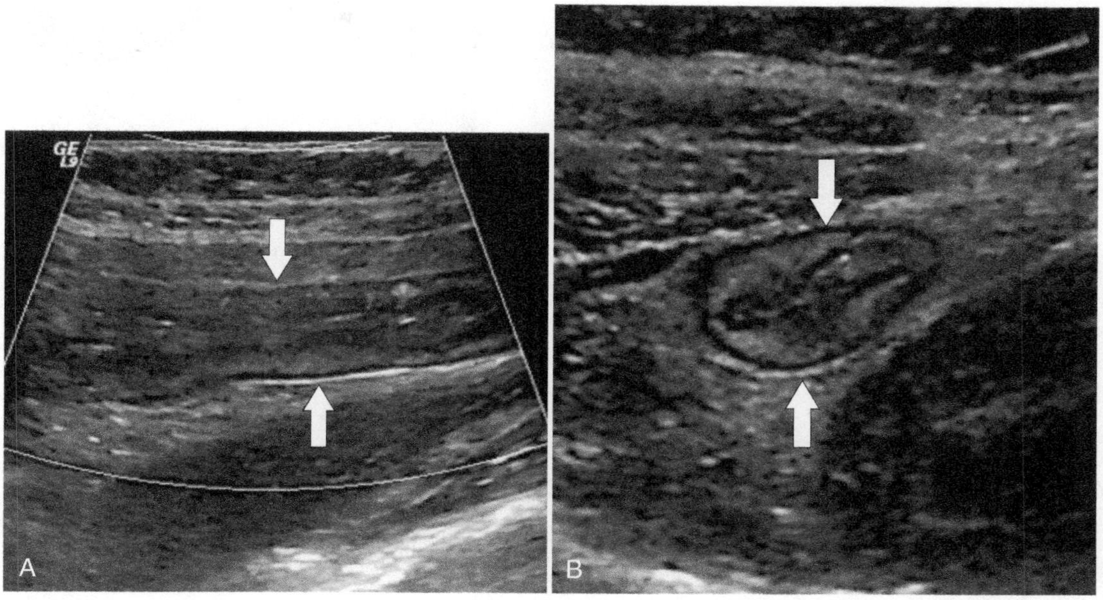

FIGURE 4-14. Sagittal (**A**) and transverse (**B**) Doppler ultrasound in a 21-year-old man with terminal ileal thickening and mural hyperemia (*arrows*). *See ExpertConsult.com for color image.*

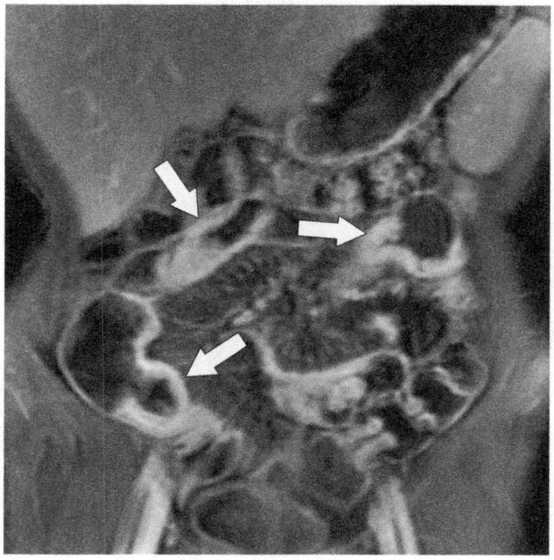

FIGURE 4-15. Coronal contrast-enhanced fat-saturated T1-weighted MRI in a 23-year-old woman with terminal ileal thickening and skip lesions (*arrows*).

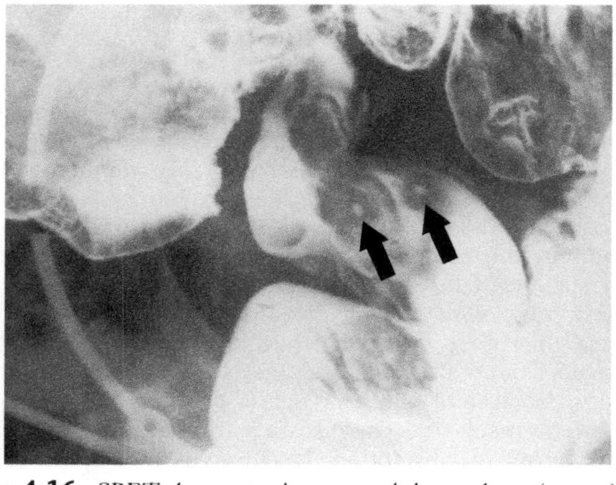

FIGURE 4-16. SBFT demonstrating two aphthous ulcers (*arrows*) from Crohn disease.

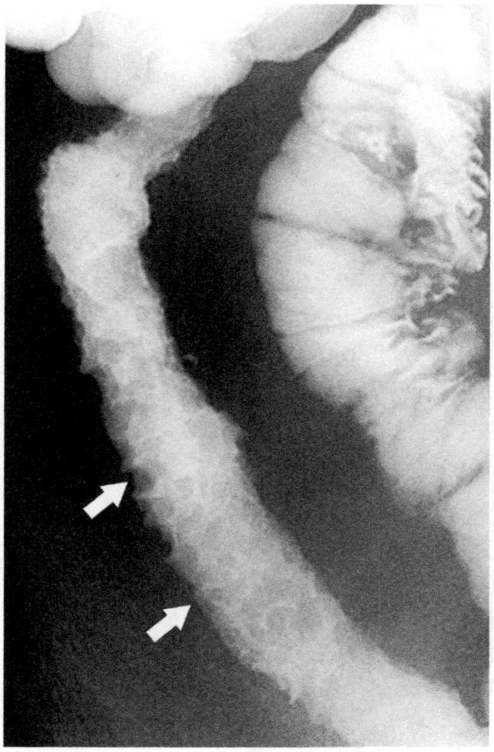

FIGURE 4-17. SBFT in a 36-year-old woman with diffuse terminal ileal mucosal irregularity (cobblestoning) (*arrows*) in Crohn disease.

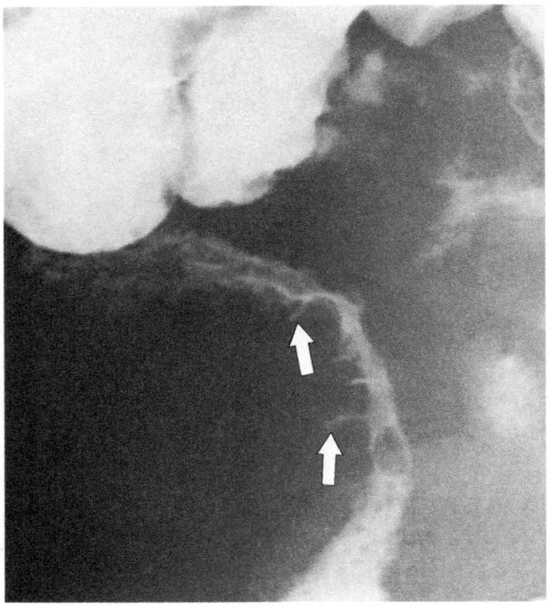

FIGURE 4-18. SBFT in a 39-year-old woman with several terminal ileal fissures (*arrows*) from acute Crohn disease.

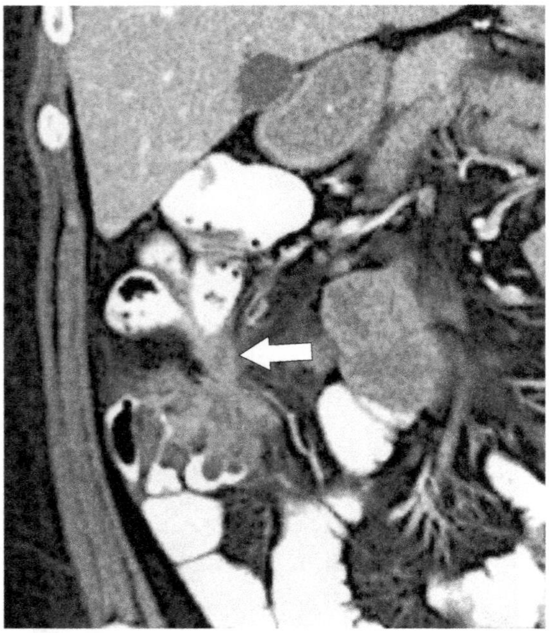

FIGURE 4-19. Coronal contrast-enhanced CT in a 36-year-old woman with angulated small and large bowel due to retraction from an intervening enterocolic fistula (*arrow*).

just gastric irritation, but also enterocolitis, with healing by fibrosis and stricturing, particularly of the midbowel and distal bowel (Fig. 4-33). These strictures can be numerous, and most are abrupt and short, unlike Crohn disease, which typically has longer strictures. Surgery may be required to remove the localized obstruction, although the cessation of the drug may be sufficient. Chemotherapeutic drugs may have a direct cytotoxic effect on the small mesenteric vasculature, causing ischemia and fibrosis with a similar mechanism to radiation enteritis and fibrosis (Fig. 4-33).

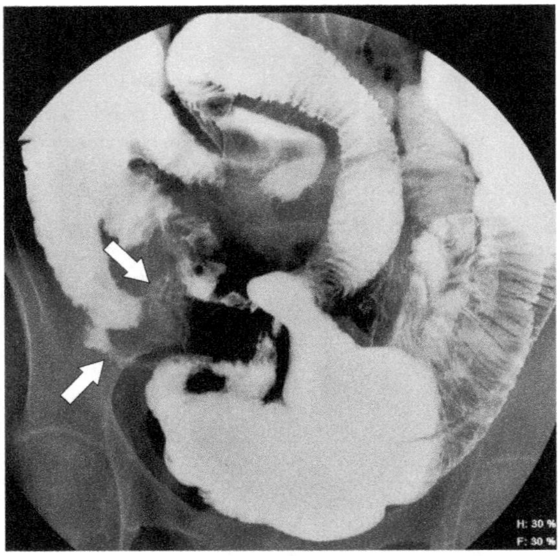

FIGURE 4-20. SBFT in a 53-year-old woman with multiple small bowel fistulas from Crohn disease (*arrows*).

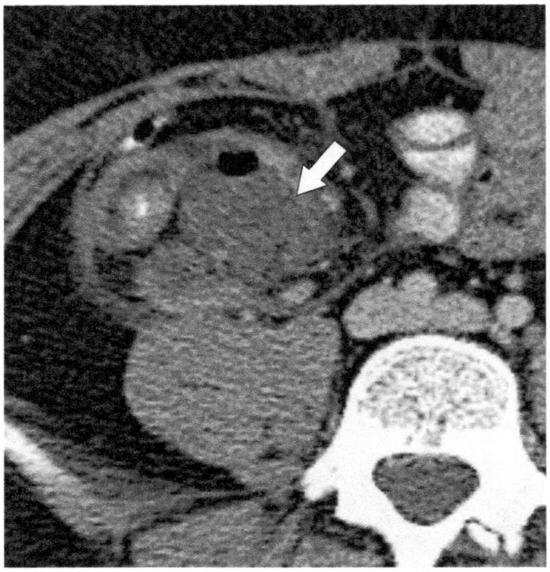

FIGURE 4-21. Axial contrast-enhanced CT in a 38-year-old woman with a 4-cm right lower quadrant gas- and fluid-containing abscess (*arrow*) that is a result of complications from Crohn disease.

Celiac Disease (Sprue)

Celiac disease is an autoimmune disorder resulting from a reaction to gliadin (a gluten protein) found in wheat products. It is associated with other conditions including immunoglobulin A (IgA) deficiency. Clinically, patients as young as 2 can have symptoms, and there is a second peak between ages 20 and 40. The autoimmune reaction to the gluten product leads to inflammatory changes that truncates and atrophies the intestinal villi. The resulting villous atrophy results in a malabsorption picture, particularly fat and steatorrhea, which is common. As the villi become more affected, a degree of lactose intolerance can also occur because of a lack of lactase production. These combined effects result in celiac disease as the most common cause of small bowel malabsorption. Diagnosis is made with jejunal biopsy, which confirms the mucosal findings, in combination with

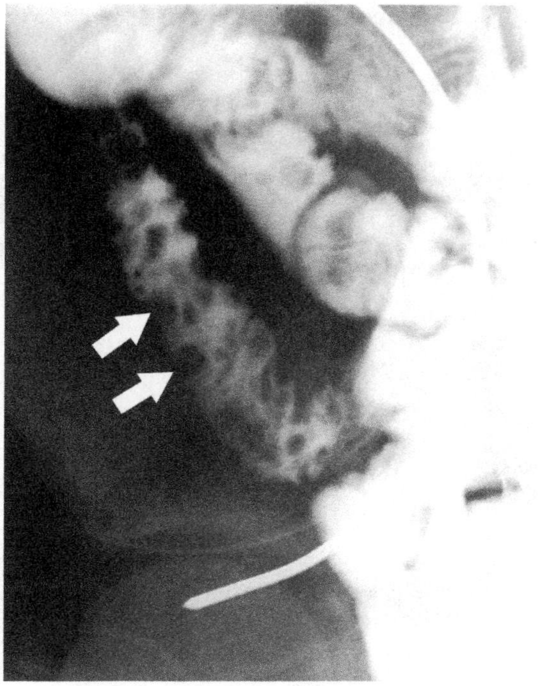

FIGURE 4-22. SBFT in a 26-year-old man with Crohn disease and lymphoid hyperplasia of the terminal ileum (*arrows*).

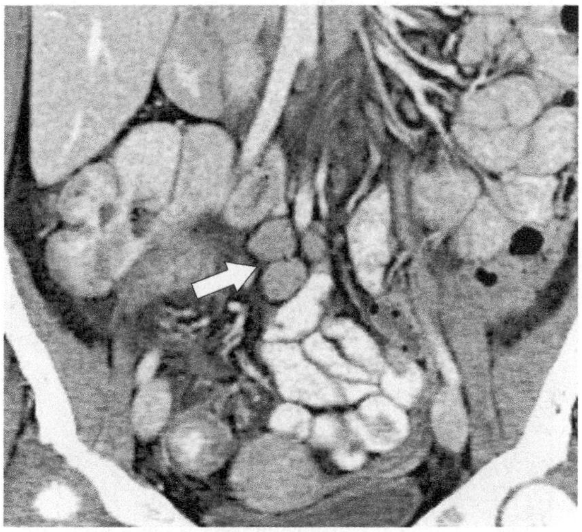

FIGURE 4-23. Coronal contrast-enhanced CT in a 48-year-old woman with multiple mesenteric lymph nodes (*arrow*) resulting from Crohn disease.

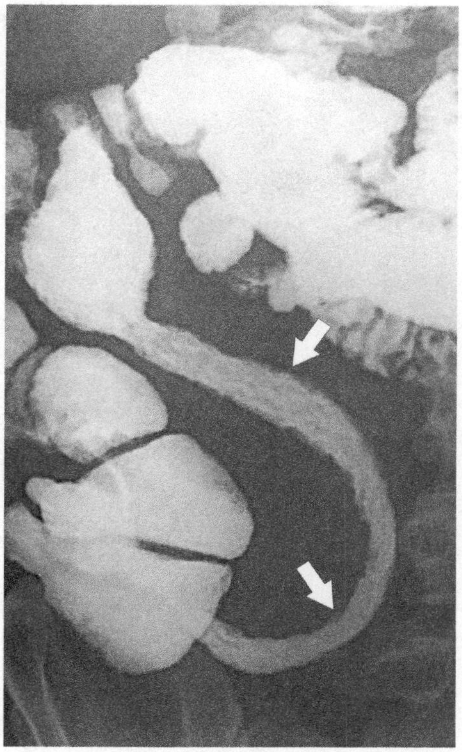

FIGURE 4-24. SBFT in a 44-year-old man with a long terminal ileal stricture ("string sign") (*arrows*) from Crohn disease.

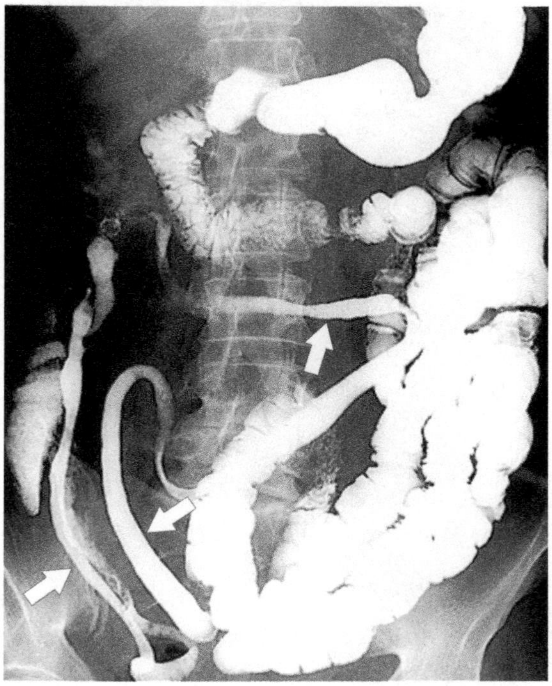

FIGURE 4-25. SBFT in a 60-year-old woman with multiple ileal strictures (*arrows*) due to chronic Crohn disease.

antibody serological testing. The removal of gluten products from the diet can treat the condition.

Certain imaging features are consistent with the diagnosis of celiac disease, mainly as a consequence of the malabsorption and excessive intestinal fluid, with flocculation (the disruption of barium into small clumps due to excessive fluid) and the segmentation of barium (the separation of the barium into relatively discrete columns, also termed *moulage*) (Fig. 4-34). The jejunum is often dilated, and there are widening and separation of the mucosal folds (valvulae conniventes) in the jejunum, better visualized by small bowel enteroclysis (preferably CT enteroclysis), which take on a colonic haustral-like pattern. Conversely, there is an increase in the number of folds and mural thickening in the ileum, which take on a jejunal fold appearance, or the "jejunization" of the ileum (Fig. 4-34). The passage of barium is often delayed with a lack of the normal peristaltic pattern. There is a propensity for jejunal intussusception, which is often asymptomatic and transitory (Fig. 4-35). At CT, there is nonspecific circumferential wall thickening with submucosal edema (Fig. 4-36). The abnormal jejunal and ileal fold pattern is less

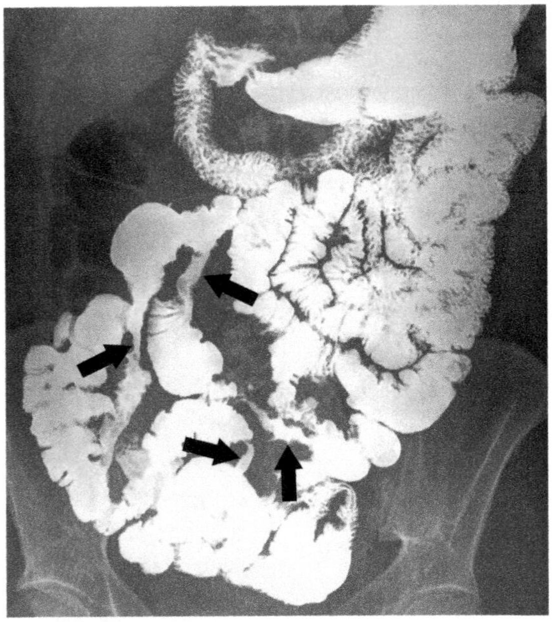

FIGURE 4-26. SBFT in a 58-year-old man with multiple "skip lesions" (*arrows*) from chronic Crohn disease.

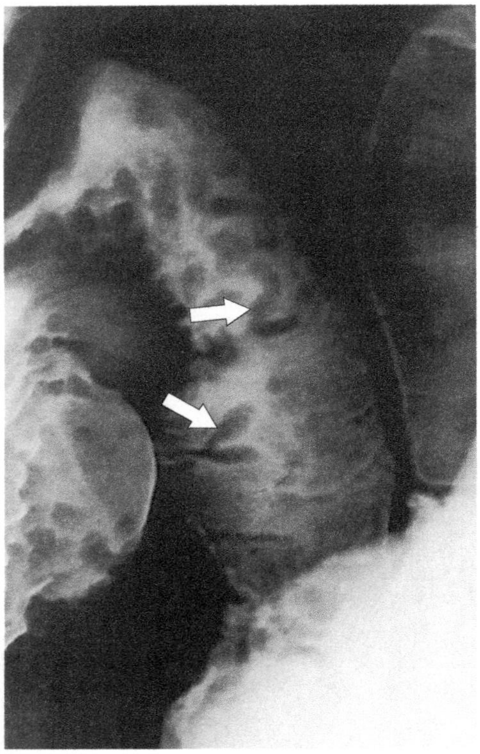

FIGURE 4-27. SBFT in a 38-year-old man with Crohn disease and multiple filiform polyps (*arrows*).

often recognized, but any intussuscepta will generally be better appreciated by CT.

Ulceration and stricturing can also be observed in the acute phase, and there is a risk of malignant degeneration with chronic disease. Both T-cell lymphoma and adenocarcinoma of the small bowel are associated with celiac disease, but the risk returns to baseline with a gluten-free diet. There is also an increased risk of squamous carcinoma of the esophagus.

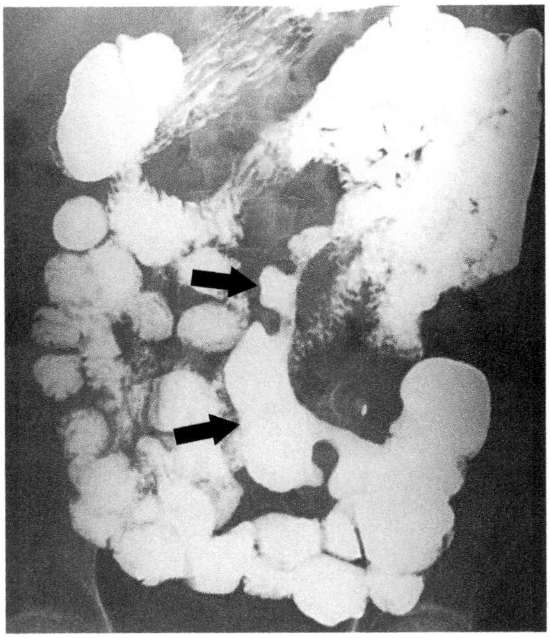

FIGURE 4-28. SBFT in a 44-year-old woman with antimesenteric jejunal pseudodiverticula (*arrows*) from Crohn disease.

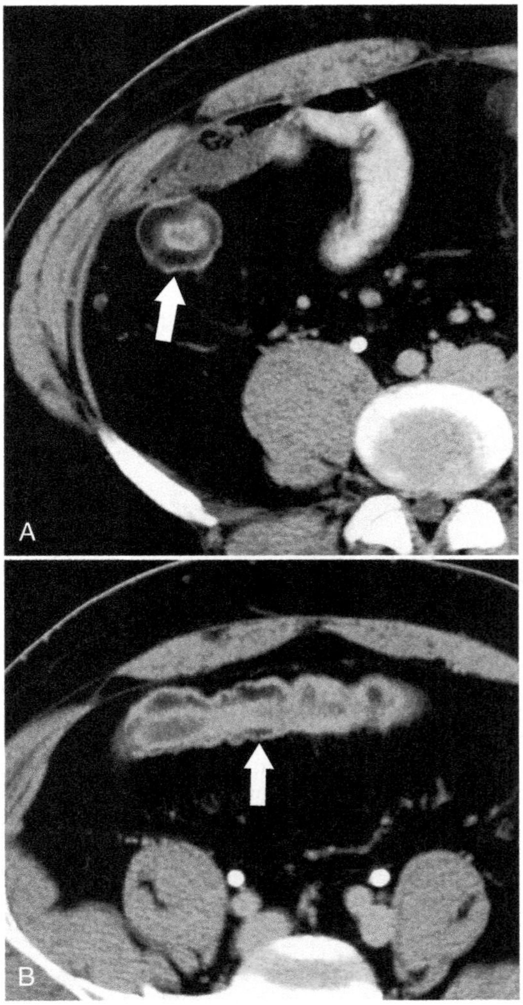

FIGURE 4-29. Axial CT (**A** and **B**) in a 44-year-old woman with a fat-halo sign (*arrows*) in a loop of terminal ileum from Crohn disease.

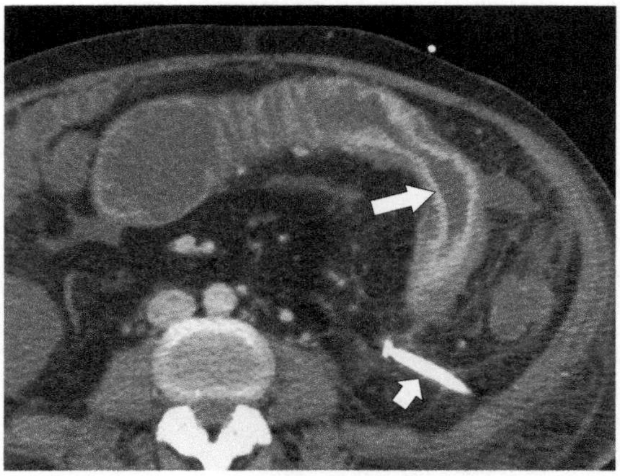

FIGURE 4-30. Axial contrast-enhanced CT in a 54-year-old man with mucosal hyperemia (*large arrow*), which at surgery and histological examination was due to underlying early adenocarcinoma. There is an abdominal drain from recent percutaneous abscess drainage (*small arrow*).

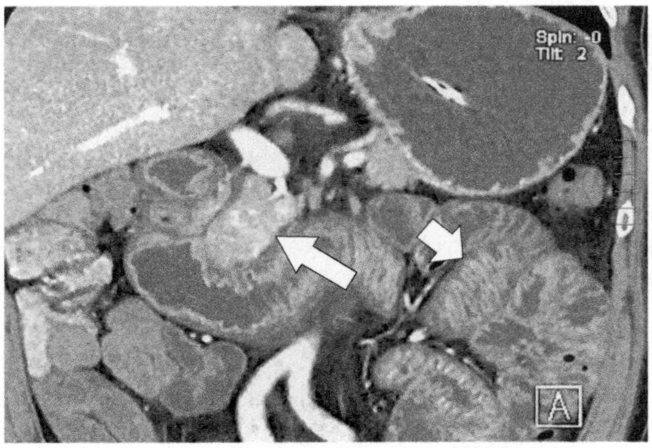

FIGURE 4-31. Coronal contrast-enhanced CT in a 36-year-old man with a duodenal gastrinoma (*large arrow*) and proximal jejunal mucosal thickening (*small arrow*).

Hyposplenia occurs in approximately 30% of cases, rendering the patient susceptible to bacterial infections. A rare complication is cavitating lymph node syndrome with multiple cystic mesenteric lymph nodes, associated with a poor clinical outcome.

Tropical Sprue

Tropical sprue is a nonhereditary form of malabsorption that is very similar to celiac disease and is seen more commonly in the tropics (hence its name) and is possibly a result of infection with *Escherichia coli*, although this is debated. It responds to antibiotics (tetracycline), vitamin B_{12}, and folic acid medication. The diagnosis of tropical sprue is also made with endoscopy and duodenal biopsy. The microscopic, clinical, and imaging findings are similar to celiac disease (Fig. 4-37). The appropriate history and response to antibiotics differentiate the two conditions.

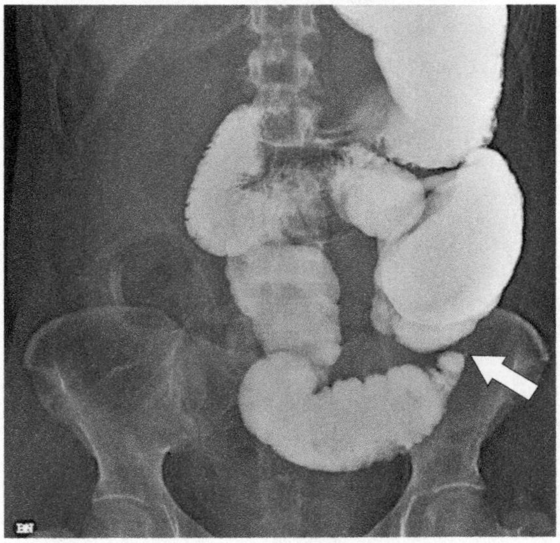

FIGURE 4-33. SBFT in a 63-year-old woman with obstruction due to a distal ileal stricture (*arrow*) from nonsteroidal drug ingestion.

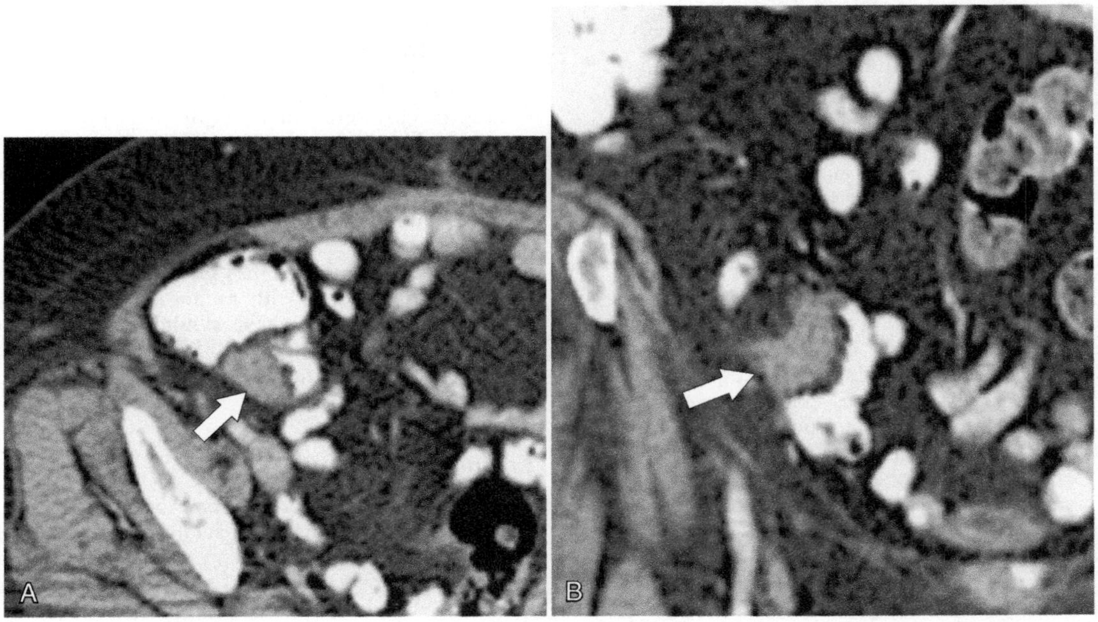

FIGURE 4-32. Axial (**A**) and coronal (**B**) contrast-enhanced CT in a 33-year-old woman with a serosal terminal ileal mass (*arrows*) due to endometriosis.

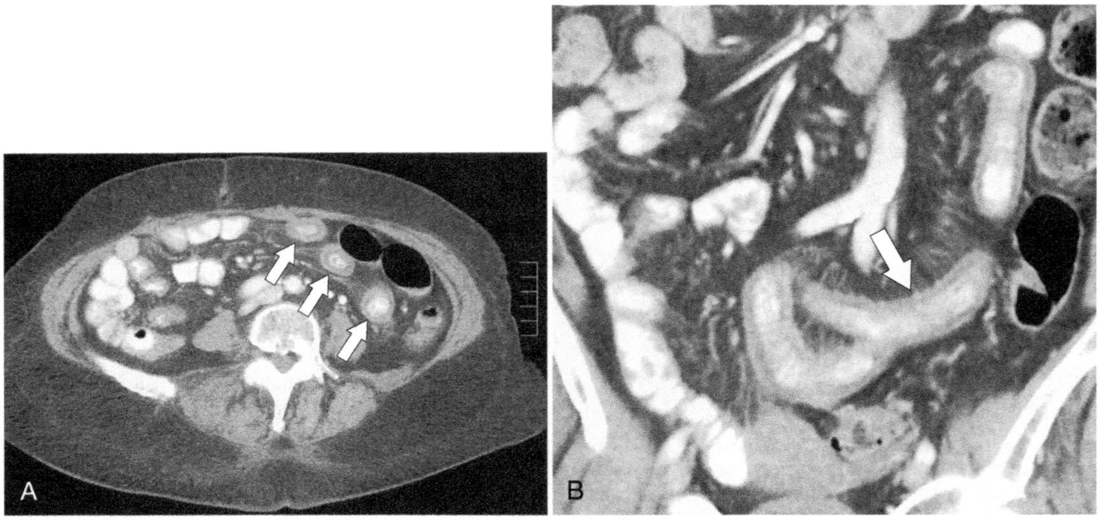

Figure 4-34. Axial (**A**) and coronal (**B**) contrast-enhanced CT in a 82-year-old woman with jejunal thickening (*arrows*) due to allergy from 5-fluorouracil administration.

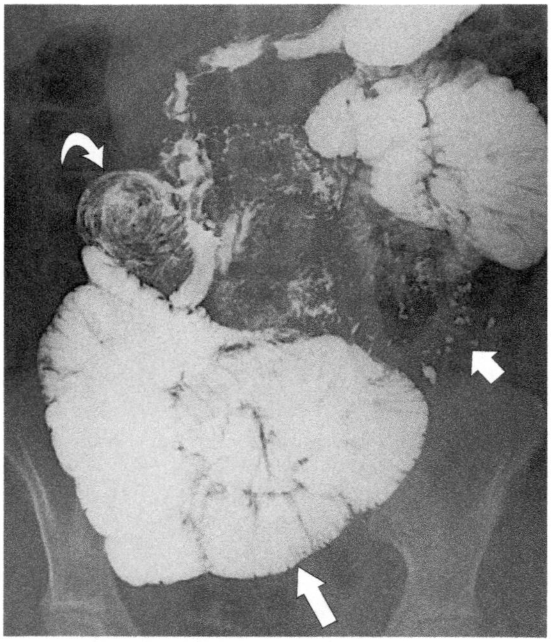

Figure 4-35. SBFT in a 39-year-old man with celiac disease. There is reversal of the normal fold pattern with prominent valvulae in the ileum (*large arrow*). There is flocculation (*small arrow*) and a jejenojejunal intussusception (*curved arrow*).

Lactose Intolerance

Lactose intolerance is primarily an adult disease caused by a progressive deficiency of the enzyme lactase (required for the metabolism of the milk sugar, lactose). The enzyme normally decreases after childhood, sometimes to such low levels that lactase deficiency can ensue in the adult. There is also a rare congenital lactase deficiency that appears in early infancy.

The most common form is primary lactose intolerance, although the secondary form can develop after GI infections, particularly giardiasis, but also after the more common gastroenteritides (e.g., rotavirus). Patients with celiac disease often have concomitant lactase deficiency due to the villous atrophy and the destruction of small bowel mucosal cells that produce lactase.

It is a surprisingly common disease, with up to 75% of adults worldwide demonstrating some degree of lactose intolerance, although most cases are subclinical. Symptoms vary markedly and occur from 30 minutes to 2 hours after the ingestion of dairy products. Symptoms include nausea, abdominal cramps, bloating, excessive gas, and sometimes diarrhea. Because the patient cannot metabolize lactose, there is some osmotic hypersecretion of fluid into the small bowel lumen, resulting in small bowel distention, pain, and cramps. Excessive lactose then enters the colon, which is metabolized and fermented by colonic flora, leading to excessive gas and bloating. The diagnosis is readily made by challenging the patient with excessive dairy products or by administering a hydrogen breath test (patients with lactose intolerance have higher hydrogen levels). Lactose intolerance can be treated by the patient's avoiding products that contain lactose (mainly dairy products) or by lactase enzyme supplementation. The imaging findings at SBFT are similar to those of celiac disease in that the column of barium is diluted by excessive fluid and the barium becomes flocculated and segmented. There is often small bowel dilatation due to the excess fluid.

Nodular Lymphoid Hyperplasia

Nodular lymphoid hyperplasia is more common and a normal finding in children, but in adults it is idiopathic and is less common. Although it is a benign finding in itself, it is associated with immune deficiency, particularly IgA deficiency associated with *Giardia lamblia* or lymphoma. Therefore these diseases should be excluded in the presence of nodular lymphoid hyperplasia.

The whole small bowel may be affected, or it may be confined to the terminal ileum with numerous small (<5 mm) mucosal nodules (Fig. 4-38). Polyposis syndromes can also develop multiple small bowel nodules, but SBFT can generally differentiate between the two by their smaller size compared with other polyposis syndromes.

Eosinophilic Enteritis

Eosinophilic enteritis can affect any aspect of the UGI tract from the esophagus, stomach, and small bowel, the latter being the most commonly affected. It may simply affect the mucosa only, or the muscularis and serosa. Fold thickening is common in the small bowel and can be either uniform or irregular, focal or diffuse. Although the imaging findings are common to many causes

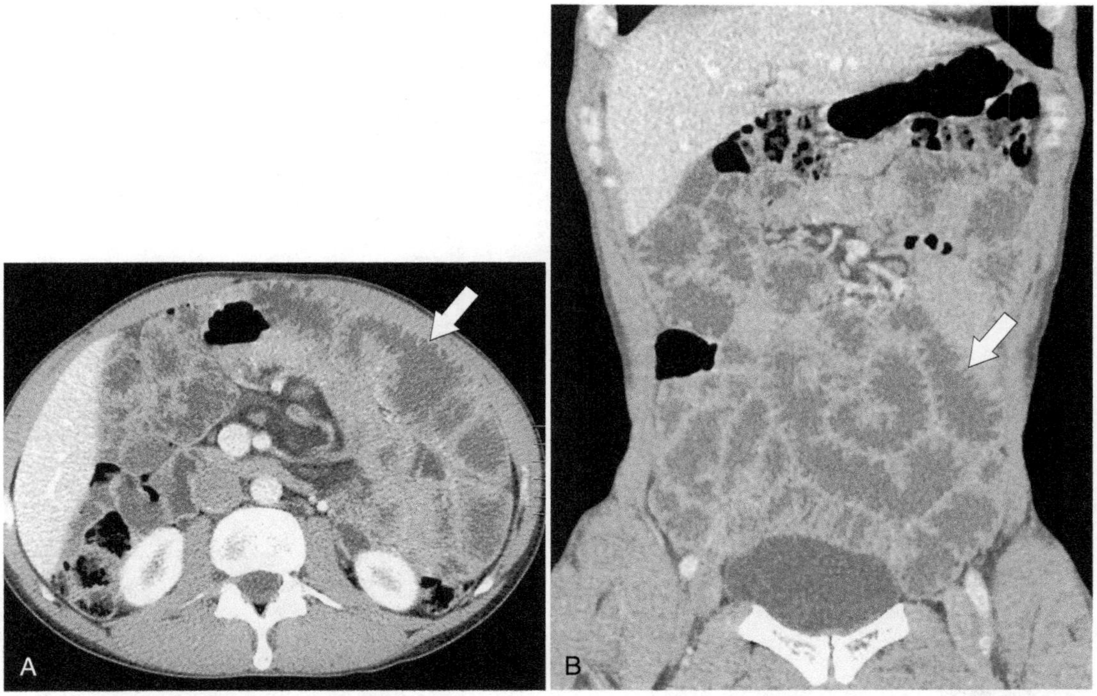

FIGURE 4-36. Axial (**A**) and coronal (**B**) contrast-enhanced CT performed with water-based oral contrast medium in a 43-year-old man with diffuse small bowel mucosal thickening (*arrows*) from celiac disease.

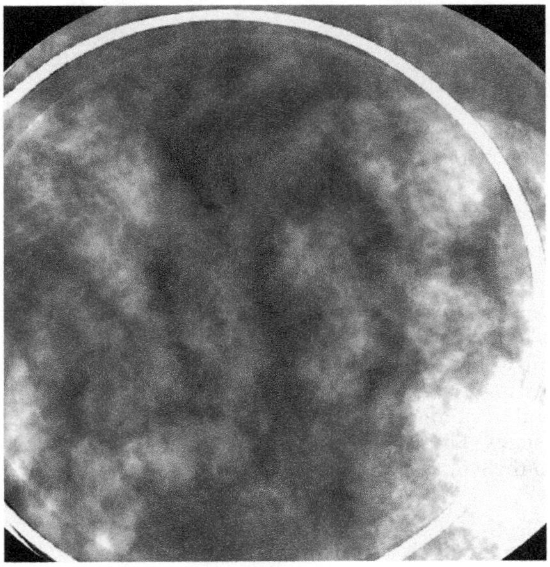

FIGURE 4-37. SBFT in a 50-year-old man with multiple nodular thickened small bowel folds due to tropical sprue.

of small bowel fold thickening, the disease is characterized by peripheral eosinophilia and prolonged history of allergy.

Graft-Versus-Host-Disease

Graft-versus-host disease (GVHD) results from an immune response by donor lymphocytes, usually after allogeneic bone marrow transplantation. The liver, skin, and GI tract are typically involved. The small bowel is frequently involved with a severe edema and mucosal inflammatory change (Fig. 4-39). The inflamed mucosa may demonstrate intense enhancement, and strictures and loss of fold pattern can be present in healing (Figs. 4-40 and 4-41).

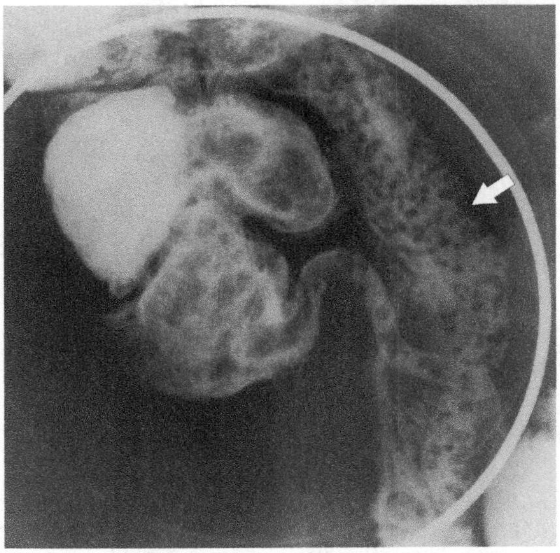

FIGURE 4-38. SBFT in a 38-year-old woman with multiple nodular terminal ileal nodules due to nodular lymphoid hyperplasia (*arrow*).

Mastocytosis

This disease results from excessive systemic histamine release from mast cells (hence, mastocytosis) and affects multiple sites and organs—including the skin (urticaria pigmentosa), lymph nodes (lymphadenopathy), liver (hepatomegaly), spleen (splenomegaly with focal deposits), and bone (sclerotic and lytic lesions in the axial skeleton)—not just the small bowel. Symptoms are expected and related to the histamine release. Patients have headache, flushing, urticaria and pruritus, and sometimes profuse diarrhea.

There is often associated peptic ulcer disease, but it more commonly affects the small bowel with diffusely thickened folds, usually in an irregular pattern but they can also be uniform. There is fine mucosal nodularity (up to 3 mm), which may be identified at SBFT, but identification by CT is unlikely. CT may demonstrate other findings of mesenteric disease, including lymphadenopathy (Fig. 4-42).

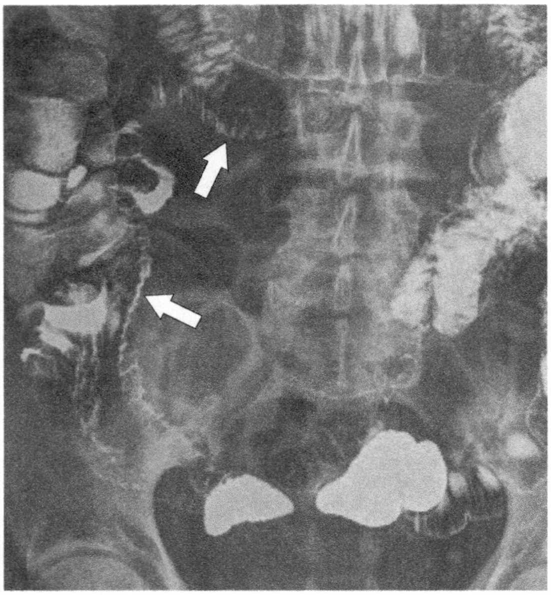

FIGURE 4-39. SBFT in a 61-year-old woman with a long ileal stricture and mucosal thickening (*arrows*) due to GVHD.

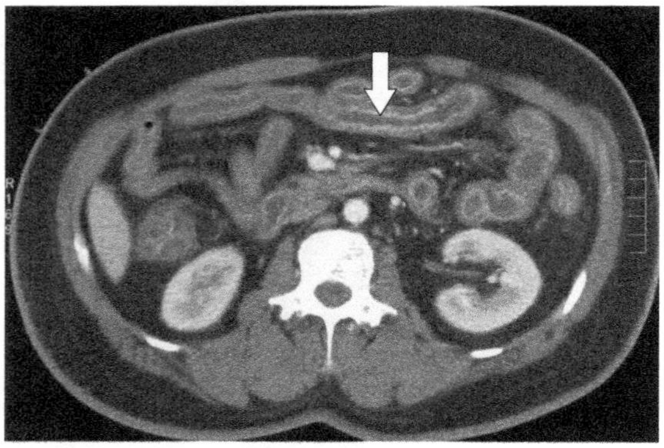

FIGURE 4-40. Axial contrast-enhanced CT in a 44-year-old man with diffuse small bowel narrowing and mucosal hyperemia (*arrow*) due to GVHD.

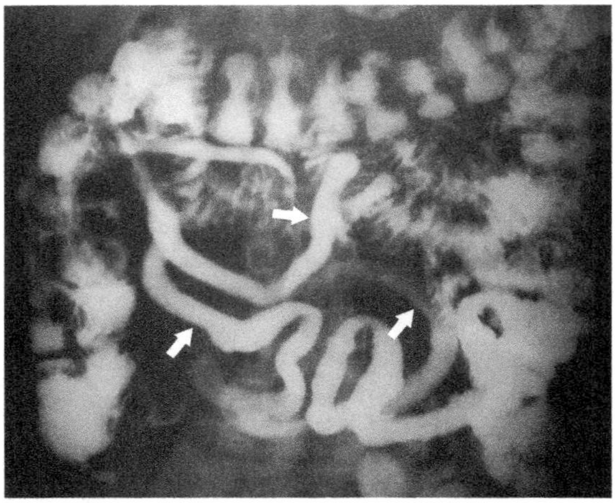

FIGURE 4-41. SBFT in a 55-year-old man with a long ileal stricture (*arrows*) resulting from prior GVHD.

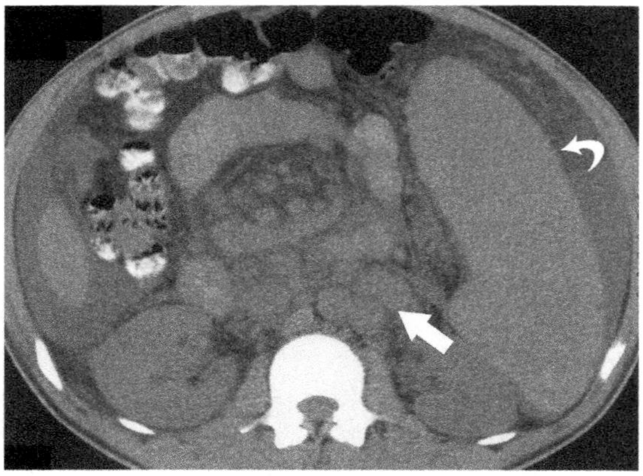

FIGURE 4-42. Axial noncontrast CT in a 43-year-old man with mastocytosis and multiple intraabdominal nodes (*arrow*). There is associated splenomegaly (*curved arrow*) and ascites.

Angioneurotic Edema

Angioneurotic edema is congenital (autosomal dominant hereditary angioneurotic edema) or acquired and is the result of a specific allergen or drug. It is potentially life threatening because of airway edema and obstruction. In an acute attack, there is marked elevation of bradykinin and mast cell tryptase with deficiency of complement factors and C1 esterase, resulting in widespread vasodilatation. These potent vasodilators produce widespread interstitial edema and in the small bowel diffuse small bowel mucosal edema (Fig. 4-43). Drug-induced angioedema is increasingly recognized, particularly that caused by angiotensin-converting enzyme (ACE) inhibitors (African Americans are more susceptible). ACE inhibitors, which prevent bradykinin metabolism in susceptible individuals, accumulate systemically and causes the angioedema (Fig. 4-44).

Waldenström Macroglobulinemia

Waldenström* macroglobulinemia, also known as lymphoplasmacytic lymphoma with excessive B-cell proliferation, is predominantly in the bone marrow and lymph nodes. There are large concentrations of the paraprotein IgM in the peripheral blood, which is readily identified by electrophoresis. The IgM proliferation can cause hyperviscosity in the intestinal lymphatics, leading to intestinal malabsorption. Imaging features are nonspecific with mucosal thickening, similar to lymphangiectasia or hypoproteinemic states. There may be associated retroperitoneal adenopathy due to the lymphoproliferative disorder.

*Jan G. Waldenström (1906-1996), Swedish oncologist.

Hemorrhage

Intramural hemorrhage from any cause typically causes uniform small bowel mucosal thickening with the valvulae conniventes having a "picket fence" or "stacked coin" appearance on SBFT and nonspecific mucosal and submucosal thickening at CT, which may be hyperdense depending on disease acuity (Figs. 4-45 and 4-46). It is generally impossible to differentiate the causes by imaging, so clinical history is the key to the diagnosis once the abnormality is identified. Hemorrhages can result from several causes, listed in Table 4-3.

Henoch-Schönlein Purpura

Henoch-Schönlein purpura (HSP) disease usually affects children and young adults. It is of uncertain etiology, generally follows viral or bacterial infections, and causes symptoms such as hemorrhagic skin rash, joint and abdominal pain, and melena. It is due to a systemic vasculitis that results from immune complex

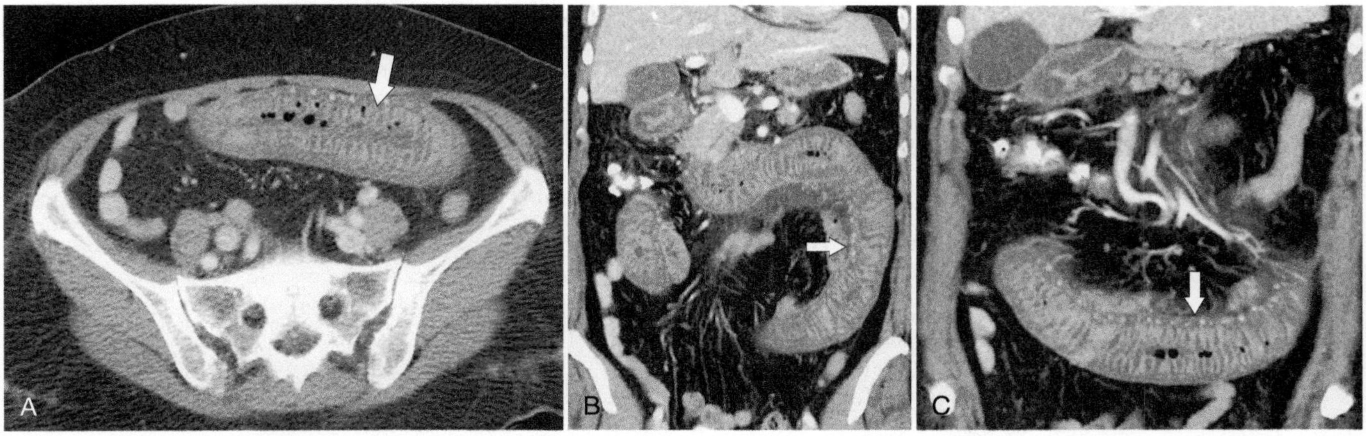

Figure 4-43. Axial (**A**) and coronal (**B** and **C**) contrast-enhanced CT in a 70-year-old man with marked duoedenal and jejunal thickening (*arrows*) caused by hereditary angioneurotic edema.

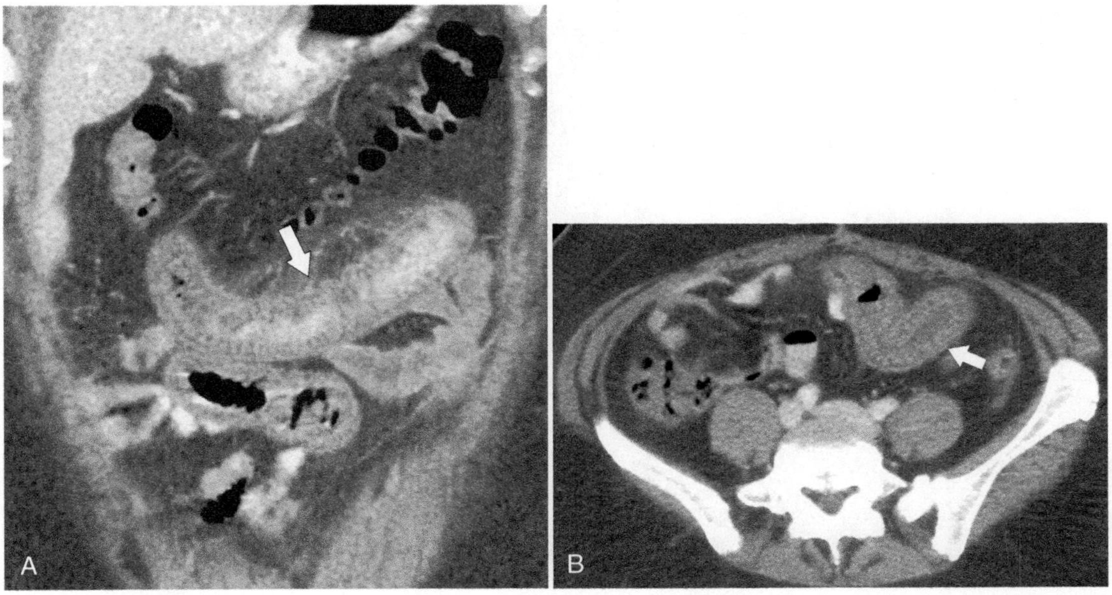

Figure 4-44. Coronal (**A**) and axial (**B**) contrast-enhanced CT in a 31-year-old woman with marked mucosal and wall thickening (*arrows*) and inflammation (stranding) caused by angioneurotic edema from lisinopril administration.

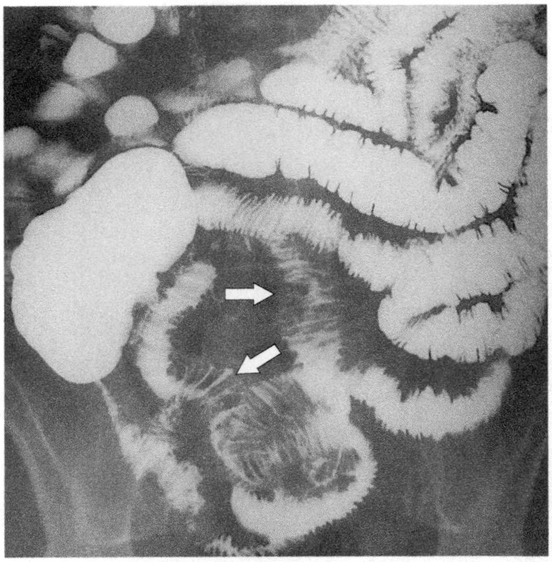

Figure 4-45. SBFT in a 37-year-old woman with small bowel hemorrhage with a "picket-fence"–appearing mucosa (*arrows*).

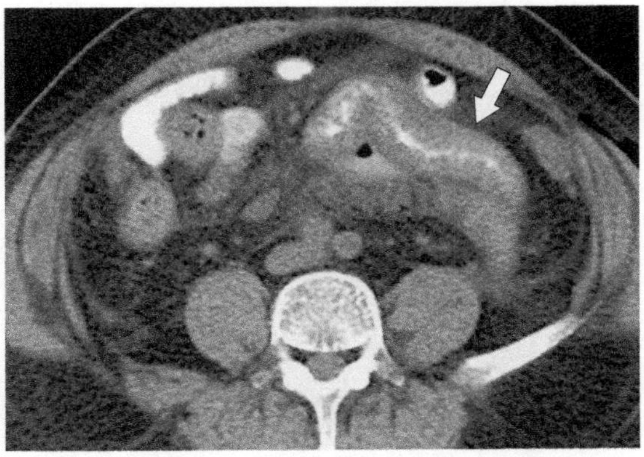

Figure 4-46. Axial contrast-enhanced CT in a 40-year-old man with recent motor vehicle accident and jejunal wall thickening (*arrow*) caused by jejunal hemorrhage. There is also diffuse mesenteric edema (stranding).

TABLE 4-3 Intramural Hemorrhage

Bleeding diatheses	Diffuse intravascular coagulation Anticoagulants Hemophilia
Vasculitis	Systemic lupus erythematosus Churg-Strauss syndrome Granulomatosis with polyangiitis Radiation
Trauma	
Mesenteric ischemia/infarction	
Congenital	Idiopathic thrombocytopenia Henoch-Schönlein purpura
Malignancy	Lymphoma

deposition containing IgA. In the small bowel, the vasculitis can cause edema, intramural hemorrhage, intussusception, necrosis, and perforation, particularly of the upper small bowel, but it can occur anywhere in the small bowel and colon. Imaging can be of a nonspecific vasculitis with wall and mucosal thickening but with increased density due to intramural hemorrhage, which may be visualized by CT (Fig. 4-47). The mucosal folds in intramural hemorrhage have a "picket fence" appearance at SBFT. The mucosal and wall thickening are readily identified at CT. The intramural hemorrhage can also be visualized by ultrasound, and because the disease often occurs in younger patients, ultrasound is the investigation of choice in this age group (Fig. 4-48).

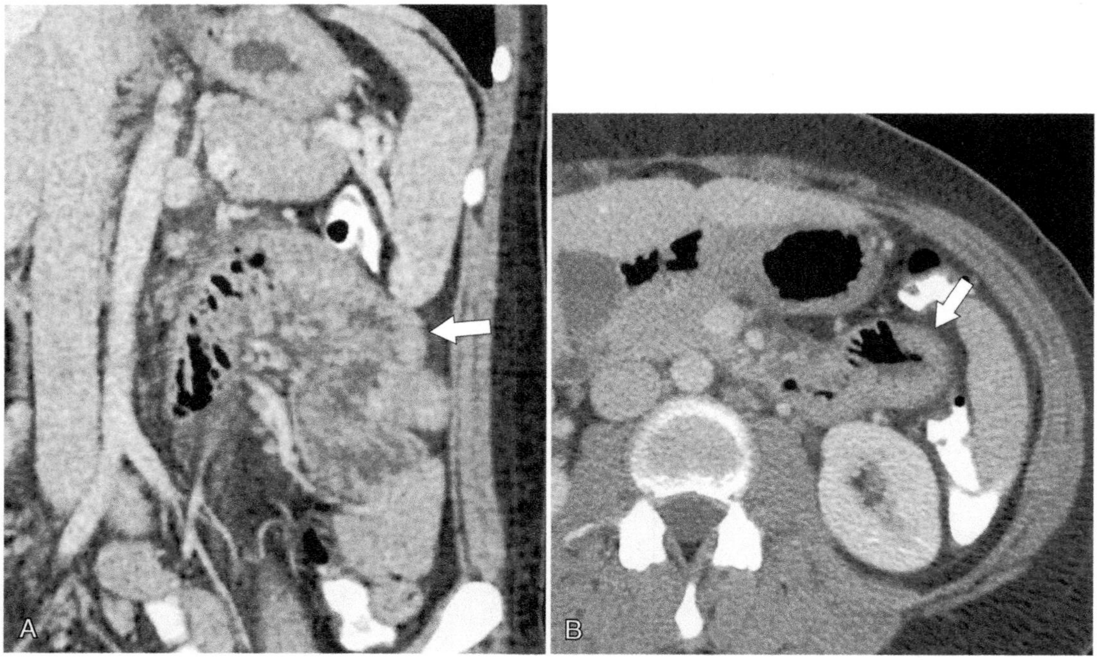

FIGURE 4-47. Coronal (**A**) and axial (**B**) CT in a 23-year-old woman with jejunal thickening due to intramural hemorrhage (*arrows*) from Henoch-Schönlein purpura.

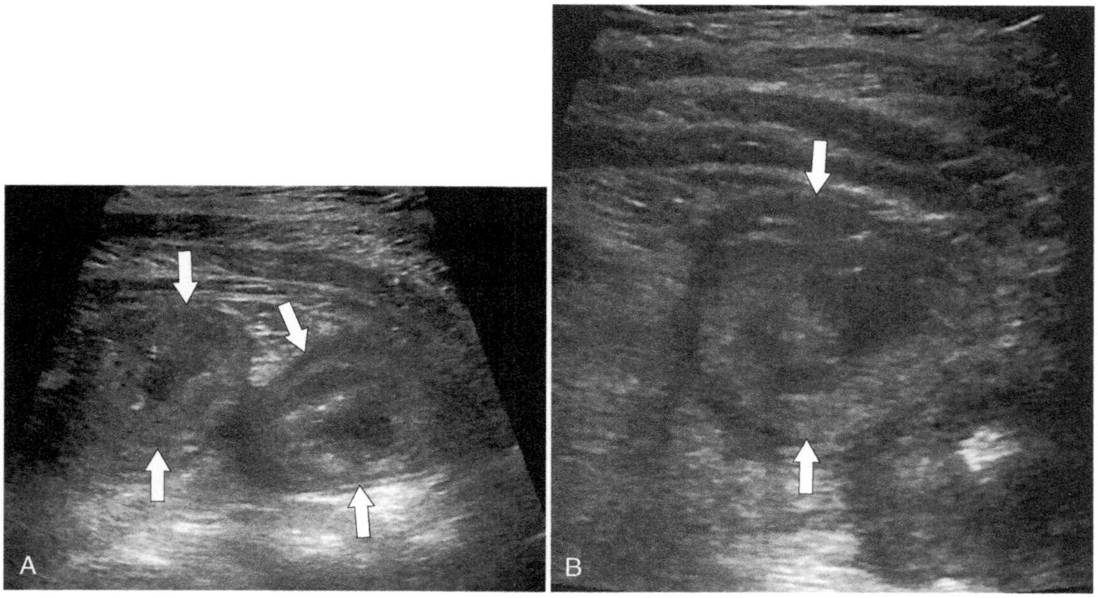

FIGURE 4-48. Transverse ultrasound (**A** and **B**) in a 21-year-old woman with Henoch-Schönlein purpura with marked jejunal wall and mucosal thickening (*arrows*).

Vasculitis

A range of autoimmune disease, such as systemic lupus erythematosus, Churg-Strauss syndrome, and granulomatosis with polyangiitis, causes small bowel edema through vasculitis. The small bowel is often affected, given the rich mesenteric vascular supply, which can affect both small and large vessels (arteries and veins). The inflammatory effect on small mesenteric vessels leads to localized ischemia with small bowel wall and mucosal thickening, which is often widespread (Figs. 4-49 and 4-50).

Idiopathic Thrombocytopenia

Idiopathic thrombocytopenia (ITP) is a disease characterized by platelet depletion from antibody destruction, predominantly in the spleen, which, when severe, can cause widespread hemorrhage in different organs, including the small or large bowel. In the small bowel, the features are of submucosal bleeding with thickened, crowded picket fence–like folds, similar to other causes of intramural small bowel hemorrhage.

Small Bowel Varices

Small bowel varices are rare but can produce a smooth submucosal serpiginous defect similar to that seen in esophageal varices.

Ischemic Enteritis

Ischemic enteritis can be acute (with sudden onset of abdominal pain, diarrhea, and vomiting) or chronic with symptoms of intestinal

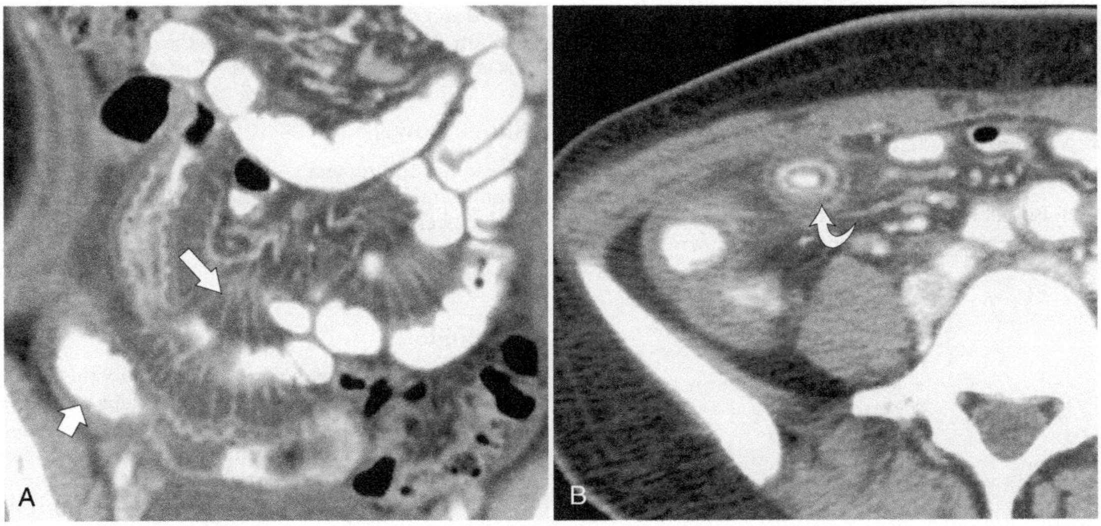

FIGURE 4-49. Coronal (**A**) and axial (**B**) contrast-enhanced CT in a 29-year-old woman with mesenteric hyperermia (*large arrow*), thickened ileum (*small arrow*), and mural stratification (*curved arrow*) from acute systemic lupus erythematosus.

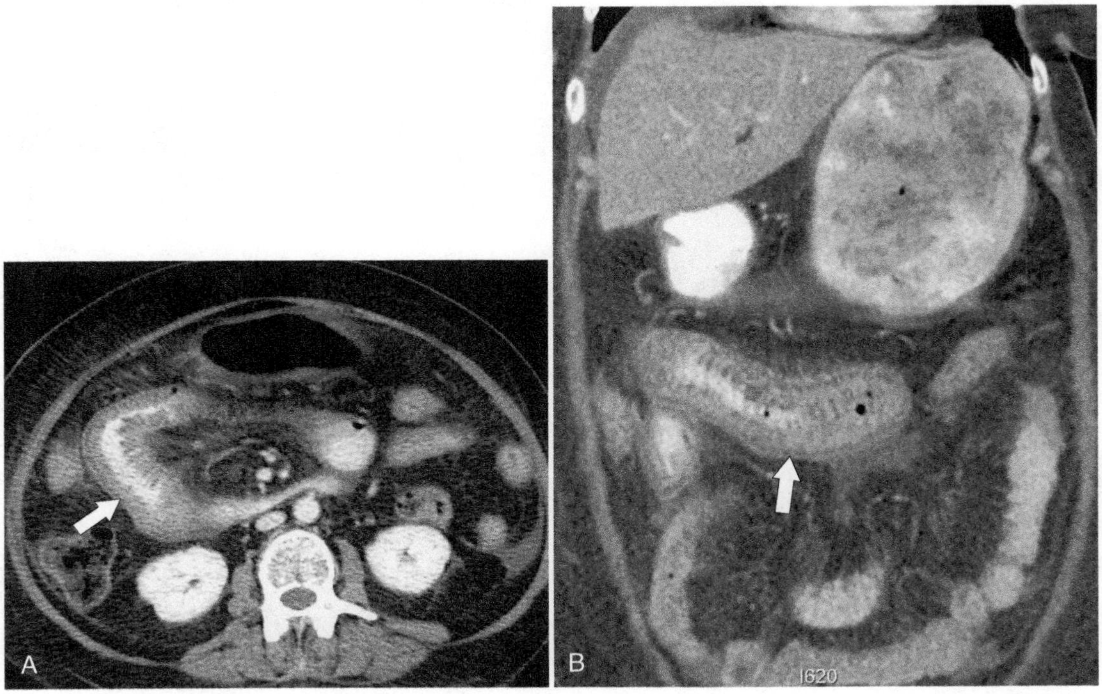

FIGURE 4-50. Axial (**A**) and coronal (**B**) contrast-enhanced CT in a 60-year-old woman with marked diffuse small bowel wall thickening (*arrows*) due to Churg-Strauss disease (autoimmune vasculitis).

angina (postprandial abdominal pain), weight loss, vomiting, and diarrhea. Acute forms usually result from vascular occlusion (emboli, thrombosis), which can be arterial or venous, although the former is far more common. However, up to 30% of acute ischemic events are nonocclusive. Given that acute ischemia carries a high mortality if it is left untreated (50% to 90%), most patients should be considered a surgical emergency to rescue the affected bowel from infarction and necrosis. Patients with cardiac disease are particularly susceptible to mesenteric ischemia because the combined effect of poor cardiac output and vascular stenosis can result in marked low-flow mesenteric vascular states. Other causes of ischemic enteritis are listed in Table 4-4 and can be inflammatory or caused by the cytotoxic vascular effects of radiation or drugs.

Plain radiographs often demonstrate an ileus and thickened bowel wall if severe. In delayed cases, intramural gas can be identified, representing profound ischemia as intraluminal gas permeates the mucosa and then through the bowel wall and subsequently into the mesenteric venous system and liver in advanced cases. A small bowel follow-through examination, which is now rarely performed, will demonstrate thickening and crowding of the valvulae conniventes ("stacked coin" appearance) caused by submucosal edema and hemorrhage (Fig. 4-51). It usually heals by stricture formation, which is generally "fixed" at SBFT (Fig. 4-52).

TABLE 4-4 Small Bowel Ischemic Enteritis

Vascular occlusion	Emboli Thrombosis Hypercoagulable states Volvulus/closed-loop obstruction
Inflammatory	Pancreatitis Systemic lupus erythematosus Polyarteritis nodosa chemotherapy
Hypoperfusion	Sepsis Heart failure
Amyloid	
Radiation	Endarteritis obliterans
Drugs	Chemotherapy Heroin/cocaine Digoxin Dopamine Vasopressive agents

A multitude of findings can be demonstrated at CT, which is the investigation of choice. This requires contrast-enhanced CT, which should include arterial and venous phases to evaluate both the arterial and venous supply. This may identify arterial occlusive disease in the superior mesenteric artery or superior mesenteric vein. Because of the low-flow states, the small bowel mucosa enhances poorly and the bowel wall is thickened. There is a propensity for submucosal hemorrhage, which is identified as high-density material in the bowel wall at CT. The surrounding small bowel mesentery is edematous (stranding), and the affected bowel will demonstrate mucosal and mural thickening (Fig. 4-53). Severe ischemia will ultimately cause small bowel infarction, which at CT can be recognized as an area of poorly enhancing or nonenhancing bowel, which has an ominous "dusky" appearance, usually with adjacent edema (Fig. 4-54). Pneumatosis may also develop in severe cases with gas in the bowel wall, mesenteric vessels, or hepatic portal venous system (Fig. 4-55). The finding of intraluminal or mesenteric gas may be subtle and only be appreciated by viewing CT images with "lung windows" contrast settings to maximize the contrast between the gas and surrounding soft tissues (Fig. 4-55).

Shock Bowel

Shock bowel is reversible ischemic small bowel, usually caused by hypovolemic states. The transitory hypoperfusion results in diffuse bowel wall thickening and characteristic increased mucosal enhancement due to the capillary low-flow states combined with increased vascular permeability induced by the ischemia (Fig. 4-56).

Amyloidosis

Amyloidosis is a systemic disease caused by the deposit of amyloid proteins. There are multiple designations of amyloid, depending on the protein type. For instance, AL is amyloid light chain, seen in multiple myeloma and can also be classified as primary amyloidosis. Other forms are familial (ATTR protein deposition). Secondary amyloidosis (AA protein deposition) is due to protein production from chronic, particularly infective, disease (e.g., bronchiectasis). Amyloid can deposit almost anywhere, including the heart, lungs, joints, brain, skin, and GI tract. Disease in the small bowel is often due to ischemia resulting from amyloid deposition within submucosal vessels. This can result in an edematous and thickened small bowel wall, which can also ulcerate and even

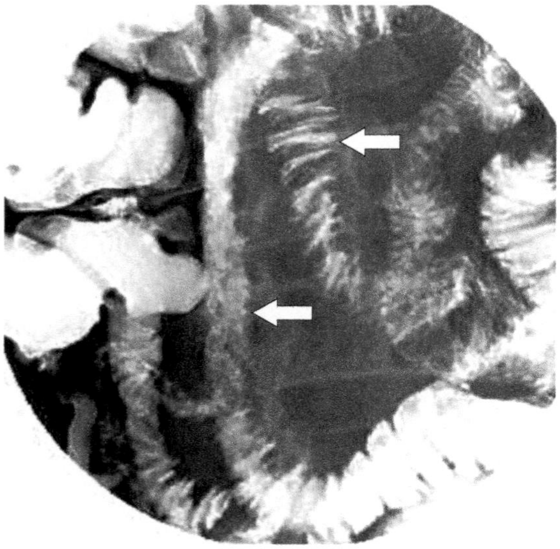

FIGURE 4-51. SBFT in a 68-year-old woman with ischemic ileal strictures and mucosal edema (*arrows*).

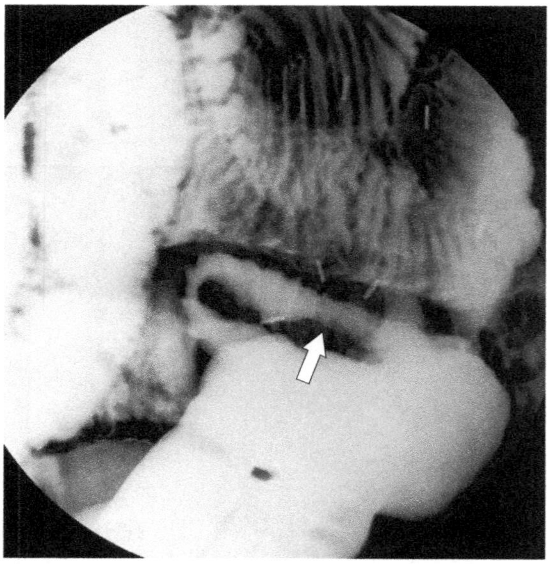

FIGURE 4-52. SBFT in a 61-year-old man with ischemic postsurgical stricture (*arrow*).

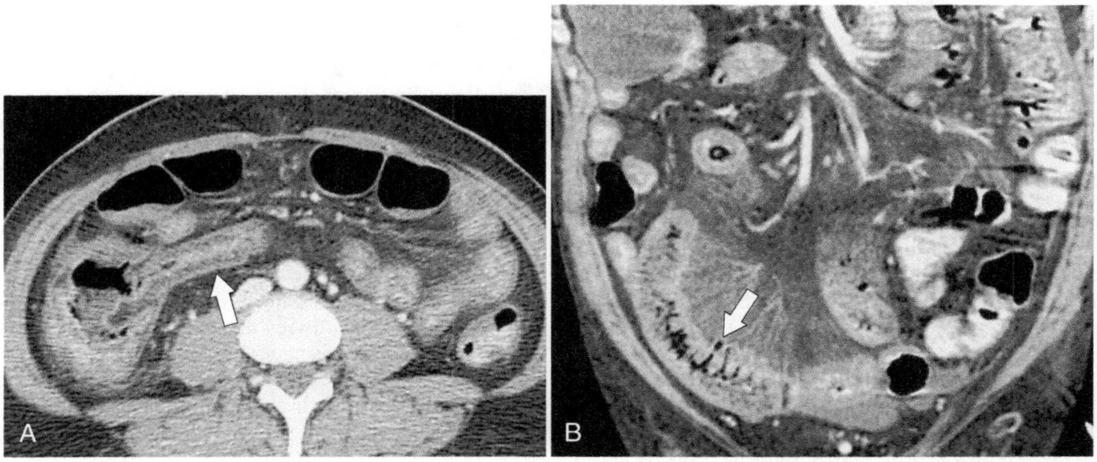

FIGURE 4-53. Axial (**A**) and coronal (**B**) contrast-enhanced CT in a 68-year-old woman with distal ileal thickening (*arrows*) due to ischemia.

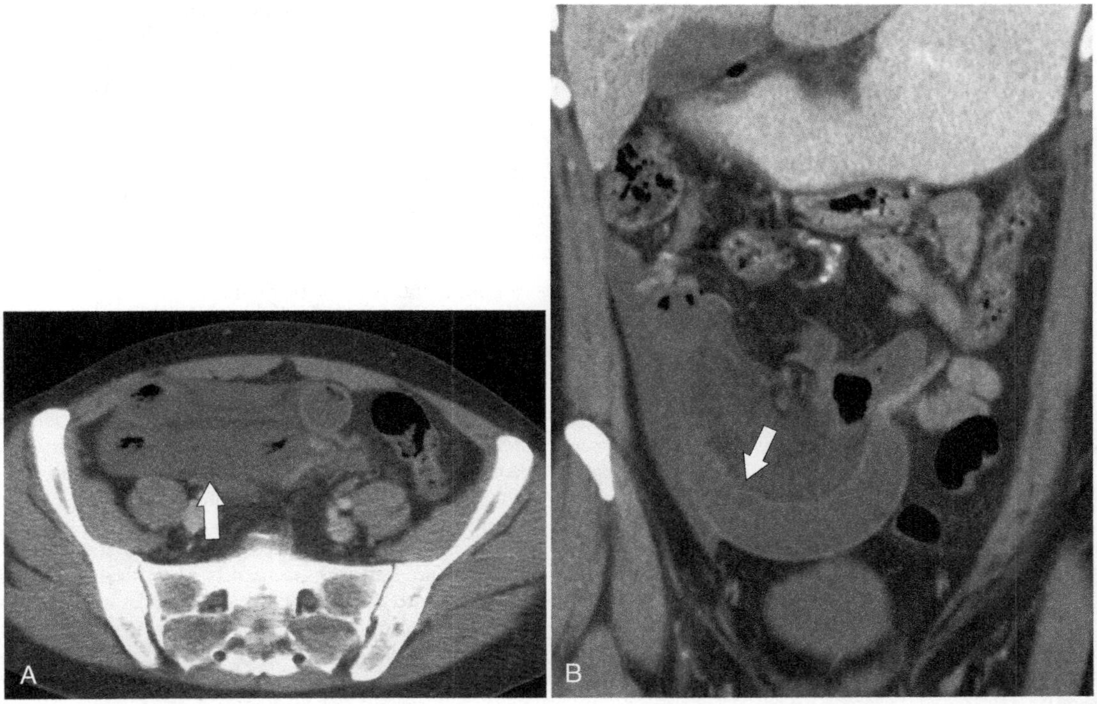

FIGURE 4-54. Axial (**A**) and coronal (**B**) contrast-enhanced CT in a 46-year-old woman with an incarcerated closed-loop obstruction with a dusky appearance due to lack of normal bowel enhancement (*arrows*) signifying pending infarction.

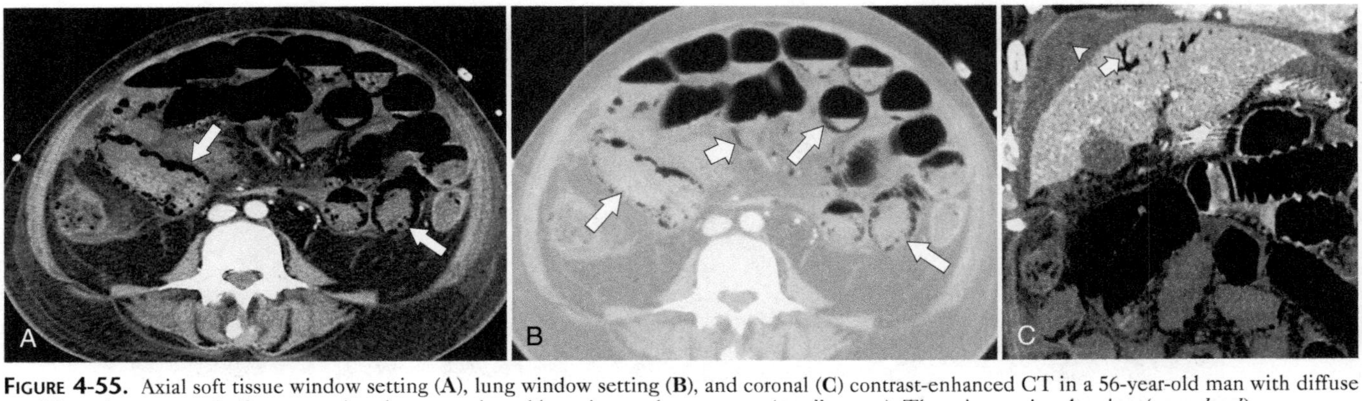

FIGURE 4-55. Axial soft tissue window setting (**A**), lung window setting (**B**), and coronal (**C**) contrast-enhanced CT in a 56-year-old man with diffuse small bowel pneumatosis (*large arrows*) and mesenteric and hepatic portal venous gas (*small arrows*). There is associated ascites (*arrowhead*).

perforate. Patients will usually have symptoms of diarrhea, malabsorption, and sometimes perforation. Multiple small mucosal nodular densities, which are granular, can be identified by SBFT. At CT there is nonspecific wall thickening, and the clue to the diagnosis will be the clinical history (Fig. 4-57).

Radiation Enteritis

Modern radiation therapy protocols have significantly reduced the complications from radiation therapy, but given its frequent use, radiation enteritis is unavoidable for some patients. Its mechanism is by either direct cytotoxic cell death from free radical production or endarteritis and vascular occlusion. Different parts of the bowel better tolerate the effects of radiation than others, with the rectum and the esophagus being least tolerant and the small bowel being the most tolerant.

Patients present with either acute or subacute/chronic disease. In the acute phase (typically less than 2 months after therapy), there is hyperemia, mucosal thickening, or ulceration. These may produce pain, diarrhea, and bleeding. In the subacute/chronic phase, there is intermittent colicky abdominal pain with diarrhea and sometimes steatorrhea.

Although SBFT can demonstrate many findings, it is performed less often. In the acute phase, there are mucosal edema and thickening of the valvulae conniventes with the picket fence configuration at SBFT. Depending on the severity, there is evidence of stricture formation in the chronic phase, and the bowel may become acutely angulated from adhesion formation. Chronic ulcers and fistulas can occur, particularly at any surgical anastomotic site. CT findings demonstrate similar features with bowel wall and mucosal thickening in the acute phase (there may be associated mucosal hyperemia and enhancement). Stricture and fistula formation may be harder to identify by CT than by SBFT.

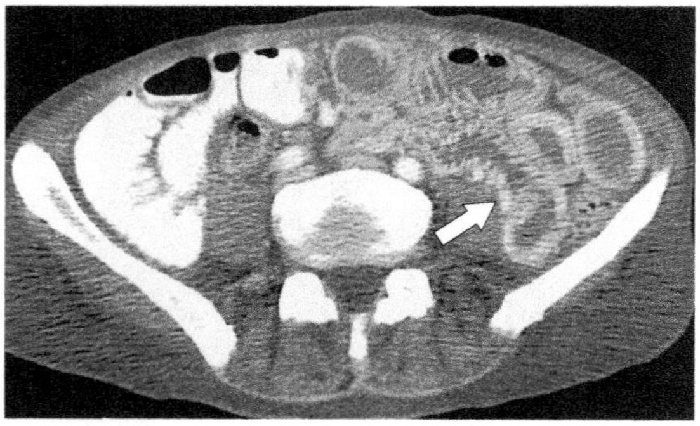

FIGURE 4-56. Axial contrast-enhanced CT in a 58-year-old man in a motor vehicle accident with hyperenhancing thickened distal jejunum (*arrow*) caused by shock bowel.

Small Bowel Edematous States

Although most inflammatory diseases (e.g., Crohn disease) will produce small bowel edema, particularly in their acute forms, some diseases produce diffuse bowel wall thickening (primarily mucosal) because of marked edema, also known as wet bowel. There are often edematous findings elsewhere (ascites, pleural effusion, and anasarca).

Venous Pressure

Increased venous pressure causes uniform small bowel fold thickening. Edema usually results from low-flow states from increased downstream intravascular venous pressure, including severe congestive heart failure, portal venous hypertension from any cause, mesenteric vessel ischemia, or thrombosis (Fig. 4-58).

Hypoproteinemic States

Hypoproteinemic states result from renal, GI, and particularly hepatic disease. GI diseases (e.g., giardiasis) can cause malabsorption syndromes that contribute to a hypoproteinemic state and subsequent anasarca. The findings at imaging are nonspecific and common to other causes of "wet" bowel with widespread mucosal edema that can usually be identified at CT (Fig. 4-59).

Lymphangiectasia

Lymphangiectasia is a rare disease characterized by hypoproteinemia, diffuse edema, and nutritional and immune deficiency from the loss of lymphatic fluid into the small intestine. There is a congenital form with malformation of lymphatics, resulting in ineffective lymphatic flow that causes regular thickening of the small bowel mucosa resulting from increased lymphatic pressure. It can also be acquired with lymphatic obstruction from inflammatory disease (particularly tuberculosis [TB]) or invasion from adjacent malignancies. Both congenital and acquired forms also lead to a protein-losing enteropathy, further exacerbating the small bowel thickening because of the edema and anasarca produced by the hypoproteinemia.

At SBFT there is diffuse, nonspecific, mucosal thickening from the edematous hypoproteinemic state (Fig. 4-60). These nonspecific features are readily identified at CT, which may also demonstrate the cause of obstruction from retroperitoneal masses in the acquired form. The dilated lymphatics are usually identified within the mesentery (Fig. 4-61).

Abetalipoproteinemia

Abetalipoproteinemia is a rare genetic autosomal recessive disorder of lipid metabolism that usually appears in infancy and

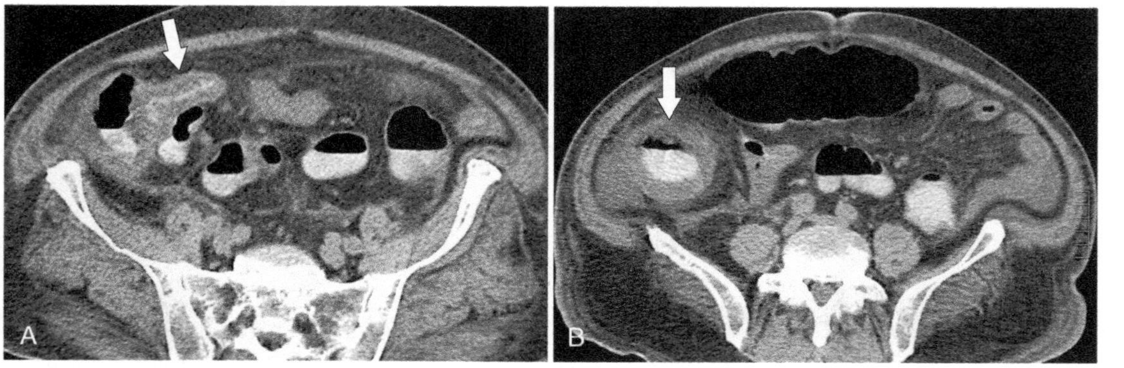

FIGURE 4-57. Axial (**A** and **B**) noncontrast CT in a 64-year-old man with diffuse small and large bowel thickening (*arrows*) due to amyloid deposition.

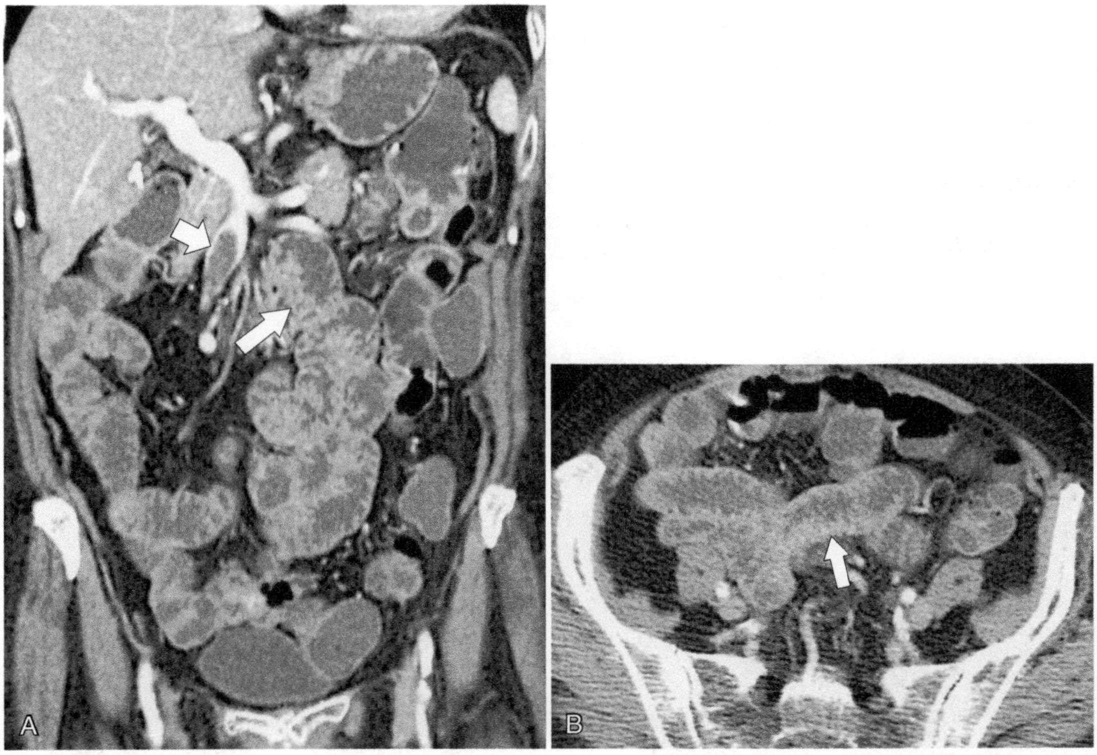

FIGURE 4-58. Coronal (**A**) and axial (**B**) contrast-enhanced CT in a 54-year-old man with diffuse small bowel mucosal thickening (*large arrows*) due to portal hypertension from a superior mesenteric vein thrombus (*small arrow*).

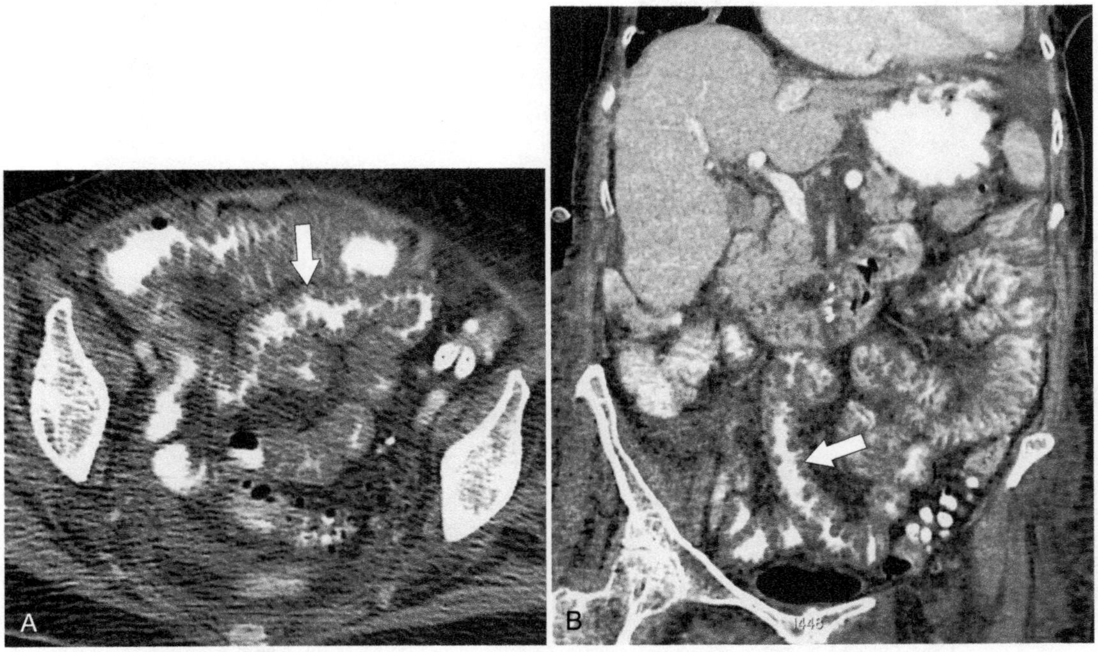

FIGURE 4-59. Axial (**A**) and coronal (**B**) contrast-enhanced CT in a 79-year-old woman with hyperproteinemia from protein-losing enteropathy, as well as "wet" bowel appearance from diffuse small bowel mucosal thickening (*arrows*) and mesenteric edema.

childhood and results in fat and fat-soluble vitamin malabsorption, producing steatorrhea and excessive fat deposition in mucosal cells. These conditions can then produce nonspecific uniformly thickened folds. There are associated cerebellar degeneration and acanthocytosis (star-shaped red blood cells).

Small Bowel Xanthomatosis

Small bowel xanthomatosis is a very rare disease with widespread lipid-laden macrophage deposition, particularly of the skin. It more commonly affects the stomach, but in the small bowel there is diffuse regular mucosal thickening caused by macrophage deposition. There is usually an associated hyperlipidemia.

INFECTIONS

Whipple disease

Whipple* disease predominantly affects middle-aged men, primarily in the proximal small bowel, and is recognized by

*George Hoyt Whipple (1878-1976), American pathologist.

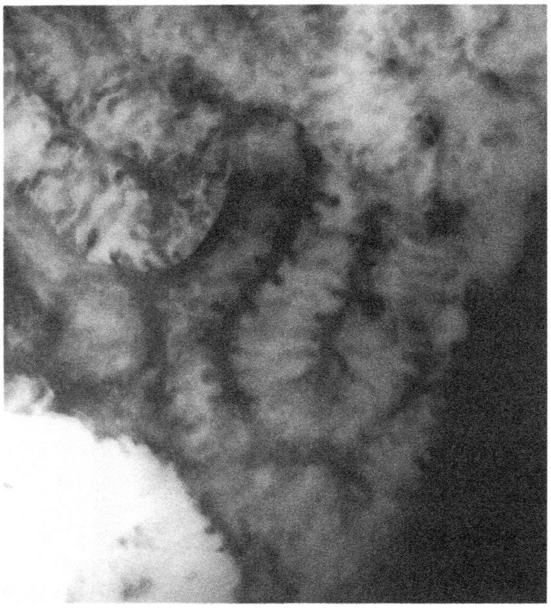

FIGURE 4-60. SBFT demonstrating uniformly thickened small bowel folds from lymphangiectasia.

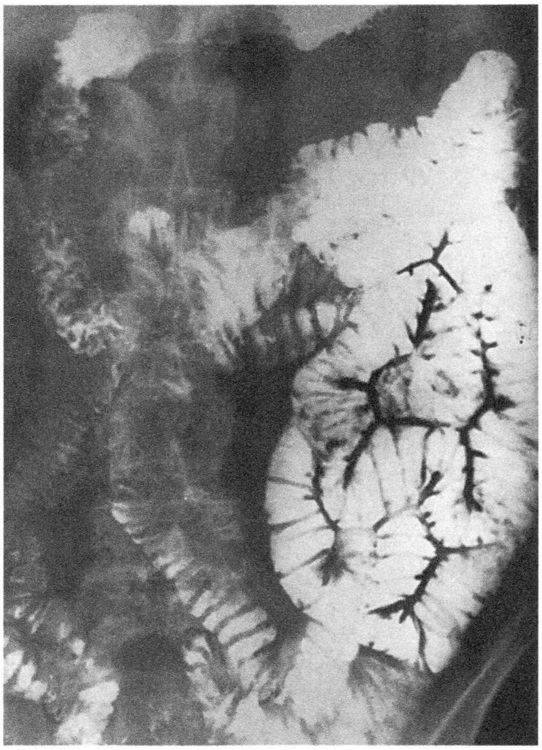

FIGURE 4-62. Diffuse small bowel thickening in Whipple disease.

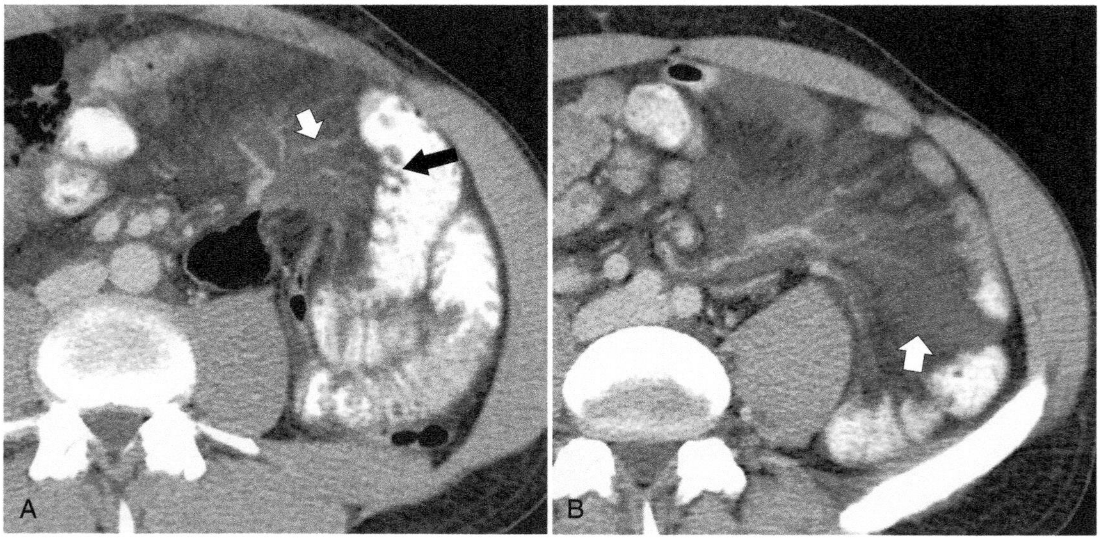

FIGURE 4-61. Axial (**A** and **B**) contrast-enhanced CT in a 47-year-old man with mucosal small bowel thickening (*black arrow*) due to intestinal lymphangiectasia (*white arrows*).

TABLE 4-5 Small Bowel Infections

Cause	Location	Specific Features
Bacteria		
Mycobacterium tuberculosis	Distal small bowel	Coned-shaped cecum Mesenteric and retroperitoneal adenopathy
Mycobacterium avium-intracellulare	Entire small bowel	Low-density adenopathy
Yersinia enterocolitica	Terminal ileum	Nonspecific wall thickening
Salmonella typhi	Distal small bowel	Nonspecific wall thickening
Shigella dysenteriae	Distal small bowel	Nonspecific wall thickening
Campylobacter jejuni	Small bowel	Usually no imaging findings, possible colonic focal thickening
Helicobacter pylori	Stomach and duodenum	Responsible for gastritis/duodenitis and peptic ulcer disease
Virus		
Herpes simplex	Distal small bowel	Mucosal thickening and ulceration
Cytomegalovirus	Entire small bowel	Mucosal thickening and ulceration Colonic infection more common
Human immunodeficiency virus	Entire small bowel	Mucosal thickening and ulceration
Fungus		
Paracoccidioides brasiliensis (blastomycosis)	Distal small bowel	Wall thickening and ulceration
Histoplasma capsulatum (histoplasmosis)	Entire small bowel	Wall thickening and ulceration
Candida albicans	Entire small bowel	Wall thickening and ulceration
Actinomycetes	Terminal ileum and colon	Wall thickening and ulceration
Aspergillosis	Entire small bowel	Wall thickening and ulceration
Coccidioidomycosis	Entire small bowel	Wall thickening and ulceration
Protozoa		
Giardia lamblia	Proximal small bowel	Mucosal thickening and flocculation
Cryptosporidium enteritis	Proximal small bowel	Mucosal thickening and flocculation
Isospora belli	Proximal small bowel	Mucosal thickening and flocculation
Entamoeba histolytica (amebiasis)	Terminal ileum and cecum	Chronic disease results in ameboma
Parasitic worm infection (see Table 4-6)	Entire small bowel	Some organisms can be identified at imaging (e.g., *Ascaris*).

macrophages laden with periodic acid–Schiff* material and gram-positive rods (*Tropheryma whipplei*) in the lamina propria of the bowel wall. Despite this, an infectious cause of this disease has not been fully established, although antibiotics are usually curative. Other clinical features include pleural and pericardial effusions, arthralgias, and central nervous system symptoms.

At imaging, thickened, nonspecific proximal small bowel folds are identified, either at SBFT or CT. There is often associated submucosal edema caused by an associated hypoproteinemic state (Fig. 4-62). CT will identify large mesenteric and retroperitoneal low-density nodes secondary to fatty replacement. There may be ascites and splenomegaly.

Box 4-1. Nodular Small Bowel Mucosal Thickening

Whipple disease
Yersinia
MAI
Histoplasmosis
Mastocytosis
Waldenström macroglobulinemia
Nodular lymphoid hyperplasia

MAI, Mycobacterium avium-intracellulare.

BACTERIAL INFECTIONS

Most infectious processes of the small bowel are indistinguishable from one another by imaging, although some affect certain regions of the small bowel more than others (Table 4-5). The infections that primarily affect the proximal small bowel include cryptosporidiosis, *Isospora* infections, giardiasis, and amebiasis. Those affecting the distal small bowel include *Yersinia* infections, TB, *Salmonella, Shigella,* herpes, and blastomycoses. The remaining infections can affect any aspect of the small bowel and include *Mycobacterium avium-intracellulare,* cytomegalovirus, human immunodeficiency virus (HIV), histoplasmosis, and *Candida* infection.

Before CT imaging was available, SBFT was common for the evaluation of the small bowel for the disparate disease listed in Table 4-5. Familiarity with different patterns of mucosal thickening was recognized, with uniform thickening, nodular thickening or a combination of both (Box 4-1). Some diseases produced reduced or effaced folds, representing profound mucosal thickening and fold coalescence and signaling more severe disease (Table 4-6).

*Hugo Schiff (1834-1915), German chemist

Mycobacteria

Mycobacterium tuberculosis remains very common worldwide, with a recent increase resulting from high HIV infection rates in some developing countries. In addition to the risk posed by underlying HIV or acquired immune deficiency syndrome (AIDS), patients are at greater risk with underlying type 2 diabetes, alcoholism, or any immunosuppressed state. Infection with the bovine strain is rare because of widespread milk pasteurization,* so most patients have gastrointestinal TB through the ingestion of infected sputum of the pulmonary strain. Despite this, concomitant pulmonary TB is seen only in about 30% of cases. Gastrointestinal TB predominantly affects the terminal ileum and colon, mainly because the bacterium is protected by a fatty capsule in the stomach and UGI tract, which becomes less protective the further it travels down the GI tract. With higher doses, however, gastric or duodenal infection can also occur. Patients may be asymptomatic or complain of ill-defined abdominal pain. Other symptoms are in keeping with TB infection elsewhere, including night sweats, fever, and weight loss. In more severe cases, patients will also have diarrhea and melena.

Infection is predominantly hypertrophic (70% of cases). This represents a fibroblastic reaction to the bacilli, which heals by fibrosis and stricturing. Ulcerative forms occur in 30% of patients, which are irregular and circumferential. Combined forms can appear similar to carcinoma and are more difficult to diagnose by imaging. Overwhelming infection can cause tuberculous peritonitis (usually follows perforation of the terminal ileum or colon) with widespread disease throughout the peritoneum. Imaging features will depend on the type and severity of disease and the timing of diagnosis. Acute ulcerative disease can be observed at SBFT by ulcerative disease in the ileocecal region and may be confused with Crohn disease. More commonly, there is ileocecal wall thickening along a length of bowel (which helps distinguish it from carcinoma, which is usually more focal) with or without stricture formation (Fig. 4-63). There is frequently regional or mesenteric lymphadenopathy. Chronic disease may result in a narrowed fibrotic cecum, sometimes termed a *coned cecum* (see Chapter 5). Patients with tuberculous peritonitis will generally be sicker and demonstrate thickening of the affected bowel, ascites, and mesenteric lymphadenopathy and can produce omental "caking," whereby the omentum is studded with tuberculous deposits and granulomata (Fig. 4-64).

*Louis Pasteur (1822-1895), French chemist and microbiologist.

TABLE 4-6 Small Bowel Fold Effacement

Infections	CMV Cryptosporidiosis Strongyloidiasis
Immune	GVHD Sprue
Inflammatory	Crohn disease Scleroderma Backwash ileitis (UC)
Vascular	Ischemia Radiation
Toxins	KCl Chemotherapeutic agents Cathartic abuse
	Amyloid
Neoplastic	Lymphoma

CMV, Cytomegalovirus; *GVHD*, graft-versus-host disease; *KCl*, potassium chloride; *UC*, ulcerative colitis.

Other Bacterial Enteritides

Shigella and *Salmonella* are gram-negative rods, acquired through the fecal-oral route, that can cause debilitating dysenteric GI infections, primarily of the ileocecal region. *Shigella*, of which there are many species, is responsible for shigellosis or shigella dysentery with symptoms of diarrhea, nausea, vomiting, pain, and sometimes bloody stool. With severe infections, nonspecific terminal ileal thickening can be observed by CT, but the diagnosis between this and other terminal ileal diseases (infectious or Crohn disease) can be difficult (Fig. 4-65).

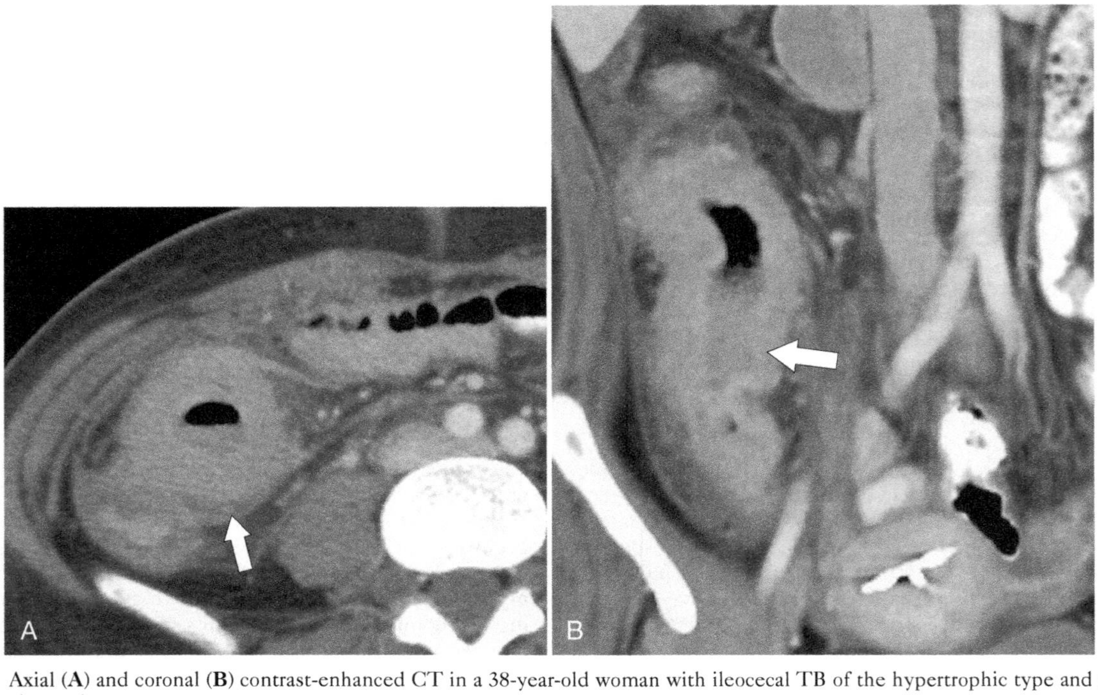

FIGURE 4-63. Axial (**A**) and coronal (**B**) contrast-enhanced CT in a 38-year-old woman with ileocecal TB of the hypertrophic type and marked bowel wall thickening (*arrows*).

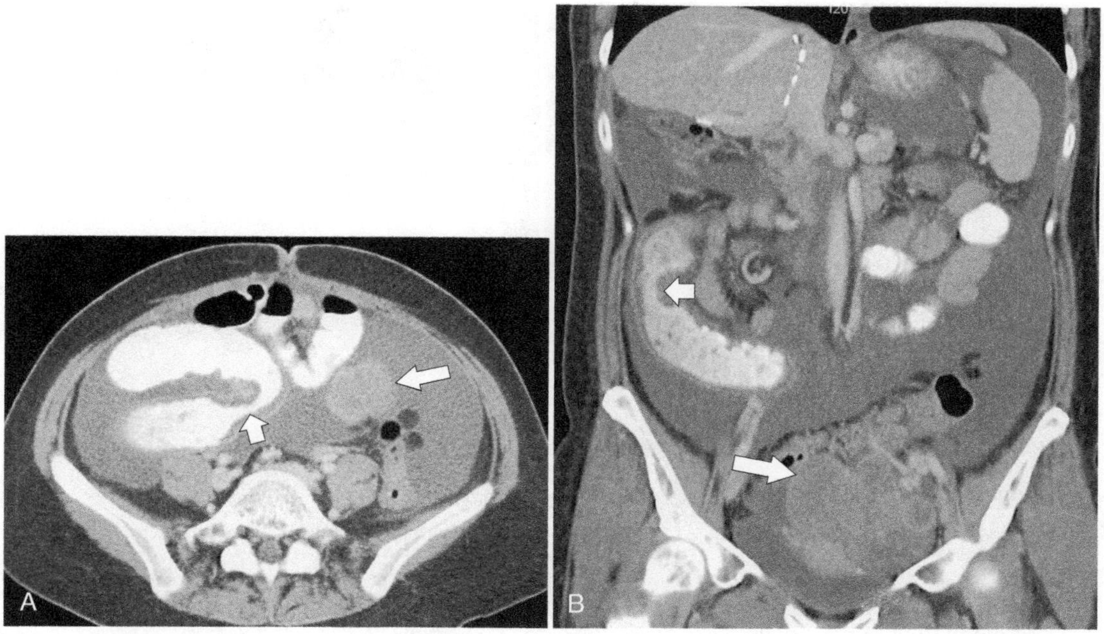

FIGURE 4-64. Axial (**A**) and coronal (**B**) contrast-enhanced CT in an immunosuppressed 51-year-old man with tuberculous peritonitis. There are terminal ileal thickening and stricturing (*small arrows*), ascites, and peritoneal masses caused by tuberculous adenopathy (*large arrows*).

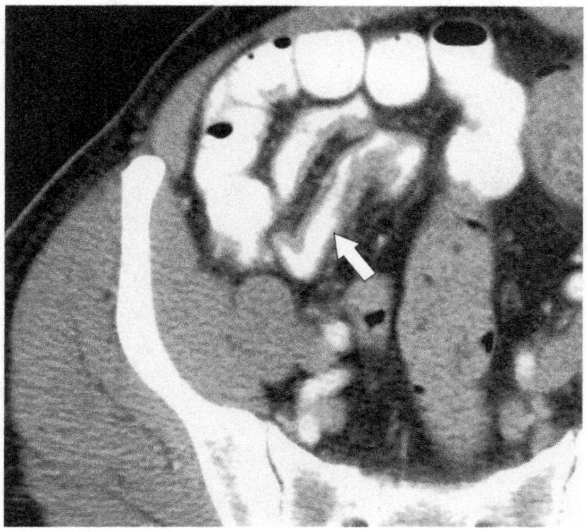

FIGURE 4-65. Axial contrast-enhanced CT in a 39-year-old man with terminal ileal wall thickening (*arrow*) caused by shigellosis.

Salmonella, of which there are also many species, is another dysenteric disease, ranging from a mild diarrheal food poisoning–type illness to typhoid fever and responsible for millions of deaths through the ages. Most patients with simple food poisoning have few or no imaging findings. *Salmonella typhi* infection, on the other hand, is responsible for typhoid fever, which is often a chronic, systemic disease with terminal ileal changes at imaging. Patients have a progressively high fever, cough, headache, bradycardia, and profound malaise. Although there is marked terminal ileal disease, there is little, if any, diarrhea. Terminal ileal hemorrhage may occur and appear with melena and perforation, and septicemia is often fatal. Ultimately, patients become severely dehydrated because of their fever and delirium. Most patients survive, though, with adequate rehydration alone, and antibiotics will expedite recovery. At imaging, there is nonspecific terminal ileal thickening, and splenomegaly is noted in severe cases (Fig. 4-66).

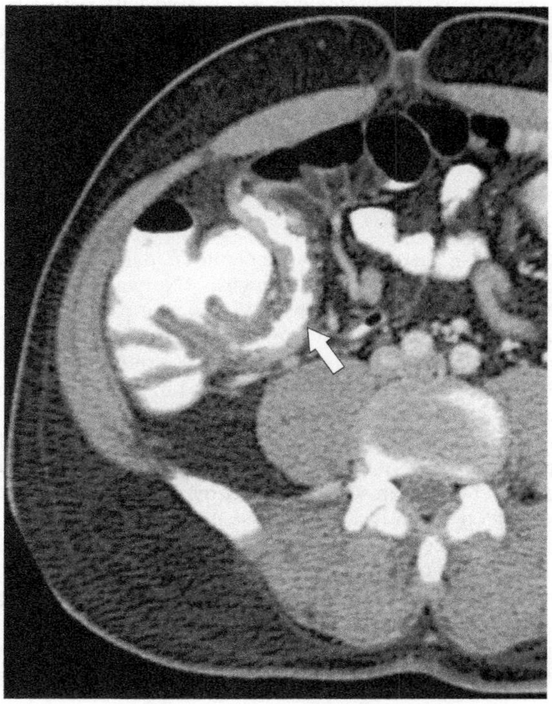

FIGURE 4-66. Axial contrast-enhanced CT in a 41-year-old man with terminal ileal mural thickening (*arrow*) due to *Salmonella typhi* infection.

Yersinia enterocolitica, also a gram-negative bacillus, can cause a self-limiting enterocolitis of the terminal ileum and cecum. The disease can be confused with acute appendicitis, given that patients often have right-sided abdominal pain and fever. At imaging there is nonspecific terminal ileal and/or cecal or ascending colonic thickness, but there may be regional lymphadenopathy because the disease can also invade Peyer patches and extend beyond to local lymph nodes (Fig. 4-67).

Campylobacter jejuni is a gram-negative helical organism, commonly responsible for gastroenteritis, usually by food poisoning.

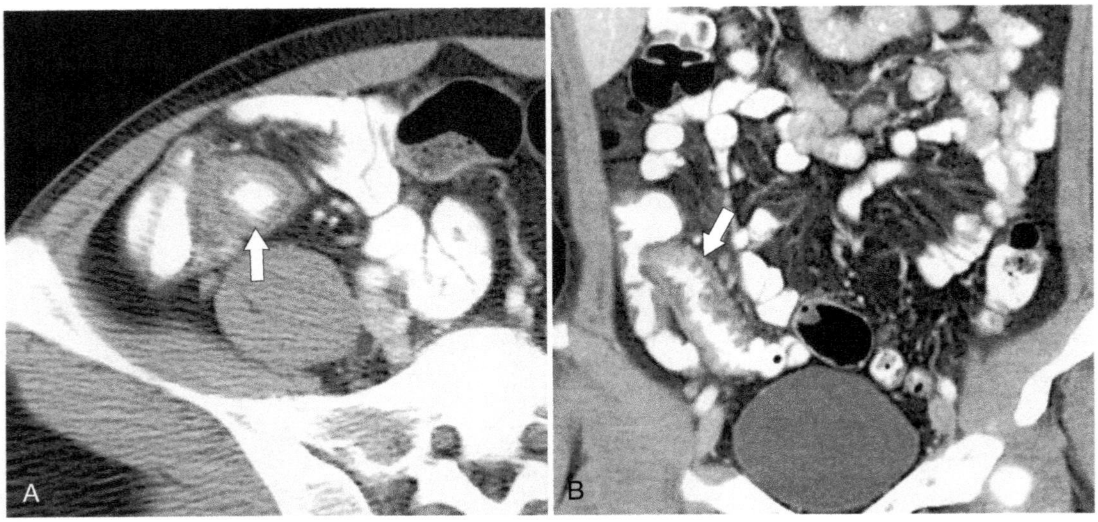

FIGURE 4-67. Axial (A) and coronal (B) contrast-enhanced CT in a 38-year-old man with terminal ileal mucosal thickening (*arrows*) caused by *Yersinia enterocolitica*.

It can be quite debilitating but is not usually fatal. It is, however, commonly associated with Guillain-Barré* syndrome, which starts 2 to 3 weeks after the initial infection. Patients with straightforward gastroenteritis complain of pain, diarrhea, and fever, but these symptoms can be aborted with early antibiotic treatment. *C. jejuni* affects the jejunum, ileum, and colon, and imaging findings are usually not present, partly because it is a self-limiting disease and imaging is not indicated. However, with more severe disease, some mural thickening can be visualized, particularly in the colon (see Chapter 5). *Helicobacter* infection is discussed in Chapters 2 and 3.

VIRAL ENTERITIS

Viral causes of gastroenteritis are common, particularly with rotavirus and norovirus (formerly known as "Norwalk agent"). These are usually UGI infections with vomiting a prominent feature, although many patients have some element of diarrhea. The disease is usually self-limiting, so imaging is rarely performed.

Other viruses are more sinister and can produce a more profound illness, particularly because they are more prevalent in immunocompromised patients. These include cytomegalovirus, herpes simplex, and HIV infections, and patients have a significantly higher mortality than with infection by other viral agents. Small bowel infection can result in diffuse mucosal edema with chronic diarrhea, which can ultimately lead to mucosal atrophy, ulceration, and malabsorption. Most patients also have a severe colitis. Imaging of the small bowel is rarely performed because specific features are generally not visible, but imaging of the colonic viral infection may demonstrate florid bowel wall thickening and even toxic megacolon (see Chapter 5).

FUNGAL ENTERITIS

The most common cause is *Candida* species, and infection typically occurs in the immunocompromised patient. Infection is far more common in the esophagus, and sometimes the stomach, but gastric hyperacidity often neutralizes the yeast. Other diseases are listed in Table 4-5. Patients complain of diarrhea, which can be bloody and profuse because colitis is often associated with small bowel disease in these patients. Many patients, in fact, have evidence of yeast infection in other organs as part of the immunocompromised systemic infection. Patients with small bowel enteritis are rarely imaged, and the diagnosis is made from stool analysis in the appropriate clinical setting and evidence of fungal disease elsewhere.

*Georges Guillain (1876-1961), French neurologist; Jean Barré (1880-1967), French neurologist.

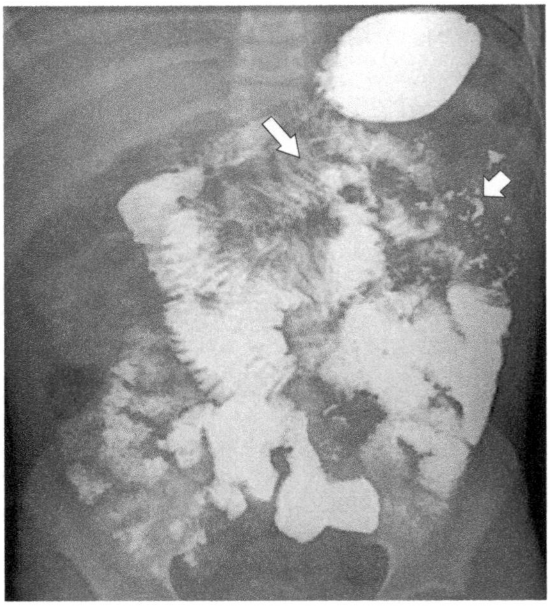

FIGURE 4-68. SBFT in a 9-year-old boy with giardiasis and small bowel mucosal thickening (*large arrow*) and flocculation (*small arrow*).

Protozoal Enteritis

Protozoal enteritis is a worldwide infectious process (up to 25% prevalence in some countries) of the small intestine due to ingestion and proliferation of the parasite *G. lamblia*. Infection is via ingestion of giardial cysts, usually via the fecal-oral route. Symptoms are the abrupt onset of watery diarrhea and excessive foul-smelling gas. There is nonspecific mucosal thickening, particularly of the distal duodenum and upper jejunum. At SBFT, there is the characteristically rapid transit of the barium from the small bowel into the colon and mucosal thickening of the duodenum and jejunum (Figure 4-68). There may be flocculation

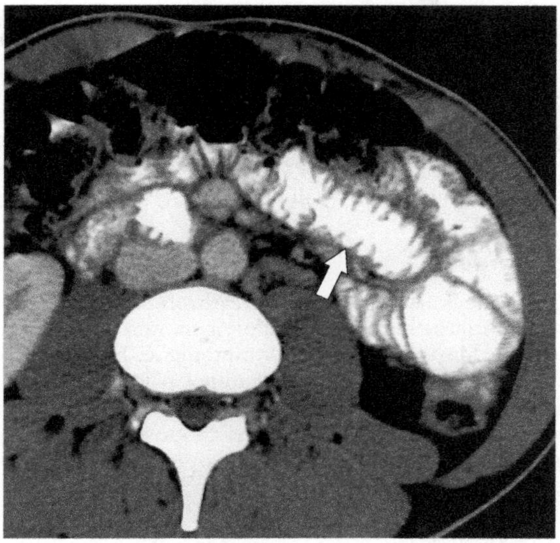

FIGURE 4-69. Axial contrast-enhanced CT in a 23-year-old man with giardiasis and thickened jejunal mucosa (*arrow*).

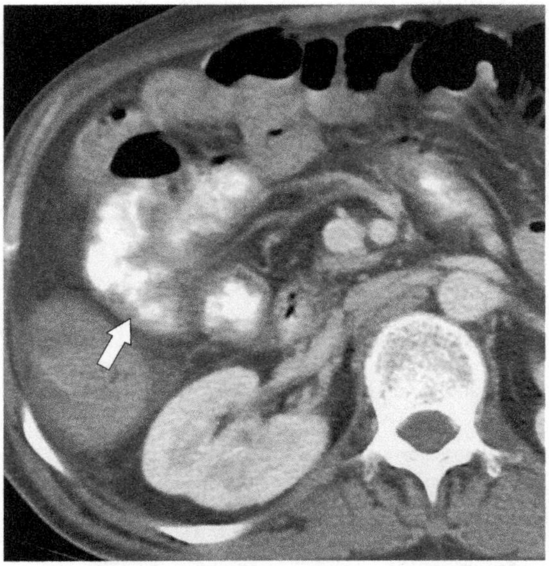

FIGURE 4-70. Axial contrast-enhanced CT in a 38-year-old man with small bowel wall thckening (*arrow*) due to *Isospora* infection.

of the barium as seen in celiac disease, consistent with the malabsorptive process. If CT is performed, which should be unnecessary, mucosal thickening, particularly of the duodenum and jejunum, can be observed (Figure 4-69). It is diagnosed by the identification of stool parasites or ELISA (enzyme-linked immunosorbent assay) testing.

Infection with *Isospora belli* causes clinical symptoms and imaging signs similar to giardiasis, and the disease can last for weeks (Fig. 4-70). Immunosuppressed patients are at risk for more severe disease, producing a concomitant colitis (Fig. 4-71).

Cryptosporidium enteritis is typically a short-term illness, but it can be severe in immunocompromised patients, particularly those with HIV infection, where coexistent infection is common. Patients are not usually imaged, but if they are, they may demonstrate mild small bowel wall thickening, similar to that seen with isosporal infections.

Entamoeba histolytica, or amebiasis, is a common protozoal infection, with perhaps up to 10% of the world's population being infected. Infection is via the fecal-oral route. The cysts

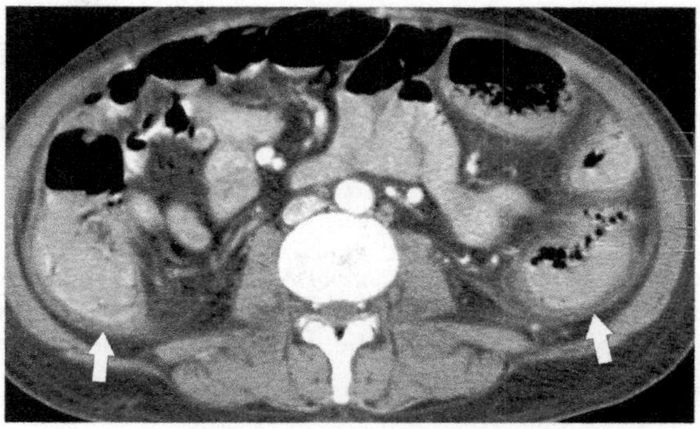

FIGURE 4-71. Axial contrast-enhanced CT in a 50-year-old man with *Isospora* infection with a pancolitis (*arrows*).

TABLE 4-7 Small Bowel Worms

Common Name	Scientific Name	Origin	Location in Small Bowel
Hookworm	*Necator americanus* *Ancylostoma duodenale*	Soil Soil	Proximal Proximal
Tapeworm	*Taenia saginata* *Taenia solium* *Diphyllobothrium latum*	Beef Pork Fish	Entire Entire Entire
Roundworm	*Ascaris lumbricoides*	Water	Entire
Strongyloidiasis	*Strongyloides stercoralis*	Water	Entire
Anisakiasis	*Anisakis*	Raw fish	Entire

are ingested, and they release trophozoites that invade the large intestine and can infect the lungs, brain, and liver. Intestinal evidence of disease is usually confined to the ileocecal region, producing bloody diarrhea. An ameboma may develop, representing ileocolic complex amebic fibrotic mass from chronic infection that can distort the cecal architecture and is one of the causes of a "coned" cecum. Patients may have large hepatic abscesses without any obvious imaging evidence of GI disease.

PARASITIC WORMS

Parasitic worms are also referred to as *helminth infection* and are endemic worldwide, with millions of patients infected (Table 4-7). Patients are generally asymptomatic, but severe infestation can result in abdominal pain, malabsorption, and anemia.

Hookworm

There are two species of this parasitic nematode that infests humans, *Necator americanus* and *Ancylostoma duodenale.* They are found mainly in the duodenum and proximal small bowel. They are thought to infect more than 500 million people worldwide and are very common outside the industrialized West. An infection is usually unrecognized unless the resulting iron deficiency anemia caused by parasitic small bowel mucosal damage, microscopic hemorrhage, and engorgement by the parasites are severe. A diagnosis is usually made by detecting eggs in the stool because adult worms are rarely seen by imaging or endoscopy. Antihelminthic therapy is highly effective at eradicating host infection.

Tapeworm

Tapeworms are parasitic flatworms (cestodes) with three main species—*Taenia saginata, Taenia solium* and *Diphyllobothrium latum*—that originate from uncooked beef, pork, and fish, respectively. The worm anchors its head anywhere in the small bowel, and aside from absorbing ingested nutrients, they produce no major complications. These worms also can occasionally be visualized by imaging, particularly because they can grow up to enormous lengths (12 m long).

Roundworm

Another nematode, the *Ascaris lumbricoides*, or giant roundworm, is the most common parasitic worm to infect humans; more than 1 billion people are thought to be infected worldwide. Patients are usually asymptomatic, but a heavy infestation can cause nutritional deficiency or obstructive symptoms because of the mass effect from the entangled worms. They can also obstruct the pancreatic/bile duct and induce pancreatitis or biliary obstruction. Given their size (they can be up to 30 cm), roundworms can be identified by imaging, particularly with a large worm load, either by plain radiographs, SBFT, or CT (Figs. 4-72 and 4-73). They reside anywhere along the small bowel tract.

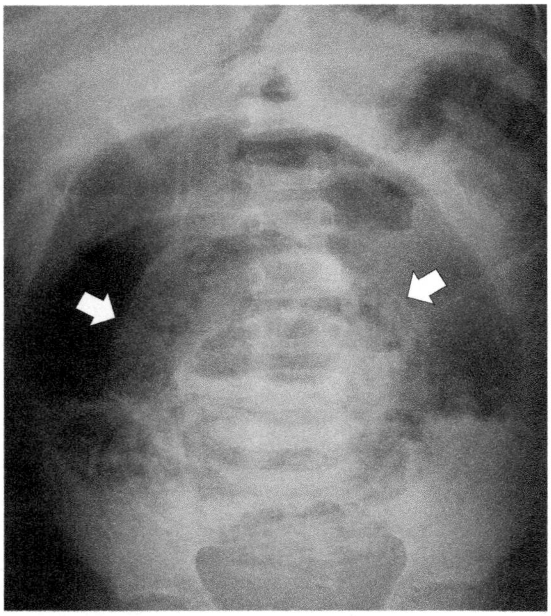

FIGURE 4-72. Plain abdominal radiograph in a 17-year-old boy with a mottled central abdominal mass (*arrows*) caused by hundreds of small bowel matted *Ascaris* worms.

Strongyloides

This nematode is also known as a threadworm and lives throughout the small intestine, but it is more common in the proximal small bowel. Most patients are asymptomatic, but severe small bowel infestation can lead to abdominal pain, ulceration, and bleeding. Worms will be harder than others to identify; males are only about 1 cm in length, and females grow to up to 2.5 cm. Rarely, patients can have a severe colitis, similar to acute ulcerative colitis (see Chapter 5).

Anisakiasis

Anisakiasis is a nematodal infection with the *Anisakis* worm from uncooked fish. These worms can grow to 2 cm and so may be hard to identify with imaging. They can reside anywhere along the small bowel tract. Infection causes abdominal pain and eosinophilic granulomatous-type disease with features mimicking Crohn disease. In the colon, they can also cause a localized colitis with focal bowel wall thickening at the site of worm penetration.

SMALL BOWEL TUMORS

Many small bowel tumors are also recognized elsewhere in the esophagus and stomach and colon (Table 4-8).

Benign Small Bowel Tumors

Gastrointestinal Stromal Tumors (see Chapter 2)

Gastrointestinal stromal tumors (GISTs) occur most commonly in the stomach and next most commonly in the duodenum but are

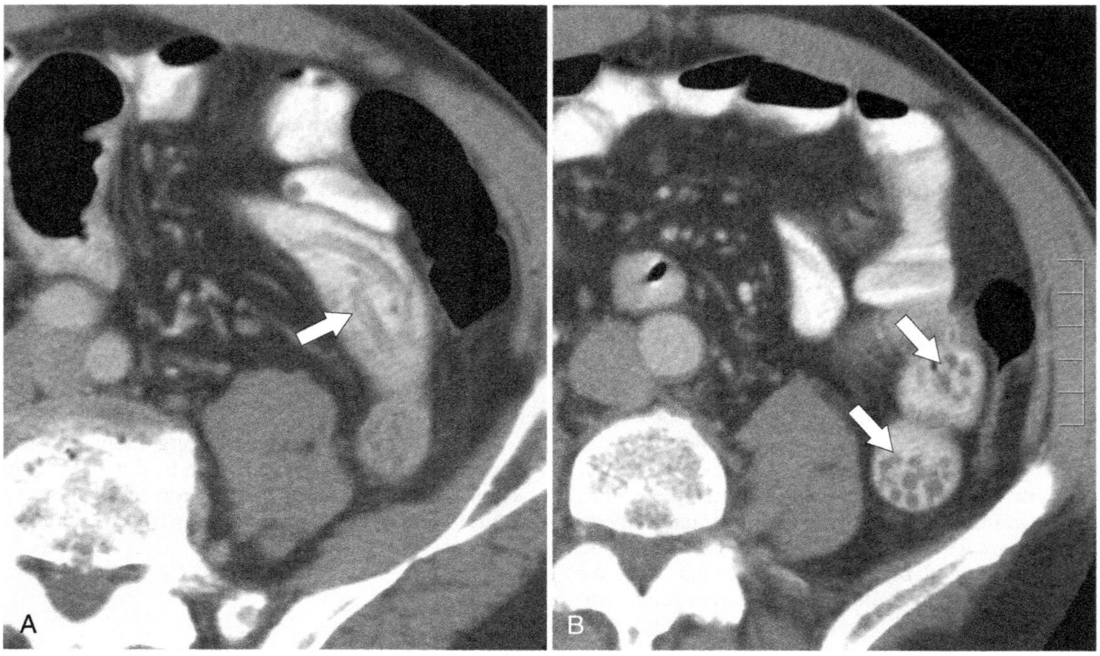

FIGURE 4-73. **A** and **B**, Axial contrast-enhanced CT in a 73-year-old woman with multiple tubular filling defects in the jejunum due to *Ascaris* infiltration (*arrows*).

recognized throughout the rest of the GI tract. If they are small, it may be difficult to differentiate them from other intramural tumors. When the tumors are larger, they are often exophytic, sometimes with ulceration, and necrosis may occur. The latter features, however, are more common with malignant GIST. At imaging, the features are nonspecific and may present as a soft tissue mass, sometimes in an eccentric position to the small bowel (Fig. 4-74).

Small Bowel Neurofibromatosis

Small bowel neurofibromatosis is associated with the systemic manifestations of neurofibromatosis 1, an inherited disorder due to a mutation on chromosome 17, also known as von Recklinghausen* disease. There are numerous clinical manifestations, including cutaneous neurofibromas, freckling, café au lait spots (light brown macules), optic glioma, skeletal anomalies, and hamartomas of the iris. In the small bowel, there can be multiple neurofibromas, typically on the antimesenteric border, yielding imaging findings of multiple smooth extramucosal masses within the affected small bowel segment.

Other rare submucosal benign lesions include schwannoma and paraganglioma, which are indistinguishable at SBFT or CT. The diagnosis will usually be made only during histological examination.

Small Bowel Lipoma and Lipomatosis

Single small bowel lipomas are the most common small bowel tumor and are identified at CT as generally small, smooth, fat-density masses, often within the small bowel lumen, even though they are submucosal in origin (Fig. 4-75). Their only significance is that they can act as the lead point for intussusception.

Small bowel lipomatosis is a very rare condition demonstrating multiple submucosal intestinal lipomas, which can ulcerate, hemorrhage, intussuscept, obstruct, and even cause volvulus. It is often asymptomatic and should be differentiated from other multiple polyposis syndromes. The diagnosis should be readily made at CT with multiple fat-density masses associated with the small bowel.

*Friedrich Daniel von Recklinghausen (1833-1910), German pathologist.

TABLE 4-8 Small Bowel Neoplasms

	Typical Location	Characteristics
Benign		
GIST	Jejunum	Mass ± ulceration
Neurofibroma	Ileum	Smooth submucosal mass
Hemangioma	Anywhere	Smooth submucosal mass
Lipoma	Ileum	Changeable mass
Carcinoid	Ileum	Usually not identified
Adenoma	Ileum	Variable size, villous or tubulovillous
Hamartoma	Anywhere	Usually multiple
Malignant		
GIST	Anywhere	Mass with large extraluminal component
Lymphoma	Terminal ileum	Variable mass, diffuse thickening, strictures, nodules
Carcinoid	Ileum	Nodule or mass
Metastases	Anywhere	Single or multiple, serosal or submucosal masses, ulceration, intussusception
Adenocarcinoma	Jejunum	Mass or annular constricting lesion

GIST, Gastrointestinal stromal tumor.

Lipomatous Infiltration of the Ileocecal Valve

Lipomatous infiltration of the ileocecal valve is not strictly a neoplasm because it is a normal finding in most patients. It should be distinguished from lipoma in the region of the ileocecal valve. Lipomatous infiltration refers to fat proliferation of the ileocecal valve itself, a normal finding identified at CT by irregular submucosal circumferential fatty replacement at the ileocecal valve (Fig. 4-76).

Hemangioma

Hemangiomas are generally small and will only be recognized by multiple small phleboliths that form within the dilated vasculature.

Carcinoid

After lipoma, carcinoid is the most common benign neoplasm of the small bowel (but is also recognized in the lungs, rectum, small bowel, pancreas, liver and biliary system) and is typically located in the terminal ileum and appendix. It is an indolent neuroendocrine tumor, arising from argentaffin cells of the crypts of Lieberkühn.* Most carcinoids are asymptomatic and discovered incidentally during operations performed for other reasons. All carcinoids are potentially malignant, although most remain benign. Malignancy mostly depends on size; the smaller they are, the more likely

*Johann Nathanael Lieberkühn (1711-1756), German physician.

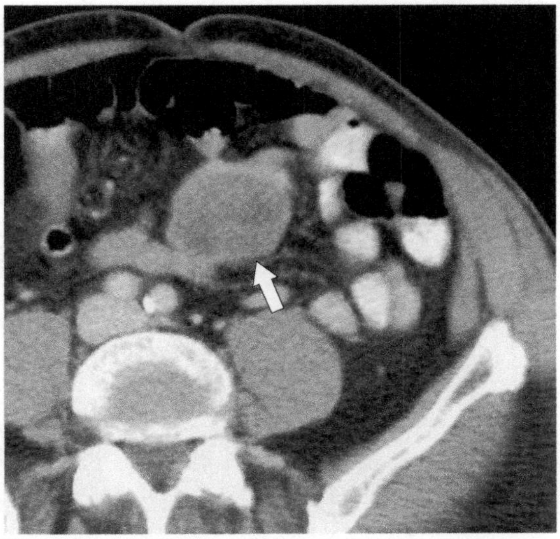

FIGURE 4-74. Axial contrast-enhanced CT in a 44-year-old woman with a homogeneous 4-cm mass (*arrow*) in the left mesentery due to a benign GIST.

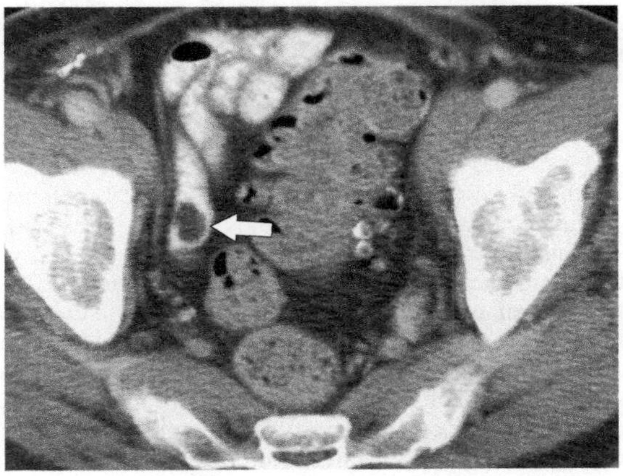

FIGURE 4-75. Axial contrast-enhanced CT in a 70-year-old man with a small intraluminal fatty mass due to a small bowel lipoma (*arrow*).

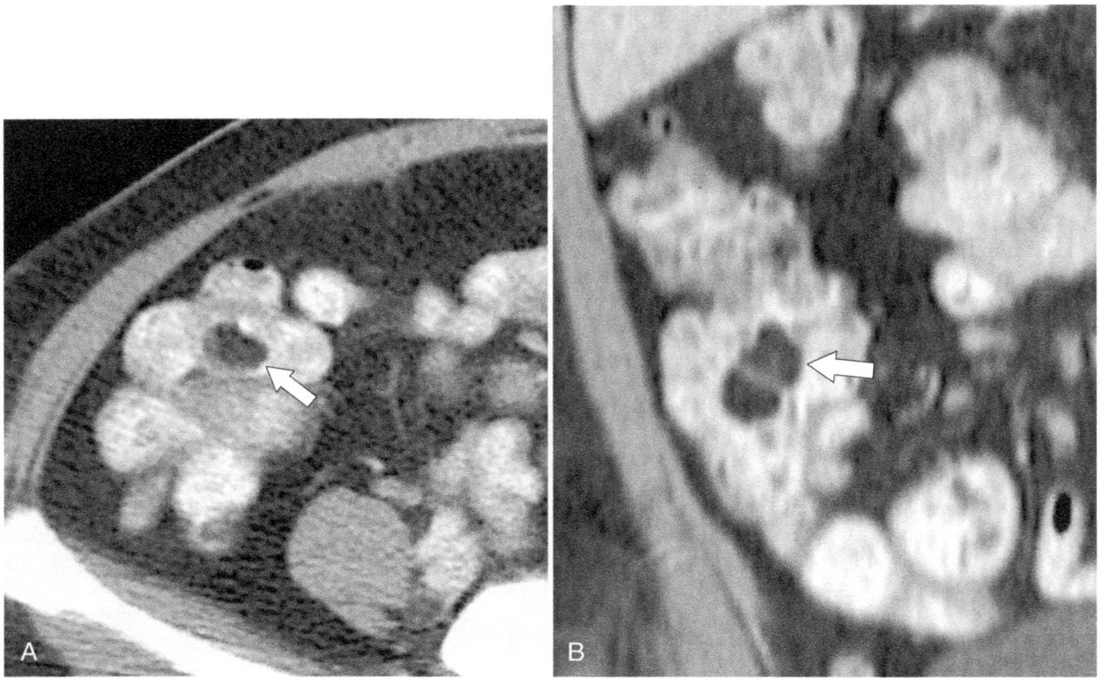

FIGURE 4-76. Axial (**A**) and coronal (**B**) contrast-enhanced CT in a 43-year-old woman with a normal fat-containing ileocecal valve (*arrows*).

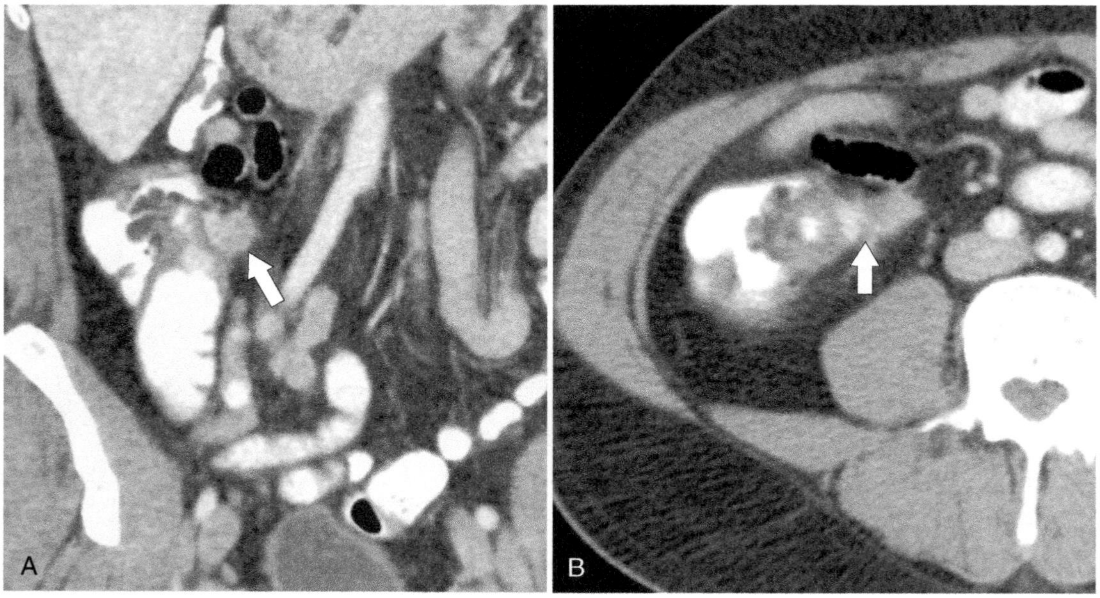

FIGURE 4-77. Coronal (**A**) and axial (**B**) contrast-enhanced CT in a 36-year-old man with terminal ileal dilatation and a 1-cm enhancing mass (*arrows*) due to ileal carcinoid.

they are to be benign (90% metastasize when they are larger than 2 cm). Duodenal and jejunal carcinoids are associated with multiple endocrine neoplasia (MEN) type I.

Most benign lesions are likely never discovered by imaging because of their small size, although at barium examination they may appear as a smooth submucosal mass, or with thickened mucosal folds. As they grow, they can penetrate into the mucosa and ulcerate or may be large enough to act as a lead point for intussusception. At CT, they are also difficult to identify because of their small size, but typically they avidly enhance in the arterial phase after intravenous contrast administration (similar to other neuroendocrine tumors) and therefore may be missed by portal venous–phase imaging or if positive oral contrast agents are used (as the hyperenhancing mass is obscured by surrounding dense contrast media) (Fig. 4-77). Therefore, if CT is being performed to specifically evaluate for carcinoid, a neutral oral contrast agent (e.g., water) should be used with arterial phase scanning to maximize the possibility of identifying the mass. Despite this, many masses, being too small, are not identified unless they are malignant and they have metastasized either to the mesentery or to the liver (see Chapter 6).

Adenoma

The detection of adenomas will mostly be missed at imaging because of their small size, difficulty in visualization by imaging

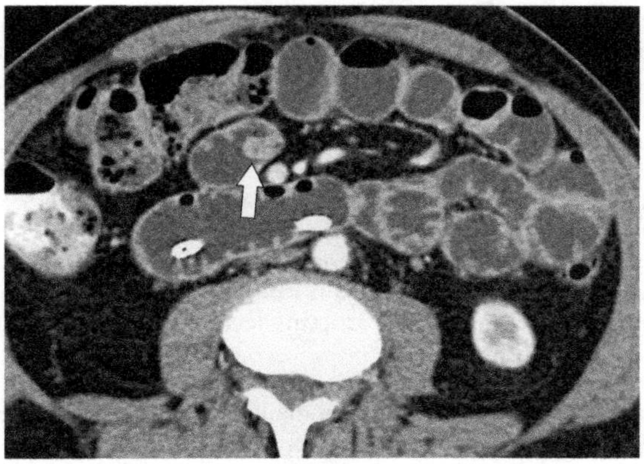

FIGURE 4-78. Small bowel CT enteroclysis in a 41-year-old woman with a small jejunal adenomatous polyp (*arrow*).

or endoscopy, and their rarity. Detection, when possible, is important, though, because their natural history follows the course of adenomas elsewhere (e.g., the colon). Depending on their size, there is a propensity for adenomas to undergo metaplasia and frank malignant degeneration, the so-called adenoma-carcinoma sequence. They may occasionally be identified incidentally at CT as smooth, rounded intraluminal filling defects within the small bowel (Fig. 4-78). Mostly, however, they will not be detected until the patient has adenocarcinoma. Adenomatous polyps are associated with some polyposis syndromes, and patients with these syndromes undergo heightened surveillance because of the risk of adenocarcinoma developing.

Polyposis Syndromes

A number of familial and nonfamilial polyposis syndromes are recognized (Table 4-9).

TABLE 4-9 Polyposis Syndromes

Name	Polyp Type	Other Clinical Features
Familial polyposis	Adenomas	Mainly colon, sometimes small bowel
Gardner syndrome	Adenomas	Small and large bowel polyps, osteomas, desmoid tumors
Peutz-Jeghers syndrome	Hamartomas	Small and large bowel polyps Mucocutaneous pigmentation
Cronkhite-Canada syndrome	Hamartomas	Protein malabsorption, alopecia, nail dystrophy
Juvenile polyposis	Hamartomas	Small and large bowel polyps
Cowden's disease	Hamartomas	Small and large bowel
Neurofibromatosis	Neurofibromas	Café au lait spots, cutaneous nodules

Familial Adenomatous Polyposis (see Chapter 5)

Familial adenomatous polyposis can be inherited as either an autosomal dominant or a recessive trait and is characterized by numerous (can be many thousands) adenomatous polyps. These polyps are located mainly in the large intestine but can also be seen throughout the small bowel. They often bleed, leading to anemia, and they are also at a high risk of malignant degeneration, so aggressive screening is warranted with early colectomy for patients with 100 or more identified polyps. Malignant degeneration can also occur from small bowel adenomatous polyps, but far less commonly than those in the colon. These polyps should be identifiable by SBFT or barium enema, usually as a carpet of numerous small mucosal polyps, if barium refluxes into the small bowel. Patients are also at risk of having other unrelated malignancies.

Gardner Syndrome

Gardner* syndrome is an inherited autosomal dominant disorder caused by mutation on the chromosome 5 gene and is now more commonly considered a variant of familial adenomatous polyposis coli. Affected patients have diffuse polyposis mainly in the colon and to a lesser extent in the small bowel, but they are most common in the stomach. The syndrome is also associated with skull osteomas, epidermoid and sebaceous cysts, fibromas, and thyroid cancer. Approximately 15% of patients have desmoid tumors (slow-growing benign mesenteric fibrous tumors; see Chapter 5), but more important, they are at high risk for having malignant degeneration of both small and large bowel polyps to adenocarcinoma, similar to familial adenomatous polyposis.

*Eldon J. Gardner (1909-1989), American geneticist.

Peutz-Jeghers Syndrome

Peutz-Jeghers* syndrome either is inherited as an autosomal dominant disorder or occurs as a spontaneous mutation, due to a possible mutation on chromosome 19. It is characterized by multiple benign hamartomatous polyps throughout the small bowel combined with mucocutaneous pigmentation. The polyps are sometimes recognized because they commonly produce intussusception. Although the polyps themselves have low malignancy potential, patients are susceptible to malignancies in multiple organs elsewhere (anywhere in the GI tract, pancreas, breast, ovary, testes, cervix, thyroid). The lifetime cumulative risk of having a malignancy is approximately 70%. The polyps can be identified at SBFT (Fig. 4-79). CT is more likely to identify any intussuscepta. They are most commonly identified in the small bowel but can be seen throughout the bowel, including the colon.

Cronkhite-Canada Syndrome

Cronkhite-Canada† syndrome is a very rare disorder, possibly inherited, characterized by multiple hamartomatous polyps, most commonly in the stomach and colon, and less commonly in the small bowel and esophagus. Malignant degeneration is unlikely.

Juvenile Polyposis Syndrome

Juvenile polyposis syndrome is usually an autosomal dominant inherited disorder of younger adults, characterized by multiple hamartomatous polyps, typically in the stomach and colon but sometimes in the small bowel. Unlike most other hamartomatous syndromes, there is an increased risk of adenocarcinoma developing in some of, but not all, the polyps. Patients usually have a family history and have symptoms including GI bleeding, pain, and anemia. The polyps are difficult to distinguish from other polyposis syndromes at SBFT, and the diagnosis is usually made with an appropriate family history.

Cowden's Disease

Cowden's‡ disease is an autosomal inherited disorder characterized by widespread hamartomatous polyp formation and an increased risk of malignancies elsewhere, unrelated to the

*Johannes Peutz (1864-1940), Dutch physician; Harold Jeghers (1904-1990), American physician.
†Leonard W. Cronkhite, Jr. (1919-), American pediatrician; Wilma J. Canada (1926-), American radiologist.
‡Disease named after the first recognized patient with the disease.

hamartomas themselves. Hamartomas can be found in the mouth and throughout the GI tract.

Malignant Small Bowel Tumors

Adenocarcinoma

Adenocarcinomas are relatively rare and likely follow the adenoma-carcinoma sequence (see Chapter 5). Predisposing factors include celiac disease, Crohn disease, polyposis, and Peutz-Jeghers syndrome. Most lesions occur in the jejunum and appear as an infiltrating mass that produces circumferential thickening and sometimes apple core–type lesions, which ulcerate as they enlarge. The mass is best imaged by CT and may occlude the small bowel lumen or may act as a lead point for intussusception, both of which may present with small bowel obstruction (Fig. 4-80). Extramural extension to regional lymph nodes is common. These features are mostly identifiable by CT, which is the optimal imaging tool. An SBFT is uncommonly performed but may demonstrate an annular constricting lesion or intussusception.

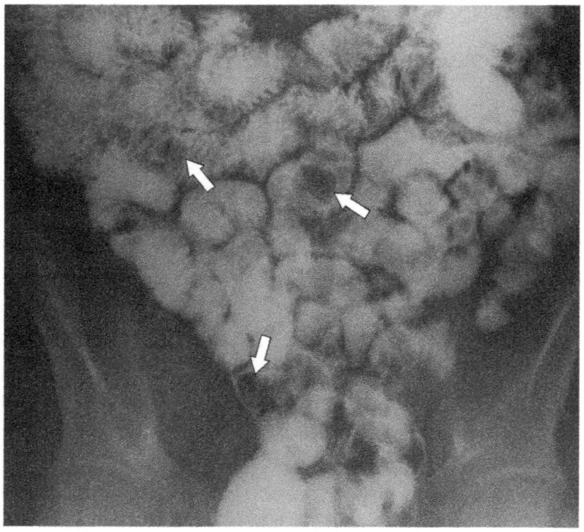

FIGURE 4-79. SBFT in a 35-year-old man with Peutz-Jeghers syndrome and small bowel polyps (*arrows*) due to hamartomas.

Lymphoma

Lymphoma is the most common malignant neoplasm to affect the small bowel and is mostly the non-Hodgkin diffuse large B-cell type. It is more common in immunosuppressed patients. Other lymphomas are recognized, including enteropathy-associated T-cell lymphoma (EATL), which is a long-term complication of celiac disease, and mucosa-associated lymphoid tissue (MALT) lymphoma. The latter disease usually affects the terminal ileum because of the greater concentration of lymphoid tissue. Various macroscopic types are recognized, including infiltrating, polypoid, nodular, cavitary and mesenteric forms.

The most common presentation is with an infiltrating mass and circumferential, irregular bowel wall thickening, which typically leaves the lumen preserved or even dilated (aneurysmal dilation) because of destruction of the myenteric plexus by the lymphomatous tissue (Fig. 4-81). The lymphomatous mass may be relatively subtle or may appear similar to other small bowel benign disease (e.g., Crohn disease or infective enteritis) (Fig. 4-82). Sometimes, the disease is bulkier, but both types should

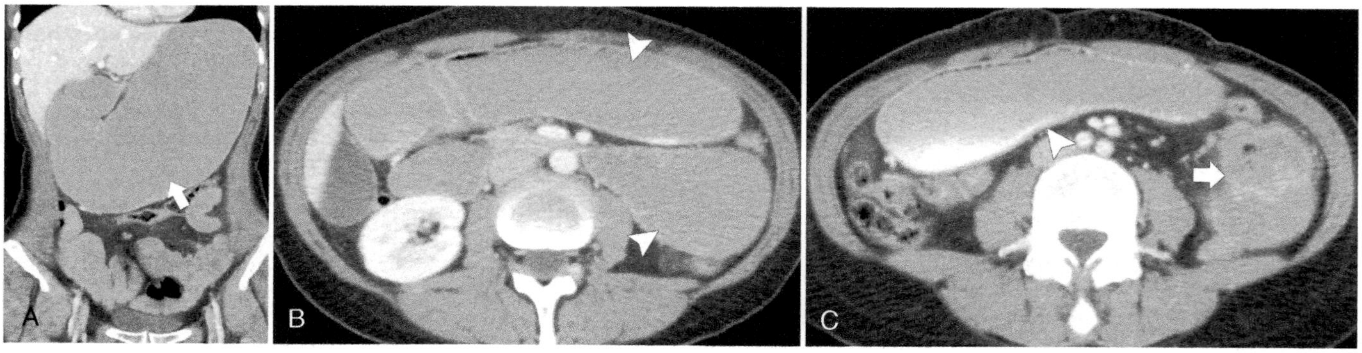

FIGURE 4-80. Coronal (**A**) and axial (**B** and **C**) contrast-enhanced CT in a 55-year-old woman and upper gastric distention and small bowel obstruction (*arrows*) due to an obstructing mass in the mid jejunum, confirmed to be jejunal adenocarcinoma (*arrow* in **C**).

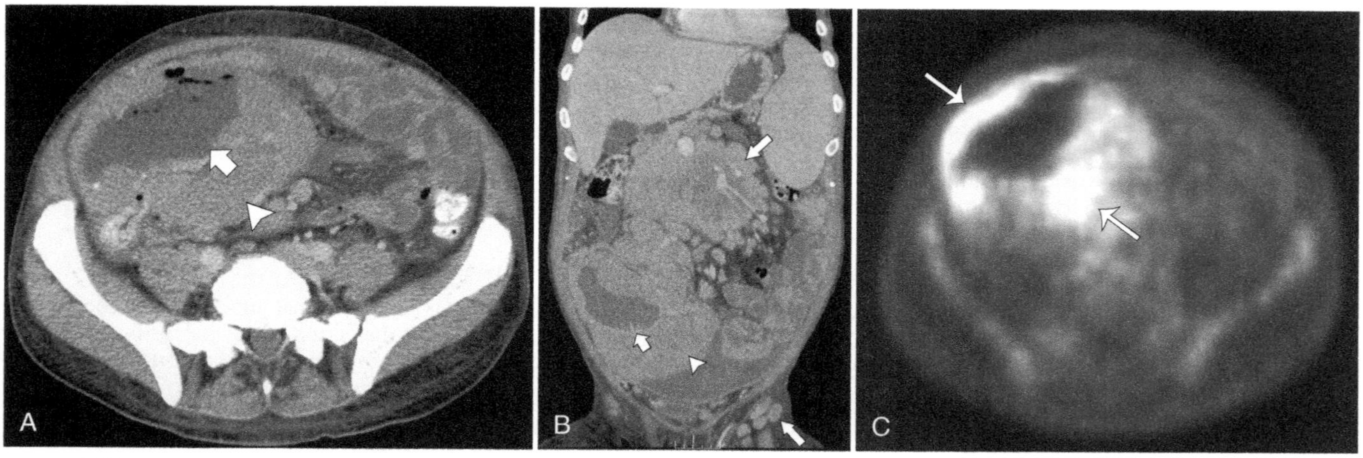

FIGURE 4-81. Axial (**A**) and coronal (**B**) contrast-enhanced PET/CT (**C**) in a 40-year-old man with diffuse abdominal and inguinal adenopathy (*long arrows*) and aneurysmal dilatation of the terminal ileum (*small arrows*) due to lymphomatous involvement (*arrowhead*). PET demonstrates increased FDG uptake (*thin arrows*).

be readily identified at CT, which often demonstrates associated mesenteric lymphadenopathy (Fig. 4-83).

Less commonly, polypoid lymphomatous deposition appears as multiple small submucosal filling defects, which can ulcerate and appear similar to hematogenous small bowel metastases. A rare variant presents as multiple small nodular submucosal lesions, often in the terminal ileum, and may be difficult to distinguish from lymphoid nodular hyperplasia (Fig. 4-84).

Cavitary lymphoma is represented by a large lymphomatous mass with a small bowel perforation and the extravasation of contents into a relatively large cavitary space (Fig. 4-85). This may sometimes be difficult to distinguish from larger forms of aneurysmal dilatation caused by the infiltrating types. In the mesenteric form, lymphoma most often appears in the abdomen as large mesenteric masses associated with bulky retroperitoneal adenopathy (see Fig. 4-83). Typically these lymphomas do not invade and obstruct the small or large bowel, but if they are large enough, they may cause displacement and external compression, which can occasionally cause small bowel obstruction.

Abdominal lymphoma is more often being evaluated by positron emission tomography/computed tomography (PET/CT) for the location and extent of disease and its response to chemotherapy, which may demonstrate a therapeutic response before macroscopic changes (Figs 4-81 and 4-85).

Mediterranean Lymphoma

Mediterranean lymphoma has two variants, immunoproliferative small intestinal disease or late-stage alpha chain heavy disease, and is the most common lymphoma identified in the Middle East, usually in patients younger than age 30. Most patients have progressive malabsorption with or without abdominal pain. They have variable appearances at imaging, including a mass, a polyp or polyps, and mural infiltration, similar to the more commonly recognized non-Hodgkin types of lymphoma.

Malignant Gastrointestinal Stromal Tumor (see Chapter 2)

Malignant GISTs are most common in the stomach, followed by the duodenum, jejunum, and ileum. As with a GIST elsewhere,

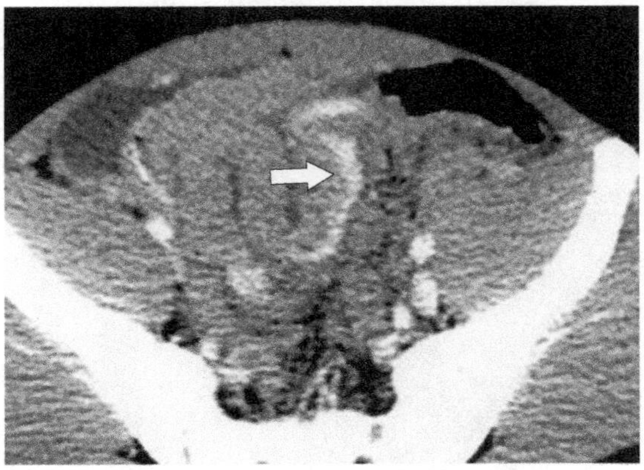

FIGURE 4-82. Axial contrast-enhanced CT in a 58-year-old woman with ileal mural thickening (*arrow*) due to small bowel lymphoma.

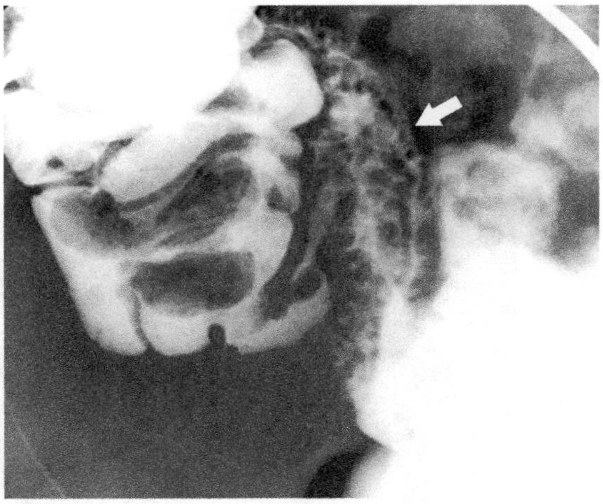

FIGURE 4-84. SBFT in a 48-year-old woman with multiple lymphoid nodules in the terminal ileum (*arrow*) due to early lymphoma. This can appear similar to lymphoid nodular hyperplasia.

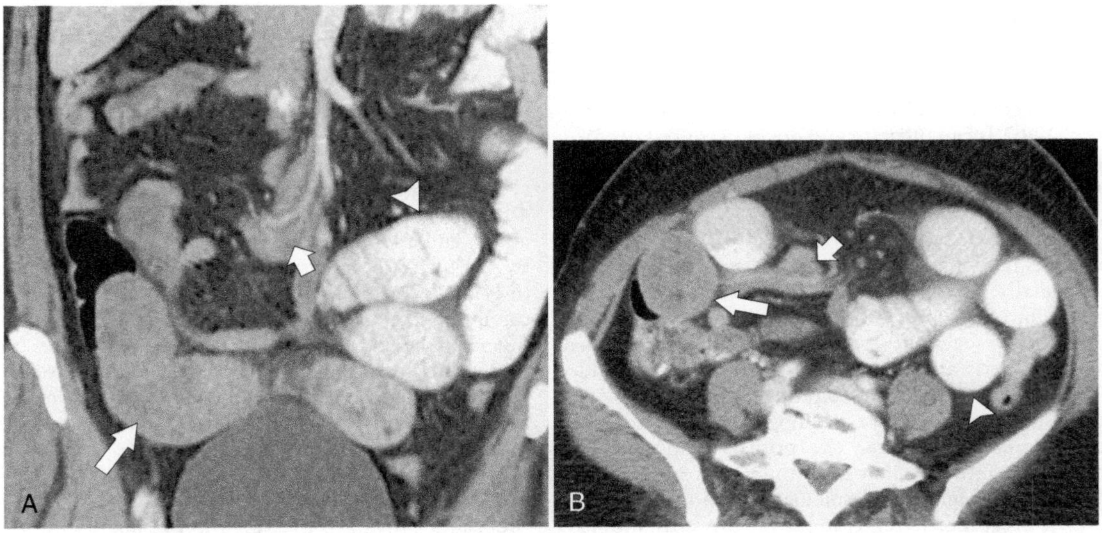

FIGURE 4-83. Coronal (**A**) and axial (**B**) contrast-enhanced CT in a 43-year-old man with ileal lymphoma (*large arrows*) giving partial small bowel obstruction (*arrowheads*) and lymphomatous extension along the small bowel mesentery (*small arrows*).

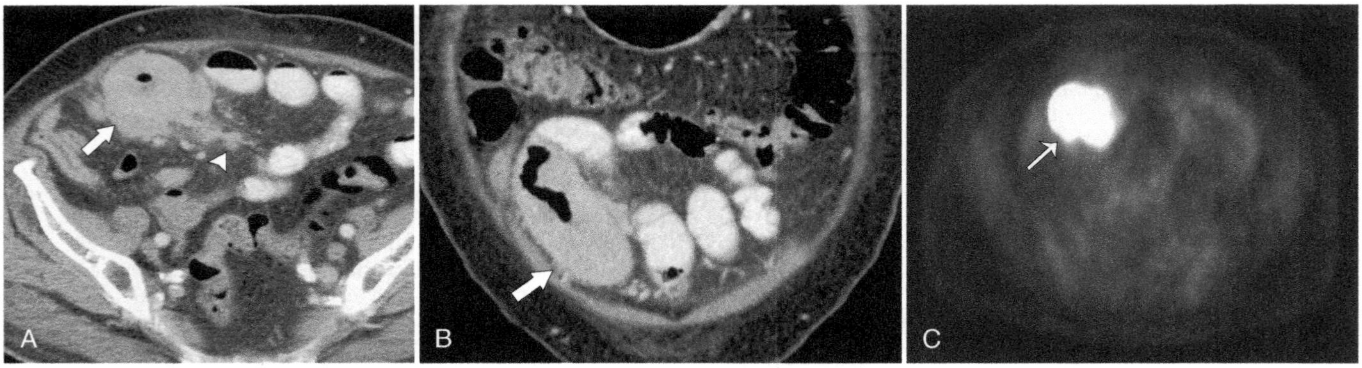

FIGURE 4-85. Axial (**A**) and coronal (**B**) CT and PET (**C**) in a 57-year-old woman with a large circumferential terminal ileal mass (*arrows*) with adjacent lymphadenopathy (*arrowhead*) due to lymphoma. The lesion demonstrates increased FDG activity at PET (*thin arrow*).

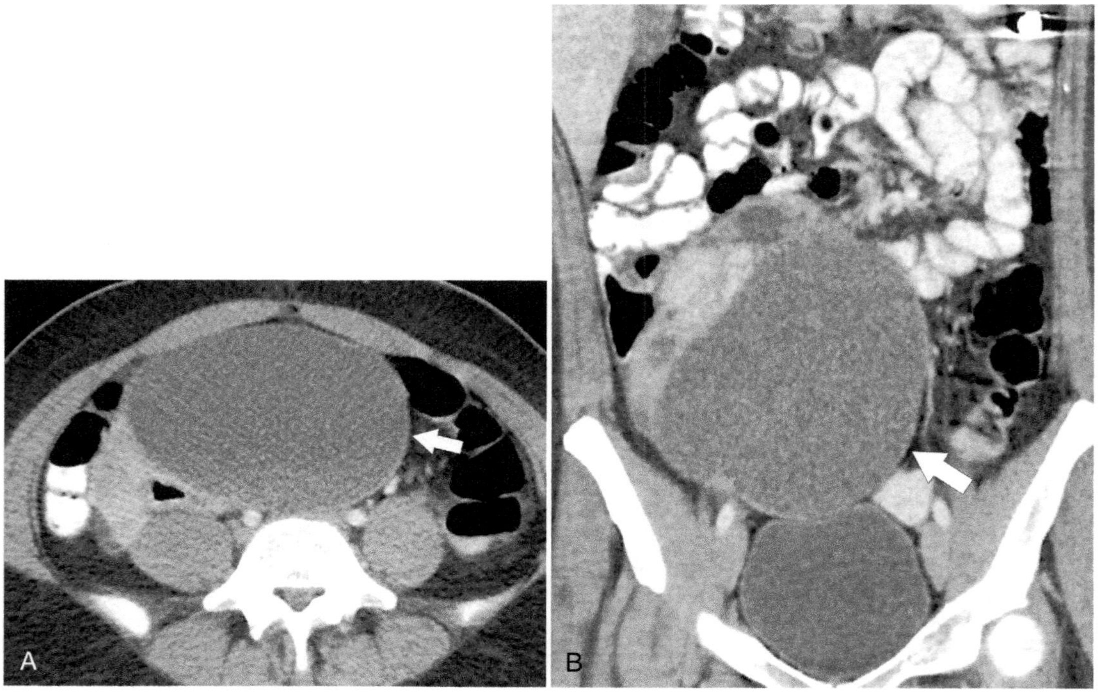

FIGURE 4-86. Axial (**A**) and coronal (**B**) contrast-enhanced CT in a 28-year-old woman with a predominantly cystic mass in the terminal ileum (*arrows*) due to a malignant GIST.

the mass may be eccentric and exophytic, and sometimes partially cystic (Fig. 4-86). It can ulcerate and develop central necrosis as it enlarges (Fig. 4-87). Metastatic spread to the peritoneum or liver, often as cystic metastases, is common.

Malignant Carcinoid

Most carcinoids are benign and too small to be recognized by imaging. They usually become evident, however, when metastatic. Extension into the local adjacent mesentery tends to induce a desmoplastic reaction resulting from serotonin production in the muscularis and serosa with the constriction and angulation of the bowel wall and subsequent small bowel strictures. Local metastases usually extend to regional lymph nodes, which are usually much larger than the primary tumor itself. These mesenteric lymph nodes may also undergo a desmoplastic reaction, becoming irregular and spiculated and often calcified (up to 70%). This response tends to retract the surrounding mesentery, giving its characteristic CT appearances, with either small or larger metastatic disease (Figs. 4-88 and 4-89). These mesenteric appearances can appear identical to retractile (fibrotic) mesenteritis.

Further metastatic extension is usually to the liver, which is characteristically recognized by hypervascular masses (see Fig. 4-88). When there are enough masses to overwhelm the liver's ability to metabolize the overproduction of serotonin (produced by about 10% of carcinoids) into 5-hydroxyindoleacetic acid (5-HIAA), serotonin enters the systemic circulation, producing carcinoid syndrome of flushing, diarrhea, abdominal pain, sweating and wheezing, and right-sided heart failure. Nuclear medicine techniques can also demonstrate either the primary mass or metastatic disease with indium-111 (^{111}In) or somatostatin. PET imaging can also identify local or distant disease, depending on the size of the mass.

Metastatic Disease

Metastatic spread to the small bowel results from either peritoneal seeding or direct, lymphatic, or hematogenous spreading. Most metastatic involvement of the small bowel is thought to be

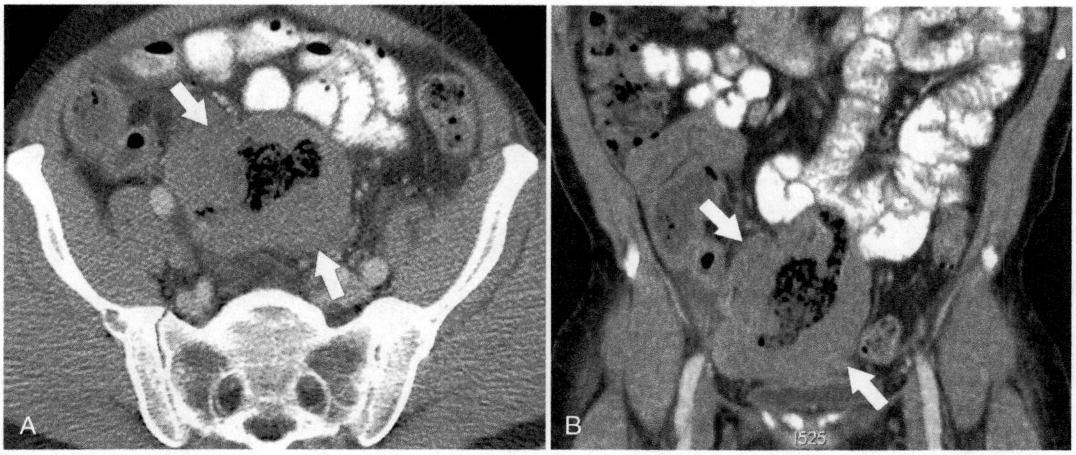

FIGURE 4-87. Axial (**A**) and coronal (**B**) contrast-enhanced CT in a 52-year-old man with a circumferential terminal ileal mass (*arrows*) due to a GIST. The appearances can be similar to some forms of lymphoma.

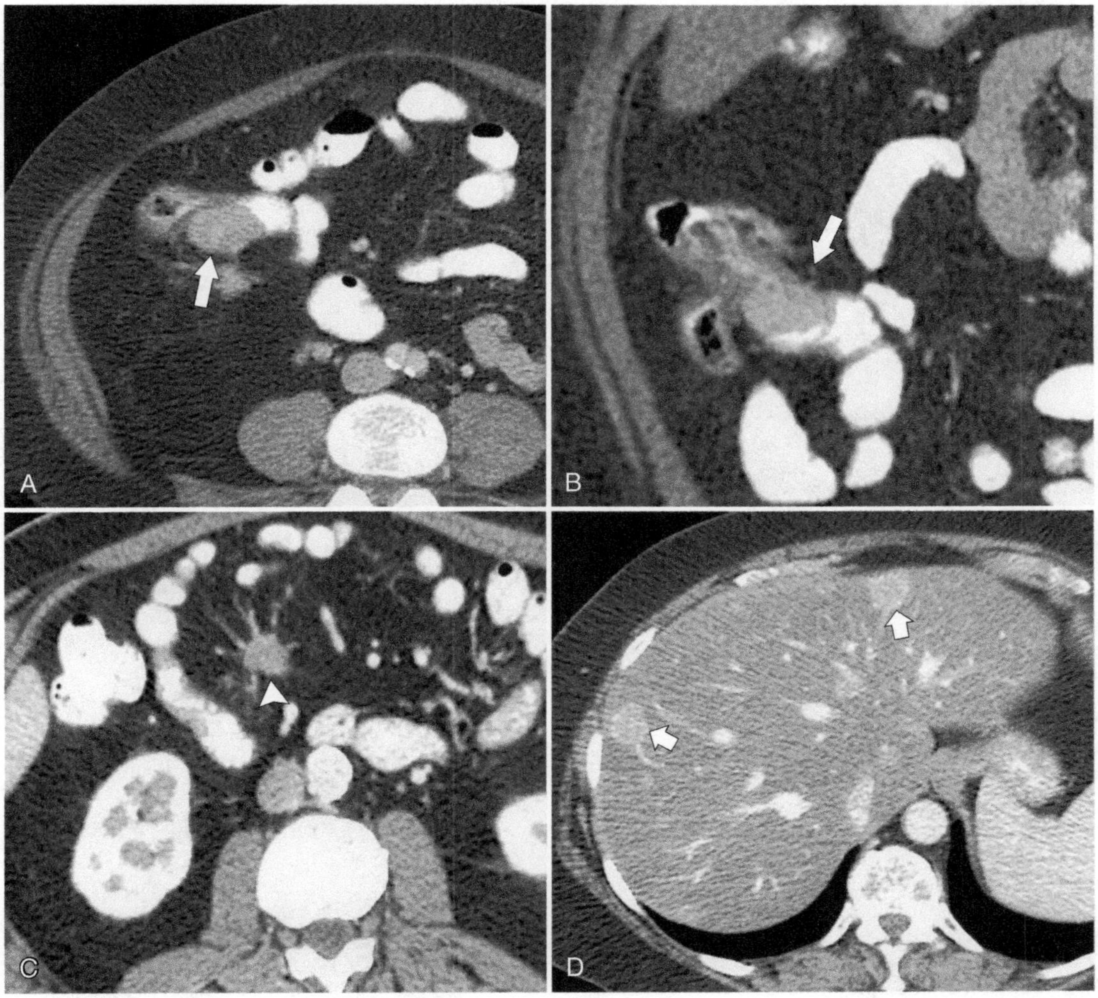

FIGURE 4-88. Axial (**A**, **C**, and **D**) and coronal (**B**) contrast-enhanced CT in a 55-year-old man with a 1.8-cm terminal ileal mass (*large arrows*) due to carcinoid tumor. There are a spiculated mesenteric metastasis (*arrowhead*) and hypervascular liver metastases (*small arrows*) in a fatty liver.

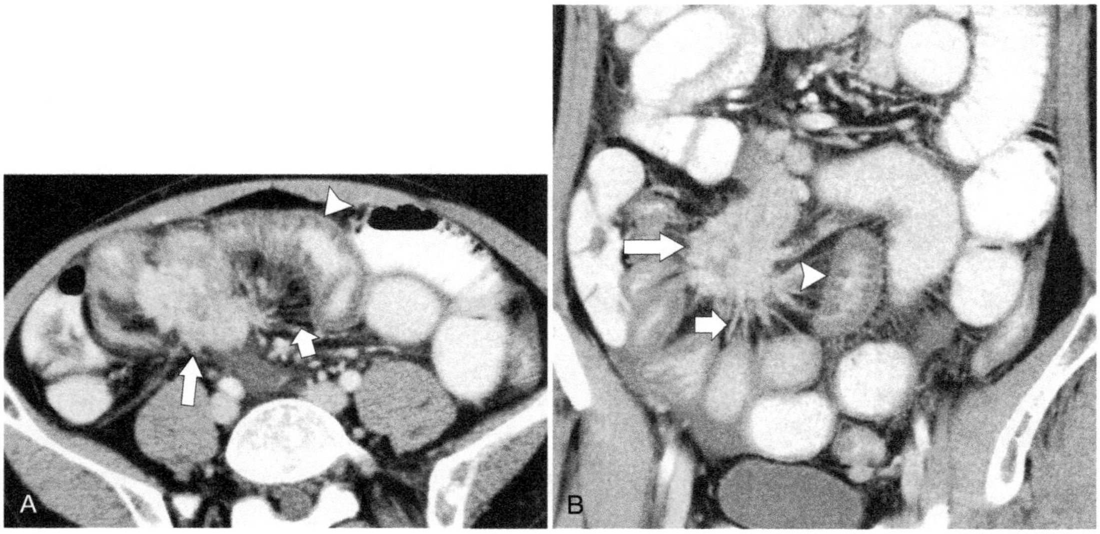

FIGURE 4-89. Axial (**A**) and coronal (**B**) contrast-enhanced CT in a 49-year-old woman with metastatic carcinoid. There is a lower mesenteric mass (*large arrows*) with radiating vessels (*small arrows*) due to the desmoplastic reaction with edema of the ileal mucosa (*arrowheads*) due to vascular obstruction from the mass.

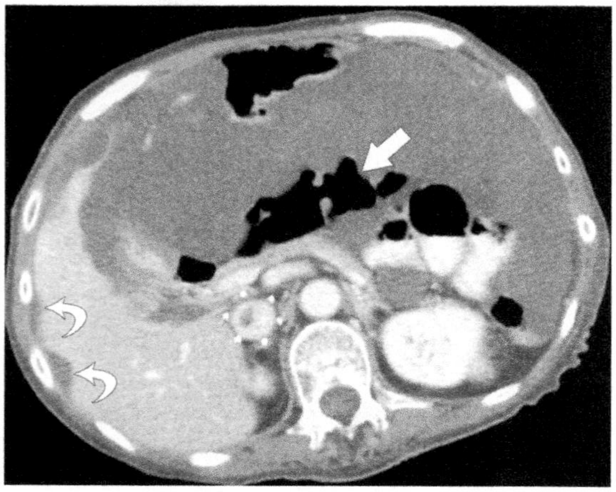

FIGURE 4-90. Axial CT in a 56-year-old woman with widespread peritoneal mucinous deposits in pseudomyxoma peritonei (*arrow*). The small bowel wall is distorted and compressed by the malignant process and there is capsular hepatic scalloping (*curved arrows*).

peritoneal seeding and spreads from the ovary, colon, stomach, appendix, pancreas, and cervix. Tumor deposition tends to follow peritoneal malignant fluid deposits in dependent peritoneal recesses, including the cul-de-sac and ileocecal region. At imaging, either SBFT or CT, the small bowel may be fixed and angulated, mainly on the mesenteric border. Pseudomyxoma peritonei commonly causes small bowel narrowing and stricture formation as the metastatic mucinous material deposits throughout the peritoneum (Fig. 4-90).

Because the small bowel covers a large volume of the abdomen, many primary tumors can directly invade the small bowel. The small bowel then becomes fixed within the larger primary mass, which may ulcerate and become necrotic as identified by CT (Fig. 4-91). Hematogenous spread occurs most commonly from melanoma, but breast, lung, and cervical cancer are also recognized. They generally deposit on the antimesenteric borders at the site of vascular penetration into the small bowel. These may be identified at SBFT (uncommonly performed) as single or multiple submucosal filling defects. They may have a classic bull's-eye or target appearance, particularly with melanoma, representing a smooth rounded submucosal mass with a central

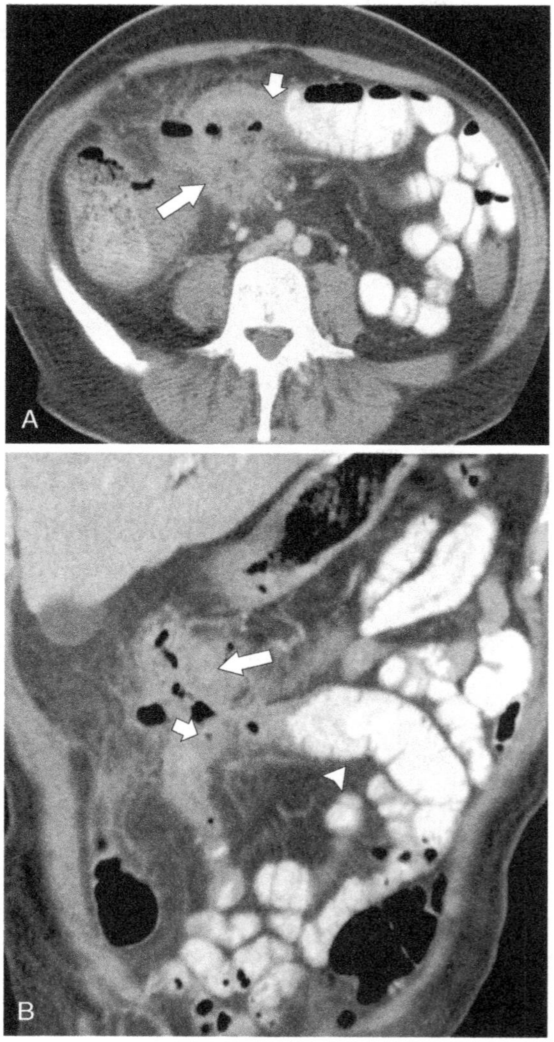

FIGURE 4-91. Axial (**A**) and coronal (**B**) contrast-enhanced CT in 66-year-old man with carcinoma of the transverse colon (*large arrows*) invading the jejunum (*small arrows*) causing partial small bowel obstruction (*arrowhead*).

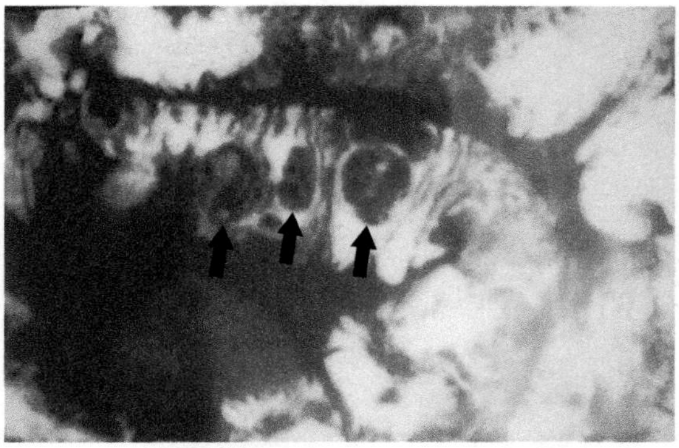

FIGURE 4-92. SBFT in a 66-year-old woman with jejunal bull's-eye target lesions (*arrows*) from submucosal breast metastases.

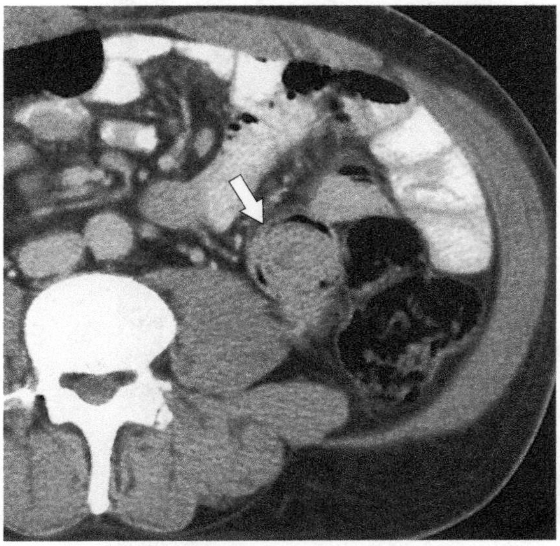

FIGURE 4-93. Axial contrast-enhanced CT in a 60-year-old man with a small bowel mass filling the jejunum due to metastasis from melanoma (*arrow*).

ulceration, which can be identified in the dependent position by a small pool of barium (Fig. 4-92). These metastases are generally too small to be recognized at CT, but larger lesions can be identified (Fig. 4-93). Submucosal melanoma metastases are prone to act as a lead point for intussusception, which may be the only clue to the submucosal metastasis (Fig. 4-94).

Kaposi Sarcoma

Kaposi* sarcoma is a virally induced systemic tumor (human herpesvirus 8), most commonly associated with immunosuppressed states, particularly AIDS-related illnesses. Its primary features are purple macular cutaneous lesions, and it can produce duodenal and less commonly more distal small bowel ulcerations. Lesions can appear similar to the hematogenous (bull's-eye appearing) lesions seen from melanoma.

SMALL BOWEL DILATATION

The normal small bowel diameter is up to 3 cm, although it is not possible to categorically state that the bowel is abnormally distended if it is larger because many patients will have no symptoms and further investigation will be fruitless. Given the right set of clinical symptoms and signs, though, a distended and dilated small bowel larger than 3 cm may be significant, certainly becoming more significant the greater the distention is. Any dilution of barium at SBFT should be considered abnormal and indicative of fluid retention and stasis because there usually is little residual fluid in the small bowel.

There is a large variation from one individual to another in the transit time of barium from the duodenum/jejunum to the ileocecal valve, ranging from less than 30 minutes to more than an hour. However, barium transit times longer than 1 hour to the ileocecal valve are usually abnormal and indicative of stasis due to obstruction or ileus.

ADYNAMIC ILEUS

Adynamic ileus refers to functional obstruction of the small and large bowel, when it becomes flaccid and atonic. These changes lead to dilatation as peristalsis ceases and gas, fluid, and food are not propagated along the bowel. There is both small and large bowel distention with no evidence of mechanical obstruction. There are numerous causes, the most common being recent abdominal surgery (Box 4-2). This cause is multifactorial, due partly to the trauma to the small bowel (i.e., handling by the surgeon) combined with the numerous anesthetic and pain medications, which render the small bowel relatively functionless. Typically bowel sounds are absent, and gentle feeding starts once bowel sounds are heard and flatus is passed. Neuropathic causes are generally irreversible, but others, including hypovolemia, electrolyte disturbances, and ischemia, are reversible. Acute peritoneal inflammatory disorders (e.g., pancreatitis, appendicitis) commonly cause adynamic ileus, but the bowel dilatation may be more localized to the general area of inflammation.

At imaging, there is dilatation of both large and small bowel by plain radiographs, SBFT, and CT, accompanied by air-fluid levels on the upright plain radiograph or sagittal CT view (Fig. 4-95). If SBFT is performed, there is delayed transit time of contrast through the small bowel (more than an hour to reach the ileocecal valve), which appears relatively functionless and motionless at dynamic fluoroscopy. It can be difficult to differentiate this from mechanical obstruction, but the large bowel is commonly collapsed in the presence of mechanical obstruction. Sometimes there is little air in the distal colon, yet the remaining colon and small bowel appear distended. Confirmation that this is adynamic rather than a mechanical obstruction can be made by performing a prone abdominal plain radiograph. If the cause is adynamic ileus, gas will pass freely into the rectum (as it is less dependent in the prone position), ruling out obstruction. Occasionally a single-contrast barium enema is performed for the same purpose, during which contrast is observed freely passing throughout a relatively atonic colon. Other times, a predominantly fluid-filled small bowel and colon may appear relatively normal at abdominal plain radiograph but markedly distended on CT (Fig. 4-96).

Neurogenic and Myopathic Disease

Neurogenic and myopathic disease is secondary to conditions that induce neuropathic or myopathic injury to the small bowel. The affected bowel becomes relatively functionless and dilated. Diseases associated with these features include scleroderma, muscular dystrophy, and degenerative neurological disorders.

Ogilvie Syndrome

Ogilvie* syndrome typically affects the large rather than small bowel and causes chronic and steady dilatation, which can be massive. However, the small bowel can become distended, usually less so than the colon. An obstructive cause is sometimes

*Moritz Kaposi (1837-1902), Hungarian physician and dermatologist.

*William Heneage Ogilvie (1887-1971), British surgeon.

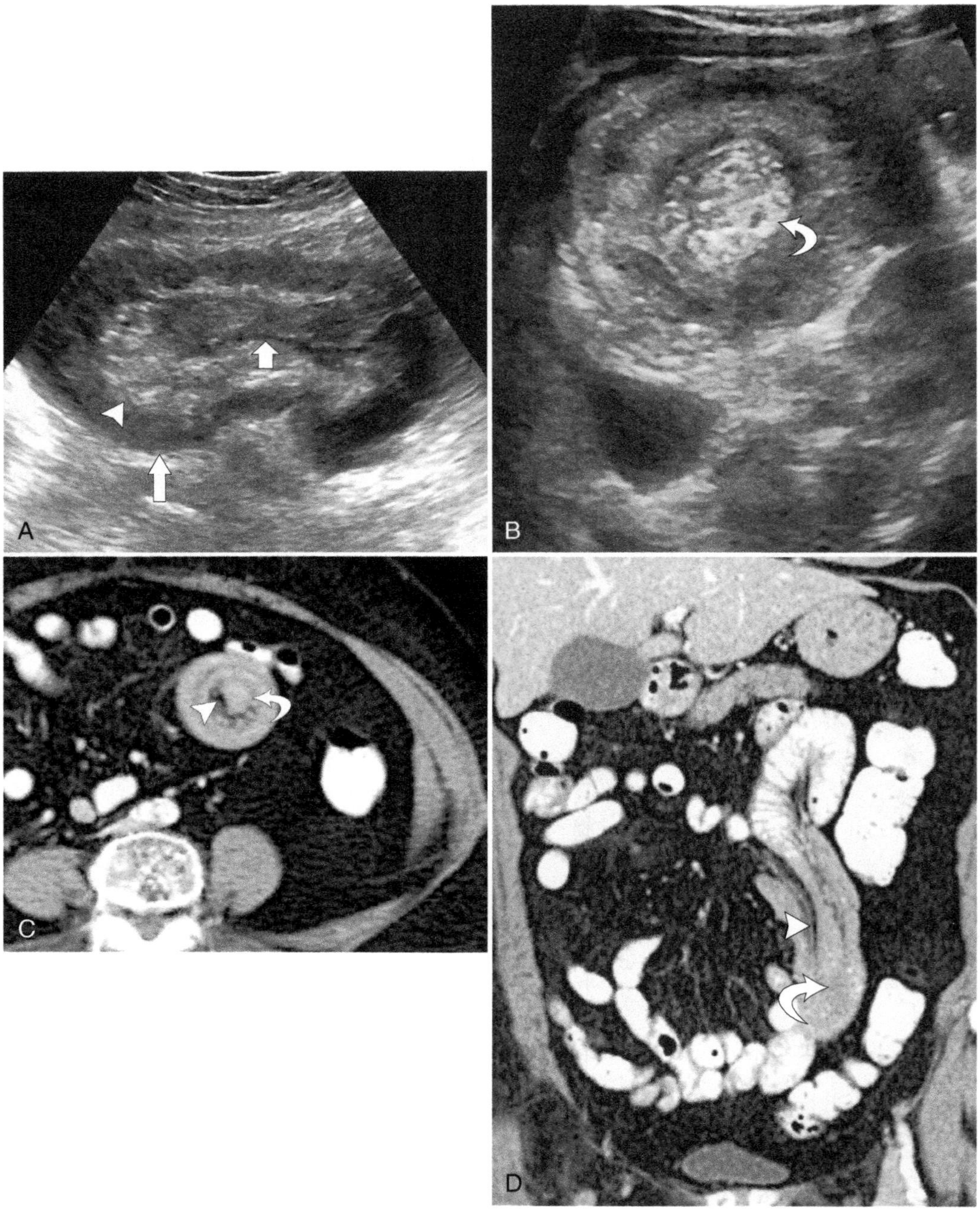

FIGURE 4-94. Sagittal (**A**) and transverse (**B**) ultrasound and axial (**C**) and coronal (**D**) contrast-enhanced CT in a 38-year-old man with intussusception due to a jejunal submucosal melanoma metastasis (*curved arrows*). At ultrasound there is hypoechoic inner intussusceptum (*small arrow*) separated from the outer intussuscipiens (*large arrow*) by hyperechoic mesenteric fat (*arrowhead*). At CT, the intussusceptum is immediately surrounded by mesenteric fat and the intussuscipiens.

Box 4-2. Causes of Adynamic Ileus

Posttraumatic (surgery)
Peritonitis
Electrolyte disturbance
Drugs (anticholinergics, morphine)
Prior vagotomy
Ischemia (thromboembolism, vasculitis, hypovolemia)
Idiopathic pseudoobstruction
Neuromuscular disorders (scleroderma, Chagas disease)
Sprue
Lactose intolerance

suspected, and the passage of a rectal tube to deflate the colon or a single-contrast enema to exclude obstruction may be required.

Scleroderma (see Chapter 1)

Scleroderma is an autoimmune disorder of uncertain etiology that is a chronic systemic disease. It affects the skin, lungs, heart, kidneys, central nervous system, and GI tract (the second most common manifestation after the skin). It is part of the CREST (calcinosis cutis, Raynaud* phenomenon, esophageal dysmotility, sclerodactyly, and telangiectasia) syndrome.

*Maurice Raynaud (1834-1881), French internal medicine physician.

Within the GI tract, the esophagus is most commonly affected (approximately 90% of cases), although small bowel involvement occurs in approximately 50% of cases. There is a progressive smooth muscular atrophy of the small bowel wall resulting from a chronic fibrosing process. The bowel becomes variably functionless and dilated with loss of normal peristaltic activity. The atonic small bowel can also encourage the proliferation of bacteria that are not usually present, resulting in a malabsorptive pattern. Other features of progressive small bowel changes, which can also occur in the colon, are wide-mouthed diverticula or sacculations, which also harbor bacteria, and these can further exacerbate the malabsorptive pattern. Ultimately, if the fibrosis is severe enough, permanent small bowel dilatation occurs and the mucosal folds are crowded together resulting in the classic hidebound appearance, which can be recognized by SBFT examination (Fig. 4-97).

Chagas Disease

Chagas* disease is caused by the protozoan *Trypanosoma cruzi*, which is endemic in Central and South America. In those regions, it is estimated that approximately 10 million people are infected, most of them being asymptomatic. The disease is transferred to humans via the reduviid bug, which becomes infected with *T. cruzi* by feeding on the blood of infected humans. The bugs infect other humans by defecating into the bites they cause. In the acute phase, it can be recognized by the Romaña† sign, which is periorbital redness and swelling that appear after the reduviid bug has bitten. Despite treatment, the infection may enter a chronic phase, with most patients being asymptomatic,

*Carlos Chagas (1879-1934), Brazilian physician.
†Cecílio Romaña (1899-1997), Argentinean epidemiologist and physician.

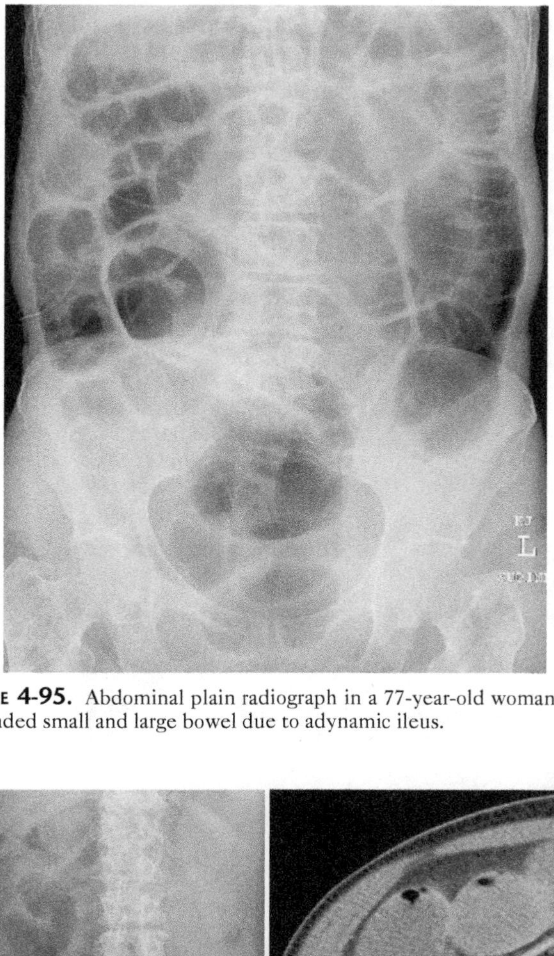

FIGURE 4-95. Abdominal plain radiograph in a 77-year-old woman with distended small and large bowel due to adynamic ileus.

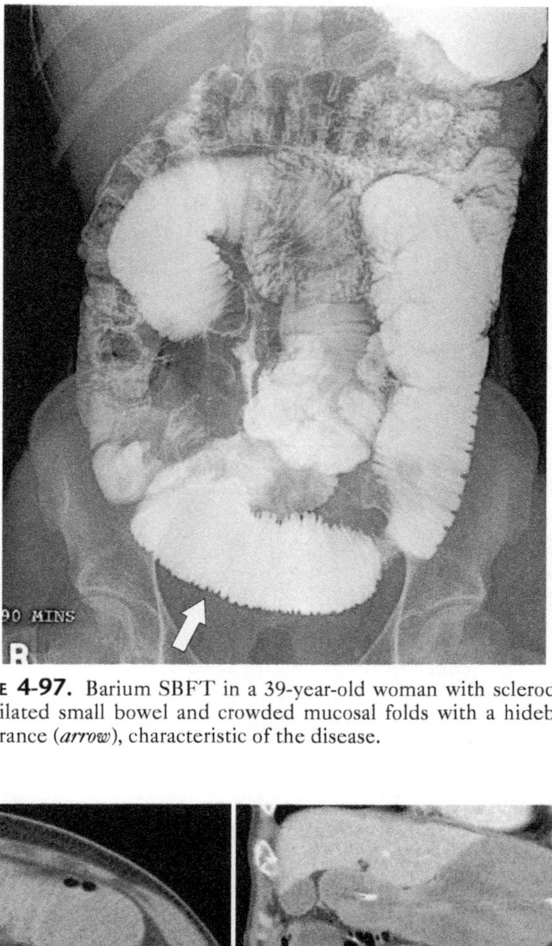

FIGURE 4-97. Barium SBFT in a 39-year-old woman with scleroderma and dilated small bowel and crowded mucosal folds with a hidebound appearance (*arrow*), characteristic of the disease.

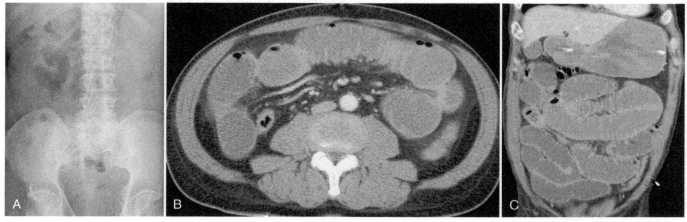

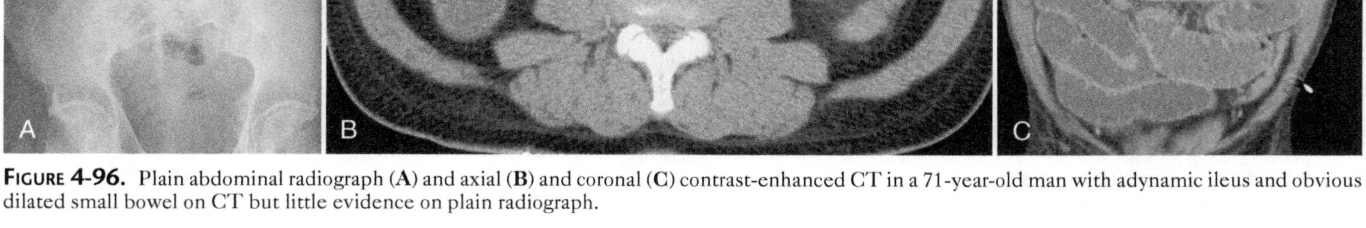

FIGURE 4-96. Plain abdominal radiograph (**A**) and axial (**B**) and coronal (**C**) contrast-enhanced CT in a 71-year-old man with adynamic ileus and obvious dilated small bowel on CT but little evidence on plain radiograph.

but some will have potentially fatal complications that result from progressive neural plexal destruction, which can result in dilated cardiomyopathy and marked dilatation of the esophagus and colon (megaesophagus and megacolon) and sometimes the small bowel.

TABLE 4-10 Causes of Small Bowel Obstruction

Inflammatory	Crohn disease GVHD Postoperative edema
Vascular	Ischemia Radiation
Drugs	NSAIDs
Infectious	*Giardia lamblia* *Strongyloides stercoralis* TB *Campylobacter* *Yersinia enterocolitica* *Salmonella typhi* *Anisakis* Cytomegalovirus HIV
Neoplastic	Primary: adenocarcinoma, lymphoma, carcinoid Secondary: hematogenous, lymphatic, peritoneal, local invasion
Extraluminal	Volvulus Adhesions Hernias
Intraluminal	Intussception Foreign body Gallstone *Ascaris* worms Meconium ileus

GVHD, Graft-versus-host disease; *HIV*, human immunodeficiency virus; *NSAIDs*, nonsteroidal antiinflammatory drugs; *TB*, tuberculosis.

SMALL BOWEL OBSTRUCTION

Small bowel obstruction (SBO) can be total when there is complete obstruction of the small bowel lumen, or partial when the small bowel lumen is significantly narrowed, but does allow the passage of some visceral contents. Mechanical SBO should be differentiated from nonmechanical obstruction or ileus; in the former there is a physical obstruction to the bowel lumen due to masses or strictures, and in the latter no obstruction can be identified. It is generally not possible, even with CT, to differentiate between the different causes of SBO, but the clinical history can point to the appropriate diagnosis (Table 4-10). For instance, the patient may have a history of abdominal surgery (adhesions), pain in the inguinal region (inguinal/femoral hernia), or acute onset of pain (possible volvulus). SBO may also result from large bowel obstruction (Fig. 4-98).

The imaging findings of SBO are similar on plain radiographs and CT, but the location of the obstruction can often be difficult using plain radiographs alone and either contrast studies or, preferably, CT, will be required (Fig. 4-99). The colon will typically be collapsed when the obstruction originates in the small bowel (Fig. 4-100). When small bowel is dilated secondary to large bowel obstruction, there will be both small and large bowel dilatation proximal from the point of obstruction. Supine plain radiographs will typically demonstrate dilated loops of air and fluid-filled small bowel. An upright (erect) plain radiograph is usually performed because it will often demonstrate air-fluid levels (Fig. 4-101). Sometimes the dilated bowel is almost completely fluid filled, and the dilated bowel may not be appreciated on the supine view because of insufficient contrast between the fluid and bowel wall. However, a few small air-fluid levels are to be expected on the upright view and sometimes can be seen as a "string of pearls" representing multiple beads of nondependent gas positioned just under the nondependent wall of the small bowel (Fig. 4-102). Depending on the degree of obstruction there is a variable appearance of the small bowel, but in severe obstruction, the dilated small bowel is positioned toward the center of the abdomen, often with a characteristic whorled appearance (Figs. 4-100 and 4-103). There

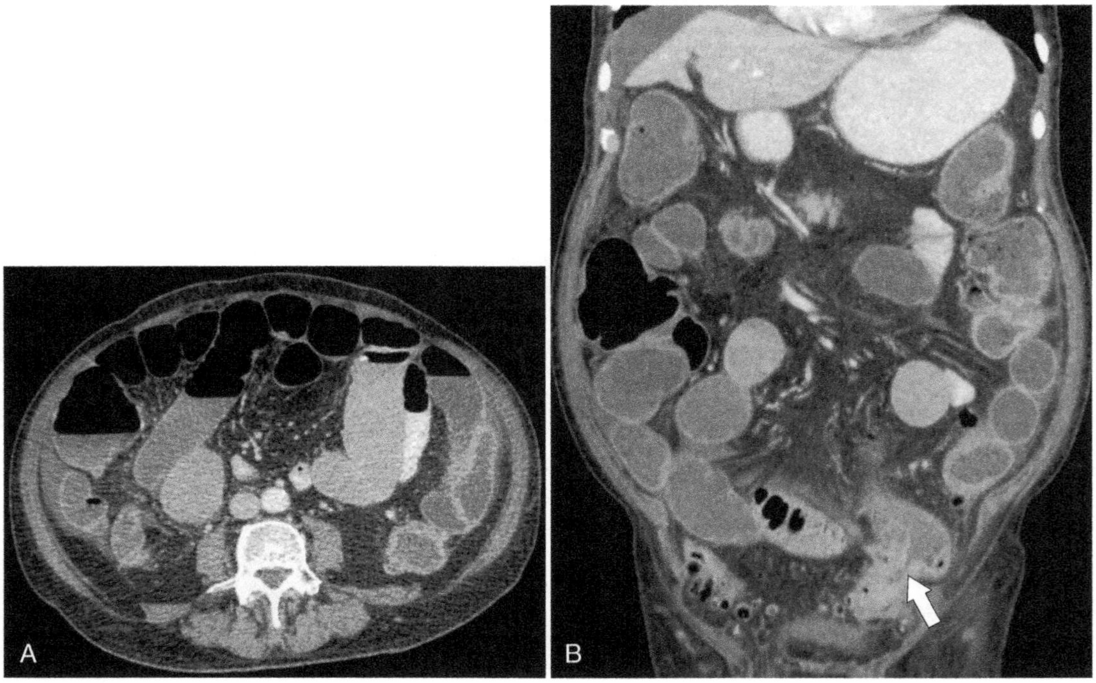

FIGURE 4-98. Axial (**A**) and coronal (**B**) contrast-enhanced CT in a 62-year-old man with small and large bowel dilated loops caused by obstruction from a sigmoid adenocarcinoma (*arrow*).

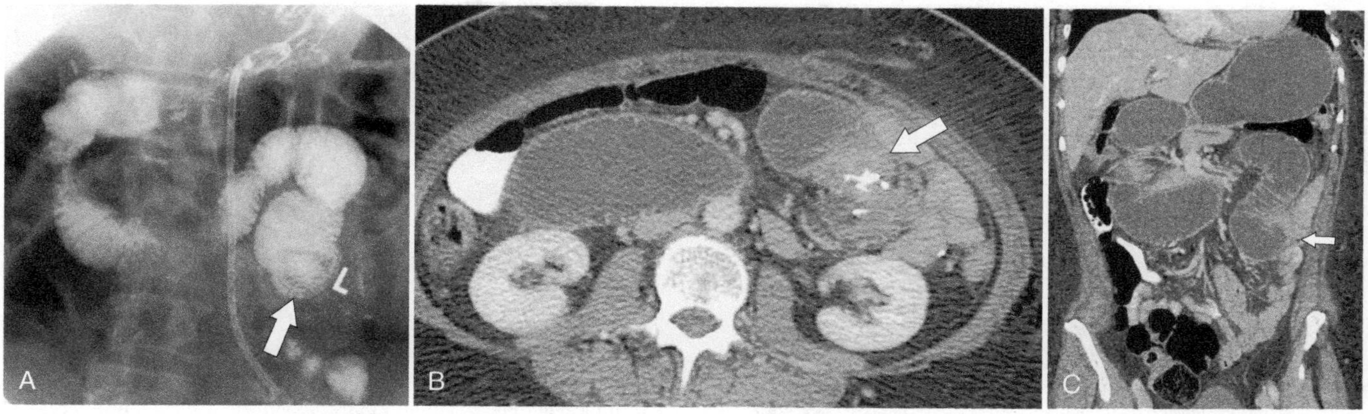

FIGURE 4-99. Gastric catheter contrast injection (**A**) and axial (**B**) and coronal (**C**) constrast-enhanced CT in a 56-year-old man demonstrates duodenal and jejunal dilatation produced when a recurrence of jejunal adenocarcinoma caused an obstruction by a mass (*arrows*) at the jejunojejunal anastomosis.

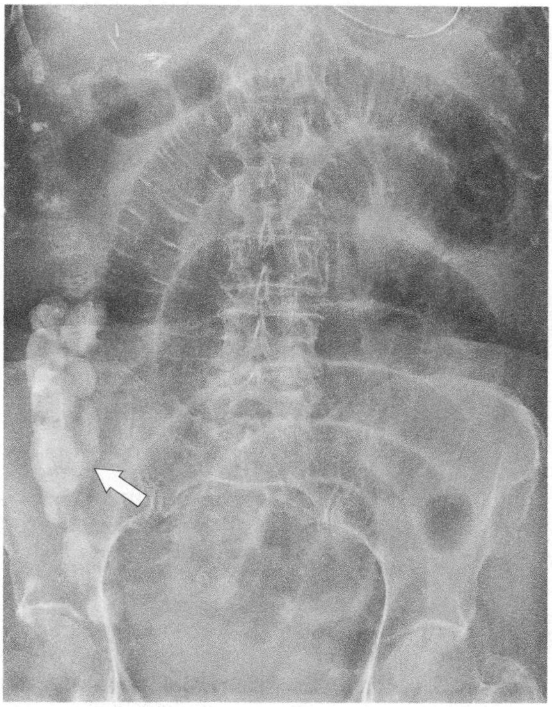

FIGURE 4-100. Plain abdominal supine radiograph in a 77-year-old woman with small bowel obstruction and multiple centrally placed loops of small bowel. There is residual contrast from a recent barium enema (performed to exclude larger bowel obstruction) demonstrating a collapsed colon (*arrow*).

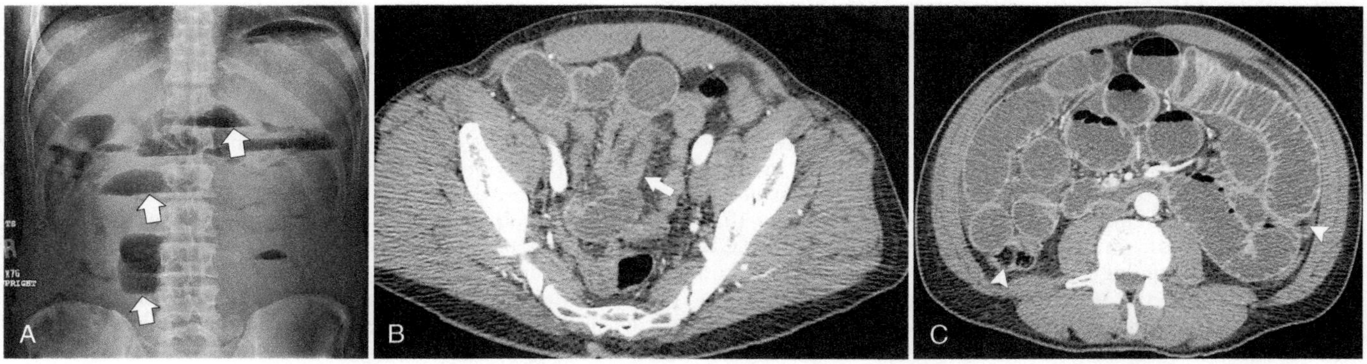

FIGURE 4-101. Plain abdominal radiograph (**A**) and axial (**B** and **C**) contrast-enhanced CT in a 44-year-old woman with multiple air-fluid levels (*arrows* in **A**) due to small bowel obstruction from adhesions. CT confirms the marked small bowel distention and collapsed ileum beyond the obstruction (*arrow* in **B**). The colon is also collapsed (*arrowheads*).

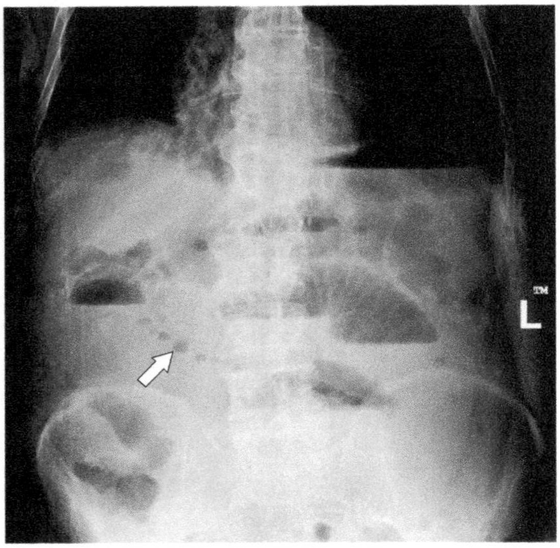

FIGURE 4-102. Plain abdominal radiograph in an 80-year-old woman with small bowel obtruction and a "string of pearls" sign (*arrow*).

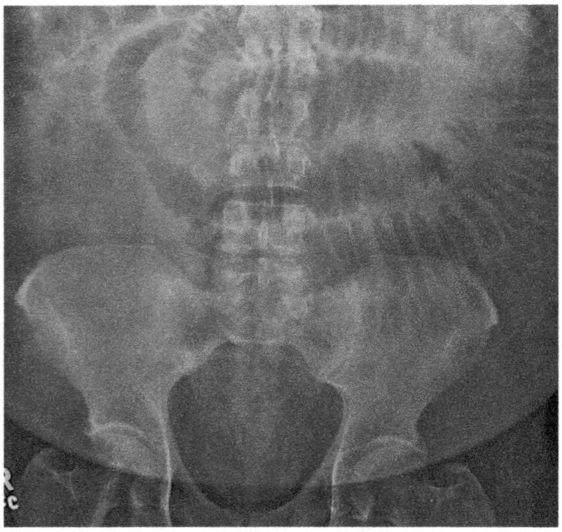

FIGURE 4-103. Abdominal supine plain radiograph demonstrating small bowel obstructon with predominantly centrally located obstructed loops. Presence of small bowel valvulae conniventes helps differentiate the distention from large bowel obstruction.

may be a variable amount of gas in the colon, depending on the degree of obstruction, and this should not deter the diagnosis of SBO unless either there is concurrent large bowel obstruction or the colon is moderately to significantly distended with air. Sometimes it can be challenging to differentiate SBO from large bowel obstruction, but the small bowel obstructed loops tend to lie centrally within the abdomen as described, the dilatation is often less than that observed with colonic obstruction alone, and valvulae conniventes can be identified (Fig. 4-103). Prolonged SBO can result in a small bowel feces sign at CT, a characteristic imaging sign for SBO. This occurs after fluid reabsorption from the stagnant visceral material deposited in the obstructed small bowel, resulting in the luminal contents appearing similar to colonic stool (Fig. 4-104). The appearances can be identical to meconium ileus seen in patients with cystic fibrosis, whereby thick, mucoid visceral contents also stagnate within a relatively functionless small bowel (Fig. 4-105).

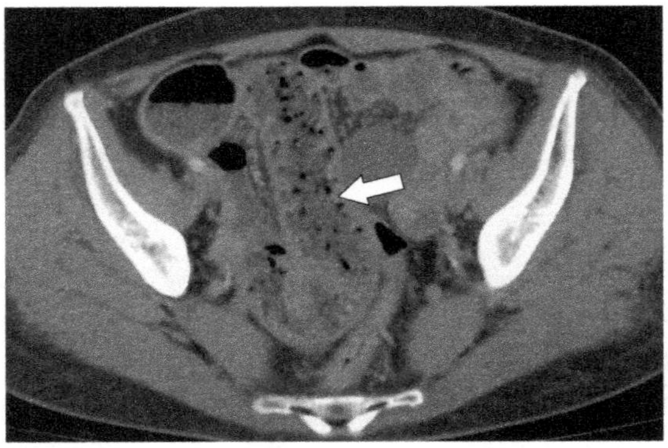

FIGURE 4-104. Axial contrast-enhanced CT in a 54-year-old woman with focal chronic small bowel obstruction and a small bowel feces sign (*arrow*) due to serosal metastases (not shown).

Extraluminal Causes of Small Bowel Obstruction

Adhesions

Adhesions are by far the most common cause of SBO and usually are a result of prior abdominal surgery. Any insult to the mesentery, whether from trauma, such as surgery, or peritonitis, can heal by fibrosis and adhesion formation. The obstruction (acute and subacute) by adhesions can spontaneously resolve, but persistent symptoms will require further investigation. Contrast small bowel series can be used to identify the site of obstruction, but CT after the administration of oral contrast media is now the first-line investigation to delineate the site, and quite often the cause, of obstruction. The adhesions will not be seen by SBFT or CT per se, but the small bowel dilatation and site obstruction should be visible. Given the appropriate history, SBO due to adhesion formation can be inferred (Figs. 4-106 and 4-107). When more than a single adhesion is present, a closed-loop obstruction may result. This entraps bowel and can rapidly lead to bowel ischemia and infarction as its vascular supply is compromised (Fig. 4-108).

Abdominal Hernias

There are many types of hernias that occur in the abdomen, some of little clinical significance, whereas others are potentially fatal if complications are left untreated. Diaphragmatic, hiatal, and paraesophageal hernias are discussed in Chapters 1 and 2.

Abdominal hernias are either internal or external. Together they are the second most common causes of SBO after adhesion formation. Internal hernias are less common and usually result from defects in the mesentery or peritoneum and include transmesenteric, paraduodenal, pericecal, and intersigmoid hernias. Rarely, small bowel can enter the epiploic foramen, producing a lesser sac hernia. Far more common are external hernias (Table 4-11). The specific type of hernia is usually identified at CT, along with any signs of obstruction, although it can be difficult to differentiate inguinal from femoral hernias. Intravenous contrast should be administered to assess for any evidence of bowel ischemia (reduction in normal bowel enhancement when compromised or avascular bowel when infarcted), which is generally a surgical emergency. Oral contrast media may pass into the hernia and should not deter a diagnosis of at least partial SBO if other bowel loops are dilated.

Inguinal hernias are the most common abdominal hernia (75%) and are either direct (occurring in the floor of the inguinal canal) or, more commonly, indirect (passing along the inguinal canal through both the internal and external inguinal ring). Inguinal and femoral hernias are readily identified at CT but can be difficult to differentiate. Inguinal hernias are confirmed if the herniated contents, fat, or bowel passes from lateral to medial toward the scrotum, into which these contents can present if large enough (Fig. 4-109).

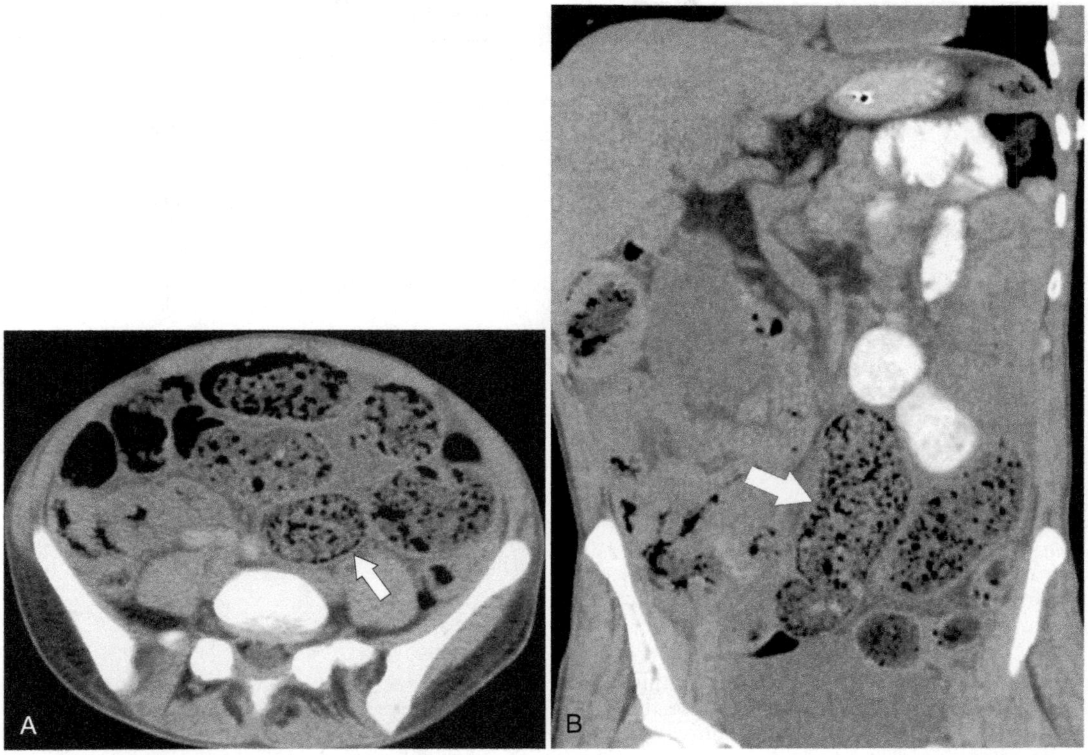

FIGURE 4-105. Axial (**A**) and coronal (**B**) noncontrast CT in a 47-year-old man with cystic fibrosis and small bowel feces sign (*arrows*) due to meconium ileus leading to small bowel obstruction.

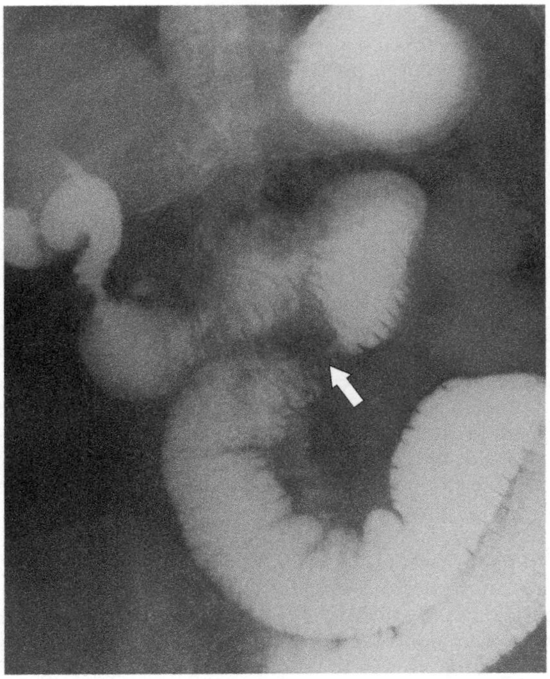

FIGURE 4-106. SBFT in a 67-year-old woman with small bowel obstruction due to adhesions (*arrow*). The small bowel is dilated beyond the stricture because of a more distal adhesion (not shown).

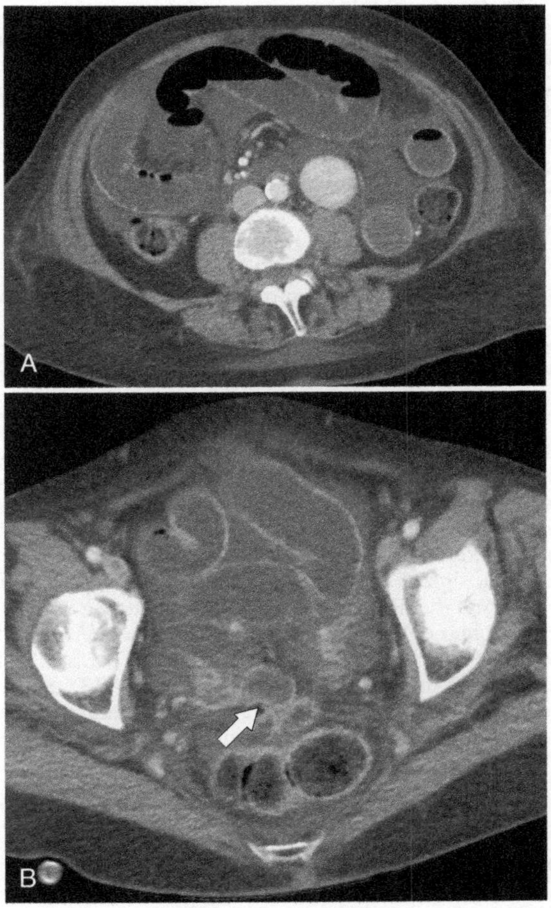

FIGURE 4-107. Axial contrast-enhanced CT (**A** and **B**) in an 83-year-old woman with small bowel obstruction and ascites due to small bowel adhesions (*arrow*).

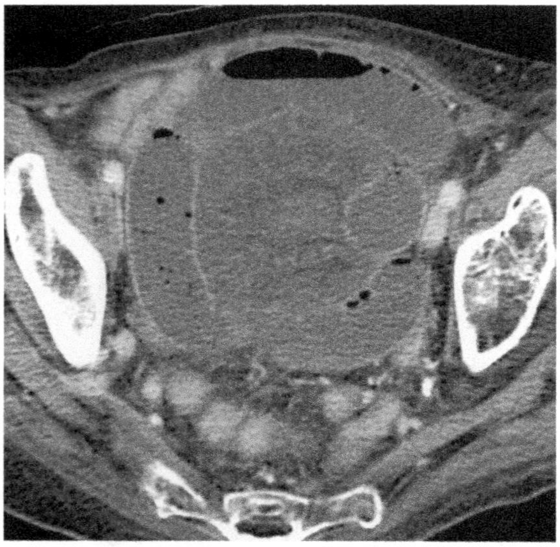

FIGURE 4-108. Axial contrast-enhanced CT in a 54-year-old man after colectomy, now with a closed-loop small bowel obstruction with circular loops of incarcerated ischemic small bowel and edematous mesentery.

TABLE 4-11 External Abdominal Hernias

Type	Features
Inguinal (Figs. 4-109, 4-111, 4-112)	Most common external abdominal hernia
Femoral (Fig. 4-110)	Often obstructs
Richter* hernia (Fig. 4-115)	Herniation of one side of the bowel wall, which does not obstruct but may infarct
Ventral hernia (Fig. 4-113)	Occurs along the midline through the linea alba
Epigastric hernia	(Variant of ventral hernia) herniation through the linea alba above the umbilicus
Spigelian† hernia (Fig. 4-116)	Herniation between oblique and transverse abdominal muscles
Incisional hernia (Fig. 4-114)	Herniation through weakness and defect from surgical or laparoscopic incision
Obturator hernia	Herniation of fat or bowel (ileum most common) between pectineus and obturator muscle
Lumbar hernia	Posterolateral herniation of fat or viscera
Umbilical hernia (Figs. 4-117, 4-118)	Herniation of fat or bowel through the umbilical ring

*August G. Richter (1742-1812), German surgeon.
†Adriaan van den Spiegel (1578-1625), Flemish anatomist.

Femoral hernias are generally lower than inguinal hernias and pass medial to the femoral vein. They result from intraabdominal contents (fat, vessels, or bowel) extending into the femoral canal, which is below the inguinal canal and lateral to the pubic tubercle (Fig. 4-110). Femoral hernias are more likely to obstruct than their inguinal counterparts because of their narrower orifice, but they are far less common than inguinal hernias. Obstructing inguinal hernias are actually observed more frequently in clinical practice. As with adhesions, the obstruction can be transient and intermittent, but complete obstruction usually warrants surgical intervention, particularly because the bowel can rapidly become ischemic from vascular compromise due to restricted blood flow. Incarcerated hernias refer to any type of abdominal hernia that becomes irreducible and may or may not be symptomatic.

When symptomatic, these hernias typically cause localized pain. Patients with incarcerated hernias are at risk of obstruction (Fig. 4-111). Initially there is no ischemia, but as the stricture at the hernial orifice worsens, the bowel can become ischemic. This may progress to strangulation, a serious complication because of the imminent possibility of bowel perforation. The dilated bowel compresses the arterial blood supply as it passes through the narrowed hiatal orifice, resulting in bowel ischemia, which is prolonged and can lead to necrosis and perforation. At CT, the bowel wall is usually thickened, and there is little or no enhancement because of the arterial impingement. The bowel itself is "dusky," an ominous sign (Fig. 4-112). There is often associated mesenteric edema or ascites. As ischemia progresses, pneumatosis develops (an imminent sign of bowel necrosis), and the gas is transported distally through the mesenteric venous system to the liver.

There are numerous other abdominal hernias, some of which involve abdominal viscera and others that that do not, and include peritoneal fat (Table 4-11 and Figs. 4-113 to 4-118). Some are more at risk of obstruction, incarceration, and strangulation than others, mostly depending on the width of the hernial orifices. Those with wide orifices are unlikely to be problematic. Others have a narrow neck and bowel can become readily incarcerated and ischemic (Figs. 4-113 and 4-114).

Internal Hernias

The small bowel can protrude or invaginate into mesenteric and peritoneal spaces, either because there is incomplete congenital formation of the peritoneum in utero or because protrusion or invagination can develop after surgical procedures. These can be transient and asymptomatic or incarcerate and be life threatening because of strangulation and ischemia.

Paraduodenal Hernia

Paraduodenal hernias are usually left sided (although they can also occur on the right) because of a congenital defect in the descending mesocolon. They can also result from postsurgical defects in the mesocolon. At imaging, there is an abnormal cluster of small bowel loops between the tail of pancreas and stomach and just medial to the upper descending colon when left sided. When they are right sided, they are identified at CT lateral and inferior to the second part of the duodenum and medial to the ascending colon. Many are asymptomatic but can become incarcerated or strangulated if the hernial orifice is too tight and the vascular supply is compromised (Fig. 4-119). This may be either due to simple compression or due to volvulus of the herniated bowel and mesentery. Either will cause a closed-loop obstruction (see later) requiring surgical fixation.

Transmesenteric Hernia

Transmesenteric hernias result from herniation of bowel contents through a surgically created defect within small bowel mesentery or, less commonly, a congenital defect. The small bowel herniation can range from a few to many centimeters (Fig. 4-120). Similar to other internal hernias observed by CT imaging, bowel loops will be recognized as clustered and enclosed adjacent to the location of the hernia (Fig. 4-121). These loops can undergo volvulus formation and obstruct at the hernial orifice, and a transient point should be identified at CT. Small bowel vasculature can twist as the small bowel mesentery is forced through the hiatus. Incarceration and strangulation can then occur, with bowel wall thickening and hypoperfused bowel, with or without ascites (Fig. 4-122). These require immediate surgical intervention to prevent bowel infarction.

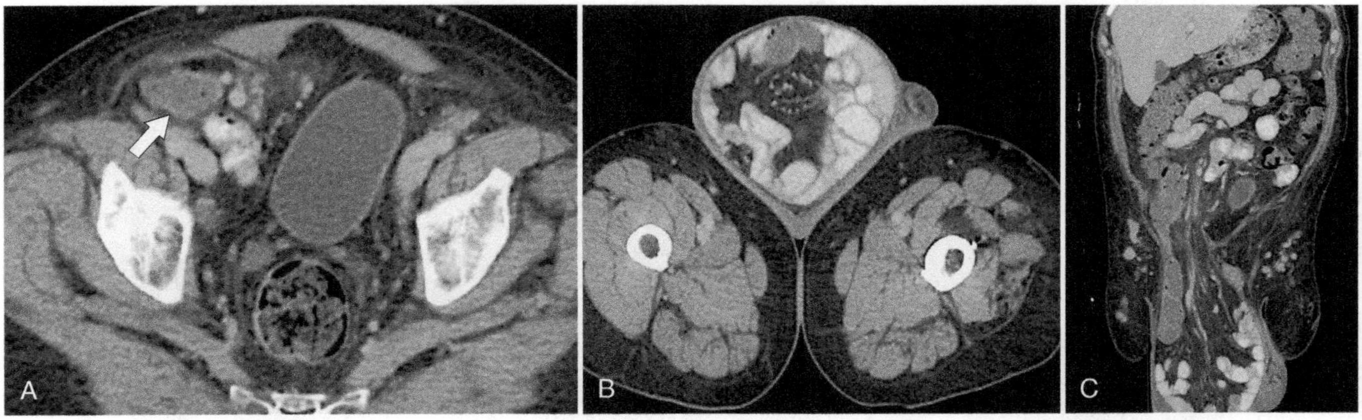

FIGURE 4-109. Axial (**A** and **B**) and coronal (**C**) contrast-enhanced CT in an 81-year-old man with massive herniation (*arrow*) of small and large bowel through a right inguinal hernia.

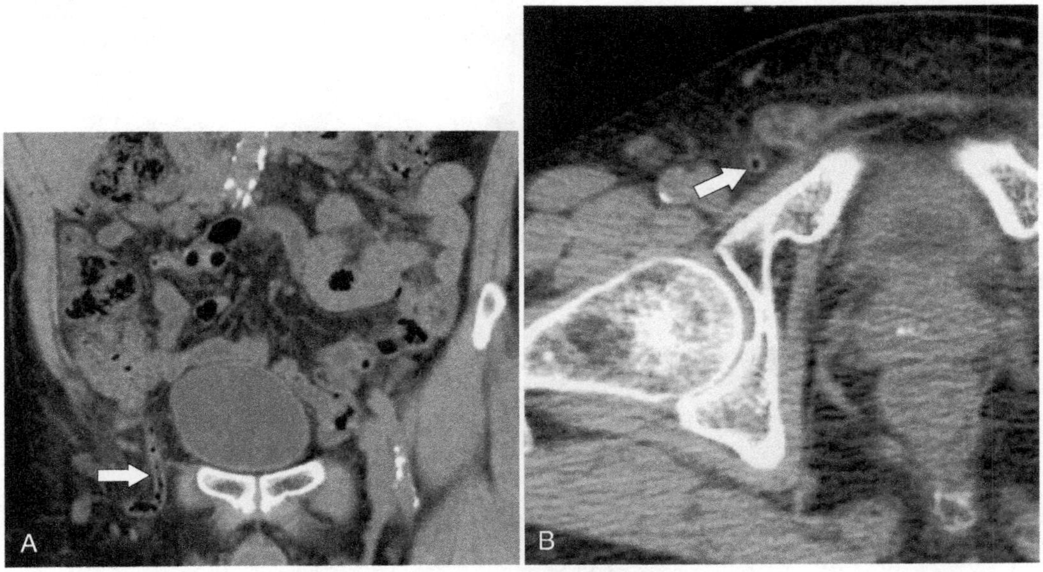

FIGURE 4-110. Coronal (**A**) and axial (**B**) noncontrast CT in an 80-year-old woman with herniation of the appendix through a right-sided femoral hernia (*arrows*), also known as Amyand hernia. (Claudius Amyand 1680-1740, British surgeon.)

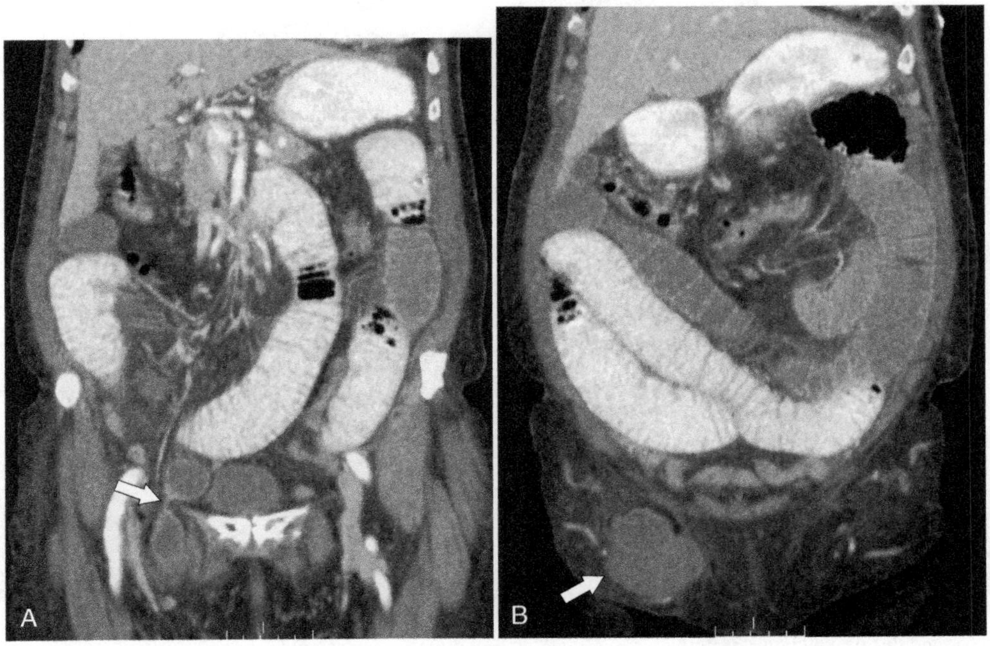

FIGURE 4-111. **A** and **B**, Coronal contrast-enhanced CT in a 59-year-old woman with small bowel obstruction due to an obstructing right inguinal hernia (*arrows*).

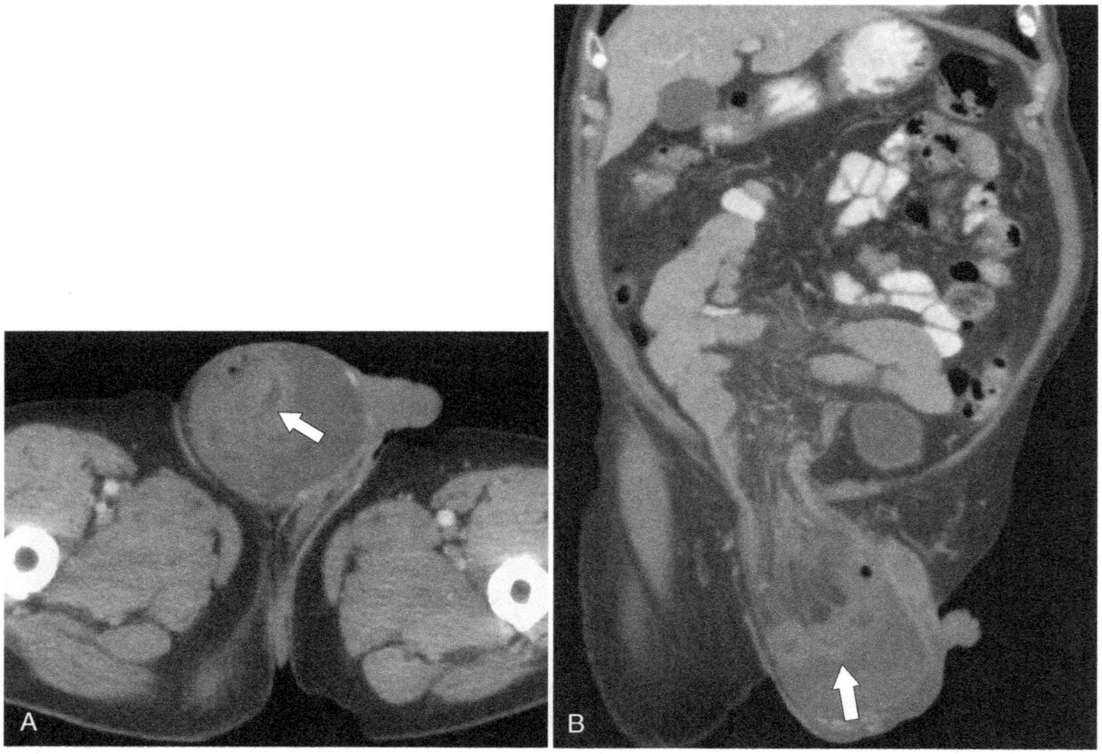

Figure 4-112. Axial (**A**) and coronal (**B**) CT in a 76-year-old man with a strangulated inguinal hernia with infarcted small bowel (*arrows*).

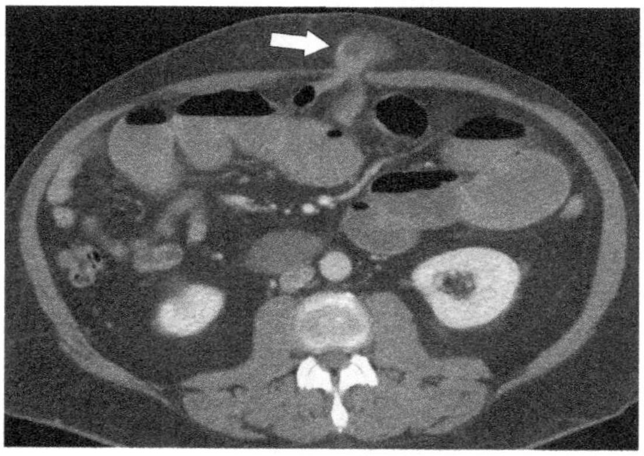

Figure 4-113. Axial CT in a 66-year-old woman with a ventral hernia that is incarcerated and partial small bowel obstruction (*arrow*).

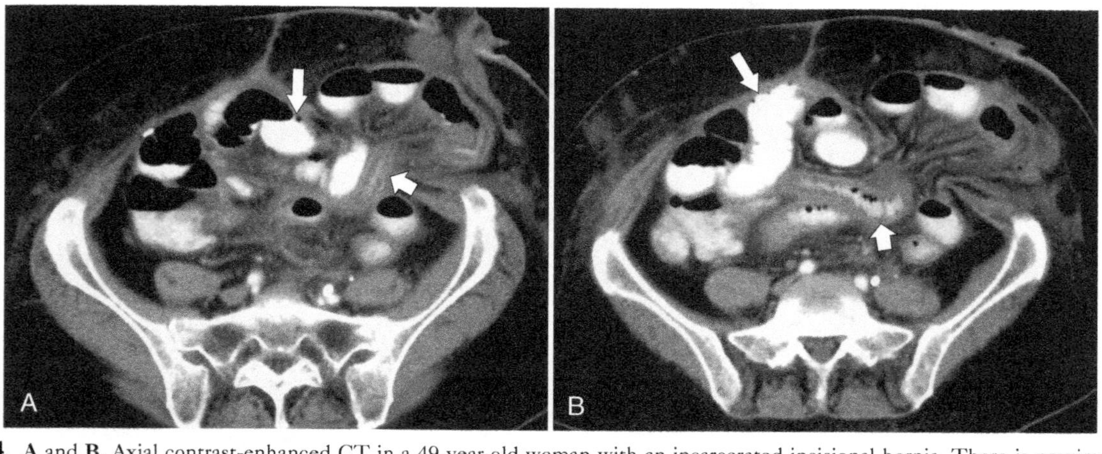

Figure 4-114. **A** and **B**, Axial contrast-enhanced CT in a 49-year-old woman with an incarcerated incisional hernia. There is proximal small bowel obstruction (*large arrows*) and distal small bowel wall thickening (*small arrows*) due to vascular compromise.

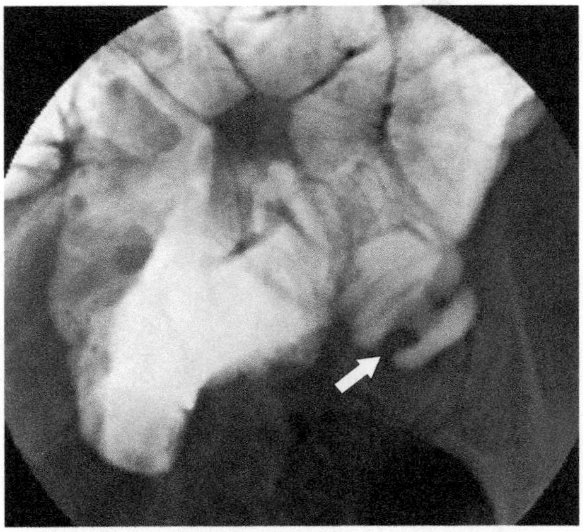

FIGURE 4-115. SBFT in a 56-year-old man with a Richter hernia (*arrow*).

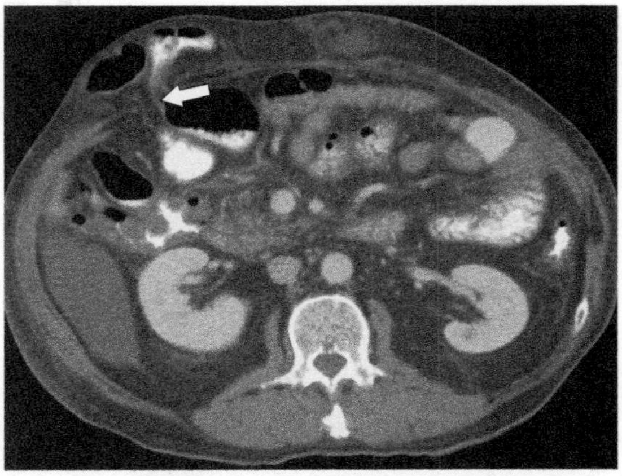

FIGURE 4-116. Axial noncontrast CT in a 71-year-old man with a Spigelian hernia (*arrow*). Herniated small bowel is prone to incarceration and obstruction because of the narrow hiatal orifice.

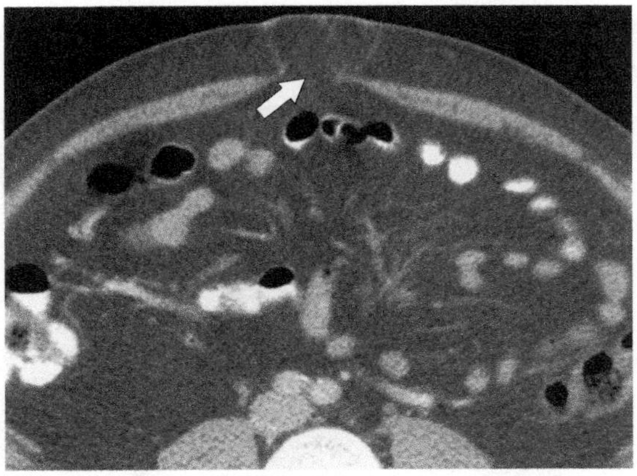

FIGURE 4-117. Axial contrast-enhanced CT in a 53-year-old man with a fat-containing umbilical hernia (*arrow*).

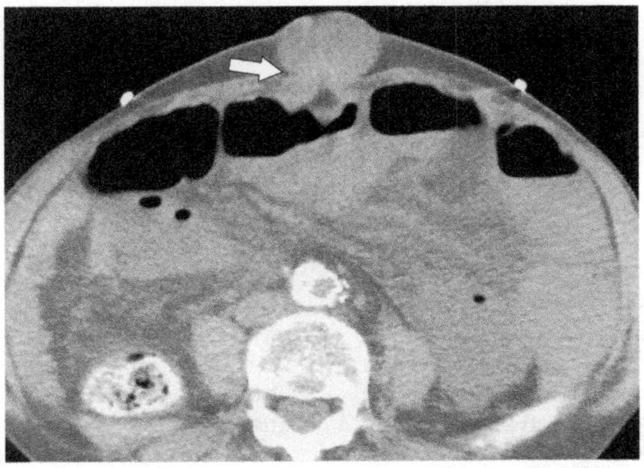

FIGURE 4-118. Axial contrast-enhanced CT in a 73-year-old man with an incarcerated umbilical hernia and small bowel obstruction (*arrow*).

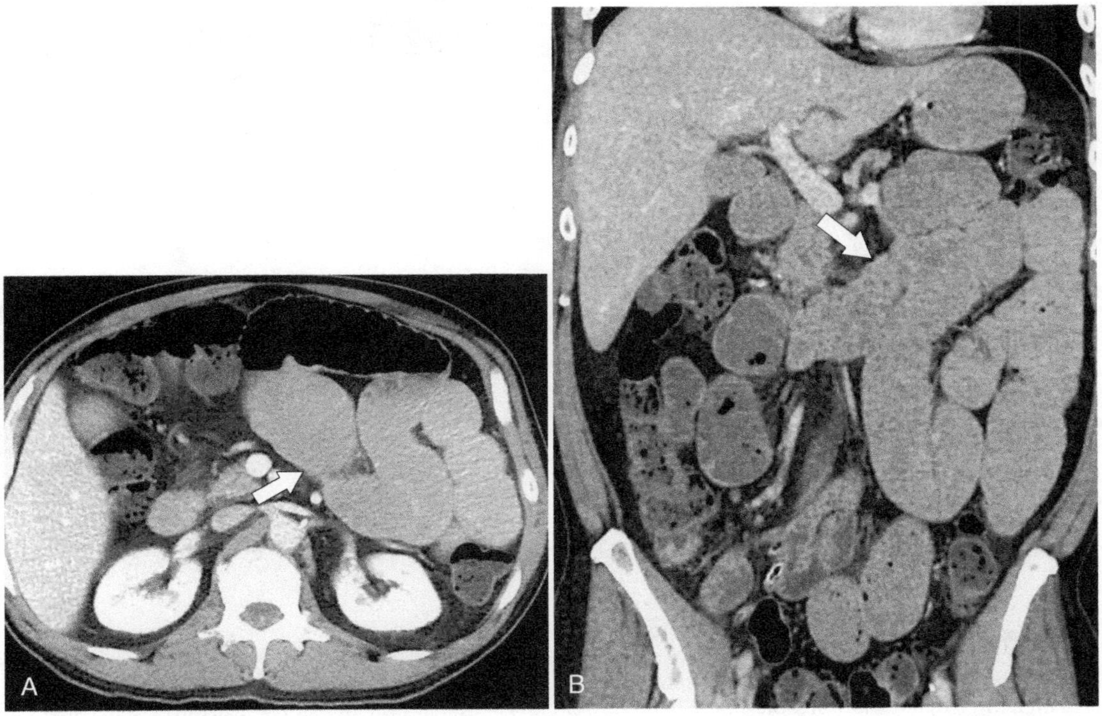

FIGURE 4-119. Axial (**A**) and coronal (**B**) contrast-enhanced CT in a 50-year-old man with a left-sided paraduodenal internal obstructed hernia (*arrows*) secondary to prior colonic surgery.

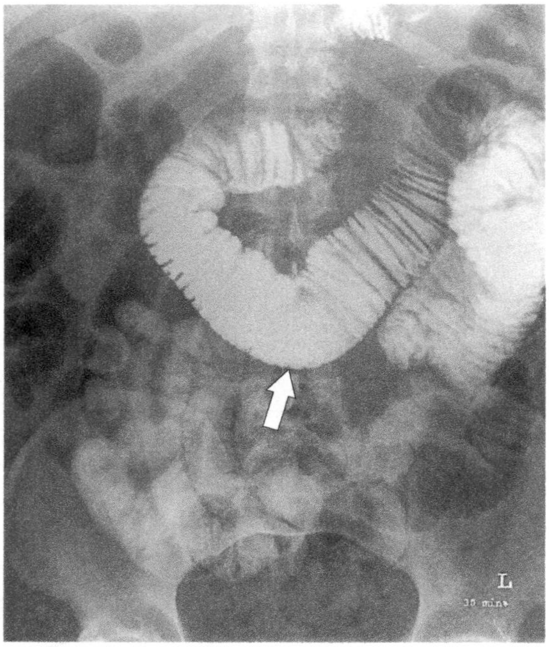

FIGURE 4-120. SBFT in a 44-year-old woman after bariatric surgery and now with a closed-loop obstruction (*arrow*).

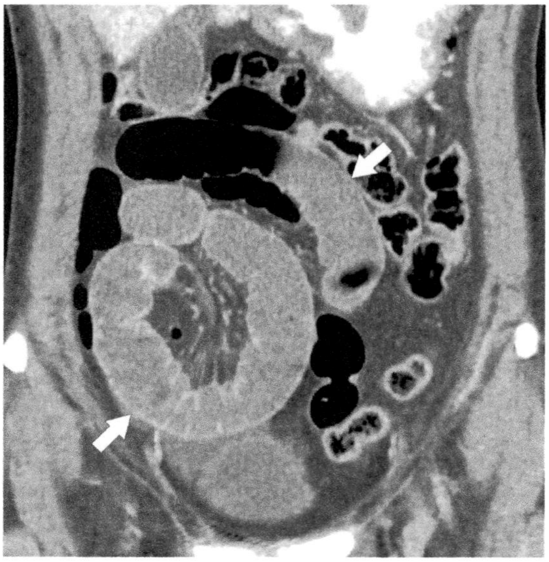

FIGURE 4-121. Coronal contrast-enhanced CT in a 43-year-old woman with a transmesenteric hernia and closed-loop obstruction (*arrows*).

Closed-Loop Obstruction

Closed-loop obstruction simply refers to SBO at two points. The obstruction may be simply due to impingement of the small bowel at a tight hernia orifice (as in paraduodenal and transmesenteric hernias) but often results from a small bowel volvulus, usually caused by adhesions. The small bowel twists at the anchor point so that bowel contents can neither enter nor exit the closed loop. The closed loop then distends with fluid because of existing bowel contents and continuing mucosal secretions. Vessels and fat also twist, potentially leading to vascular compromise, and consequently volvulus is a major complication and is the most common cause of small bowel strangulation.

At imaging by CT, the distended closed loop, which is narrowed or tapered at its apex, is identified. Although upstream SBO occurs, the dilatation is usually less impressive than the dilatation of the closed loop. Mesentery within the closed loop is twisted and recognized at CT by observing mesenteric vessels in a whorled configuration (Fig. 4-123). These findings usually indicate a surgical emergency because the bowel is at significant risk of infarction.

Small Bowel Volvulus

A volvulus means a twisting of the bowel, usually around its mesentery. It is more common in children, mostly as a result of congenital malrotation anomalies (e.g., midgut volvulus), but when it is present in adults, it is usually a result of an underlying acquired abnormality, including internal hernias, adhesions, and neoplasms. The volvulus can constrict vascular supply or cut off blood flow completely, rendering it a surgical emergency to prevent bowel infarction. The investigation of choice is CT, which will demonstrate multiple loops of dilated small bowel converging to a narrowing and constriction often to a circular loop (Fig. 4-124).

Mural Causes of Small Bowel Obstruction

Mural causes are most commonly due to benign inflammatory strictures or malignant small bowel neoplasms. Small bowel inflammatory strictures are caused by the fibrotic reparative

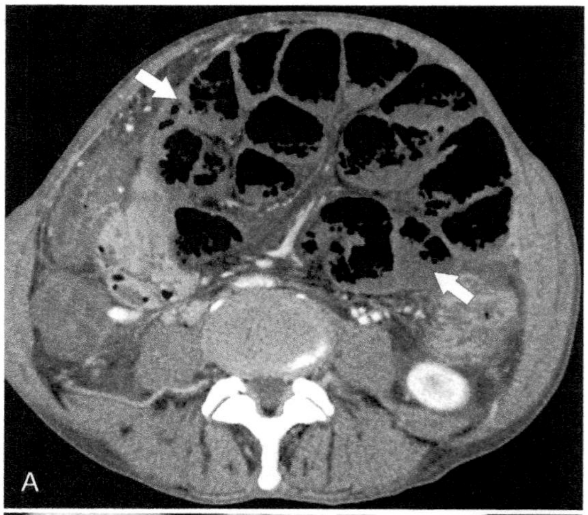

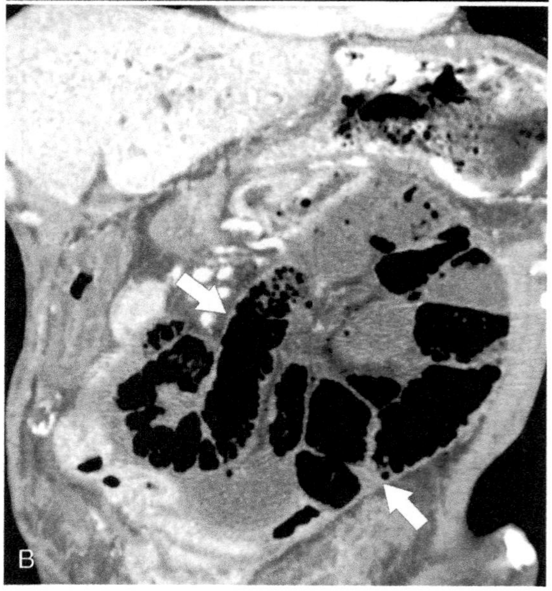

FIGURE 4-122. Axial (**A**) and coronal (**B**) contrast-enhanced CT in a 71-year-old man and an internal volvulus and absence of small bowel enhancement resulting from ischemia (*arrows*).

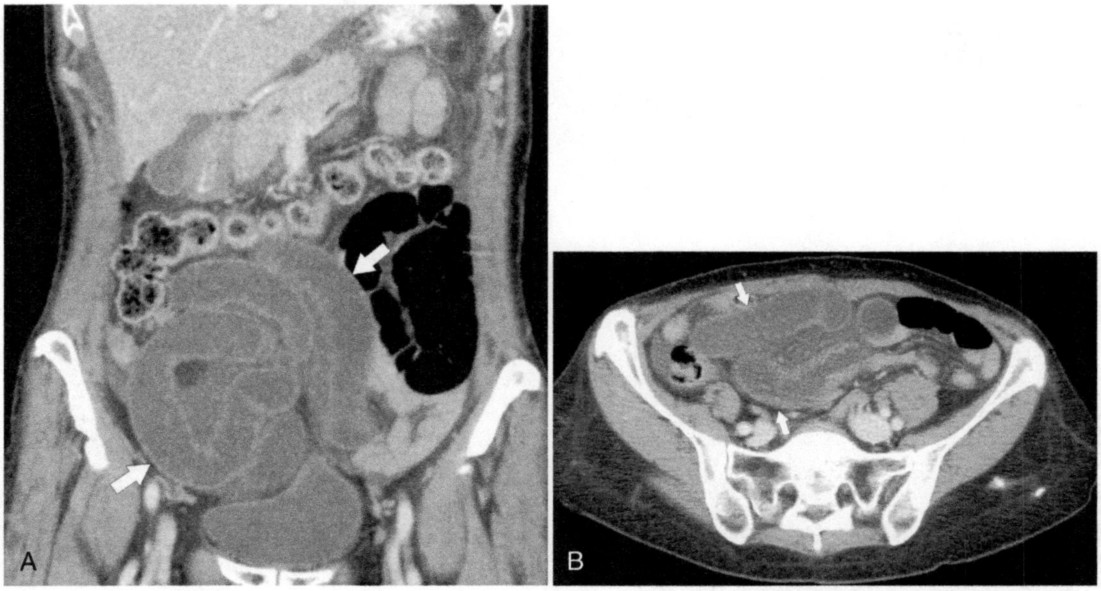

FIGURE 4-123. Coronal (**A**) and axial (**B**) CT in a 53-year-old man with a closed-loop obstruction from adhesions, which has undergone volvulus, rendering the bowel wall ischemic.

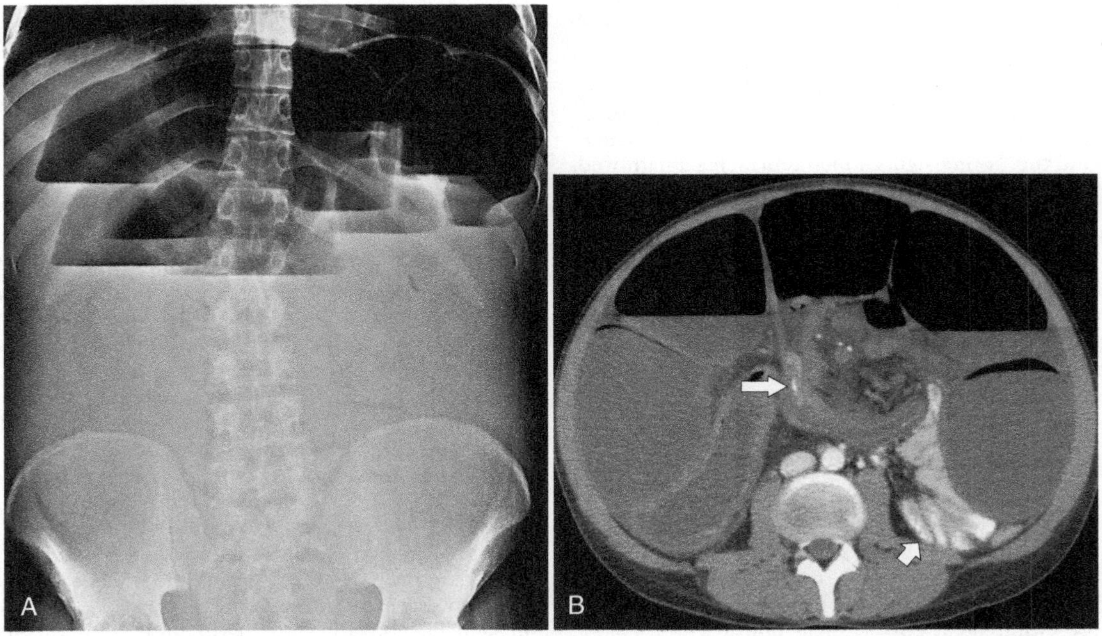

FIGURE 4-124. Plain abdominal radiograph (**A**) and axial contrast-enhanced CT (**B**) in a 23-year-old man with gross small bowel obstruction (air-fluid levels in **A** and dilated small bowel in **B**) due to a small bowel volvulus (*large arrow*) and collapsed distal small bowel (*small arrow*).

process and are discussed in detail earlier in this chapter. Most fibrotic strictures do not cause complete SBO but rather a variable degree of incomplete or partial SBO. Patient symptoms range from none to repetitive bouts of nausea, bloating, fullness, and vomiting. At imaging, there may or may not be signs of SBO because this is intermittent. More acute or severe forms will usually cause small bowel distention and be observed even on plain imaging. CT is the investigation of choice to evaluate the site of obstruction, but SBFT will generally demonstrate the stricture itself to better effect, assuming sufficient contrast material reaches the point of obstruction (Fig. 4-125).

All malignant small bowel disease may cause obstruction once the mass becomes large enough, whether because of primary or metastatic tumors (Fig. 4-126).

Terminal Ileal Strictures

The differential diagnosis for terminal ileal strictures is relatively limited (Table 4-12). A clinical history is important to determine appropriate diagnosis. Crohn disease is by far the most common cause of terminal ileal narrowing and should always be considered, particularly in younger patients with an appropriate history. All manifestations of Crohn disease can be found in the terminal

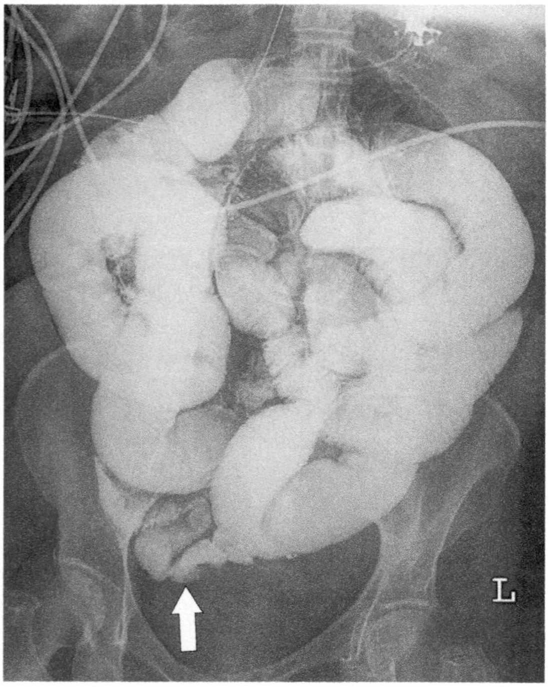

FIGURE 4-125. SBFT in a 70-year-old man with an ischemic stricture of the distal ileum causing small bowel obstruction (*arrow*).

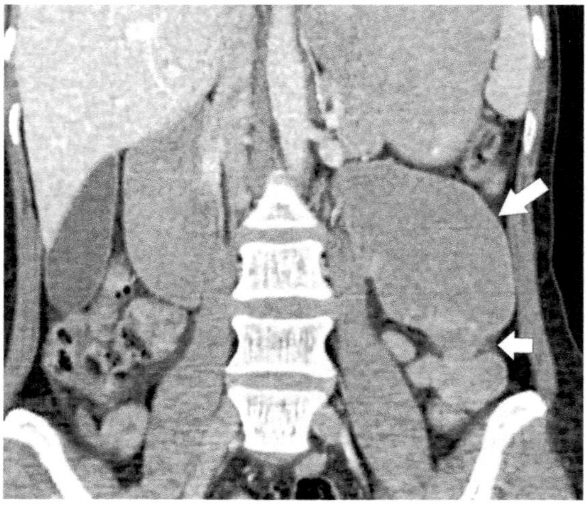

FIGURE 4-126. Coronal contrast-enhanced CT in a 55-year-old woman with complete small bowel obstruction (*large arrow*) due to jejunal adenocarcinoma (*small arrow*). There are dilated loops of small bowel.

TABLE 4-12 Terminal Ileal Stricture

Inflammatory	Crohn disease Extrinsic abscess (i.e., appendiceal)
Infection	Tuberculosis *Yersinia*
Neoplasia	Lymphoma Carcinoid Appendix mucinous tumor Colonic adenocarcinoma Ileal carcinoma Metastases

ileum, including stricture formation, ulceration, fistula, abscess formation, and, rarely, adenocarcinoma or lymphoma (Fig. 4-127). Specific signs include cobblestone formation representing deep mucosal ulcers separated by more normal, but edematous mucosa, and the "string sign," which represents a narrowed length of terminal ileum and displaced adjacent folds due to wall thickening and fibrosis.

Focal narrowing of the terminal ileum is a relatively common complication of several infectious processes, particularly TB and *Yersinia enterocolitis* (see earlier in chapter). Patients with ileal tuberculosis can have almost identical appearances to terminal ileal Crohn disease with ulcers, strictures, fistula, and abscess formation. Other specific causes of terminal ileal strictures are discussed earlier in this chapter.

Intraluminal Causes of Small Bowel Obstruction

Intussusception

Intussusception occurs when a loop of bowel invaginates into another, pulling its mesentery along with it. The resulting forward peristalsis "pushes" the proximal (intussusceptum) bowel further into the distal (intussuscipiens). The intussusceptum can be small bowel within small bowel, small bowel within colon, colon within colon, and even jejunum into stomach or vice versa (jejunogastric or gastrojejunal), which are observed after gastrojejunal anastomoses. Many cases are transitory and asymptomatic, particularly in younger patients, or can cause pain and bleeding (Fig. 4-128). Patients with celiac disease are also known to have transient episodes of intussusception without an obvious recognized mechanism (see Fig.4-35). Although smaller intussusceptions are transitory and asymptomatic, an intussusception in older patients is often due to an underlying mass that acts as a "lead point," being propelled distally by peristalsis, which pulls the more proximal bowel with it into the distal bowel. These are usually due to polypoid benign neoplasms, including lipoma or adenoma, that promote the process, whereas more malignant "fixed" lesions (lymphoma or carcinoma) usually render the bowel too firm for the process to occur. Some smaller metastatic lesions, particularly small bowel melanoma, also have a propensity to cause intussusception (Figs. 4-93 and 4-129). Sometimes a small bowel feeding tube or catheter, particularly if it has a balloon tip, precipitates intussusception. Meckel diverticula can sometimes present with an intussusception (see Fig. 4-6). Depending on the length and severity of the intussusception, there is variable bowel obstruction, ischemia, and if advanced, perforation.

Most intussusceptions are now detected by CT, although SBFT can demonstrate an intussusception as a "coiled spring" of crowded mucosal folds within the intussusception (see Fig. 4-35). Ultrasound, however, is the investigating tool of choice in children to avoid radiation exposure (see Fig. 4-94). The cardinal sign with both CT and ultrasound is a soft tissue mass with a target-like appearance representing, from outer to inner, the outer bowel wall of the intussuscipiens, then mesenteric fat that has invaginated into the intussuscipiens, within which is the inner bowel (intussusceptum) (see Figs. 4-94 and 4-129).

The treatment of childhood ileocolic or colocolonic intussusceptions is usually with air or contrast enema, but in adults, surgery may sometimes be required to disengage the bowel from itself.

Gallstone Ileus

A consequence of chronic cholecystitis with inflammatory weakening of the gallbladder wall, the gallstone erodes through the wall into the duodenum and is propelled usually as far as the ileocecal valve, the narrowest point in the small bowel. If the stone is large enough, it can become lodged in the narrow lumen, causing SBO. Smaller stones may pass through the ileocecal valve without causing any obstruction. Ingested foreign bodies may also become lodged in the narrow ileocecal valve region with similar results.

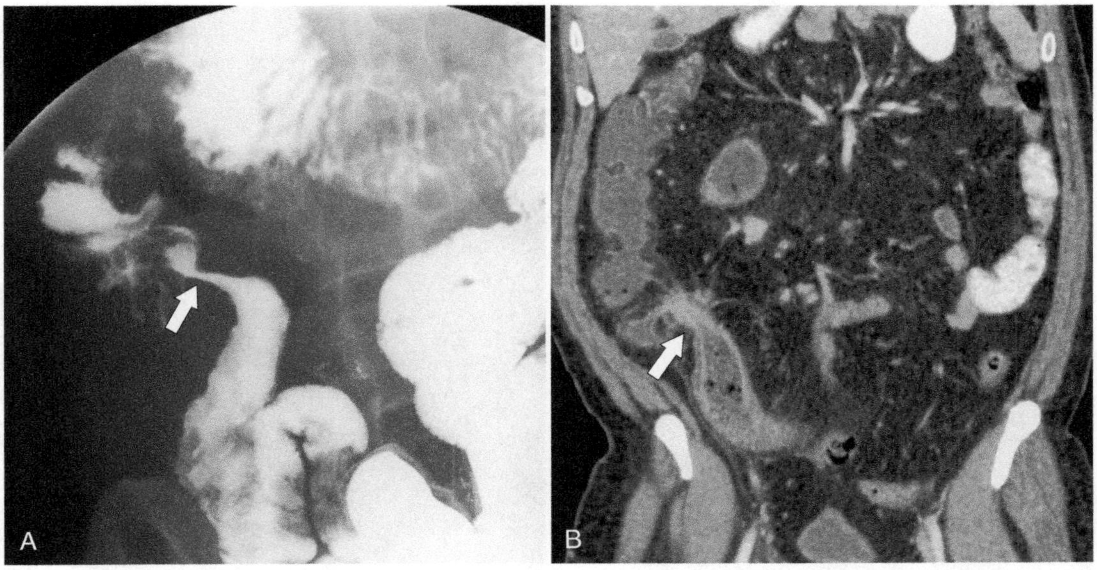

FIGURE 4-127. SBFT examination (**A**) and coronal CT (**B**) in a 20-year-old man with a terminal ileal stricture (*arrows*) due to Crohn disease.

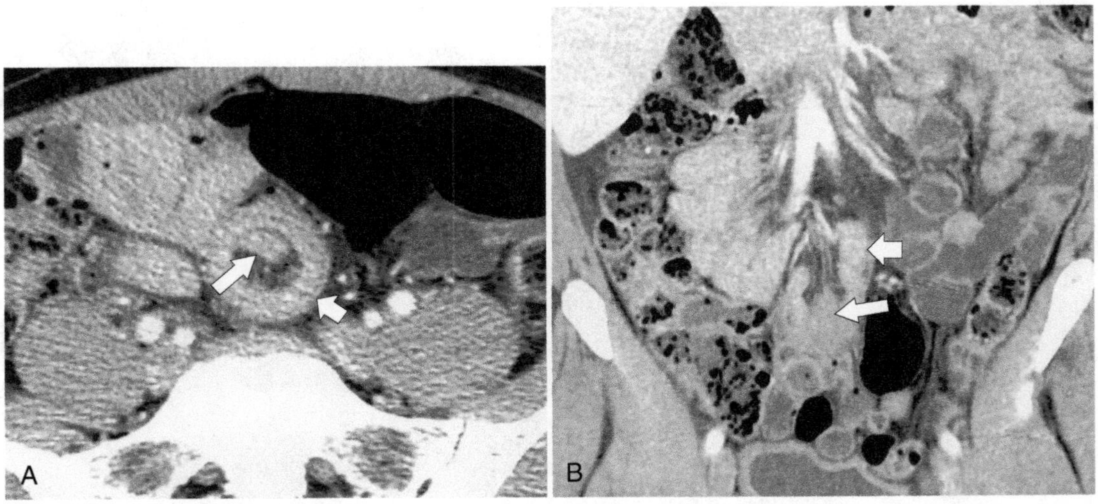

FIGURE 4-128. Axial (**A**) and coronal (**B**) contrast-enhanced CT in a 54-year-old man with a transient ileal intussusception. The intussusceptum (*long arrows*) is surrounded by mesenteric fat within the intussuscipiens (*short arrows*).

At CT, there is evidence of a thickened gallbladder wall that adheres to the duodenum. There is often gas in the gallbladder and common bile duct due to the fistula between the duodenum and gallbladder. There is small bowel dilatation, with the offending gallstone identified at or near the ileocecal valve (Fig. 4-130).

Foreign Bodies

Ingested foreign bodies usually pass via the rectum asymptomatically but can become lodged within the small bowel, particularly at its narrowest point at, or near, the ileocecal valve (Fig. 4-131). Larger material may cause more proximal obstruction (Fig. 4-132). The most commonly ingested foreign bodies are fruit pits (e.g., peach, prune), but more bizarre objects can be found, particularly in psychiatric patients. Many are identified on plain radiographs if metallic (Fig. 4-133). Drug dealers can transport their drugs by packing narcotics into condoms and swallowing them. Sometimes the load is sufficient to cause obstruction. They can usually be identified on plain radiographs as oval opacities, possibly with air surrounding them (double condom sign). These can be fatal if they rupture, causing a massive drug overdose. Iatrogenic material can become dislodged (e.g., parts of feeding tubes) and migrate down the GI tract and may sometimes cause obstruction (see Fig. 4-131).

Small Bowel Bezoars

Small bowel bezoars are uncommon, and like stomach bezoars, can be caused by the overingestion of vegetable matter (phytobezoar), which, when severe, can lead to SBO. The diagnosis can be made at SBFT with an appearance of an irregular mass with barium interspersed among the vegetable matter. At CT, it may be harder to identify the specific cause of SBO unless large enough, although the obstruction itself is readily identified (Fig. 4-134).

Diverticula

The most common small bowel diverticulum is in the duodenum (see Chapter 2) and is of no significance except for causing difficulties with ampullary cannulation at endoscopic retrograde

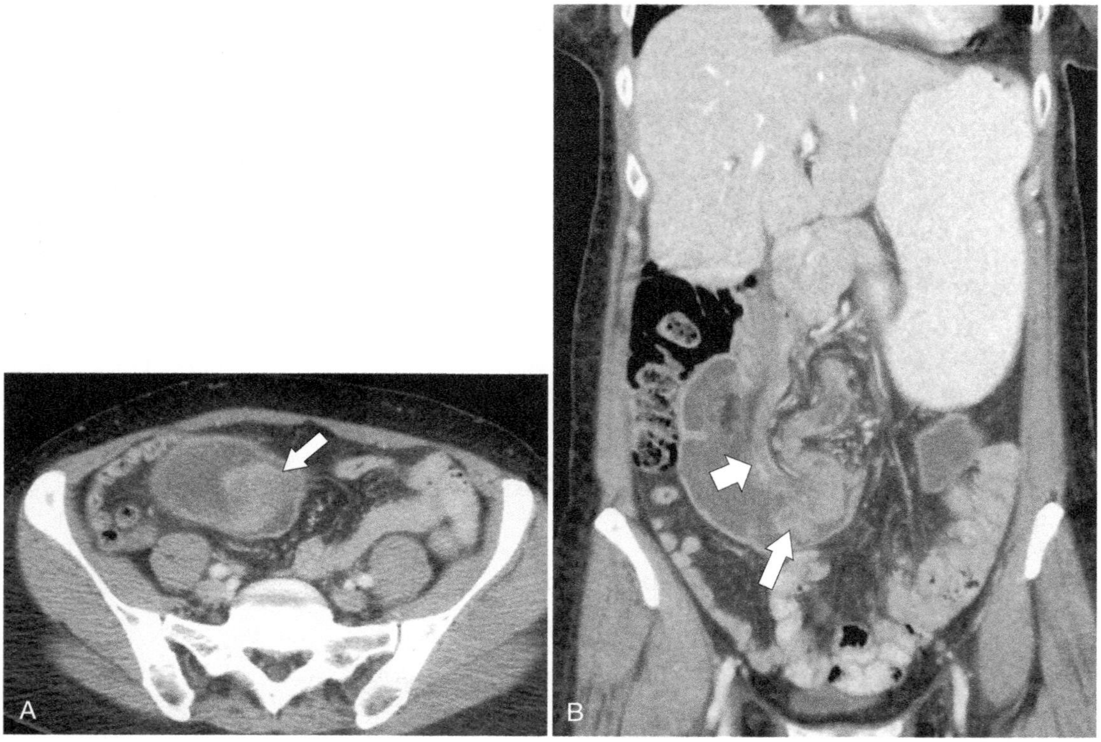

FIGURE 4-129. Axial (**A**) and coronal (**B**) CT in a 61-year-old man with a distal jejunal melanoma deposit (*large arrows*) acting as the lead point for a jejunal intussusception (*small arrow*).

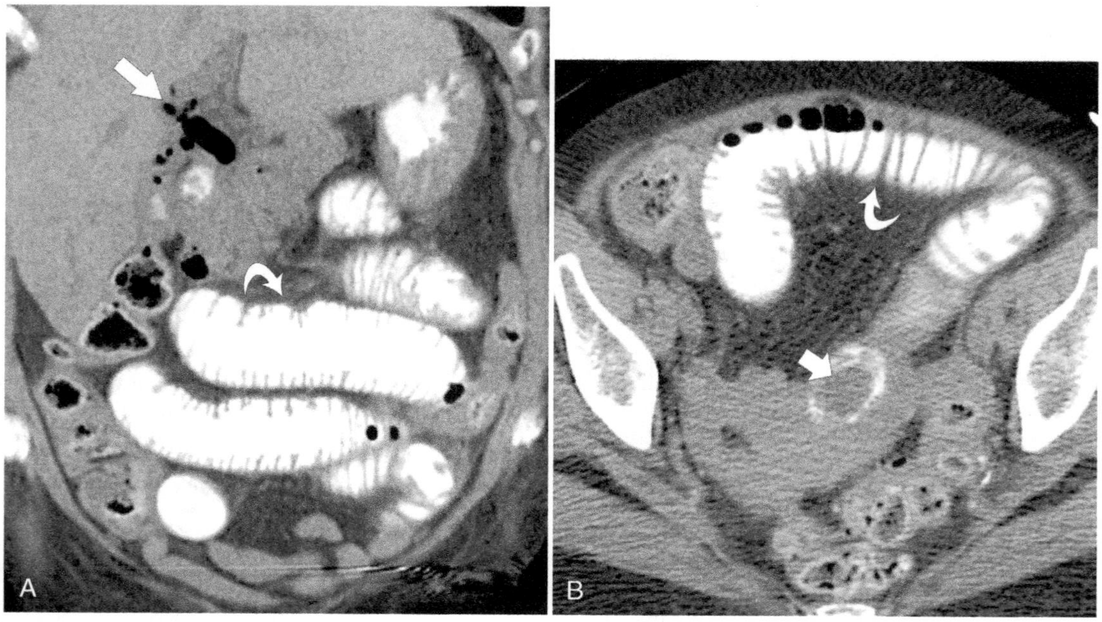

FIGURE 4-130. Coronal (**A**) and axial (**B**) noncontrast CT in a 67-year-old woman with biliary gas (*large arrow*) and a contracted gallbladder and small bowel obstruction (*curved arrows*). There is an obstructing gallstone in the distal ileum (*small arrow*).

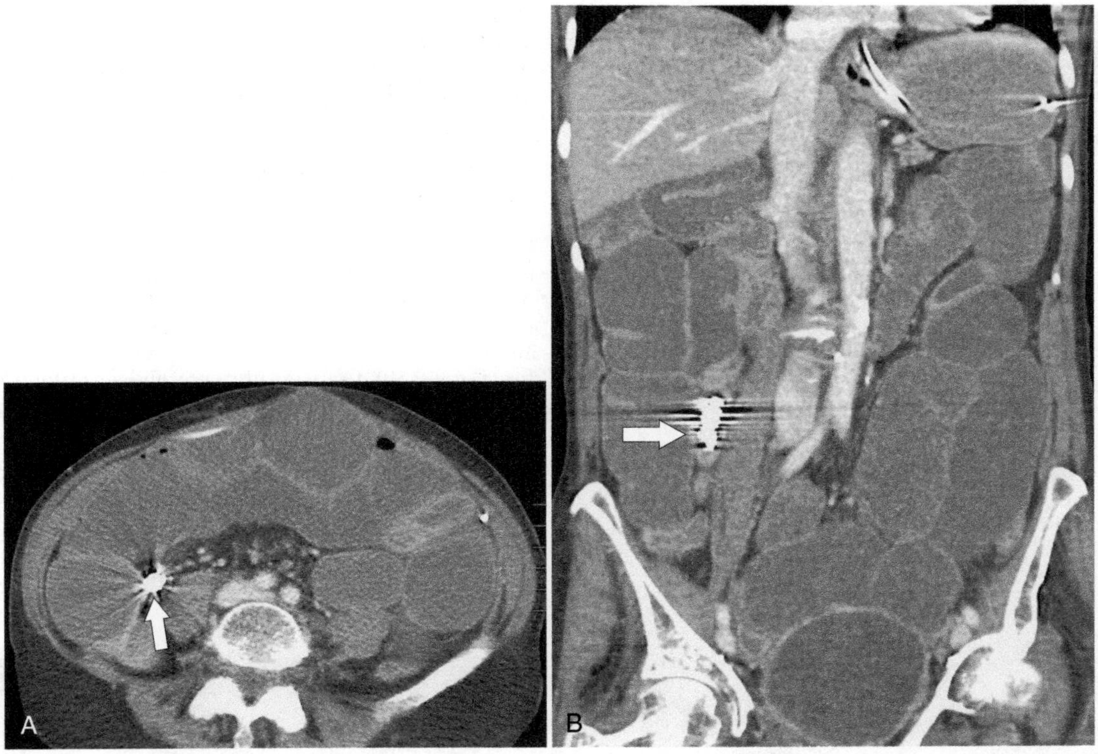

FIGURE 4-131. Axial (**A**) and coronal (**B**) contrast-enhanced CT in a 32-year-old woman with gross small bowel dilation due to obstruction near the ileocecal valve from an endoscopic capsule (*arrows*).

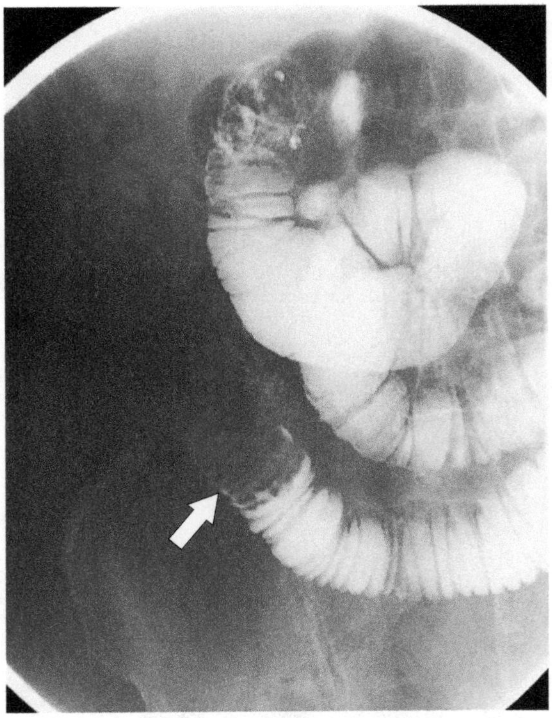

FIGURE 4-132. Barium SBFT in a 66-year-old man with small bowel obstruction due to an ingested foreign body (*arrow*).

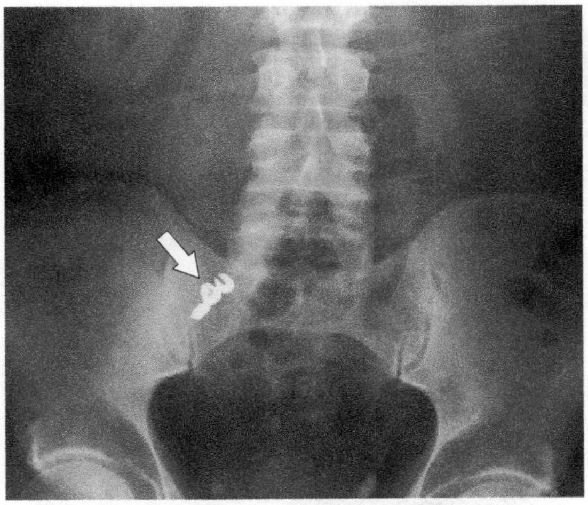

FIGURE 4-133. Plain abdominal radiograph in a 59-year-old woman with swallowed dentures (*arrow*).

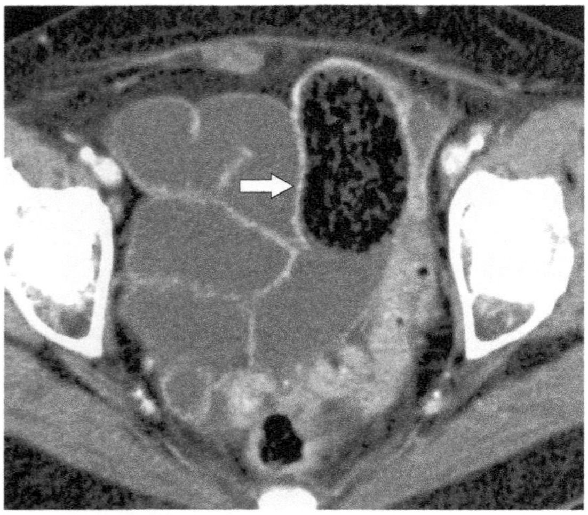

FIGURE 4-134. Axial contrast-enhanced CT in a 55-year-old man with small bowel obstruction due to a phytobezoar (*arrow*).

cholangiopancreatography (ERCP). Jejunal and ileal diverticula occur in about 2% of the elderly population and typically along the mesenteric border from a site of weakness at the point where mesenteric vessels penetrate the bowel wall. They are often multiple and large, particularly in the jejunum (Figure 4-135). Their main significance is that bacterial overgrowth within the diverticula can occur, feeding off the stagnant food that accumulates within them. Bacterial overgrowth can cause a malabsorption syndrome with diarrhea (especially steatorrhea), pain, and bloating. The diverticula are relatively easy to identify at SBFT or enteroclysis but are harder to identify at CT, being confused with adjacent loops of small bowel. However, close scrutiny of the small bowel should identify them as partially contrast- or air-filled, circular or ovoid strictures without valvulae conniventes (Fig. 4-136). Occasionally, enteroliths can form within them and, similar to the appendix, can become inflamed and present acutely, sometimes with perforation.

Pseudodiverticula

Inflammatory conditions such as Crohn disease and scleroderma can distort the bowel to such an extent that the small bowel has the appearance of a diverticulum, hence the term *pseudodiverticula* or *sacculations* (Figs 4-28 and 4-137). Other false diverticula

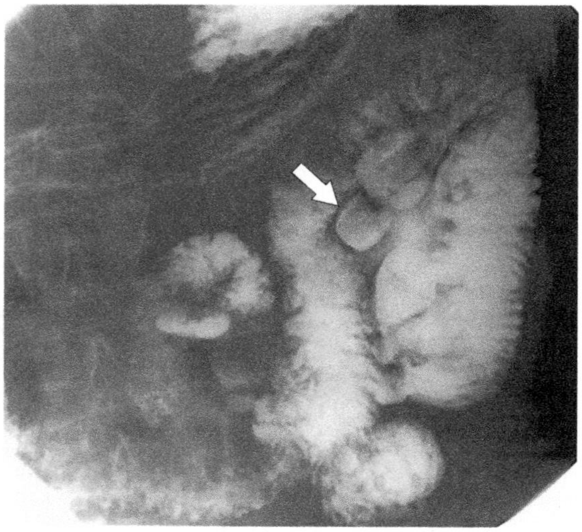

FIGURE 4-135. SBFT in a 68-year-old man with several jejunal diverticula (*arrow*).

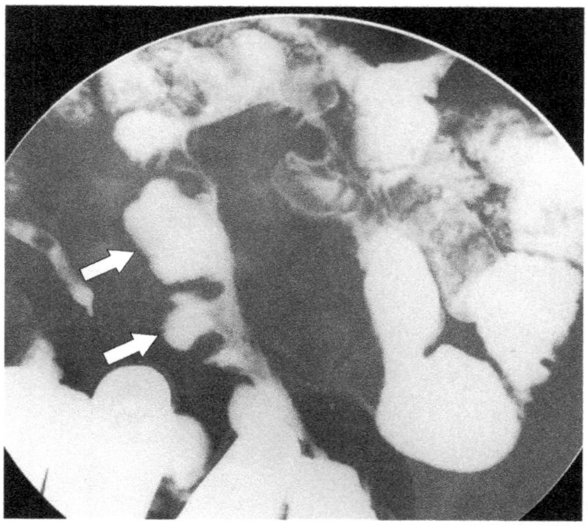

FIGURE 4-137. SBFT in a 63-year-old woman with Crohn disease and terminal ileal pseudosacculation (*arrows*).

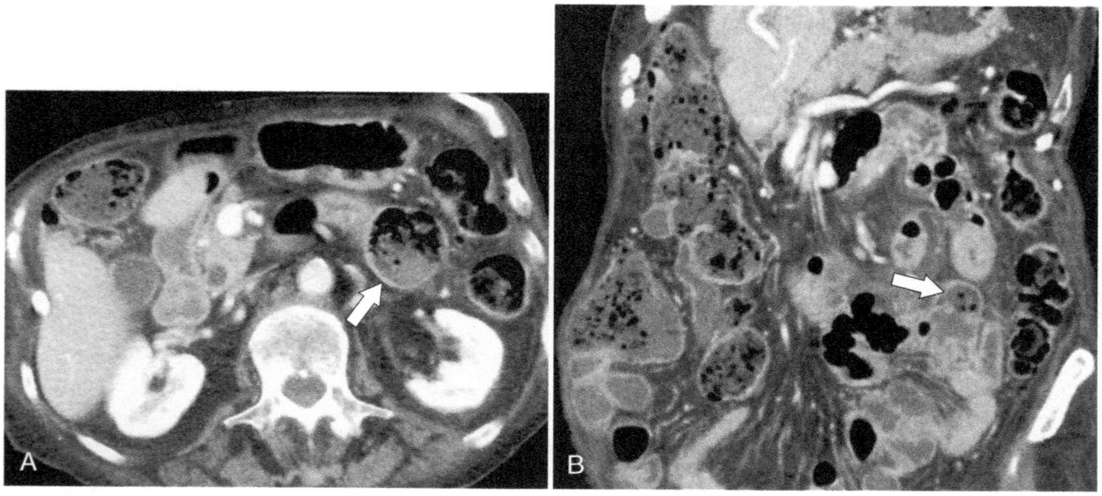

FIGURE 4-136. Axial (**A**) and coronal (**B**) contrast-enhanced CT in a 75-year-old man with multiple jejunal diverticula (*arrows*) and diverticulitis as evidenced by mesenteric inflammation (stranding).

can be created surgically from bowel anastomoses. Lymphoma often invades and destroys the bowel myenteric plexuses leading to aneurysmal dilation of the small bowel, sometimes with a diverticulum-like configuration.

Pneumatosis Intestinalis

Pneumatosis intestinalis can be idiopathic and asymptomatic in approximately 15% of cases. The gas in the bowel wall is typically cystic and present in both the small and large bowel (Fig. 4-138). The findings are better observed at CT, particularly on "lung window" contrast settings (Fig. 4-139). Obstructive airways disease, if severe, can cause retroperitoneal air, peritoneal air, and pneumatosis intestinalis as leaked air from ruptured lung alveoli tracks into the abdomen through diaphragmatic defects.

However, many causes are far more sinister, usually because of bowel ischemia or inflammatory perforation. Pneumatosis resulting from ischemia is often preterminal, and gas may be seen tracking up the mesenteric veins and into the portal hepatic veins (Fig. 4-140). Infections with gas-forming organisms also carry a high mortality.

Pneumatosis can also be seen with infectious enteritides or inflammatory bowel disease, especially if associated with multiple mucosal ulcers (Fig. 4-141). Occasionally gross bowel distention proximal to an obstruction can also demonstrate gas within the bowel wall. Other causes include iatrogenic instrumentation, particularly from catheter insertion or enteric anastomoses.

Fistulae and Sinuses

A fistula is an abnormal connection between two epithelium-lined organs. A sinus is a blind-ending cavity or sac. Fistulas and sinuses often have the same underlying causes (Table 4-13). Fistulas are best observed at SBFT, which may identify a subtle track of contrast connecting the small bowel loop to an adjacent enteric or colonic loop or to the bladder or skin (Fig. 4-142). However, the retrograde catheter injection of water-soluble contrast media may be required for fistulas that emerge onto the skin, because this has a greater chance of identifying the fistulous track and its origin. Enteroenteric or enterocolic fistulas can be identified at CT as two contiguous viscera that are drawn together within an inflammatory mass (Fig. 4-143).

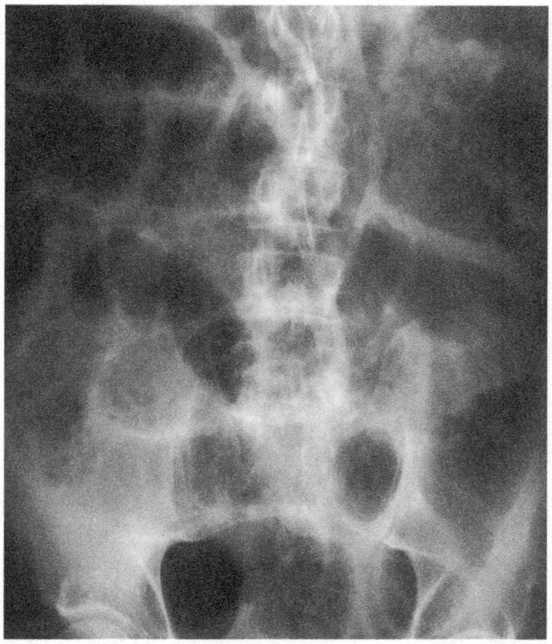

FIGURE 4-138. Plain abdominal radiograph in a 78-year-old man demonstrating ill-defined small bowel due to small bowel pneumatosis. The cause was idiopathic.

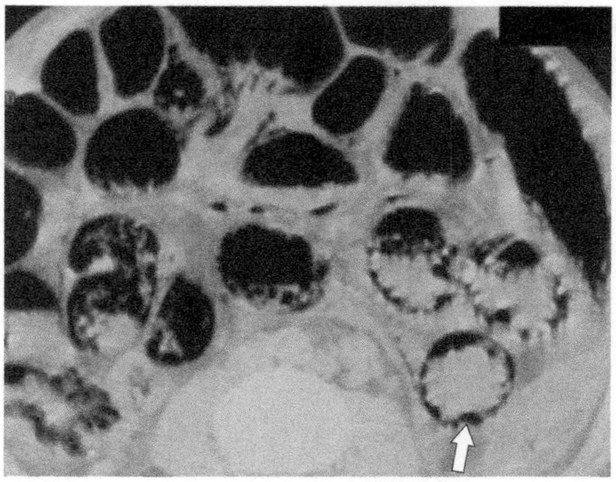

FIGURE 4-140. Axial CT on "lung window" contrast settings with small bowel pneumatosis secondary to ischemia (*arrow*).

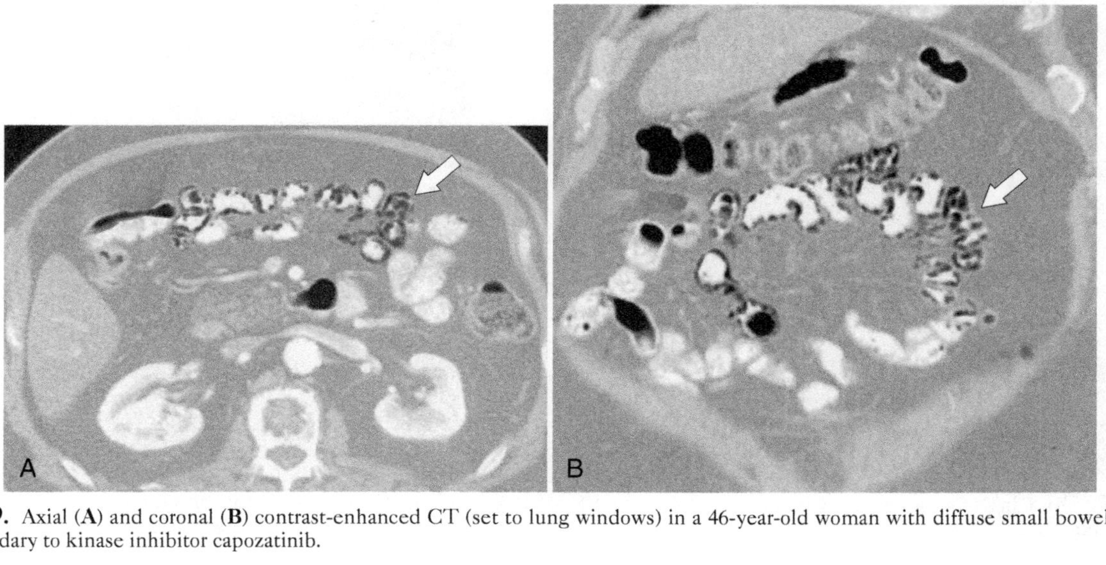

FIGURE 4-139. Axial (**A**) and coronal (**B**) contrast-enhanced CT (set to lung windows) in a 46-year-old woman with diffuse small bowel pneumatosis (*arrows*) secondary to kinase inhibitor capozatinib.

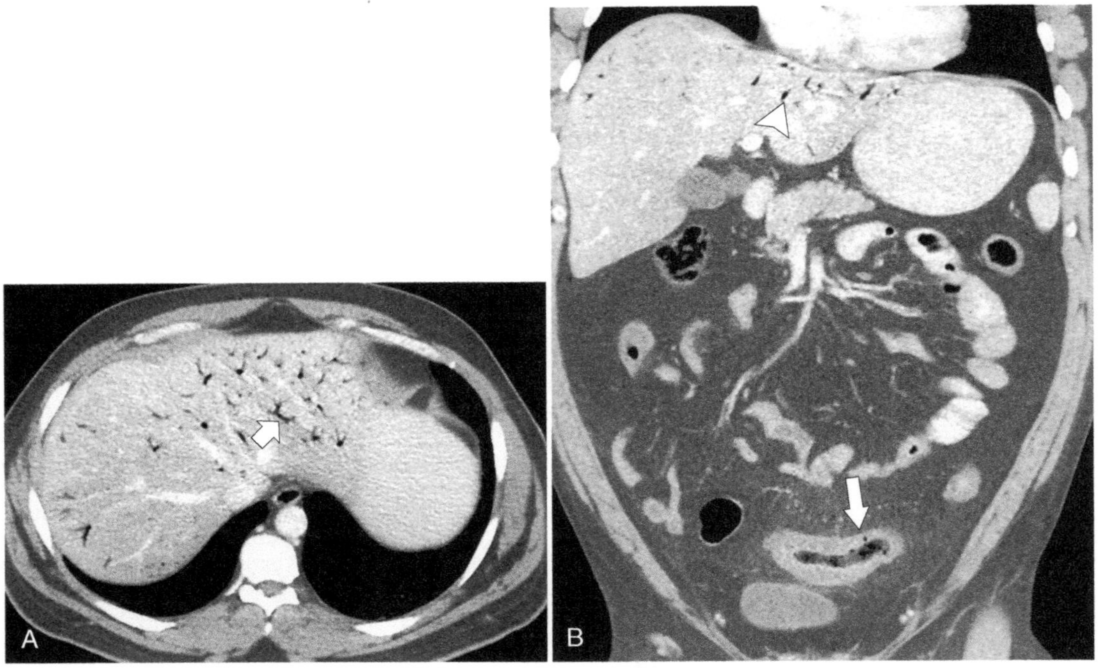

Figure 4-141. Axial (**A**) and coronal (**B**) contrast-enhanced CT in a 41-year-old man with a loop of thickened ileum (*arrow*) due to active Crohn disease and perforation as evidenced by portal venous gas in the liver (*arrow* in **A** and *arrowhead* in **B**).

Table 4-13 Causes of Fistulas and Sinuses

Inflammatory	Crohn disease Adjacent organ inflammatory process (e.g., cholecystitis, pancreatitis)
Infectious	Tuberculosis
Ischemia	Radiation Vascular Bowel necrosis Postsurgical
Neoplastic	Lymphoma Adenocarcinoma (small and large bowel) Serosal metastatic disease

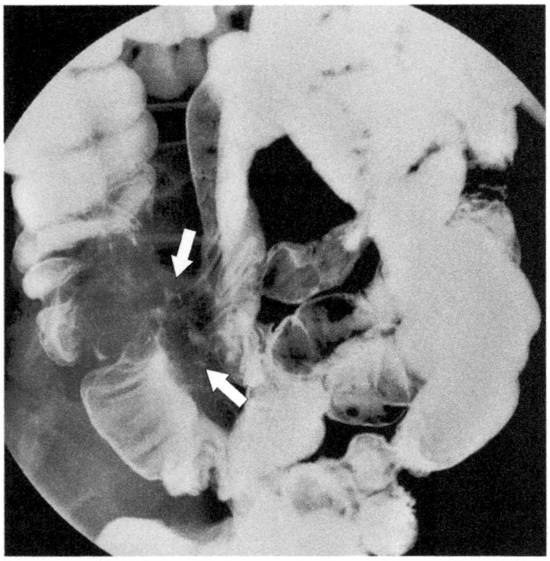

Figure 4-142. SBFT in a 55-year-old man with multiple enteroenteric and enterocolonic fistulas (*arrows*).

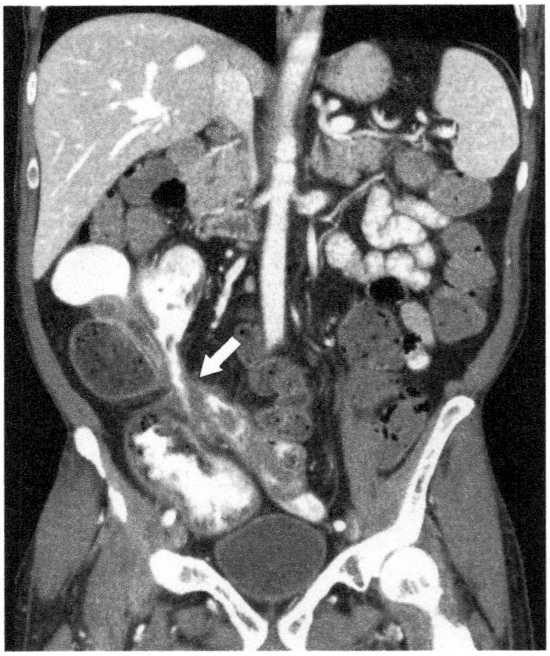

Figure 4-143. Coronal contrast-enhanced CT in a 40–year-old woman with Crohn disease and a enteroenteric and coloenteric fistula (*arrow*).

POSTOPERATIVE SMALL BOWEL

Small bowel resection is relatively common given the incidence of hernia and small bowel disease. Adhesion formation is a common secondary result, which may require further surgery and small bowel resection. A resection for Crohn disease can be performed but is often withheld unless absolutely necessary because of the frequent complication of fistula and recurrent disease at the anastomotic site, but sometimes the disease is too severe to avoid it.

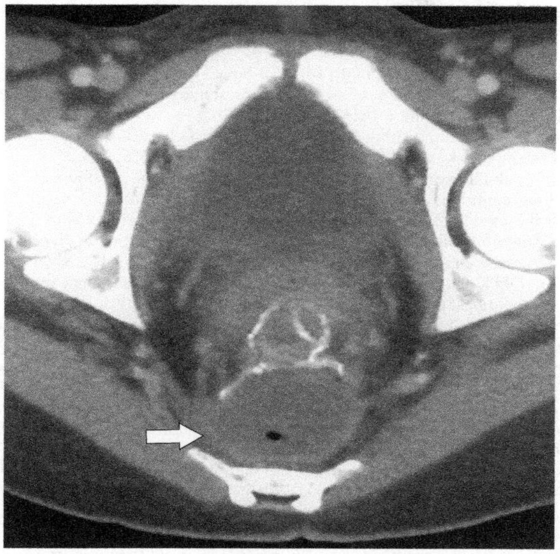

FIGURE 4-144. Axial CT in a 20-year-old woman with ileoanal pouch performed after colectomy for ulcerative colitis and a postoperative leakage into the presacral space and abscess formation (*arrow*).

Stomas and Reservoirs

Ileal Conduit Urinary Diversion

Ileal conduit urinary diversion is a procedure that is performed after cystectomy for bladder cancer, whereby the ureters are inserted into a detached length of ileum, which retains its own vascularity, and are brought to the skin as a stoma.

Hartmann Procedure

The Hartmann* procedure is a rectosigmoid resection (usually for rectocolonic cancer or diverticulitis), with the formation of a blind-ending rectal stump and creation of proximal colostomy or ileostomy. It is most commonly used as a temporizing procedure when immediate colonic anastomosis is not possible (or for palliative bypass for advanced lower malignancies).

Kock Ileostomy

Kock* ileostomy is an uncommon procedure with creation of an internal ileal reservoir after colectomy, usually for inflammatory bowel disease (ulcerative colitis), which can be emptied by catheter insertion via a stoma when desired. The major complication is a "slipped valve," whereby patients have incontinence of the pouch, although newer surgical procedural modifications to the pouch have reduced the frequency of this complication. Other complications include fistulas and pelvic abscess formation.

Diverting Ileostomy

Diverting ileostomy is usually a temporizing procedure performed to protect distal bowel anastomosis from surgical resection for malignancy or inflammatory disease. The anastomotic site can be evaluated for leaks, strictures, or adhesions by fluoroscopic evaluation after the injection of contrast via a balloon-secured catheter into the distal ileal loop.

Ileoanal Pouch

Ileoanal pouch is the most common postcolectomy reservoir procedure. The reservoir is formed by stitching or stapling several loops of ileum together, removing their intervening walls, and then anastomosing them to the perineum. This pouch is then attached to the rectal remnant or anal sphincter. A pouchogram is injection of contrast material via the anus to evaluate the pouch for strictures or leaks. Leaks can also be evaluated by CT (Fig. 4-144).

Small Bowel Transplantation

Small bowel transplantation is usually performed to avoid the need for parenteral nutrition in patients who have had large sections of small bowel removed ("short gut") and is sometimes combined with pancreatic or liver transplant. The most common anastomosis is with the duodenal or proximal jejunum proximally and ileum to sigmoid colon distally. Numerous complications are recognized, including graft-versus-host rejection, postoperative infection, complications of immunosuppression, vascular thromboses, anastomotic strictures, motility disorders, and mesenteritis. Pneumatosis is observed frequently and is generally not a pathological finding.

Choledochojejunostomy

Choledochojejunostomy is anastomosis of the common bile duct into a loop of jejunum, usually as an efferent loop as part of a Roux-en-Y procedure from gastric surgery. Complications include infection, anastomotic leakage, stricture, and afferent loop syndrome (see Chapter 2).

*Henri A. Hartmann (1860-1952), French surgeon.

*Nils Kock (1924-2011), Finnish surgeon.

SUGGESTED READINGS

AJR 196:577-584, 2011.

Alfisher MM et al: Radiology of ileal pouch-anal anastomosis: normal findings, examination pitfalls, and complications. Radiographics 17(1):81-98, 1997. discussion 98-99.

Balthazar EJ et al: Ileocecal tuberculosis: CT and radiologic evaluation. AJR Am J Roentgenol 154:499-503, 1990.

Bartnicke BJ et al: CT appearance of intestinal ischemia and intramural hemorrhage. Radiol Clin North Am 32:845, 1994.

Bennett GL et al: CT of Meckel's diverticulitis in 11 patients. AJR Am J Roentgenol 182(3):625-629, 2004.

Bhatnagar A et al: Scintigraphic detection of localized small bowel abnormality. Clin Nucl Med 20:367, 1995.

Birgisson H et al: Late gastrointestinal disorders after rectal cancer surgery with and without preoperative radiation therapy. Br J Surg 95(2):206-213, 2008.

Boudiaf M et al: Small-bowel diseases: prospective evaluation of multi-detector row helical CT enteroclysis in 107 consecutive patients. Radiology 233(2):338-344, 2004.

Broder JC et al: Ileal pouch–anal anastomosis surgery: imaging and intervention for post-operative complications. Radiographics 30(1):221-233, 2010.

Buck JL et al: Carcinoids of the gastrointestinal tract. Radiographics 10:1081-1095, 1990.

Buckley JA et al: CT evaluation of small bowel neoplasms: spectrum of disease. Radiographics 18(2):379-392, 1998.

Buckley O et al: The imaging of celiac disease and its complications. Eur J Radiol 65(3):483-490, 2008.

Burkhardt JH et al: Diagnosis of inguinal region hernias with axial CT: the lateral crescent sign and other key findings. Radiographics 31(2):E1-E12, 2011.

Burkill GJ et al: Malignant gastrointestinal stromal tumor: distribution, imaging features, and pattern of metastatic spread. Radiology 226(2):527-532, 2003.

Butela ST et al: Performance of CT in detection of bowel injury. AJR Am J Roentgenol 176(1):129-135, 2001.

Byun JH et al: CT findings in peripheral T-cell lymphoma involving the gastrointestinal tract. Radiology 227(1):59-67, 2003.

Cherian PT et al: Radiologic anatomy of the inguinofermal region: insights from MDCT. AJR Am J Roentgenol 189(4):W177-W183, 2007.

Cherian PT et al: The diagnosis and classification of inguinal and femoral hernia on multisection spiral CT. Clin Radiol 63(2):184-192, 2008.

Choi SH et al: Intussusception in adults: from stomach to rectum. AJR Am J Roentgenol 183:691-698, 2004.

Chopra S: Small-bowel obstruction: CT features with plain film and US correlations. Radiology 252(3):662, 2009.

Crema MD et al: Pouchography, CT, MRI features of ileal J pouch-anal anastomosis. AJR Am J Roentgenol 187(6):W594-W603, 2006.

Darge K et al: MR imaging of the abdomen and pelvis in infants, children, and adolescents. Radiology 261(1):12-29, 2011.

Delabrousse E et al: Small-bowel obstruction from adhesive bands and matted adhesions: CT differentiation. AJR Am J Roentgenol 192(3):693-697, 2009.

Delabrousse E et al: Small-bowel obstruction from adhesive bands and matted adhesions: CT differentiation. AJR Am J Roentgenol 192:693-697, 2009.

Doherty M et al: Afferent loop syndrome. AJR Am J Roengenol 171(852):856-857, 1998.

Duda JB et al: Utility of CT whirl sign in guiding management of small-bowel obstruction. AJR Am J Roentgenol 191:743-747, 2008.

El Mouhadi S et al: Pictorial Essay: CT and MRI Features of Ileostomies.
Elsayes KM et al: CT enterography: principles, trends, and interpretation of findings. Radiographics 30(7):1955-1970, 2010.
Mouhadi El et al: CT and MRI features of ileostomies. AJR Am J Roentgenol 196:577-584, 2011.
Fanso A et al: Current approaches to diagnosis and treatment of celiac disease: an evolving spectrum. Gastroenterology 120:635-651, 2001.
Frager D et al: Detection of intestinal ischemia in patients with acute small-bowel obstruction due to adhesions or hernia:efficacy of CT. AJR Am J Roentgenol 166:67-71, 1996.
Furukawa A, Saotome T, Yamaski M: Cross-sectional imaging in Crohn disease. Radiographics 24:689-702, 2004.
Gastrointestinal Imaging AJR 198, 2012. 198_5_Supplement_047.
Gastrointestinal Imaging AJR 198, 2012. 198_5_Supplement_098.
Gastrointestinal Imaging AJR 198, 2012. 198_5_Supplement_E130.
Gayer G et al: CT diagnosis of afferent loop syndrome. Clin Radiol 57(9):835-839, 2002.
Gayer G et al: Pictorial review: adult intussusception—a CT diagnosis. Br J Radiol 75(890):185-190, 2002.
Gervais DA et al: Percutaneous abscess drainage in Crohn disease: technical success and short- and long-term outcomes during 14 years. Radiology 222(3):645-651, 2002.
Ha AS et al: Radiographic examination of the small bowel: survey of the practice patterns in the United States. Radiology 231:407-412, 2004.
Ha CS et al: Primary non-Hodgkin lymphoma of the small bowel. Radiology 211(1):183-187, 1999.
Hanks PW et al: Blunt injury to mesentery and small bowel: CT evaluation. Radiol Clin North Am 41(6):1171-1182, 2003.
Hazelwood S et al: Images in clinical medicine, Colonic ileus. N Engl J Med 354(7):e6, 2006.
Hernanz-Schulman M: CT as an outcome surrogate in patients with cystic fibrosis: does the effort justify the risks? Radiology 262(3):746-749, 2012.
Hong SS et al: MDCT of small-bowel disease: value of 3D imaging. AJR Am J Roentgenol 187(5):1212-1221, 2006.
Horton KM et al: Multidetector-row computed tomography and 3-dimensional computed tomography imaging of small bowel neoplasms: current concept in diagnosis. J Comput Assist Tomogr 28(1):106-116, 2004.
Huang BY et al: Adult intussusceptions: diagnosis and clinical relevance. Radiol Clin North Am 41(6):1137-1151, 2003.
Hyland R et al: CT features of jejunal pathology. Clin Radiol 62(12):1154-1162, 2007.
Ishida T et al: The management of gastrointestinal infections caused by cytomegalovirus. J Gastroenterol 38(7):712-713, 2003.
Jaffe TA et al: Small-bowel obstruction: coronal reformations from isotropic voxels at 16-section multi–detector row CT. Radiology 238(1):135-142, 2006.
Jancelelwicz T et al: Predicting strangulated small bowel obstruction: an old problem revisited. J Gastrointest Surg 13(1):93-99, 2009.
Jang KM et al: Diagnostic performance of CT in the detection of intestinal ischemia associated with small-bowel obstruction using maximal attenuation of region of interest. AJR Am J Roengenol 194:957-963, 2012.
Johnson PT et al: Case 127: Henoch-Schonlein purpura. Radiology 245(3):909-913, 2007.
Kalanteri BN et al: CT features with pathologic correlation of acute gastrointestinal graft-versus-host disease after bone marrow transplants in adults. AJR Am J Roentgenol 181:1621-1625, 2003.
Kandpal H et al: Combined transmesocolic and left paraduodenal hernia: barium, CT and MRI features. Abdom Imaging 32(2):224-227, 2007.
Kao S et al: Education and imaging. Gastrointestinal: Amebic colitis. J Gastroenterol Hepatol 24(1):167, 2009.
Kim JH et al: Case 156: Inverted Meckel Diverticulum Radiology 255(1):303-306, 2012.
Kiran RP et al: Complications and functional results after ileoanal pouch formation in obese patients. J Gastrointest Surg 12(4):668-674, 2008.
Kiratli PO et al: Detection of ectopic gastric mucosa using 99mTc pertechnetate: review of the literature. Ann Nucl Med 23(2):97-105, 2009.
Lappas JC et al: Abdominal radiography findings in small-bowel obstruction: relevance to triage for additional diagnostic imaging. AJR Am J Roentgenol 176:167-174, 2001.
Lazarus DE et al: Frequency and relevance of the "small-bowel feces" sign on CT in patients with small-bowel obstruction. AJR Am J Roentgenol 183(5):1361-1366, 2004.
Lee MW et al: Sonography of acute right lower quadrant pain: importance of increased intraabdominal fat echo. AJR Am J Roentgenol 192(1):174-179, 2009.
Lee SS et al: Crohn disease of the small bowel: comparison of CT enterography, MR enterography, and small-bowel follow-through as diagnostic techniques. Radiology 251(3):751-761, 2009.
Lee SS et al: Obscure gastrointestinal bleeding: diagnostic performance of multidetector CT Enterography. Radiology 259(3):739-748, 2011.
Levine MS et al: Pattern Approach for Diseases of Mesenteric Small Bowel on Barium Studies. Radiology 249(2):445-460, 2008.
Linsenmaier U et al: Diagnosis and classification of pancreatic and duodenal injuries in emergency radiology. Radiographics 28(6):1591-1602, 2008.
Lockhart ME et al: Internal hernia after gastric bypass: sensitivity and specificity of seven CT signs with surgical correlation and controls. AJR Am J Roentgenol 188:745-750, 2007.
Loh S et al: Delayed adverse reaction to contrast-enhanced CT: a prospective single-center study comparison to control group without enhancement. Radiology 255(3):764-771, 2010.
Lohan DG et al: MR enterography of small-bowel lymphoma: potential for suggestion of histologic subtype and the presence of underlying celiac disease. AJR Am J Roentgenol 190:287-293, 2008.
Low RN et al: Distinguishing benign from malignant bowel obstruction in patients with malignancy at MR imaging. Radiology 228:157-165, 2003.
Lvoff N et al: Distinguishing features of self-limiting adult small-bowel intussusception identified at CT. Radiology 227(1):68-72, 2003.
Maccioni F et al: MR imaging in patients with Crohn disease: value of T2- versus T1-weighted gadolinium-enhanced MR sequences with use of an oral superparamagnetic contrast agent. Radiology 238(2):517-530, 2006.
Maglinte DDT et al: Small-bowel obstruction: optimizing radiologic investigation and nonsurgical management. Radiology 218(1):39-46, 2001.
Marmery H et al: Angiotensin-converting enzyme inhibitor-induced visceral angioedema. Clin Radiol 61(11):979-982, 2006.
Martin LC et al: Review of internal hernias: radiographic and clinical findings. AJR AM J Roentgenol 186(3):703-717, 2006.
Maturen KE et al: Pictorial essay: ultrasound imaging of bowel pathology: technique and keys to diagnosis in the acute abdomen. AJR Am J Roentgenol 197:W1067-W1075, 2011.
Masselli G et al: Celiac disease: evaluation with dynamic contrast-enhanced MR imaging. Radiology 256(3):783-790, 2010.
Mateen MA et al: Transient small bowel intussusceptions: ultrasound findings and clinical significance. Abdom Imaging 31:410-416, 2006.
Menke J: Diagnostic accuracy of multidetector CT in acute mesenteric ischemia: systematic review and meta-analysis. Radiology 256(1):93-101, 2010.
Mullan CP et al: Pattern of the month: small bowel obstruction. AJR Am J Roentgenol 198:W105-W117, 2012.
Neef B et al: Image of the month: "hide-bound" bowel sign in scleroderma. Gastroenterology 124(5), 2003. 1179, 1567.
O'Connor OJ et al: Role of radiologic imaging in irritable bowel syndrome: evidence-based review. Radiology 262(2):485-494, 2012.
Olson DE et al: CT predictors for differentiating benign and clinically worrisome pneumatosis intestinalis in children beyond the neonatal period. Radiology 253(2):513-519, 2009.
Osadchy A et al: Small bowel obstruction related to leftside paraduodenal hernia: CT findings. Abdom Imaging 30(1):53-55, 2005.
Pantongrag-Brown L: Gastrointestinal manifestations of acquired immunodeficiency syndrome: radiologic-pathologic correlation. Radiographics 15(5):1155-1178, 1995.
Pantongrag-Brown L et al: Inverted Meckel diverticulum: clinical, radiologic, and pathologic findings. Radiology 199(3):693-696, 1996.
Parodi A et al: Small intestinal bacterial overgrowth in patients suffering from scleroderma: clinical effectiveness of its eradication. Am J Gastroenterol 103(5):1257-1262, 2008.
Paulsen SR et al: CT enterography as a diagnostic tool in evaluating small bowel disorders: review of clinical experience with over 700 cases. Radiographics 26(3):641-657, 2006. discussion 657-662.
Pickhardt PJ et al: Asymptomatic pneumatosis at CT colonography: a benign self-limited imaging finding distinct from perforation. AJR Am J Roentgenol 190(2):W112-W117, 2008.
Pickhardt PJ et al: Evaluation of submucosal lesions of the large intestine: part 1. Neoplasms. Radiographics 27(6):1681-1692, 2007.
Pickhardt PJ et al: Unusual nonneoplastic peritoneal and subperitoneal conditions: CT findings. Radiographics 25(3):719-730, 2005.
Pilleul F et al: Possible small-bowel neoplasms: contrast-enhanced and water-enhanced multidetector CT enteroclysis. Radiology 241(3):796-801, 2006.
Power N et al: CT assessment of anastomotic bowel leak. Clin Radiol 62(1):37-42, 2007.
Rao PM et al: CT diagnosis of mesenteric adenitis. Radiology 202(1):145-149, 1997.
Raptospoulos V et al: Mutiplanar helical CT enterography in patients with Crohn's disease. AJR Am J Roentgenol 169:1545-1550, 1997.
Reddy SA et al: Diagnosis of transmesocolic internal hernia as a complication of retrocolic gastric bypass: CT imaging criteria. AJR Am J Roentgenol 189:52-55, 2007.
Romano S et al: Small bowel vascular disorders from arterial etiology and impaired venous drainage. Radiol Clin North Am 46(5):891-908, 2008. vi.
Rossi P et al: Meckel's diverticulum: imaging diagnosis. AJR Am J Roentgenol 166:567-573, 1996.
Saba L et al: Computed tomographic imaging findings of bowel ischemia. J Comput Assist Tomogr 32(3):329-340, 2008.
Sandrasegaran K et al: CT findings for postsurgical blind pouch of small bowel. AJR Am J Roentgenol 186(1):110-113, 2006.
Sandrasegaran K et al: Small-bowel complications of major gastrointestinal tract surgery. AJR Am J Roentgenol 185(3):671-681, 2005.
Scholz FJ et al: Diaphragmlike strictures of the small bowel associated with the use of nonsteroidal antiinflammatory drugs. AJR Am J Roentgenol 162(1):49-50, 1994.
Scholz FJ et al: Intramural fat in the duodenum and proximal small intestine in patients with celiac disease. AJR Am J Roentgenol 189(4):786-790, 2007.
Shanbhogue AKP et al: Comprehensive update on select immune-mediated gastroenterocolitis syndromes: implications for diagnosis and management. Radiographics 30(6):1465-1487, 2010.

Silva AC et al: Small bowel obstruction: what to look for. Radiographics 29(2):423-439, 2009.
Sinha R et al: Utility of high-resolution MR imaging in demonstrating transmural pathologic changes in Crohn disease. Radiographics 29(6):1847-1867, 2009.
Soyer P et al: Celiac disease in adults: evaluation with MDCT enteroclysis. AJR Am J Roentgenol 191(5):1483-1492, 2008.
Soyer P et al: CT enteroclysis features of uncomplicated celiac disease: retrospective analysis of 44 patients. Radiology 253(2):416-424, 2009.
Soyer P et al: Suspected anastomotic recurrence of Crohn disease after ileocolic resection: evaluation with CT enteroclysis. Radiology 254(3):755-764, 2010.
Stoker J et al: Imaging Patients with Acute Abdominal Pain Radiology 253(1):31-46, 2009.
Sunnapwar A et al: Taxonomy and imaging spectrum of small bowel obstruction after Roux-en-Y gastric bypass surgery. AJR Am J Roengenol 194:120-128, 2010.
Taylor SA et al: Mural Crohn disease: correlation of dynamic contrast-enhanced MR imaging findings with angiogenesis and inflammation at histologic examination—pilot study. Radiology 251(2):369-379, 2009.
Thurley PD et al: Radiological features of Meckel's diverticulum and its complications. Clin Radiol 64(2):109-118, 2009.
Timpone VM et al: Abdominal twists and turns: part I, gastrointestinal tract torsions with pathologic correlation. AJR Am J Roentgenol 197:86-96, 2011.
Umphrey H et al: Differential diagnosis of small bowel ischemia. Radiol Clin North Am 46(5):943-952, 2008. vi-vii.
Van Weyenberg SJB et al: MR enteroclysis in refractory celiac disease: proposal and validation of a severity scoring system. Radiology 259(1):151-161, 2011.
Van Weyenberg SJB et al: MR enteroclysis in the diagnosis of small-bowel neoplasms. Radiology 254(3):765-773, 2010.
Warshauer DM et al: Imaging manifestations of abdominal sarcoidosis. AJR Am J Roentgenol 182:15-28, 2004.
Wei SC et al: CT findings in small bowel angioedema: a cause of acute abdominal pain. Emerg Radiol 13(5):281-283, 2007.
Werneck-Silva AL et al: Gastroduodenal opportunistic infections and dyspepsia in HIV-infected patients in the era of Highly Active Antiretroviral Therapy. J Gastroenterol Hepatol 24(1):135-139, 2009.
Yang DM et al: Localized intestinal lymphangiectasia: CT findings. AJR Am J Roentgenol 180(1):213-214, 2004.

CHAPTER 5

Colon and Appendix

COLON

Anatomy

The colon starts at the ileocecal valve and is made up anatomically of the cecum; appendix (which is discussed separately below); ascending, transverse, descending, and sigmoid colon; and rectum. The ascending and transverse colon develops along with the small bowel as part of the embryologic midgut. As such, its vascular supply is from the superior mesenteric artery (right and middle colic branches), ending approximately in the distal two thirds of the transverse colon. The remainder of the colon and rectum is supplied predominantly by the inferior mesenteric artery. The junction between the two arterial supplies around the region of the splenic flexure is sometimes known as the watershed area, a territory that is most at risk from colonic ischemic episodes.

The colonic wall has an outer longitudinal muscle layer that is separated into three separate longitudinal bands, or teniae, between which are sacculations caused by contractions of the longitudinal muscle layers. The rectum has a continuous circumferential muscle layer. The whole colon has a uniform circumferential submucosa and mucosa that can penetrate the outer muscle layer as diverticula. The whole colon is suspended by a mesentery, although the ascending colon and descending colon become fixed to the posterior abdominal wall in utero and lose their suspended mesentery. Abnormal rotations occur in utero, leaving a spectrum of anomalies.

Examination Techniques

Barium Enema

The barium enema (BE) is performed either as a double-contrast barium enema (DCBE) technique with the instillation of barium and air or as a single-contrast technique. The latter is usually reserved for patients who may not be able to move or roll as required for the DCBE or for the evaluation of postsurgical abnormalities or emergency conditions, typically after the administration of water-soluble contrast material, rather than barium. If there is any suspicion of perforation, barium must not be used because it can cause a lethal peritonitis if present within the peritoneum.

The goal of the DCBE is to fully coat the colonic mucosa initially with barium, after which air is insufflated. The patient is maneuvered into variable positions to distend the colonic lumen by air so that mucosal relief images can be taken of the nondependent wall distended with gas. When the DCBE is performed properly, small (5-mm) polyps can be well visualized. Spot radiographic images in orthogonal planes should be taken of any fluoroscopically observed abnormality to maximize the radiologist's ability to characterize lesions once the examination is finished.

Adequate bowel cleansing is important for all colonic evaluation (whether by optical colonoscopy, CT colonoscopy [CTC], or BE) to exclude polyp or malignancy. However, it is a particular problem with the BE because stool residue (especially if adherent to the mucosa) can be difficult to distinguish from true lesions. Sometimes a decubitus view in the DCBE will dislodge less adherent feces, but not always. Extensive diverticular disease also hampers detection of smaller lesions because of bowel distortion. Detection of tumors at the ileocecal valve can be challenging because the valve has a variable and occasionally masslike appearance. Compounding these potential problems is the necessity to pay meticulous attention to technique, particularly for the DCBE. Often insufficient air is insufflated, perhaps from inexperience or because the patient reports discomfort. Antispasmodics are useful in this regard to reduce motility and spasm temporarily. Even in a high-quality examination with good bowel cleansing and a well-distended colon, the detection of small polyps can be challenging for the less experienced. Regardless of whether a single-contrast or DCBE technique is performed, close scrutiny during the fluoroscopic phase is required and any suspect lesion should be analyzed in multiple planes (with spot images) to increase the diagnostic confidence of lesion detection and subsequent characterization. Given that BE has been largely superseded by other techniques for the detection of colonic neoplastic lesions (most notably by direct optical colonoscopy, which also permits immediate biopsy results of any detected lesion, and to some extent by CTC), BE will most likely be reserved for other specific indications such as evaluation of postoperative patients with either barium or water-soluble contrast media depending on the clinical circumstance.

Computed Tomography

Imaging of mural disease in the colon is largely performed via computed tomography (CT), which enables visualization of transmural processes (e.g., Crohn disease). Mucosal abnormalities are generally better observed at DCBE, optical, or virtual CT colonoscopy, but inflammatory colonic mucosa shows a variable degree of enhancement after the administration of intravenous (IV) contrast material, which can be helpful in evaluating the acuity and extent of colonic disease. CT also offers the opportunity to evaluate for any associated mesenteric concomitant disease (e.g., pericolonic inflammation or "fat-stranding") or for regional lymph nodes, as might be seen with Crohn disease or malignancy. In general, the administration of oral contrast material to outline the colonic lumen is warranted, although water-based compounds may help show mucosal hyperemia better after the administration of IV contrast medium.

It is important for the radiologist to evaluate the whole colon carefully at CT performed for other indications because in busy practices incidental colonic malignancies are occasionally detected. Sometimes small tumors are difficult to detect because of colonic spasm, feces, or a collapsed colon. The ileocecal valve is a particularly difficult area to evaluate because there is often the spurious appearance of colonic wall thickening. Inevitably, some patients who have been referred for optical colonoscopy to confirm disease seen on CT turn out to have normal findings.

Magnetic Resonance Imaging

In general, MRI has been less useful for evaluating the bowel and colon, although fast single-shot, fat-saturated scanning techniques are now being used to evaluate colonic disease. The technique (sometimes also referred to as MR enterography) is particularly useful for evaluating younger patients with chronic colonic disease (e.g., ulcerative colitis or Crohn disease) to avoid the potentially large lifetime radiation burden they might incur if serial imaging were performed by CT. MRI is also highly effective in evaluating rectal extension of tumor and is now routinely performed in many centers to help determine if patients require chemotherapy or radiation (chemoradiation) preceding surgical removal.

Positron Emission Tomography

Positron emission tomography (PET scanning) has little role in the evaluation of the colon itself, although rectal tumors

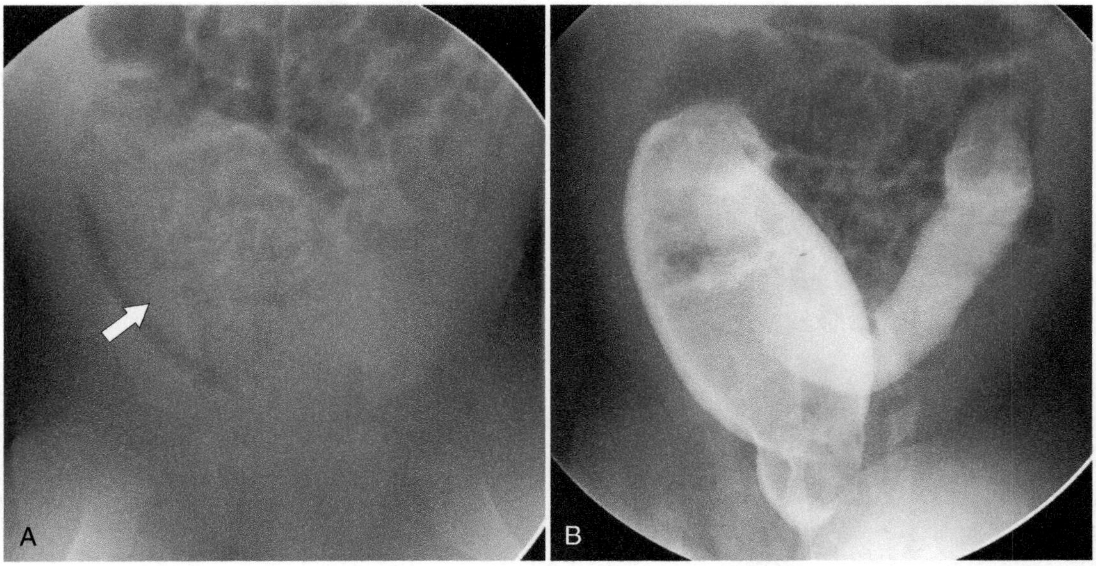

FIGURE 5-1. Plain abdominal radiograph (**A**) and contrast enema (**B**) in a 4-month-old male infant with constipation (*arrow*) due to Hirschsprung disease.

(adenoma or cancer) are sometimes detected by PET performed for the evaluation of metastatic disease in other diseases. The role of PET is primarily to evaluate for distant metastatic disease, but it is more commonly used for other malignancies (e.g., lung cancer and lymphoma).

CT Colonoscopy

CT colonoscopy (CTC) offers the potential to replace optical colonoscopy for the screening of colorectal cancer. The detection of small polyps (5 to 10 mm) is equivalent by both techniques. CTC is used widely in some practices for the evaluation of colonic polyps but in other practices is reserved for patients in whom optical colonoscopy has been indeterminate or because of patient preference. Many patients older than 50 years of age decline optical colonoscopic screening for various reasons. Therefore it is hoped that a substantial proportion of these patients may benefit from CTC. Once a polyp is detected at CTC screening, the patient can be referred for optical colonoscopy for polyp removal and histological analysis.

Congenital Colonic Anomalies

Hirschsprung Disease*

Also known as hypoganglionosis or aganglionic megacolon, Hirschsprung disease is typically diagnosed in the neonatal period (failure to pass meconium within 24 hours) or early childhood, but less severe forms with profound constipation, abdominal distention, and weight loss are occasionally present in late childhood or early adulthood. The disease is more common in males and is caused by a focal aganglionic segment of the large bowel as a result of failure of enteric ganglion cells to migrate to myenteric plexus to the lower colon (Fig. 5-1). However, it can rarely affect the whole colon (Fig. 5-2). The disease is associated with other very rare congenital syndromes.

The aganglionic segment is usually located in the upper rectum or rectosigmoid junction, with the proximal large bowel becoming grossly dilated over many years of partial obstruction. The diagnosis is usually best made by contrast enema studies (Fig. 5-2), even in the neonate, but definitive diagnosis requires rectal biopsy. The stricture is usually identified at contrast enema in the rectosigmoid regions with variable colonic distention proximal to the stricture. The aganglionic segment may not appear as an abrupt transition but rather as an irregular serrated or "sawtooth" appearance, which is characteristic of the disease (Fig. 5-3). Some patients develop an associated colitis, termed "Hirschsprung-associated enterocolitis," that is characterized by foul-smelling diarrhea. These patients are at risk of perforation because of acute colitis, but subacute forms exist, and contrast enema studies may show the characteristic rectal sawtooth finding.

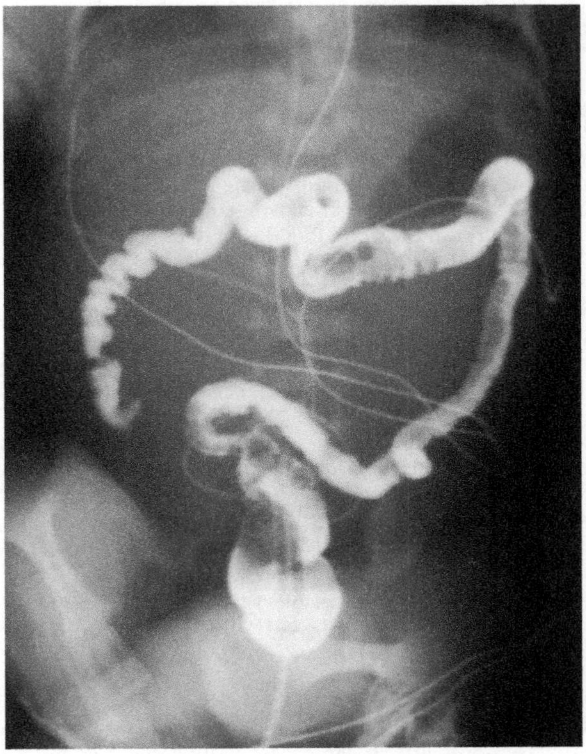

FIGURE 5-2. Contrast enema in a male neonate with a hypoplastic colon.

*Harald Hirschsprung (1830-1916), Danish pediatrician.

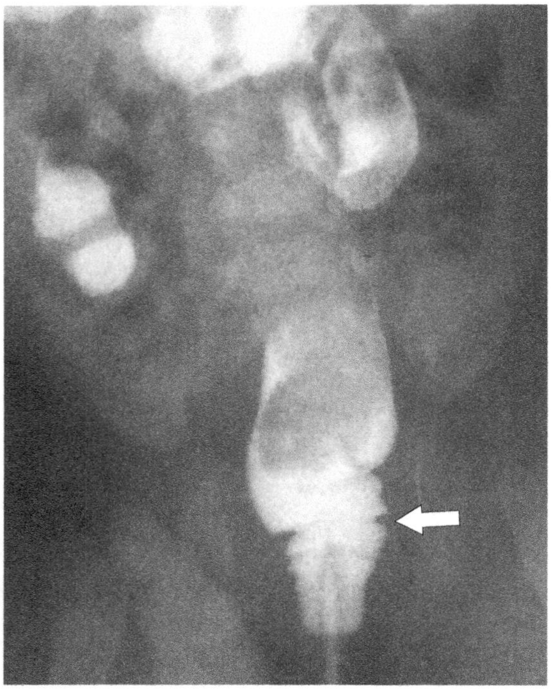

FIGURE 5-3. BE in a 3-week-old male neonate with Hirschsprung disease as evidenced by a "sawtooth" rectum (*arrow*).

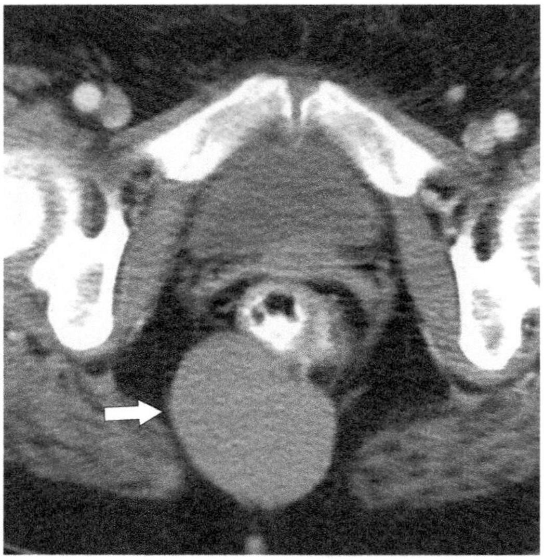

FIGURE 5-4. Axial contrast-enhanced CT in a 46-year-old woman with a 4.5-cm homogeneous pararectal mass (*arrow*) caused by rectal enteric duplication.

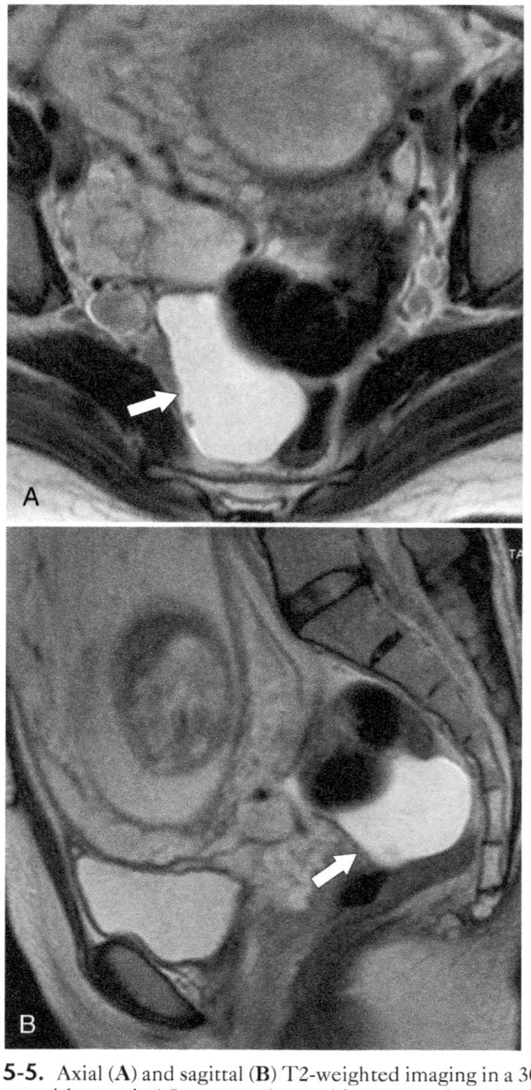

FIGURE 5-5. Axial (A) and sagittal (B) T2-weighted imaging in a 30-year-old woman with a cystic 4.5-cm mass (*arrows*) in a posterolateral perirectal location resulting from a rectal duplication cyst.

Enteric Duplication Cysts

Rare congenital anomalies occur on the mesenteric border anywhere along the gastrointestinal (GI) tract, but most commonly in the ileum and less commonly in the colon. They can be associated with other extraintestinal congenital malformations. Most patients present in early childhood with pain, bleeding, volvulus, intussusception, perforation, or obstruction. Malignant degeneration of the cysts has been reported, mostly within colonic duplication cysts, and is usually an adenocarcinoma on histological examination.

Ultrasound (US) sometimes shows a hypoechoic cystic mass with a thick wall, which has an echogenic outer layer and hypoechoic inner layer. On BE the cyst produces a mass effect of adjacent bowel and on CT appears as a nonenhancing mass, compressing or displacing the adjacent bowel, which may contain simple fluid, hemorrhage, or proteinaceous fluid (Fig. 5-4). On MRI the enteric cysts are usually hyperintense on T2-weighted imaging, reflecting their cystic nature (Fig. 5-5). Because many duplication cysts contain ectopic gastric mucosa, a Tc-99m pertechnetate radionuclide study can often show radionuclide uptake, which can also be observed within a Meckel diverticulum for the same reason.

Colonic Duplication

Colonic duplication is a very rare congenital anomaly that is usually asymptomatic. It can occasionally present in childhood, however, with symptoms of obstruction, bleeding, and perforation resulting from ectopic gastric mucosa, which is commonly present. It may be cystic or tubular, occur for the whole or partial length of any segment of the colon or rectum, and communicate or not with the other lumen. It is extremely rare in adults and will most likely be detected by CT, although contrast enema examination may show the two lumens should they communicate.

Malrotation

As the midgut returns from the umbilical sac into the abdomen between 6 and 12 weeks in utero, it usually rotates 270 degrees

TABLE 5-1 Colitis

Classification	Type	Etiology	Typical Features
Inflammatory bowel disease	Ulcerative colitis Crohn disease		Variable colitis extending proximally from rectum Variable—skip lesions or pancolitis
Ischemic		Emboli or low-flow states	Watershed areas—splenic flexure
Radiation		Dose dependent	Usually pelvic
Infectious	Viral	Norwalk Rotavirus *E. coli* CMV Herpes	Diffuse colitis Diffuse colitis Often severe, predominantly transverse colon Pancolitis in immunosuppressed patients Rectosigmoid region
	Bacterial	*Shigella* sp. *Salmonella* sp. *Campylobacter* sp. *Yersinia* sp. *Clostridia* sp. *Chlamydia* sp. Actinomycetes Gonococcus TB	Ileocecal region ± lymphadenopathy Left colon Colon and small bowel Ileocecal region Pancolitis—diffuse thickening Rectosigmoid—causes lymphogranuloma venereum Ileocecal and rectosigmoid Rectosigmoid Late-onset—right colon and ileocecal region
	Parasitic	Amebiasis *Anisakis* *Schistosoma* *Strongyloides* Trichuriasis	Right colon and ileocecal region Right colon Left colon and sigmoid Skip or pancolitis, mimics ulcerative colitis Localized thickening at site of whipworm penetration
	Fungal	*Histoplasma* *Mucor*	Ileocecal region Right colon
Solitary rectal ulcer		Unknown	Anterior rectal wall
Trauma			
Iatrogenic	Diversion colitis; chemical colitis		

CMV, Cytomegalovirus; *TB*, tuberculosis.

in a counterclockwise direction, but many failures of full rotation occur, resulting in various degrees of colonic malrotation. The cecum and ascending colon may fail to fixate to their normal position in the right side of the abdomen, becoming quite mobile and at risk for volvulus or torsion. Most malrotations, even when complete with the colon residing in the left side of the abdomen, are asymptomatic.

Inflammatory Colonic Disease

Colitis

Colonic and rectal inflammatory disease has multiple causes (Table 5-1), of which some are self-limiting, others produce lifelong morbidity, and some are potentially fatal.

Ulcerative Colitis

Ulcerative colitis (UC), like Crohn disease, is an inflammatory bowel disease (IBD), but unlike Crohn disease, its intestinal manifestations are limited to the colonic mucosa. It can, however, present with widespread additional clinical manifestations in the mouth (aphthous ulcers), eyes (iritis, uveitis, and episcleritis), musculoskeletal system (arthritis, ankylosing spondylitis, and sacroileitis), skin (erythema nodosum and pyoderma gangrenosum), and biliary tree (primary sclerosing cholangitis). It is a disease usually found in young adults (although symptoms may persist for many years), and symptoms may include pain, diarrhea, and rectal bleeding. UC in its milder forms can be confused with irritable bowel syndrome. UC is familial, being more common in first-degree relatives; is thought to be autoimmune in origin; and is treated as such with immunosuppressive therapy.

The colonic mucosal disease always starts in the rectum and extends proximally to a variable degree, sometimes affecting the whole colon (pancolitis) and sometimes even a short segment of ileum, so-called backwash ileitis. The extent of colonic involvement typically directs the symptoms and seriousness of the disease. Some patients have only one short episode confined to the rectum, and others have recurring disease, sometimes with a life-threatening toxic megacolon. This usually necessitates aggressive medical or surgical therapy, often requiring an emergency total colectomy as the diffusely involved colonic mucosa becomes so thickened, friable, and distended that perforation is imminent.

The imaging features depend on the stage of the disease (Table 5-2), and many of these features are shared by Crohn disease (Table 5-3). They can sometimes be identified by plain abdominal radiography as thickened haustra, particularly when caused by a pancolitis (Fig. 5-5). Severe disease can almost certainly be recognized on plain radiography as can toxic megacolon, with marked colonic distention resulting from ileus (Fig. 5-6) and wall and mucosal thickening (Fig. 5-7). The wall thickening is sometimes referred to as "thumb-printing" because of the polypoid soft tissue nature of the mucosal edema and thickening. BE demonstrates typical features but has largely been replaced by optical colonoscopy for diagnosis. When BE is performed, the features depend on the severity and acuity of disease. In acute disease a variable length of colon (starting in the rectum) shows a granular mucosal pattern representing edema and ulcer formation, sometimes of the whole colon (Fig. 5-8), which may also affect the last few centimeters of the terminal ileum ("backwash ileitis") (Fig. 5-9). "Collar-button ulcer" formation has been described, which represents acute ulceration of the colon with submucosal extension (Fig. 5-10), with further ulceration prevented by the

TABLE 5-2 Imaging Features of Ulcerative Colitis

Imaging Finding	Mechanism
Barium enema	
Mucosal granular pattern	Edema
Luminal narrowing	Spasm and edema in acute phase Fibrosis in chronic phase
Ulcer formation	Mucosal stippling—crypt abscess formation Collar-button ulcers—mucosal islands and polyps
Inflammatory pseudopolyps	Normal mucosa surrounded by deep crypt ulceration
Backwash ileitis	Distal ileal involvement
Shortened colon	Fibrosis with chronic healing—lead pipe
Haustral loss and strictures	Fibrosis with chronic healing
Toxic megacolon	Acute severe inflammation
Computed tomography	
Mucosal thickening and luminal narrowing—accordion pattern	Edema in acute phase (thumb-printing) Fibrosis in chronic phase
Mucosal enhancement and muscularis enhancement—mural stratification	Active inflammation—hyperemia
Mesenteric hypervascular changes	Hyperemic changes
Pericolonic inflammation	Stranding
Increased submucosal fat—fat halo sign	Submucosa surrounded by enhancing mucosa and muscularis (halo or target sign), particularly chronic disease
Widened presacral space (>20 mm)	Extramural fat deposition
Toxic megacolon	Acute severe inflammation

TABLE 5-3 Distinguishing Features Between Ulcerative Colitis and Crohn Disease

Feature	Ulcerative Colitis	Crohn Disease
Small bowel involvement	Terminal ileum only	Common
Aphthous ulceration	No	Yes
Anal involvement	Rare	Common
Colorectal involvement	Always	Sometimes
Skip lesions	No	Yes
Stenosis	Rare	Common
Fistula	No	Common

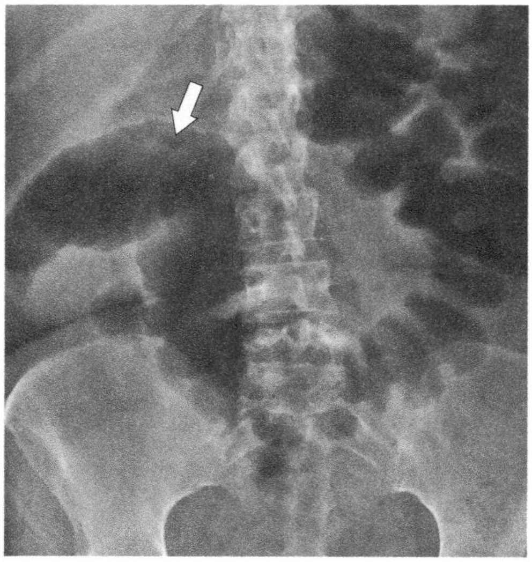

FIGURE 5-6. Plain abdominal radiograph in a 29-year-old man with friable colonic mucosa (*arrow*) and a toxic megacolon.

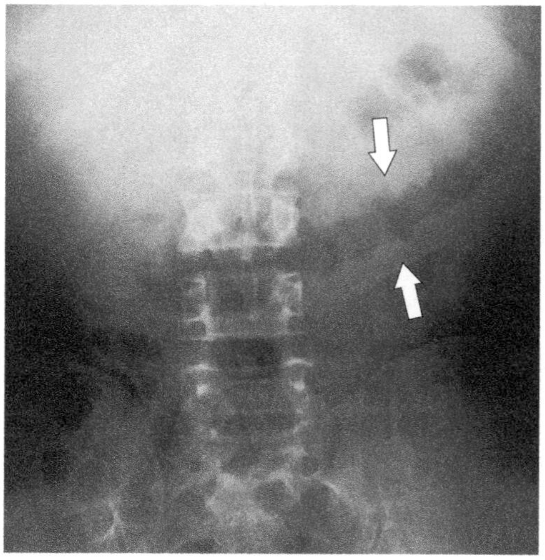

FIGURE 5-7. Plain abdominal radiograph in a 33-year-old woman with marked colonic haustral thickening (*arrows*) due to an acute pancolitis from ulcerative colitis.

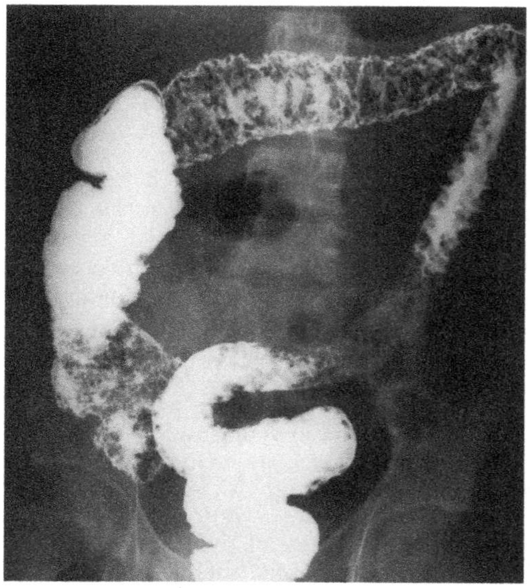

FIGURE 5-8. BE in a 23-year-old man with pancolitic granular appearance due to acute ulceration from ulcerative colitis.

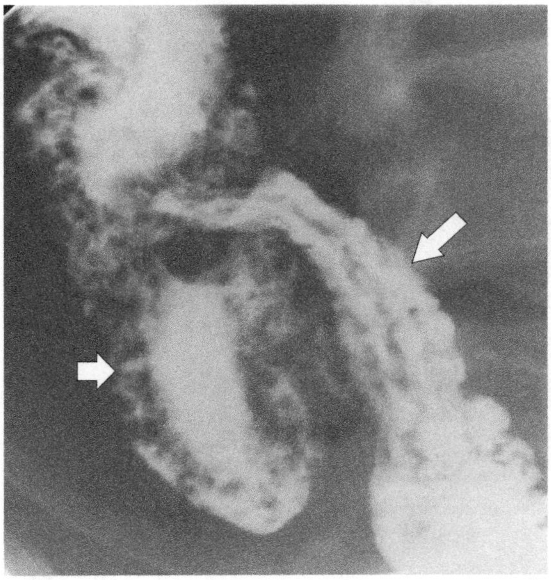

FIGURE 5-9. Single-contrast BE with nodular mucosal irregularity (*small arrow*) due to acute ulcerative colitis. There is associated fold thickening (*arrow*) in the terminal ileum due to backwash ileitis.

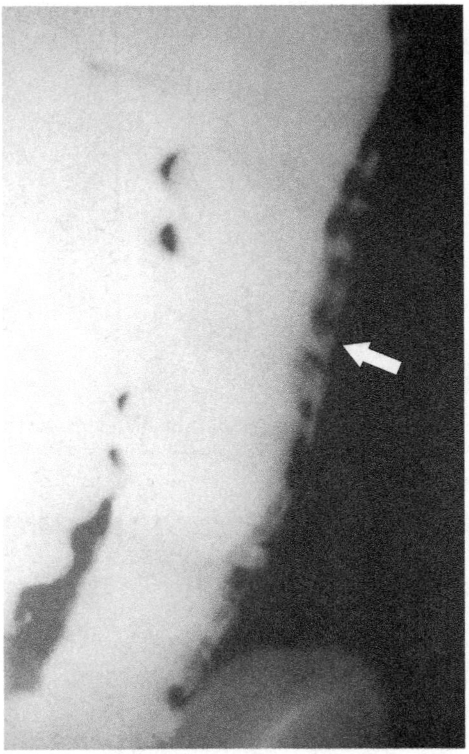

FIGURE 5-10. Single-contrast BE in a 30-year-old woman with ulcerative colitis and multiple "collar button" ulcers (*arrow*).

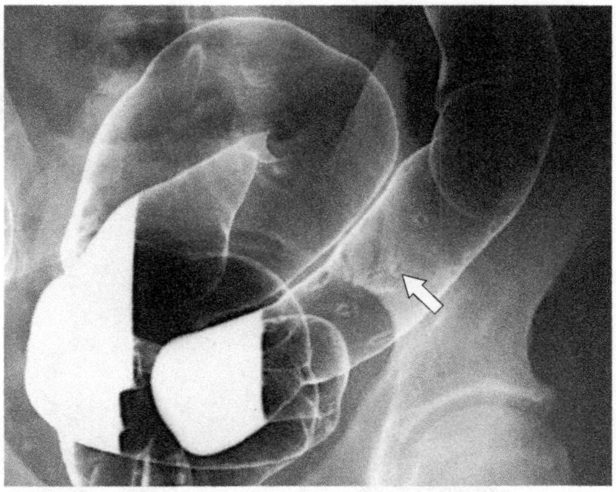

FIGURE 5-11. DCBE in 38-year-old man with chronic ulcerative colitis and filiform polyp formation (*arrow*).

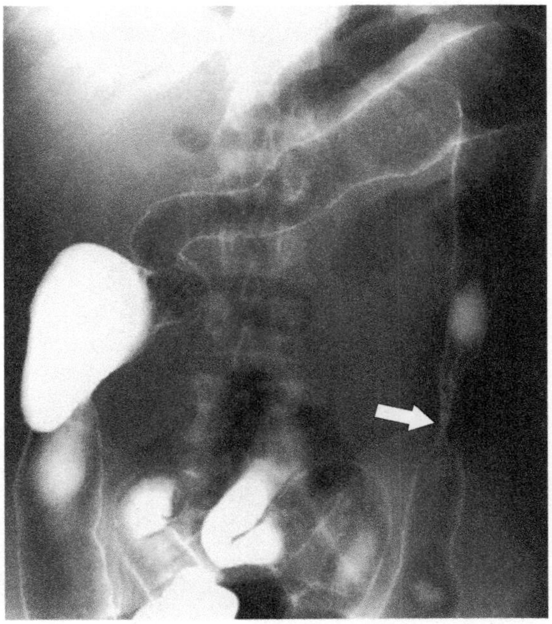

FIGURE 5-12. DCBE in a 41-year-old woman with chronic ulcerative colitis and diffuse colonic lead-piping. There is also a descending colon benign inflammatory stricture (*arrow*).

relatively impermeable bowel wall. This sign is three times as common in UC as in Crohn disease. Pseudopolyp formation, which can also be recognized in Crohn disease, can occur with more chronic disease and represents areas of reparative mucosa between areas of ulceration (Fig. 5-11). As the disease progresses, the affected length of colon becomes featureless and shortened, termed "lead piping" (Fig. 5-12).

The presence and extent of disease are more readily evaluated by CT than by contrast enema, whose features also mirror the clinical disease. These include bowel wall thickening and luminal narrowing with a variable amount of pericolonic edema and mesenteric vascular hyperemia (Fig. 5-13). The degree of inflammation may be reflected by ^{18}F-fluorodeoxyglucose (FDG) uptake at PET imaging (Fig. 5-13). Mural stratification or double-halo sign, which is common with an acute presentation, is a nonspecific sign for inflammatory bowel disease representing hyperemic mucosa and serosa with intervening submucosal edema (Fig. 5-14). If the acute disease worsens, the mucosa becomes progressively thickened and inflamed (Fig. 5-15), which can ultimately lead to a toxic megacolon, whose CT features include a distended colon with profusely thickened mucosal tissue, sometimes referred to as an "accordion pattern" (see Fig. 5-52).

More chronic features of the disease at CT are similar to those observed at BE with colonic shortening and luminal fibrotic narrowing. However, CT may identify widening of the presacral fat space and a characteristic "fat halo" sign consisting of inner mucosal and outer muscularis enhancement with a nonenhancing middle submucosal ring. This ring is composed of increased

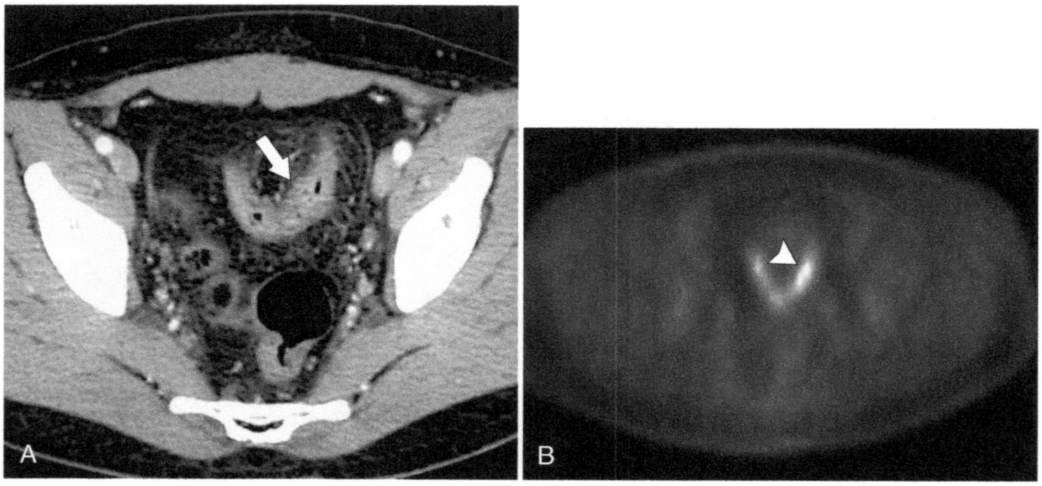

FIGURE 5-13. Axial contrast-enhanced CT (**A**) and PET (**B**) in a 36-year-old man with acute ulcerative colitis with sigmoid thickening (*arrow*) and pericolonic inflammation (stranding) and increased FDG activity (*arrowhead*) indicative of acute inflammation.

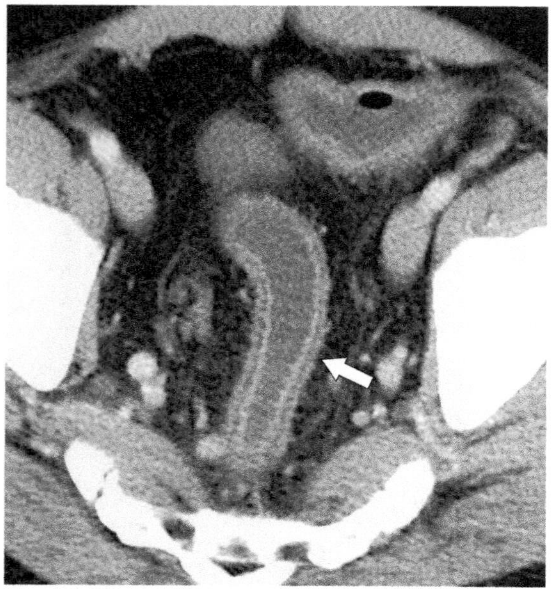

FIGURE 5-14. Axial contrast-enhanced CT in a 45-year-old man with sigmoid mural stratification (*arrow*) due to acute ulcerative colitis.

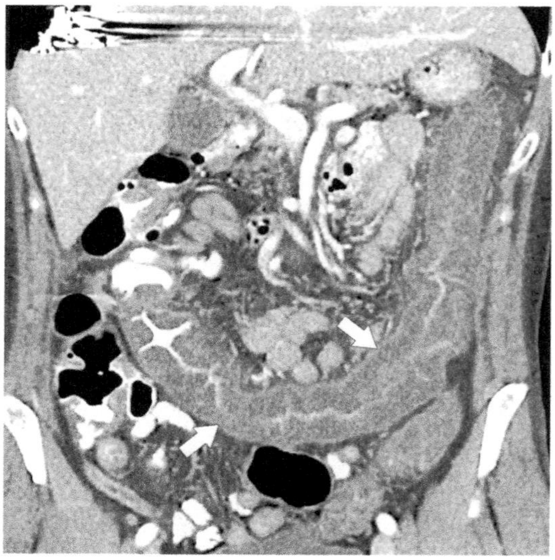

FIGURE 5-15. Coronal contrast-enhanced CT in a 61-year-old woman with marked colonic mucosal thickening due to acute ulcerative colitis.

submucosal fat deposition (Fig. 5-16). There may be mesenteric adenopathy, but this is less common in UC than in Crohn disease. Stricture formation may be seen but is also less common than in Crohn disease (Figs. 5-12 and 5-17).

In addition to perforation from toxic megacolon, the greatest risk to patients with chronic UC is the late development of adenocarcinoma of the colon, for which they have an increased risk of 5% to 30% over the general population (Fig. 5-18). The risk increases by 10% for each decade of disease. Patients with more extensive disease may therefore undergo prophylactic colectomy.

Crohn Disease (see Chapter 4)

Crohn disease is an inflammatory bowel disease that can affect any aspect of the GI tract from the mouth to the anus but most commonly affects the ileocolic region (50%), terminal ileum alone (30%), or colon (20%). It is considered an autoimmune disease, but the etiology is still unknown despite its relatively common presentation, particularly in young adults. Patients usually present with pain; diarrhea, sometimes bloody; weight loss; and

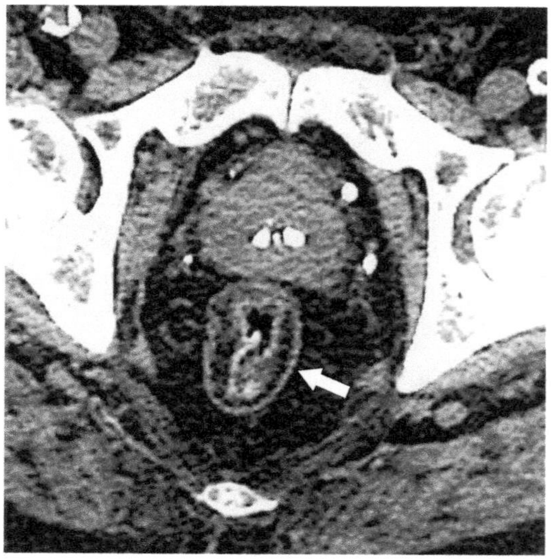

FIGURE 5-16. Axial contrast-enhanced CT in a 70-year-old man with a fat halo sign from chronic ulcerative colitis (*arrow*).

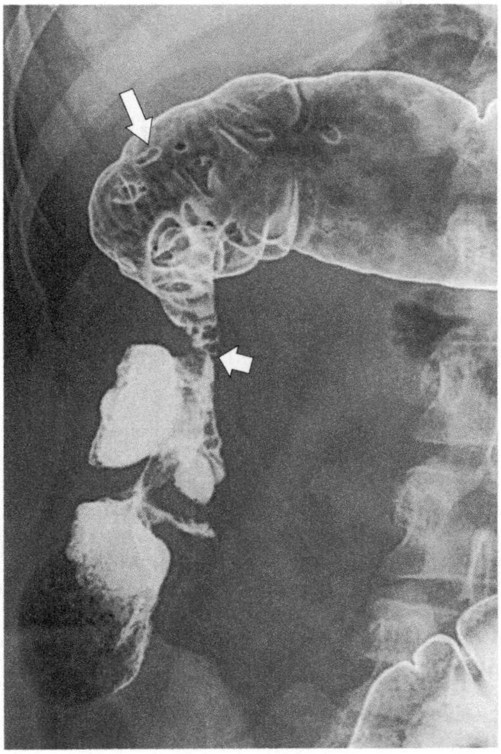

FIGURE 5-17. BE in a 40-year-old woman with a chronic ascending colon stricture (*arrow*) and filiform pseudopolyps (*small arrow*) due to chronic ulcerative colitis.

accompanying associated systemic symptoms of skin rash, iritis, and arthritis. As with UC, the patient may have only one brief, relatively low-grade presentation; may present with severe, life-threatening disease; or may have repeated bouts for many years, if not for life.

As in the small bowel, transmural inflammation and thickening of the bowel wall occur during the acute phase with pericolonic inflammatory change, which can be almost impossible to distinguish from other forms of acute colitis, especially if a large segment of colon is involved. Repetitive inflammatory disease causes deep ulceration with localized perforation and abscess formation or fistulization with adjacent small bowel. Because these repetitive bouts of acute disease heal, luminal narrowing and stricture formation often occur. Perianal disease with fistula and abscess formation is common in Crohn disease.

The imaging features are similar to those described in the small bowel, although the imaging of colonic Crohn disease can, at times, mimic those of UC. However, there are a number of distinguishing features that help to differentiate the two diseases (Table 5-3). Plain radiography may demonstrate mucosal thickening (Fig. 5-19) or toxic megacolon. Contrast enema studies (usually barium) may demonstrate involvement of the whole colon (which is therefore difficult to distinguish from UC), but this is uncommon. More commonly a variable segment of the colon is affected (Fig. 5-20, *A*), and the disease may or may not involve the rectum. Acute disease at CT may present with mural stratification similar to that in the small bowel, representing mucosal and serosal hyperemia with submucosal inflammation or simple mural thickening and mesenteric edema (Fig. 5-20, *B*). Aphthous ulceration is characteristic of Crohn disease (Fig. 5-21). As in the small bowel, the mucosa in active disease enhances avidly after the administration of IV gadolinium. Although CT is easier and faster to perform, many patients with Crohn disease are young and may require repetitive assessment of the extent of their disease, so avoiding the radiation dose from multiple CT images is preferable. Therefore MRI is often advised, and newer MR enterographic techniques, particularly of the small bowel, have proved highly effective for evaluating the extent of disease (Fig. 5-22). Furthermore, the extent of

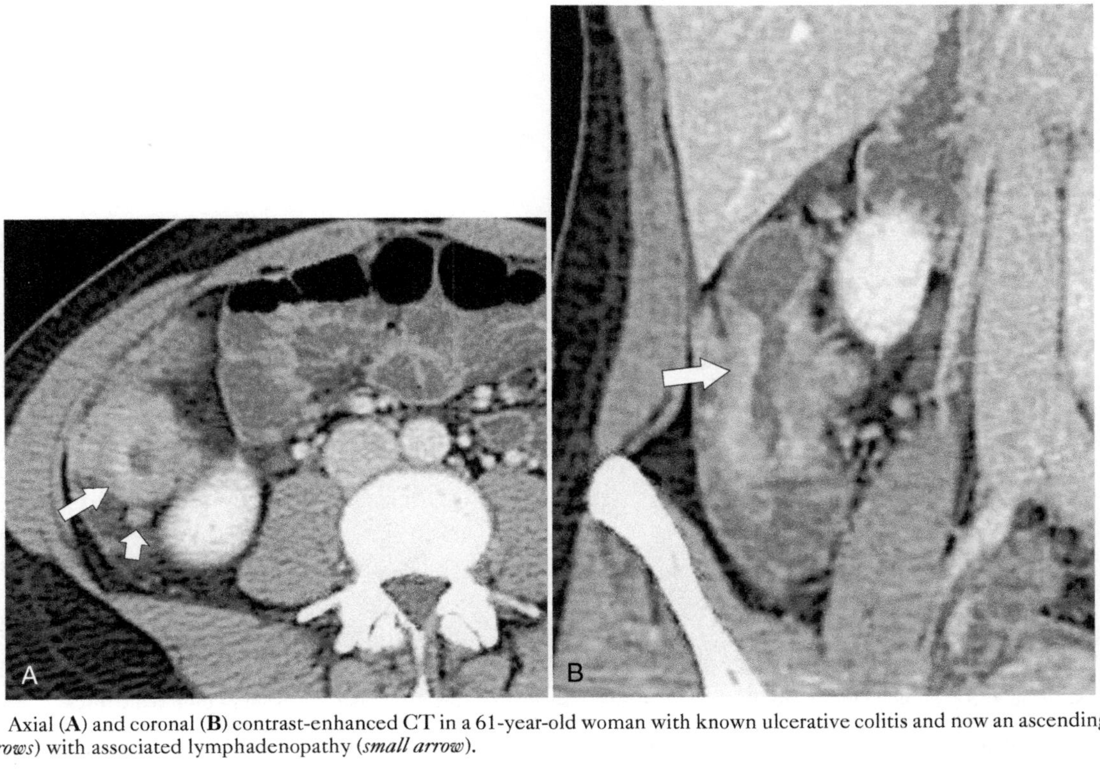

FIGURE 5-18. Axial (**A**) and coronal (**B**) contrast-enhanced CT in a 61-year-old woman with known ulcerative colitis and now an ascending colon adenocarcinoma (*arrows*) with associated lymphadenopathy (*small arrow*).

perianal disease is best imaged with MRI, which can outline the relationship of inflammatory disease to the internal and external anal sphincters; this is important to determine whether surgical repair is needed.

Other differentiating features of UC include a propensity for Crohn disease to fistulize with the small bowel, with adjacent organs, or to the skin. This can be assessed by CT (Fig. 5-23), BE (Figs. 5-24 and 5-25), or MRI (Fig. 5-26). Abscess formation is also recognized in Crohn disease rather than UC (Fig. 5-27). An increased risk of small and large bowel malignancies, predominantly adenocarcinomas, is associated with Crohn disease (Fig. 5-28).

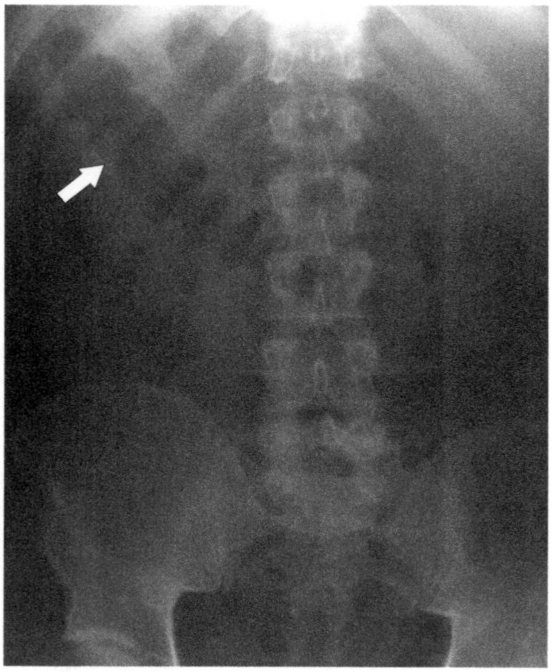

FIGURE 5-19. Plain abdominal radiograph in a 40-year-old man with acute Crohn disease and transmural transverse colonic wall thickening (*arrow*).

Eosinophilic Colitis

Eosinophilic colitis is a disease of uncertain etiology. It is associated with marked peripheral eosinophilia in the blood (although not always) and may be mediated via immunoglobulin E (IgE)-related food allergies. Eosinophilic esophagitis, gastritis, and enteritis also occur, but eosinophilic colitis is rather rare. Symptoms are nonspecific and include pain, diarrhea, and melena. Patients respond well to steroid therapy. At imaging, there are nonspecific features of colitis such as wall thickening, mucosal edema, and, if severe, pericolonic edema (Fig. 5-29). The differentiation from other causes of colitis is generally not possible by imaging alone.

Endometriosis

Ectopic endometrial tissue can reside anywhere within the peritoneum but is most often found in the pelvis and sometimes on the serosal surface of the large bowel, usually in the rectosigmoid region. In general, the patient has crampy abdominal pain that coincides with menses, which should be a key to the diagnosis, although many patients are asymptomatic. The imaging findings, particularly in the correct clinical setting, should ultimately give the diagnosis away. At BE, the bowel wall mucosa is eccentrically spiculated and puckered adjacent to the endometrial tissue.

Behçet Disease

Behçet disease is a multisystem disorder that can affect the colon with severe ulceration mimicking UC. Given that patients with IBD also manifest noncolonic manifestations (e.g., skin, joints, eyes), the correct diagnosis can be delayed.

Diversion Colitis

Diversion colitis is a poorly understood condition in which the extruded distal colon and rectum that remain redundant from a more proximal colostomy or ileostomy develop colitis that is not dissimilar to UC. Diversion colitis can be severe but resolves once the ostomy is reversed and normal fecal flow resumes.

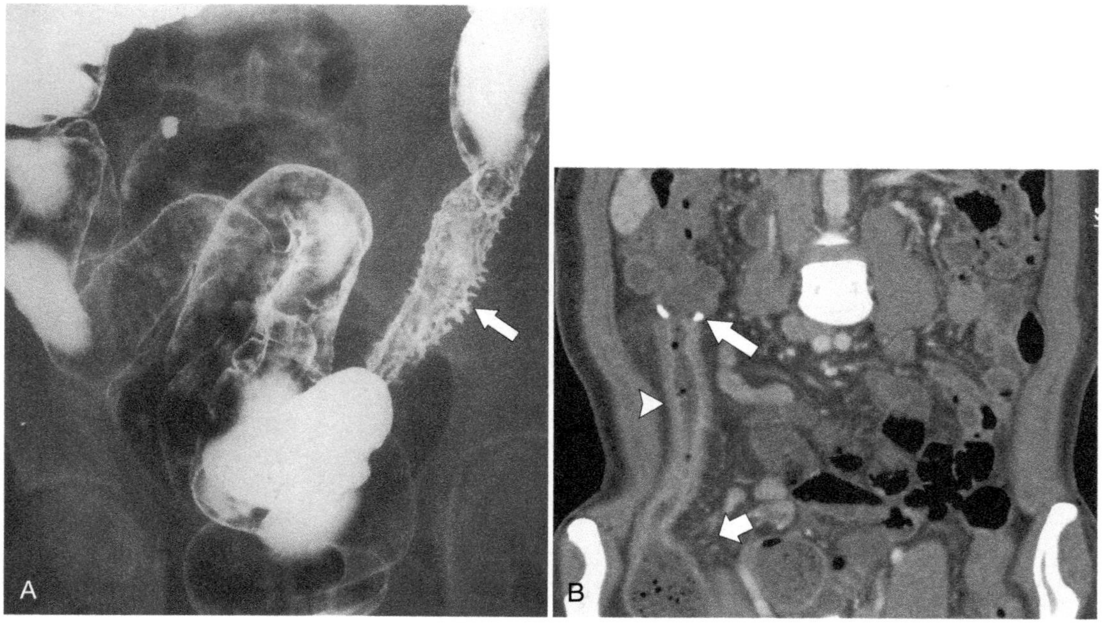

FIGURE 5-20. **A,** BE in a 33-year-old man with focal left-sided Crohn disease with spiculated mucosal changes from acute disease (*arrow*). **B,** Coronal contrast-enhanced CT in a 44-year-old woman with prior surgery for Crohn disease (*arrow*) and now acute disease in the ascending colon (*arrowhead*) with wall thickening and mucosal and mesenteric hyperemia (*small arrow*).

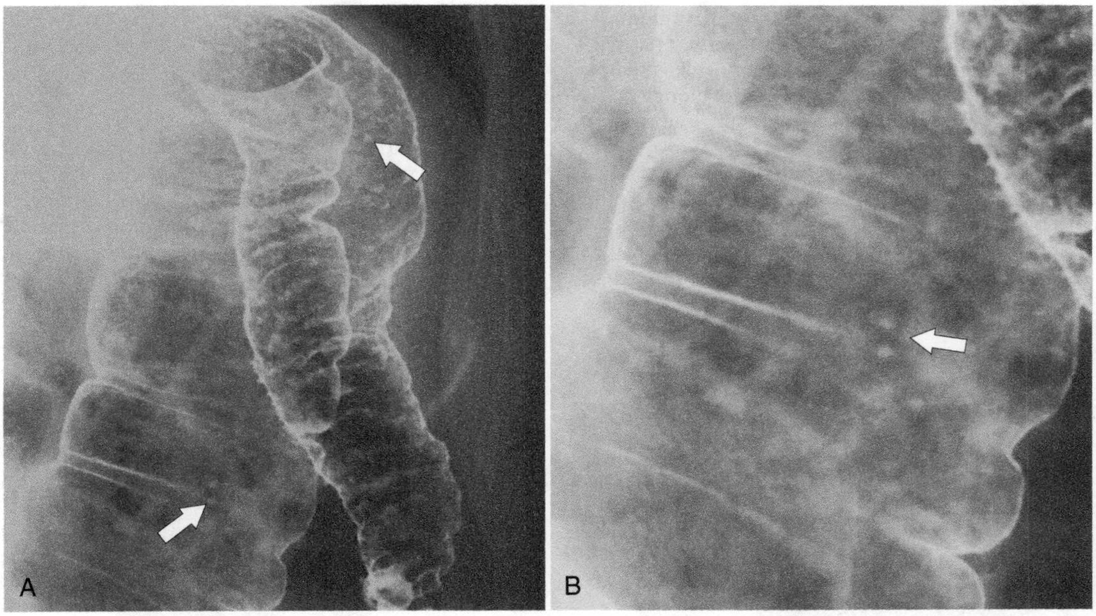

FIGURE 5-21. A, BE in a 36-year-old woman with numerous apthous ulcers (*arrows*) in the left colon from Crohn disease. B, Magnified view of apthous ulcers (*arrow*) in the distal transverse colon.

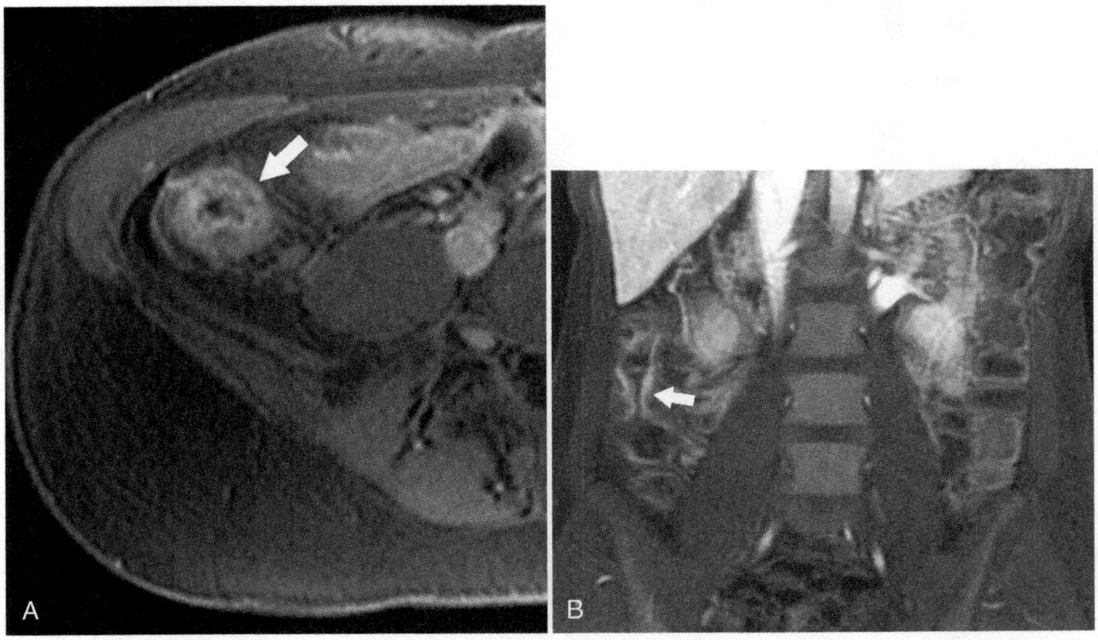

FIGURE 5-22. Axial fat-saturated postcontrast T1-weighted images in a 22-year-old woman with focal Crohn disease of the ascending colon (A, *arrows*). B, Coronal view demonstrates mucosal enhancement and mural thickening (*arrow*).

Graft-Versus-Host Disease

Graft-versus-host disease usually develops after allogeneic bone marrow transplantation (and rarely thymic transplantation) and is caused by immunological destruction of host tissue, characterized on histological examination by apoptosis, a form of cell death. This disease particularly affects the GI tract but also the liver and dermis. In the colon there are nonspecific features of colitis with bowel wall and mucosal thickening, often involving the whole colon as a pancolitis (Fig. 5-30).

Drug-Induced Colitis

Drugs can cause colitis via various mechanisms, including direct mucosal necrosis, ischemia, lymphocytic colitis, and a particular form, pseudomembranous colitis (see page 174). Direct colitis may be secondary to some sorbitol enema formulations and chemotherapeutic regimens (Fig. 5-31). Ischemic colitis may manifest after the administration of drugs that cause thrombosis (e.g., oral contraceptive pill) or spasm (e.g., cocaine and amphetamines). Lymphocytic colitis is of uncertain etiology and is associated with some H_2 blockers and cholesterol-lowering agents. At imaging, the colitis is nonspecific with a variable length of colonic thickening (which may be in a vascular territorial distribution if caused by ischemia) with or without pericolonic edema, depending on the severity (Fig. 5-32).

Typhlitis

Sometimes known as neutropenic colitis because it is an acute inflammatory condition (mainly of the terminal ileum, cecum, and ascending colon), typhlitis is identified in patients with neutropenia from any cause, but particularly those with hematologic malignancies. It is most commonly seen in younger patients with aplastic anemia, patients with lymphoma, transplant recipients, and those infected with human immunodeficiency virus (HIV). Patients present with right lower quadrant pain, fever, and diarrhea.

Typhlitis is readily identified at CT by circumferential cecal wall thickening, sometimes marked, that is thought to be caused by a combination of infection, hemorrhage, and ischemia. Bowel wall enhancement in common with other colitides is present, and there is often pericolonic inflammatory change (fat-stranding). Typhlitis may affect a variable length of the ascending colon, and the adjacent terminal ileum or appendix may be affected (Fig. 5-33).

Ischemic Colitis

Ischemic colitis is the most common vascular disease of the GI tract, occurring mainly in the elderly, either from occlusive disease (typically the inferior mesenteric artery) or from low-perfusion states caused by atherosclerotic disease. Patients with atherosclerosis are particularly susceptible after any additional insult that may lead to hypoperfusion, such as surgery, trauma, or low–cardiac output states. The colonic mucosa is particularly susceptible to ischemic events and will rapidly become edematous,

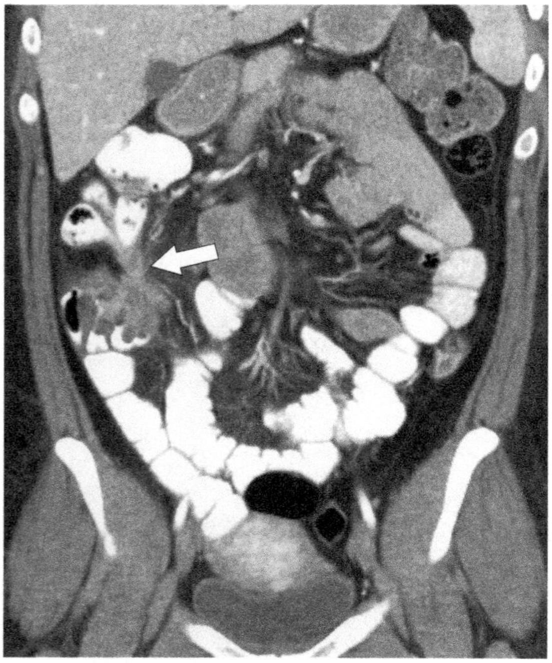

FIGURE 5-23. Coronal CT in a 38-year-old woman with a coloenteric fistula (*arrow*) due to Crohn disease.

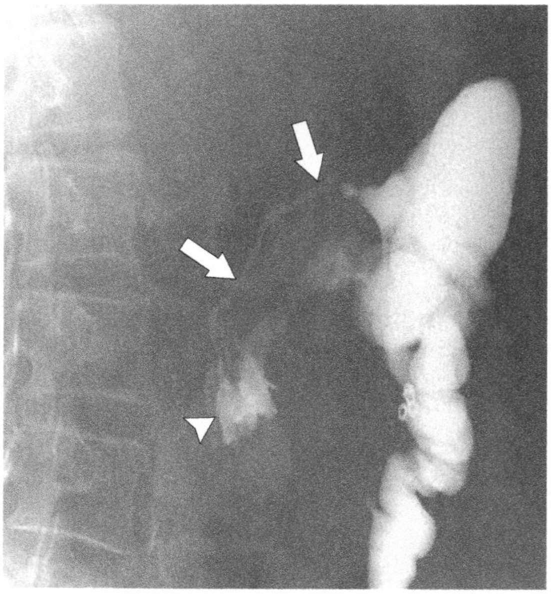

FIGURE 5-25. BE in a 44-year-old woman with a coloenteric fistula (*arrows*) with a segment of jejunum (*arrowhead*) due to Crohn disease.

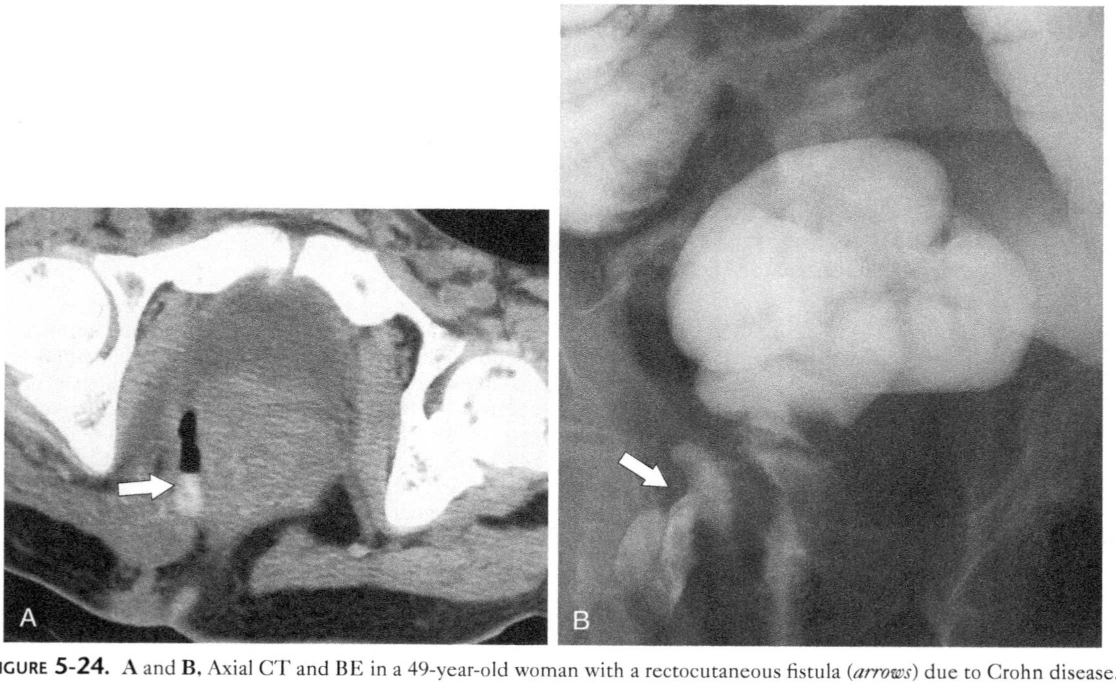

FIGURE 5-24. **A** and **B**, Axial CT and BE in a 49-year-old woman with a rectocutaneous fistula (*arrows*) due to Crohn disease.

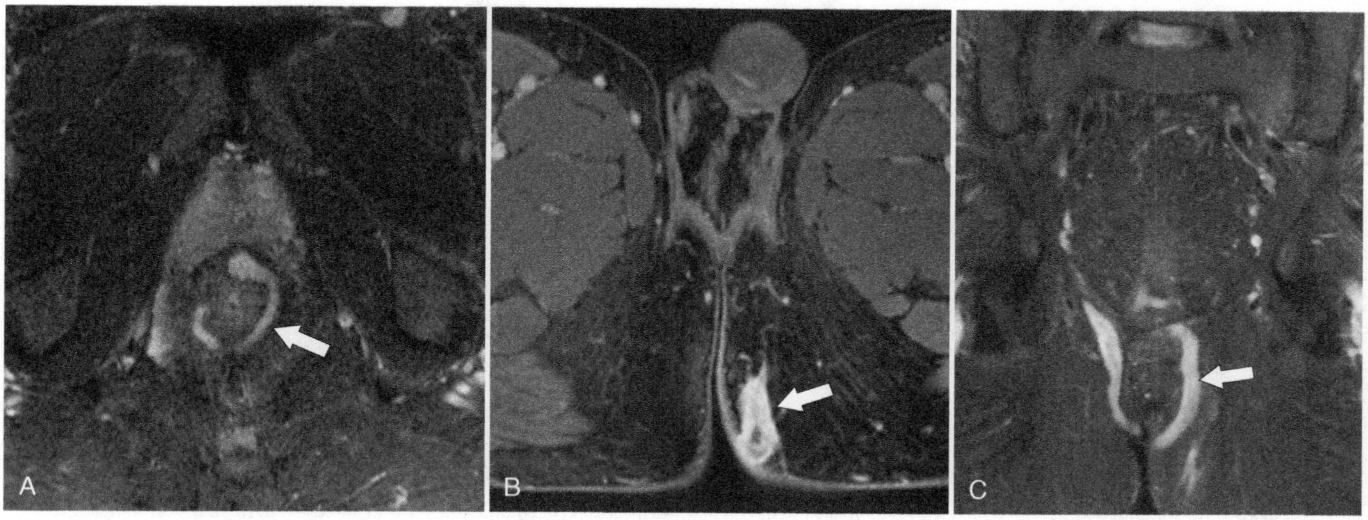

FIGURE 5-26. Axial (**A** and **B**) T2-weighted and coronal (**C**) T1-weighted fat-saturated postcontrast MRI in a 43-year-old man with a perianal fistula with an almost circumferential perianal fistula (*arrows*) tracking to the left medial buttock.

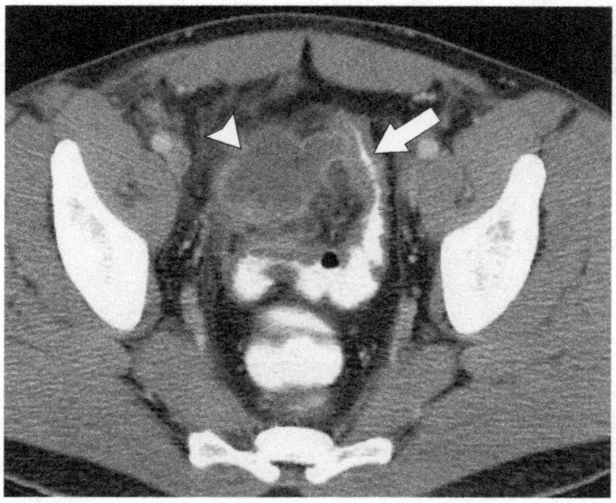

FIGURE 5-27. Axial contrast-enhanced CT in a 38-year-old man with sigmoid mural thickening (*arrow*) and a 4-cm pericolonic Crohn abscess (*arrowhead*).

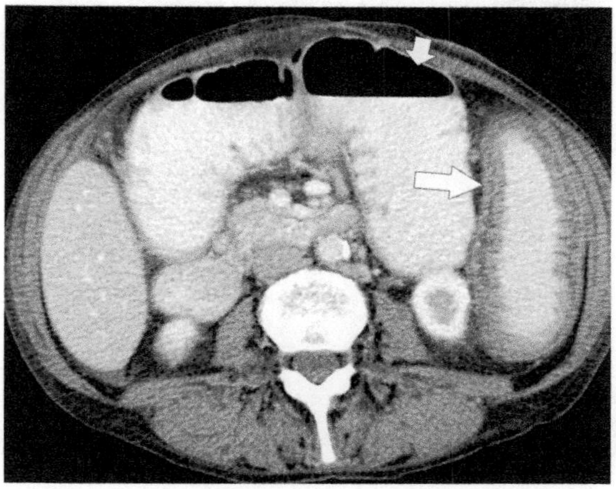

FIGURE 5-29. Axial contrast-enhanced CT in a 66-year-old woman with colonic dilatation (*short arrow*) and mural thickening of the descending colon (*arrow*) due to eosinophilic colitis.

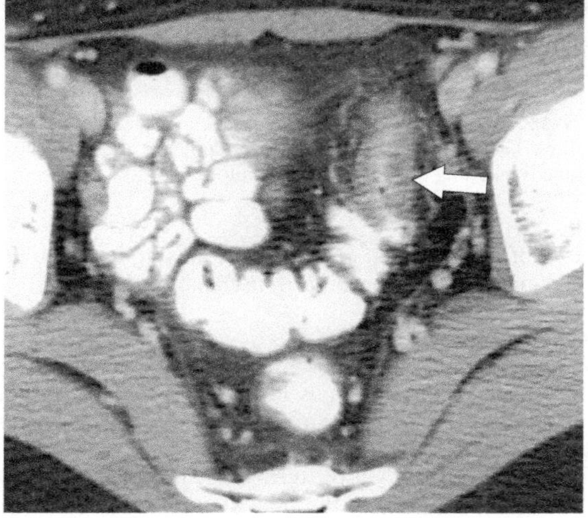

FIGURE 5-28. Axial contrast-enhanced CT in a 28-year-old woman with circumferential sigmoid thickening (*arrow*) due to adenocarcinoma as a complication of Crohn disease.

hyperemic, and markedly thickened ("thumb-printing"), which can occur within 24 hours of the ischemic onset. Patients may be relatively asymptomatic early in the process, but as the severity increases, symptoms similar to other colitides, including diarrhea, pain, and rectal bleeding, develop.

Most disease is segmental in the colonic "watershed" areas, with the splenic flexure (i.e., arterial vascular transition between the superior mesenteric and inferior mesenteric arteries) and rectosigmoid region (i.e., junction between the inferior mesenteric and hypogastric arteries) most at risk. More extensive disease is, however, well recognized, particularly if the superior mesenteric artery is also affected and a pancolitis ensues, which is difficult to differentiate from other colitides.

Plain radiography may demonstrate an ileus, sometimes confined to the left colon. As the disease progresses, bowel wall thickening develops (Fig. 5-34) with a toxic megacolon if severe (Fig. 5-35). BE is now rarely performed, but results demonstrate thickened folds and ulceration, either linear or with mucosal sloughing. Healing can lead to stricture formation (Fig. 5-36). The findings are now usually made by CT and are similar to other forms of colitis (inflammatory bowel disease, infectious colitides, and radiation colitis if the radiation field included the colon). The disease is suggested in the appropriate clinical setting and by the left-sided

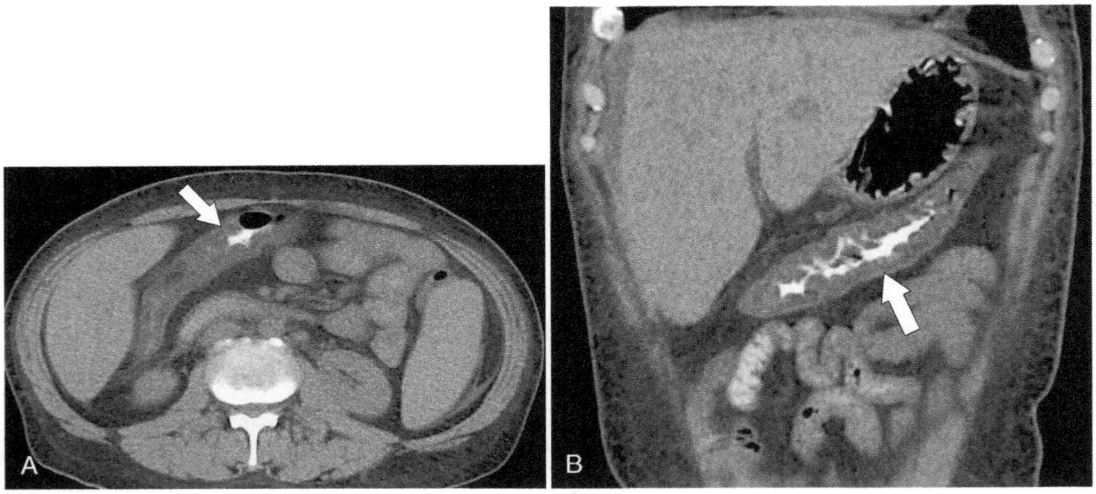

FIGURE 5-30. Axial (**A**) and coronal (**B**) noncontrast CT in a 44-year-old man with transverse colonic thickening (*arrows*) due to graft-versus-host disease.

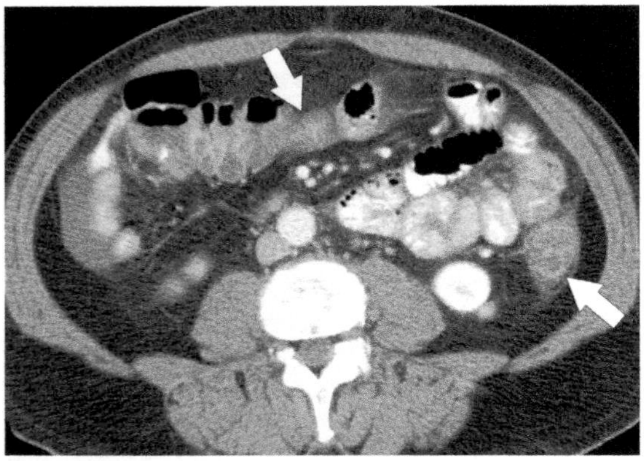

FIGURE 5-31. Axial contrast-enhanced CT in a 58-year-old man with recent right colectomy for colon adenocarcinoma and now with a chemotherapy-induced pancolitis (*arrows*).

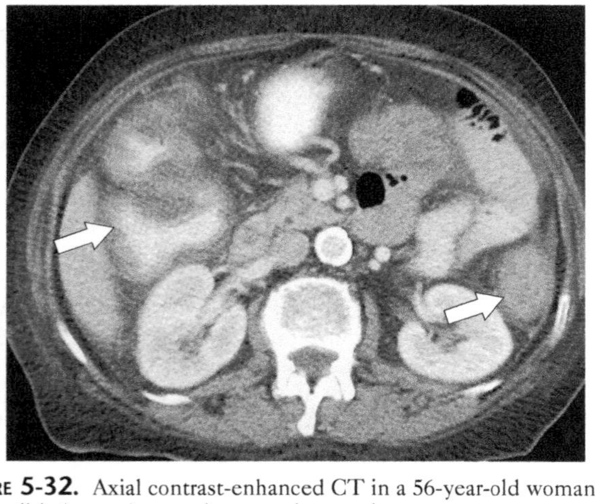

FIGURE 5-32. Axial contrast-enhanced CT in a 56-year-old woman with a pancolitis (*arrows*) secondary to quinones therapy.

distribution of the colonic changes (Fig. 5-37). Severely affected patients show colonic pneumatosis as the gas permeates the damaged mucosa, which can then enter the mesenteric venous system and be recognized as mesenteric venous gas (particularly at CT) and ultimately intrahepatic portal venous gas. Occasionally, ischemia occurs proximal to an obstructing colonic stricture, such as colonic adenocarcinoma. The obstruction causes marked

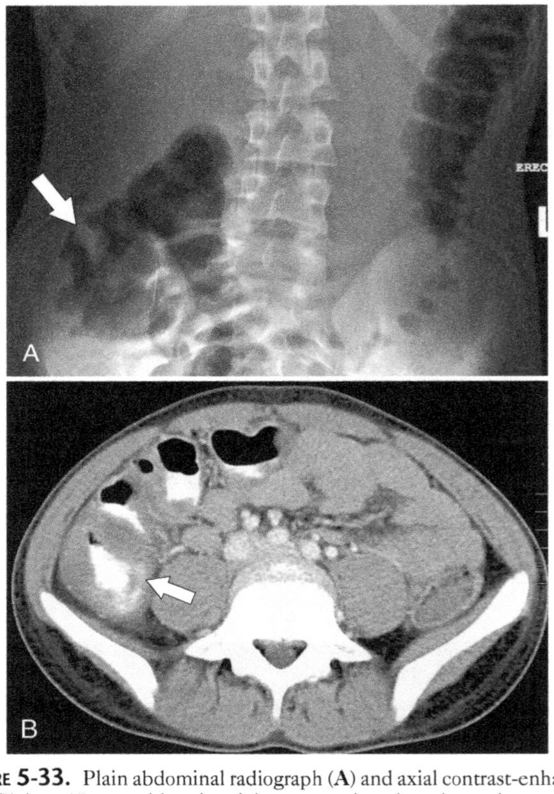

FIGURE 5-33. Plain abdominal radiograph (**A**) and axial contrast-enhanced CT (**B**) in a 17-year-old male adolescent undergoing chemotherapy with cecal mural thickening (*arrows*) due to typhlitis.

distention of the proximal colon, compromising its vascular supply or directly invading mesenteric vasculature (Fig. 5-38).

Reversible Ischemic Colitis

Reversible ischemic colitis is sometimes referred to as jogger's or runner's colitis because it is observed in otherwise healthy patients in whom colitis develops (with pain and diarrhea, which is rarely bloody) either during or soon after long-distance running and resolves shortly after termination of the exercise. The mechanism of injury is poorly understood but is a nonocclusive ischemia thought to be caused by low mesenteric flow states from arterial shunting to extremity musculature away from the mesentery combined with marked dehydration. Both the superior and

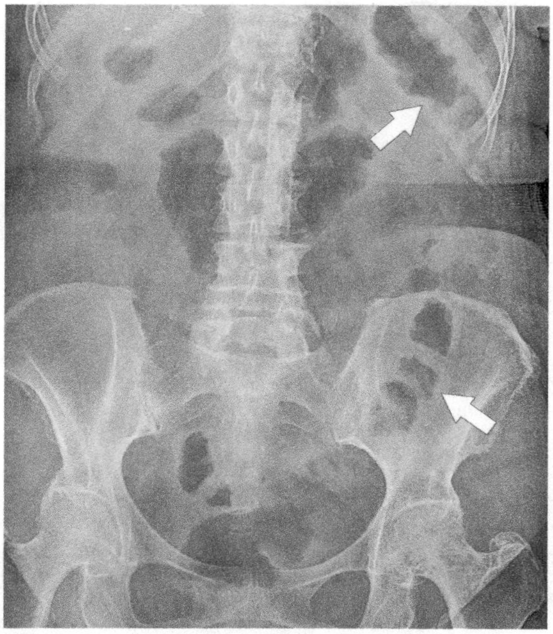

FIGURE 5-34. Plain abdominal radiograph in a 78-year-old woman with left-sided colonic wall thickening (*arrows*) due to ischemic colitis.

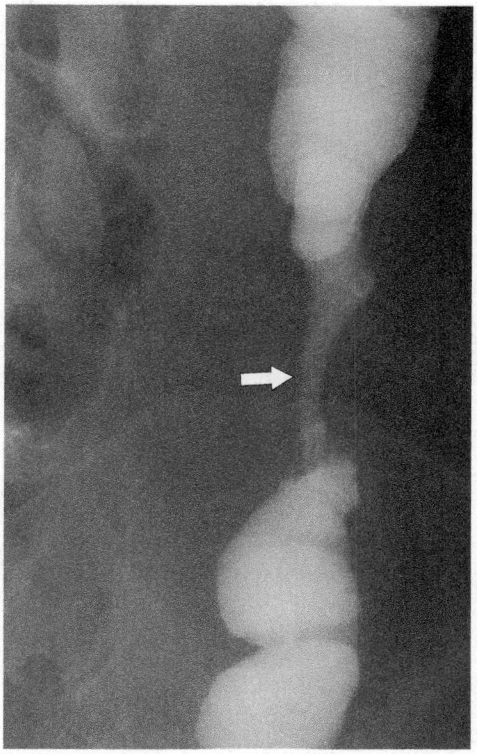

FIGURE 5-36. BE in a 71-year-old man with a left mid-descending colon stricture (*arrow*) secondary to fibrosis from prior ischemic colitis.

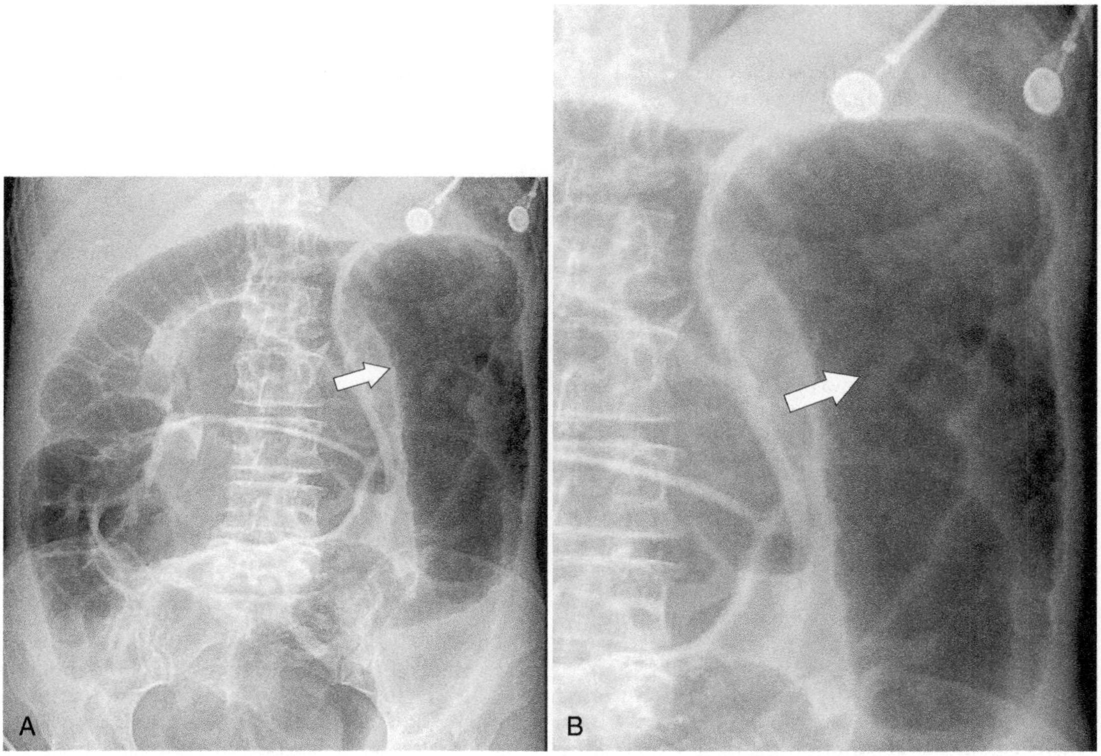

FIGURE 5-35. **A** and **B**, Plain abdominal radiograph (**A**) and magnified view (**B**) in a 56-year-old man with a left-sided toxic megacolon due to ischemic colitis. There is thumb-printing of the colonic mucosa at the splenic flexure (*arrows*).

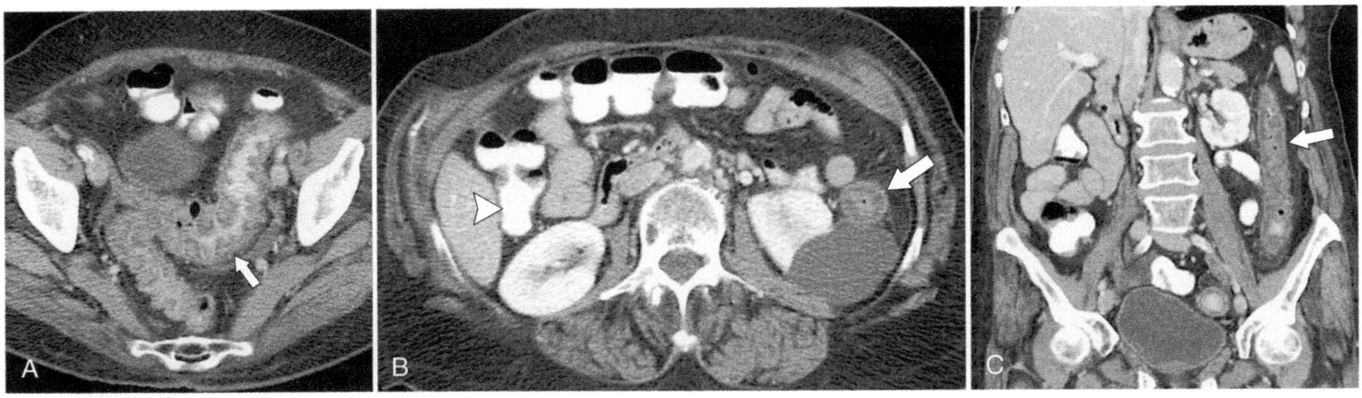

FIGURE 5-37. Axial (**A** and **B**) and coronal (**C**) contrast-enhanced CT in a 66-year-old woman with diffuse left colonic mucosal thickening (*arrows*) due to ischemic colitis. Note the normal right colon (*arrowhead*).

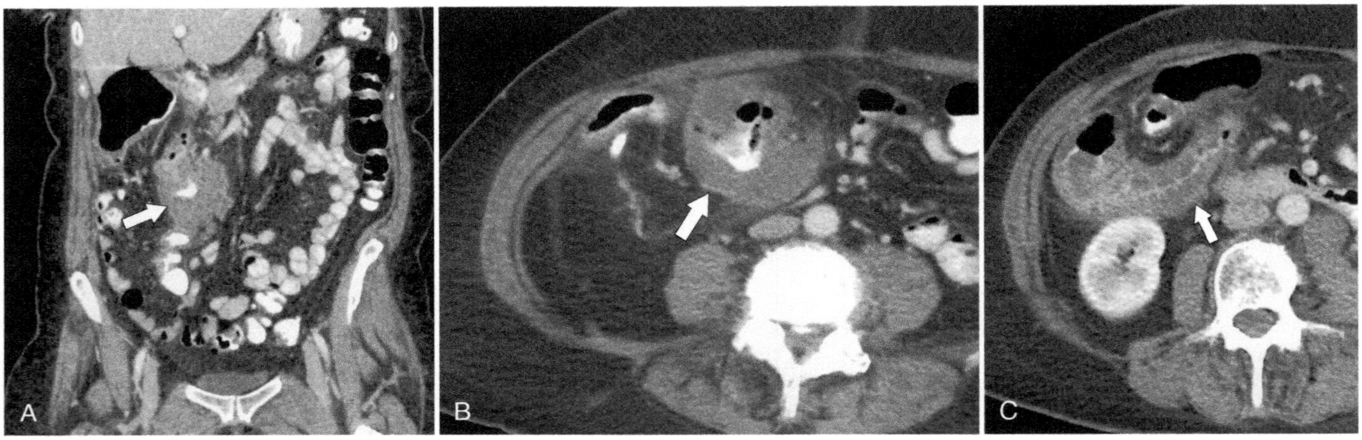

FIGURE 5-38. **A** through **C**, Coronal and axial contrast-enhanced CT in a 62-year-old man with a transverse colon adenocarcinoma (*arrows*) with proximal ascending colon mucosal thickening due to secondary ischemia.

inferior mesenteric territories are at risk, so the entire colon may be affected. The disease more commonly occurs in unconditioned athletes, and it seems to improve with training. The diagnosis is made with the relevant history, and if imaging is performed, there will often be no findings because the colitis has resolved or mild colitic changes of bowel wall thickening may be seen (Fig. 5-39). More severe wall thickening suggests an alternative diagnosis.

Radiation Colitis

Radiation colitis is less commonly seen today because of more sophisticated radiation treatment protocols, which attempt to remove the bowel from the radiation field. This may include the placement of spacers to push bowel and other anatomy away from the radiation field. However, with pelvic radiation for local malignancies (e.g., cervical cancer) the rectosigmoid may unavoidably be in the radiation field. Similar to radiation bowel changes elsewhere, the acute changes include mucosal thickening and edema and ulceration. In the chronic form of radiation colitis there may be stricture formation from endarteritis obliterans and loss of the normal haustral pattern, such that the bowel appears featureless, not dissimilar to UC.

The findings are most often visualized by CT, particularly because patients are often serially imaged to evaluate for any local cancer recurrence or metastatic disease, although MRI often detects more subtle changes (Fig. 5-40). Associated inflammatory changes are often observed in the surrounding mesentery (fat-stranding). This is commonly seen in the presacral region after radiation for rectal cancer preceding attempted surgical removal of the tumor. Radiation changes can sometimes be difficult to differentiate from local recurrence, but awareness that the patient has undergone radiation should alert the radiologist that the changes are benign rather than malignant recurrence. Increasingly, PET imaging is used to differentiate postradiation changes from recurrent disease (Fig. 5-41).

Portal Colopathy

Portal colopathy is not strictly an inflammatory disease but is included here for completeness. Chronic liver disease with secondary portal venous hypertension can affect almost the whole GI tract from the esophagus and stomach (varices) to the small bowel (diffuse mucosal thickening) and colon. In the colon there may be variceal formation (similar to the mechanism in the stomach and esophagus) or diffuse vascular ectasia, which has a propensity for hemorrhage. Imaging may demonstrate diffuse colonic thickening secondary to increased venous pressure or hypoproteinemia (Fig. 5-42). Direct evidence of variceal formation (Fig. 5-43) may appear throughout the colon or be limited to the rectum, where it may present as hemorrhoids or rectal bleeding (Fig. 5-44).

Infectious Colitis

Numerous infectious agents (Table 5-1) result in colitis. Acute presentation, usually bacterial or viral, is with profuse watery or bloody diarrhea, abdominal pain and cramping, fever, and arthralgia. Bacterial organisms include *Salmonella* sp., *Shigella* sp., *Staphylococcus* sp., *Campylobacter* sp., *Yersinia* sp., *Escherichia coli*, *Chlamydia* sp., and actinomycetes, among others. Viruses include herpes, cytomegalovirus (CMV), rotavirus, and Norwalk

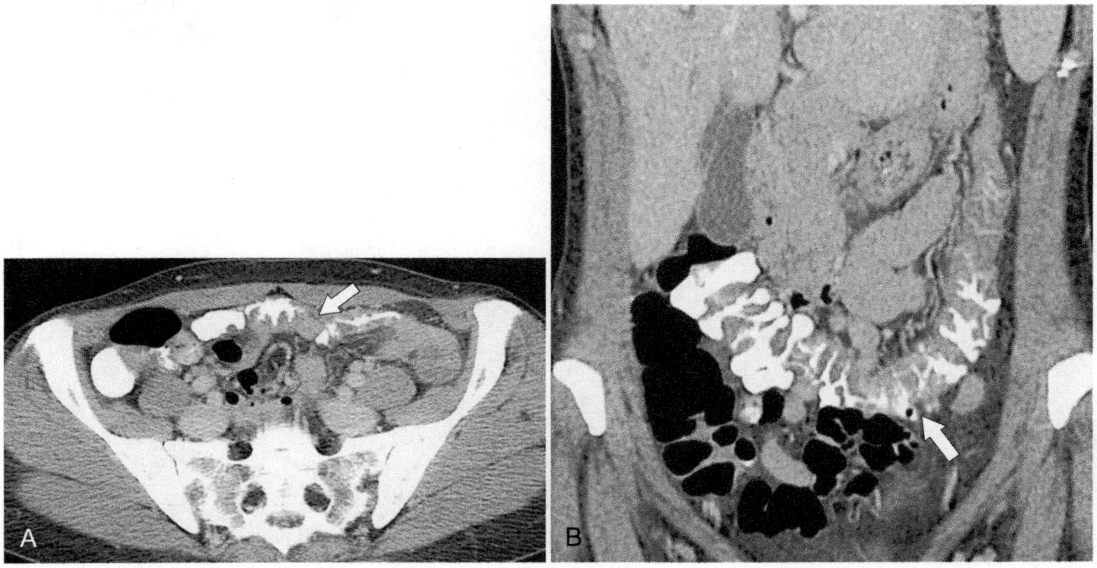

FIGURE 5-39. Axial (**A**) and coronal (**B**) contrast-enhanced fat-saturated CT in a 37-year-old female marathon runner with transverse colon mucosal thickening (*arrows*) due to "runner's" colitis.

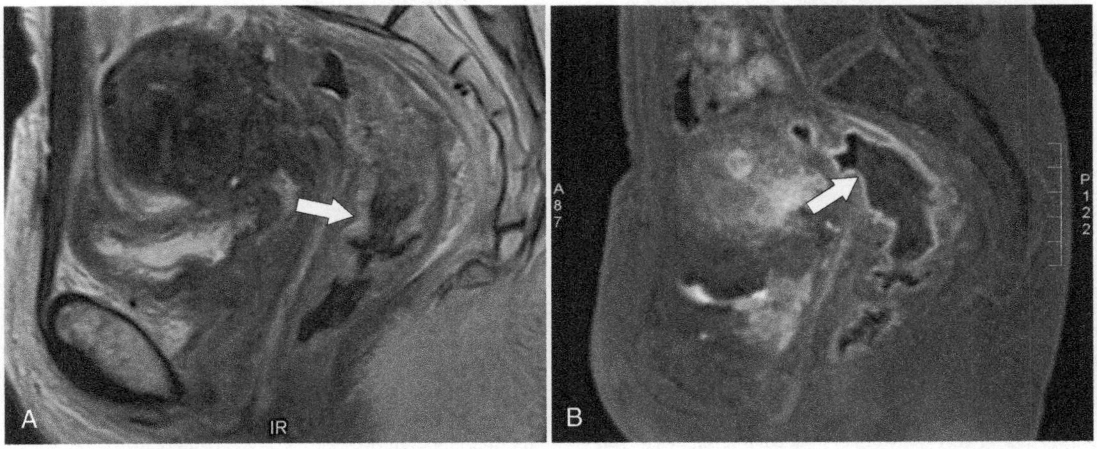

FIGURE 5-40. Sagittal T2-weighted (**A**) and contrast-enhanced MRI (**B**) in a 47-year-old woman with rectal wall thickening (*arrow*) and mucosal hyperenhancement due to radiation colitis (*arrows*).

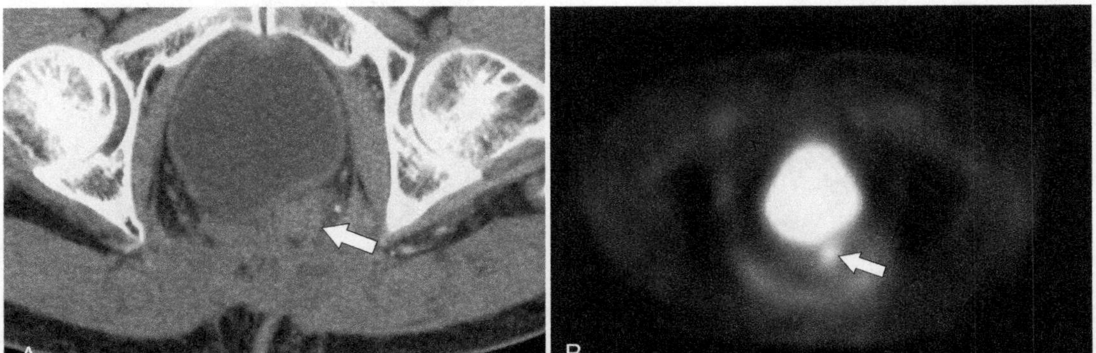

FIGURE 5-41. Axial CT (**A**) and PET (**B**) in a 73-year-old man with prior colectomy for rectal cancer and question of postoperative pelvic changes versus recurrence. PET imaging confirms tumor recurrence (*arrows*).

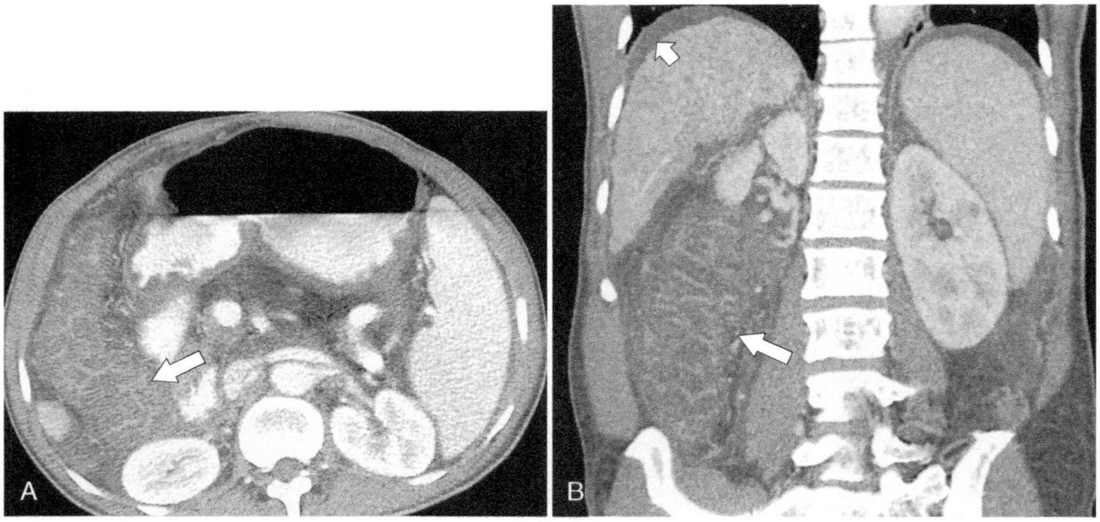

FIGURE 5-42. Axial (**A**) and coronal (**B**) contrast-enhanced CT in a 44-year-old man with cirrhosis and portal colopathy (*arrows*). There is associated ascites and splenomegaly (*small arrow*).

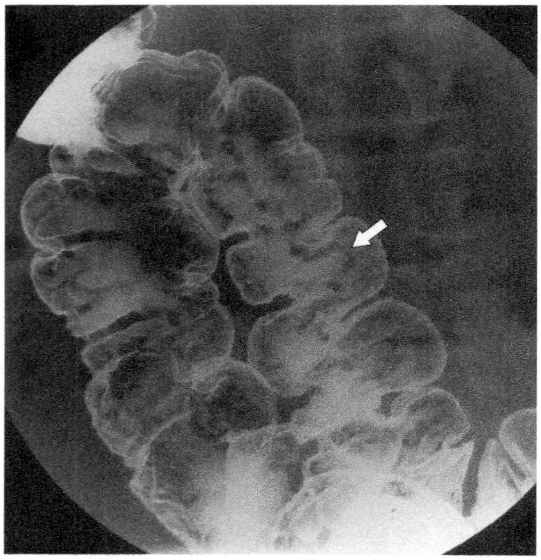

FIGURE 5-43. DCBE in a 56-year-old woman with colonic varices (*arrow*).

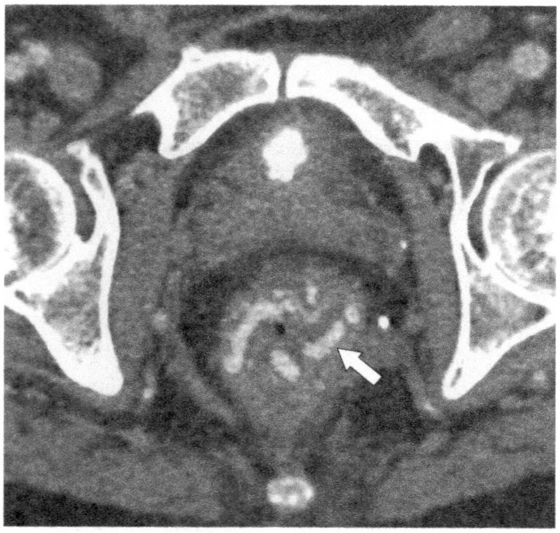

FIGURE 5-44. Axial contrast-enhanced CT in a 64-year-old man with rectal varices (*arrow*).

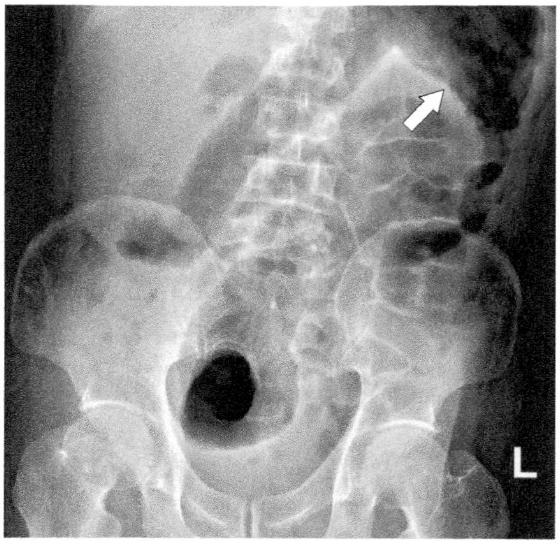

FIGURE 5-45. Plain abdominal radiograph in a 36-year-old woman with nodular mucosal thickening (*arrow*) due to pseudomembranes from pseudomembranous colitis.

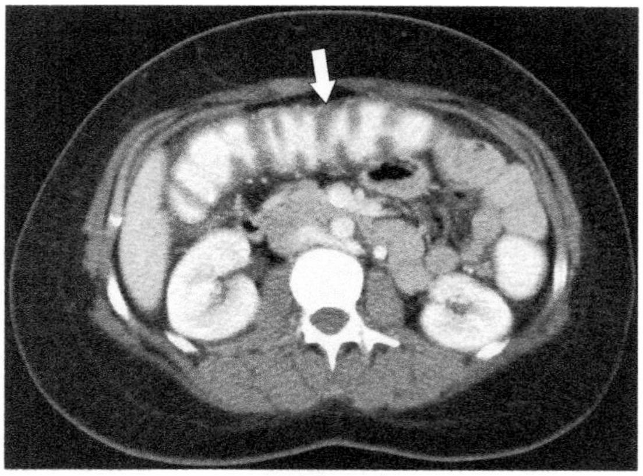

FIGURE 5-46. Axial contrast-enhanced CT in a 73-year-old woman with haustral thickening of the transverse colon caused by pseudomembranous pancolitis (*arrow*).

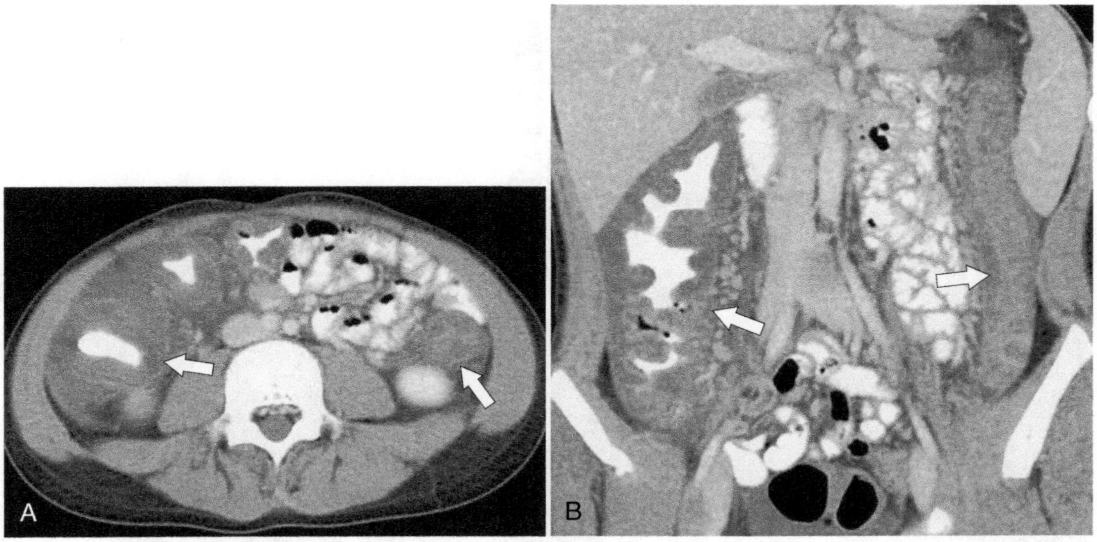

FIGURE 5-47. Axial (**A**) and coronal (**B**) contrast-enhanced CT in a 12-year-old boy with marked colonic thickening (*arrows*), particularly the right colon due to *E. coli* colitis.

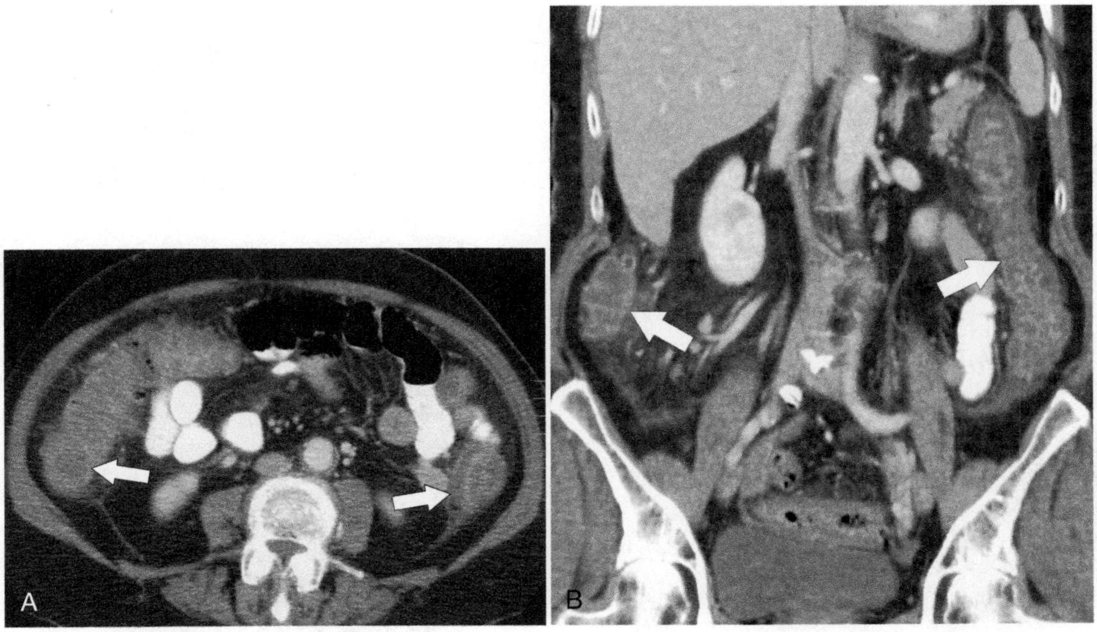

FIGURE 5-48. Axial (**A**) and coronal (**B**) contrast-enhanced CT in a 64-year-old woman with pancolitic mucosal thickening (*arrows*) due to traveler's diarrhea.

gastroenteritis virus. Less acute presentations include histoplasmosis (a fungus) and several parasites (*Ascaris*, *Amoeba*, *Schistosoma*, *Strongyloides*, *Trichuris*, and *Anisakis* species). A prolonged chronic presentation is recognized with tuberculosis.

Most patients with infectious diarrhea are not imaged because the diagnosis is made clinically, sometimes by means of stool specimens or serological analysis. However, severely affected patients, particularly those hospitalized, may have imaging, usually CT, performed to evaluate for evidence of colitis or its complications. Plain radiography often demonstrates an ileus, and mucosal thickening may be recognized and, if severe, may demonstrate thumb-printing and toxic megacolon (Fig. 5-45). The features of colitis are better appreciated with CT (Fig. 5-46), including the ileus and wall thickening, as well as mucosal and serosal enhancement with hyperattenuating submucosa (target sign), pericolonic edema (stranding), and ascites.

Often the infectious etiology cannot be determined by imaging alone because all the agents cause nonspecific colonic wall thickening and some cause a pancolitis, including *Escherichia coli* (although this colitis can be severe [Fig. 5-47]) and those involved in traveler's diarrhea (Fig. 5-48). Other pathogens tend to affect specific colonic areas more than others. *Campylobacter* sp. is sometimes indistinguishable from UC (Fig. 5-49), but is often confined to the rectum. Other rectal colitides include gonococcal and herpes colitis. *Shigella* sp. primarily affects the left side of the colon, whereas *Salmonella typhi*, tuberculosis, *Yersinia*, and amebiasis are focally confined to the ileocecal region with or without local adenopathy.

Strongyloides infection can mimic UC in its diffuse form but can also present with focal right colonic disease (Fig. 5-50). *Actinomyces* infection is usually secondary to pelvic colonization of intrauterine contraceptive devices and may cause a focal, either cecal

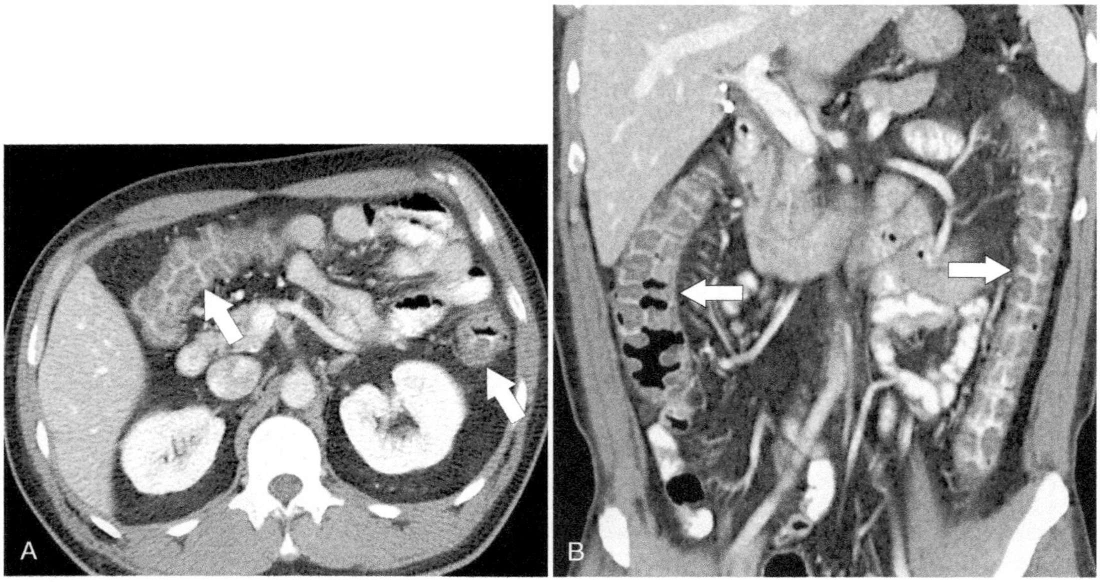

FIGURE 5-49. Axial (**A**) and coronal (**B**) contrast-enhanced CT in a 39-year-old man with marked pancolitic mucosal thickening (*arrows*) due to *Campylobacter* sp. infection. The appearances are similar to most other infectious colitides.

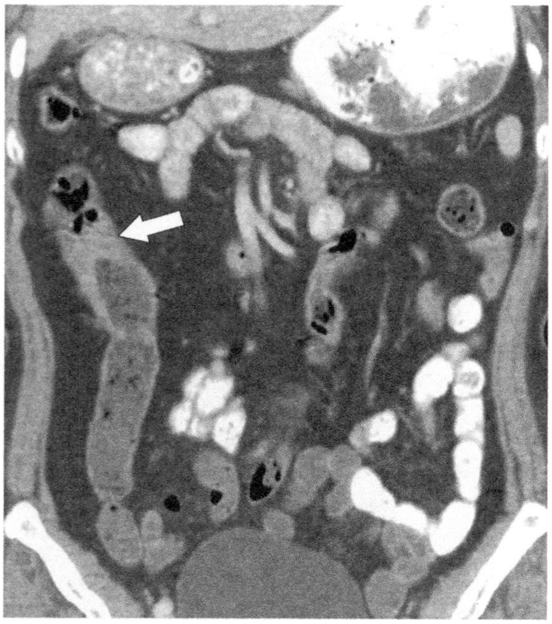

FIGURE 5-50. Coronal contrast-enhanced CT in a 49-year-old woman with focal mucosal thickening (*arrow*) of the ascending colon due to *Strongyloides* sp. infection.

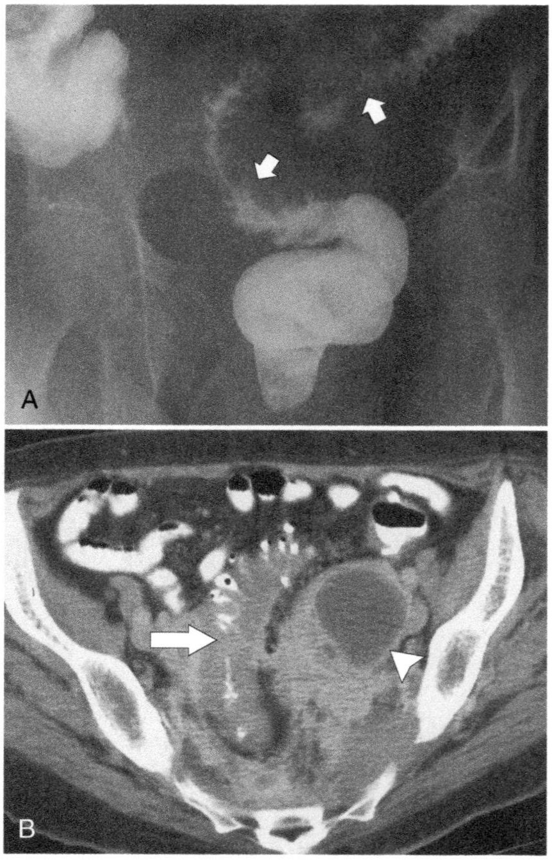

FIGURE 5-51. BE (**A**) and axial contrast-enhanced CT (**B**) in a 39-year-old woman with pelvic actinomycetes infection with sigmoid wall thickening (*arrow*) and narrowing (*small arrows*) and a pelvic abscess (*arrowhead*).

or rectosigmoid, colitis (Fig. 5-51). *Actinomyces* may also be associated with right-sided ileocecal infection after secondary infection following appendectomy.

The infectious colitides that are more likely to be recognized at imaging include *Clostridium difficile* (pseudomembranous) colitis, less commonly CMV colitis, and sometimes tuberculous and amebic colitis. These will be specifically addressed.

Clostridium difficile *(Pseudomembranous Colitis)*

Pseudomembranous colitis, also known as antibiotic-associated diarrhea, is secondary to *Clostridium difficile* infection and is relatively common, particularly in the hospital setting, given the widespread use of antibiotics. Use of these drugs predisposes the patient to colonic *C. difficile* overgrowth after the antibiotics have eliminated normal bacterial flora. Toxin production ensues, leading to an acute inflammatory colitis. Clindamycin is most commonly implicated, but many antibiotics are responsible, including cephalosporins and amoxicillin. The disease may develop with even relatively remote antibiotic usage (up to several months prior). Patients present with the typical features of colitis, including bloody diarrhea, pain, and fever. The disease owes its notoriety to its marked propensity in untreated patients to progress to fulminant colitis and toxic megacolon with marked haustral and mucosal thickening. Pseudomembranes are characteristic of the disease and are best visualized endoscopically as yellow exudates representing the inflammatory detritus in the colon or rectum.

The imaging findings may lag behind the clinical features, and patients may have pronounced clinical disease without obvious imaging findings. When observed, the imaging features are similar to most other colitides. Plain radiography often demonstrates ileus and, as the disease progresses, nodular haustral thickening, often over a long segment because the disease usually presents as a pancolitis. There may be polypoid mucosal thickening representing the pseudomembranes, but this is not often observed (Fig. 5-45). The disease can progress readily to frank toxic megacolon. However, it is optimally evaluated by CT, which demonstrates bowel wall thickening, mucosal enhancement, often with a mural stratification (or target sign representing unenhanced thickened submucosa surrounded by enhancing mucosa and muscularis propria), pericolonic edema, and mild ascites. The bowel wall thickening is often pronounced, more so than in other colitides, with the thickened haustra giving the appearance of an accordion pattern (also found with CMV colitis) over a relatively long segment of bowel (Fig. 5-52), representing oral contrast material trapped between the bulbous-thickened haustra.

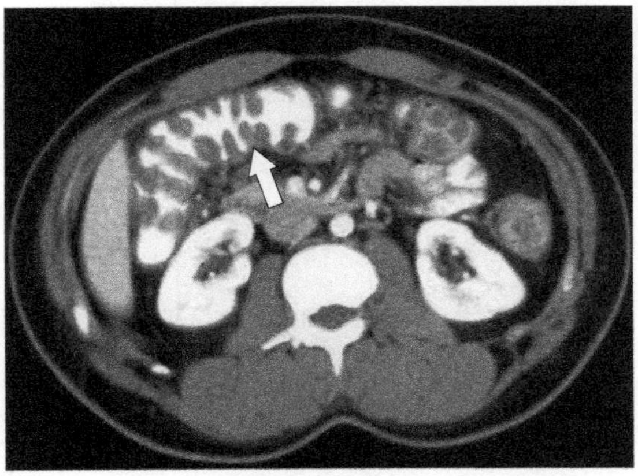

FIGURE 5-52. Axial contrast-enhanced CT in a 46-year-old woman with pancolitic mucosal thickening (*arrow*) due to *Clostridium difficile* colitis. The haustral thickening in the right colon conforms to the "accordion pattern."

Cytomegalovirus

Cytomegalovirus is a herpesvirus that has well-recognized somatic complications from congenital fetal infection but is usually asymptomatic in adults. However, CMV is potentially life threatening in an immune-compromised patient, who can develop severe hepatitis and colitis. Its colitic imaging appearances (usually by CT) are almost identical to the much more common *C. difficile* colitis or IBD, producing a diffuse colitis (Fig. 5-53) and sometimes an accordion-type pattern. The colonic wall thickening can be profound, as in *C. difficile* colitis, and toxic megacolon is a recognized complication.

Tuberculosis

The abdomen is the second most common region affected by the *Mycobacterium tuberculosis* (TB) organism and usually is secondary to pulmonary infection. *Mycobacterium bovium* can result in direct infection of the alimentary tract, sometimes the small bowel, in preference to the colon. Tuberculosis remains remarkably common worldwide, with up to a third of the world population affected. Most infected persons are relatively asymptomatic. In many countries, therefore, the diagnosis of TB would be at or close to the top of any differential diagnosis for many abnormal imaging findings. In the West, TB is most likely secondary to immunosuppressed states from any cause, including primary disease and iatrogenic causes (immunosuppressive drugs). Abdominal tuberculous infection most commonly produces hypodense mesenteric and retroperitoneal adenopathy, best appreciated after administration of IV contrast material. Healing is by nodal calcification, which is a clue to prior infection. When the infection is florid, diffuse peritoneal and omental thickening can occur, usually with ascites (see Chapter 10).

Mycobacterium avium intracellulare (MAI) infection is an atypical mycobacterial infection most commonly seen in patients in the

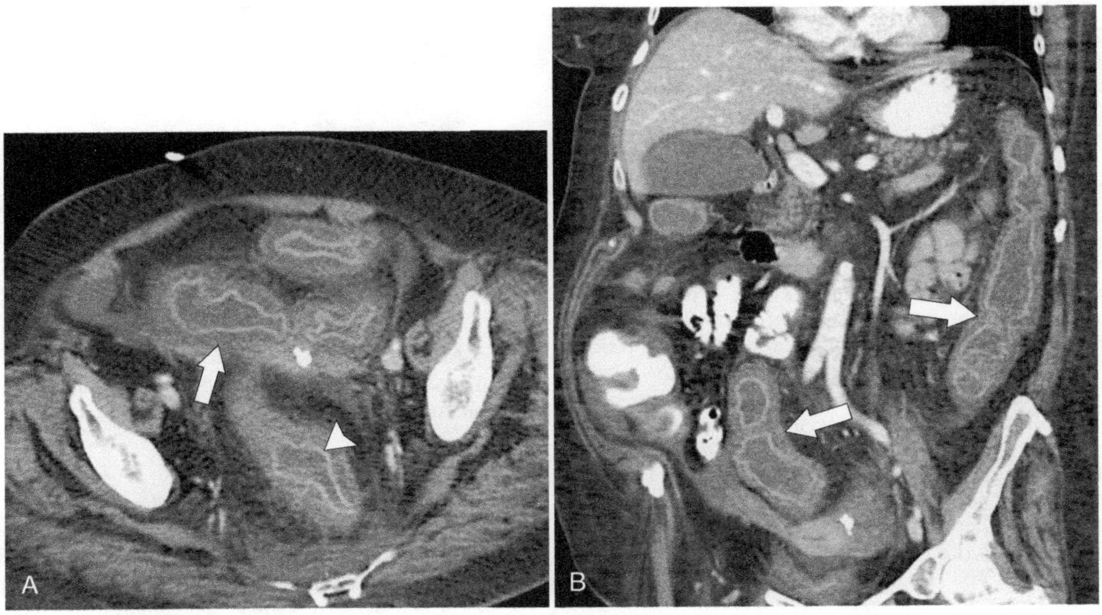

FIGURE 5-53. Axial (**A**) and coronal (**B**) contrast-enhanced CT in a 46-year-old man with marked pancolitic mucosal thickening (*arrows*) with mucosal hyperenhancement (*arrowhead*) due to CMV colitis.

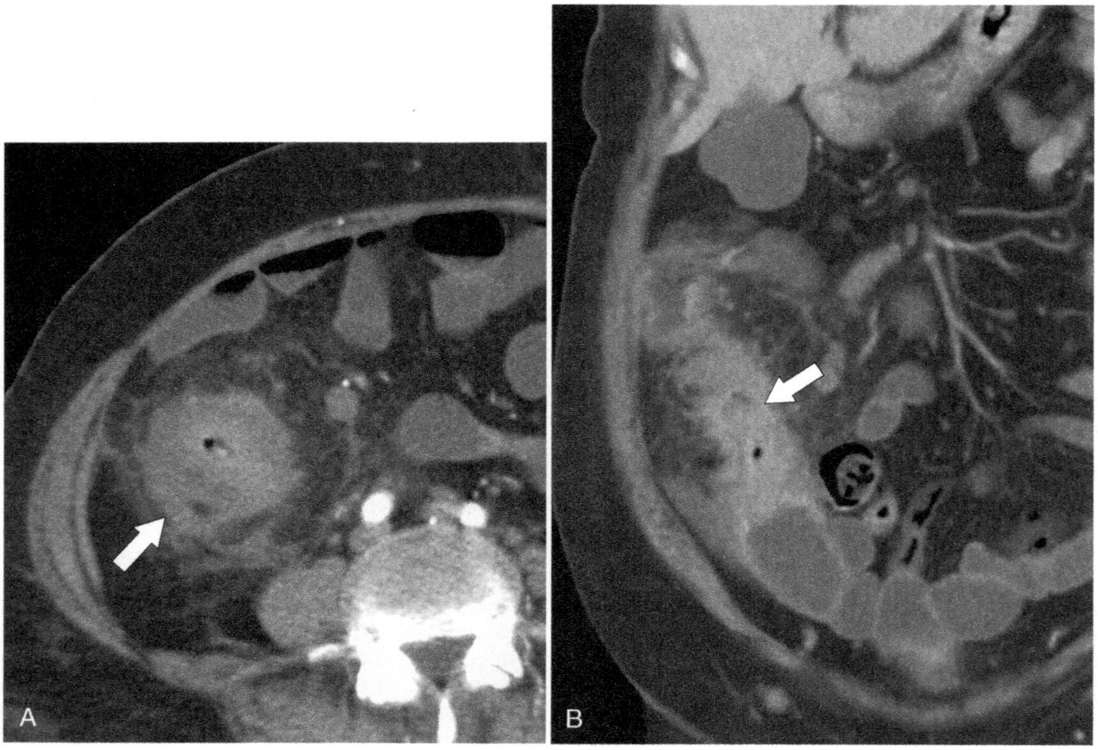

FIGURE 5-54. Axial (**A**) and coronal (**B**) contrast-enhanced CT in a 31-year-old woman with marked colonic wall thickening and irregularity (*arrows*) and pericolonic inflammation or (stranding) due to acute colitic tuberculosis.

latter stages of acquired immunodeficiency syndrome (AIDS). It can also be a multisystem disease, often producing multiple enlarged hypoattenuating nodes in the abdomen and retroperitoneum. MAI can be difficult to distinguish from the more common forms of TB but should be strongly considered in a patient with AIDS.

TB most commonly affects the ileocecal region when involving the GI tract. In the acute phase, there is an edematous thick-walled inflammatory mass of the terminal ileum and cecum, which can be identified at BE or CT imaging (Fig. 5-54). Because TB is a chronic disease, there may be fibrotic changes with contraction and distortion of colonic mucosa and wall, producing focal right-sided colonic strictures (Fig. 5-55). The fibrotic process may cause a fixed, distorted, or narrowed cecum, a so-called coned cecum (Fig. 5-56; Table 5-4). CT usually demonstrates associated regional adenopathy.

Actinomyces

Actinomyces is a gram*-positive anaerobic bacterium, recognized by characteristic sulfur granules on histological examination. It normally resides in the GI tract but can become invasive in patients debilitated by other disease or surgery. It is more commonly observed in the lungs or the endometrium, particularly in patients using intrauterine contraceptive devices. This predisposes patients to *Actinomyces* endometritis, which can develop into a more florid tuboovarian abscess.

In the bowel, *Actinomyces* usually occurs in the appendix or cecum, although any part of the GI tract may be affected. Acute disease leads to ulceration and multiple small and larger abscess formation, which can be recognized by CT (Fig. 5-51). As the disease progresses, numerous small sinus tracts can develop, and the healing process with the granulation tissue can cause stricture formation.

*Hans C. Gram (1850-1938), Danish bacteriologist.

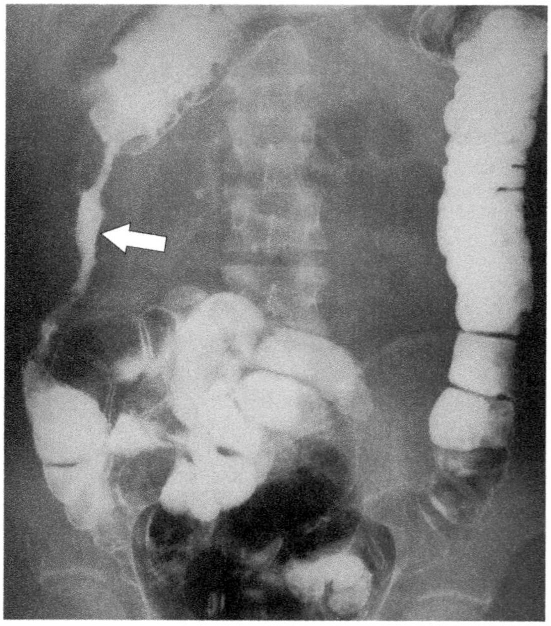

FIGURE 5-55. BE in a 37-year-old man with an ascending colon stricture (*arrow*) and irregular lumen due to colonic tuberculosis.

Amebiasis

Amebiasis is primarily a colonic disease, usually of the right side of the colon, caused by the protozoan *Entomoeba histolytica*, which is endemic in the developing world but rarely seen in the West. Patients are infected through oral ingestion of the amebic cysts, which dissolve in the distal small bowel colon, releasing a trophozoite that then invades the colonic mucosa. This causes an inflammatory, usually focal, response with hyperemia and

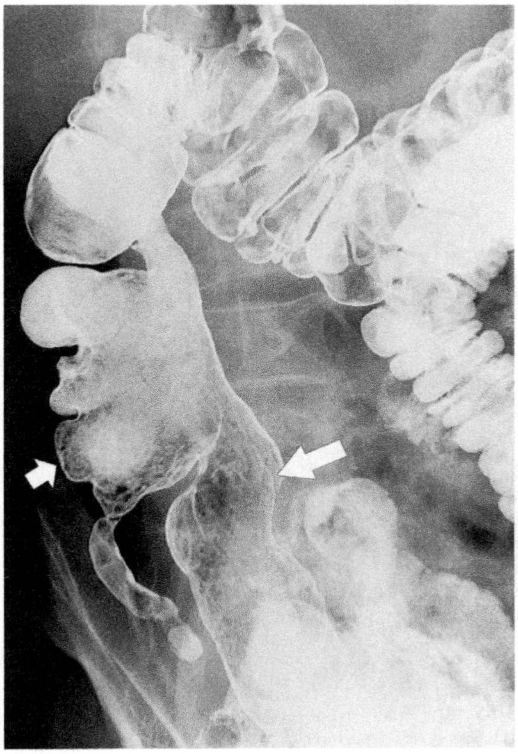

FIGURE 5-56. BE in a 39-year-old man with marked distortion of the cecum (coned cecum) (*small arrow*) and terminal ileum (*arrow*) due to chronic ileocecal TB.

TABLE 5-4 Causes of Coned Cecum

Type	Disease
Infectious	Amebiasis Tuberculosis Actinomycetes
Inflammation	Crohn disease Adjacent appendiceal disease
Neoplastic	Adenocarcinoma Lymphoma

edematous mucosa. Eventually, ulceration occurs and further extension of the disease results in an ameboma, a relatively large mass that develops from a granulomatous reaction to the infestation. This can cause luminal narrowing, can appear similar to colon carcinoma, and is a recognized cause of colonic obstruction. Amebae can then infest the liver and are a well-recognized cause of hepatic abscess with an "anchovy paste" color at percutaneous drainage.

The imaging features are not specific to amebiasis and include mucosal thickening, sometimes severe with "thumb-printing" (Fig. 5-57). The disease may progress to toxic megacolon. Unless amebiasis is considered, the disease may be mistakenly diagnosed as IBD, which has a very different treatment regimen. The diagnosis is readily made by identifying stool cysts or by antibody detection at serological testing. Amebomas are recognized at CT as heterogeneous masses, either single or multiple, and are one of the recognized causes of a "coned" cecum, in which the cecum takes on the shape of an inverted cone because of circumferential diffuse inflammation. Other causes of a coned cecum are listed in Table 5-4.

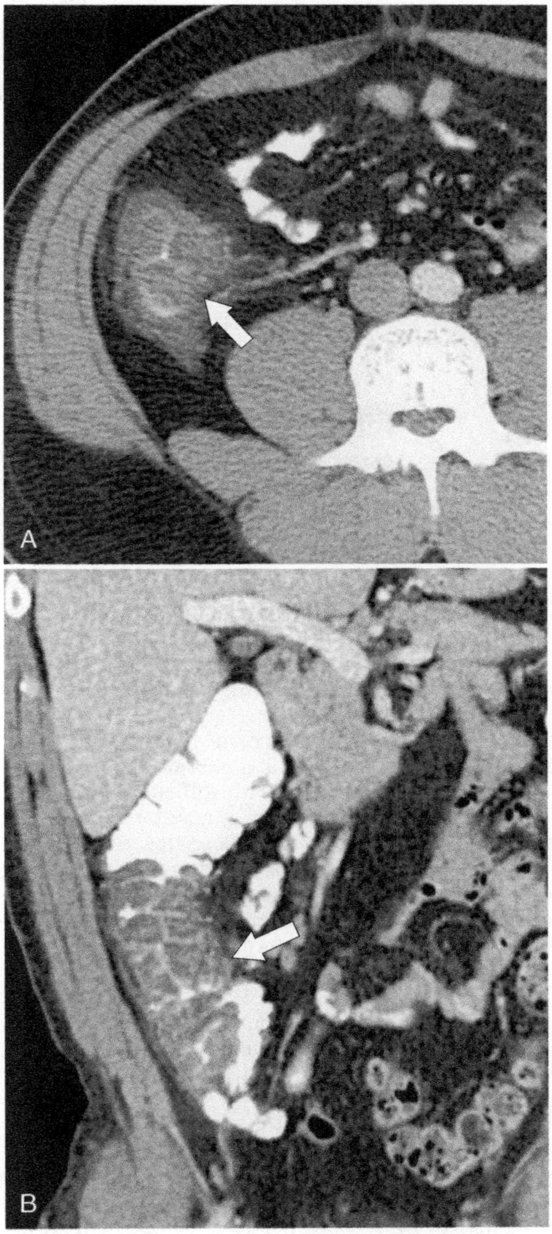

FIGURE 5-57. Axial (**A**) and coronal (**B**) contrast-enhanced CT in a 33-year-old man with cecal mucosal thickening (*arrows*) due to amebic colitis.

Colonic Schistosomiasis

Colonic schistosomiasis is usually due to *Schistosoma mansoni* or *Schistosoma hematobium* (rather than *Schistosoma japonicum*), which can infect the genitourinary tract and liver, but chronic infection can result in granulomatous polyps, particularly in the rectosigmoid region. Pericolonic abscess may form, resulting in left colonic fibrotic strictures, not dissimilar to UC. Large granulomatous masses (bilharziomas*) can develop, mimicking adenocarcinoma. The diagnosis should be suspected in patients traveling from endemic regions.

Colonic Gonorrhea

Colonic gonorrhea in women arises either from secondary urethral, vaginal, and cervical infection or from direct infection

*Theodore Maximilian Bilharz (1825-1862), German physician.

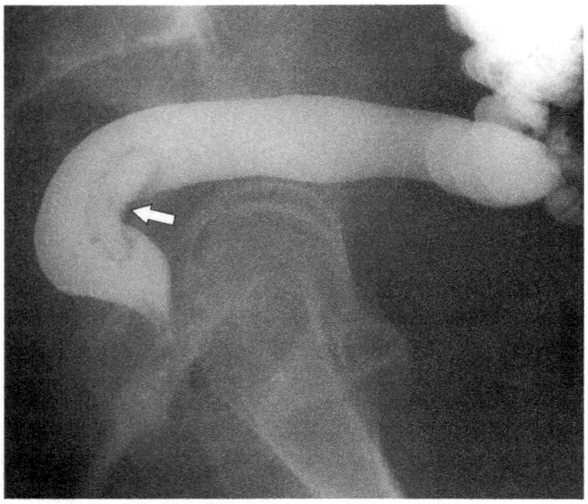

FIGURE 5-58. BE in a 51-year-old man with an anterior rectal wall solitary rectal ulcer (*arrow*).

during anal intercourse. In men, it almost always results from direct anal intercourse. The rectal mucosa becomes inflamed and may show small ulcerations, which may mimic UC. Infection with *Campylobacter* sp. may have similar appearances.

Solitary Rectal Ulcer Syndrome

Solitary rectal ulcer syndrome is a chronic benign disorder of unknown cause but associated with difficulty with defecation and repetitive straining. Therefore it may be related to trauma or localized ischemia. The rectal ulceration occurs mostly on the anterior rectal wall. Some patients present with hyperemic mucosa or broad-based polyps rather than ulcers. The disease is thought to be part of a spectrum with colitis cystica profunda, particularly the nonulcerating forms. The diagnosis is usually made by direct visualization, but the rectal ulceration or polyps can be visualized at BE (Fig. 5-58). The ulcers or polypoid masses are to be distinguished from early rectal cancer. There is often associated rectal mucosal prolapse because of the straining associated with the condition, which can be identified with defecography.

Lymphogranuloma Venereum

A sexually transmitted disease, lymphogranuloma venereum (LGV) affects the rectal lymphatics and is caused by the bacterium *Chlamydia trachomatis*. It mostly causes marked inguinal lymphadenopathy, which may suppurate, but when it involves the rectal region, it causes ulceration, abscess, fistula, and stricture formation (Fig. 5-59).

Postinflammatory Strictures and Coned Cecum

Approximately 10% of patients with UC develop colonic strictures in the chronic phase, although usually they do not obstruct the colon. Stricture formation can be focal (Fig. 5-17) or involve a relatively long length of bowel. Stricture formation is more common, however, with Crohn disease, primarily because the disease process involves the full thickness of the bowel wall, unlike UC. These strictures are asymmetrical and can be multiple (Fig. 5-60). Radiation and ischemic colitis can heal by fibrosis and secondary stricture formation.

A coned cecum refers to a conical cecal shape that results from the inflammatory and fibrotic response to a number of limited right lower quadrant diseases (Table 5-4). The most common cause worldwide is TB (Figs. 5-56 and 5-61) and in the West is Crohn disease (Fig. 5-62). Occasionally, neoplastic infiltration of the cecum produces a coned cecum (Fig. 5-63).

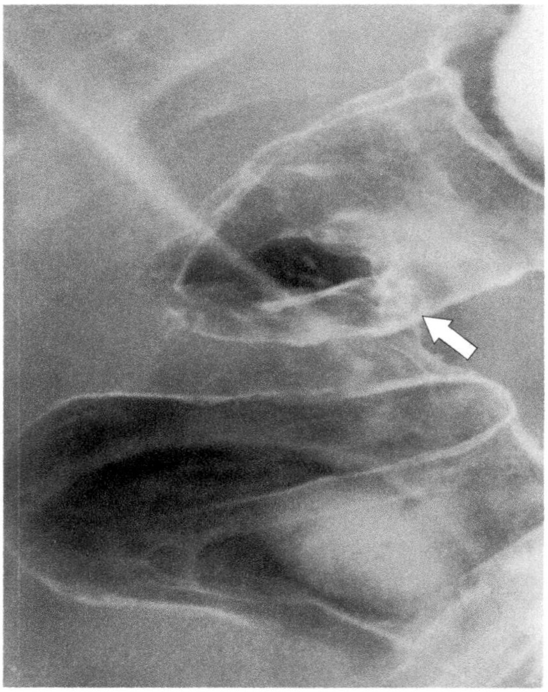

FIGURE 5-59. BE in a 33-year-old man with irregular rectal irregularity (*arrow*) and stricture formation due to lymphogranuloma venereum.

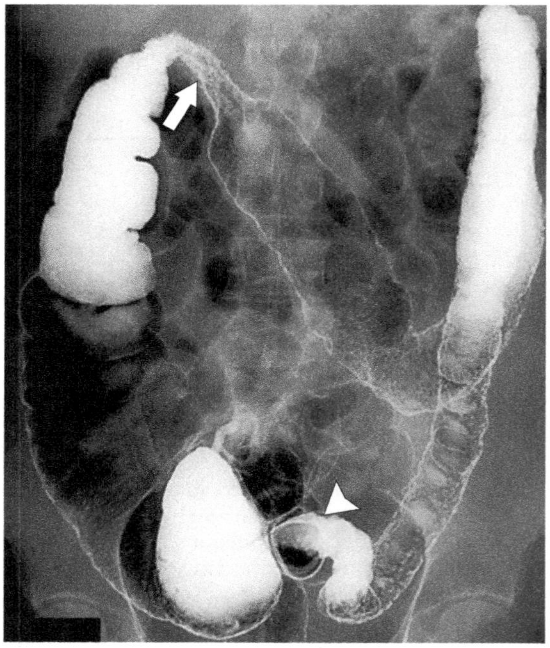

FIGURE 5-60. DCBE in a 47-year-old woman with transverse colonic rigidity and stricture (*arrow*) due to chronic Crohn disease. There is another stricture in the sigmoid colon (*arrowhead*) representative of a "skip lesion," characteristic of the disease.

Thumb-Printing and Toxic Megacolon

Thumb-printing (Table 5-5) represents severe thickening of colonic haustral folds owing to edema, hemorrhage, or malignancy. The term derives from the observation on plain radiography that the haustral thickening resembles a thumb-print (Figs. 5-34 and 5-64). The CT equivalent feature is the accordion pattern (Fig. 5-52). Thumb-printing is most commonly secondary to IBD, either Crohn disease or UC, but is also commonly caused by infectious

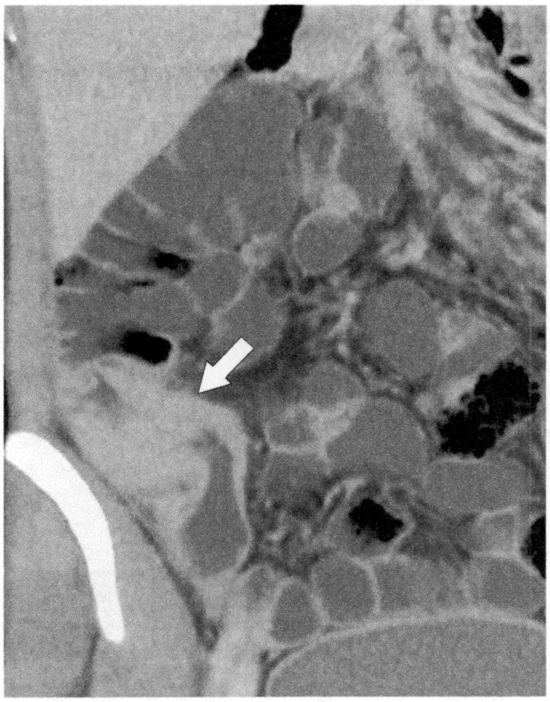

FIGURE 5-61. Coronal contrast-enhanced CT in a 44-year-old woman with terminal ileal and cecal wall thickening (*arrow*) producing a "coned cecum" due to ileocecal tuberculosis.

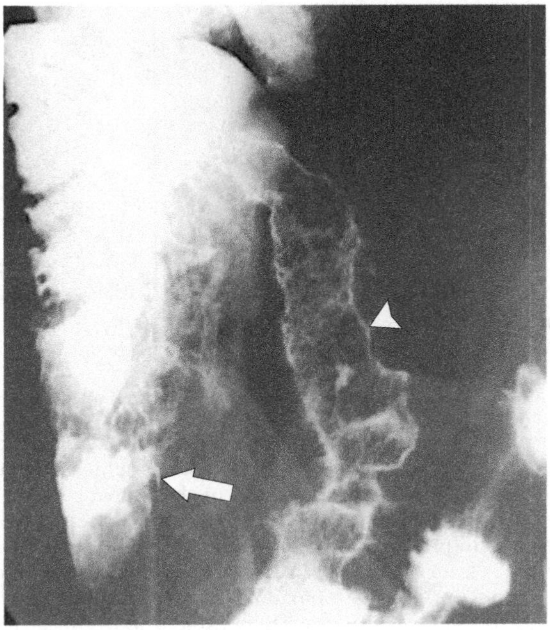

FIGURE 5-62. Small bowel follow-through in a 46-year-old man with acute terminal ileitis (*arrowhead*) and a "coned" cecum (*arrow*) due to Crohn disease.

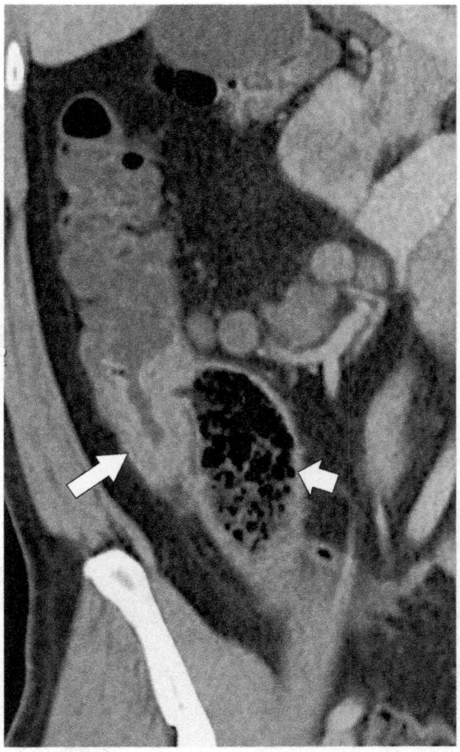

FIGURE 5-63. Coronal CT in a 78-year-old man with a cecal carcinoma (*arrow*) with a conical appearance and small bowel obstruction as evidenced by small bowel feces sign in the terminal ileum (*small arrow*).

TABLE 5-5 Causes of Diffuse Haustral Thickening (Thumb-Printing)

Type	Disease
Inflammatory bowel disease*	Crohn disease Ulcerative colitis Behçet disease
Ischemia*	Usually atherosclerotic disease and/or cardiac disease
Neutropenic colitis	Typhlitis
Infectious colitis*	*Clostridium difficile* colitis Cytomegalovirus Amebiasis Strongyloidosis Bacillary dysentery Typhoid Cholera
Neoplasm lymphoma	Lymphoma Adenocarcinoma Serosal metastases
Infiltrative	Amyloid

*Also causes of toxic megacolon.

colitides (especially CMV and *C. difficile*). Other, less common causes are listed in Table 5-5. Thumb-printing is most often identified in the transverse and proximal descending colon. Many cases resolve spontaneously with or without later stricture formation, but it should be considered a potential prequel to bowel necrosis and colonic perforation and therefore a potential surgical emergency.

Toxic megacolon is a progression beyond simple thumb-printing and is a serious clinical finding, potentially fatal if not treated urgently and appropriately. The diagnosis is usually straightforward when x-ray or CT demonstrates gross colonic distention (often >9 cm), particularly of the transverse colon, which is the most anterior colonic structure in the supine position and readily distends with the nondependent colonic gas. The haustra are markedly thickened and nodular (and some even slough off) and are better appreciated on CT, particularly on "lung window" contrast settings (Fig. 5-64).

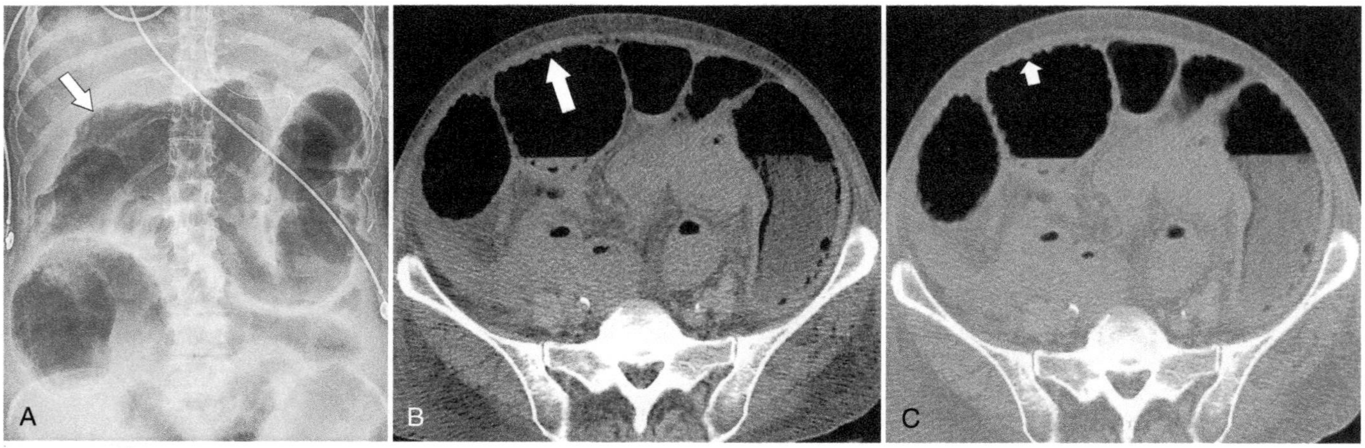

FIGURE 5-64. A through C, Plain radiograph of the abdomen and axial non-contrast-enhanced CT in a 66-year-old woman with toxic megacolon due to ulcerative colitis. There is dilatation of the whole colon with nodular mucosal thickening throughout (*arrows*). The mural nodules are seen to better effect on bone or lung windows (*small arrow*).

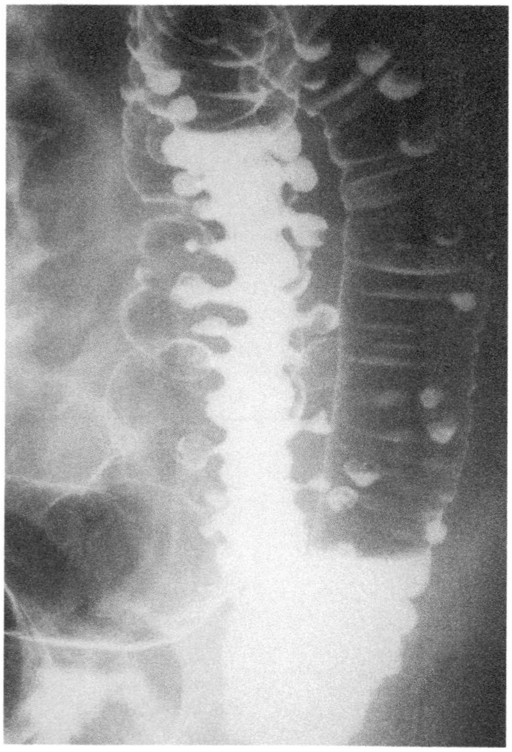

FIGURE 5-65. DCBE in a 70-year-old man demonstrating numerous colonic outpouchings due to diverticula.

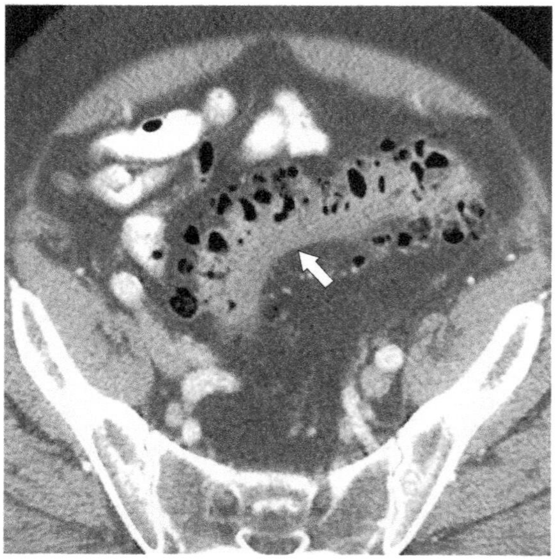

FIGURE 5-66. Axial contrast-enhanced CT in a 60-year-old man with multiple gas-filled sigmoid outpouchings due to marked diverticular disease. There is associated muscular hypertrophy (*arrow*).

Diverticulosis and Diverticulitis

Diverticular disease is common among Westerners (affecting the majority of the elderly) but far less common in developing nations. It is thought to be secondary to less roughage in the diet with a resultant higher intraluminal colonic pressure, although this theory has recently been disputed. Herniations of colonic submucosa penetrate through areas of wall weakness created by the incoming vasculature (vasa recta). They are most common in the rectosigmoid area, thought to be due to its higher intraluminal pressure and smaller luminal diameter (as per LaPlace's* law), but can occur anywhere along the colon. In most patients they go unnoticed and are asymptomatic, even when muscular hypertrophy, bowel wall thickening, and spasm occur from chronically raised intraluminal pressure. In some patients, however, the colonic spasm causes repeated bouts of abdominal pain.

At imaging, diverticula are readily identified by either contrast enema technique (Fig. 5-65) as numerous gas- or contrast-filled outpouches from the normal colonic wall. With CT the diverticula are easy to identify (Fig. 5-66). There is no pericolonic edema in simple diverticulosis. Mucosal hypertrophy and a focally thickened colonic wall are often present (Fig. 5-66). Sometimes the diverticula are isolated and few in number and can be difficult to differentiate from small mucosal polyps at BE, especially if viewed end on. Polyps and diverticula, however, can be differentiated using the "bowler hat" sign at BE. With polyps, the apex of the bowler hat points into the lumen if viewed en face (i.e., sideways) (Fig. 5-67), whereas if the apex points outward from the colonic wall, it represents a diverticulum (Fig. 5-68). If viewed end on, polyps and diverticula can be almost impossible to differentiate from one another. Here the outer margin with a barium ring can help because a sharper outer barium margin suggests a diverticulum, whereas a less well-defined border suggests a polyp. Furthermore, when barium pools in the colon, polyps are less

*Pierre-Simon Laplace (1749-1827), French mathematician.

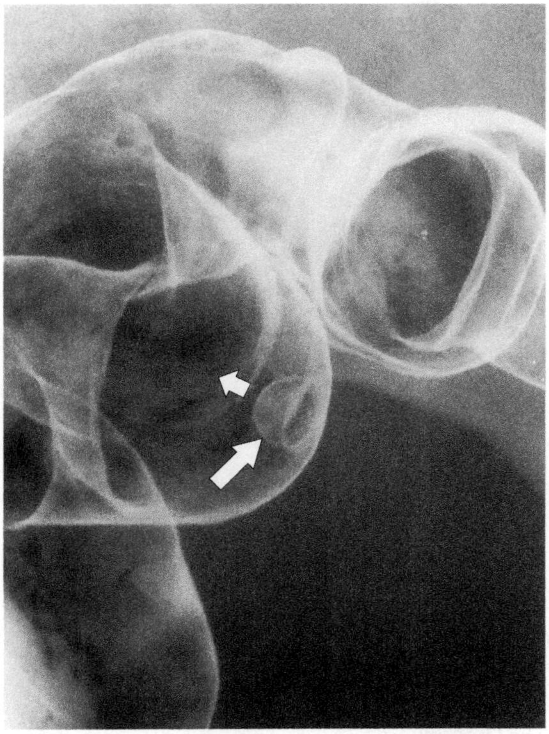

FIGURE 5-67. DCBE in a 55-year-old man with a colonic polyp and bowler hat sign (*long arrow*). The apex of the bowler hat points toward the colonic lumen (*short arrow*).

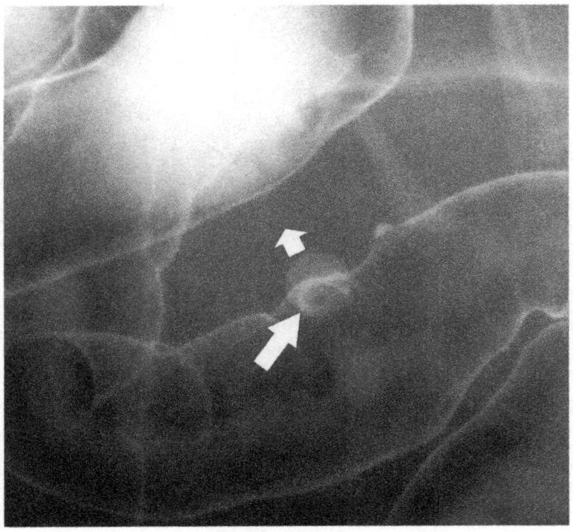

FIGURE 5-68. DCBE in a 70-year-old woman and a bowler hat sign (*arrow*), where its apex points out from the colonic lumen (*short arrow*), consistent with a diverticulum.

dense within the pool (negative shadow), and they do not show fluid levels when the patient is upright, as do diverticula. Very large diverticula are termed "giant diverticula." They are uncommon, but characteristic on plain radiography or CT (Fig. 5-69).

Although simple diverticula are of little significance for the majority of patients, some may develop diverticulitis in a mode similar to the development of appendicitis in the appendix. A stool pellet becomes impacted in a diverticulum and sets up a local inflammatory reaction and often a microperforation. The resulting inflammatory changes lead to colonic spasm with luminal narrowing, wall thickening, and pericolonic edema (stranding) (Figs. 5-70 and 5-71). These findings can be subtle

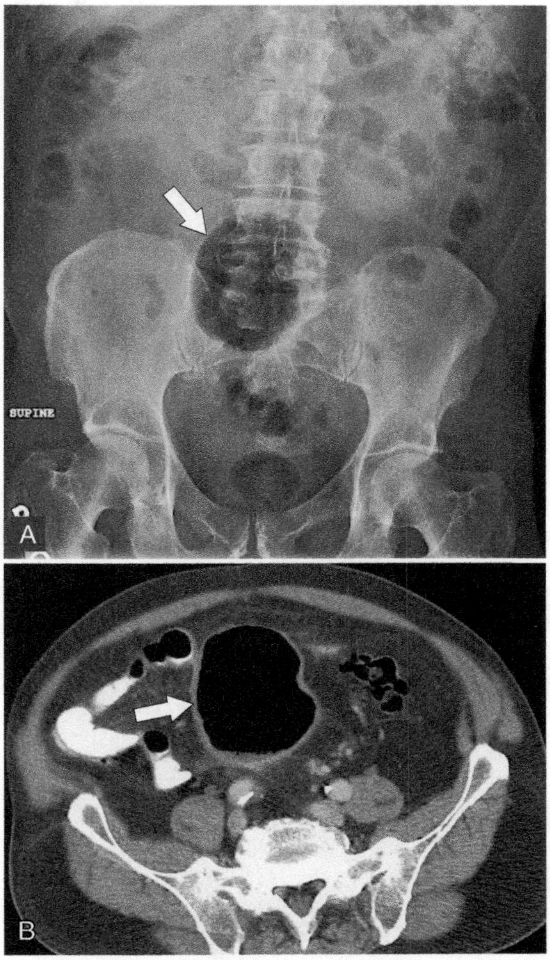

FIGURE 5-69. Plain abdominal radiograph (**A**) and axial contrast-enhanced CT (**B**) in a 70-year-old man with a rounded, gas-filled central abdominal structure (*arrows*) due to a giant diverticulum.

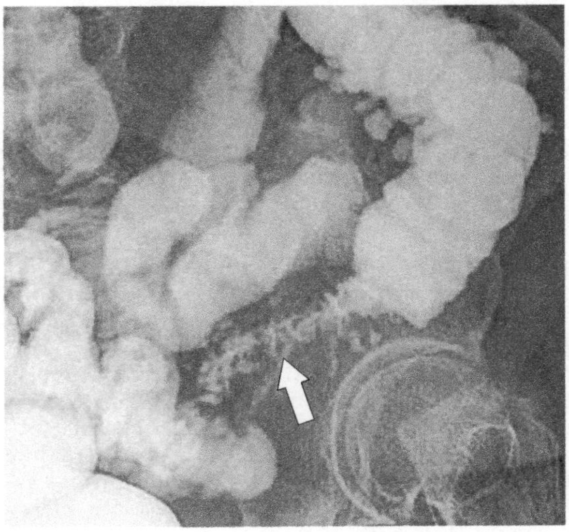

FIGURE 5-70. BE in a 66-year-old woman with diverticular disease and spasm (*arrow*) in the lower descending colon due to diverticulitis.

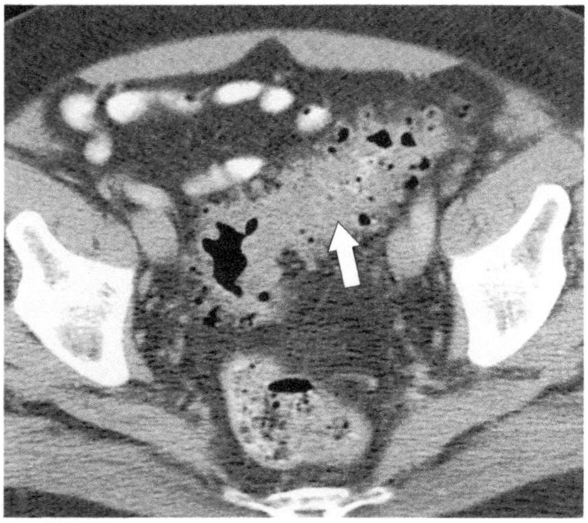

FIGURE 5-71. Axial contrast-enhanced CT in a 72-year-old man with multiple sigmoid diverticula and wall thickening (*arrow*) due to diverticulitis.

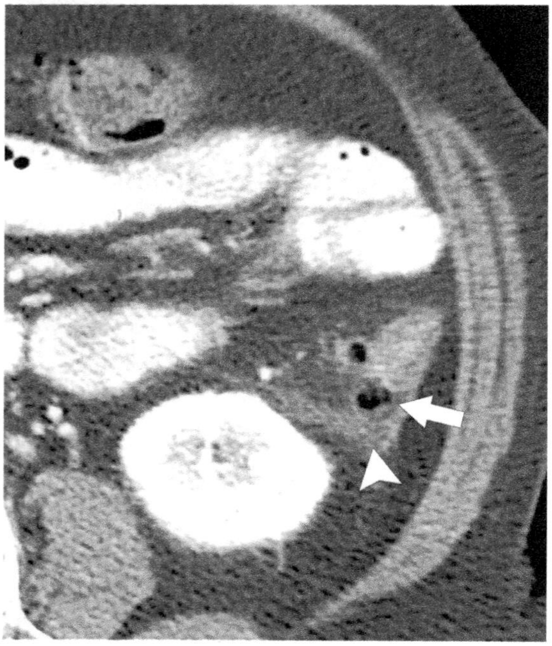

FIGURE 5-72. Axial contrast-enhanced CT in a 70-year-old man with descending colon diverticula (*arrow*) and mild pericolonic edema (stranding) (*arrowhead*) due to mild diverticulitis.

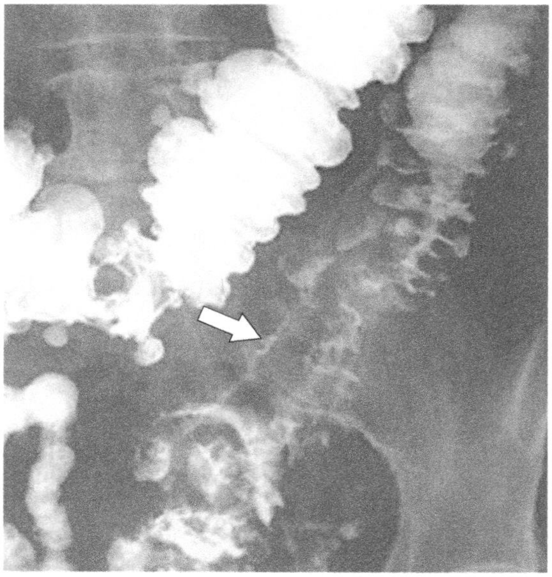

FIGURE 5-73. Single-contrast BE in a 70-year-old woman with multiple diverticula, distal descending colon stricture formation due to diverticulitis, and pericolonic "tram-tracking" (*arrow*) of contrast due to perforation from diverticulitis.

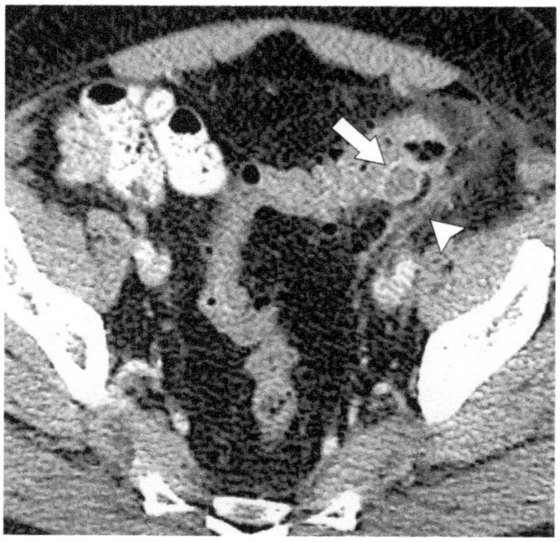

FIGURE 5-74. Axial contrast-enhanced CT in a 56-year-old man with sigmoid wall thickening, pericolonic edema (stranding) (*arrowhead*) due to diverticulitis, and a small pericolonic abscess (*arrow*).

and confined to one diverticulum or multiple (Fig. 5-72). The inflammatory reaction may cause a larger local perforation, which can be identified at BE by contrast tracking outside the colonic lumen, often in a linear "tram-track" fashion (Fig. 5-73). The perforation, however, is preferably imaged by CT and visualized as a linear gas pocket or fluid collection outside the colonic wall, representing an abscess, which can be either small or large, depending on the degree of perforation (Fig. 5-74). More distant effects may include mesenteric and portal venous gas and hepatic abscess formation after seeding via the mesenteric venous system (Fig. 5-75). Larger abscesses generally do not respond to antibiotic treatment alone, and percutaneous image-guided catheter placement is often required.

Hemorrhage is relatively common with diverticulitis because of mural inflammation and vascular erosion with consequent rectal bleeding, which at times can be profuse, requiring emergency surgery to prevent further profound blood loss. This occurs more frequently with the less commonly observed right-sided diverticula (Fig. 5-76). Severe diverticulitis can cause such an inflammatory reaction that fistulas with adjacent bowel, bladder, or vagina can form. This can be observed with BE (Fig. 5-77), but because of the risk of peritoneal barium leakage (although slight) and the greater ease of CT imaging, it is better evaluated by CT (Fig. 5-78). Giant diverticula are also at risk of diverticulitis (Fig. 5-79) and its complications (hemorrhage, abscess, and fistula formation).

On occasion, an attack of diverticulitis can mask an underlying adenocarcinoma (Fig. 5-80), and the radiologist should always consider the possibility of underlying colon cancer in the presence of diverticulitis. Features that suggest an underlying malignancy include a short segmental mass, shouldering (abrupt cutoff of colonic wall thickening), a large mass, pericolonic soft tissue

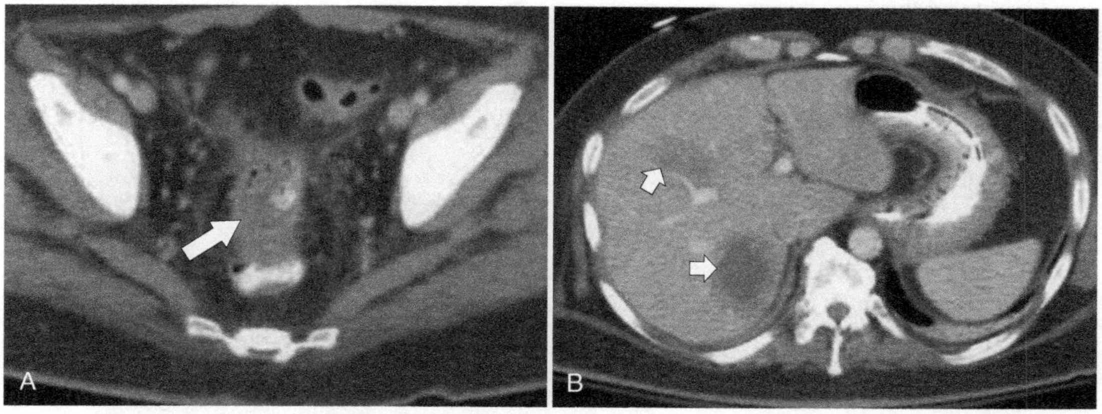

FIGURE 5-75. A and B, Axial contrast-enhanced CT in a 56-year-old man with pelvic diverticulitis (*arrow*) and two liver abscesses (*small arrows*) secondary to mesenteric seeding from the pelvic infection.

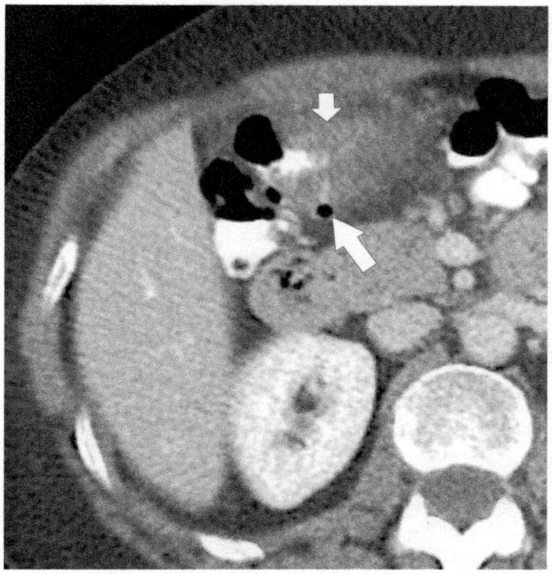

FIGURE 5-76. Axial contrast-enhanced CT in a 52-year-old man with thickening of the ascending colon (*short arrow*) and pericolonic edema (stranding) due to right-sided diverticulitis. A single diverticulum is identified (*long arrow*).

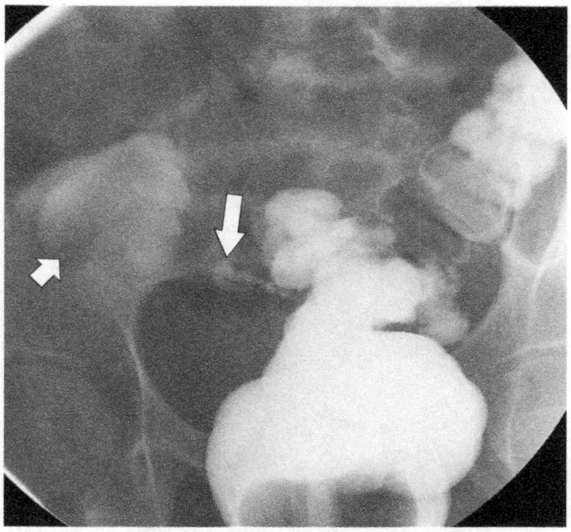

FIGURE 5-77. Single contrast BE in a 56-year-old woman with sigmoid narrowing due to diverticulitis and a colocolonic fistula (*arrow*) connected to the cecum (*small arrow*).

extension of the mass, and regional lymphadenopathy. In practice, it can be very difficult to differentiate between the two (Figs. 5-71 and 5-80), and the radiologist should have a relatively low threshold for recommending repeat imaging after antibiotic treatment or follow-up endoscopy.

Epiploic Appendagitis

Epiploic appendagitis is an uncommon inflammatory process of the colonic epiloic appendices, which are peritoneal globule-like fatty appendages attached to the serosal colonic wall. These can undergo torsion or venous infarction, become inflamed, and cause acute abdominal pain, not unlike diverticulitis, appendicitis, or cholecystitis. Epiploic appendagitis is more commonly left sided, and so the main clinical differentiation is with diverticulitis. The appearances at CT imaging are diagnostic with a small (between 1 and 4 cm) fat density lesion surrounded by a circular (Fig. 5-81) or oval (Fig. 5-82) inflammatory ring. Its recognition is important because it is a self-limiting disease and does not require surgery.

Colonic Polyps

Adenomatous Polyps

Adenomatous polyps are relatively common (incidence between 10% and 30% of the population, increasing with age). Most develop spontaneously and arise in the rectosigmoid region. They are far less commonly associated with congenital disease (Table 5-6). They are classified into tubular (most common), villous, and tubulovillous. More recently, a variant of villous and tubulovillous adenomas has been described as the serrated adenoma. Tubular polyps occur anywhere in the colon, whereas villous lesions are more common in the rectosigmoid region. Their main significance is that all adenomatous polyps are premalignant. The risk of malignancy increases as the proportion of villous change increases, so tubular polyps have the least risk of developing adenocarcinoma and villous the most. This is known as the adenoma-carcinoma sequence, which takes approximately 10 years to develop in the colon (the risk is highest in the stomach). In the colon the risk is low (approximately 5%) for polyps less than 1 cm, increasing to 10% for adenomas between 1 and 2 cm and 50% for tumors greater than 2 cm. Polyps themselves are usually asymptomatic but may present with pain, diarrhea, and rectal bleeding. Rarely, larger villous

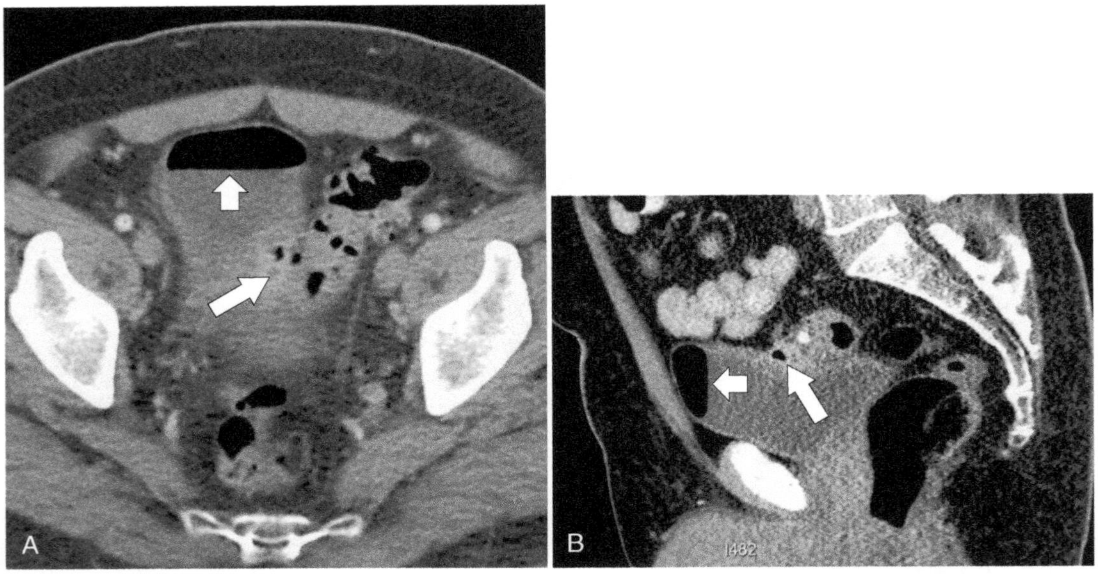

FIGURE 5-78. Axial (**A**) and sagittal (**B**) contrast-enhanced CT in a 58-year-old man with diverticulitis (*arrows*) with fistulization to the bladder and intracystic gas (*small arrows*).

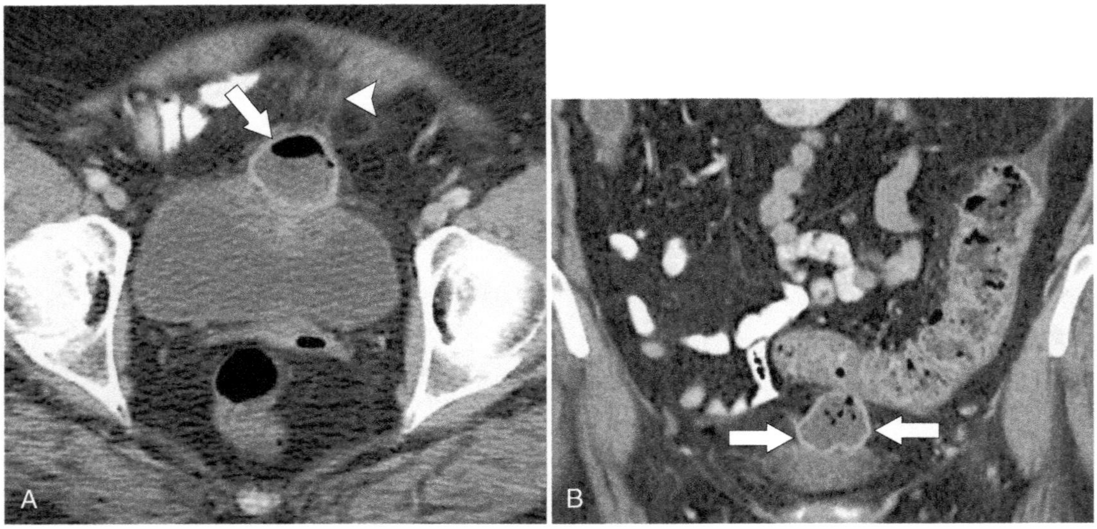

FIGURE 5-79. Axial (**A**) and coronal (**B**) contrast-enhanced CT in a 71-year-old woman with a giant diverticulum (*arrows*) of the sigmoid colon with mild diverticulitis as evidenced by slight mesenteric inflammation (stranding) (*arrowhead*).

polyps can cause profuse mucus-like diarrhea and hypokalemia or intussusception.

Because of the well-recognized risk that polyps will transform into adenocarcinoma, colonic screening with fecal occult blood after the age of 40 years and colonoscopy after the age of 50 years are recommended to reduce the incidence of colorectal cancers in the general population. Computed tomographic colonoscopy (CTC) has performed well in clinical trials compared with optical colonoscopy, although the latter is performed far more often. However, substantial numbers of the population are still not screened, and it is hoped that CTC might increase the number of patients who undergo colonic screening to prevent the development of larger polyps and malignant degeneration. Once a polyp is discovered by CTC, the patient is referred for optical colonoscopy and polyp removal.

The primary imaging investigation for colonic abnormalities was formerly DCBE but has now been largely superseded by optical colonoscopy. However, the imaging features are well described. Good colonic preparation and fluoroscopic technique are critical to reduce the number of false-positive findings, primarily because of stool residue. This requires good distention at DCBE and multiple views to evaluate the whole colonic wall. Polyps are recognized as filling defects, and the larger they are, the better they are appreciated. As with any contrast fluoroscopic technique, once an abnormality is detected, it is vital to take spot views in multiple planes to maximize the radiologist's ability to classify the lesion. All features of the polyps can be identified, from sessile to pedunculated. Tubular adenomatous polyps usually have a smooth surface with or without polypoid features and are pedunculated (i.e., arise from a stalk). This stalk can be hard to identify unless orthogonal views are obtained, which will increase the chance of its detection. The stalk can be short (Fig. 5-83) or long (Fig. 5-84). When the tubular stalk is seen end-on, a characteristic "Mexican hat" sign is noted, representing the outer ring of the polyp and the inner ring of the stalk (Fig. 5-85). Most tubular polyps are not identified with conventional CT but can be with CTC (Fig. 5-86).

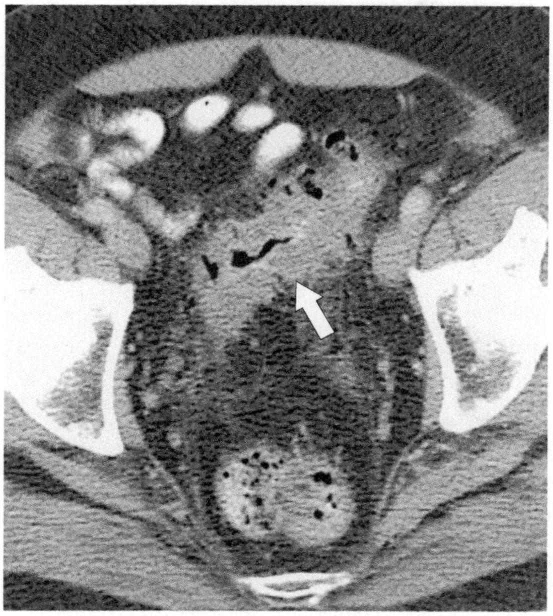

FIGURE 5-80. Axial CT with contrast with multiple sigmoid diverticula, diffuse wall thickening (*arrow*), and mild pericolonic edema consistent with diverticulitis. Colonoscopy also identified an underlying adenocarcinoma.

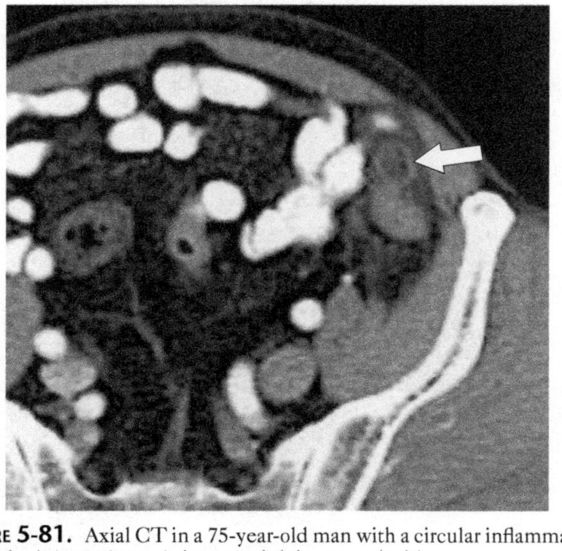

FIGURE 5-81. Axial CT in a 75-year-old man with a circular inflammatory paracolonic mass (*arrow*) due to epiploic appendagitis.

Sessile polyps are typically radiolucent when visualized on the dependent wall but when on a nondependent wall may demonstrate a barium-coated barium ring. A "bowler hat" sign, representing the base and tip of the polyp, may be seen when the polyp is viewed en face or side on (Fig. 5-66). Most sessile polyps larger than 5 mm can be detected with CTC (Fig. 5-87).

Villous polyps are almost always sessile and are usually multilobulated (frond or cauliflower like) on DCBE (Fig. 5-88) or CTC (Fig. 5-89). They can be carpet like where they "coat" the mucosal lining (Fig. 5-90). Tubulovillous polyps are a combination of tubular and villous adenomas and so have a stalk of variable length and a villous frond-like tip. Adenomatous polyps are occasionally detected by CT or MRI (Fig. 5-91), but most are not unless they are large enough (Fig. 5-92) or unless FDG avidity (some adenomas are hypermetabolic) points the radiologist to what was otherwise thought to be normal bowel (Fig. 5-93).

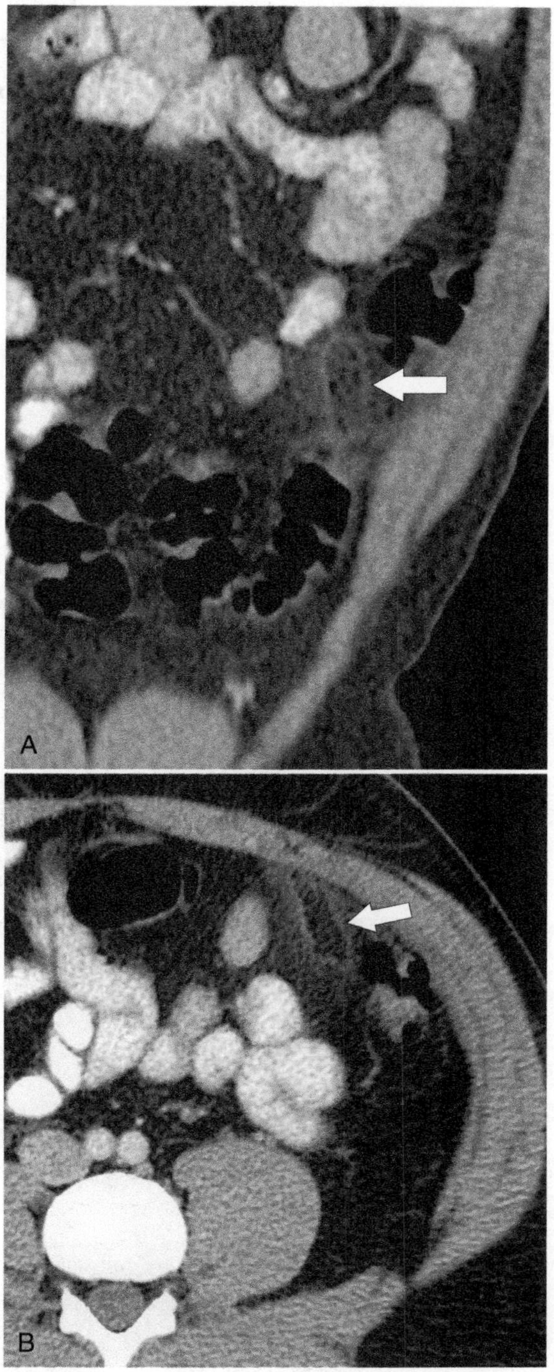

FIGURE 5-82. Coronal (**A**) and axial (**B**) contrast-enhanced CT in a 33-year-old man with an ovoid inflammatory mass (*arrows*) adjacent to the descending colon due to epiploic appendagitis.

Mismatch Repair Cancer Syndrome (Turcot Syndrome)

Mismatch repair cancer syndrome, or Turcot* syndrome, is an inherited disorder in which genetic mutations, primarily of *MSH1* and *MSH2* genes (the same genes as those of Lynch syndrome; see below), cause a DNA mismatch repair. Adenomatous polyps develop in patients, who are at high risk of developing adenocarcinoma of the colon and cerebral glioma.

*Jacques Turcot (1914-1977), Canadian surgeon.

TABLE 5-6 Colonic Polyps

Type	Malignant Potential	Subtype
Adenoma	Yes	Spontaneous (common) Congenital (uncommon) Mismatch repair cancer syndrome (Turcot) Hereditary nonpolyposis colorectal cancer (Lynch syndrome) Familial polyposis Gardner syndrome
Hamartoma	Yes	Juvenile polyposis Peutz-Jeghers syndrome Cronkhite-Canada syndrome
Hyperplastic	No	
Inflammatory	No	Usually secondary to ulcerative colitis

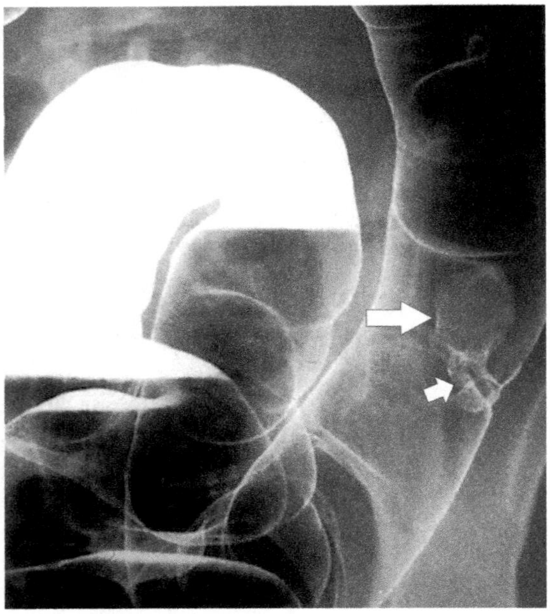

FIGURE 5-83. DCBE in a 53-year-old man with a tubular adenoma (*arrow*) with a short stalk (*short arrow*).

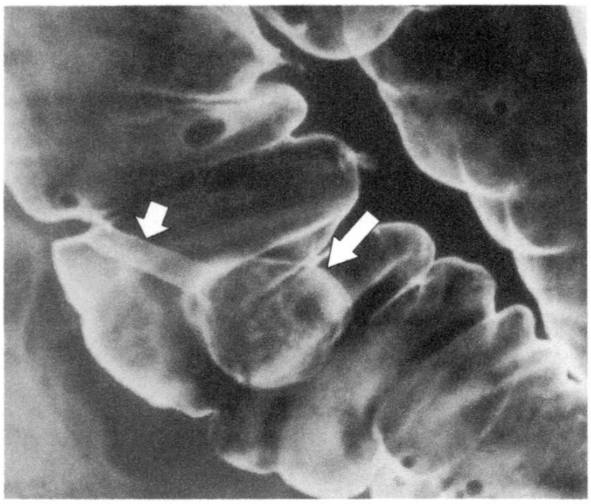

FIGURE 5-84. DCBE in a 59-year-old man with a tubulovillous (*arrow*) polyp in the ascending colon. The stalk is observed originating from the lateral wall (*small arrow*).

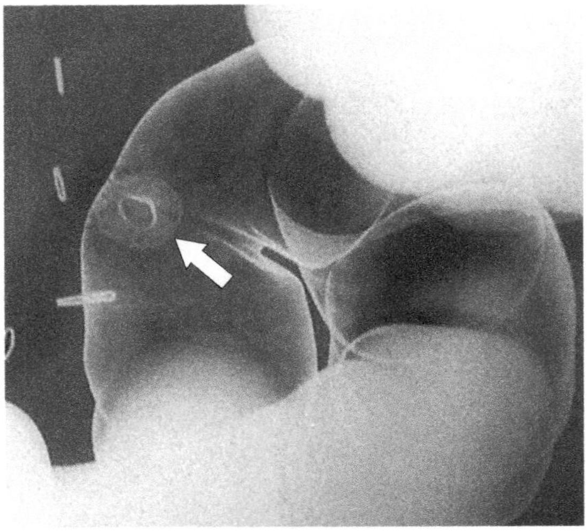

FIGURE 5-85. DCBE in a 64-year-old woman with a "Mexican hat" sign from a polyp observed end on (*arrow*). Surgical clips from prior surgery are visualized.

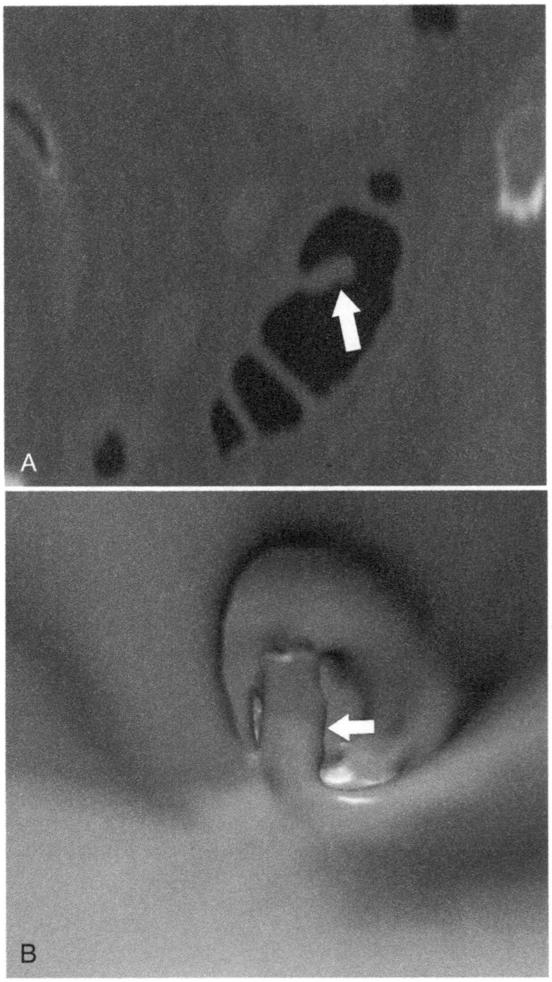

FIGURE 5-86. A and B, CTC in a 53-year-old woman with a tubular colonic polyp (*arrows*). *See ExpertConsult.com for color image.*

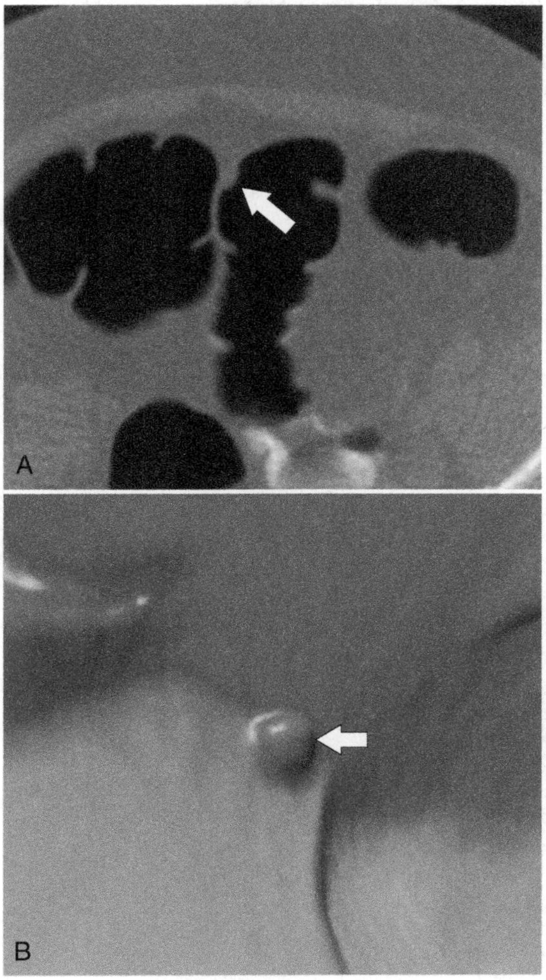

FIGURE 5-87. **A** and **B**, CTC in a 51-year-old man with a sessile polyp (*arrows*). *See ExpertConsult.com for color image.*

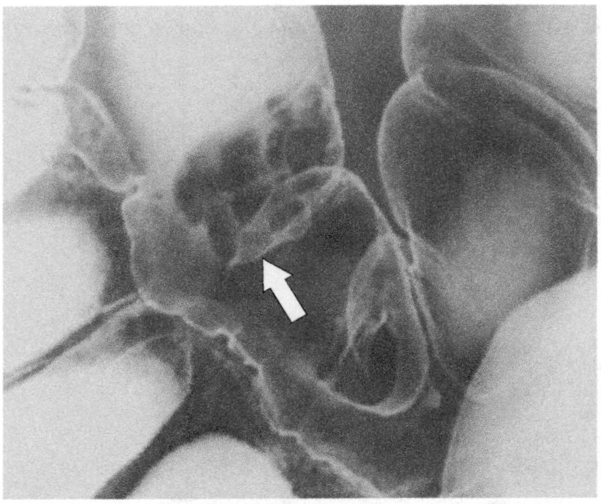

FIGURE 5-88. DCBE in a 66-year-old man with a hepatic flexure villous adenoma (*arrow*).

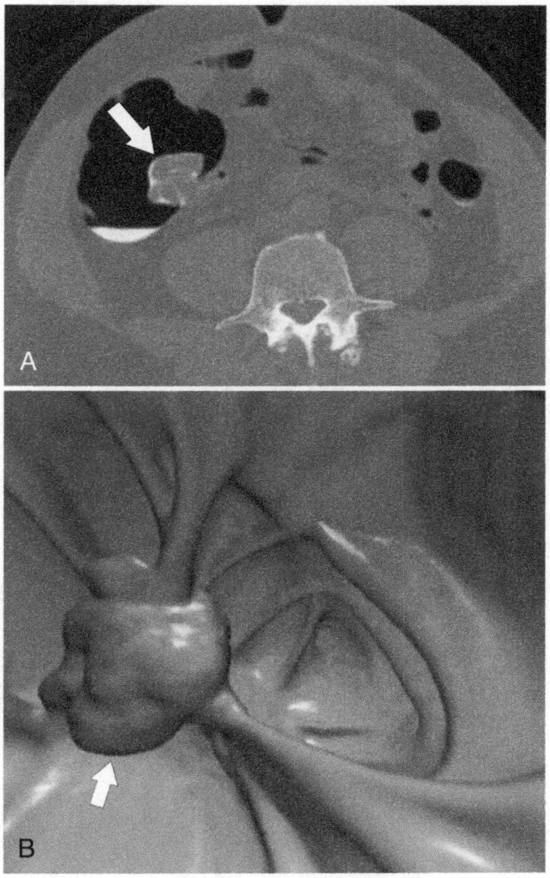

FIGURE 5-89. **A** and **B**, CTC demonstrating a villous adenomatous polyp (*arrows*). *See ExpertConsult.com for color image.*

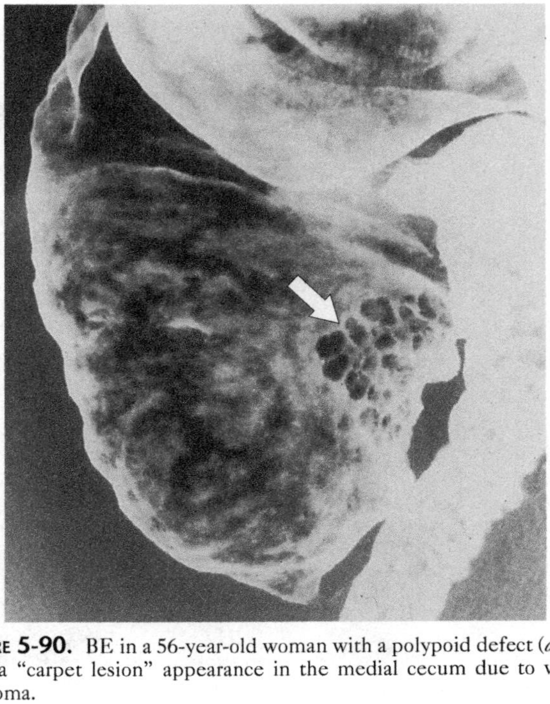

FIGURE 5-90. BE in a 56-year-old woman with a polypoid defect (*arrow*) with a "carpet lesion" appearance in the medial cecum due to villous adenoma.

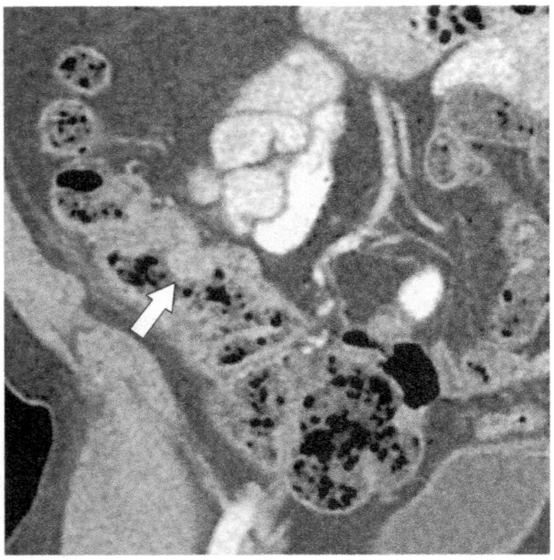

FIGURE 5-91. Coronal contrast-enhanced CT in a 55-year-old man with a medial ascending colon villous polyp (*arrow*).

Hereditary Nonpolyposis Colorectal Cancer—Lynch Syndrome

Hereditary nonpolyposis colorectal cancer, or Lynch* syndrome, is an autosomal-dominant disease caused by a DNA mismatch repair from a variety of genetic mutations, mainly the *MSH2* gene. Adenomatous polyps develop in patients, placing them at a high (80% lifetime) risk of colorectal cancer. Cancer occurs mostly in the proximal colon, but also in the stomach and small bowel, ovary, endometrium, brain, hepatic, renal tract, and skin.

Hyperplastic Polyps

Hyperplastic polyps have no malignant potential, although there is a slight increase in concomitant adenomatous polyps (and therefore carcinoma). They are more common in the elderly and usually quite small (2 to 10 mm). They are usually sessile polyps, mostly in the distal colon, and generally cannot be distinguished from small sessile adenomatous polyps. However, larger right-sided hyperplastic polyps may be associated with serrated adenomatous polyps, which do have malignant potential. Because they

*Henry T. Lynch (1928-), American physician.

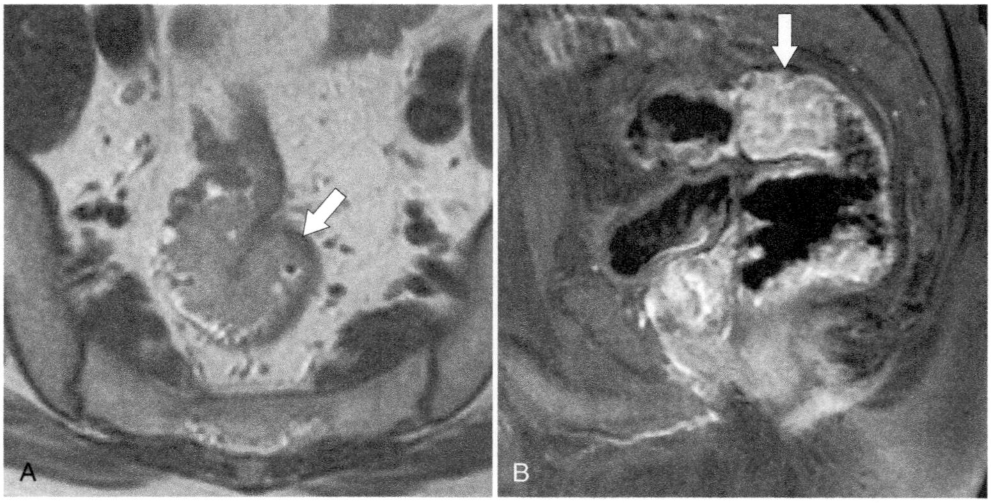

FIGURE 5-92. Axial precontrast (**A**) and sagittal postcontrast MRI (**B**) in a 51-year-old man with a 3.8-cm enhancing villous polyp at the rectosigmoid junction (*arrows*).

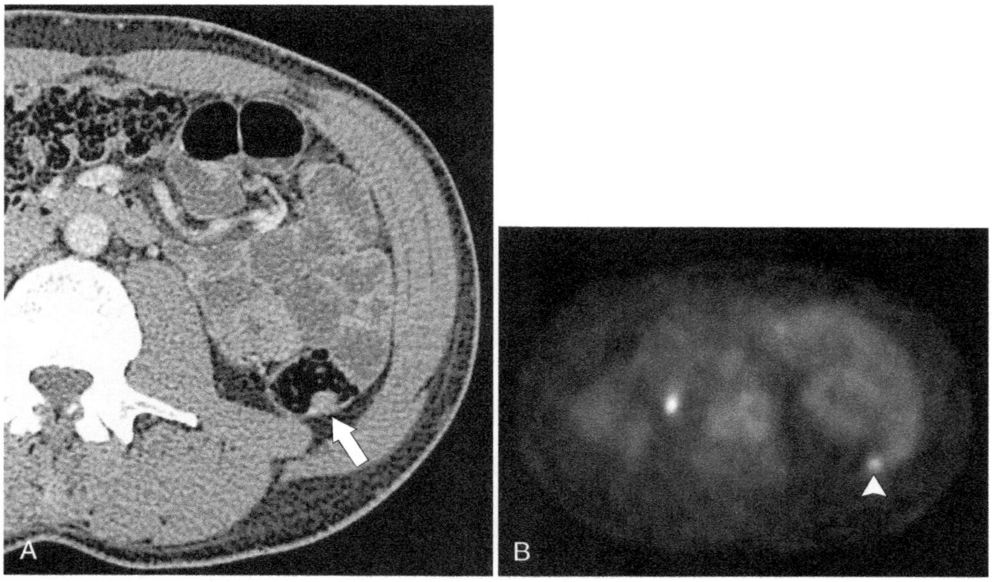

FIGURE 5-93. Axial contrast-enhanced CT (**A**) and PET (**B**) in a 55-year-old woman with a 1-cm villous adenoma of the descending colon (*arrow*) only identified after increased FDG activity (*arrowhead*) was recognized on PET. There is also normal activity in the right ureter.

are small, hyperplastic polyps are almost never seen with CT but can be identified with DCBE, CTC, and OC.

Polyposis Syndromes

Polyposis syndromes represent a variety of inherited disorders (see Chapters 2 and 4), most producing either adenomatous (familial polyposis coli, Gardner syndrome) or hamartomatous (Peutz-Jeghers syndrome, Cronkhite-Canada syndrome, juvenile polyposis, Cowden's disease) polyps. Rarely, neurofibromatosis produces multiple colonic neurofibromas.

Patients with familial adenomatous polyposis (FAP) usually undergo prophylactic colectomy because of the sheer number of colonic polyps, all of which are at risk of malignant transformation. The polyps are readily identifiable by BE, CTC, and OC and may even be found with conventional CT (Fig. 5-94). Detection of malignant transformation can be harder because of the overwhelming number of polyps, which may easily obscure early malignant colon cancer, although larger lesions should be detected (Fig. 5-95).

Gardner syndrome is now considered a variant of FAP because there are numerous colonic adenomatous polyps, but not as many as are observed in FAP. They are more commonly identified in the stomach (unlike those of FAP). The disease is also associated with desmoid tumors, osteomas, epidermoid and sebaceous cysts, fibromas, and thyroid cancer. With imaging, Gardner adenomatous polyps generally cannot be distinguished from those of FAP, except perhaps that they are usually fewer in number (Fig. 5-96).

Other polyposis syndromes can produce hamartomatous colonic polyps, but they are far more common in the small bowel and only very rarely cause colonic polyps (see Chapter 4).

Pseudopolyps

Pseudopolyps are almost exclusively secondary to IBD, particularly UC. They represent edematous mucosa that appears to project into the bowel but really is not a polyp at all. Rather, the second effect of deep ulceration and undermining of adjacent mucosa gives the spurious appearance that the normal mucosa is a polyp. Given that IBD can affect any bowel length, pseudopolyps are often multiple (Fig. 5-8). They are readily observed with CTC (Fig. 5-97).

Pseudoinflammatory Polyps

In similarity to pseudopolyps, pseudoinflammatory polyps are also secondary to IBD, usually occur in the distal colon, and are more common with UC. They represent the healed stage of a pseudopolyp, when the ulcerated portions of the bowel heal by reepithelialization. This also gives rise to the spurious appearance of the polyps, with a filiform rather than a villiform shape. Their features are fairly characteristic, and usually, but not always, they are identified in the left side of the colon, sometimes for a variable length (Figs. 5-11 and 5-17). Concomitant active colitis may or may not be present in other areas of the colon.

Lymphoid Hyperplasia

Lymphoid hyperplasia is usually a normal finding observed with DCBE rather than CT because the polyps are typically only 1 to 3 mm. They are usually adjacent to more concentrated lymphoid

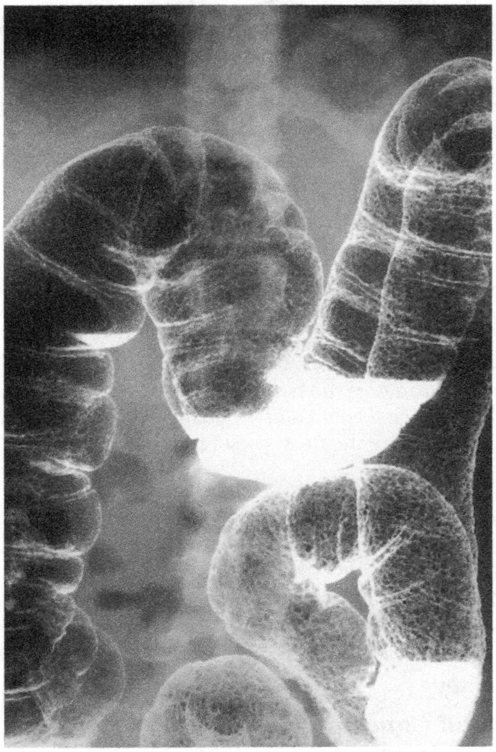

FIGURE 5-94. DCBE in a 38-year-old woman with numerous small, rounded filling defects throughout the colon due to multiple polyposis from familial adenomatous polyposis.

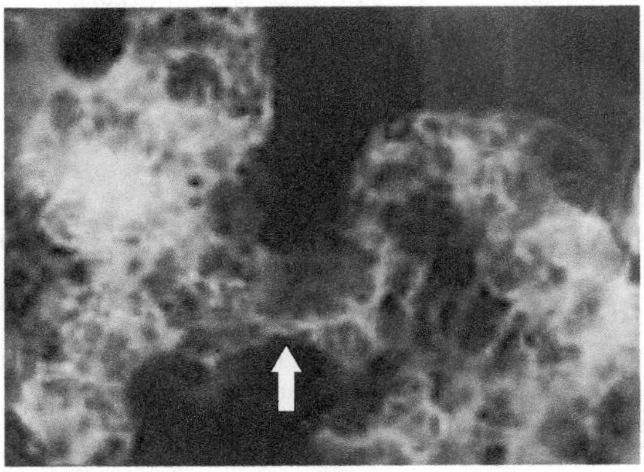

FIGURE 5-95. BE in a 45-year-old man with familial adenomatous polyposis and an annular constricting lesion of the transverse colon (*arrow*) due to adenocarcinoma.

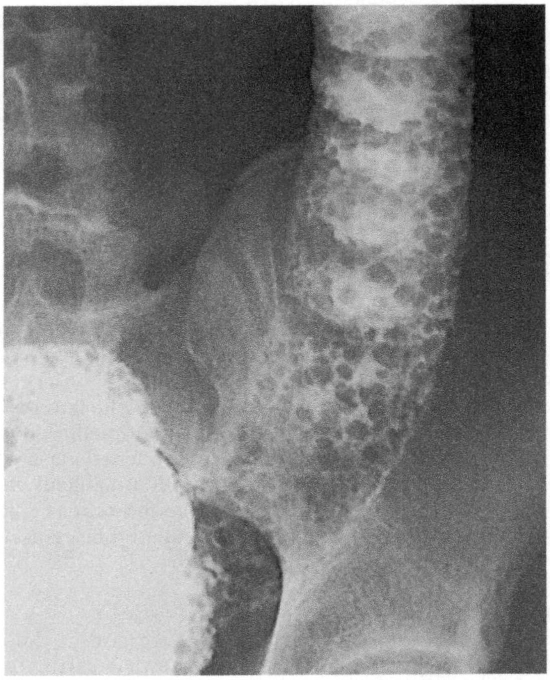

FIGURE 5-96. BE in a 38-year-old man with Gardner syndrome and multiple adenomatous colonic polyps.

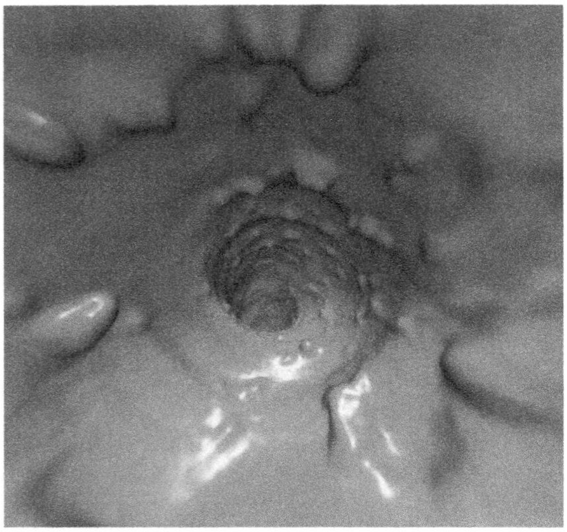

Figure 5-97. CTC in a 38-year-old woman with multiple intraluminal filling defects due to pseudopolyps. *See ExpertConsult.com for color image.*

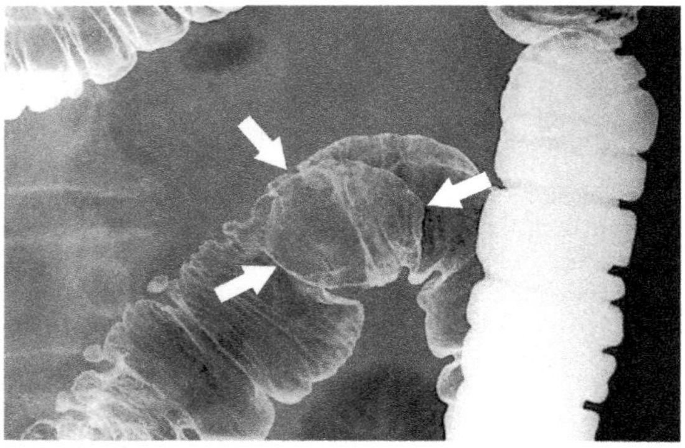

Figure 5-98. DCBE in a 77-year-old man with a smooth filling defect (*arrows*) in the transverse colon due to a lipoma.

areas (i.e., the ileocecal and rectal areas) (see Chapter 4). Sometimes a much larger segment of the colon is affected or even the whole colon, particularly in children, in whom this is a normal variant. Lymphoid hyperplasia has also been identified in giardiasis associated with hypogammaglobulinema. There is no malignant potential.

Other Benign Colonic Neoplastic Lesions

Lipoma

Lipomas are the second most common benign tumors of the colon after adenomas and are usually identified incidentally at abdominal CT imaging performed for other reasons. As elsewhere in the small bowel, they have submucosal appearances at imaging (Fig. 5-98) and may show ulceration of erosions on its surface, which can result in a variable degree of hemorrhage. The latter findings will most likely be identified only with a high-quality DCBE or with optical colonoscopy. The smooth submucosal masses rarely are larger than 4 cm, but many are readily identifiable by their fat density at CT (Fig. 5-99). Sometimes they possess a stalk (Fig. 5-99) or are large enough to act as a lead point for intussusception (Fig. 5-100).

Gastrointestinal Stromal Tumor (GIST)

Gastrointestinal stromal tumors (GISTs) are rare in the colon. They have features similar to the more common gastric or small bowel GISTs, often presenting with an exophytic submucosal

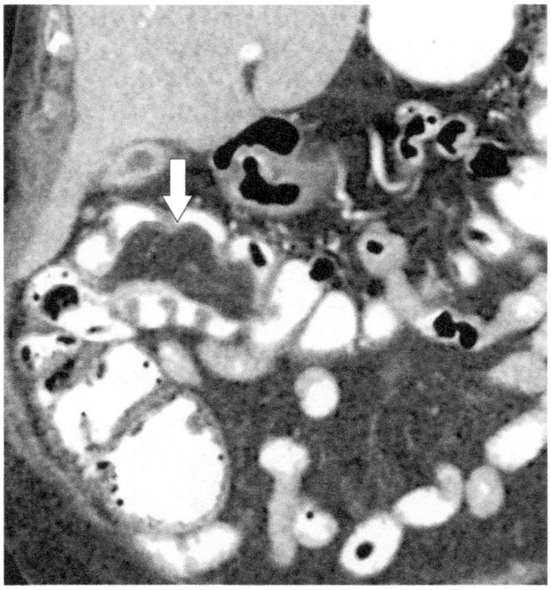

Figure 5-99. Coronal contrast-enhanced CT in a 55-year-old woman with a transverse colonic lipoma with a stalk (*arrow*).

mass (Fig. 5-101) that can be quite necrotic. As they enlarge, GISTs tend to ulcerate through the mucosa and therefore bleed and present with rectal bleeding or anemia.

Hemangioma

An even rarer tumor is the hemangioma, which is most commonly present in the distal colon and is usually multiple. Hemangiomas are characterized by the presence of phleboliths, which should be identifiable by CT.

Carcinoid (see Chapter 4)

Primary carcinoids appear most commonly in the appendix or terminal ileum (approximately 90%) and only rarely in the remaining large bowel, where they are usually confined to the rectum or cecum. Most are benign, asymptomatic, and never detected.

Malignancy

Colorectal Cancer

Colorectal cancer is responsible for up to 1.5 million cases diagnosed annually worldwide with as many as 600,000 deaths. It therefore remains a major killer even though the comprehensive colonic screening widely available in the West (where the disease is most common) could reduce this number to a small fraction. Survival is therefore related to early detection. Once colorectal cancer is detected, survival is predicted by TNM staging (Table 5-7), as defined by the American Joint Committee on Cancer (AJCC) and now less commonly by the Dukes* classification system.

Most tumors (95%) are adenocarcinomas (approximately 5% of tumors are squamous cell), usually mucinous, and develop secondary to the adenoma-carcinoma sequence. All adenomas, whether acquired or congenital, are at risk for the development of adenocarcinoma. Other predisposing factors include IBD (both Crohn disease and UC). There is an increased risk in patients with hamartomatous syndromes (but not because of the hamartoma itself) and rarely in cystic fibrosis. Metachronous and synchronous adenocarcinomas are well recognized. The cumulative risk for metachronous disease (presentation of another tumor at a later date) is approximately 0.3% to 0.5% per year. Risk of synchronous disease (the presence of a second

*Cuthbert Esquire Dukes (1890-1977), British physician and pathologist.

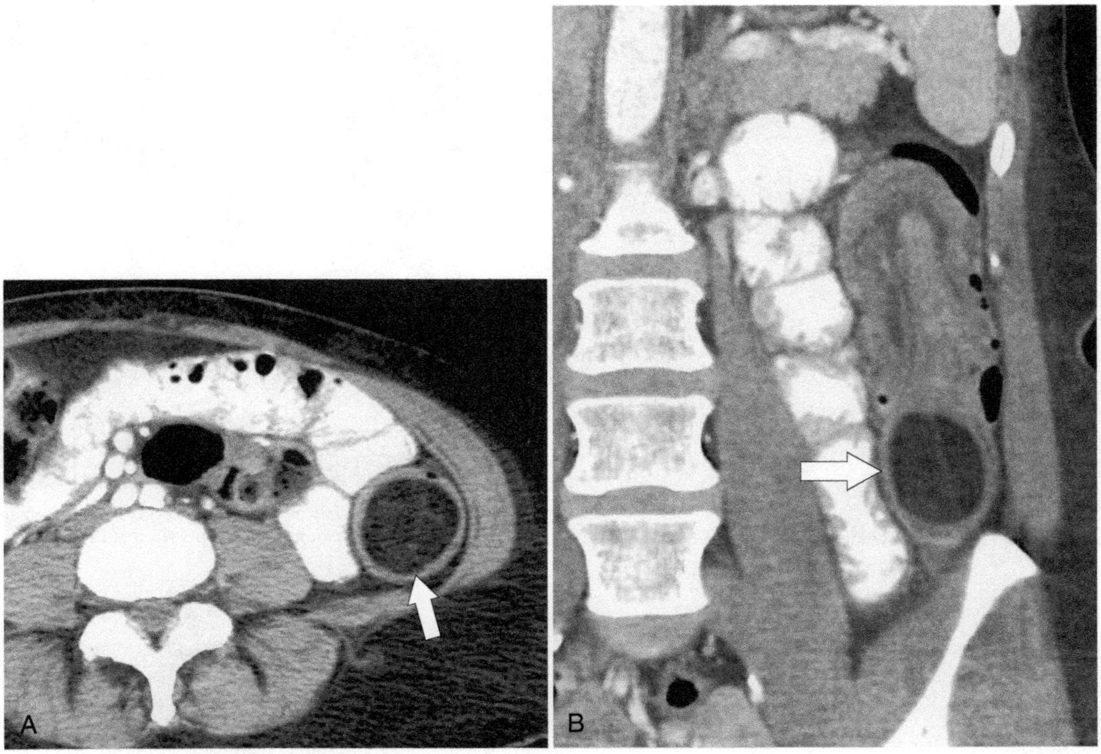

FIGURE 5-100. Axial (**A**) and coronal (**B**) contrast-enhanced CT in a 59-year-old woman with left colonic intussusception to a lipoma acting as the lead point (*arrows*).

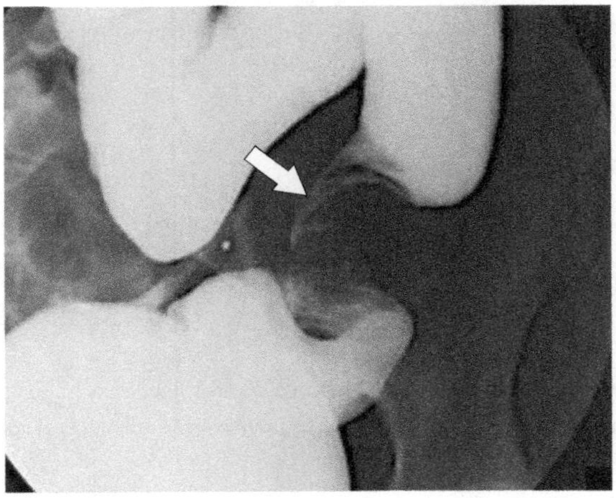

FIGURE 5-101. BE in a 45-year-old woman with a submucosal descending colonic filling defect (*arrow*) due to a benign GIST.

TABLE 5-7 Staging of Colon Cancer

AJCC Stage	TNM Stage	Criteria
0	Tis N0 M0	Confined to mucosa—cancer in situ
I	T1 N0 M0	Submucosal invasion
I	T2 N0 M0	Muscularis propria invasion
II-A	T3 N0 M0	Serosal invasion
II-B	T4 N0 M0	Invades adjacent organs
III-A	T1-2 N1 M0	T1-2 + 1-3 regional nodes involved
III-B	T3-4 N1 M0	T3-4 + 1-3 regional nodes involved
III-C	T1-4 N2 M0	T1-4 + 4 regional nodes involved
IV	T1-4 N1-2 M1	T1-4 N1-2 M1

AJCC, American Joint Committee on Cancer; *T* (*in TNM*), extent of tumor invasion of colorectal wall; *N* (*in TNM*), nearby lymph nodes that are involved; *M* (*in TNM*), distant metastases.

primary adenocarcinoma at the initial primary diagnosis) is approximately 5% (Fig. 5-102).

Squamous cell carcinoma, while representing the minority of colorectal tumors, are mostly found in the rectum. Predisposing factors include HIV and HPV infection and a rare form of rectal cancer arising from the remnant of the cloacal membrane at the anorectal junction. These tumors are usually aggressive and have metastasized at the time of presentation.

The location of the tumor usually dictates patient presentation. Tumors arising from the right side of the colon are more insidious, perhaps because the colon is wider and therefore tumors less often cause obstructive symptoms. This premise does not hold for cecal tumors that involve the ileocecal valve, which can cause early small bowel obstruction (Figs. 5-63 and 5-103). Patients may present with pain, but it is more likely that the tumor will bleed intermittently, often asymptomatically, and that the patients ultimately present with the symptoms of anemia rather than the direct local effects of the tumor. Left-sided colon tumors, in contrast, present more commonly with symptoms of obstruction because luminal narrowing is more prevalent (Fig. 5-104). Occasionally tumors are so indolent that the patient presents with a very large mass that has not yet declared itself with bleeding or obstruction.

Lesions in the rectosigmoid region commonly present with rectal bleeding (often bright red) and a change in bowel habit. They therefore tend to present earlier and consequently are associated with better survival statistics. Rarely tumors from any location in the colon can present because of perforation and peritonitis or abscess formation (Fig. 5-105). A very occasional tumor can present with intussusception, with a predominantly intraluminal mass acting as the lead point (Fig. 5-106).

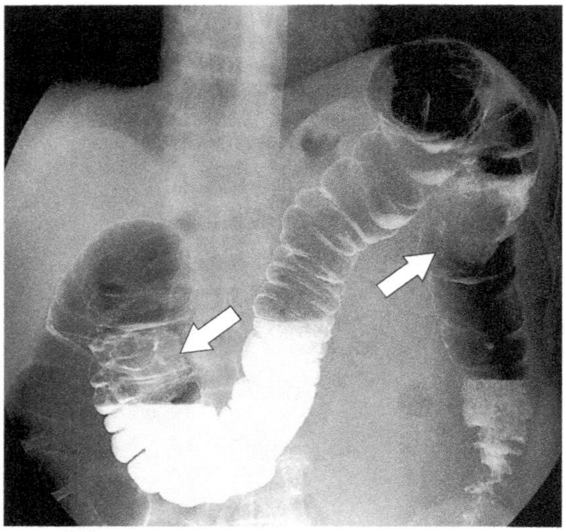

FIGURE 5-102. BE in a 71-year-old woman with synchronous carcinomas of the colon (*arrows*).

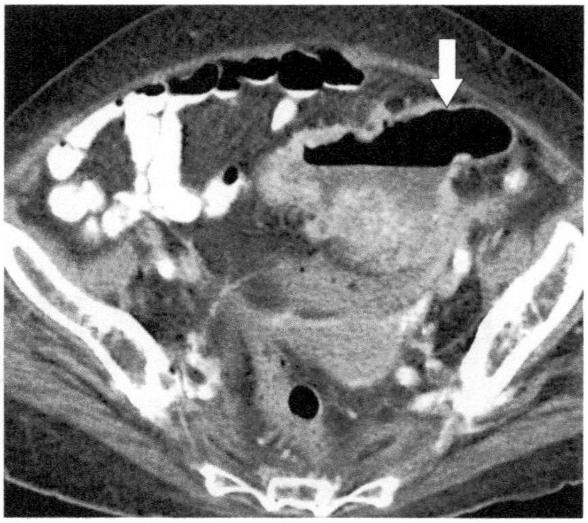

FIGURE 5-105. Axial contrast-enhanced CT in a 66-year-old man with a perforated sigmoid carcinoma and pelvic abscess (*arrow*).

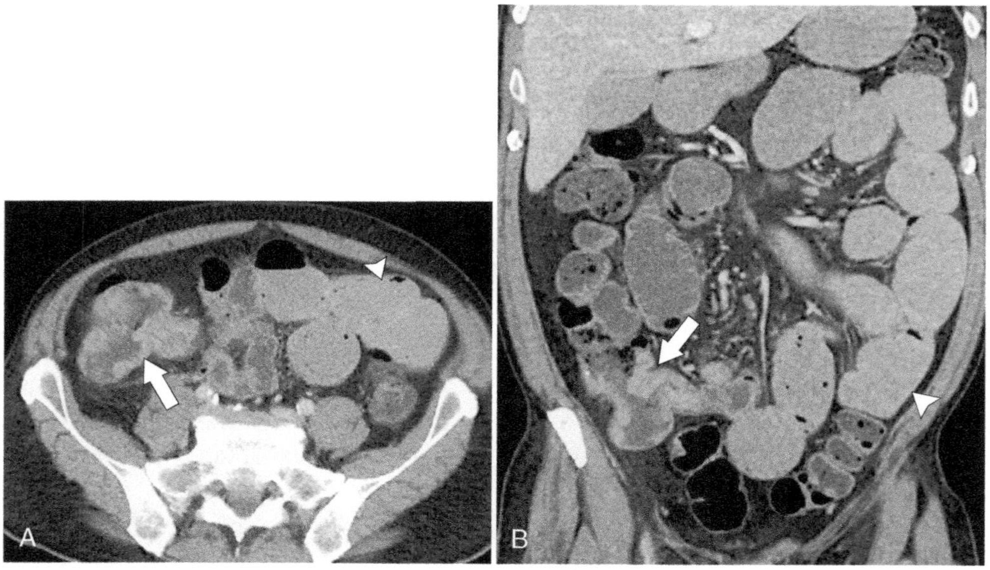

FIGURE 5-103. Axial (**A**) and coronal (**B**) contrast-enhanced CT in a 60-year-old man with small bowel obstruction (*arrowheads*) due to cecal adenocarcinoma (*arrows*).

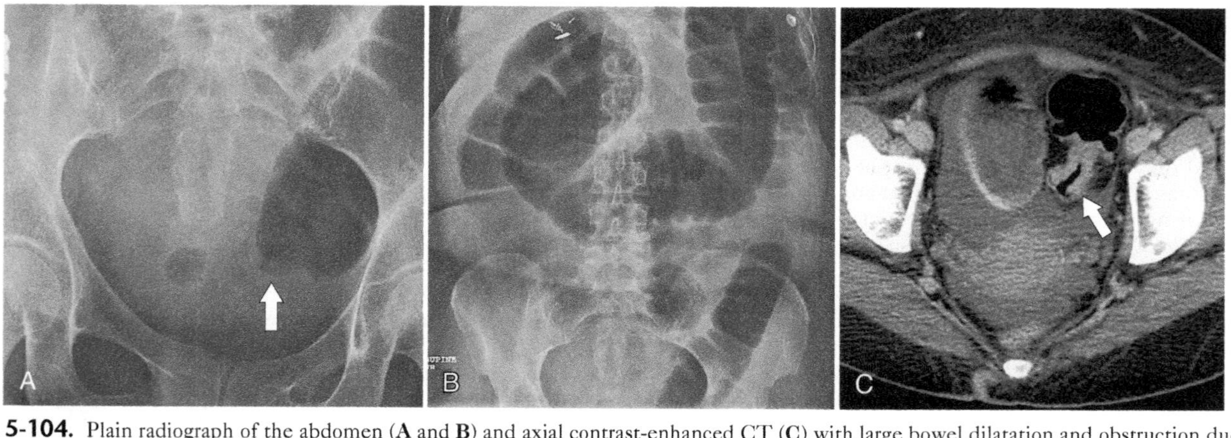

FIGURE 5-104. Plain radiograph of the abdomen (**A** and **B**) and axial contrast-enhanced CT (**C**) with large bowel dilatation and obstruction due to an obstructing sigmoid adenocarcinoma (*arrows*). There is also pelvic ascites.

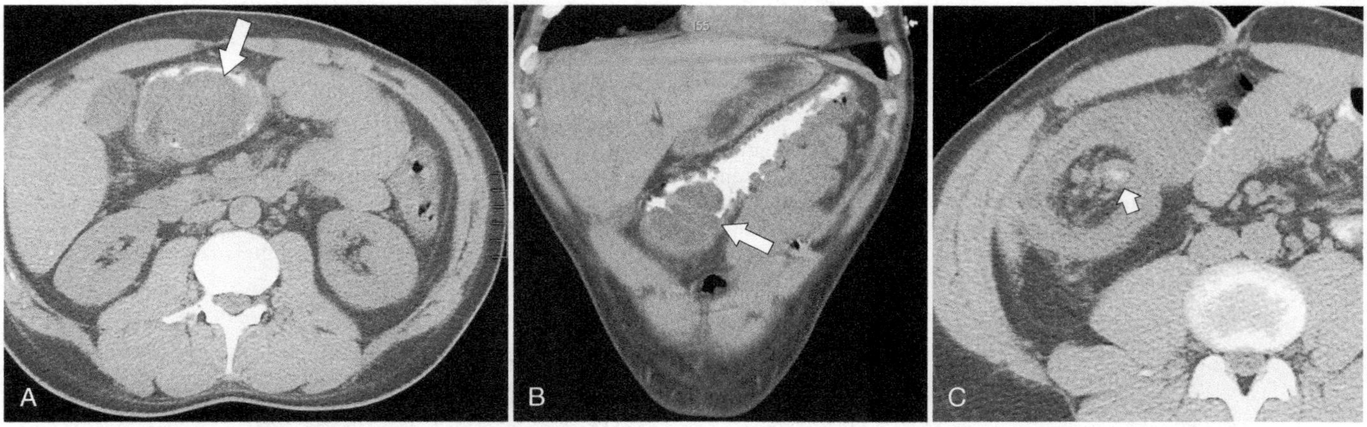

FIGURE 5-106. A through C, Axial and coronal non-contrast-enhanced CT in a 51-year-old man with a polypoid colonic carcinoma (*arrows*) that acts as a lead point for a colocolonic intussusception (*small arrow*).

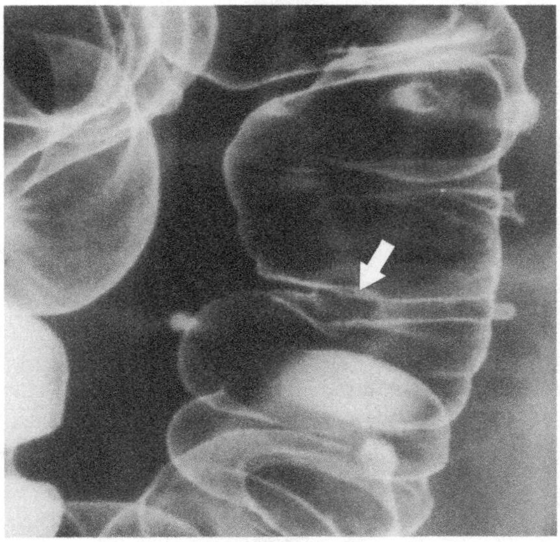

FIGURE 5-107. DCBE in a 73-year-old woman with a small plaque-like mucosal defect (*arrow*) in the left colon due to early colon adenocarcinoma.

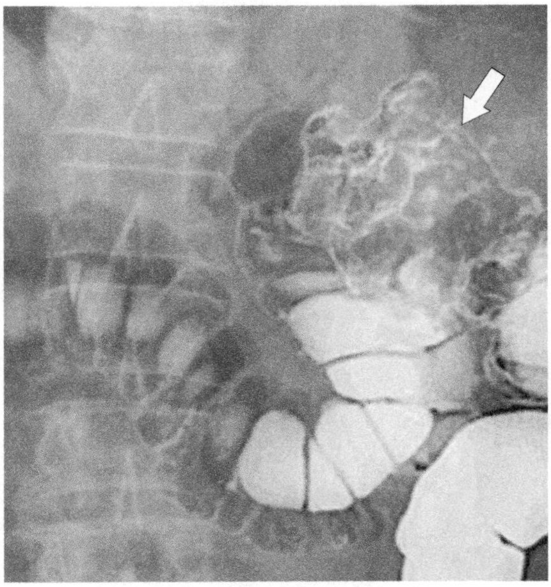

FIGURE 5-108. DCBE in a 67-year-old woman with a large polypoid mass (*arrow*) due to adenocarcinoma of the splenic flexure.

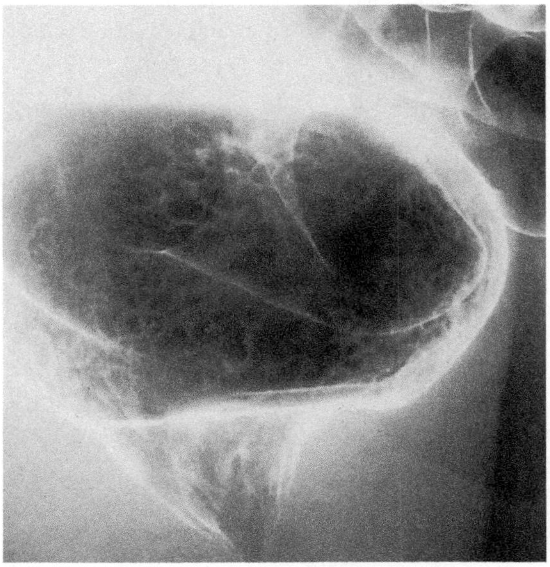

FIGURE 5-109. BE in a 77-year-old man with multiple polypoid rectal filling defects due to a superficial spreading "carpet lesion" from rectal adenocarcinoma.

Characteristics of colorectal cancer lesions at DCBE range from subtle, slightly raised, plaque-like lesions (Fig. 5-107), to smooth or irregular polypoid intraluminal lesions (Fig. 5-108), to "carpet-like" flat nodular lesions (Fig. 5-109). The classic presentation is a circumferential annular constricting appearance, which has abrupt shelf-like margins with mucosal destruction in between (Fig. 5-110). The latter (the so-called apple-core lesion) is the cardinal sign of colorectal cancer and is almost diagnostic.

The majority of colorectal cancers are now detected by optical colonoscopy, and patients are then referred for a screening metastatic CT. Less commonly, cancer might first be detected by CT if it is performed for symptoms associated with the disease (abdominal pain, weight loss, anemia, change in bowel habit) or as an incidental finding when CT is performed for other reasons. Small tumors (<2 cm) are often missed on CT because they are easily mistaken for normal stool. Masses at the ileocecal valve may be missed because the valve often has a mass-like appearance, particularly if the cecum is decompressed. A clue that a malignant mass is present at the ileocecal valve is the degree of soft tissue thickening of the cecal wall (Fig. 5-111). Multiplanar imaging can be helpful in these circumstances. Other tumors will be detected with CT based on their size (Fig. 5-112). Sometimes a CT "apple-core" equivalent can be identified (Figs. 5-104 and 5-113). Tumors may present with a more inflammatory-type mass that can be difficult to differentiate from diverticulitis (Fig. 5-114). In the diagnosis of simple diverticulitis by CT imaging, it is critical to consider any underlying carcinoma as the cause. Signs that suggest an underlying malignancy include the degree of wall thickness and regional adenopathy (Fig. 5-71). More sinister features include extension of the tumor beyond the cecal wall, with edematous changes (fat-stranding) in the surrounding mesentery or retroperitoneum or local metastatic deposits and regional lymphadenopathy (Fig. 5-112). Sometimes the tumor may perforate, usually locally, with a walled-off abscess (Fig. 5-105) or fistulize with adjacent viscera (Fig. 5-115). Ideally, however, these tumors should be detected before they have metastasized either locally or distant. Given that colorectal cancer is relatively common and early detection is critical, radiologists should evaluate the colon and rectum carefully on every CT image to exclude subtle early tumors.

Experience with CTC is sufficiently widespread that all the features identified on conventional cross-sectional CT can now be observed (Fig. 5-116). However, the main role of CTC is

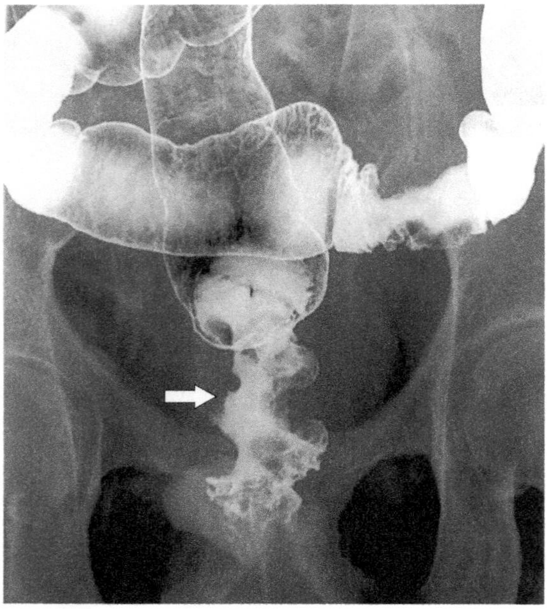

FIGURE 5-110. BE in a 61-year-old man with an "apple-core" rectal adenocarcinoma (*arrow*).

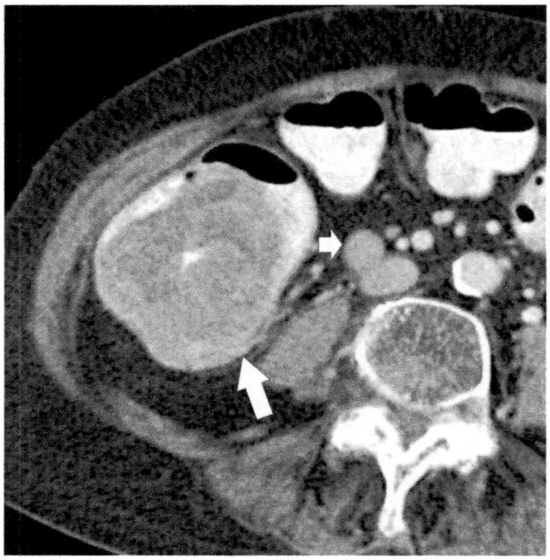

FIGURE 5-112. Axial contrast-enhanced CT in a 59-year-old woman with a large cecal mass (*arrow*) due to adenocarcinoma. There is regional metastatic adenopathy (*small arrow*).

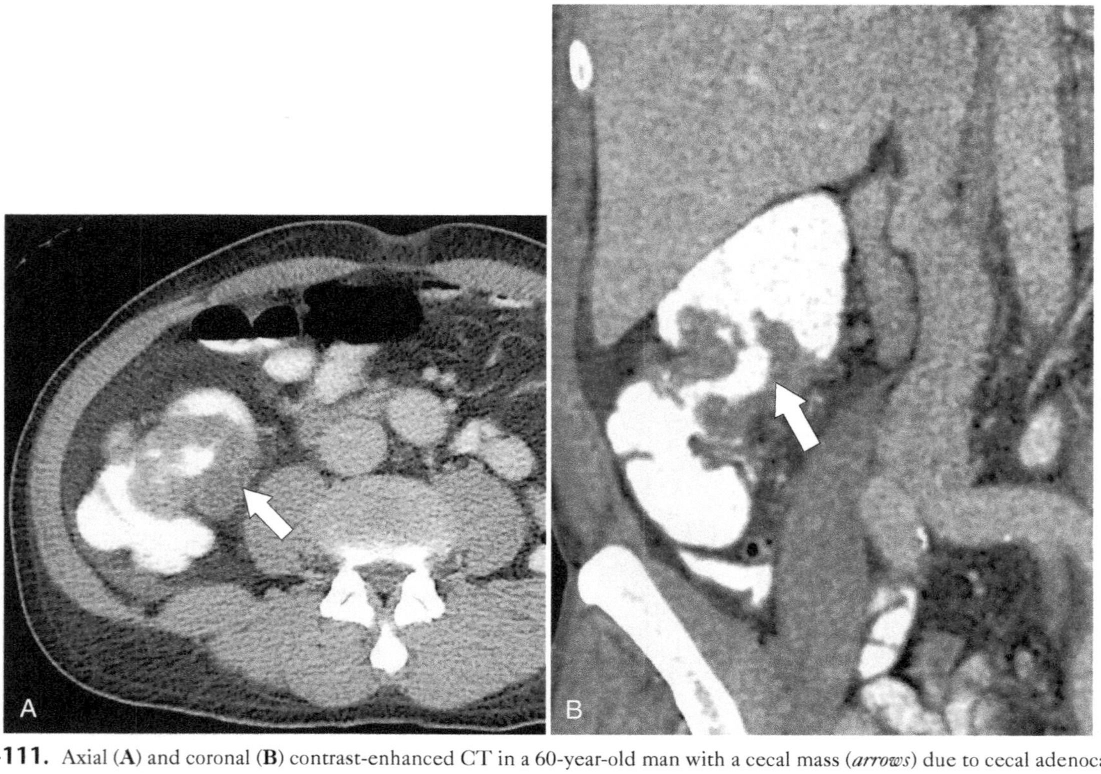

FIGURE 5-111. Axial (**A**) and coronal (**B**) contrast-enhanced CT in a 60-year-old man with a cecal mass (*arrows*) due to cecal adenocarcinoma.

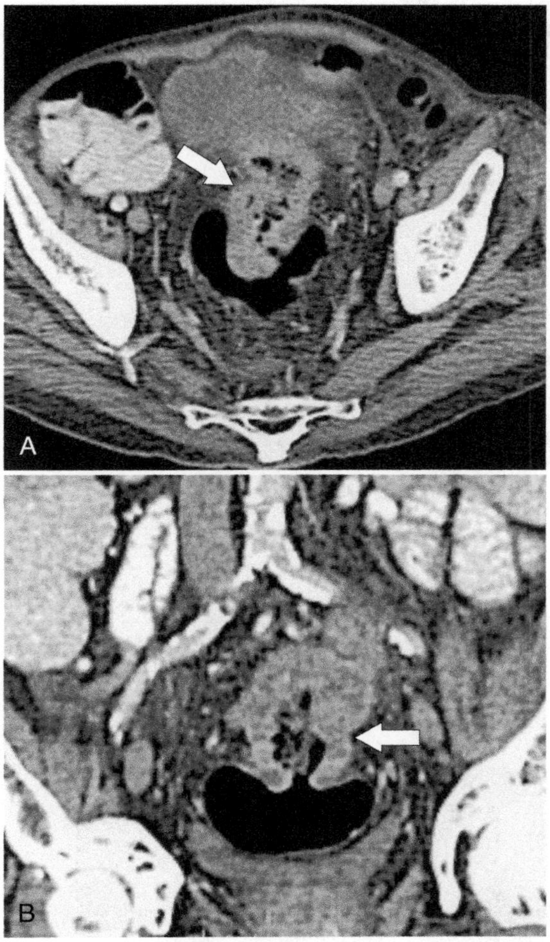

FIGURE 5-113. Axial (**A**) and coronal (**B**) contrast-enhanced CT in a 69-year-old man with a circumferential "apple-core" mass (*arrows*) of the rectosigmoid due to adenocarcinoma.

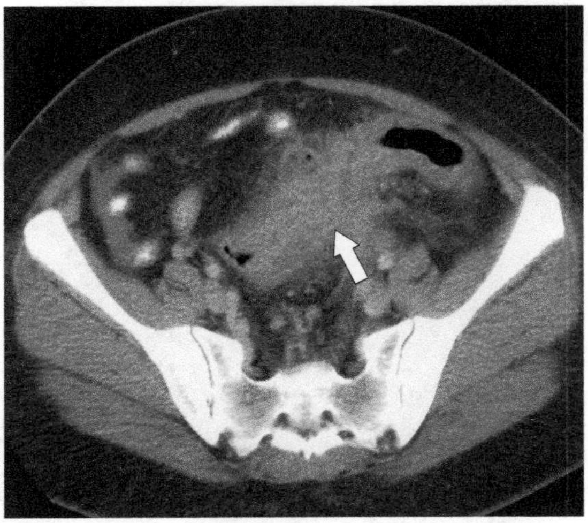

FIGURE 5-114. Axial contrast-enhanced CT in a 44-year-old woman with an inflammatory form of adenocarcinoma of the sigmoid (*arrow*).

screening, ideally to detect adenomatous polyps before they degenerate into malignant lesions. Therefore large tumors are identified only uncommonly.

PET and PET/CT are used primarily for staging and monitoring of metastatic disease, but primary colorectal tumors, if large enough, should also be visualized (Fig. 5-117). Small tumors may

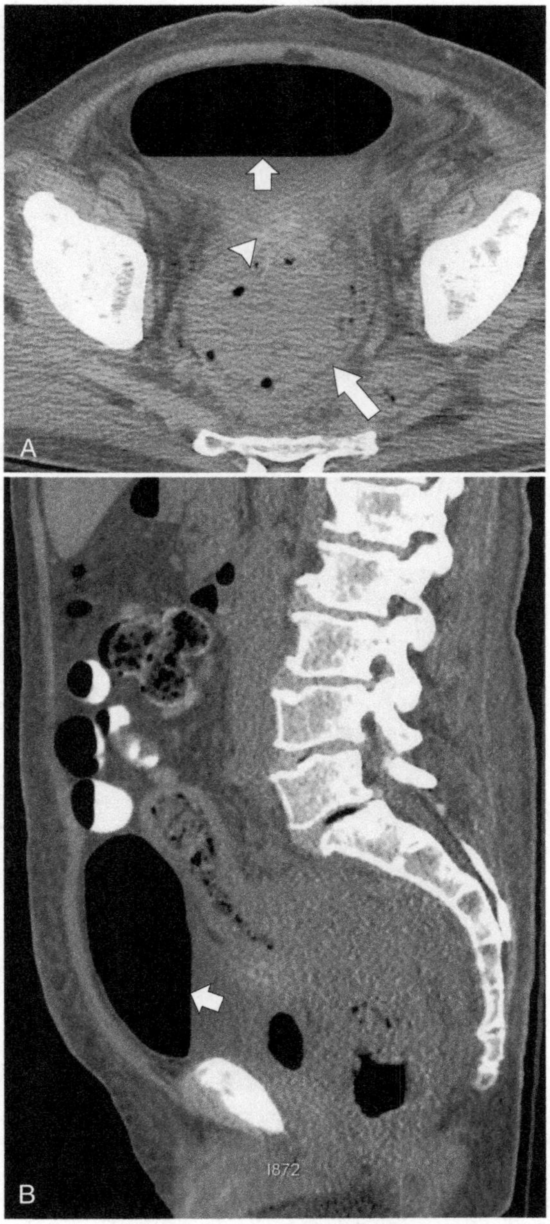

FIGURE 5-115. Axial (**A**) and sagittal (**B**) non-contrast-enhanced CT in a 76-year-old woman with a large rectal mass (*arrow*) due to rectal adenocarcinoma, which has directly invaded the posterior bladder wall (*arrowhead*) and resulted in a rectovesical fistula and gas in the bladder (*small arrows*).

not be identified, either because FDG uptake is insufficient to be visible at PET or because the normal bowel can also have some FDG activity. Determination of what constitutes normal versus abnormal uptake is also aided by PET/CT fusion software, whereby the PET uptake findings can be correlated with the anatomical CT findings. Extracolonic spread of the tumor, including spread to regional nodes or distant metastatic disease, can also be identified with PET imaging. Some adenomatous polyps are also strongly FDG avid but cannot be identified with CT alone because they are small or obscured by feces (Fig. 5-93).

Preoperative staging is increasingly being performed using MRI, particularly using an endorectal coil, which has shown benefit in determining the TNM staging of rectal adenocarcinoma. It is important preoperatively to determine whether the disease extends into the mesorectal fascia because chemoradiation treatment may be required before the surgeon contemplates

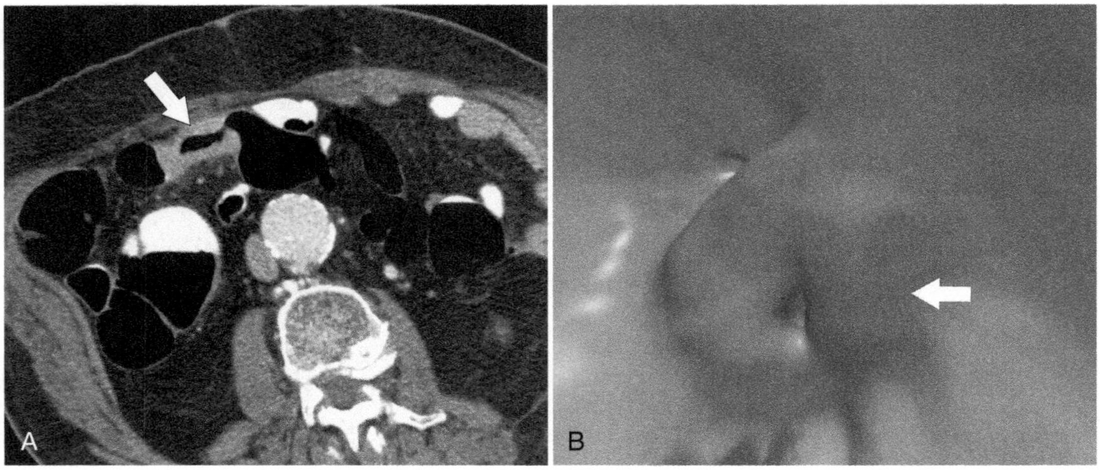

FIGURE 5-116. A and B, CTC in a 59-year-old man with an "apple-core" colon cancer in the transverse colon (*arrows*). *See ExpertConsult.com for color image.*

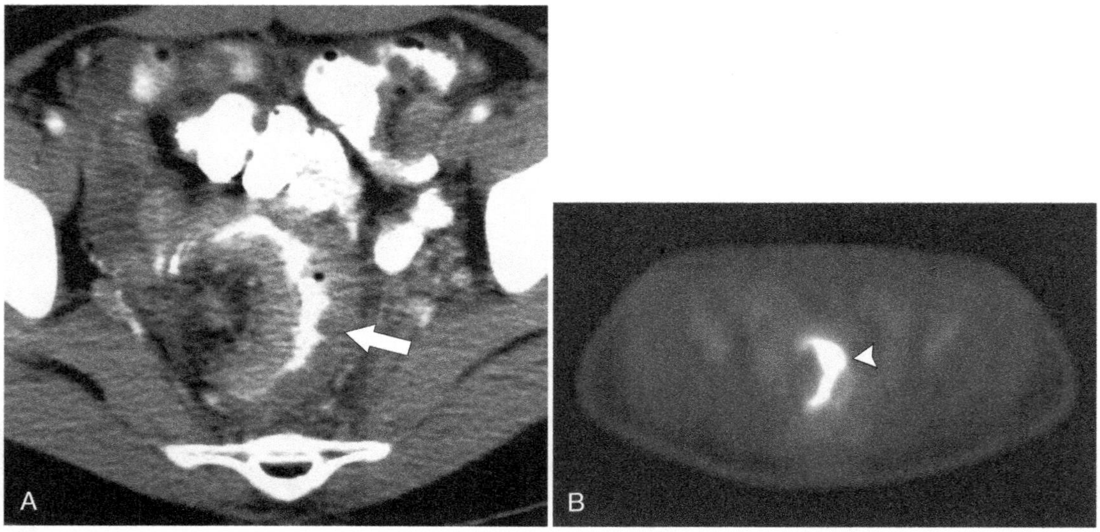

FIGURE 5-117. Axial contrast-enhanced CT (**A**) and PET (**B**) in a 35-year-old woman with rectal adenocarcinoma. There is a long segment of circumferential mural sigmoid thickening (*arrow*) that shows marked uptake on PET (*arrowhead*).

total mesorectal excision. The normal rectal submucosa has a T2 intermediate signal and hypointense serosa (Fig. 5-118). With T2 invasion, the brighter submucosa is replaced by tumor that is hypointense (Fig. 5-119). Further progression to T3 obliterates the distinction between the muscularis and serosa and extends into the perirectal fascia (Fig. 5-120). Differentiation between T2 and T3 disease can be difficult (Fig. 5-121).

Colonic Lymphoma

Lymphoma has numerous subtypes and commonly affects the GI tract by direct extension from regional disease, by metastatic disease, or less commonly as a primary colonic non-Hodgkin lymphoma. Although specific imaging features can point to the diagnosis, colonic lymphoma can appear identical to adenocarcinoma anywhere in the GI tract (Fig. 5-122). Although lymphoma is less common than adenocarcinoma, it should still be considered in the diagnosis, particularly if the lesion is focal, circumferential, or ulcerative (Fig. 5-122). Conversely, lesions can be diffuse and nodular, unlike adenocarcinoma. This rarer presentation is sometimes indistinguishable from polyposis syndromes, although the findings are usually confined to the cecum. Metastatic disease from either lymphomatous type is common, with local lymph node involvement.

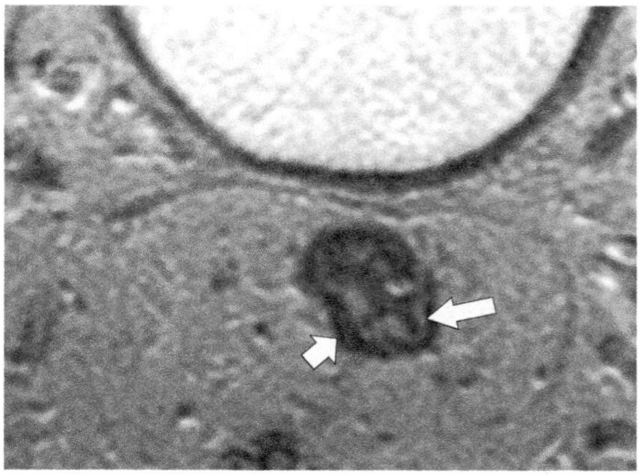

FIGURE 5-118. Axial T2-weighted MRI of normal rectal mucosa with T2 bright muscularis (*arrow*) and dark serosa (*small arrow*).

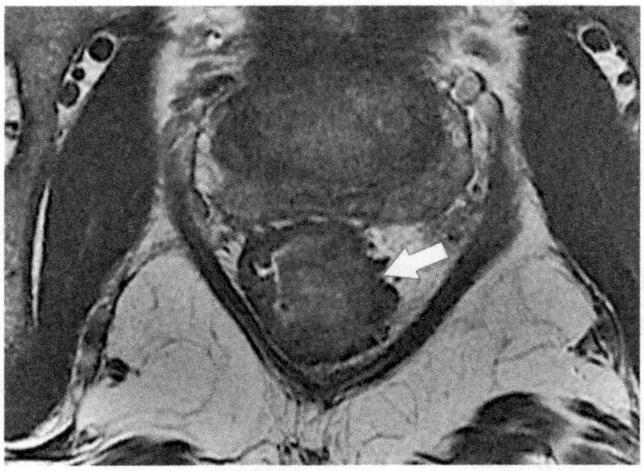

FIGURE 5-119. Axial T2-weighted MRI in a 56-year-old man with a T2 rectal adenocarcinoma. The hypointense (*arrow*) mass does not invade the serosa.

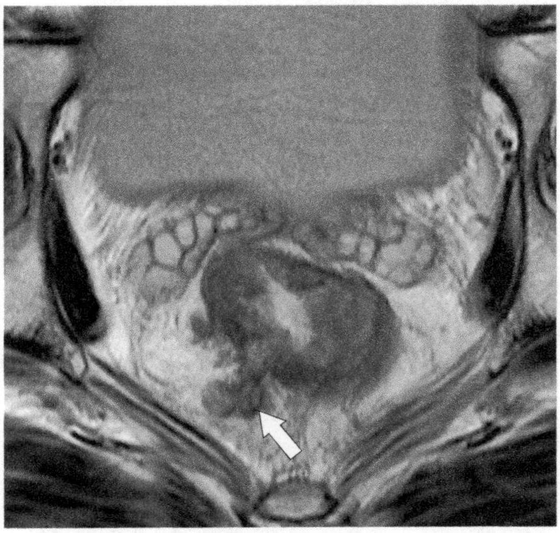

FIGURE 5-120. Axial T2-weighted MRI in a 66-year-old man with tumor extension through the serosa (*arrow*) consistent with a T3 tumor.

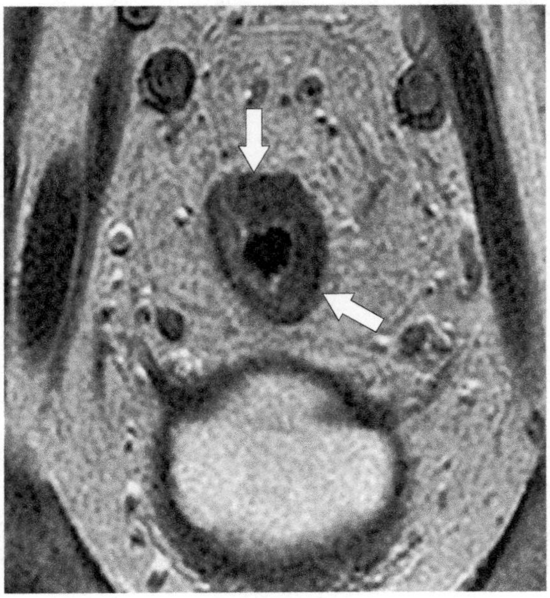

FIGURE 5-121. Coronal T2-weighted MRI in a 45-year-old man with a T2 rectal adenocarcinoma. The low signal tumor is between 11 o'clock and 5 o'clock (*arrows*), replacing the normal muscularis mucosa.

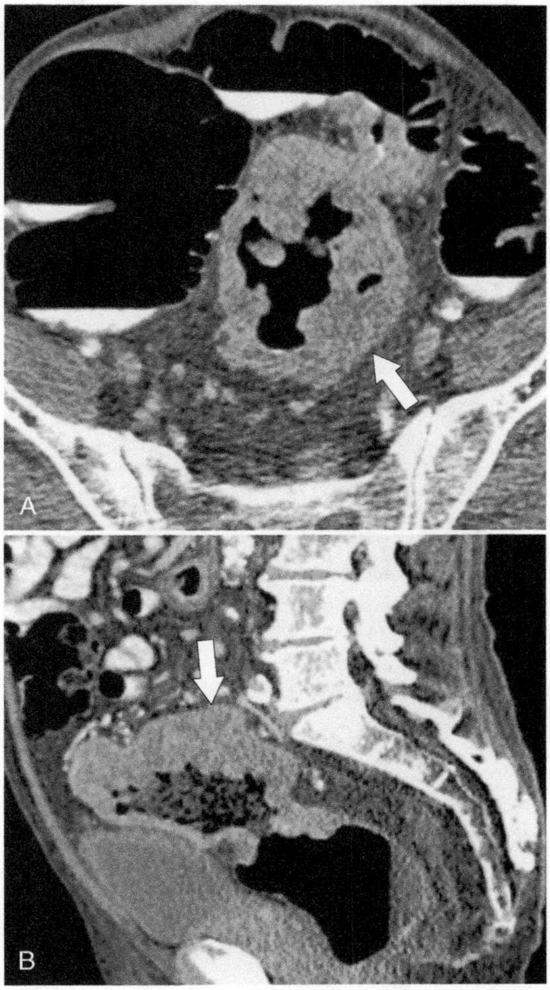

FIGURE 5-122. Axial (**A**) and sagittal (**B**) contrast-enhanced CT in a 61-year-old man with a large irregular and ulcerating mass on the sigmoid colon due to colonic lymphoma (*arrows*).

When present in the large bowel, colonic lymphoma most commonly affects the cecum. The masses are often very large with diffuse circumferential bowel wall thickening (although eccentric polypoid masses also occur) and can be associated with bulky regional lymphadenopathy. A particular feature and a strong clue to the diagnosis is "aneurysmal" dilatation of the bowel lumen, as seen in the small bowel, because of destruction by lymphomatous cells of the myenteric plexus. It would be highly unusual, particularly if large, for an adenocarcinoma to show luminal dilatation. Rather, adenocarcinomas constrict the lumen and present with luminal narrowing and, if large enough, obstruction. Lymphoma typically does not present with bowel obstruction in either the small or large bowel. Increasingly, PET/CT is being used to evaluate the extent of disease and response to chemotherapy. Residual disease identified by CT may no longer represent active tumor by PET, termed a "metabolic response."

Anal Cancer

Anal cancer should be considered a different disease from colorectal cancer because it has different risk factors, histological features, and treatment. Risk factors include human papillomavirus, immunosuppression, and Crohn disease. Histologically, these tumors are mostly squamous cell, although adenocarcinoma, lymphoma, melanoma, and sarcoma have been described. The diagnosis is relatively straightforward given the location of the

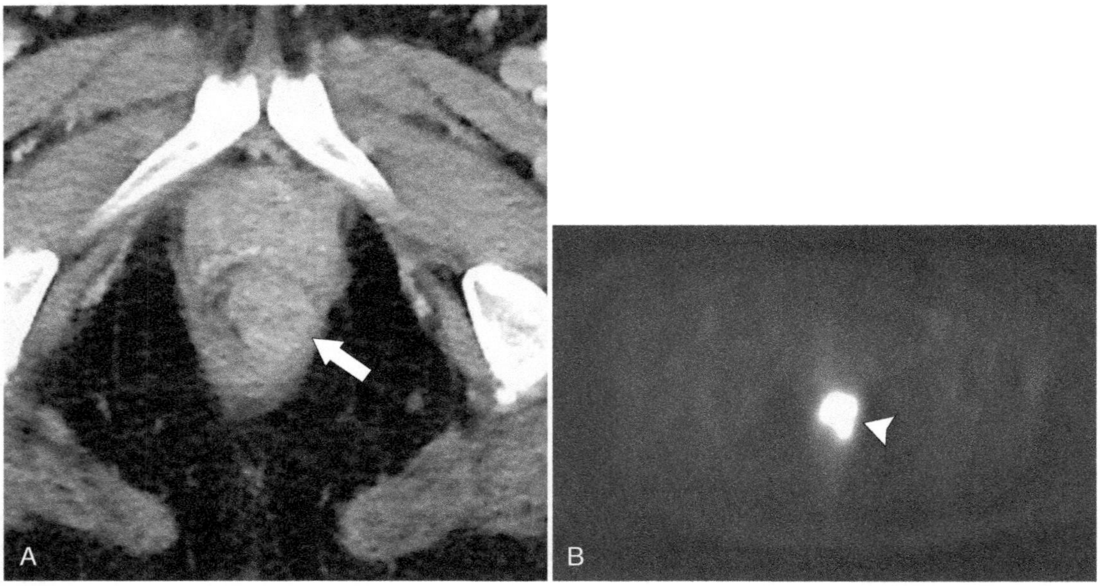

FIGURE 5-123. Axial contrast-enhanced CT (**A**) and PET (**B**) in a 62-year-old woman with a 2.5-cm anal mass (*arrow*) due to squamous cell carcinoma that shows marked FDG uptake at PET (*arrowhead*).

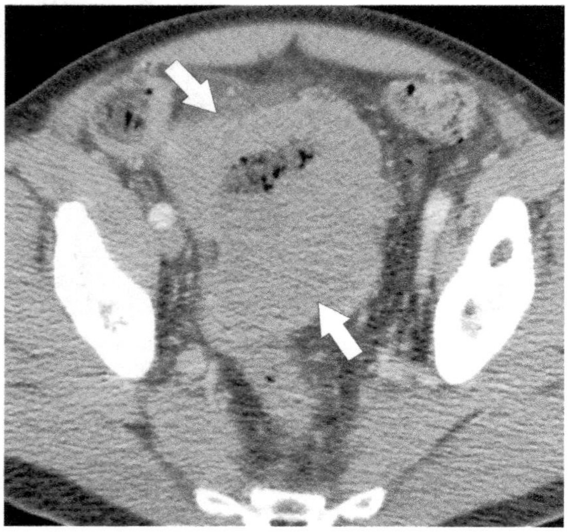

FIGURE 5-124. Axial contrast-enhanced CT in a 50-year-old woman with a large irregular sigmoid mass (*arrows*) due to a malignant GIST.

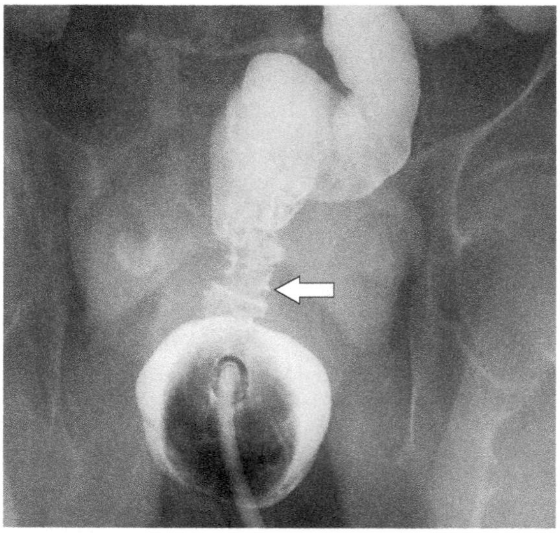

FIGURE 5-125. Single-contrast BE in a patient with metastatic gastric cancer and a circumferential upper rectal narrowing (*arrow*) due to serosal gastric metastases.

tumor, but cross-sectional imaging (e.g., MRI, CT, or PET/CT) is usually performed for staging purposes (Fig. 5-123). Metastatic disease is less common than with colorectal cancer, so patients with anal cancer have a better prognosis.

Malignant Gastrointestinal Stromal Tumor (see Chapter 2)

GISTs are very uncommon in the colon, but when present, they demonstrate features similar to those of malignant GISTs elsewhere in the GI tract. These include a large soft tissue mass, often eccentric, that tends to produce mucosal ulceration and central necrosis as the tumor enlarges (Fig. 5-124).

Kaposi Sarcoma (see Chapters 2 and 3)

Kaposi sarcoma is either an AIDS-related disease or secondary to prolonged immunosuppression. It is caused by herpesvirus 8 (HHV8) and usually presents with mucocutaneous violaceous lesions. It rarely affects the colon, but when it does, it produces lesions similar to those elsewhere in the GI tract, with submucosal "bulls-eye" or target lesions or larger ulcerating intraluminal masses. Lesions can be multiple, which is sometimes a clue to the diagnosis.

Metastatic Disease

Metastases from noncolonic sites can invade the colon by one of three routes: intraperitoneal along the mesentery (e.g., stomach, pancreas), hematogenous (e.g., melanoma, breast, stomach, lung), or direct local extension (e.g., ovarian, bladder). The imaging appearances differ according to the form of metastatic spread. These range from small target-like (or bulls-eye) submucosal lesions, such as that seen in hematogenous spread from melanoma elsewhere in the GI tract, to a more substantial eccentric or circumferential mass from peritoneal seeding from stomach cancer (Fig. 5-125). Direct spread from adnexal malignancies generally causes luminal distortion and stricture (Fig. 5-126). Small submucosal lesions are unlikely to be identified by CT, but larger lesions should be (Fig. 5-127). Metachronous or synchronous colorectal cancer should be considered in the diagnosis because of their frequency in patients with a known history of this disease (Fig. 5-102).

Large Bowel Dilatation

Nonmechanical Dilatation

By far the most common cause of large bowel dilatation is colonic ileus (Table 5-8), which like small bowel ileus is most common after surgery, particularly abdominal surgery, because bowel manipulation results in a lack of peristalsis lasting up to a few days. Other intraabdominal events (peritonitis, abscess) often cause an ileus. Patients with severe nonabdominal insults (myocardial infarction, sepsis, electrolyte disturbances) are also at risk for bowel dilatation. The colon is usually moderately distended along with the small bowel (see Chapter 4), which helps differentiate nonmechanical from mechanical large bowel obstruction, although mechanical large bowel obstruction often ultimately causes small bowel obstruction. A form of nonmechanical chronic dilatation occurs in institutionalized patients, perhaps because of their regimen of multiple medications, many of which have anticholinergic side effects. Patients with large bowel dilatation are also at risk of volvulus.

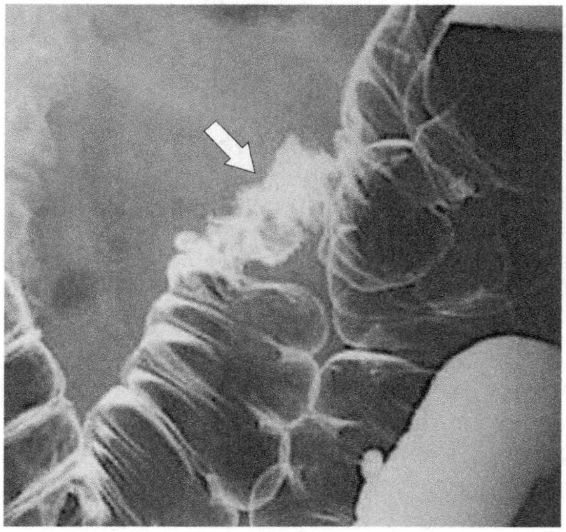

FIGURE 5-126. DCBE in a 56-year-old man with a stricture (*arrow*) of the distal transverse colon due to direct invasion from gastic cancer.

Ogilvie Syndrome

In Ogilvie* syndrome, also termed "colonic pseudoobstruction," patients (who are almost always elderly) have gross colonic dilatation without any mechanical obstruction. Causes of the condition are similar to those of colonic ileus (postsurgery, peritonitis, narcotics, and antispasmodic drugs), but the large bowel dilatation is more severe (colonic diameter >10 cm) and there is a risk of perforation from ischemic necrosis or volvulus. Treatment, however, is usually conservative, including withdrawal of the precipitating causes (i.e., narcotic or antispasmodic drugs). Colonic decompression measures may be required in severe, more prolonged cases. At imaging, there is usually impressive large bowel dilatation, which may require confirmation with contrast enema (or rectal tube) to exclude large bowel obstruction (Fig. 5-128).

Psychogenic Megacolon

Psychogenic megacolon is a rare disease of childhood associated with behavioral issues and failure to develop normal bowel elimination habits. The result is gross stool impaction, further exacerbating the colonic dilatation with a combination of mechanical and nonmechanical obstruction.

Toxic Megacolon

The megacolon aspect of toxic megacolon refers to gross colonic dilatation, and the toxic component refers to the fact that

*William Heneage Ogilvie (1887-1971), British surgeon.

TABLE 5-8 Causes of Nonmechanical Large Bowel Obstruction

Cause	Description
Ileus	Drugs, surgery, trauma, peritonitis
Ogilvie syndrome	Usually in elderly after surgery or severe illness
Psychogenic megacolon	Rare childhood phenomenon
Toxic megacolon	Inflammatory bowel disease, ischemia, infectious
Scleroderma	Muscularis atrophy and fibrosis
Chagas disease	Destruction of myenteric plexus
Cystic fibrosis	Meconium ileus equivalent syndrome
Myotonic dystrophy	Atonic bowel
Idiopathic intestinal pseudoobstruction	Congenital or acquired

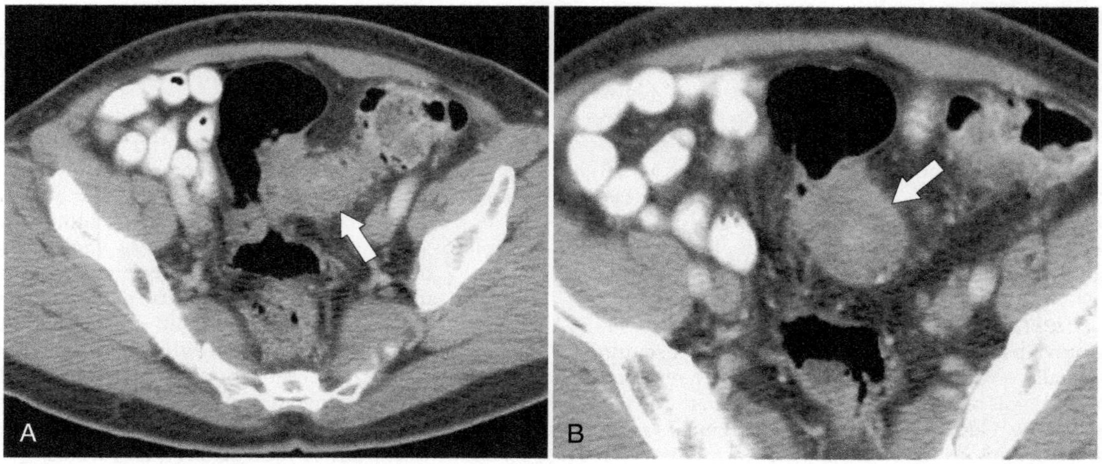

FIGURE 5-127. Axial contrast-enhanced CT (**A** and **B**) in a 39-year-old man with a 4-cm parasigmoid mass (*arrows*) due to a carcinoid metastasis.

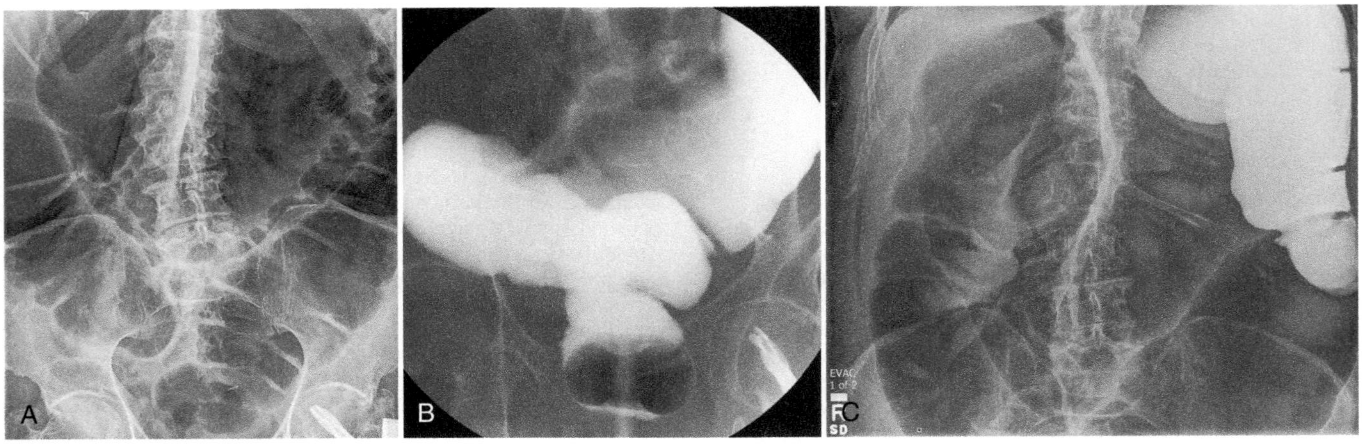

FIGURE 5-128. Plain radiograph of the abdomen (**A**) and BE (**B, C**) in a 70-year-old man with Ogilvie syndrome. The large bowel is grossly dilated, but there is no evidence of obstruction as evidenced by free passage of contrast medium up the colon.

perforation is imminent and is often a surgical emergency. This is discussed in more detail earlier in the chapter. The causes are mostly inflammatory or infectious, including IBD, certain bacterial or viral pathogens, or ischemic bowel.

Scleroderma

Scleroderma is a multisystemic autoimmune disease that commonly affects any aspect of the GI tract and progressively leads to atonic bowel and dilatation. This is caused by collagen deposition in the muscularis mucosae layer of the affected bowel with smooth muscle atrophy and fibrosis. The colon ultimately becomes functionless and can be grossly dilated.

Chagas Disease

Often acute and self-limiting, Chagas disease can proceed to a chronic, sometimes debilitating and fatal disease. Chagas disease is caused by the parasite *Trypansoma cruzi*, which can cause chronic neuronal inflammation and destruction of the myenteric plexus, leading to an atonic viscus that usually affects the esophagus or colon. This can cause marked distention of the esophagus or colon, with the latter at risk of volvulus. The GI symptoms are often secondary to the more serious effects of a dilated cardiomyopathy and heart failure.

Cystic Fibrosis

Cystic fibrosis has a number of GI complications, mostly resulting from the viscous mucoid inspissated material that occupies the small and large bowel. These include meconium ileus, intussusception, and appendicitis. The colon can also become occupied by the viscoid material, leading to meconium ileus equivalent syndrome, which resembles meconium ileus and predominantly affects the cecum and ascending colon. Colonic strictures have also been reported in children because of a submucosal fibrosis, termed "fibrosing colopathy." In some patients a colitis-type picture with wall thickening and pericolonic inflammation (fat-stranding) develops and can be difficult to distinguish from IBD (Fig. 5-129). Patients with cystic fibrosis are at a slight increased risk of adenocarcinoma in the small or large bowel (Fig. 5-130), although there is dispute as to whether this simply reflects the expected normal frequency of cancer in the general population.

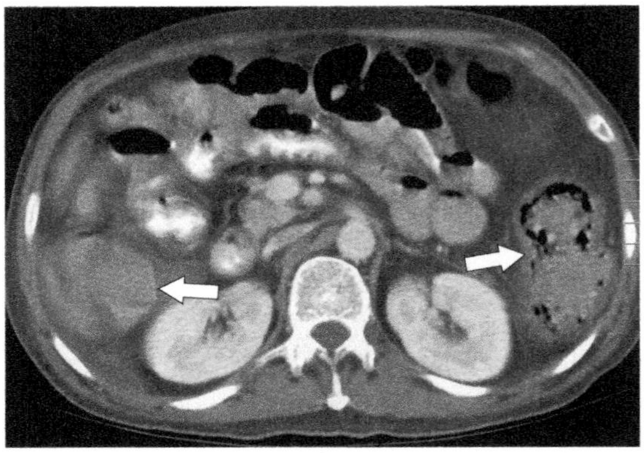

FIGURE 5-129. Axial CT in a 34-year-old man with colonic colopathy (*arrows*) due to cystic fibrosis.

Idiopathic Intestinal Pseudoobstruction

Idiopathic intestinal pseudoobstruction is a congenital or acquired rare disorder usually observed in children. Patients have repetitive symptoms and signs of large bowel obstruction in the absence of a mechanical cause. Congenital causes are extremely rare and are caused by myopathic or neuropathic disease and associated with other dilated structures (i.e., megaureters). The secondary or acquired form is more common because of a variety of metabolic, infectious, endocrinological, muscular, and neuropathic disorders.

Extracolonic Causes of Colonic Stricture

Adjacent inflammatory disease (e.g., pancreatitis) or abscess formation anywhere along the length of the bowel (i.e., secondary to tuboovarian abscess or appendiceal abscess) may cause localized stricture formation from the secondary inflammatory change.

Malignant invasion of the colonic serosa, usually via direct peritoneal spread, may cause localized stricture formation and marked spasm (Fig. 5-125). Other malignant causes are secondary to direct colonic invasion from adjacent malignancy (Fig. 5-126).

Mechanical Large Bowel Obstruction

In common with mechanical obstruction in any viscera or vessel, the cause of mechanical large bowel obstruction can be outside the bowel (extraluminal), within the bowel wall (mucosal or submucosal), or within the bowel lumen (intraluminal) (Table 5-9). The imaging appearances vary according to the cause. Extraluminal obstruction generally causes a smooth, shallow, angled stricture, unless caused by hernia or volvulus, where the stricture is tight and abrupt. Intramural causes produce a more obtuse angled filling defect within the bowel lumen, whereas mucosal strictures generally produce sharply marginated strictures, either polypoid or shouldering (abrupt transition between normal mucosa and stricture) (see Chapter 1). Mechanical obstruction is often assessed initially with the abdominal plain radiography to determine whether the large

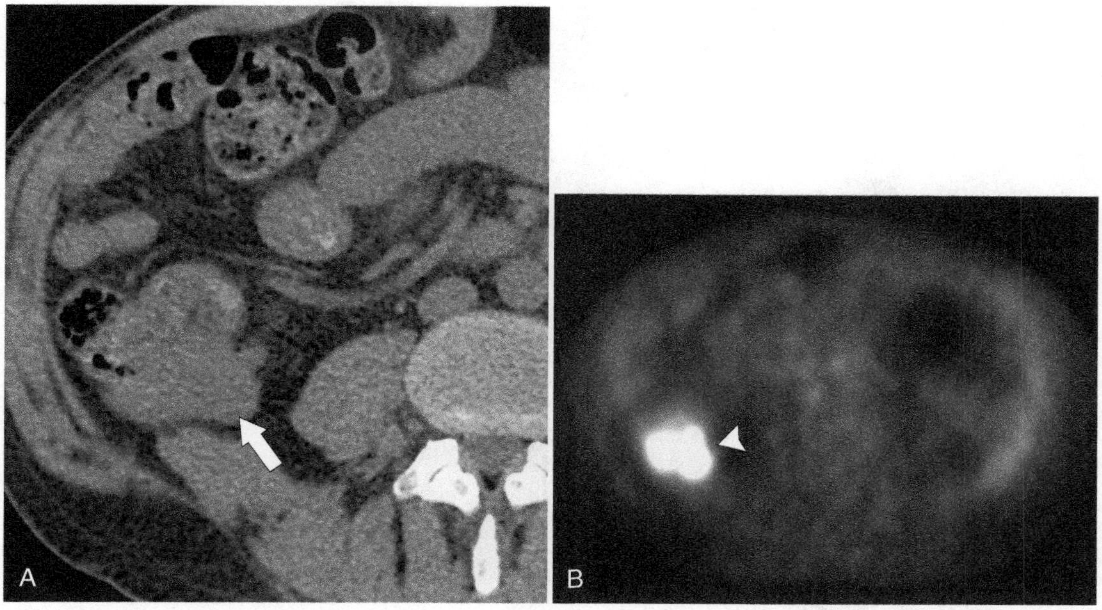

FIGURE 5-130. Axial non-contrast-enhanced CT (**A**) and PET (**B**) in a 44-year-old woman with cystic fibrosis with a 4-cm mass in the cecum (*arrow*) with marked PET uptake (*arrowhead*) due to colon adenocarcinoma.

TABLE 5-9 Causes of Colonic Mechanical Obstruction

Type	Disease
Extraluminal	
Abdominal masses	Direct metastatic spread Adjacent disease (fibroid, distended bladder) Pelvic lipomatosis Neurofibromatosis
Volvulus	
Hernia	
Adhesions	
Endometriosis	
Intramural	
Mucosal and submucosal disease	Carcinoma GIST Lymphoma Benign neoplasia
Inflammatory	Inflammatory bowel disease Infectious (TB, hydatid) Diverticulitis
Vascular	Ischemia
Congenital	Hirschsprung Imperforate anus
Intraluminal	
Foreign body Gallstones Fecal impaction Meconium plug Intussusception	

GIST, Gastrointestinal stromal tumor; *TB*, tuberculosis.

bowel is distended and to determine any abrupt transition points (Fig. 5-104). The differentiation between mechanical obstruction and ileus can often be challenging, particularly if the obstruction is located in the distal colon and there is an absence of rectal gas. Under these circumstances, prone imaging of the abdomen can often be helpful to distinguish between the two. The rectum is ante-dependent in the prone position, so gas readily flows into the rectum in the presence of an ileus, excluding a mechanical cause for the obstruction (Fig. 5-131). Conversely, the presence of gas in the rectum on supine imaging does not totally exclude a mechanical obstruction because small amounts of gas can pass through a stricture that causes near, but not total, obstruction.

Extramural Large Bowel Obstruction

Given the presence of the colon throughout the abdomen and pelvis, many organs can normally impinge on it, including the liver, gallbladder, and spleen. Similarly, many abnormal processes can produce mass effect on the colon, such as masses from almost any abdominal or pelvic organ, including the peritoneum. Direct compression by adjacent disease (e.g., fibroids, abscess) may cause a smooth colonic stricture (Fig. 5-132), whereas direct invasion of the colon by adjacent malignancies (e.g., gallbladder, stomach, ovarian) tends to produce more irregular strictures because they often invade through the wall to the colonic mucosa (Fig. 5-126). Pelvic lipomatosis is an uncommon disease, usually identified in African American men with prolific fat deposition in the pelvis (particularly perirectal area), which can compress the bladder and the small and large bowel sufficiently to cause urinary symptoms as well as constipation, tenesmus, and even bowel obstruction.

Volvulus

A volvulus is a twisting or torsion of a viscus around its mesentery, which can then develop a closed-loop obstruction. In the colon, both cecal and sigmoid volvuli occur in the bowel with an abnormally long or redundant mesentery, resulting in relative colonic mobility of the affected viscus. Most patients with redundant mesentery do not undergo torsion and volvulus, but twisting may occur if the mesentery is fixed from prior inflammatory disease or the presence of a mass. Both are potentially life threatening because of the closed-loop obstruction and ischemic necrosis and perforation.

Cecal volvulus

The cecal volvulus must be differentiated from the more common sigmoid volvulus. The cecal volvulus typically twists up and to the left (Fig. 5-133), whereas the sigmoid volvulus typically twists up and to the right, although sometimes these can be difficult to

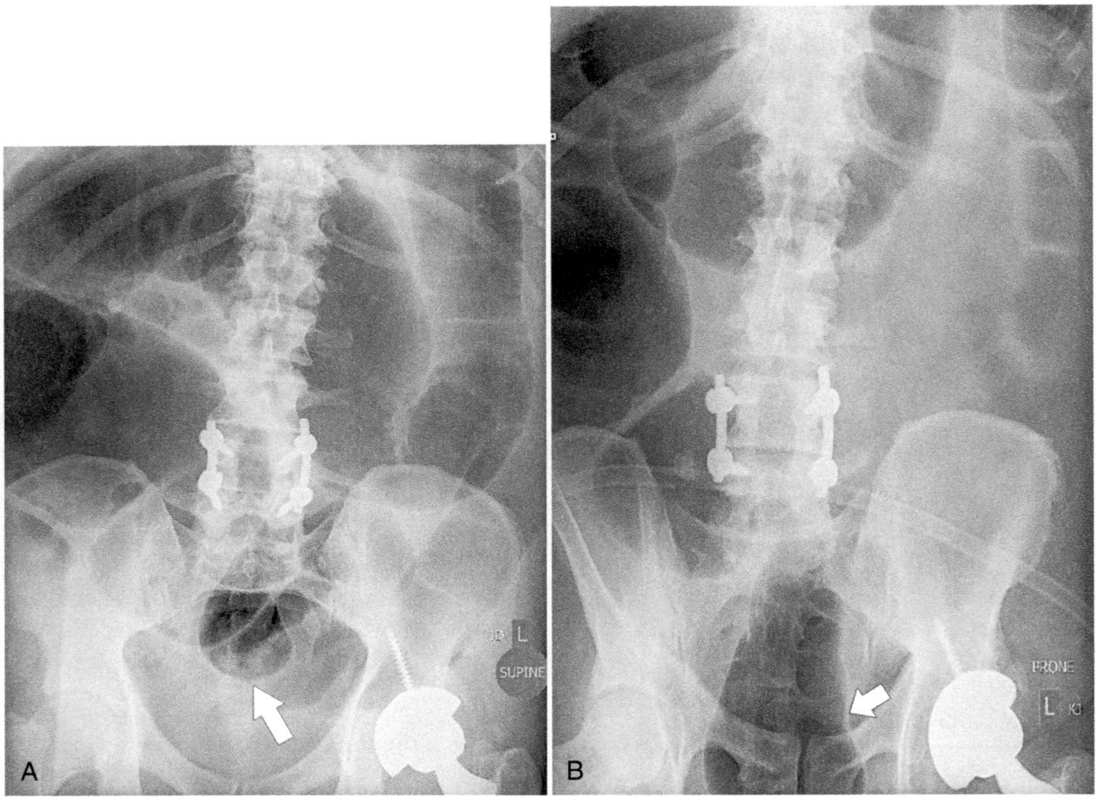

FIGURE 5-131. Supine (**A**) and prone (**B**) abdominal plain radiograph in a 68-year-old man with marked large bowel dilatation, thought initially to be caused by distal mechanical obstruction (*arrow*). However, prone imaging demonstrates free flow of gas into the rectum (*small arrow*), confirming ileus.

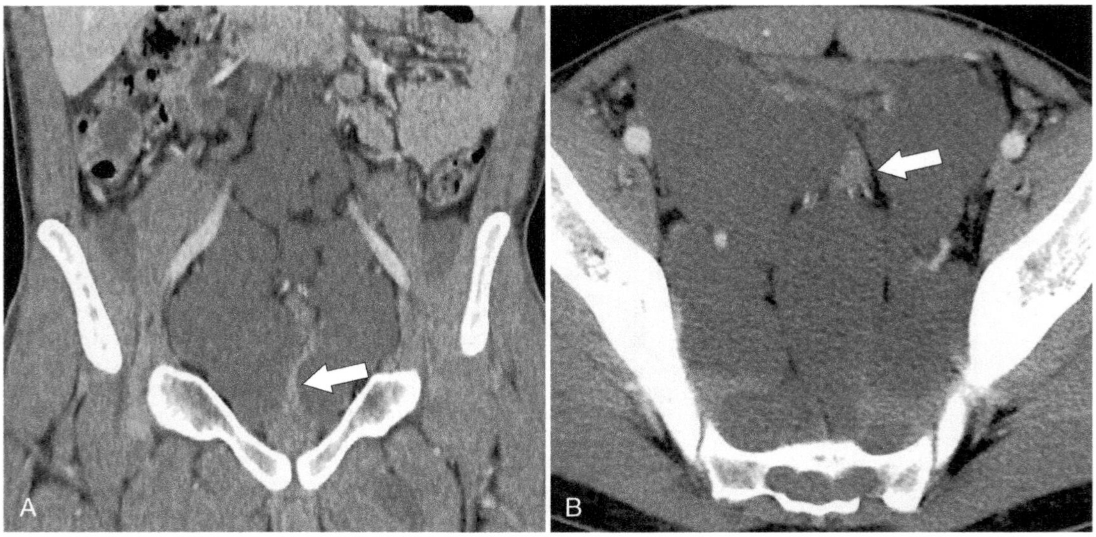

FIGURE 5-132. Coronal (**A**) and axial (**B**) contrast-enhanced CT in a 21-year-old man with neurofibromatosis and multiple abdominopelvic neurofibromas compressing the sigmoid colon (*arrows*).

differentiate by either plain radiography or CT. Previously, cecal volvulus was diagnosed with BE (water-soluble contrast material because of the risk of perforation), which demonstrated the abrupt and tight stricture as a so-called bird beak sign (Fig. 5-134), but it is now more commonly diagnosed with CT. The cecum is generally grossly distended, and careful evaluation of the cecal mesentery should demonstrate the mesenteric torsion (Fig. 5-133). Given that the cecal volvulus represents an acute colonic obstruction, it is often associated with small bowel dilatation. A cecal volvulus must be differentiated from a cecal bascule. This represents a distended cecum, often pointing in the same direction as a cecal volvulus, but not due to volvulus or cecal obstruction; rather, it is a normal cecum with a long and redundant mesentery (Fig. 5-135). Cecal bascules are, however, at risk of volvulus because of their long mesenteric pedicle. The differentiation is made on clinical grounds (the patient is generally well and asymptomatic). If necessary, a contrast enema can be performed, which will fail to identify any torsion, volvulus, or cecal obstruction.

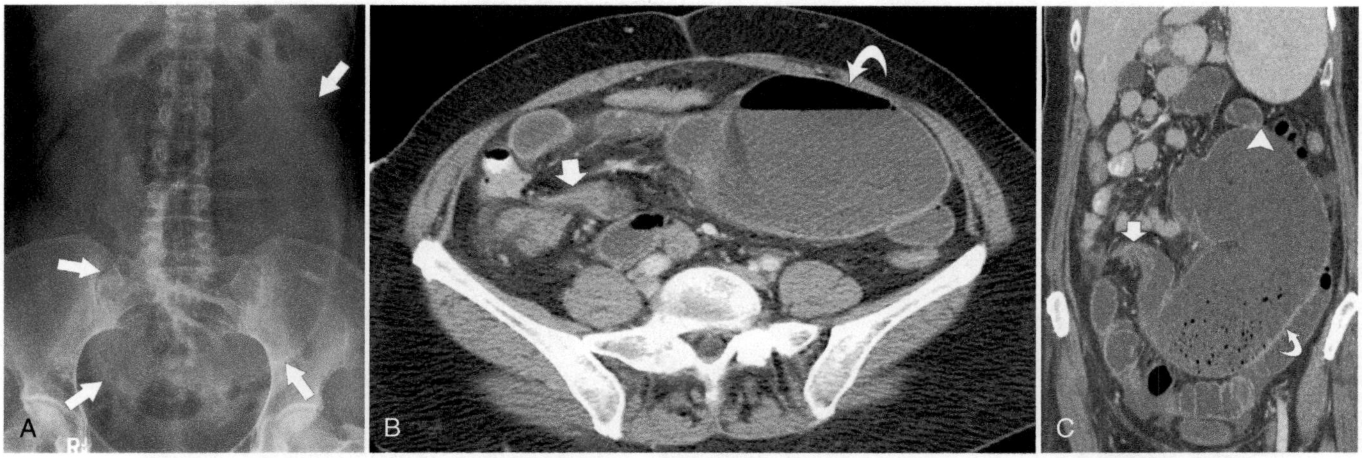

FIGURE 5-133. Plain radiography of the abdomen (**A**) and axial (**B**) and coronal (**C**) contrast-enhanced CT in a 74-year-old woman with a grossly distended cecum (*arrows*) whose tip points cephalad and to the left upper quadrant (*arrowhead*). CT demonstrates the dilated cecum (*curved arrows*) and stricture at the point of the cecal volvulus (*small arrows*).

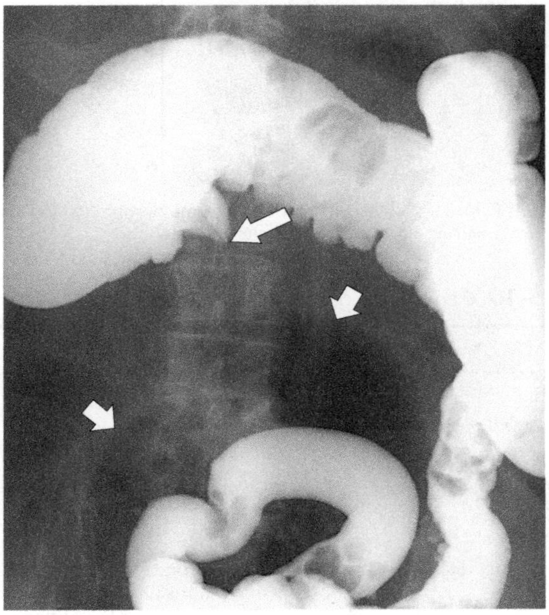

FIGURE 5-134. Single-contrast BE in a 66-year-old woman with cecal vovlulus and a "bird beak" sign (*arrow*) representing the point of torsion. Gas can be identified in the vovlulized cecum (*small arrows*).

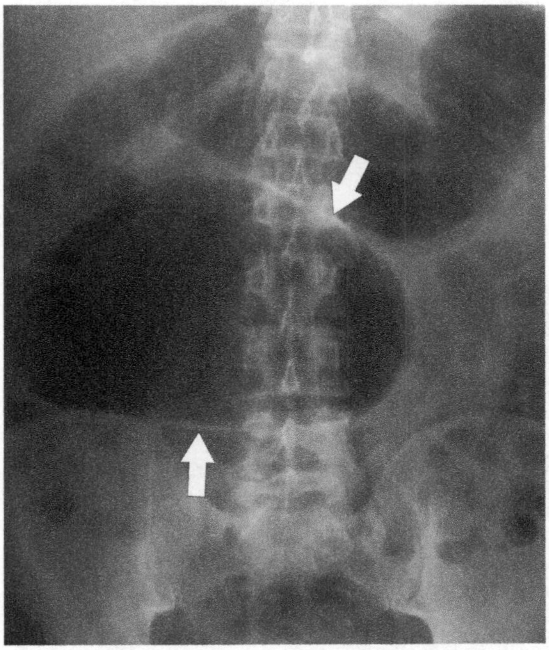

FIGURE 5-135. Abdominal plain radiograph demonstrating a distended, medially pointing cecum (*arrows*) due to cecal bascule.

Sigmoid volvulus

The sigmoid volvulus occurs when a tortuous sigmoid twists on its mesentery, usually upward and to the right (Fig. 5-136), resulting in a closed-loop obstruction in which the closed loop is distended and cannot deflate because of the "pinch" at its base. The dilated closed loop has been described as having a "coffee-bean" appearance on plain radiography and may extend all the way up to the right hemidiaphragm. There will be a similar beak-like obstructive appearance at BE, although this is rarely performed; instead the diagnosis is made with CT imaging (Fig. 5-136).

Hernias (see Chapter 4)

Colonic herniation is far less common than small bowel herniation but can occur into inguinal, anterior abdominal wall, incisional, or lateral rectus sheath hernias (Fig. 5-137). Other colonic hernias can occur through the diaphragm, as either a Bochdalek* hernia (anterior diaphragmatic hernia) or a Morgagni* hernia (posterior diaphragmatic hernia; see Chapter 10).

Intramural Causes of Large Bowel Obstruction

The causes of large bowel obstruction are listed in Table 5-10 and have been discussed earlier in this chapter. Most inflammatory, ischemic, and infectious causes do not produce complete obstruction. Large adenomatous lesions may also cause partial obstruction. Complete obstruction is most commonly associated with colorectal cancer (Fig. 5-103).

Intraluminal Causes of Large Bowel Obstruction

Intussusception

Colocolonic intussusception (as opposed to ileocolic) is much more common in childhood and rare in adulthood. Usually

*Vincent Alexander Bochdalek (1801-1883), Czech anatomist.

*Giovanni Batista Morgagni (1682-1771), Italian anatomist.

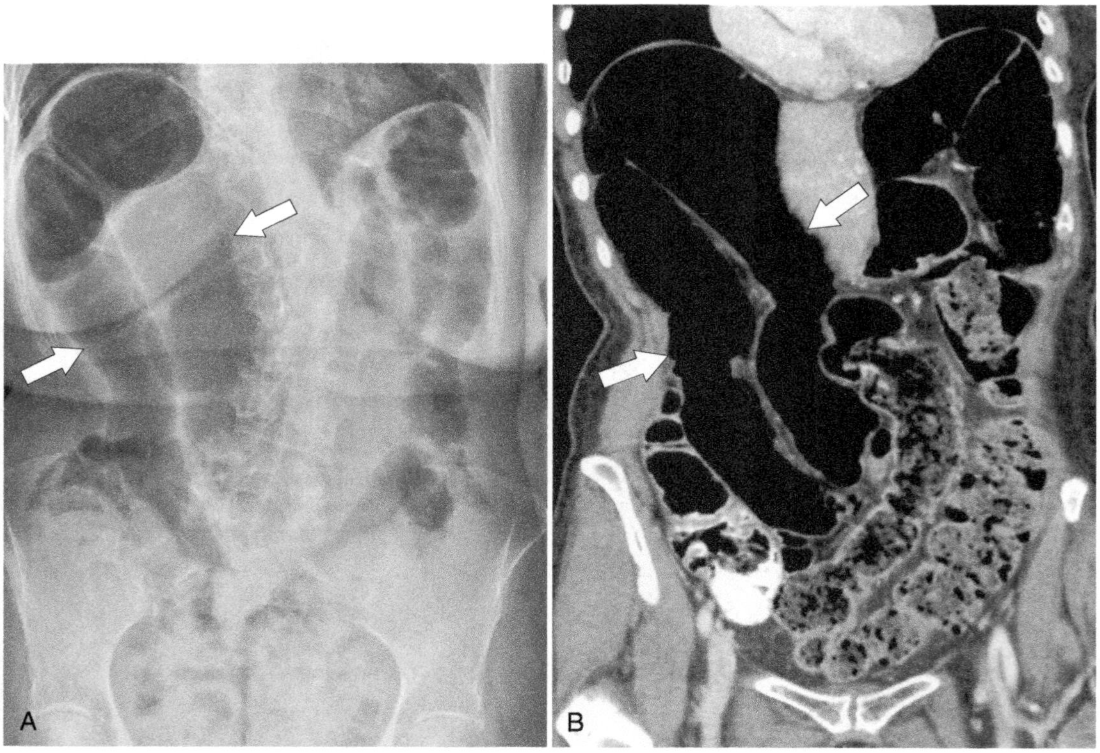

FIGURE 5-136. Plain radiograph of the abdomen (**A**) and coronal (**B**) contrast-enhanced CT in a 76-year-old man with sigmoid volvulus and marked distention of the sigmoid that points to the right upper quadrant (*arrows*) with large bowel obstruction of the remaining colon.

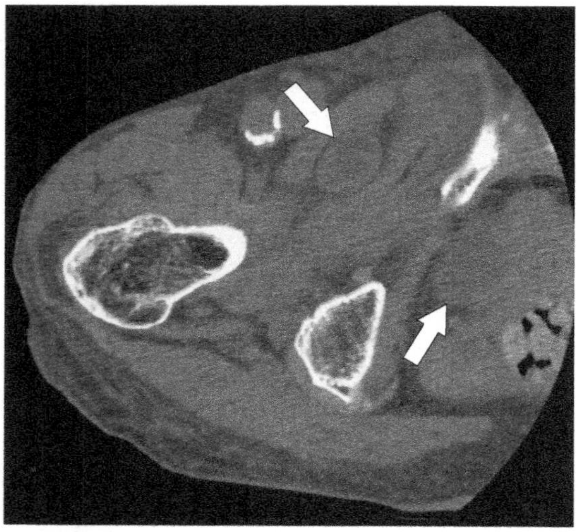

FIGURE 5-137. Axial noncontrast CT in a 71-year-old man with an obturator hernia. The colon has herniated through the right pelvic wall (*arrows*).

a pathological lesion acts as a lead point, unlike ileoileal intussusception, which is often transitory and of little significance. Both benign (Fig. 5-100) and malignant lesions (Fig. 5-106) can act as the lead point (Fig. 5-100). The diagnosis can be made with BE but is now almost always made with CT imaging in adults, but US in children. In children, ileocolic or colocolic intussusception can often be reduced without surgery by using rectal air or water, monitored fluoroscopically or by US, whereas surgery is generally required in adult forms.

Foreign Bodies

Foreign bodies are usually ingested orally, either accidentally or purposely, and should be visualized by BE or CT, particularly if metallic. Some undigested medication tablets can occasionally be identified and show their expected shape. Rectal foreign bodies are sometimes rectally self-inserted and may require general anesthesia or surgery or both for removal. Sharp foreign bodies may perforate the mucosa (Fig. 5-138).

TABLE 5-10 Causes of Colonic Pneumatosis

Type	Disease
Primary pneumatosis	Pneumatosis cystoides coli
Large bowel obstruction	Volvulus Neoplastic obstruction
Pulmonary disease	Chronic obstructive airways disease Asthma Cystic fibrosis
Inflammatory disease	Inflammatory bowel disease Infectious colitis (especially pseudomembranous and CMV colitis) Diverticulitis
Vascular	Ischemia (embolus or atheroma) Vasculitis (SLE, polyangiitis)
Neoplastic	Malignancies (carcinoma, lymphoma) Direct metastatic invasion
Trauma	Iatrogenic (colonoscopy) Enema studies Self-induced trauma
Drugs	Chemotherapy (colitis) Steroids
Graft-versus-host disease	Posttransplantation

CMV, Cytomegalovirus, *SLE*, systemic lupus erythematosus.

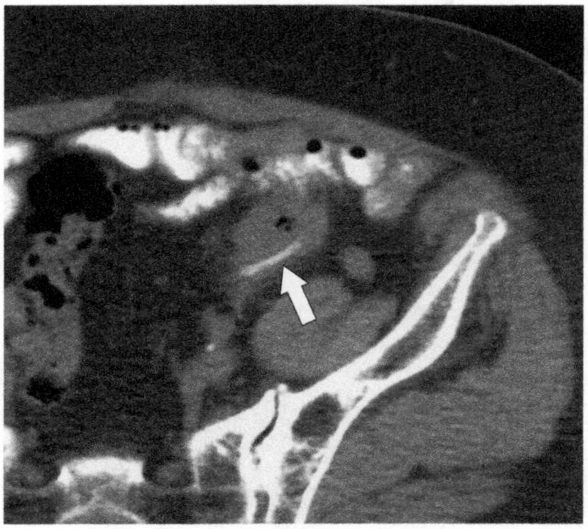

FIGURE 5-138. Axial noncontrast CT in a 71-year-old woman with mild sigmoid thickening and pericolonic edema or stranding associated with a linear density (*arrow*), found to be a chicken bone at surgery.

Fecal Impaction

Fecal impaction is usually caused by poor dietary habits (poor fluid intake, low roughage); inactivity; antispasmodic drugs, including narcotics; and anticholinergic medications. Profound constipation occurs in some institutionalized and psychiatric patients. In children, the causes may be psychological or due to congenital anomalies. Patients usually report constipation, but some may also report encopresis, which is overflow diarrhea around the fecal obstruction.

The imaging findings are usually straightforward, with fecal impaction, sometimes severe, noted on plain radiography (Fig. 5-139). Fecal impaction also is commonly identified at CT.

Stercoral Ulcer

Sometimes fecal impacted stool causes abrasive damage to the colonic mucosa, ischemia, and ulceration. Stercoral ulceration most commonly occurs in the rectum, but when constipation is severe, it can be identified in the more proximal colon (Fig. 5-140).

Gallstone Ileus (see Chapter 4)

The pericholecystic inflammation from chronic cholecystitis can sometimes create fistulae between adjacent viscera, usually the

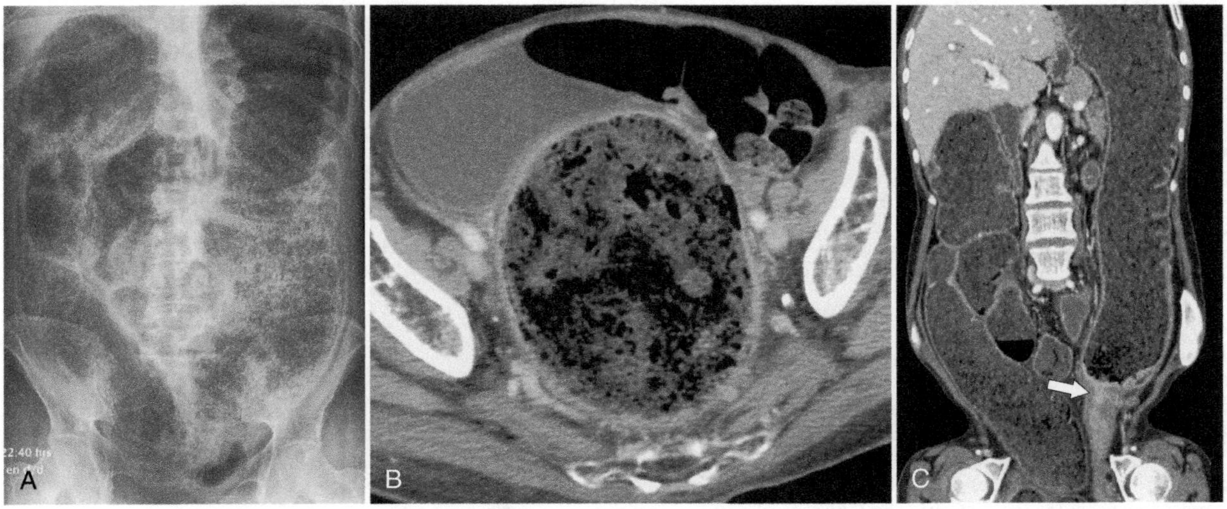

FIGURE 5-139. Plain abdominal radiograph (**A**) and axial (**B**) and coronal (**C**) contrast-enhanced CT in a 45-year-old man with upper sigmoid Crohn stricture (*arrow*) and gross fecal impaction due to chronic obstruction.

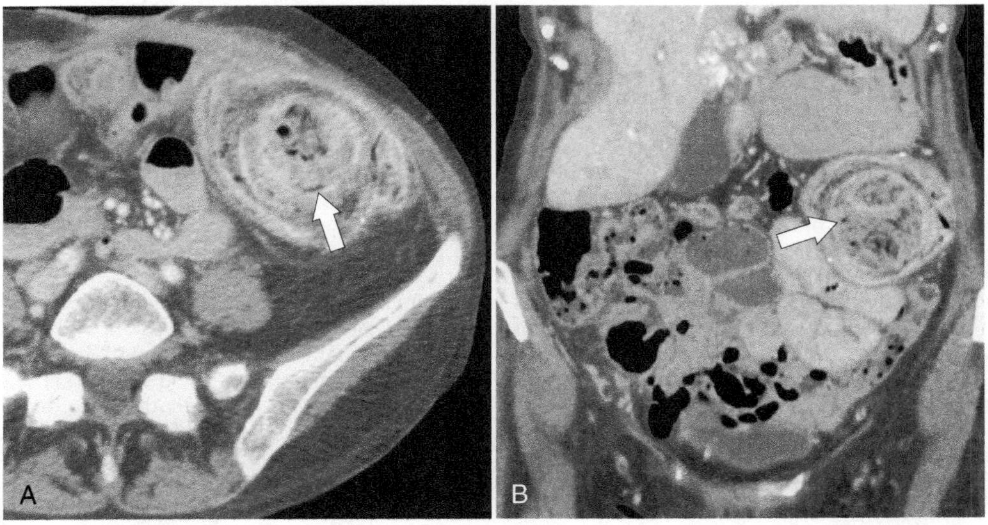

FIGURE 5-140. Axial (**A**) and coronal (**B**) contrast-enhanced CT in a 53-year-old woman with left colonic stool ball (*arrows*) with colonic wall thickening due to abrasive inflammation.

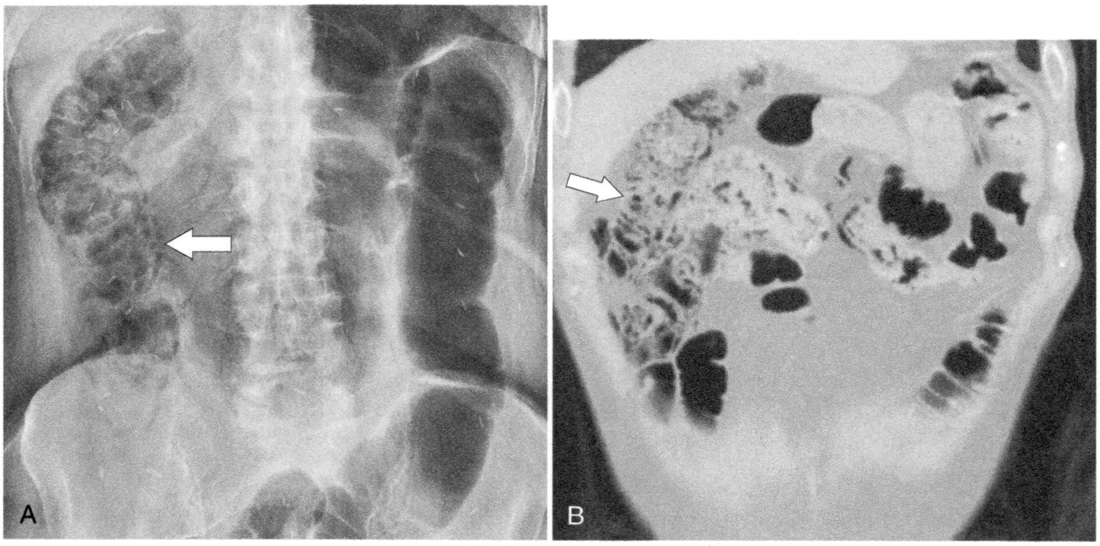

FIGURE 5-141. Plain radiograph (**A**) of the abdomen and coronal CT (**B**) in a 66-year-old man with multiple submucosal gas lucencies of the ascending (*arrows*) and transverse colon due to colonic pneumatosis.

small bowel, but also the colon, and rarely the stomach. Gallstones (which are almost always present in patients with chronic cholecystitis) then can pass through the fistula into the lumen of the small bowel or colon. Most of these stones pass spontaneously via the rectum, but larger stones may cause bowel obstruction, mainly in the small bowel (particularly at the ileocecal valve) because of the smaller luminal caliber. Colonic gallstones are usually excreted via the rectum because of the larger colonic caliber, but rarely gallstones are so large that they may even cause large bowel obstruction.

Colonic Pneumatosis

Colonic pneumatosis is defined as gas in the bowel wall and can be an incidental and asymptomatic finding or a harbinger of impending bowel perforation from ischemia and overwhelming sepsis (Table 5-10). The disease can be considered primary (approximately 15% of large bowel pneumatosis), and this is termed "pneumatosis cystoides coli." This is the colonic variant of pneumatosis cystoides intestinalis (see Chapter 4) and is more common in the large bowel. This is a benign condition (although rarely it may cause obstruction or pneumoperitoneum) and is sometimes termed "primary pneumatosis intestinalis." It is usually detected incidentally at CT (Fig. 5-141) with multiple thin-walled submucosal or subserosal cysts in the colonic wall, which may mimic polyps at BE.

Pneumatosis cystoides coli is to be distinguished from the more common secondary forms of pneumatosis intestinalis resulting from chronic obstructive airway disease and necrotic conditions of the bowel wall, which affect the small bowel much more often than the large bowel. Any inflammatory large bowel disease can result in colonic pneumatosis once the mucosa has been breached. On plain radiography and CT, the gas is more linear or curvilinear (Fig. 5-142) than the gas cysts seen in pneumatosis cystoides coli (Fig. 5-143), and gas is often identified in the mesenteric venous system or liver or both (Fig. 5-144).

Colitis Cystica Profunda

Colitis cystica profunda is a rare benign condition characterized by multiple smooth rectosigmoid mucous cysts. It is to be distinguished from colitis cystica superficialis, which also produces cystic dilatation of rectosigmoid mucous glands but is always associated with pellagra. The mucous cysts can be multiple when colitis cystica profunda is associated with solitary rectal ulcer syndrome or with colitis from any cause. On occasion, the cysts may coalesce and give the appearance of a larger mass that is difficult to distinguish from carcinoma. More commonly, they appear as multiple intraluminal filling defects in the rectosigmoid region on BE. They are usually identified incidentally when cross-sectional imaging is performed for other reasons (Fig. 5-145).

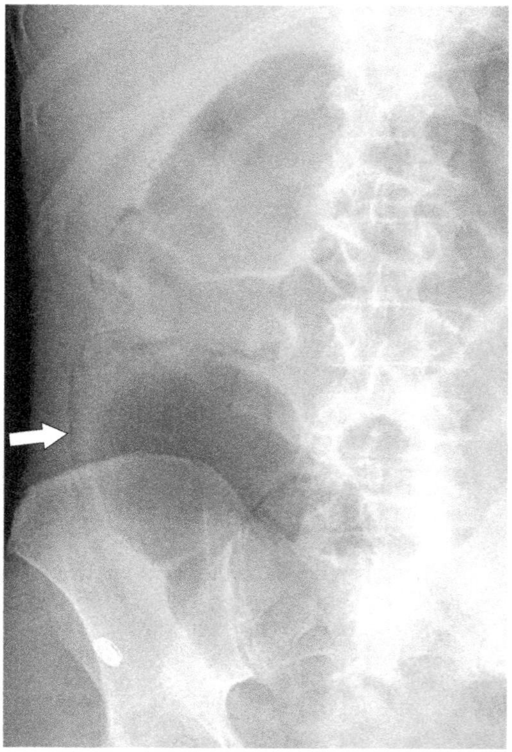

FIGURE 5-142. Plain abdominal radiograph in a 69-year-old man with subtle ascending colon linear pneumatosis (*arrow*).

Colonic Trauma

Most colonic trauma is iatrogenic, usually as a complication from surgery or instrumentation, particularly colonoscopy (Figs. 5-146 and 5-147). Rectal perforation can occur after forceful BE tube

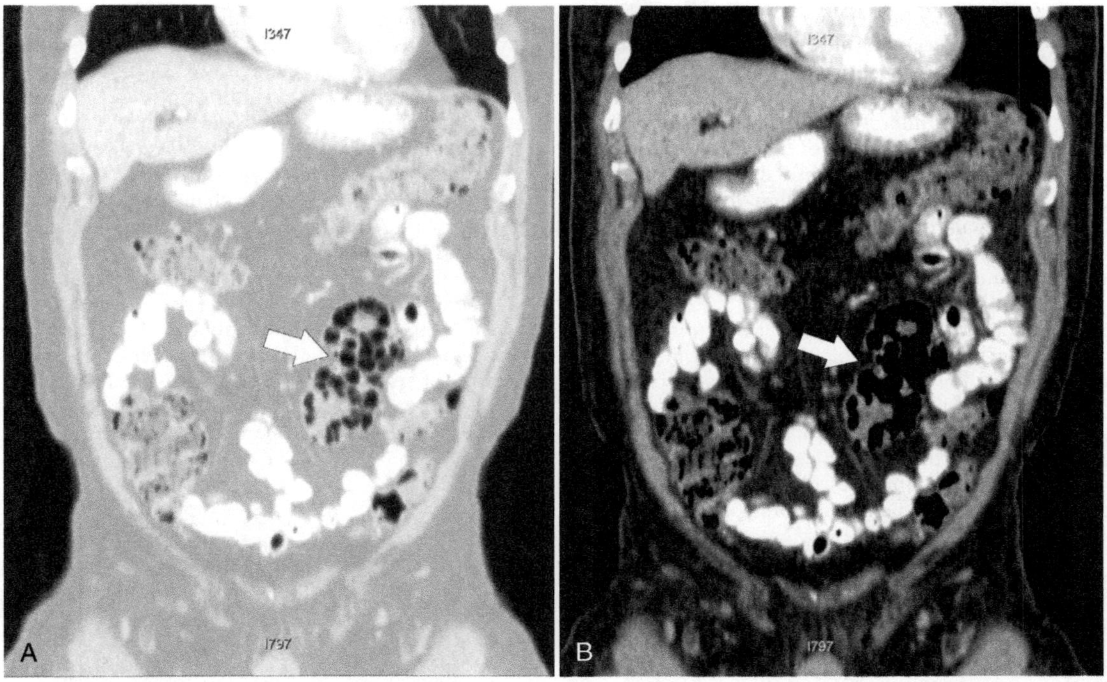

FIGURE 5-143. **A** and **B**, Coronal CT with soft-tissue and lung window settings in a 68-year-old man with pneumatosis cystoides (*arrows*).

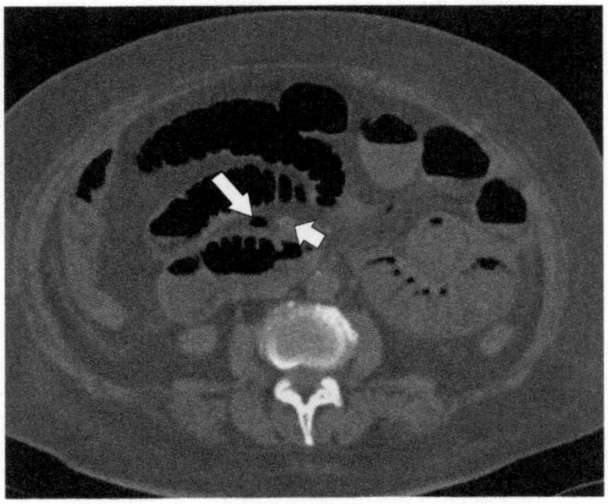

FIGURE 5-144. Axial noncontrast CT (on bone window settings) in a 69-year-old man with both small bowel and colonic ischemia due to a calcified and partially occluded superior mesenteric artery (*small arrow*) and gas within the superior mesenteric vein (*arrow*).

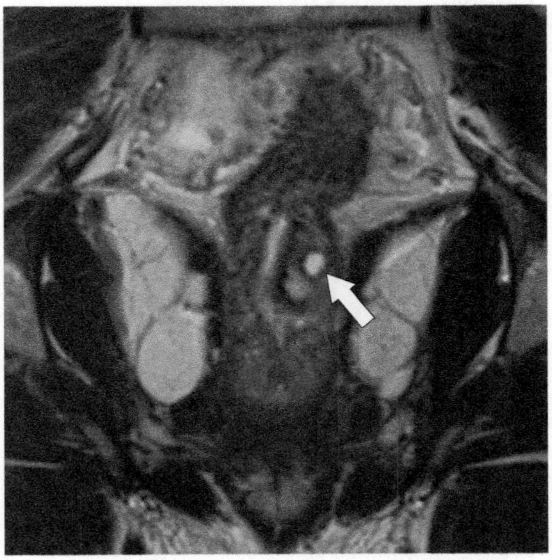

FIGURE 5-145. Coronal T2-weighted MRI in a 36-year-old woman with small T2 bright submucosal cysts (*arrow*) due to colitis cystica.

insertion, and if the rupture is intraperitoneal, the extravasated colonic contents can cause a severe, life-threatening peritonitis. If patients survive the initial insult, they are likely to have long-term complications of multiple adhesions secondary to the original peritonitis.

Most rectal perforation with BE rectal tubes is confined below the peritoneal reflection, so diffuse peritonitis is unlikely. Colonic perforation caused by overdistention with gas, whether iatrogenic or obstructive, is most likely to occur in the cecum because this region distends the most with equal pressure applied throughout the colon (Laplace's* law).

Other colonic trauma may result from self-induced trauma caused by objects inserted into the rectum, which can perforate and lead to either local abscess formation or more diffuse peritonitis if the peritoneal reflection is perforated.

*Pierre-Simon Laplace (1749-1827), French mathematician and astronomer.

Pelvic Floor Anomalies

Pelvic floor anomalies are common in middle-aged and elderly women, particularly after multiple childbirths. Diagnostic imaging, including video fluoroscopy and MRI, plays an increasing role in the evaluation of pelvic floor dysfunction. Endoanal US can also be used to evaluate anal sphincter rupture or tears. Imaging referral is mainly to evaluate pelvic floor prolapse and incontinence. Pelvic floor anatomy is complex, and a comprehensive understanding is necessary to perform and provide accurate diagnosis of these abnormalities. It is divided into three compartments: anterior (bladder, urethra), middle (vagina), and posterior (rectum). They are supported by the levator ani muscle and pelvic fascia.

MR imaging of the anal sphincter is best performed with an endorectal coil to provide better spatial resolution, but diagnostic images can be obtained with a body coil. Defecography or evacuation proctography can be used to evaluate functional abnormalities of defecation by visualizing the pelvic floor descent after the insertion of either barium paste at fluoroscopy or gel at MRI. In the former test, using video fluoroscopy, the patient is analyzed while seated upright during the process of defecation. Spot views show anatomical pelvic floor descent, but diseases are usually diagnosed by review of the fluoroscopic video. The examination has three stages: preevacuation, evacuation, and postevacuation. A line joining the posterior pubic bone margin to the lower coccyx (pubococcygeal line) defines the lower border of the pelvic floor in the healthy individual.

A rectocele is an anterior bulge of the rectal wall during evacuation (Fig. 5-148). Rectal prolapse may be internal or external. Internal prolapse is confined to the rectum and anal canal and is really a mucosal or full-thickness intrarectal intussusception. An external prolapse occurs when the rectal prolapse is visible externally beyond the anal canal. Small bowel prolapse (enterocele) occurs when the small bowel enters the rectogenital space, usually at the end of the examination from the increased intraabdominal pressure induced by the defecation process. A cystocele occurs when the bladder base descends below the inferior border of the pubic symphysis. Therefore defecography is sometimes preceded by voiding cystourethrogram to evaluate for any concomitant bladder disease.

Pelvic floor descent is defined as descent of the entire pelvic floor below the pubococcygeal line and is defined at the resting anorectal junction as greater than 3.0 cm below the ischial tuberosities or anorectal descent greater than 3.5 cm during evacuation (Fig. 5-148).

Pelvic floor descent is also observed using rapid sequence T2-weighted MRI obtained predominantly in the sagittal plane (Fig. 5-149). The pubococcygeal line (Fig. 5-149A) is used to define the pelvic floor, which extends from the inferior border of the pubic symphysis to the last joint of the coccyx. At rest, the anorectal junction normally lies at or just above this plane. Pelvic organ descent below this line generally indicates

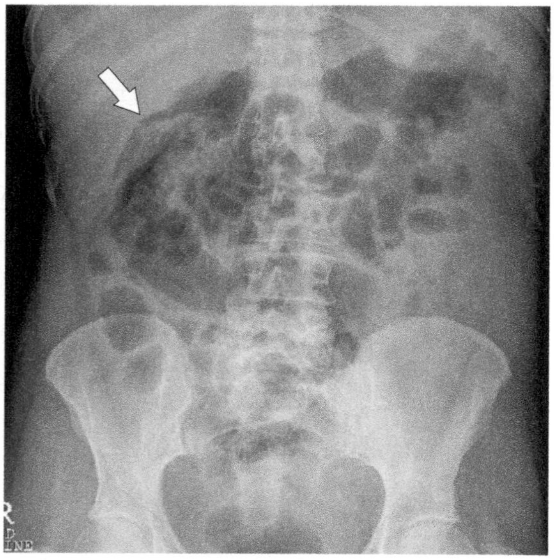

FIGURE 5-146. Plain abdominal imaging in a 56-year-old woman with extraluminal colonic gas (*arrow*) after large bowel perforation from colonoscopy.

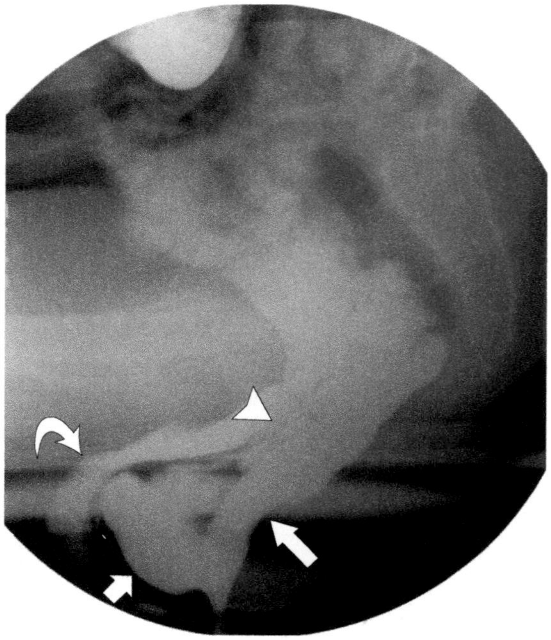

FIGURE 5-148. Defecography in a 49-year-old woman with abnormal rectal descent (*arrow*) with an anterior rectocele (*small arrow*), an enterocele (*arrowhead*), and a cystocele (*curved arrow*).

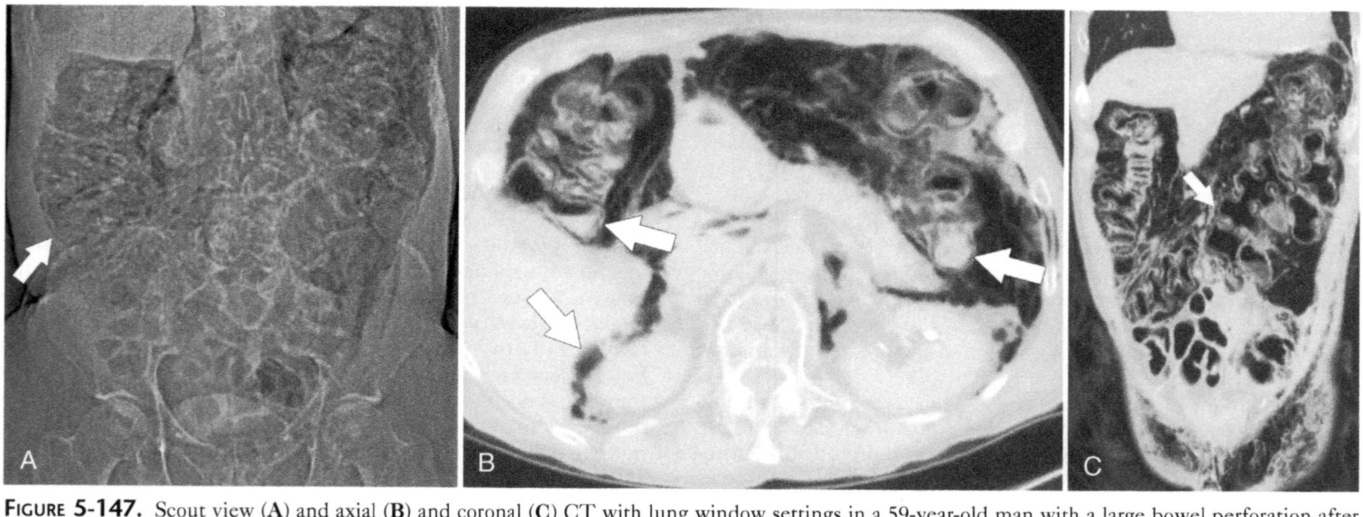

FIGURE 5-147. Scout view (**A**) and axial (**B**) and coronal (**C**) CT with lung window settings in a 59-year-old man with a large bowel perforation after colonoscopy now with diffuse gas in the colonic wall, retroperitoneal, and subcutaneous emphysema (*arrows*).

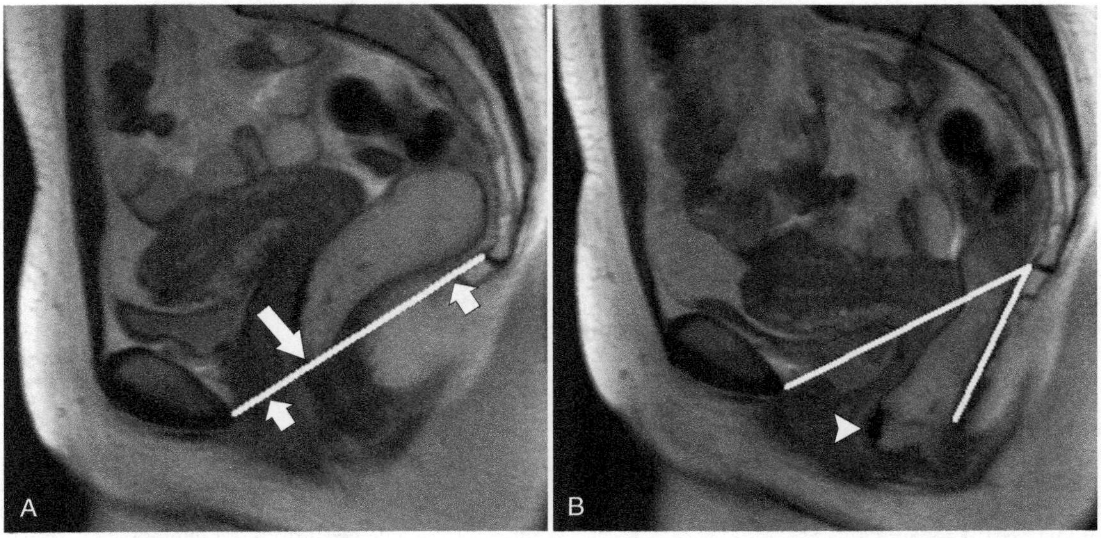

FIGURE 5-149. A, Sagittal T2-weighted MRI in a 38-year-old woman at rest with the anorectal junction (*arrow*) at the pubococcygeal line (*small arrows*). B, At straining and Valsalva, the anorectal junction descends well below the pubococcygeal line (*the rectal angle represented by lower straight line*) and a small rectocele (*arrowhead*).

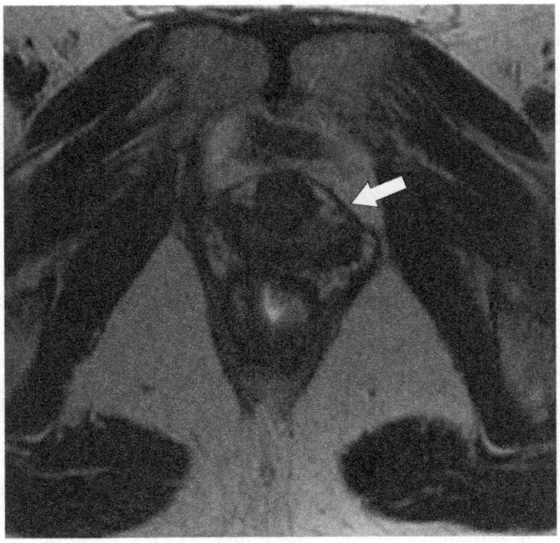

FIGURE 5-150. Axial T2-weighted MRI in a 40-year-old woman with a left-sided levator ani tear (*arrow*).

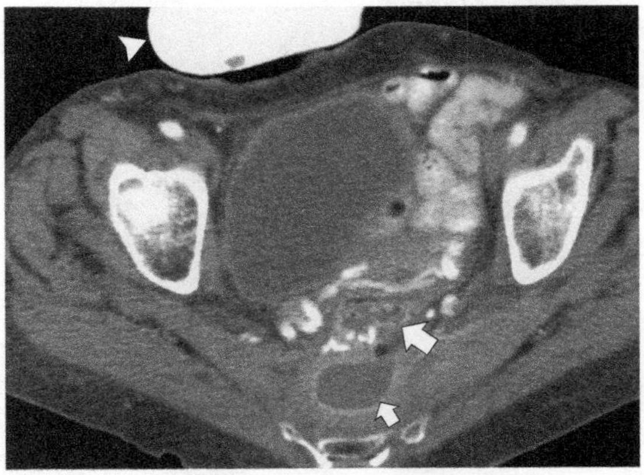

FIGURE 5-151. Axial contrast-enhanced CT in a 69-year-old man with anterior resection (*arrow*) for rectal cancer and now a postoperative fluid collection in the presacral space (*small arrow*), which was found to be infected after percutaneous aspiration. There is a defunctioning colostomy bag present (*arrowhead*).

pelvic floor descent, and if it is greater than 2 cm, the patient may benefit from corrective surgery. Other lines may be drawn, including the H line (representing the anteroposterior width of the levator hiatus) from the interior pubic symphysis to the posterior rectal wall at the level of the anorectal junction and the M line (vertical descent of levator hiatus), which represents a perpendicular line drawn from the pubococcygeal line to the posterior margin on the H line. These lines are sometimes useful to confirm pelvic floor laxity. Imaging can also demonstrate levator ani abnormalities, which contribute to pelvic floor descent (Fig. 5-150).

Postsurgical Colonic Abnormalities

There are a number of colonic surgical procedures aside from colectomy, abdominoperineal resection, and colostomy, including various colonic reanastomoses after anterior resection for rectal cancer and the creation of ileoanal pouches. As with any surgical procedure, there is a risk of hemorrhage and infection. Depending on the type of operative procedure, anastomotic leakage or fistula formation or both may occur. These complications are usually examined with CT, which should show any dehiscence of the bowel with intraperitoneal fluid (which may have formed an abscess) or pneumoperitoneum (Fig. 5-151) or both.

APPENDIX

The vermiform (meaning "worm-like") appendix is a vestigial remnant whose physiological role is still in debate. It is a thin tubular outpouching from the cecum, usually arising between its tip and the ileocecal valve, and normally is 2 to 3 mm in diameter. Its length varies remarkably, sometimes short (2 cm) and sometimes long (20 cm). Furthermore, while most are positioned to the left of the cecum, up to 25% are retrocecal, and some may extend as far as the right upper quadrant. Many appendices fill with gas or oral/rectal contrast medium as seen at CT. There are a finite number of appendiceal diseases, and despite its small size, the appendix is responsible for significant morbidity (and less often mortality), owing mainly to the complications of appendicitis.

Appendicitis

The appendix is an important factor in disease because of its propensity to be obstructed by a fecalith, usually close to its orifice. A fecalith is a small fecal concretion that often calcifies and may become quite large (Fig. 5-152). The obstructed appendix becomes distended with secreted appendiceal mucous, which is then secondarily infected, resulting in appendicitis. The wall thickens because of inflammatory edema and hyperemia. When the appendiceal caliber (overall diameter) is ≥6 mm (mural thickness, >2 mm), acute appendicitis can be diagnosed with a sensitivity of 100% but lower specificity, which rises to close to 100% when the diameter is ≥7 mm. Patients typically report periumbilical pain moving to the right lower quadrant with rebound tenderness (McBurney* point). Despite these classic clinical findings, the diagnosis is notoriously difficult to make. Up to 50% of patients referred for surgery before the CT era were found to have either a normal appendix or another pathologic finding. However, since US in children and CT in adults became used routinely to evaluate for suspected appendicitis, few patients are now referred unnecessarily for surgery.

*Charles McBurney (1845-1913), American surgeon.

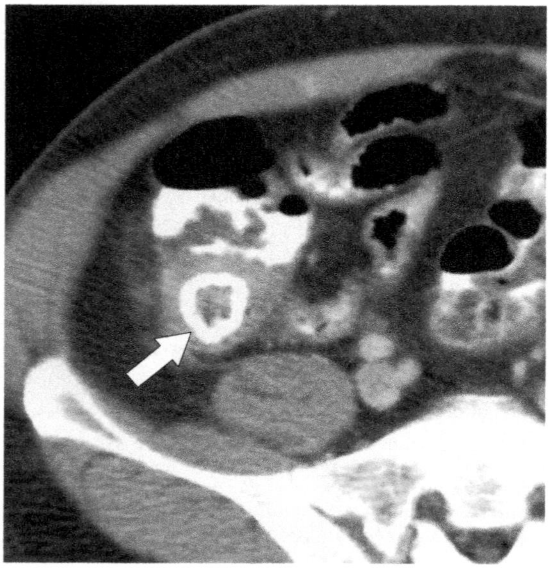

FIGURE 5-152. Axial contrast-enhanced CT in a 51-year-old woman with a large fecalith (*arrow*) that caused localized mucosal inflammation rather than appendicitis.

Plain radiography may demonstrate a fecalith in approximately 10% of patients, with possible ileus in the setting of acute appendicitis. US, the investigation of choice in children, demonstrates a noncompressible appendix dilated ≥7 mm in diameter with tenderness directly over the inflamed appendix (McBurney sign), which may also show increased Doppler* flow, although this is not necessary to make the diagnosis (Fig. 5-153). A fecalith is frequently identified as an echogenic focus with posterior acoustic shadowing. Perforation and abscess formation are seen as a complex fluid collection, with or without gas.

In adults, CT is the investigation of choice with a sensitivity and specificity approaching 100% (Fig. 5-154). The optimal technique is under debate, with some institutions recommending rectal contrast for better delineation of the cecum and appendix, but most protocols use only oral and IV contrast media (providing the patient can tolerate this). The dilated appendix (≥7 mm in diameter) should be identified, and the fecalith is frequently identified (Fig. 5-154). There is mucosal enhancement after IV contrast administration, and usually periappendiceal inflammatory change (fat-stranding) or fluid is seen, although this is variable (Figs. 5-154 and 5-155). The cecal tip often demonstrates secondary thickening, termed a "cecal bar," best observed with CT protocols using rectal contrast medium. Once perforation occurs, CT demonstrates the extraluminal collection of gas and pus (Fig. 5-156). Appendiceal perforation can lead to a localized walled-off abscess, but more extensive peritonitis may also occur. Appendicitis undiagnosed or left untreated carries high morbidity and mortality rates.

The imaging diagnosis of appendicitis is not always so straightforward. US evaluation may be compromised from overlying adipose tissue, bowel gas, and abdominal pain. Therefore CT has a higher sensitivity for the detection of an inflamed appendix (close to 100% vs. 85%). Despite this, close attention to regional anatomy may be required to identify the inflamed appendix, which can be buried between loops of small bowel, some of which may not be opacified adequately with oral contrast agent. The associated periappendiceal inflammatory change (stranding) may obliterate the normal fat planes between tissues, making evaluation of normal anatomy more challenging (Fig. 5-156). The inflamed appendix may also not be in the expected location, as explained previously. With more severe infections the appendix may not be visible at all because of a larger right lower quadrant inflammatory mass, particularly if there has been appendiceal perforation. At that point the diagnosis is inferred rather than definitive, although an acute inflammatory mass in the right lower quadrant in adulthood is likely to be appendicitis until proven otherwise. The inflammation may be confined to the appendiceal tip, known as "tip" appendicitis (Fig. 5-157), which can be an even

*Christian Doppler (1803-1853), Austrian mathematician and physicist.

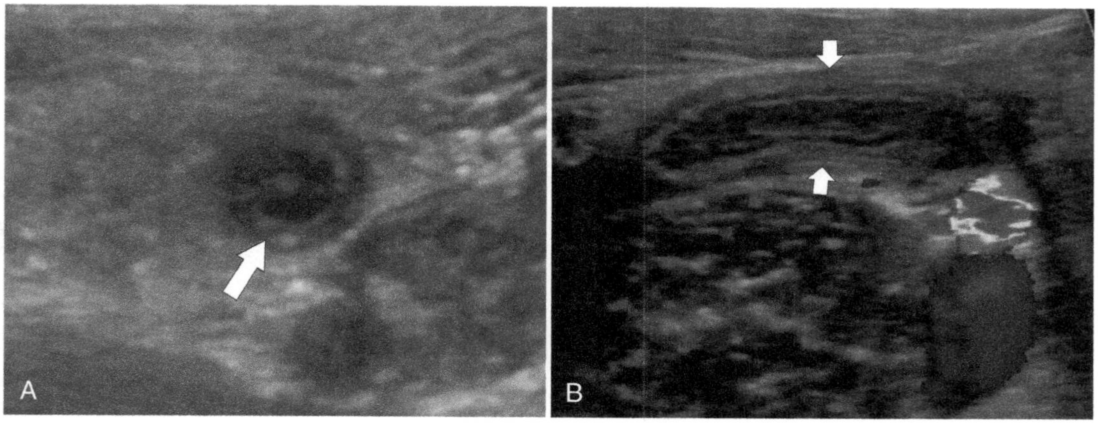

FIGURE 5-153. Transverse (**A**) and sagittal (**B**) US images in a 16-year-old girl with appendicitis demonstrating thickened walls (*arrow*) with an overall diameter (*small arrows*) of 9 mm. *See ExpertConsult.com for color image.*

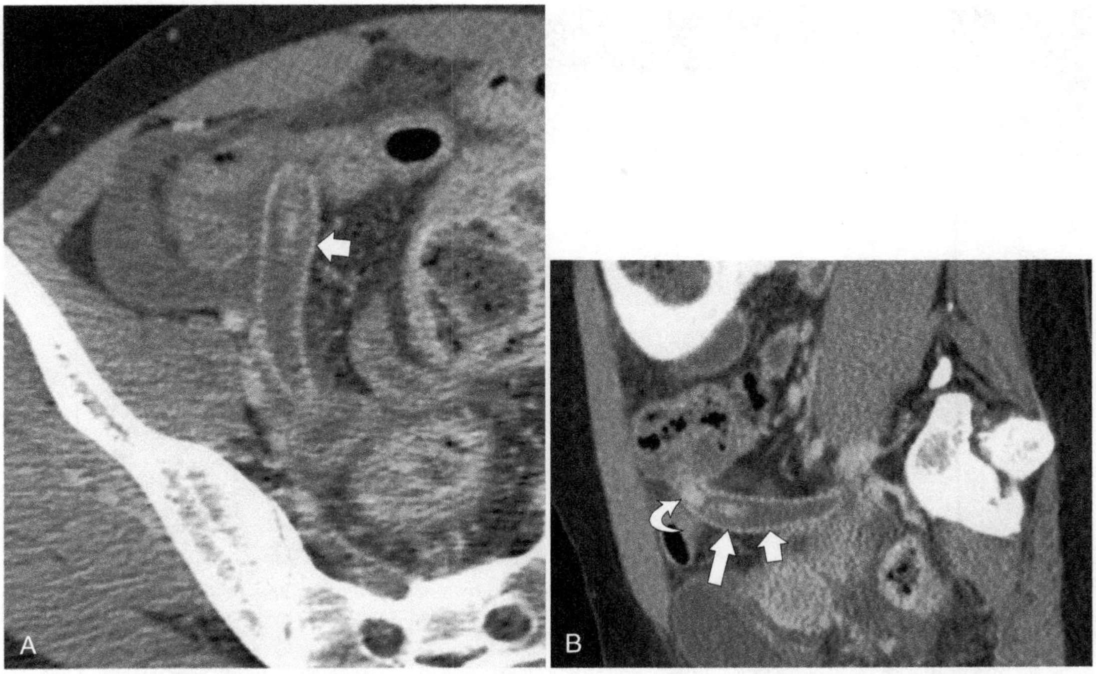

FIGURE 5-154. Axial (**A**) and sagittal (**B**) contrast-enhanced CT in a 27-year-old woman with a dilated pus-filled appendix (*arrow*) in the right lower quadrant. There is inflammatory enhancement of the appendiceal wall (*small arrows*), a fecalith at the appendiceal base (*curved arrow*), and another small fecalith in the mid appendix. There is minimal fat-stranding.

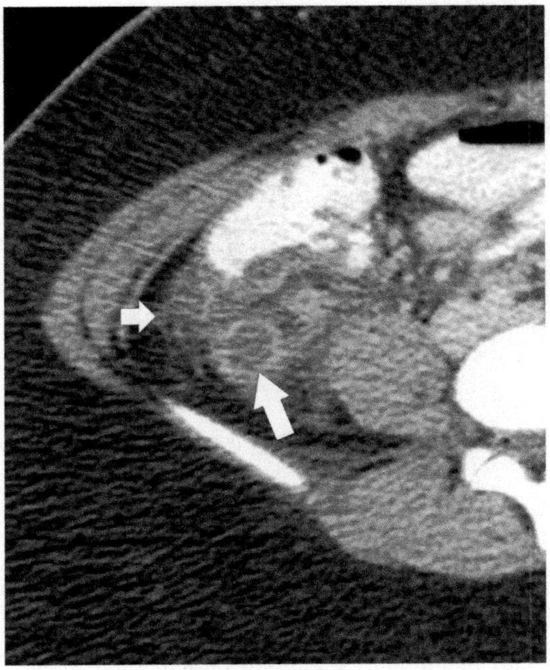

FIGURE 5-155. Axial contrast-enhanced CT in a 55-year-old man with acute appendicitis (*arrow*) and periappendiceal inflammatory change (*small arrow*).

more challenging diagnosis to make, and careful scrutiny of the whole appendiceal length is therefore warranted.

Evaluation in pregnant patients also presents challenges because of the requirement to avoid ionizing radiation (most sensitive to organogenesis in the first trimester). Patients are therefore referred for US evaluation, but if this is inconclusive, noncontrast MRI is recommended. This should identify the edematous appendix (Fig. 5-158), although the lack of IV and contrast reduces sensitivity.

Appendix Mucocele

The appendix mucocele is relatively rare and results from mucin accumulation within the appendix with resulting cystic dilatation. There are three varieties: a simple benign mucocele resulting from mucosal hypertrophy, a benign mucinous cystadenoma (the most prevalent), and malignant mucinous cystadenocarcinoma. The latter is probably secondary to the adenoma-carcinoma sequence and is prone to rupture and spread the malignant mucin throughout the peritoneum, so called pseudomyxoma peritonei.

At imaging by CT, there is a low-density cystic structure in the region of the appendix, with or without wall calcification (common in simple mucoceles) (Fig. 5-159). Cystadenomas can appear identical to simple mucoceles, although they can locally perforate with deposition of compartmentalized mucin (Fig. 5-160). Cystadenocarcinomas are usually larger, are irregular with nodular wall thickening (Fig. 5-161), and often have calcification in the solid component. These tumors rupture far more commonly than cystadenoma and readily distribute their mucin throughout the peritoneum. Pseudomyxoma peritonei is identified by loculated mucinous ascites with scalloping surrounding the internal organs, particularly the liver and spleen (Fig. 5-162). The disease is extremely difficult to treat given the widespread distribution of malignant material, and patients may require intermittent surgical removal or relief of small bowel obstruction.

Appendiceal Adenocarcinoma

Appendiceal adenocarcinomas are rare, usually develop from the adenoma-carcinoma sequence, and therefore follow the pattern of colonic adenocarcinomas in their origin and outcome. Like colon cancer, they can also be mucinous or nonmucinous (i.e., signet ring cell carcinoma). The mucinous type is now thought to be the same disease as pseudomyxoma peritonei described previously. Nonmucinous appendiceal carcinomas usually present with acute

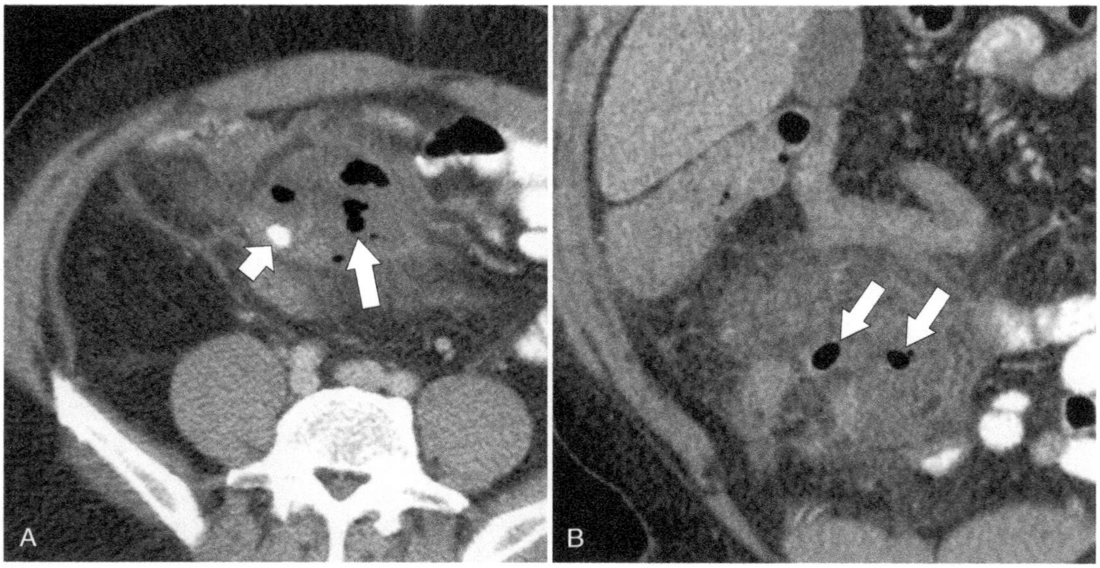

Figure 5-156. Axial (**A**) and coronal (**B**) contrast-enhanced CT in a 33-year-old man with perforated appendicitis and a pelvic abscess with pus and extraluminal gas (*arrows*). The appendix was difficult to identify, but the diagnosis was suggested by the presence of a calcified fecalith (*small arrow*).

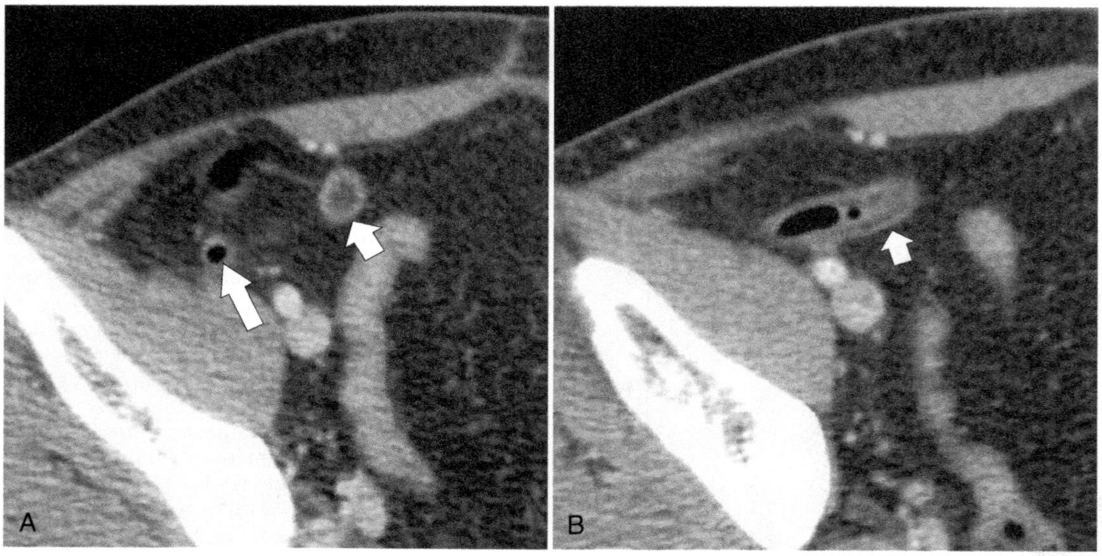

Figure 5-157. Axial contrast-enhanced (**A** and **B**) CT in a 57-year-old man with tip appendicitis. The proximal appendiceal wall is normal (*arrow*), whereas the distal wall is thickened (*small arrows*).

appendicitis, and at imaging, the differentiation between severe benign appendicitis and appendicitis secondary to malignant adenocarcinoma can be difficult. Features favoring the latter include a larger right lower quadrant solid mass (Fig. 5-163), particularly if there is regional lymphadenopathy, and distant metastases.

Appendiceal Intussusception

Appendiceal intussusception is very rare, usually presenting in the first decade of life and occurring spontaneously or secondary to benign predisposing factors (endometriosis, carcinoid, fecaliths, foreign bodies) or malignant appendiceal diseases. The clinical presentation can mimic acute appendicitis, with right lower quadrant pain. The intussusceptum becomes inflamed, enlarged, and edematous and may cause small bowel obstruction. Imaging reveals a soft tissue mass and surrounding inflammatory change in the region of the cecum and ileocecal valve, with possible CT signs of small bowel obstruction.

Carcinoid (see Chapter 4)

Carcinoids are the most common appendiceal neoplasms, accounting for approximately 1% of all appendectomy specimens. A carcinoid is a neuroendocrine tumor arising from enterochromaffin cells, which are present throughout the GI tract and bronchi. There is some debate as to whether carcinoids are more commonly located in the appendix or terminal ileum, but general consensus favors the terminal ileum. Some authorities state that benign carcinoids are more common in the appendix, whereas malignant ones more commonly occur in the terminal ileum. They are known as APUDomas because they arise from APUD cells (APUD = amine precursor [L-dopa and 5-hydroxytryptophan] and uptake decarboxylation), which produce excessive serotonin and catecholamines. Some appendiceal carcinoids are also known as goblet cell carcinoids or adenocarcinoids. Most carcinoids are asymptomatic and detected only at surgery performed for incidental reasons or because

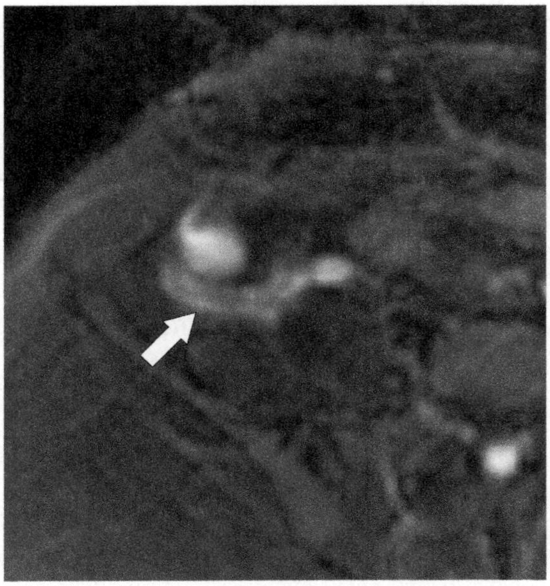

FIGURE 5-158. T2-weighted fat-saturated axial MRI in a 27-year-old pregnant woman with a T2 hyperintense inflamed appendix (*arrow*) proven to be appendicitis at surgery.

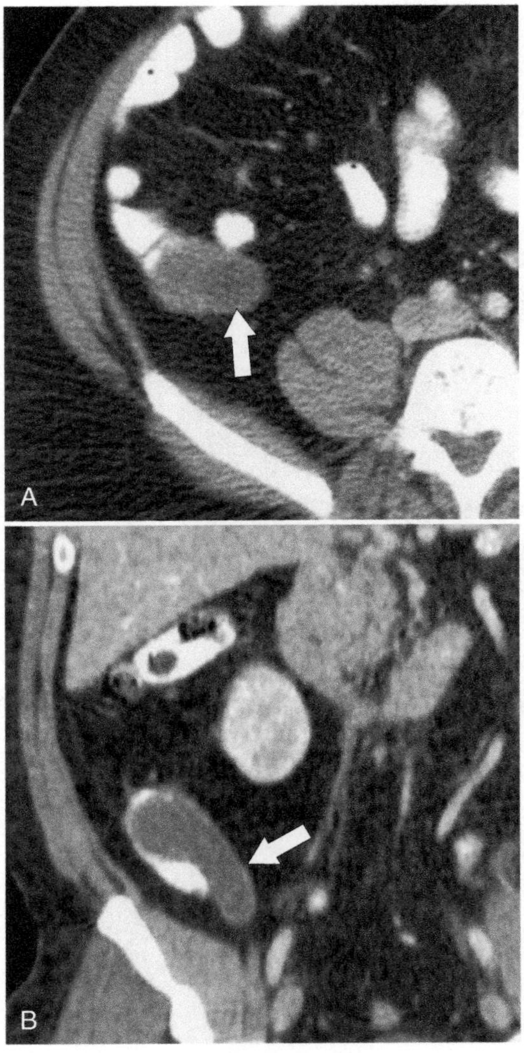

FIGURE 5-159. Axial (A) and coronal (B) CT in a 68-year-old woman and a dilated, mucus-filled appendix (*arrows*) due to a simple mucocele.

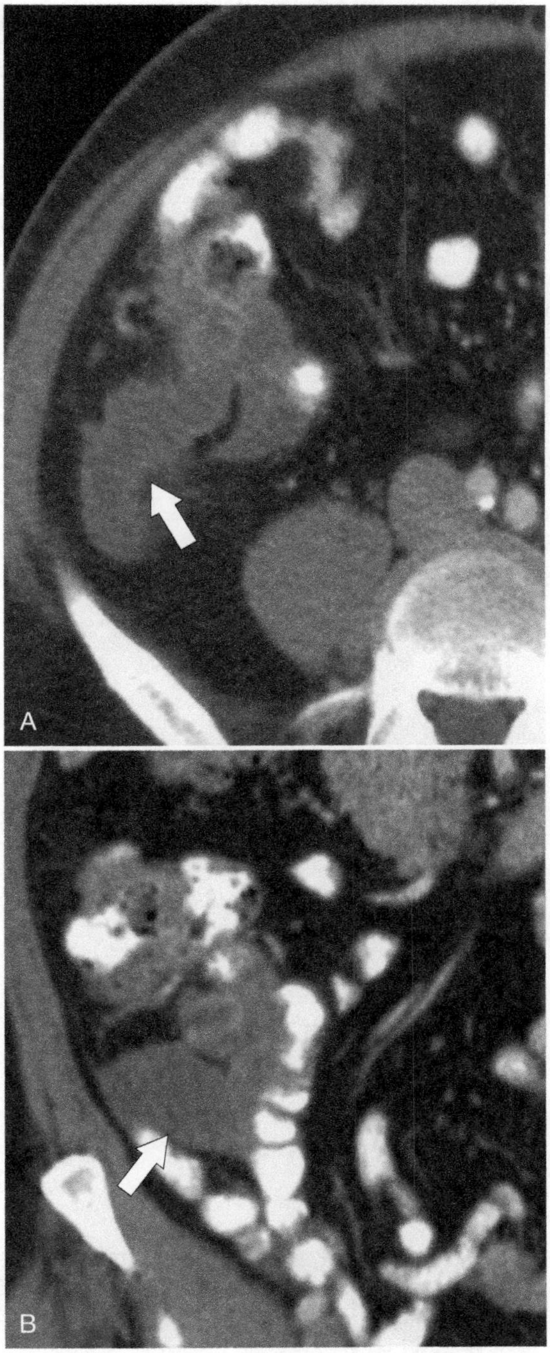

FIGURE 5-160. Axial (A) and coronal (B) contrast-enhanced CT in a 62-year-old man with an appendiceal cystadenoma. There is a complex cystic and tubular mass in the right lower quadrant that has partially ruptured but not spread throughout the peritoneum (*arrows*).

they induce appendicitis, although this is uncommon as most are confined to the distal third of the appendix. Appendiceal carcinoid tumors are usually very small (<1 cm). These tumors produce histamine, bradykinin, and serotonin but not usually in sufficient quantities to cause carcinoid syndrome. In fact, carcinoid syndrome is rare unless the tumor is larger and metastatic, which is unusual for appendiceal carcinoids. The clinical signs of the syndrome (e.g., flushing, diarrhea, tachycardia, peripheral edema) arise from carcinoids that have metastasized to the liver, usually from extraappendiceal sites (i.e., terminal ileum). If sufficiently numerous and voluminous, they can result in loss of hepatic reserve and inability to metabolize the vasoactive hormones sufficiently. Because benign lesions are small, they are almost never identified with CT unless they induce appendicitis (Fig. 5-164), but the primary malignant lesion can occasionally be identified at CT as an enhancing small mass in the expected location (see Chapter 4). They usually metastasize to the regional mesenteric lymph nodes and produce a local desmoplastic reaction, represented by spiculated mesenteric soft tissue thickening similar to that seen with other metastatic carcinoids (i.e., terminal ileum).

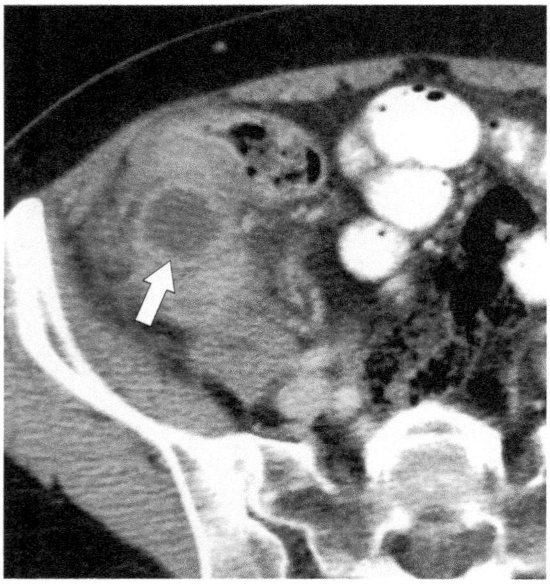

FIGURE 5-161. Axial contrast-enhanced CT in a 77-year-old man with a complex solid and cystic (*arrow*) mass in the region of the appendix proven to be a malignant mucocele.

Crohn Disease (see Chapter 4)

Primary appendiceal Crohn disease is rare. It is more common in younger patients and isolated to the appendix in most cases. It usually presents with symptoms and signs of appendicitis and is therefore diagnosed only after appendectomy. Surgical removal is usually uncomplicated with Crohn disease limited to the appendix, but if Crohn disease is elsewhere, recurrent disease is common. Appendiceal Crohn disease is most commonly part of more florid disease (Fig. 5-165); up to 50% of affected appendices are in patients with colonic disease.

Appendiceal Stump

After appendectomy, a residual appendiceal remnant known as an appendiceal stump may protrude into the cecal base and be identified at BE (Fig. 5-166). It is most likely secondary to a granulomatous reaction to retained suture material. It is usually of no clinical significance except the knowledge of its existence. Adenocarcinoma development within the stump has been reported, and because the lesions can appear similar to colonic adenomatous polyps, patients are typically referred for optical colonoscopy.

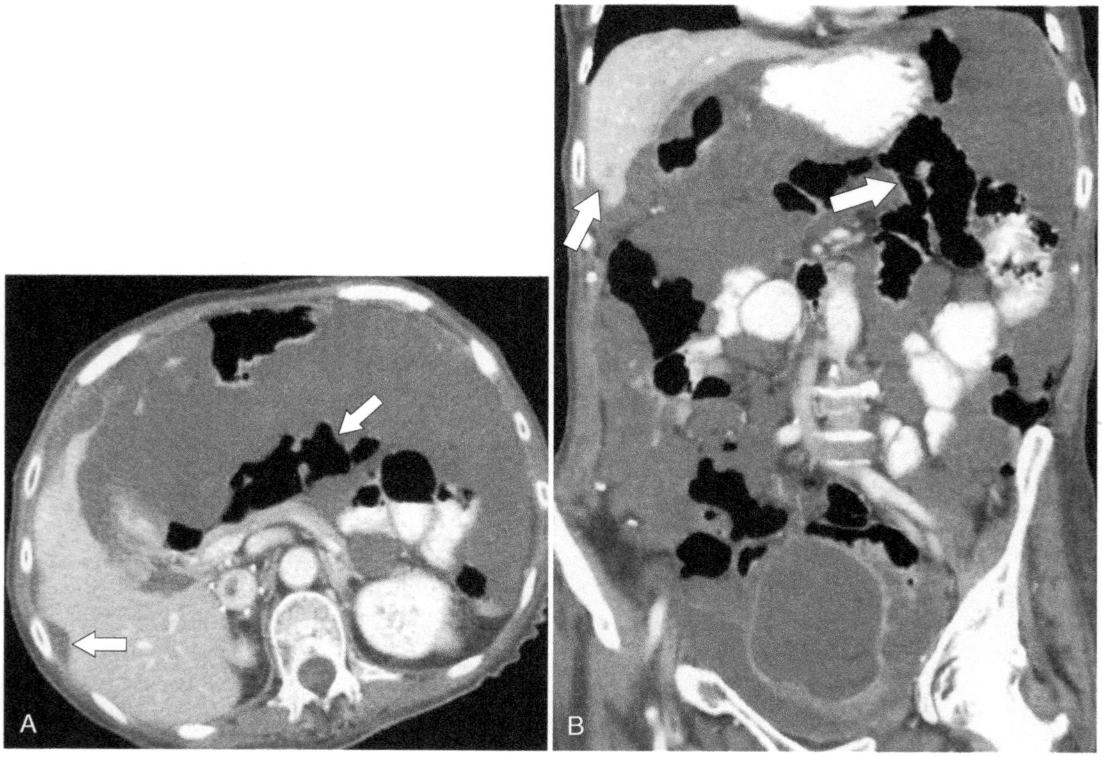

FIGURE 5-162. Axial (**A**) and coronal (**B**) contrast-enhanced CT in a 56-year-old man with pseudomyxoma peritonei. There is widespread metastatic spread of mucous material throughout the peritoneum, compressing bowel and scalloping the liver (*arrows*).

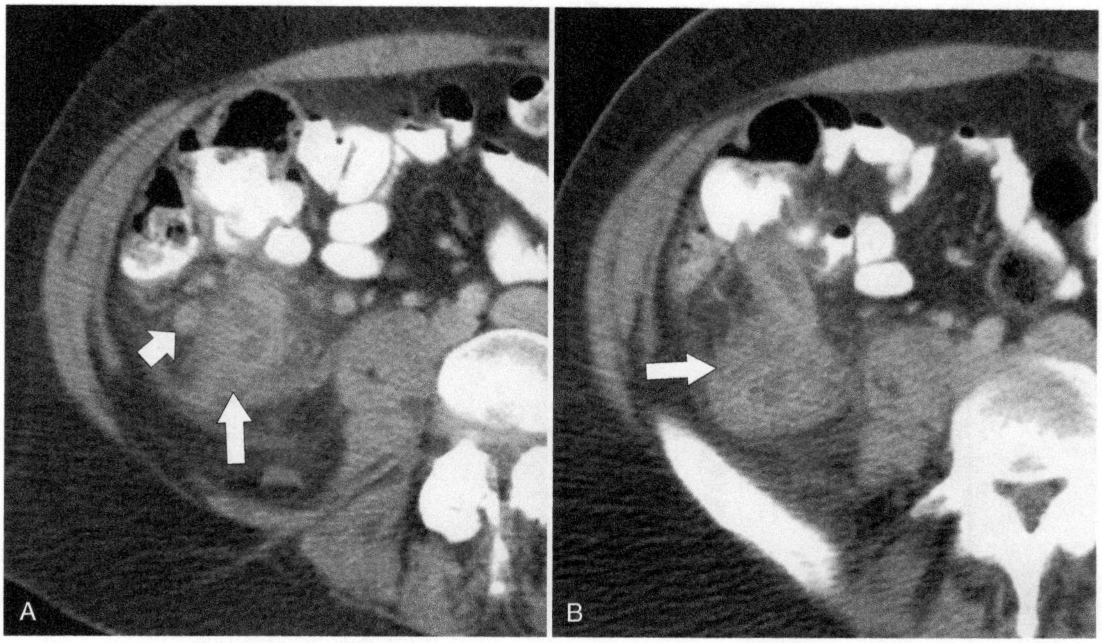

FIGURE 5-163. Axial contrast-enhanced CT (**A** and **B**) in a 50-year-old woman with clinical appendicitis due to nonmucinous appendiceal adenocarcinoma. The diagnosis should be suspected before surgery because of the irregular appendiceal mass (*arrows*) and regional lymphadenopathy (*small arrow*).

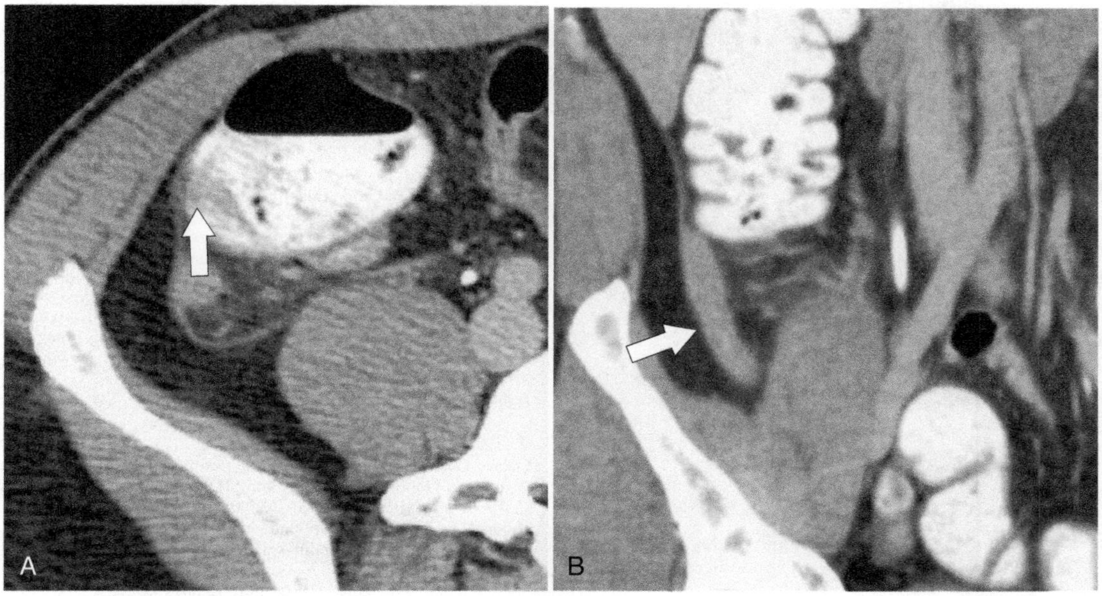

FIGURE 5-164. Axial (**A**) and coronal (**B**) contrast-enhanced CT performed with rectal contrast with appendicitis (*arrows*) due to an underlying benign carcinoid not visible at CT.

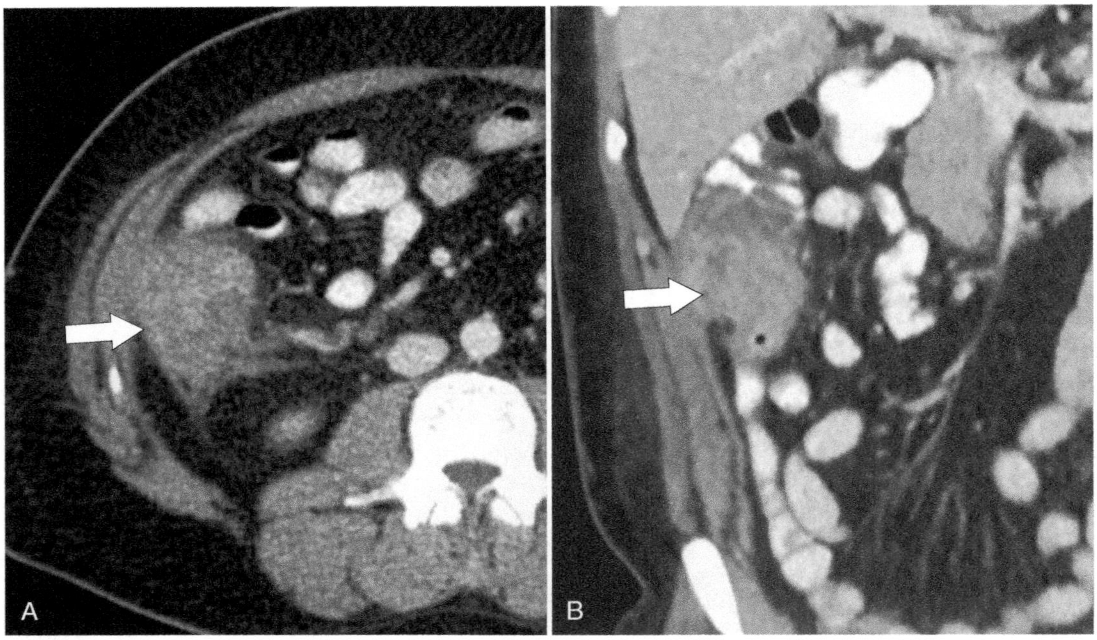

Figure 5-165. Axial (**A**) and coronal (**B**) contrast-enhanced CT in a 40-year-old man with Crohn disease. The cecal inflammatory mass (*arrows*) envelops the appendix, which cannot be identified separately.

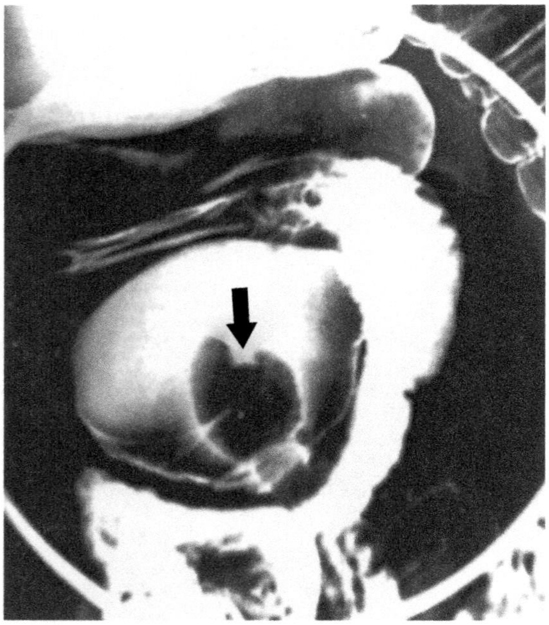

Figure 5-166. DCBE showing a polypoid colonic lesion (*arrow*) in a patient with prior appendectomy representing an appendiceal stump.

Suggested Readings

Almeida AT et al: Epiploic appendagitis: an entity frequently unknown to clinicians—diagnostic imaging, pitfalls, and look-alikes. AJR 193:1243-1251, 2009.

Ambrosini R et al: Inflammatory chronic disease of the colon: how to image. Eur J Radiol 61(3):442-448, 2007.

Anderson SW et al: Abdominal 64-MDCT for suspected appendicitis: the use of oral and IV contrast material versus IV contrast material only. AJR 193: 1282-1288, 2009.

Ash L et al: Colonic abnormalities on CT in adult hospitalized patients with *Clostridium difficile* colitis: prevalence and significance of findings. AJR 186(5):1393-1400, 2006.

Beets RGH et al: Rectal cancer: review with emphasis on MR imaging. Radiology 232(2):335-346, 2004.

Bernard A et al: Appendicitis at the millennium. Radiology 215(2):337-348, 2000.

Chintapalli KN et al: Diveriticulitis versus colon cancer: differentiation with helical CT findings. Radiology 210(2):429-435, 1999.

Choi JS et al: Colonic pseudoobstruction: CT findings. AJR 190(6):1521-1526, 2008.

Darge K et al: MR imaging of the abdomen and pelvis in infants, children, and adolescents. Radiology 261(1):12-29, 2011.

de Miguel CJ et al: MR imaging evaluation of perianal fistulas: spectrum of imaging features. Radiographics 32(1):175-194, 2012.

Doria AS et al: US or CT for diagnosis of appendicitis in children and adults? A meta-analysis. Radiology 241(1):83-94, 2006.

Dresen RC et al: Locally advanced rectal cancer: MR imaging for restaging after neoadjuvant radiation therapy with concomitant chemotherapy part I. Are we able to predict tumor confined to the rectal wall? Radiology 252(1):71-80, 2009.

Duncan JE et al: CT colonography predictably overestimates colonic length and distance to polyps compared with optical colonoscopy. AJR 193:1291-1295, 2009.

El Sayed RF et al: Pelvic floor dysfunction: assessment with combined analysis of static and dynamic MR imaging findings. Radiology 248(2):518-530, 2008.

Etzioni DA et al: Diverticulitis in the United States: 1998-2005: changing patterns of disease and treatment. Ann Surg 249(2):210-217, 2009.

Ferrucci JT: Double-contrast barium enema: use in practice and implications for CT colonography. AJR 187(1):170-173, 2006.

Gaitini D et al: Diagnosing acute appendicitis in adults: accuracy of color Doppler sonography and MDCT compared with surgery and clinical follow-up. AJR 190:1300-1306, 2008.

Gaitini D et al: Original research: diagnosing acute appendicitis in adults: accuracy of color Doppler sonography and MDCT compared with surgery and clinical follow-up. AJR 190:1300-1306, 2008.

Garcia K et al: Suspected appendicitis in children: diagnostic importance of normal abdominopelvic CT findings with nonvisualized appendix. Radiology 250(2):531-537, 2009.

Gastrointestinal imaging. AJR 5(Suppl E130):198, 2012.

Geffroy Y et al: Multidetector CT angiography in acute gastrointestinal bleeding: why, when, and how. Radiographics 31(3):E35-E46, 2011.

General and emergency radiology. AJR 198(5 Supplement E241):198, 2012.

General/emergency. AJR 194:A154-A172, 2010.

Gollub MJ: Colonic intussusception: clinical and radiographic features. AJR 196:W580-W585, 2011.

Gore RM et al: Helical CT in the evaluation of the acute abdomen. AJR 174:901-913, 2000.

Halpert RD: Toxic dilatation of the colon. Radiol Clin North Am 25(1):147-155, 1987.

Harned RK et al: The hamartomatous polyposis syndromes: clinical and radiologic features. AJR 164(3):565-571, 1995.

Hazelwood S et al: Images in clinical medicine: colonic ileus. N Engl J Med 354(7):e6, 2006.

Heffernan C et al: Stercoral colitis leading to fatal peritonitis: CT findings. AJR 184:1189-1193, 2005.
Heverhagen JT et al: MR imaging for acute lower abdominal and pelvic pain. Radiographics 29(6):1781-1796, 2009.
Hoeffel C et al: Multi-detector row CT: spectrum of diseases involving the ileocecal area. Radiographics 26(5):1373-1390, 2006.
Hoeffel CC et al: MRI of rectal disorders. AJR 187:W275-W284, 2006.
Horrow MM et al: Differentiation of perforated from nonperforated appendicitis at CT. Radiology 227(1):46-51, 2003.
Horsthuis K et al: Perianal Crohn disease: evaluation of dynamic contrast-enhanced MR imaging as an indicator of disease activity. Radiology 251(2): 380-387, 2009.
Horton KM et al: CT evaluation of the colon: inflammatory disease. Radiographics 20(2):399-418, 2000.
Horton KM et al: Volume-rendered 3D CT of the mesenteric vasculature: normal anatomy, anatomic variants, and pathologic conditions. Radiographics 22(1):161-172, 2002.
Janes SE et al: Management of diverticulitis. BMJ 332(7536):271-275, 2006.
Javors BR et al: The northern exposure sign: a newly described finding in sigmoid volvulus. AJR 173(3):571-574, 1999.
Johnson CD et al: The national CT colonography trial: assessment of accuracy in participants 65 years of age and older. Radiology 263(2):401-408, 2012.
Johnson PT et al: MDCT for suspected appendicitis: effect of reconstruction section thickness on diagnostic accuracy, rate of appendiceal visualization, and reader confidence using axial images. AJR 192:893-901, 2009.
Keeling AN et al: Limited-preparation CT colonography in frail elderly patients: a feasibility study. AJR 194:1279-1287, 2010.
Kessler N et al: Appendicitis: evaluation of sensitivity, specificity, and predictive values of US, Doppler US, and laboratory findings. Radiology 230(2):472-478, 2004.
Keyzer C et al: Acute appendicitis: comparison of low-dose and standard-dose unenhanced multi–detector row CT. Radiology 232(1):164-172, 2004.
Kim DH et al: CT colonography: performance and program outcome measures in an older screening population. Radiology 254(2):493-500, 2010.
Kirkpatrick IDC et al: Gastrointestinal complications in the neutropenic patient: characterization and differentiation with abdominal CT. Radiology 226(3): 668-674, 2003.
Lee JH et al: CT colonography in patients who have undergone sigmoid colostomy: a feasibility study. AJR 197:W653-W657, 2011.
Lee SH et al: The ileosigmoid knot: CT findings. AJR 174(3):685-687, 2000.
Levsky JM et al: CT findings of sigmoid volvulus. AJR 194:136-143, 2010.
Levsky JM et al: The coffee bean sign in sigmoid volvulus. Radiology 258(2): 651-652, 2011.
Ly JQ: The Rigler sign. Radiology 228(3):706-707, 2003.
Macari M et al: Diagnosis of familial adenomatous polyposis using two-dimensional and three-dimensional CT colonography. AJR 173(1):249-250, 1999.
Maglinte DDT et al: Functional imaging of the pelvic floor. Radiology 258(1): 23-39, 2011.
Mancuso MA et al: Case 120: ischemic colitis limited to the cecum. Radiology 244(3):919-922, 2007.
Marin D et al: Percutaneous abscess drainage in patients with perforated acute appendicitis: effectiveness, safety, and prediction of outcome. AJR 194:422-429, 2010.
Martí M et al: Acute lower intestinal bleeding: feasibility and diagnostic performance of CT angiography. Radiology 262(1):109-116, 2012.
McCarville MB et al: Typhlitis in childhood cancer. Cancer 104(2):380-387, 2005.
MERCURY Study Group: Extramural depth of tumor invasion at thin-section MR in patients with rectal cancer: results of the MERCURY study. Radiology 243(1):132-139, 2007.
Miller FH et al: Imaging features of enterohemorrhagic *Escherichia coli* colitis. AJR 177:619-623, 2001.
Moawad FJ et al: CT colonography may improve colorectal cancer screening compliance. AJR 195:1118–1112, 2010.
Moore CJ et al: CT of cecal volvulus: unraveling the image. AJR 177(1):95-98, 2001.
Ng KS et al: CT features of primary epiploic appendagitis. Eur J Radiol 59(2):284-288, 2006.
Padhani AR et al: Whole-body diffusion-weighted MR imaging in cancer: current status and research directions. Radiology 261(3):700-718, 2011.
Paulson EK et al: Acute appendicitis: added diagnostic value of coronal reformations from ositropic voxels at multi-detector row CT. Radiology 235(3):879-885, 2005.
Pedrosa I et al: Pregnant patients suspected of having acute appendicitis: effect of MR imaging on negative laparotomy rate and appendiceal perforation rate. Radiology 250(3):749-757, 2009.
Pereira JM et al: CT and MR imaging of extrahepatic fatty masses of the abdomen and pelvis: techniques, diagnosis, differential diagnosis, and pitfalls. Radiographics 25(1):69-85, 2005.
Pickhardt PJ: Differential diagnosis of polypoid lesions seen at CT colonography (virtual colonoscopy). Radiographics 24(6):1535-1556, 2004.
Pickhardt PJ: Screening CT colonography: how I do it. AJR 189:290-298, 2007.
Pickhardt PJ et al: Acquired gastrointestinal fistulas: classification, etiologies, and imaging evaluation. Radiology 224(1):9-23, 2002.
Pickhardt PJ et al: Clinical management of small (6- to 9-mm) polyps detected at screening CT colonography: a cost-effectiveness analysis. AJR 191:1509-1516, 2008.
Pickhardt PJ et al: Primary neoplasms of the appendix manifesting as acute appendicitis: CT findings with pathologic comparison. Radiology 224(3):775-781, 2002.
Poletti P-A et al: Acute left colonic diverticulitis: can CT findings be used to predict recurrence? AJR 182:1159-1165, 2004.
Punwani S et al: Mural inflammation in Crohn disease: location-matched histologic validation of MR imaging features. Radiology 252(3):712-720, 2009.
Purysko AS et al: Beyond appendicitis: common and uncommon gastrointestinal causes of right lower quadrant abdominal pain at multidetector CT. Radiographics 31(4):927-947, 2011.
Ramachandran I et al: Pseudomembranous colitis revisited: spectrum of imaging findings. Clin Radiol 61(7):535-544, 2006.
Rimola J et al: Role of 3.0-T MR colonography in the evaluation of inflammatory bowel disease. Radiographics 29(3):701-719, 2009.
Ripolles T et al: Sonographic findings in ischemic colitis in 58 patients. AJR 184(3):777-785, 2005.
Roberts CC et al: Imaging evaluation of right lower quadrant pain: self-assessment module, AJR 187:S476-S479, 2006.
Rosenblat JM et al: Findings of cecal volvulus at CT. Radiology 256(1):169-175, 2010.
Rustgi AK: Hereditary gastrointestinal polyposis and nonpolyposis syndromes. N Engl J Med 331(25):1694-1702, 1994.
Rutter MD et al: Thirty-year analysis of a colonoscopies surveillance program for neoplasia in ulcerative colitis. Gastroenterology 130(4):1030-1038, 2006.
Sayed RFE et al: Pelvic floor dysfunction: assessment with combined analysis of static and dynamic MR imaging findings. Radiology 248(2):518-530, 2008.
Shanbhogue AKP et al: Spectrum of medication-induced complications in the abdomen: role of cross-sectional imaging. AJR 197:W286-W294, 2011.
Silva AC, et al: Evaluation of benign and malignant rectal lesions with CT colonography and endoscopic correlation. Radiographics 26(4):1085-1099, 2006.
Singh AK et al: Acute epiploic appendagitis and its mimics. Radiographics 25(6):1521-1534, 2005.
Singh AK et al: CT appearance of acute appendagitis. AJR 183(5):1303-1307, 2004.
Sinha R et al: Utility of high-resolution MR imaging in demonstrating transmural pathologic changes in Crohn disease. Radiographics 29(6):1847-1867, 2009.
Sosna J et al: Critical analysis of the performance of double-contracts barium enema for detecting colorectal polyps > or = 6 mm in the era of CT colonography. AJR 190(2):374-385, 2008.
Spigelman AD: Extracolonic polyposis in familial adenomatous polyposis: so near and yet so far. Gut 53(3):322, 2004.
Stoker J et al: Imaging patients with acute abdominal pain. Radiology 253(1):31-46, 2009.
Stoker J et al: Pelvic floor imaging. Radiology 218(3):621-641, 2001.
Sultan K et al: The nature of inflammatory bowel disease in patients with coexistent colonic diverticulosis. J Clin Gastroenterol 40(4):317-321, 2006.
Summers RM: Polyp size measurement at CT colonography: what do we know and what do we need to know? Radiology 255(3):707-720, 2010.
Theilman NM et al: Clinical practice: acute infectious diarrhea. N Engl J Med 350(1):38-47, 2004.
Thoeni RF et al: CT imaging of colitis. Radiology 240(3):623-638, 2006.
Thornton E et al: Current status of MR colonography. Radiographics 30(1):201-218, 2010.
Van Randen A et al: Acute appendicitis: meta-analysis of diagnostic performance of CT and graded compression US related to prevalence of disease. Radiology 249(1):97-106, 2008.
Wan MJ et al: Acute appendicitis in young children: cost-effectiveness of US versus CT in diagnosis—a Markov decision analytic model. Radiology 250(2):378-386, 2009.
Webb EM et al: The negative appendectomy rate: who benefits from preoperative CT? AJR 197:861-866, 2011.
Wiesner W et al: CT of acute bowel ischemia. Radiology 226(3):635-650, 2003.
Wilde GE et al: Posttransplantation lymphoproliferative disorder in pediatric recipients of solid organ transplants: timing and location of disease. AJR 185:1335-1341, 2005.
Yu J et al: Helical CT evaluation of acute right lower quadrant pain. Part II, Uncommon mimics of appendicitis. AJR 184:1143-1149, 2005.

CHAPTER 6
Liver

The liver, as the largest and most complex organ in the abdomen, can present with diverse abnormalities. The most common clinical conundrum is the characterization of single or multiple hepatic lesions, primarily into benign or malignant disease, but there are many diffuse infiltrative diseases, some of which are difficult to evaluate with imaging, particularly in their early phases. However, modern imaging techniques offer the ability to characterize many, if not most, hepatic disorders, particularly if combined with the relevant clinical history. Indeed, as with imaging of other organs, a relevant clinical history is critical for the radiologist as he or she attempts to differentiate abnormalities into their disease categories. For instance, the presence of hepatic cystic lesions on computed tomography (CT) in an otherwise healthy 30-year-old is almost always benign, but similar CT findings in a 70-year-old woman with known ovarian cancer may mean metastatic disease. Furthermore, collateral biochemical, pathological, microbiological, and hematological data are often crucial in reaching the correct imaging diagnosis. As elsewhere, prior imaging is of utmost importance. In the clinical scenario outlined above, the presence of a cystic liver lesion in the 70-year-old woman many years before her ovarian cancer diagnosis would normally signify a benign cyst. Conversely, the presence of a new cystic lesion when compared with prior imaging would indicate a metastasis.

The liver is classically divided into eight lobes, or segments, according to the Couinaud* system (Fig. 6-1), and determination of lesion location can be critical if surgical resection is being considered. Each segment has portal veins, hepatic arteries, and bile ducts, and each drains into individual lobar hepatic veins (Table 6-1). The middle hepatic vein divides the liver into right and left lobes. The left lobe is then further subdivided by the left hepatic vein into medial (segment IV—sometimes further subdivided into segments IVa and IVb) and lateral components (segments II and III) (Figs. 6-1 and 6-2). Segments II and III are in turn separated by the left portal vein, with segment II above and segment III below (Figs. 6-1 and 6-2). The right hepatic vein subdivides the right lobe into anterior and posterior segments with the right portal vein further dividing these into upper and lower segments (Figs. 6-1 and 6-2). Segment VIII is upper anterior, segment VII is upper posterior, segment V is lower anterior, and segment VI is lower posterior. Segment I, or the caudate lobe, is posterior.

The liver has a dual blood supply, with approximately 80% supplied from the portal vein and 20% from the hepatic artery, and blood freely circulates into the extravascular spaces. An understanding of this paradigm is important in planning appropriate contrast-enhanced imaging protocols because different diseases have different enhancement characteristics depending on the source of their primary blood supply.

IMAGING METHODS

All imaging methods, from plain radiograph to positron emission tomography (PET), have a role in hepatic imaging. However, the majority of hepatic abnormalities are not only detected, but also characterized, by means of cross-sectional imaging.

Plain Radiograph and Fluoroscopy

Although infrequently used as a primary imaging tool, the plain radiograph is still useful to assess prosthetic positioning, intrahepatic gas, and occasionally calcification and hepatomegaly. Conventional fluoroscopy is still the primary method of choice for performing most interventional hepatic therapeutic procedures.

Ultrasound

Hepatic evaluation by ultrasound (US) is now considered less optimal than CT or magnetic resonance imaging (MRI), particularly in the United States, although the use of Doppler* harmonic and US contrast imaging has shown some advantages. However, these are not in wide clinical use. US still has a critical role in the evaluation of cirrhosis and infiltrative disease, some specific liver lesions, and some interventional procedures. US is highly operator dependent and requires extensive training, and perhaps for these reasons CT and MRI have often superseded it in clinical practice, at least in the United States. This should not deter the radiologist from using US in the appropriate setting, however, given that it is less expensive, relatively easily available, and quick, produces no ionizing radiation, and in the right hands, provides substantial opportunities for liver lesion characterization.

Computed Tomography

Multidetector CT (MDCT) is the workhorse for hepatic imaging because of its excellent spatial and contrast resolution, speed, ease of use, reproducibility, use of intravenous (IV) contrast agents, and ability to postprocess images into multiplanar formats (particularly with the newer higher detector arrays). Imaging can be tailored to coincide with maximal parenchymal, lesion, or vascular enhancement after administration of IV contrast agents, depending on the disease in question. CT provides excellent morphologic information about both the disease and its relationship to normal anatomy. Dual-energy hardware offers further opportunity to evaluate and quantify disease. Perhaps because CT is so ubiquitous and clinically useful, some have raised concerns about overuse, mainly because of cost and radiation dose.

*Christian H. Doppler (1803-1853), Austrian mathematician and physicist.

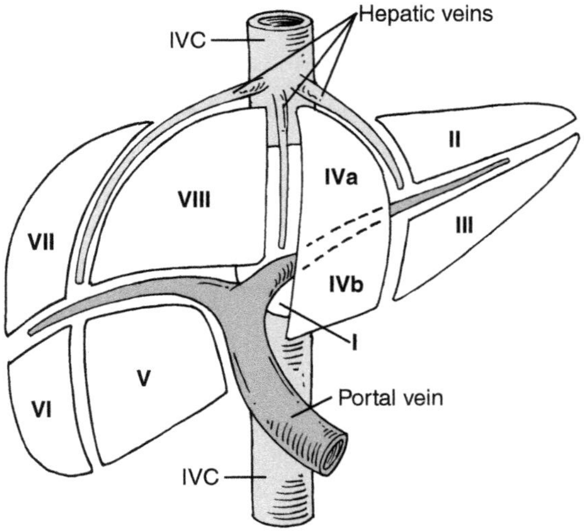

FIGURE 6-1. Schematic representation of hepatic Couinaud segments.

*Claude Couinaud (1922-2008), French surgeon.

Whether less expensive and more nonionizing radiation techniques will supersede the current demand for CT remains to be determined.

The density of the unenhanced normal liver at CT typically ranges between 55 and 65 HU. Unenhanced CT is useful for the evaluation of depositional disease (e.g., hepatic steatosis, hemochromatosis), liver calcifications, hemorrhage, and some high-contrast embolic material used for therapeutic procedures. Most patients, however, are imaged after the administration of IV iodinated contrast medium.

TABLE 6-1 Couinaud* Liver Segments

Structure	Right Lobe
Middle hepatic vein	Divides right and left lobes
Right hepatic vein	Separates right lobe into anterior (segments VIII and V) and posterior (segments VII and VI)
Right portal vein	Separates right lobe into superior (segments VII and VIII) and inferior (segments V and VI)
Left hepatic vein	Divides left lobe into medial (segment IVa and IVb) and lateral (segments II and III)
Left portal vein	Separates segment II (above) and segment III (below)
Caudate lobe	Segment I (posterior)
Falciform ligament	Divides medial and lateral segments of left lobe (segment IV from II and III)
Ligamentum venosum	Obliterated umbilical vein: extends from falciform ligament to umbilicus

Because of the dual blood supply to the liver, the liver can be imaged during multiple phases. Early imaging during the arterial phase (typically a scan delay of approximately 20 seconds from the start of IV contrast injection), when most of the hepatic normal parenchyma is not yet enhanced, visualizes the arterial structures and offers the opportunity to evaluate disease that is supplied primarily with an arterial blood supply (Table 6-2 and Fig. 6-3). Maximal opacification of the portal vein occurs at approximately 40 seconds after the initiation of IV injection, and the hepatic parenchyma is subsequently maximally enhanced during the portal or hepatic venous phase, usually at approximately 60 seconds. Most hepatic lesions are hypodense during this phase, in contrast to the relatively hyperdense liver parenchyma (Fig. 6-4). A number of lesions can be further characterized with delayed imaging (either because they retain contrast material or because they are more conspicuous against the normal liver background), usually at approximately 120 to 180 seconds after initiation of the injection (Fig. 6-5). Scan times are optimized through automatic bolus tracking techniques, which trigger scanning to coincide with the optimal arterial or portal venous phase (PVP). A fundamental understanding of these vascular dynamics is required to optimize MDCT scan protocols for the disease in question. Some diseases are best imaged with one phase, some with two phases, or some even with three phases. By the addition of a noncontrast CT, the lesions can potentially be evaluated with four phases, although because of the radiation burden this should be avoided unless clinically necessary.

Dual-Energy Computed Tomography

Two energy beams of different peak kilovoltage (kVp) provide the opportunity to maximize contrast differences between normal and abnormal tissue, particularly in high-density tissues and those affected after the use of IV contrast material. At lower energies (typically 80 kVp), there is significantly more iodine attenuation (because this energy is close to its K-edge of 33.2 keV).

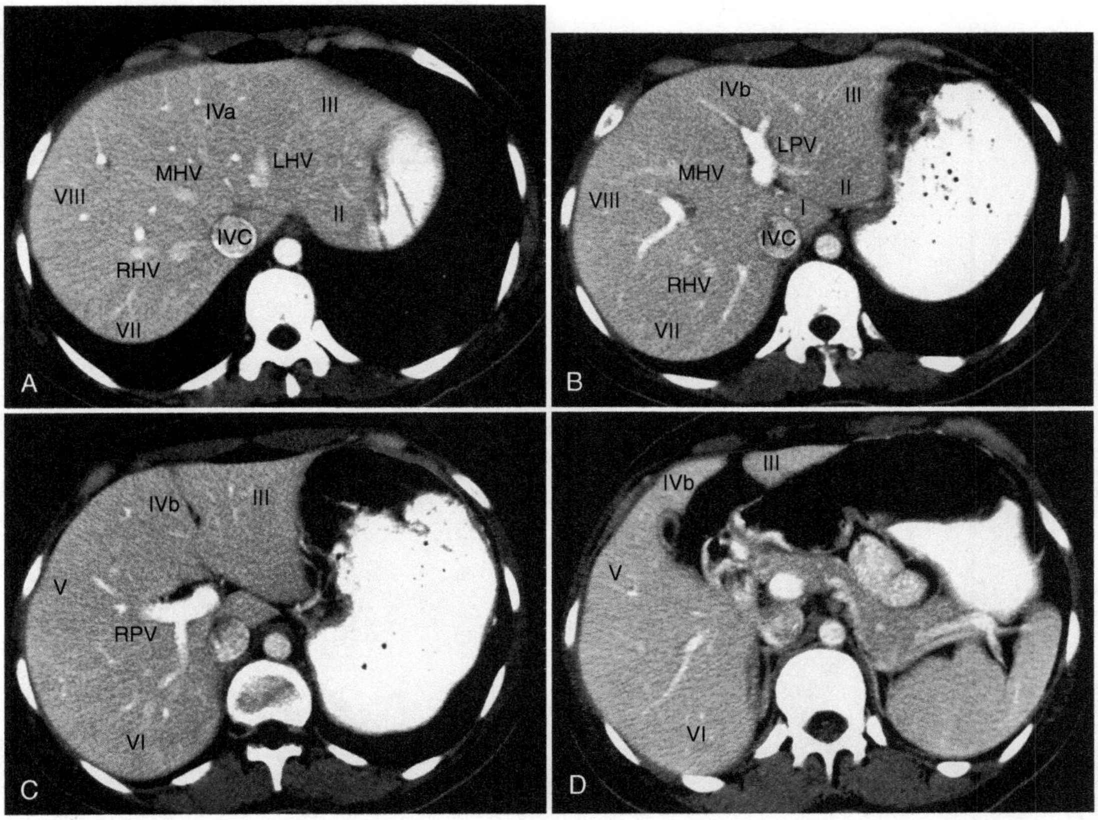

FIGURE 6-2. **A** through **D**, Axial contrast-enhanced images of hepatic segments. LHV, Left hepatic vein; LPV, left portal vein; RHV, right hepatic vein; RPV, right portal vein.

Imaging at these lower kilovoltage levels offers the opportunity to evaluate a range of high-contrast material with greater conspicuity. By subtracting images from one energy source to the other, virtual noncontrast images can also be obtained, thereby avoiding the need for standard noncontrast images (Fig. 6-6).

Magnetic Resonance Imaging

Magnetic resonance imaging (MRI) is the method of choice for evaluation of many hepatic abnormalities, mainly because of its superior contrast resolution, increasing availability, lack of ionizing radiation, use of innovative contrast agents, and multiplanar capability, as well as the development of many coils, new software, and postprocessing advances that can exploit differences in tissue characteristics. MRI can also provide more morphological and functional information than CT. Therefore, when US or CT identifies an incidental hepatic mass that cannot be characterized definitively, MRI is the next investigation of choice, despite its cost, because of its superior sensitivity and specificity. Many of the disadvantages described in the previous edition of this book are now mitigated because of technological developments, including faster scan times and respiratory gating, both of which minimize motion artifact and optimize scan times to provide the best possible tissue enhancement after the administration of IV contrast agents. There are more powerful gradients and body coils and three-dimensional data acquisitions, leading to enhanced image quality. Conversely, however, as the number of novel new protocols has increased, overall scan times have not necessarily decreased.

Table 6-2 Phase of CT Imaging in Hepatic Disease

Disease	NCCT	Arterial Phase	PVP	Delayed
Fatty liver	x			
Calcifications	x			
Hemorrhage	x			
Hemochromatosis	x			
HCC		x	x	
FNH		x	x	x
Adenoma		x	x	x
Hypervascular metastases		x	x	
Aneurysm		x	x	
Pretransplant assessment		x	x	
Most metastases			x	
Cystic disease	x		x	x
Hemangioma			x	x
Cirrhosis	x	x	x	
Cholangiocarcinoma			x	x
Confluent hepatic fibrosis				

CT, Computed tomography; *FNH*, focal nodular hyperplasia; *HCC*, hepatocellular carcinoma; *NCCT*, noncontrast CT scan; *PVP*, portal venous phase.

Conventional Magnetic Resonance Imaging Sequences

The physics and a detailed discussion of MRI pulse sequences (many of which have acronyms specific to the vendor) are beyond the scope of this book, but most abdominal MRI sequences use T1 (with or without fat saturation), in-phase (IP) and out-of-phase

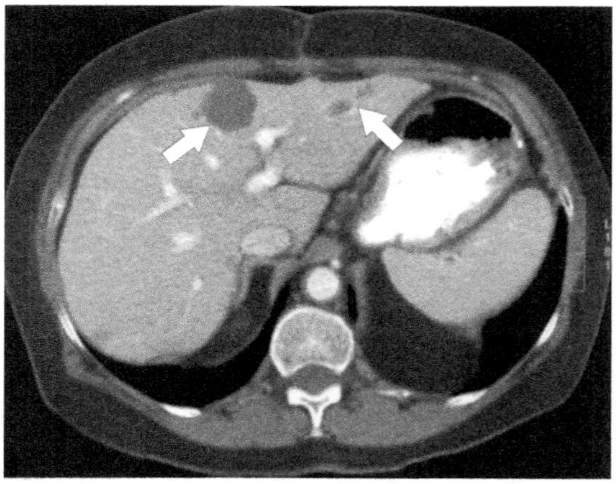

Figure 6-4. Axial contrast-enhanced CT in the PVP in a 49-year-old woman with cystic gastrointestinal stromal tumor metastases (*arrows*). These lesions are best visualized with the normal hepatic parenchyma opacified.

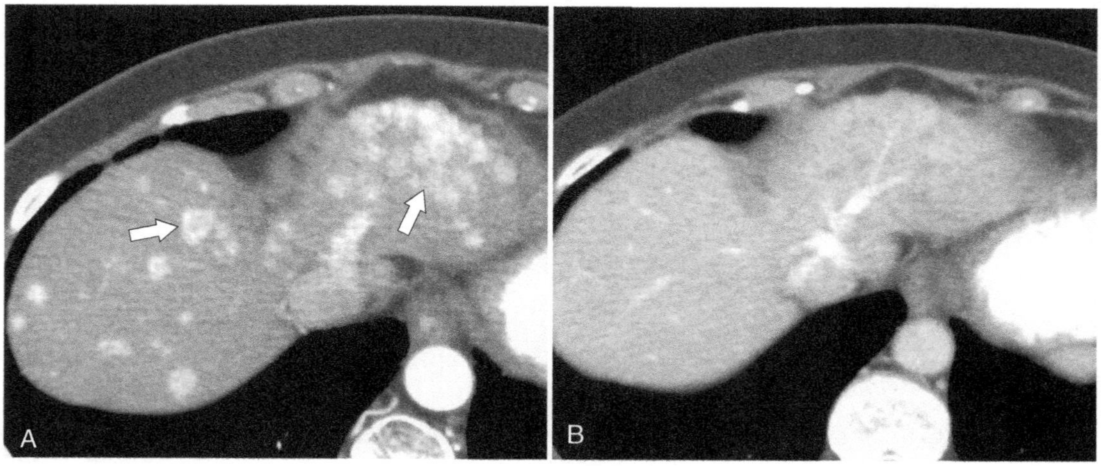

Figure 6-3. Axial contrast-enhanced CT in arterial phase (**A**) and PVP (**B**) in a 79-year-old woman with metastatic HCC (*arrows*). Their vascular supply is arterial, and the tumor burden is not appreciated during the PVP.

(OOP) imaging (or other fat-suppression techniques, e.g., Dixon), T2, and postcontrast T1 (with or without fat saturation) images. Most of these sequences are now considerably faster than those of previous MRI generations. The normal liver typically demonstrates a slightly higher T1-weighted signal and slightly lower T2-weighted signal when compared with those of the spleen. Most biliary and vascular structures are of low signal on T1-weighted images, but bile, in particular, is of high signal of T2-weighted images, hence its use in magnetic resonance cholangiopancreatography (MRCP).

Fat-Suppression Techniques

Simple fat-suppression techniques (performed on both T1 and T2 sequences) are available for all MRI scanners and null out signal in voxels with high fatty content. These techniques are most useful when evaluating disease in anatomical locations with a large amount of normal fat (e.g., peritoneum) because the resulting fat signal loss increases the contrast of any abnormal tissue with inherent higher signal (e.g., inflammatory and many benign or malignant masses that demonstrate enhancement after the administration of IV contrast agents). Furthermore, they can be used to evaluate abnormalities with substantial fatty components (fatty liver, dermoid cysts, adrenal myelolipoma, and adenomas). Alternatively, fat-containing tissue can be evaluated with IP and OOP chemical shift MRI or Dixon fat-suppression techniques, and inversion recovery sequences are also available (Fig. 6-7).

Magnetic Resonance Imaging Contrast Agents

The three main classes of MRI contrast agents are extracellular, hepatobiliary, and mononuclear phagocytic (formerly reticuloendothelial). Extracellular agents are the most common and include gadopentetate dimeglumine (Gd-DTPA). These agents behave similarly to iodinated contrast agents used in CT. They circulate freely in the extracellular spaces before being excreted predominantly in the kidneys. As with contrast-enhanced CT, the detection and characterization of liver lesions depend on the differential arterial or portal venous enhancement of liver lesions or lack of enhancement compared with that of normal hepatic parenchyma.

Hepatobiliary agents are specifically absorbed by hepatocytes and partially excreted in bile and the kidneys (Fig. 6-8), so detection and characterization of lesions depend on whether they retain hepatocyte function (e.g., focal nodular hyperplasia [FNH], some well-differentiated hepatocellular carcinoma [HCC]) or not (hemangiomas, metastases, and cysts). These agents include manganese-based mangafodipir trisodium (Mn-DPDP) and gadolinium-based gadoxetate disodium (Gd-EOB-DTPA) and

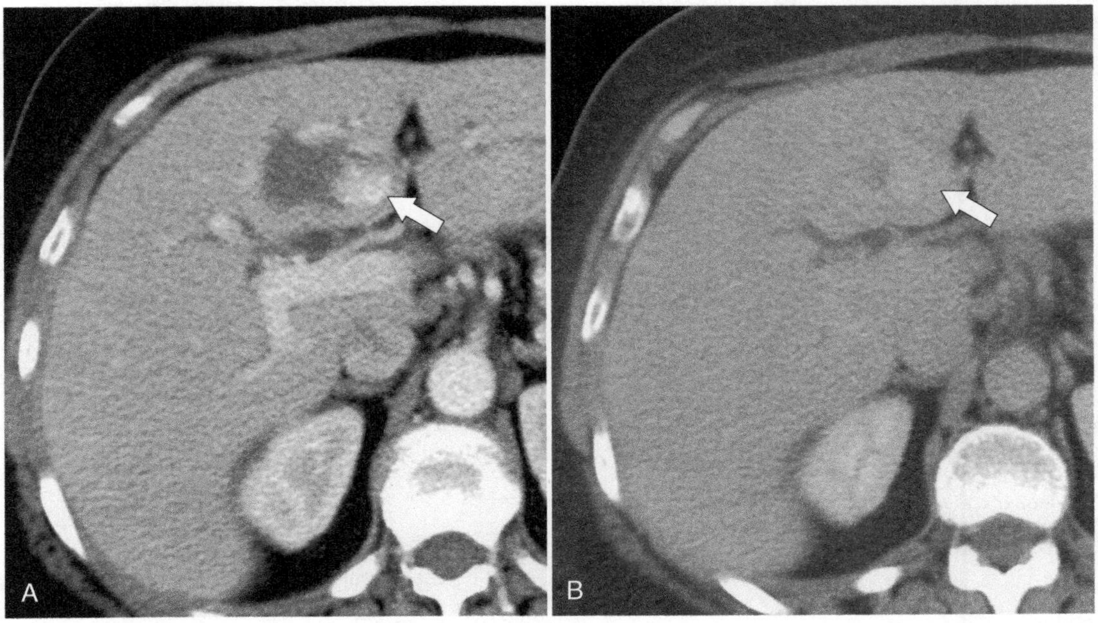

FIGURE 6-5. Axial PVP (**A**) and delayed-phase (**B**) contrast-enhanced CT in a 52-year-old woman with hemangioma. The lesion (*arrows*) demonstrates peripheral nodular enhancement that fills in on delayed imaging, characteristic of the hemangioma.

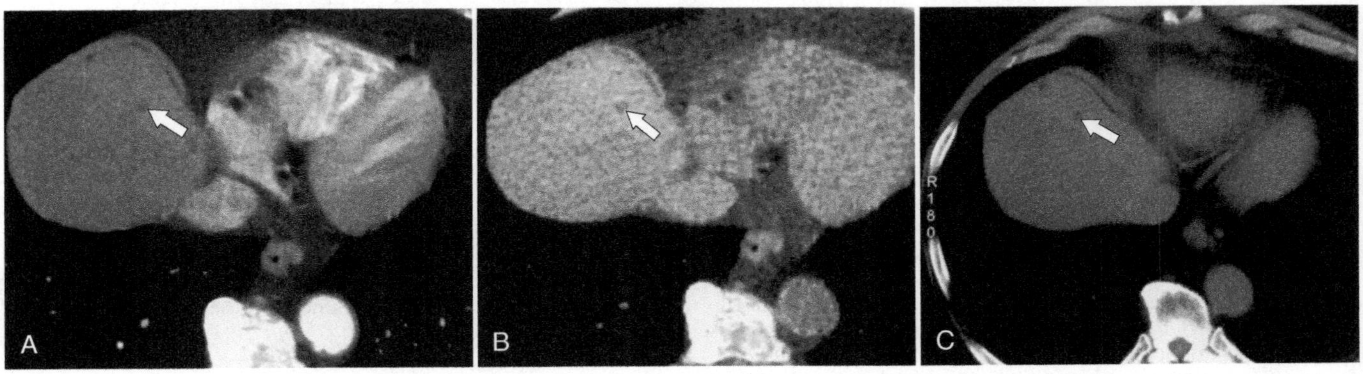

FIGURE 6-6. **A** through **C**, Virtual noncontrast CT. The original contrast-enhanced image (**A**) demonstrates a small segment VIII liver lesion (*arrow*) that can be identified on the virtual noncontrast image (*arrow*). The true noncontrast image (**C**) is shown for comparison.

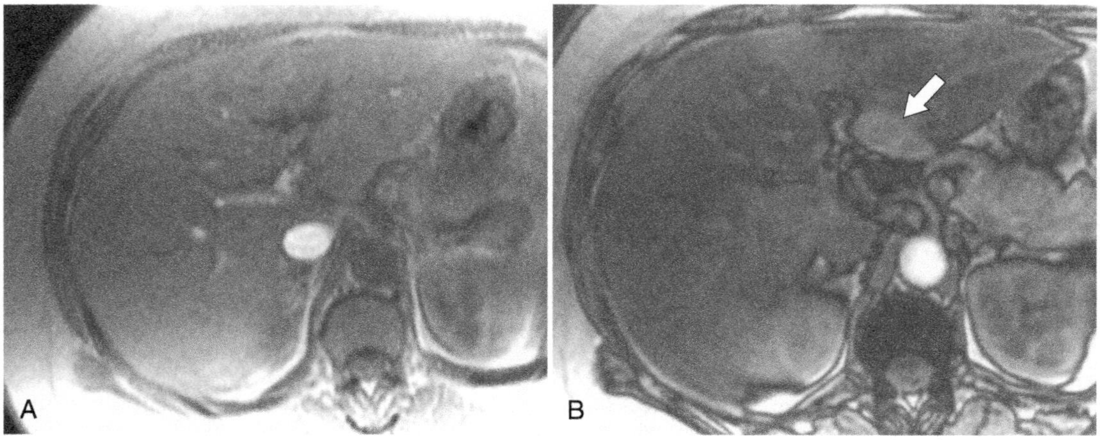

FIGURE 6-7. In-phase (**A**) and out-of-phase (**B**) MRI in a 54-year-old woman with focal fatty sparing. There is diffuse hepatic signal drop-off on out-of-phase imaging "unmasking" the normal "fat sparing" in the gallbladder fossa (*arrow*).

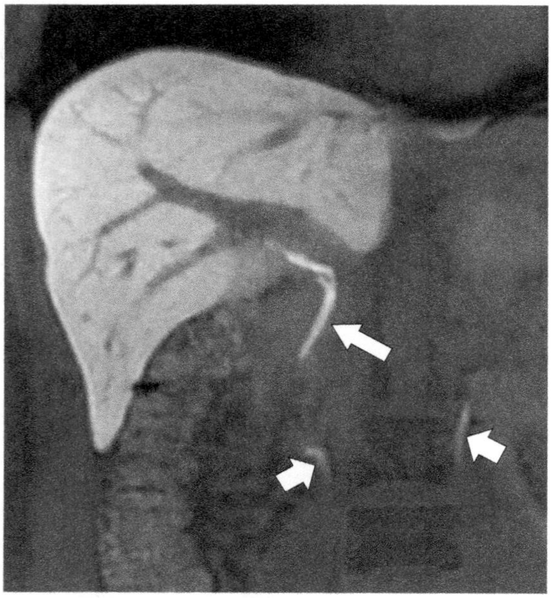

FIGURE 6-8. A 20-minute coronal T1-weighted fat-saturated postcontrast hepatobiliary MRI demonstrating marked hepatic parenchymal enhancement and biliary (*arrow*) and renal (*small arrows*) excretion of contrast material.

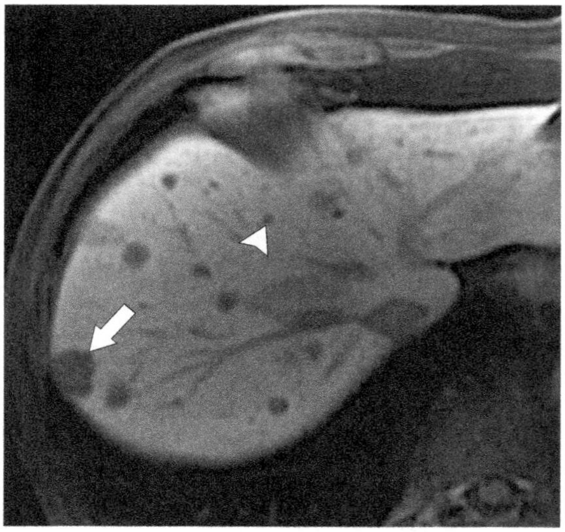

FIGURE 6-9. A 20-minute axial T1-weighted fat-saturated posthepatobiliary contrast MRI in a 61-year-old man with numerous liver metastases (*arrow*), some very small (*arrowhead*) and detected only with this technique.

gadobenate dimeglumine (Gd-BOPTA). The latter two agents permit both dynamic imaging (similar to extracellular agents) and delayed hepatocyte-phase imaging, at which point the normal liver parenchyma enhances. The superior contrast differences between normal liver and nonhepatocytic lesions (i.e., metastases) on delayed imaging can permit the detection of very small lesions compared with conventional techniques (Fig. 6-9). However, because the concentration of gadolinium in these agents is less than is used with conventional gadolinium agents, the intensity of enhancement at dynamic imaging (i.e., arterial or PVP) may be less than that observed with extracellular agents. Subtraction imaging may therefore be useful, which simply involves the digital subtraction of the unenhanced T1-weighted image from the contrast-enhanced sequence such that any remaining signal is caused only by tissue enhancement (Fig. 6-10). Delayed imaging with hepatobiliary agents has proved particularly useful in assessing whether patients with metastatic liver disease are candidates for curative resection because lesions in both right and left lobes generally preclude surgery.

The mononuclear phagocytic (reticuloendothelial) agents (or ferumoxides) contain iron and are taken up by Kupffer* phagocytic cells. Delayed imaging demonstrates loss of signal in normal anatomical structures but no loss of signal in cells that do not retain the contrast agent, either because they contain no Kupffer activity or because these tissues are replaced by the disease process (i.e., metastases). These agents are less in clinical use than extracellular and hepatobiliary agents.

Diffusion-Weighted Imaging

Diffusion-weighted imaging (DWI) is a newer technique, now gaining widespread use in clinical practice, that offers the opportunity to detect more lesions when compared with conventional MRI sequences and to aid with lesion characterization, particularly the differentiation between benign and malignant disease.

Water molecules in tissues can be thermally manipulated by using a diffusion-weighted pulse sequence and then undergo Brownian†

*Karl Wilhelm von Kupffer (1829-1902), German anatomist.
†Robert Brown (1773-1858), Scottish botanist.

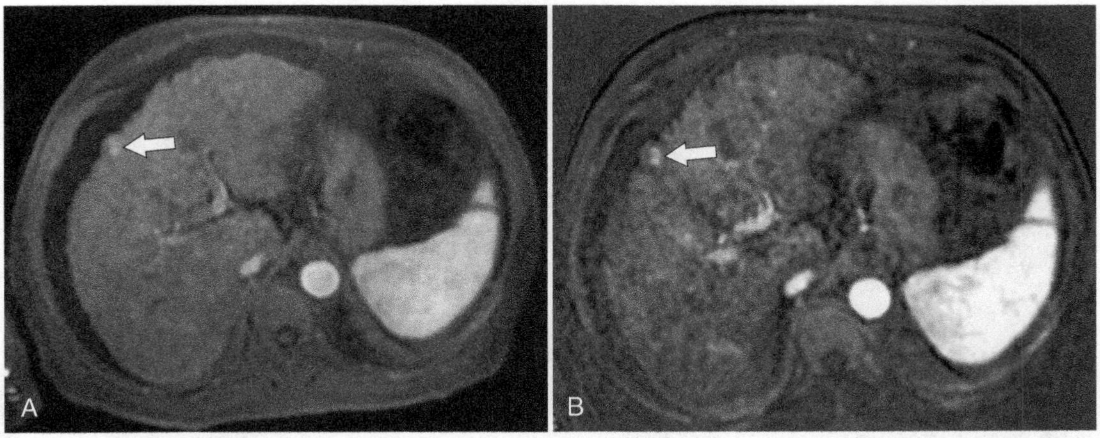

FIGURE 6-10. **A**, Axial hepatobiliary agent fat-saturated contrast-enhanced MRI and subtraction image in a 74-year-old man with cirrhosis and questionable area of enhancement in segment V (*arrow*). **B**, Subtraction images confirm enhancement in a new HCC (*arrow*).

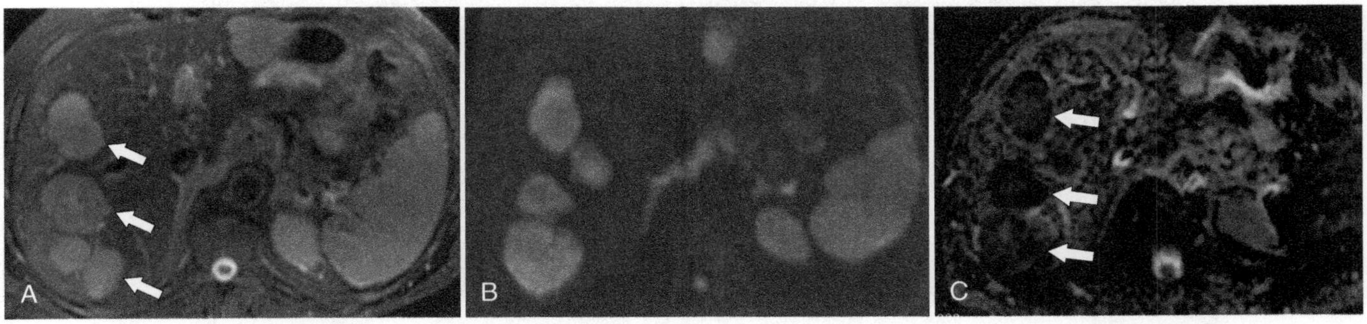

FIGURE 6-11. Axial T2-weighted (**A**), B500 (**B**), and ADC (**C**) DWI in a 73-year-old man with multiple liver metastases (*arrows*). The lesions are bright on T2-weighted and B500 imaging but dark on ADC maps.

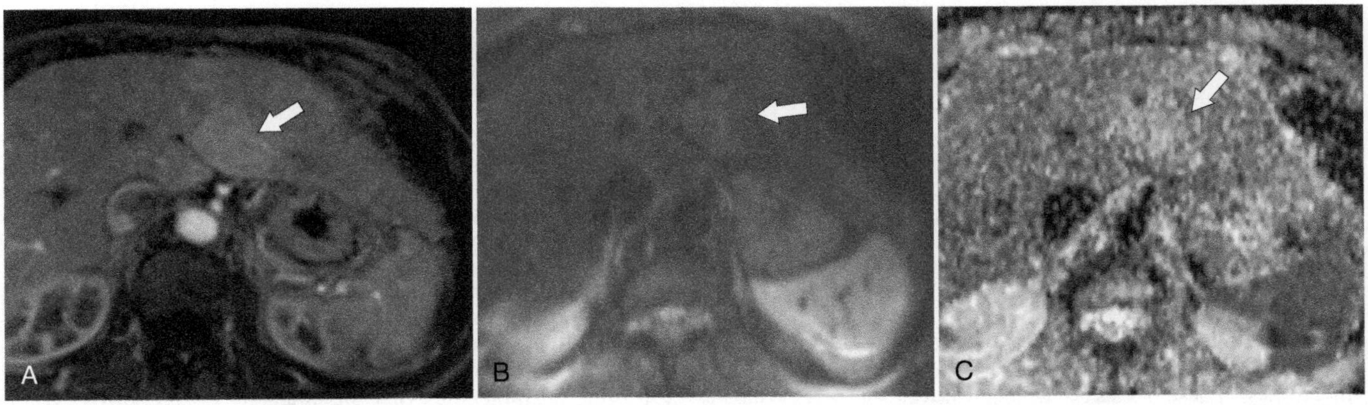

FIGURE 6-12. Axial arterial-phase hepatobiliary agent T1-weighted (**A**) MRI and B500 (**B**) and ADC (**C**) maps in a 57-year-old woman with focal nodular hyperplasia. There is mild arterial enhancement (*arrows*) and slight increased signal on DWI and ADC maps.

motion. Tissues with high cellularity (e.g., tumors) demonstrate little Brownian motion and are termed "restricted," whereas predominantly water-based tissues (e.g., simple cysts) are termed "nonrestricted." The strength of the diffusion weighting can be altered by increasing diffusion-weighted b values, which alters the signal output from these tissues. Because water molecules generally demonstrate restricted diffusion in solid lesions, they travel less distance from the time of the original pulse sequence to the rephrasing gradient, which leads to higher signal at higher diffusion-weighted b values (because the water molecules can easily be rephased by the diffusion-weighted gradient) (Fig. 6-11). In general, free-moving water (as in cystic lesions) demonstrates reduced signal on higher diffusion-weighted b values (the rephasing pulse) because the freely moving water molecules have traveled farther and are harder to rephase (Fig. 6-12).

The degree of proton motion in capillaries and tissues can be measured and quantified as the apparent diffusion coefficient (ADC). A slope can be plotted that represents the ADC, which, in turn, represents each voxel's diffusion value. Typically, the ADC is displayed pictorially as a parametric map on an axial image on which a region of interest can be placed to measure a mean ADC within the area selected. An ADC map can also reflect the signal intensities of a tissue obtained at the different b values across a range of voxels. Malignant lesions tend to demonstrate little or no signal on ADC maps (Fig. 6-11), whereas benign lesions (less water restriction) show higher signal (Fig. 6-12).

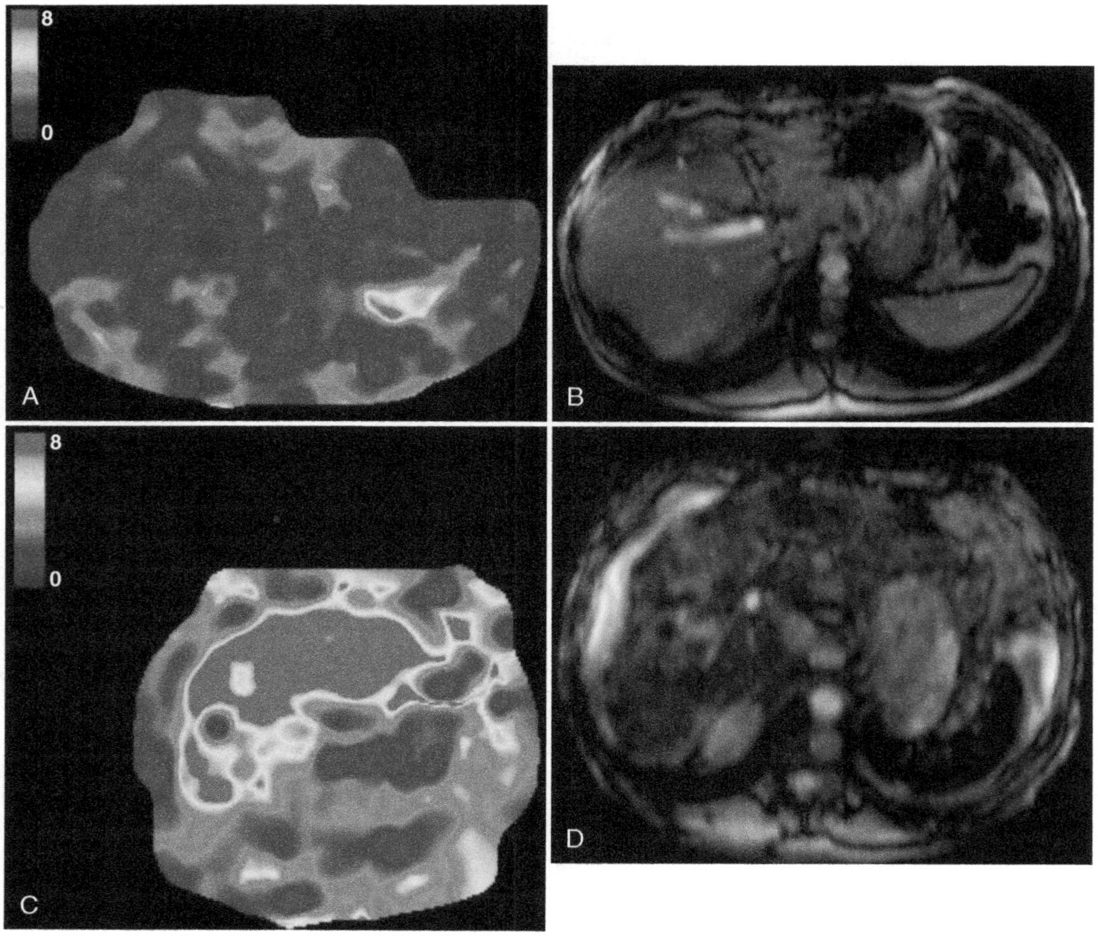

FIGURE 6-13. **A** and **B**, Normal elastography in a 38-year-old man. The raw MRI T2-weighted images demonstrate a normal liver, and sound transmission meets low impedance (0-1 kPa). **C** and **D**, Elastography in a 55-year-old man with cirrhosis and a "stiff" liver as evidenced by high impedance (7-8 kPa) to sound waves (*arrows*). *See ExpertConsult.com for color image.*

These findings are usually evaluated qualitatively, but threshold ADC cutoff values to separate benign from malignant lesions can be generated.

Care should be taken to evaluate the diffusion-weighted b value images along with the ADC map, since some cystic lesions demonstrate no increase on ADC maps because of T2 "shine-through." Furthermore, restricted diffusion can be observed in some benign lesions (some hepatic adenomas and FNH, abscess, and fibrosis) and, conversely, increased diffusion in some malignant lesions (cystic metastases). These pitfalls can generally be mitigated by evaluating conventional MRI (contrast- and non-contrast-enhanced) images.

Magnetic Resonance Elastography

An evolving technique, magnetic resonance elastography has shown that the "stiffness" of the liver (typically found in cirrhosis and fibrosis) can be measured by evaluating the shear-wave transients propagated through liver parenchyma. The images can be color coded to reflect the shear wavelength or the mean shear stiffness (in kilopascals*) of cirrhotic livers (Fig. 6-13).

Nuclear Medicine

With the relatively widespread distribution of PET and PET/CT scanners, PET body imaging has now regained much of the ground it had lost to other cross-sectional imaging techniques. Although there is still a role for more conventional nuclear medicine techniques, their hepatic applications have largely been superseded by PET. PET/CT scanners offer the unique combination of morphological (CT) and functional/metabolic (PET) imaging. PET imaging exploits the requirement for most malignant lesions to metabolize glucose at a far higher rate than normal tissue or benign disease (Fig. 6-14). Most PET applications attach the radioisotope ^{18}F-fluorodeoxyglucose (FDG) to glucose molecules that are injected intravenously. Whole body or selected scanning is performed approximately 45 minutes later. Malignant tissues typically demonstrate increased uptake, although some benign inflammatory or neoplastic conditions in the abdomen may also show mild and occasionally avid uptake.

PET imaging is now routinely used to evaluate the metabolic response of a variety of solid organ body malignancies to chemotherapy, radiation, and other interventional treatment regimens, which can often document responses earlier than the morphological features seen with CT and MRI. Furthermore, some tumors (e.g., melanoma) are highly avid for ^{18}F-FDG PET, which has increased the likelihood of detecting very small deposits, often a challenge because of surrounding muscle or peritoneum. However, PET or PET/CT is infrequently used as a front-line investigation in the liver, even to evaluate therapeutic responses, partly because of its relatively poor spatial resolution compared with MRI and also because of expense, availability, and radiation burden.

*Blaise Pascal (1623-1662), French mathematician.

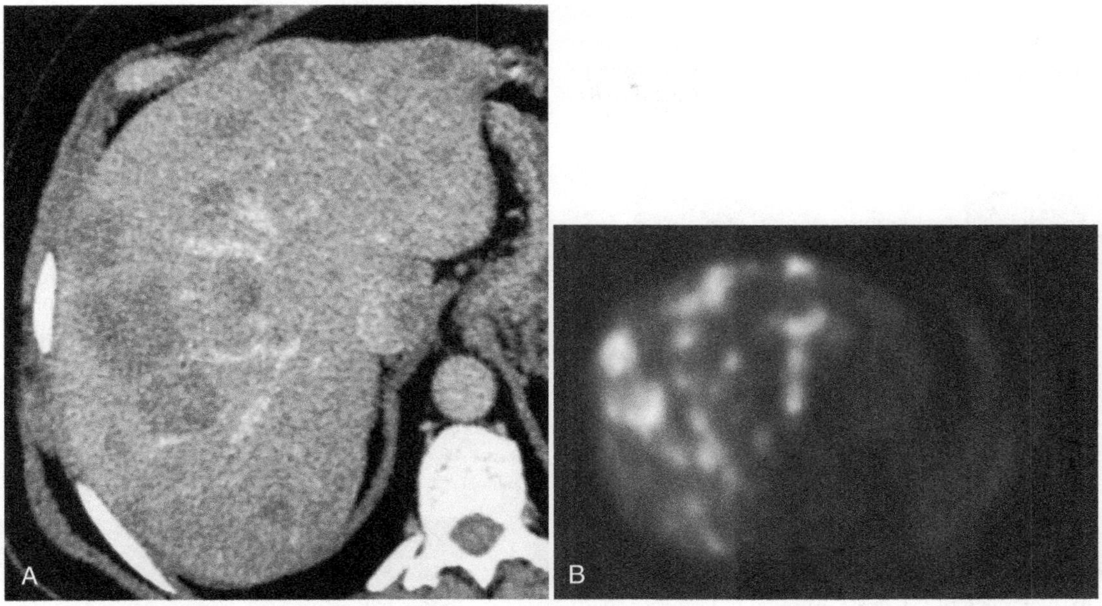

FIGURE 6-14. Axial contrast-enhanced CT (A) and PET (B) in a 50-year-old man with multiple colon metastases. More are identified at PET.

Angiography

Angiographic hepatic evaluation is confined to therapeutic procedures mainly outside the scope of this book, including treatment of arterial malformations and aneurysms, procedures to relieve portal hypertension (transjugular intrahepatic portosystemic shunting [TIPS]), and treatment of some unresectable malignancies (transarterial chemoembolization [TACE]).

CONGENITAL HEPATIC DISEASE

Congenital Hepatic Fibrosis

Congenital hepatic fibrosis is an inherited fibrocystic liver disease with variable amounts of hepatic fibrosis and hepatic and renal cystic disease. It is commonly associated with autosomal-recessive polycystic kidney disease, and some have suggested they are part of the same disease. The imaging findings are related to the effects of fibrosis with left lobe hypertrophy and a shrunken right lobe. Regenerative nodules are common, seen as multiple hypervascular lesions at CT and MRI. The bile ducts can be focally dilated, the portal tracts are fibrotic, and multiple hepatic and renal cysts are present (Fig. 6-15). The hepatic fibrosis results in portal hypertension with varices formation and splenomegaly.

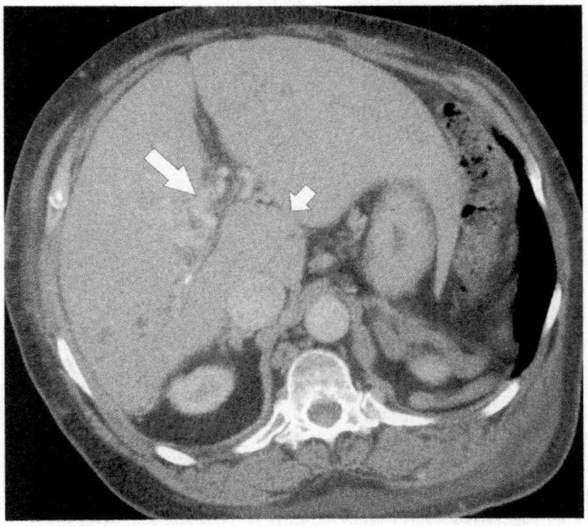

FIGURE 6-15. Axial contrast-enhanced CT in a 35-year-old man with congenital hepatic fibrosis. The caudate is enlarged (*small arrow*), and there is cavernous transformation of the portal vein (*arrow*).

Hepatic Autosomal-Dominant Polycystic Liver Disease

Hepatic autosomal-dominant (AD) polycystic liver disease is part of a spectrum with adult AD polycystic kidney disease, although it can occur in isolation. Hepatic lesions range from a few small cysts to multiple large cysts that almost replace the normal liver architecture. The cysts often hemorrhage (Fig. 6-16) and may therefore appear complex on cross-sectional imaging. Depending on the amount of hemorrhage, the cysts may appear simple or higher than water density on CT and display a reduced T2 signal on MRI. The cysts often result in wall calcification from the prior hemorrhage. The liver is frequently grossly enlarged by the cyst formation, and as hepatic function deteriorates, transplant may be needed.

Hemochromatosis

Iron overload can be congenital (autosomal recessive) or acquired, but the imaging appearances are similar. The hereditary or primary form of hemochromatosis is caused by mutation in the *HFE* gene, leading to excessive intestinal iron absorption and tissue deposition, particularly in the liver, heart, and pancreas. Patients usually present in the third to fifth decades with cirrhosis (without cardiomyopathy), diabetes mellitus, hypogonadism, arthritis, hypopituitarism, and hyperpigmentation. In the liver, the excessively absorbed iron is preferentially deposited as ferritin or hemosiderin in hepatocytes or Kupffer cells.

Secondary hemochromatosis produces parenchymal effects similar to those of primary hemochromatosis and is usually caused by excessive iron intake (iron supplements, multiple transfusions) or iron release from chronic hemolysis. It is to be distinguished from hemosiderosis, which is also caused by excessive iron intake (usually because of repeated transfusions), but with hemosiderin deposition rather than iron, so the liver fails to progress to tissue damage and hemochromatosis.

The imaging findings depend on the degree of iron deposition and tissue damage. Hemochromatosis is one of the causes of increased hepatic parenchymal density on noncontrast CT (ranging from 70 to 140 HU, normally 45 to 65 HU) (Fig. 6-17 and

Box 6-1). Because the iron deposition in the liver is paramagnetic, MRI demonstrates hypointense parenchyma on T1- and T2-weighted imaging (Fig. 6-18). The degree of iron deposition can be quantified by dual-energy CT or T2 gradient echo MRI sequences. The major complications are hepatic cirrhosis and HCC formation (Fig. 6-19).

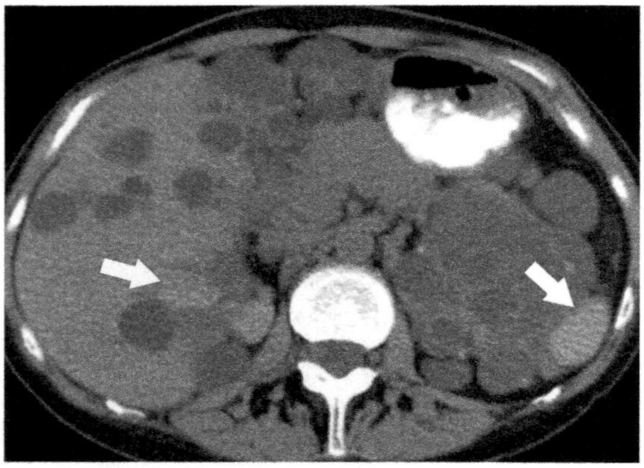

FIGURE 6-16. Axial noncontrast CT in a 37-year-old woman with adult polycystic liver and kidney disease. Some cysts have hemorrhaged (*arrows*).

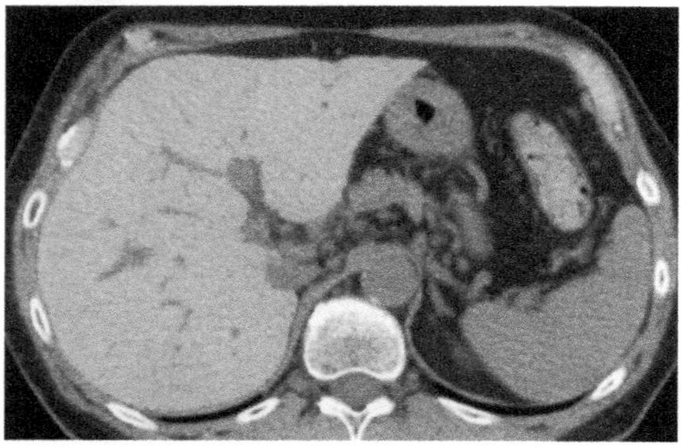

FIGURE 6-17. Axial noncontrast CT in a 49-year-old man with a dense liver (HU 96) from hemochromatosis.

***Box 6-1.* Causes of Increased Hepatic Density**

Congenital hemochromatosis
Hemosiderosis
Wilson disease
Glycogen storage diseases
Drugs (amiodarone)

Wilson Disease

Also known as hepatolenticular degeneration, Wilson* disease is an autosomal-recessive disease caused by a mutation on chromosome 13 (*ATP7B* gene). This results in defective ATPase enzyme activity that fails to effectively bind copper to ceruloplasmin (plasma protein) and failure to excrete excess copper into bile. Free copper, which is toxic, is then deposited in the liver parenchyma and causes hepatitis, fibrosis, and cirrhosis. The liver becomes overloaded with copper, which is then deposited throughout the body, but particularly in the kidney, iris, and basal ganglia of the brain. There are no specific imaging findings that manifest as cirrhosis. Because copper is not paramagnetic, it does not produce reduced T1- and T2-weighted MRI signal, but it does cause increased density at CT imaging, although generally less so than hemochromatosis. As the liver becomes cirrhotic, there is a risk of HCC.

*Samuel Alexander Kinnier Wilson (1878-1937), British neurologist.

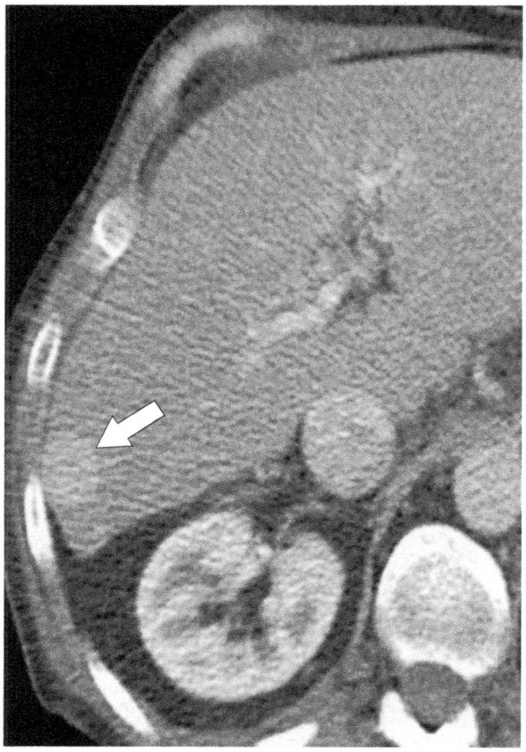

FIGURE 6-19. Axial contrast-enhanced CT in a 49-year-old woman with hemochromatosis and a 2-cm hypervascular mass (*arrow*) in segment VII of the liver, which is caused by HCC.

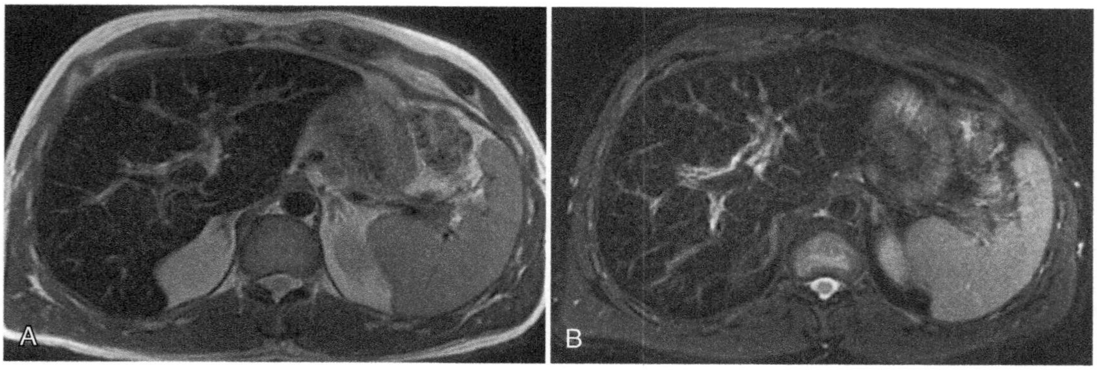

FIGURE 6-18. Axial T1-weighted (**A**) and fat-saturated T2-weighted (**B**) images in a 56-year-old man with T1 and T2 hypointense liver resulting from hemochromatosis.

DEPOSITIONAL METABOLIC DISEASE

Gaucher Disease

Gaucher* disease is due to an autosomal-recessive genetic defect of the enzyme glucosylceramidase that leads to excessive glucosylceramide accumulation, predominantly in tissues abundant in mononuclear leukocytes (macrophages), namely the spleen, lungs, kidneys, liver, brain, and bone marrow. There are three types of disease. Patients with type 2 do not usually survive into adulthood. Patients with types 1 and 3 may present with hepatosplenomegaly (the spleen is usually affected more than the liver) (Fig. 6-20) resulting from unmetabolized lipid deposition. Focal gaucheromas (i.e., focal complex glucosylceramide masses) occur particularly in the spleen but can also be observed in the liver (see Chapter 7).

Niemann-Pick Disease

Niemann-Pick† disease is a fatal lysosomal storage disorder caused by lack of the enzyme sphingomyelinase, which leads to sphingomyelin accumulation in the liver, spleen, brain, lungs, and bone marrow. Hepatosplenomegaly is common.

Mucopolysaccharidosis Disorders

The mucopolysaccharidosis (MPS) disorders are a group of often fatal lysosomal storage diseases leading to glysosaminoglycan accumulation, which in Hurler‡ (MPS I), Hunter§ (MPS II), and Sly* (MPS VII) syndromes causes hepatosplenomegaly as well as affecting other organs. All three are X-linked recessive disorders and lead to heparan and dermatan sulfate accumulation. Hurler syndrome is autosomal recessive with deficiency of alpha-L-iduronidase. Hunter is an X-linked recessive disorder leading to iduronate sulfatase deficiency. Sly syndrome is autosomal recessive and is caused by lack of beta-glucuronidase.

Langerhans† cell histiocytoses (LCH) are a group of disorders with excessive deposition of Langerhans histiocytic cells. Subtypes (now all referred to as LCH) were known as histiocytosis X, eosinophilic granuloma, Hand-Schüller-Christian‡ disease, and Letterer-Siwe§ disease. The histiocytic cells are deposited in multiple organs, including the liver, resulting in either hepatomegaly or focal lipid-rich nodular lesions.

*Phillippe Gaucher (1854-1918), French dermatologist.
†Albert Niemann (1880-1921), German physician; Ludwig Pick (1868-1944), German pathologist.
‡Gertrud Hurler (1889-1965), German pediatrician.
§Charles A. Hunter (1873-1955), Canadian physician.
*William Sly (1932-), American physician.
†Paul Langerhans (1847-1888), German pathologist.

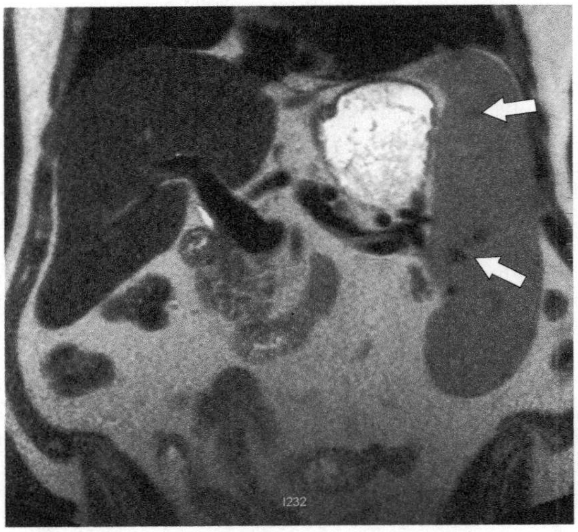

FIGURE 6-20. Coronal T2 haste image in a 76-year-old man with Gaucher disease and hepatosplenomegaly. There are small gaucheromas in the spleen (*arrows*).

Glycogen Storage Disease

Glycogen storage disease (GSD) comprises a number of genetic enzyme deficiencies in glycogen metabolism with excessive glycogen deposition, usually seen in childhood. The most common is von Gierke‖ disease (GSD type I) caused by glucose-6-phosphatase deficiency with hepatic glycogen accumulation and hepatomegaly (and, to a lesser extent, affecting the kidney and small intestine). Other GSD disorders that cause hepatomegaly include types III, VI, and IX.

Zellweger Syndrome

Zellweger¶ syndrome, also known as cerebrohepatorenal syndrome, is one of several leukodystrophic disorders. It is a rare autosomal-recessive disorder and manifests as lack of peroxisome production, which results in long-chain fatty acid deposition in multiple organs, including the liver, leading to hepatomegaly.

Alpha$_1$-Antitrypsin Deficiency

Alpha$_1$-antitrypsin deficiency is an autosomal codominant, relatively common genetic disease leading to decreased and defective production of alpha$_1$-antitrypsin (a protease inhibitor), which is deposited in the lungs and liver and causes emphysema, hepatitis, and hepatic cirrhosis.

Cystic Fibrosis (see Chapter 9)

Cystic fibrosis is a recessively inherited genetic disease resulting in sodium and chloride transepithelial transport dysfunction. Viscous secretions then develop in multiple organs. Hepatic involvement in patients with cystic fibrosis is relatively common. Focal biliary cirrhosis develops because of biliary obstruction from thickened viscous bile and subsequent periportal fibrosis.

HEPATOMEGALY

Hepatomegaly has numerous causes, many related to multisystem disorders, including genetic anomalies, infections, toxins, and vascular, neoplastic, and metabolic disorders (Table 6-3). Genetic disorders have already been discussed. The remainder are discussed initially as diffuse parenchymal and depositional diseases (hepatitis, cirrhosis, and metabolic disorders) and then separately under neoplastic, infectious, and metabolic disorders.

DIFFUSE PARENCHYMAL AND DEPOSITIONAL DISEASES

Hepatitis

Hepatitis is a diverse group of inflammatory liver diseases, most frequently resulting from viral infection but having many other causes (Table 6-3 and Box 6-2). Hepatitis can be acute or chronic, the former often self-limiting, the latter often leading to hepatic

‡Alfred Hand (1868-1949), U.S. pediatrician; Artur Schüller (1822-1884), Austrian physician; Henry A. Christian (1876-1951), U.S. internist.
§Eric Letterer (1895-1982), German pathologist; Sture A. Siwe (1897-1966), Swedish pediatrician.
‖Edgar Otto Conrad von Gierke (1877-1945), German pathologist.
¶Hans Ulrich Zellweger (1909-1990), Swiss-American pediatrician.

TABLE 6-3 Causes of Diffuse Parenchymal Disease

Diffuse Parenchymal Disease	Etiology
Genetic disorder	Glycogen storage disease, Gaucher disease, hemochromatosis, MPS, Langerhans cell histiocytosis, hemolytic anemias, Zellweger syndrome, lipid storage disorders, cystic fibrosis
Hepatitis	Viral infectious: hepatitis A, B, C, D; rubella; herpes simplex; HIV; EBV; CMV; yellow fever Drugs and toxins: alcohol, INH, halothane, chlorpromazine, acetaminophen, phenytoin, methyldopa, CCl4, steatosis
Cirrhosis	Alcoholic; hepatitis B, C; hemochromatosis; Wilson disease; alpha$_1$-antitrypsin deficiency; cystic fibrosis; biliary cirrhosis; hepatic congestions; drugs (see above)
Neoplastic	Hemangioma, metastases, myeloma, leukemia, lymphoma, HCC, polycystic disease
Other infections	Malaria, ameba, actinomycosis, hydatid, leptospirosis, TB, syphilis
Metabolic	Amyloid, sarcoidosis

CCl4, Carbon tetrachloride; *CMV*, cytomegalovirus; *EBV*, Epstein-Barr virus; *HCC*, hepatocellular carcinoma; *HIV*, human immunodeficiency virus; *INH*, isoniazid; *MPS*, mucopolysaccharidoses; *TB*, tuberculosis.

Box 6-2. **Causes of Hepatitis**

CONGENITAL
Alpha$_1$-antitrypsin deficiency
Wilson disease

INFECTIOUS
Viral: hepatitis A-E, adenovirus, yellow fever, herpes, Epstein-Barr, rubella, cytomegalovirus
Toxoplasmosis
Leptospirosis

AUTOIMMUNE
Systemic lupus erythematosus

PREGNANCY

DRUGS
Numerous, including acetaminophen, nonsteroidal antiinflammatory drugs, isoniazid, rifampicin, hormonal contraceptives, nitrofurantoin, phenytoin, methyldopa

TOXINS
Alcohol
Nonalcoholic steatohepatitis
Mushrooms
Carbon tetrachloride

VASCULAR
Ischemic hepatitis

cirrhosis. Acute hepatitis, particularly from viral sources, presents with influenza-like symptoms including fever, malaise, generalized aches and pains, nausea, and vomiting. There may be hepatic tenderness and jaundice if severe, and some patients may go on to acute fulminant hepatitis and hepatic failure. Chronic hepatitis is more insidious, often with no symptoms until cirrhosis ensues with features of portal hypertension.

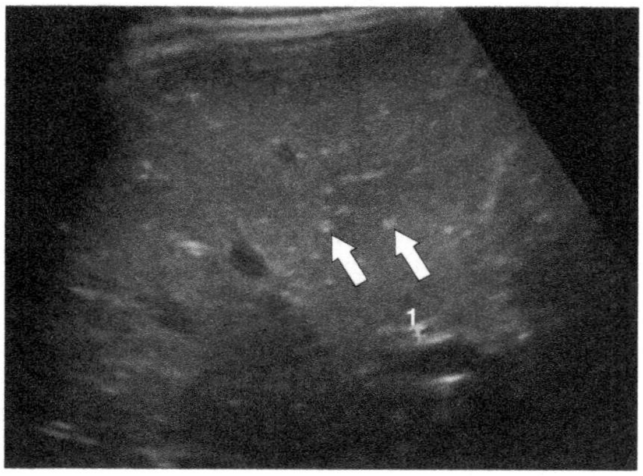

FIGURE 6-21. Sagittal US in a 55-year-old woman with hepatitis and a diffusely hypoechoic liver, giving a "starry-sky" appearance (*arrows*).

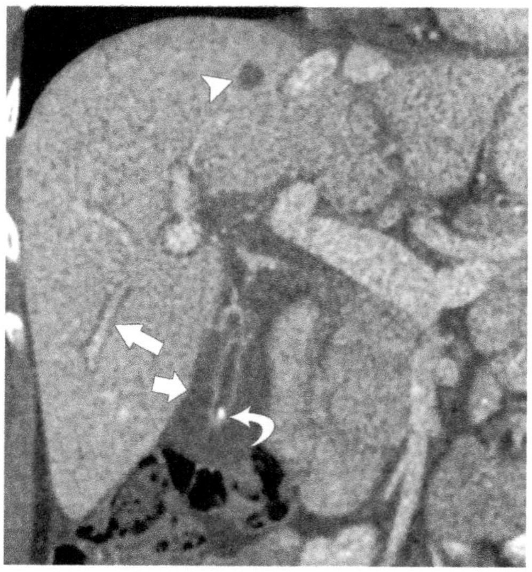

FIGURE 6-22. Coronal contrast-enhanced CT in a 36-year-old with acute viral hepatitis, mild hepatomegaly, portal tract edema (*arrow*), and diffuse gallbladder wall thickening (*small arrow*). An incidental simple hepatic cyst (*arrowhead*) and gallstone can be seen (*curved arrow*).

Viral Hepatitis

Worldwide, viral hepatitis is endemic and very common. Depending on the type of viral agent, morbidity can be immediate or prolonged or both. The five main variants are hepatitis A, B, C, D, and E, although other viruses (Epstein-Barr virus, herpes simplex, rubella, cytomegalovirus, and yellow fever) can also induce hepatitis. Hepatitis A (infectious jaundice) is usually self-limiting. Hepatitis B, conversely, is a major killer and is estimated to cause 1 million deaths annually worldwide, mainly because of chronic hepatitis, cirrhosis, and HCC development. Most patients with hepatitis C go on to develop chronic disease with similar effects to those of hepatitis B. Hepatitis D is found only in patients with preexisting hepatitis B infection and is usually acute and self-limiting, although longer term effects can develop.

At imaging, there may be hepatomegaly, and US may demonstrate sonographic features common to all hepatitis diseases, namely diffuse hypoechogenicity (Fig. 6-21), particularly in the periportal regions. There may be associated gallbladder wall thickening and increased echogenicity of the portal venules, termed a "starry-sky" appearance (these may be hypoechoic in chronic hepatitis) (Fig. 6-21). At CT, hepatomegaly and gallbladder wall thickening are also observed with heterogeneous hepatic enhancement after the administration of IV contrast material with edema of the portal tracts (Fig. 6-22). If MRI is performed, the portal tracts may demonstrate increased T2 signal secondary to periportal edema. The imaging features of chronic hepatitis are secondary to those of cirrhosis.

Because of the risk of malignant transformation from regenerative to dysplastic nodule to HCC in hepatitis B and C, most patients are subjected to serial surveillance with US. Contrast-enhanced CT and MRI are more sensitive and specific, but routine screening with these more expensive and less available methods is not considered to be warranted. Furthermore, it is proposed that even if US fails to identify small lesions (<2 cm), the patient's outcome is unaffected because most HCCs below 3 cm are still curable (US detects most lesions >2 cm).

Chemical Hepatitis (Toxins)

Chemical hepatitis is most commonly caused by acute alcoholic abuse, but a plethora of drugs can induce hepatitis, including acetaminophen, isoniazid, halothane, chlorpromazine, and phenytoin (Box 6-2). Other toxins include the *Amanita* toxin from inedible mushrooms and carbon tetrachloride. Alcoholic hepatitis is to be distinguished from alcoholic cirrhosis associated with chronic alcohol abuse. In the more acute form, symptoms can range from nothing to hepatic pain and a general feeling of malaise to a severe illness with jaundice. Severe hepatitis produces ascites and prolonged prothrombin times, which are associated with a high mortality rate. The radiological findings are similar to those of other acute forms of hepatitis with US imaging demonstrating hepatomegaly, diffuse hypoechogenicity, a "starry-sky" appearance, gallbladder wall thickening, and heterogeneous enhancement on contrast-enhanced MRI or CT.

Nonalcoholic Steatohepatitis

Nonalcoholic steatohepatitis is an acute form of nonalcoholic fatty liver disease. As its name suggests, it is not associated with alcohol, but more commonly with obesity and insulin resistance. Severe forms can lead to an acute inflammatory disease similar to alcoholic hepatitis histologically. Given that a fatty liver is already hyperechoic by US, the diagnosis of acute steatohepatitis using the same method may be difficult because the liver may not be hypoechoic as it is in other forms of acute hepatitis. The diagnosis may ultimately require percutaneous biopsy. The disease is increasingly being recognized as a major cause of hepatic cirrhosis.

Hepatic Steatosis—Fatty Liver

Hepatic steatosis or fatty liver disease is a reversible disease with multiple causes (Box 6-3). The main differentiation is between alcohol fatty liver disease and nonalcoholic fatty liver disease. Both have become epidemic, with approximately 10% to 20% of the population thought to have the disease, mainly because of obesity, diabetes mellitus, and alcohol abuse and to a lesser extent hyperlipidemia, steroid use, viral hepatitis, other viral infections (human immunodeficiency virus [HIV]), chemotherapy, lipid storage diseases and other genetic disorders (e.g., Wilson disease), pregnancy, Reye* syndrome, and kwashiorkor. Although fatty liver disease was once thought to be a relatively benign process, it is becoming increasingly recognized that long-term hepatocyte accumulation of fat (mainly triglycerides) results in steatohepatitis, hepatic cirrhosis, and, ultimately, HCC.

It is becoming increasingly important therefore not only to diagnose hepatic steatosis, but to quantify it. The degree of fatty infiltration is graded as mild when steatosis is between 5% and 33% (the fraction of hepatocytes that contain fat), moderate with 34% to 66% steatosis, and severe with ≥67% involvement. Although liver biopsy is accurate, it samples only a small portion of the liver and has recognized complications. US has a positive predictive value of between 62% and 77% for demonstrating fatty liver disease, which is typically diffusely echogenic, particular when compared with the renal cortex (Fig. 6-23). However, because of operator dependency and abdominal wall sound absorption in obese patients, CT or MRI is considered more accurate, particularly for quantification (although CT has lower sensitivity for mild steatosis). The diagnosis by noncontrast CT is made when hepatic attenuation is >10 HU less than the spleen (the liver is usually 10 HU greater than the spleen) or has an absolute value of <40 HU (Fig. 6-24). Severe forms can even be detected with contrast-enhanced CT (Fig. 6-25).

Hepatic steatosis is rapidly assessed with MRI using fat-suppression techniques, including in-phase and out-of-phase (IP and OOP) images. Increasingly fatty livers demonstrate signal drop-off on OOP images (Fig. 6-26), the degree to which can be quantified by calculating the signal loss.

*Ralph Douglas Kenneth Reye (1912-1977), Australian pathologist.

Box 6-3. Causes of Fatty Liver

TOXINS
Alcohol
Drugs: steroids, tamoxifen, methotrexate, amiodarone, chemotherapeutic agents

NUTRITIONAL
Obesity
Total parenteral nutrition
Malnutrition (kwashiorkor)
Small-bowel bypass

METABOLIC
Diabetes mellitus
Pregnancy
Hyperlipidemia
Lipodystrophy
Glycogen storage disease
Lipid-storage disease
Abetalipoproteinemia
Alpha$_1$-antitrypsin deficiency
Wilson disease
Hemochromatosis

INFECTIOUS
Hepatitis
Human immunodeficiency virus infection

INFLAMMATORY
Reye syndrome
Ulcerative colitis

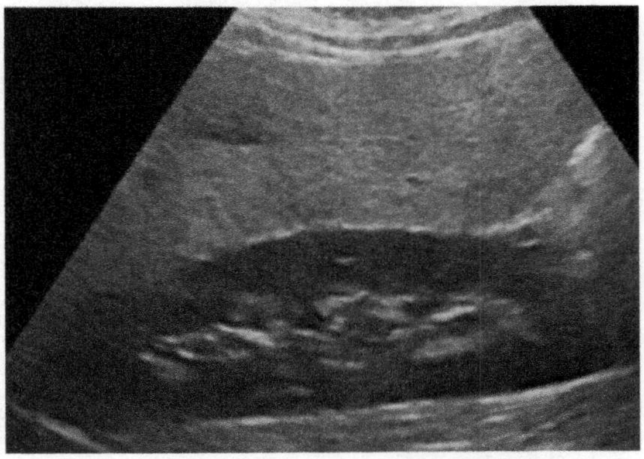

FIGURE 6-23. US in a 35-year-old woman with diffuse hepatic echogenicity resulting from fatty liver.

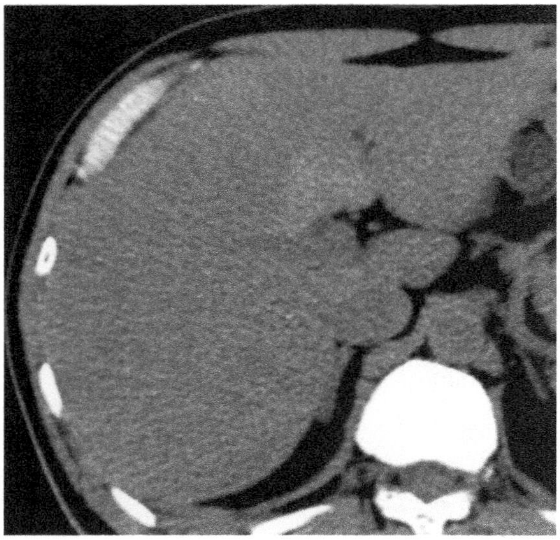

FIGURE 6-24. Axial noncontrast CT in a 56-year-old man with diffuse hypodensity, hepatic low attenuation measuring 18 HU, that is caused by hepatic steatosis.

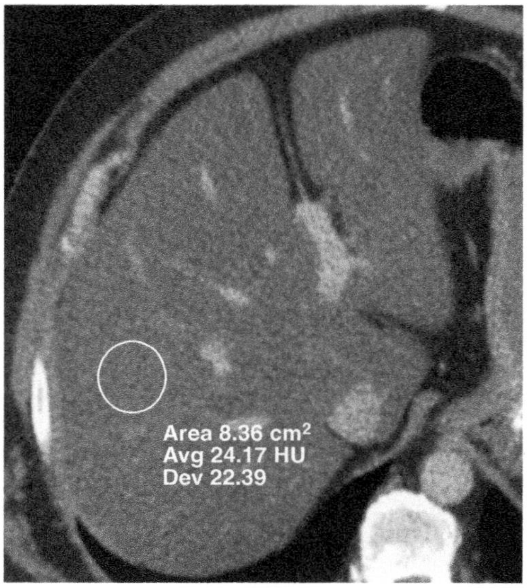

FIGURE 6-25. Axial contrast-enhanced CT in a 44-year-old woman with fatty liver. Diffuse hepatic hypodensity (24 HU) is seen, despite the use of IV contrast medium.

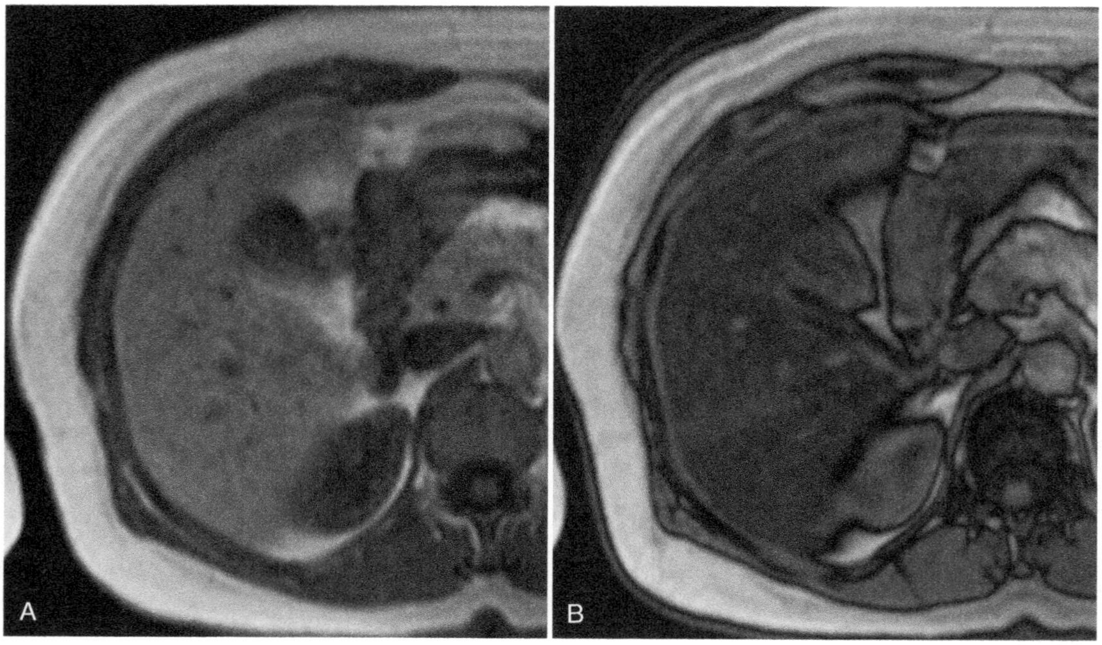

FIGURE 6-26. In-phase (**A**) and out-of-phase (**B**) MRI in a 51-year-old man demonstrating signal loss on out-of-phase images owing to a diffuse fatty liver.

Focal Fat Deposition and Focal Sparing

Hepatic steatosis can be focal or diffuse but is often confined to a segment or lobe or even a part of a segment (e.g., adjacent to the falciform ligament and ligamentum teres) (Fig. 6-27), or there may be areas of focal sparing (e.g., gallbladder bed) (Fig. 6-28). These findings must be differentiated from true mass lesions, and knowledge of their typical locations and appearances avoids unnecessary further evaluation, although in a patient with an underlying primary malignant disease, definitive characterization may be unavoidable so as to appropriately stage the disease (Fig. 6-29). This is best achieved using fat-suppressed MRI techniques (i.e., IP and OOP chemical shift imaging). Fatty liver typically loses signal on OOP images compared with IP T1-weighted images, which is diagnostic of fat. Focal fat also tends to show irregular, sometimes geographical, margins, another helpful sign because neoplastic lesions, in general, are more mass like (Figs. 6-30 and 6-31). Furthermore, focal fat shows no mass effect on vessels, nor does it distort the liver architecture.

CIRRHOSIS

Cirrhosis results from hepatocyte injury from a multiplicity of causes (Box 6-4). Cirrhosis can be caused at the presinusoidal level from extrahepatic causes (portal vein obstruction from thrombosis or external tumor compression) and congenital hepatic fibrosis, infections (malaria and schistosomiasis), sarcoidosis, and

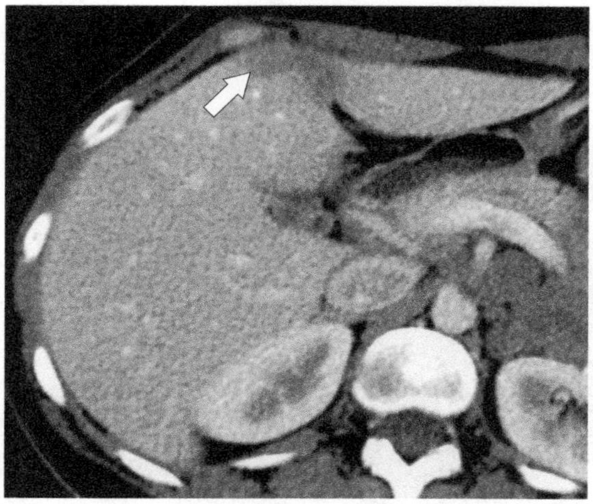

FIGURE 6-27. Axial contrast-enhanced CT in a 44-year-old woman with breast cancer. A focal hypodense area in the region of the falciform ligament is due to focal fat (*arrow*).

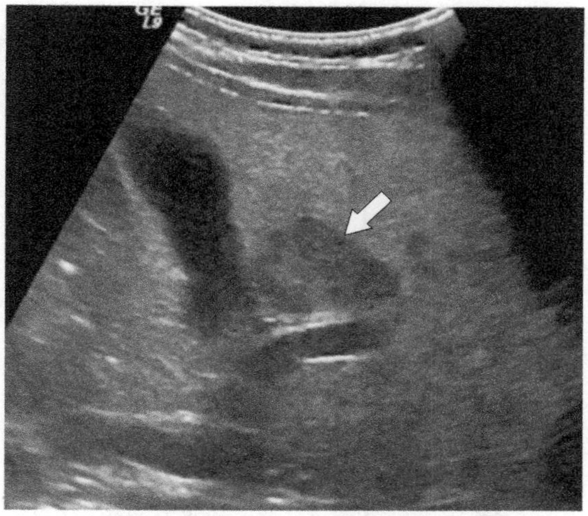

FIGURE 6-28. Sagittal US in a 53-year-old man with diffuse hepatic steatosis (echogenic liver). A hypoechoic region (*arrow*) in the gallbladder fossa is due to fatty sparing.

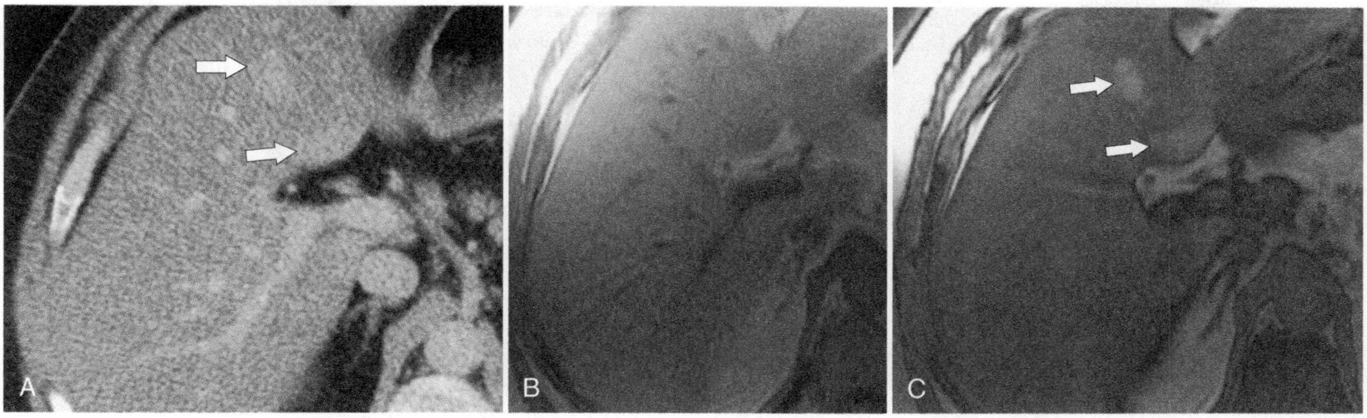

FIGURE 6-29. Axial (**A**) contrast-enhanced CT and in-phase (**B**) and out-of-phase (**C**) T1-weighted MRI in a 44-year-old woman with melanoma. Two subtle, small, hyperdense regions (*arrows*) in segment V of the liver become more evident as normal hyperintense liver surrounded by hypointense fatty liver on out-of-phase MRI.

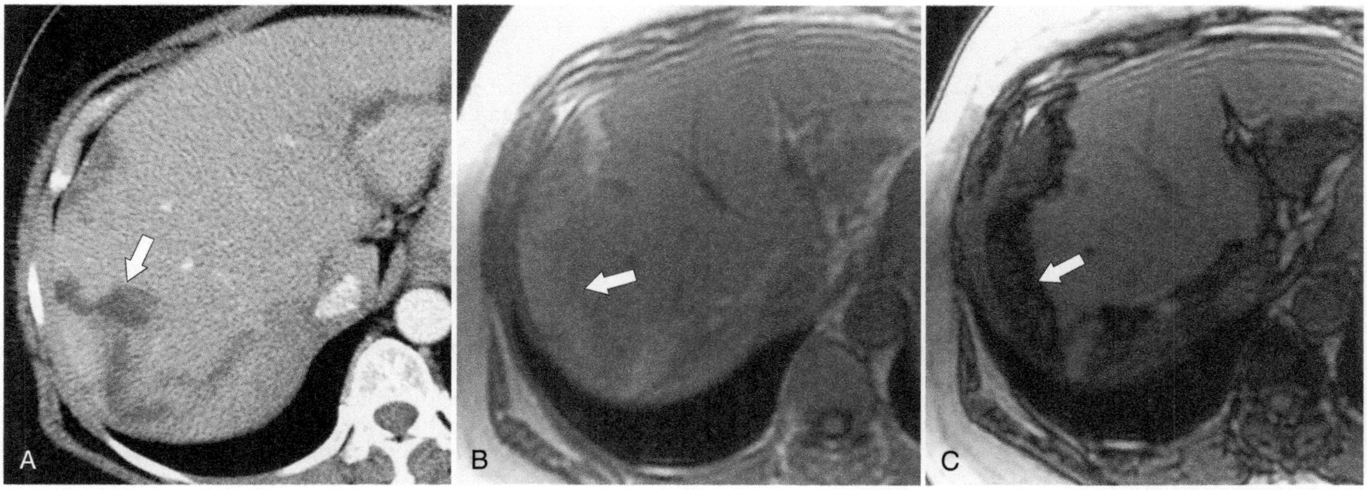

FIGURE 6-30. Axial (**A**) contrast-enhanced CT and in-phase (**B**) and out-of-phase (**C**) T1-weighted MRI in a 60-year-old woman with serpiginous and geographical hypodense regions (*arrows*) in segments VII and VIII that demonstrate increased in-phase but decreased out-of-phase signal consistent with focal fat.

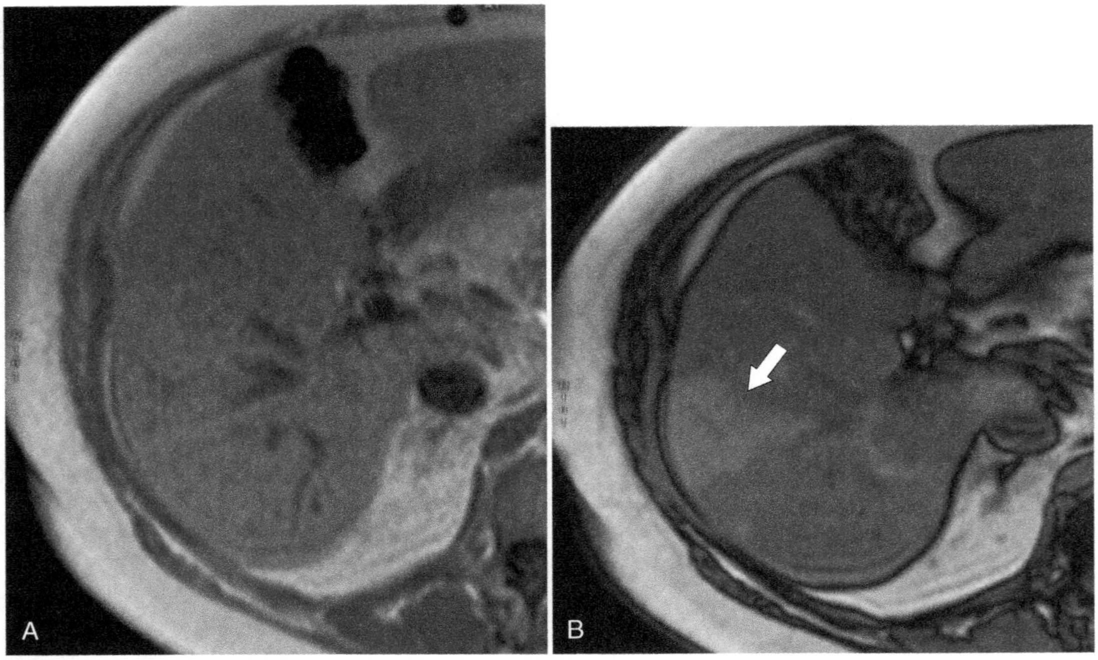

FIGURE 6-31. In-phase (**A**) and out-of-phase (**B**) T1-weighted MRI in an 80-year-old woman with a geographical region of fat in segment VI (*arrow*) of the liver.

Box 6-4. Causes of Cirrhosis

CONGENITAL
Biliary atresia
Hemochromatosis
Wilson disease
Alpha$_1$-antitrypsin deficiency
Glycogen storage disease
Cystic fibrosis
Lysosomal acid lipase deficiency
Galactosemia
Primary biliary cirrhosis
Cystic fibrosis

TOXINS
Alcohol
Drugs

INFECTIONS
Hepatitis B and C
Schistosomiasis

METABOLIC
Nonalcoholic steatohepatitis

AUTOIMMUNE
Autoimmune hepatitis
Primary sclerosing cholangitis
Primary biliary cirrhosis
Postinfantile giant cell hepatitis

VASCULAR
Venoocclusive disease
Budd-Chiari
Cardiac cirrhosis

deposition diseases (e.g., Wilson disease). Postsinusoidal causes include Budd-Chiari* syndrome and passive venous congestion from heart failure, so-called cardiac cirrhosis. The most common causes, however, are at the sinusoidal level, mainly viral or toxin in origin.

The histological hallmark of cirrhosis is fibrosis and nodule formation, representing the results of the liver attempting to repair hepatocytic damage. Macroscopically there are three types that reflect the size of nodule formation. Micronodular (Laennec*) cirrhosis is defined as nodules typically <3 mm (usual findings in alcoholic cirrhosis) (Fig. 6-32). Macronodular cirrhosis is nodule formation >3 mm (Fig. 6-33). Mixed cirrhosis has nodules of differing sizes. These regenerative nodules can, over a variable period, increase in size and develop into dysplastic nodules, which are premalignant, degenerating into HCC that, depending on the grade, can then enlarge rapidly (see later in this chapter). Often small HCCs cannot be distinguished from dysplastic nodules by either imaging or histological analysis.

Ultimately, the fibrotic process overwhelms the liver architecture, resulting in generalized hepatic contraction and shrinkage. Some lobes, particularly segment I (caudate lobe), often retain normal volume or even undergo compensatory hypertrophy, which is a relatively specific sign for cirrhosis (Fig. 6-34). Segments II and III can also be spared and compensate for liver atrophy in other lobes. This is most likely explained by their variable blood supply. The caudate lobe drains into the inferior vena cava (IVC) directly rather than via hepatic veins, thereby preserving vascular outflow and parenchymal function. As fibrosis progresses in other lobes, it impinges on vascular structures, which become attenuated, leading to degrees of portal venous occlusion. This results in portal hypertension, reversal of venous flow, variceal and collateral vessel formation, splenomegaly, and ascites (Fig. 6-35).

*George Budd (1808-1882), British physician; Hans Chiari (1851-1916), Austrian pathologist.
*René Laennec (1781-1826), French physician.

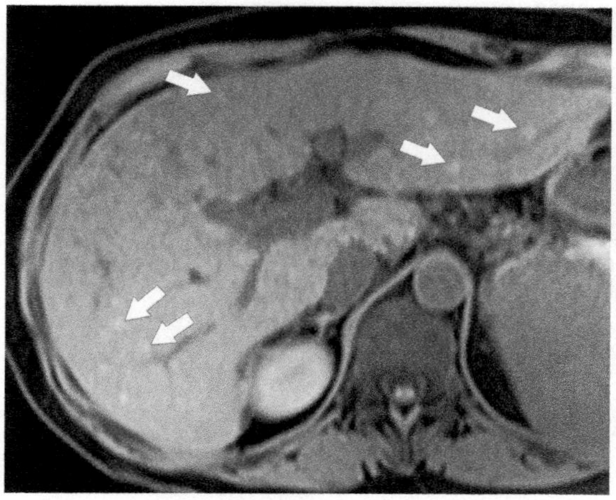

FIGURE 6-32. Axial fat-saturated T1-weighted image in a 63-year-old man with multiple T1 bright regenerative nodules scattered in both lobes (*arrows*).

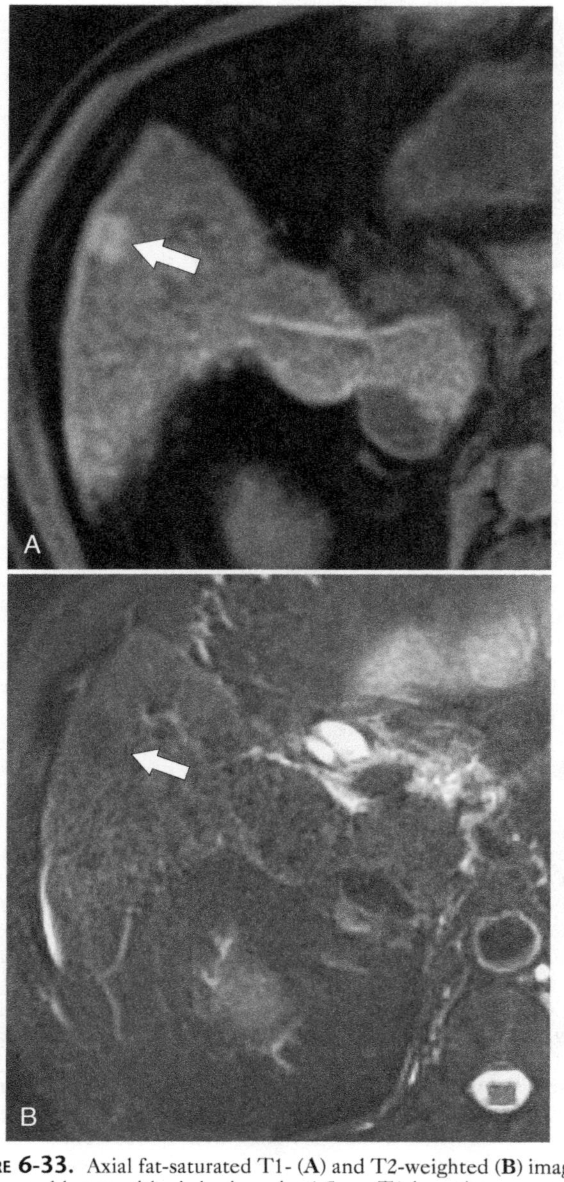

FIGURE 6-33. Axial fat-saturated T1- (**A**) and T2-weighted (**B**) image in a 69-year-old man with cirrhosis and a 1.5-cm T1 hyperintense and T2 hypointense regenerative nodule (*arrows*) from macronodular cirrhosis.

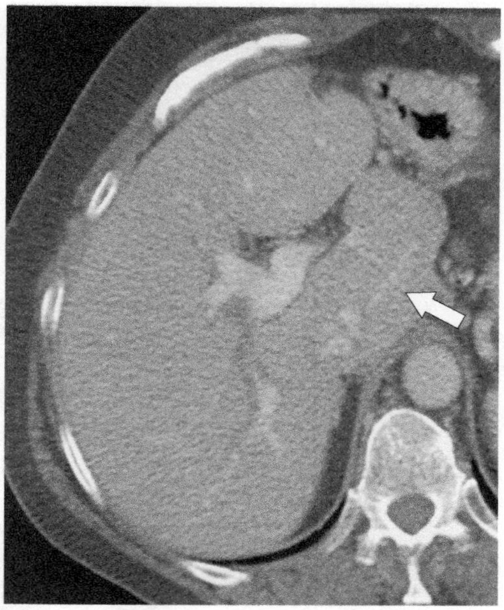

FIGURE 6-34. Axial CT in a 38-year-old woman with primary biliary cirrhosis and a markedly enlarged caudate lobe (*arrow*), specific for cirrhosis.

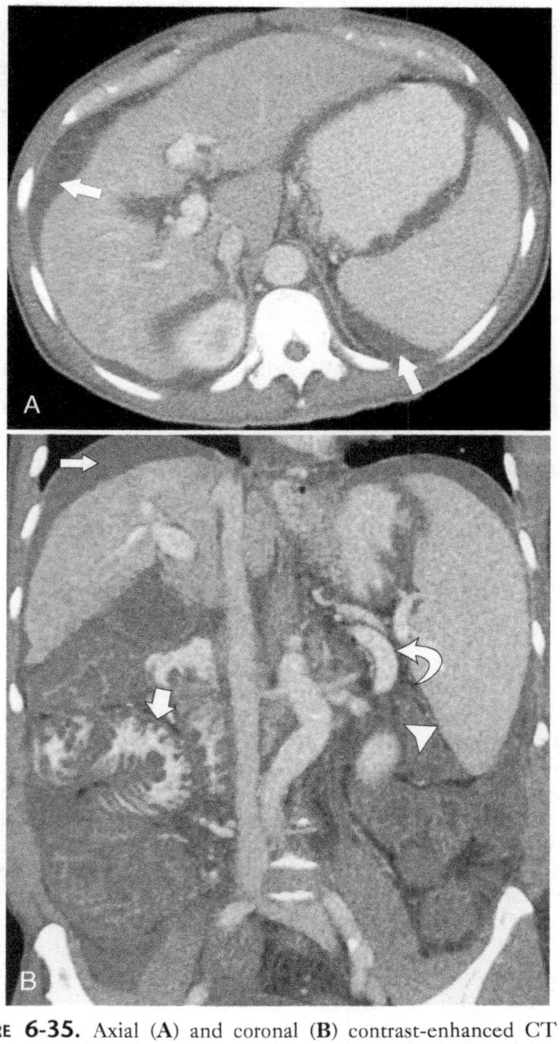

FIGURE 6-35. Axial (**A**) and coronal (**B**) contrast-enhanced CT in a 50-year-old man with end-stage cirrhotic changes, including a shrunken distorted liver, ascites (*arrows*), splenic varices (*curved arrow*), splenomegaly (*arrowhead*), and small bowel edema (*small arrow*).

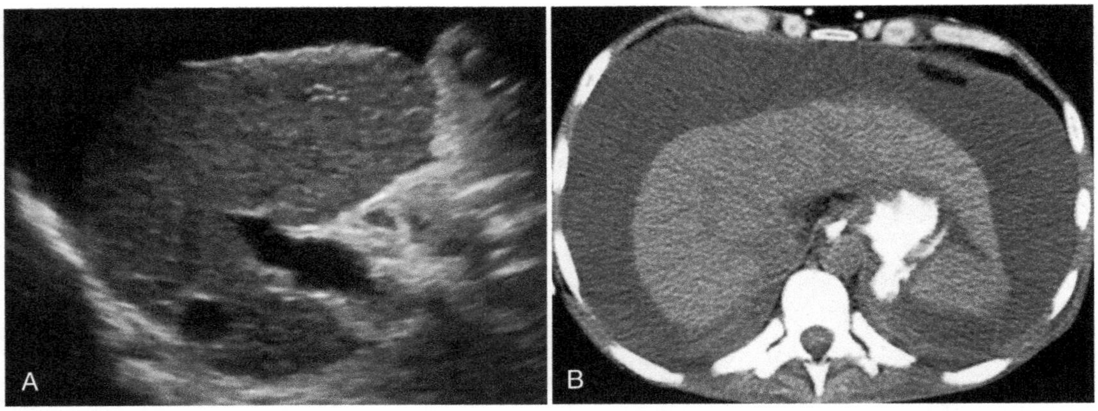

FIGURE 6-36. US (A) and CT (B) in a 70-year-old with end-stage cirrhosis. The liver has a coarse echotexture at US and is irregular and shrunken, with marked ascites also demonstrated at CT.

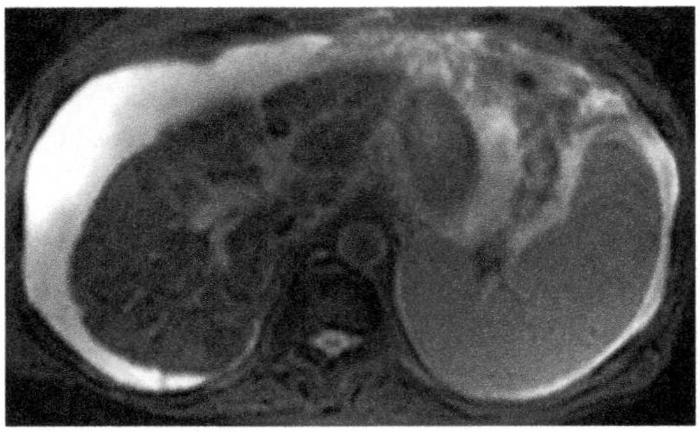

FIGURE 6-37. Axial T2-weighted MRI in a 60-year-old man with end-stage cirrhosis, including a small shrunken liver, splenomegaly, and T2 bright ascites.

TABLE 6-4 MRI Appearances of Hepatic Nodules in Cirrhosis

Nodule	T1-Weighted	T2-Weighted	Dynamic Imaging with Gadolinium Contrast Agents	Delayed Imaging with Hepatobiliary Contrast Agents
Regenerative nodule	Isointense or hypointense	Hypointense (siderotic)	Do not enhance	Enhances—isointense to hyperintense
Dysplastic nodules	Isointense to hyperintense	Well differentiated: hypointense Poorly differentiated: hyperintense	Enhance: hyperintense	Well differentiated: enhanced Poorly differentiated: variable to no enhancement
Hepatocellular carcinoma	Isointense/hypointense/hyperintense	Hyperintense	Enhance: hyperintense	Well differentiated: variable Poorly differentiated: no enhancement

From an imaging perspective, the different classifications of cirrhosis cannot generally be distinguished. The liver is often small, whatever imaging method is performed, with an irregular and nodular surface. On US, echo texture is heterogeneous but generally echogenic and coarse (Fig. 6-36). CT and MRI features reflect the histological features and consequences of cirrhosis (Fig. 6-37). The liver is irregular, usually with a nodular and irregular border, atrophy of the right lobe, and hypertrophy of the caudate lobe (segment I) and sometimes left lobe (Figs. 6-34 and 6-35). There may be areas of fat replacement and a reticular parenchymal pattern (better identified after contrast administration), representing the fibrotic process.

Nodule formation is common in cirrhosis and can usually be differentiated by imaging (Table 6-4). Siderotic (iron-laden) regenerative nodules are typically hyperdense on noncontrast CT and isodense after the administration of IV contrast medium. Because they are paramagnetic, they are hypointense on both T1- and T2-weighted MRI (Fig. 6-38). These are better delineated after the administration of IV gadolinium, which outlines the hypointense nodules (Fig. 6-39). Dysplastic nodules (premalignant for HCC), conversely, are typically hyperintense on T1-weighted imaging but hypointense on T2-weighted imaging and enhance after the administration of IV contrast material (Fig. 6-40). HCC, conversely, is typically T2 hyperintense (Fig. 6-41), which distinguishes it from dysplastic nodules, since both generally avidly enhance after IV contrast medium administration (Figs. 6-40 and 6-41). As regenerative nodules retain normal hepatocyte function, they enhance with hepatocellular contrast agents and mononuclear phagocytic agents, whereas some dysplastic nodules and HCCs do not (Fig. 6-42). MRI therefore is

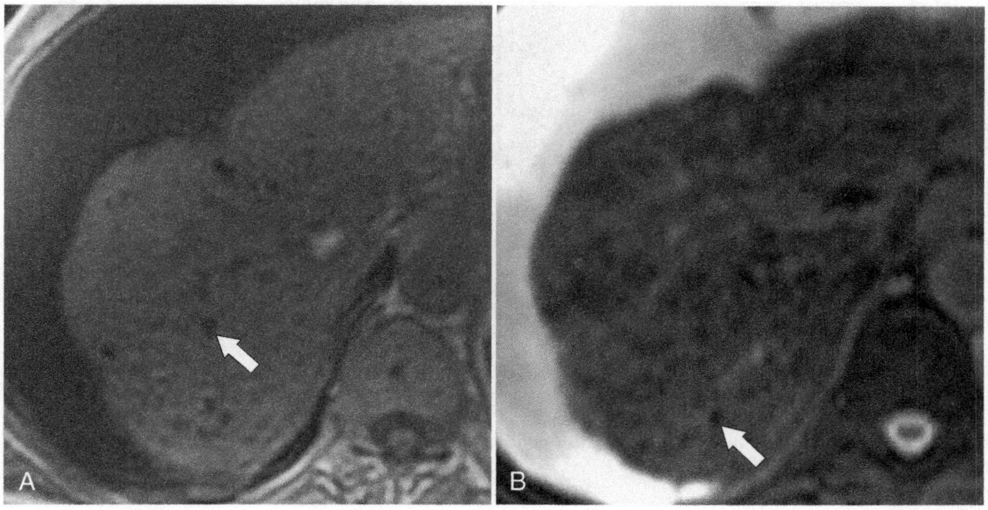

FIGURE 6-38. Axial T1- (A) and T2-weighted (B) MRI in a 63-year-old man with multiple small T1 and T2 hyperintense siderotic regenerative nodules (*arrows*).

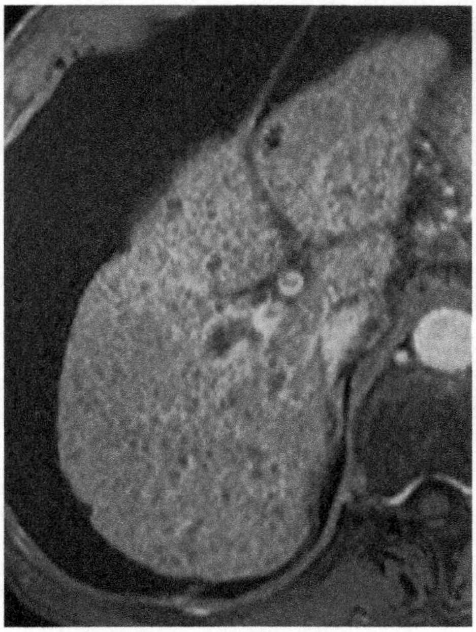

FIGURE 6-39. Axial postcontrast MRI in a 63-year-old man with numerous small hypointense regenerative nodules present throughout the cirrhotic liver.

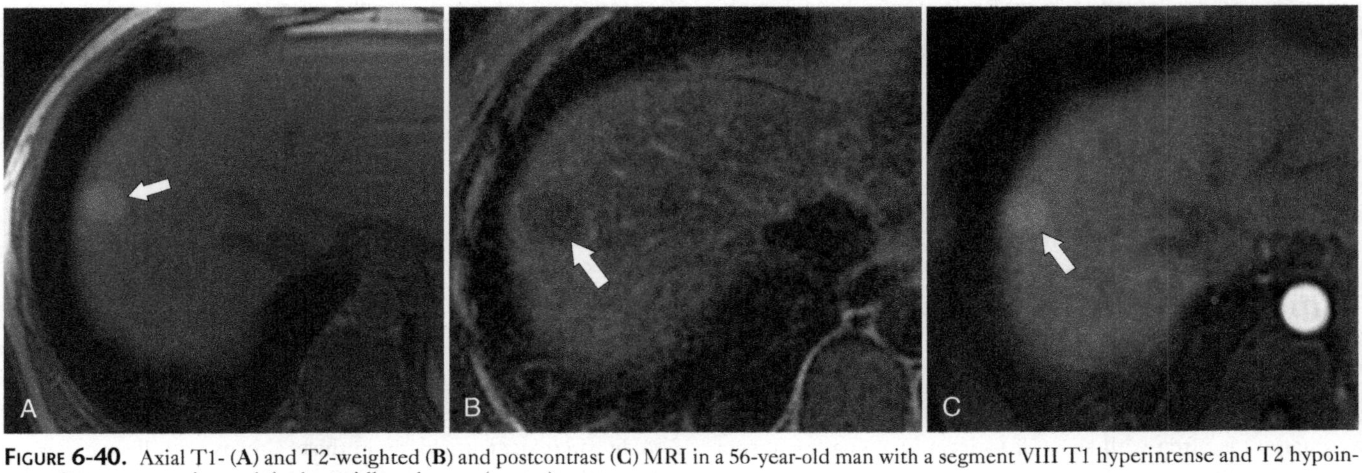

FIGURE 6-40. Axial T1- (A) and T2-weighted (B) and postcontrast (C) MRI in a 56-year-old man with a segment VIII T1 hyperintense and T2 hypointense 2-cm regenerative nodule that avidly enhances (*arrows*).

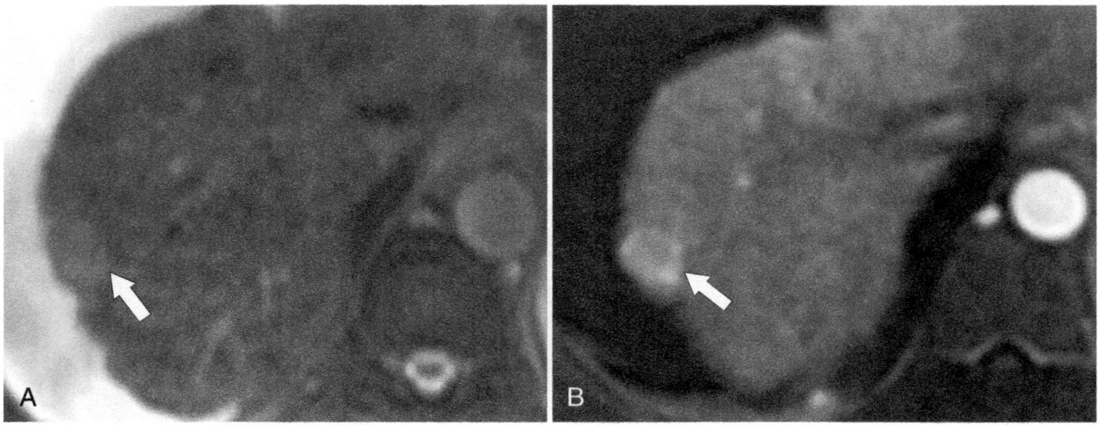

FIGURE 6-41. Axial T2-weighted (**A**) and postcontrast (**B**) MRI in a 69-year-old man with a 2-cm T2 hyperintense HCC (*arrows*) in segment VIII that avidly enhances in the arterial phase.

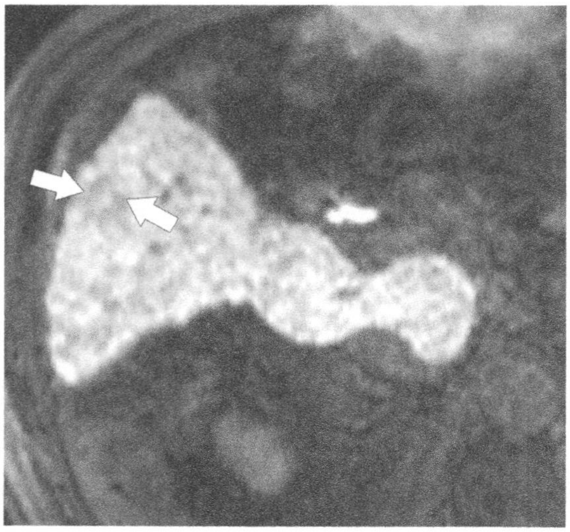

FIGURE 6-42. Delayed hepatobiliary agent imaging in a 69-year-old man. The regenerative nodule has moderate hepatocyte activity (*arrows*).

generally a more sensitive and specific imaging method than multidetector CT to evaluate the cirrhotic liver for regenerative and dysplastic nodules and HCC.

Nodular Regenerative Hyperplasia

A rare disease of unknown cause, also known as nodular transformation, nodular regenerative hyperplasia is to be differentiated from regenerative nodules in cirrhosis and is characterized by multiple and diffuse micronodules throughout the hepatic parenchyma, but without intervening fibrosis (in contradistinction to cirrhosis). Larger lesions are known as multiacinar regenerative nodules. There is no malignant potential, unlike the regenerative-to-dysplastic nodule sequence seen in cirrhosis. Nodular regenerative hyperplasia is associated with myeloproliferative disorders, bone marrow and solid organ transplants, various drugs (particularly chemotherapeutic agents), and autoimmune diseases (sarcoidosis, systemic sclerosis, systemic lupus erythematosus, rheumatoid arthritis).

Nodular regenerative hyperplasia is more commonly identified in Budd-Chiari syndrome, which may explain the finding of reduced hepatic and portal venous flow, with the frequently associated finding of small portal venous thrombosis. It is therefore a recognized cause of noncirrhotic portal hypertension, and presentation is often with signs of variceal bleeding, ascites, or hypersplenism.

Lesions are generally isodense on noncontrast CT, or no CT abnormality may be discernible, although portal hypertension is common. Multiple tiny nodules may be observed on contrast-enhanced CT, and larger lesions (up to several centimeters) that enhance avidly on contrast-enhanced CT are known to occur. Unlike HCC, these larger nodules do not wash out (i.e., they retain contrast material on delayed imaging). Some may demonstrate a characteristic "halo" sign around the avidly enhancing lesion. Some have a central scar, and these may be difficult to differentiate from FNH. There may be associated features of Budd-Chiari syndrome (hepatic venous thrombosis, central hepatic hypertrophy with peripheral atrophy and irregular reticular enhancement of the parenchyma, and portal hypertension). At MRI, small regenerative nodules are mostly not visualized but large regenerative nodules are hyperintense on T1-weighted imaging and isointense or hypointense on T2-weighted imaging. They avidly enhance after administration of gadolinium agents and, because they retain their hepatocellular function, are hyperintense on delayed imaging with hepatobiliary contrast agents (Fig. 6-43).

Confluent Hepatic Fibrosis

Sometimes only a portion of the hepatic parenchyma is cirrhotic (from any cause), leading to confluent hepatic fibrosis. This is usually observed in the anterior and medial hepatic segments (segments IV and V) with focal atrophy, irregularity, and capsular retraction. Most are isodense on contrast-enhanced CT, although sometimes they are hyperdense on delayed imaging. At MRI the affected region is hypointense on T1-weighted imaging, relatively hyperintense (sometimes subtle) on T2-weighted imaging, and less enhanced than the normal liver, although delayed imaging may show irregular patches of fibrotic enhancement (Fig. 6-44).

Postinfantile Giant Cell Hepatitis

Postinfantile giant cell hepatitis, also known as giant cell hepatitis in infancy, is usually the result of hepatocyte injury from cholestasis. Numerous viruses (especially hepatitis viruses and parvoviruses) and drugs (methotrexate, chlorpromazine) are associated with the disease, but it is thought to be an autoimmune response to these agents. The cardinal feature is giant cell hepatocyte transformation. At imaging, there are multiple large, irregular, hepatic nodules (Fig. 6-45). The diagnosis is usually made by biopsy.

Chemotherapy-Induced Cirrhosis

Many chemotherapeutic agents used in the treatment of cancer are hepatotoxic, particularly in those already with liver metastases, perhaps because of reduced hepatic functional reserve. As

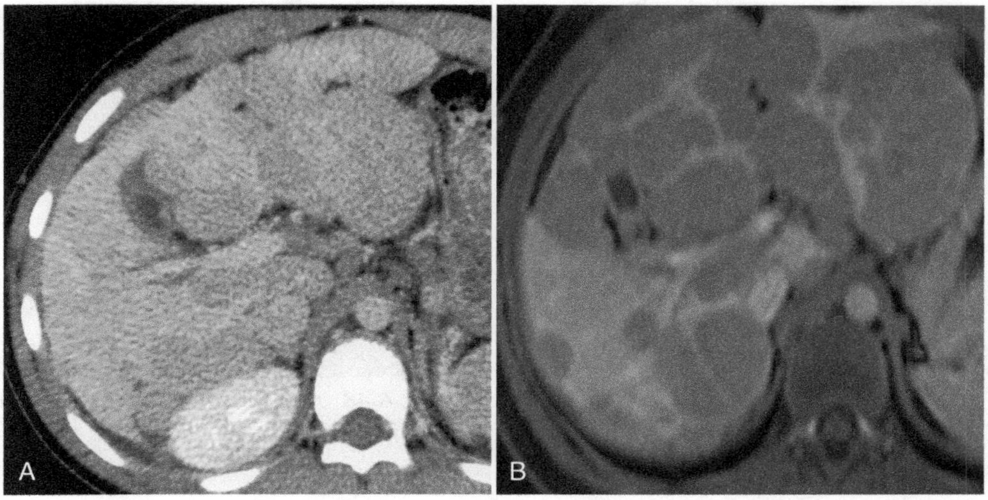

FIGURE 6-43. Axial postcontrast CT (**A**) and MRI (**B**) in an 8-year-old boy with nodular regenerative hyperplasia. The liver is replaced by multiple lobular regenerative lesions.

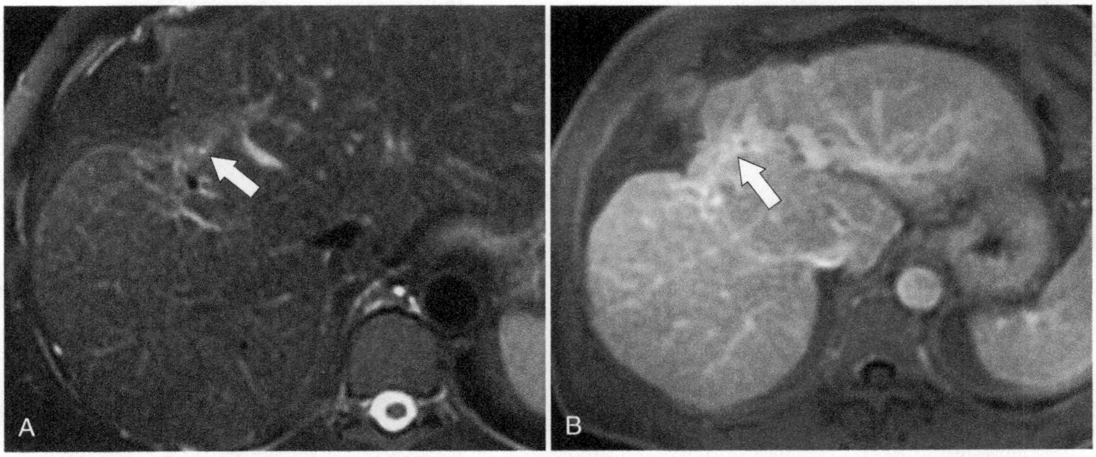

FIGURE 6-44. Axial T2-weighted (**A**) and postcontrast (**B**) fat-saturated images in a 57-year-old man with subtle T2 bright peripheral parenchyma (*arrows*) that enhances slightly at delayed postcontrast imaging due to confluent hepatic fibrosis.

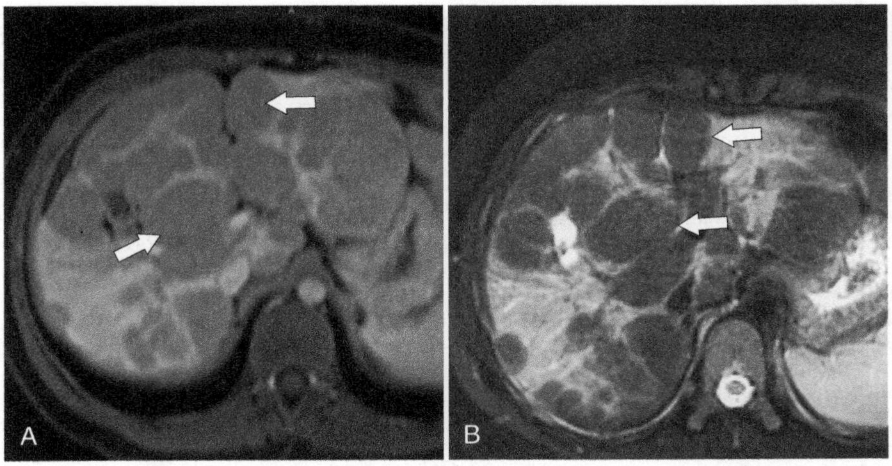

FIGURE 6-45. Axial T1-weighted (**A**) and postcontrast (**B**) MRI in an 11-year-old boy with diffuse T1 and T2 dark, nonenhancing hepatic nodular formation from postinfantile giant cell hepatitis (*arrows*).

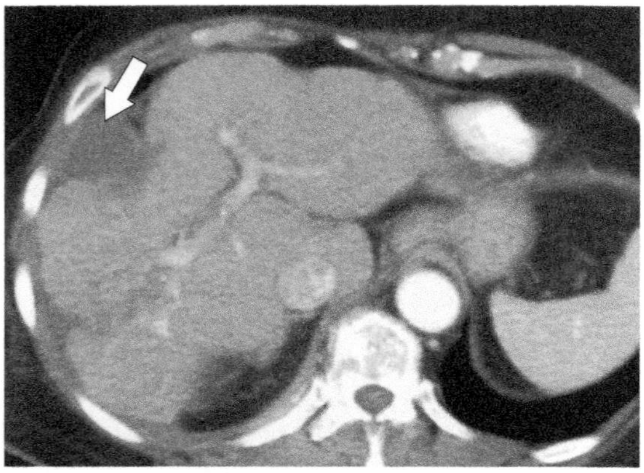

FIGURE 6-46. Axial contrast-enhanced CT in a 79-year-old woman who underwent chemotherapy for breast cancer and now has a cirrhotic irregular liver and some ascites (*arrow*).

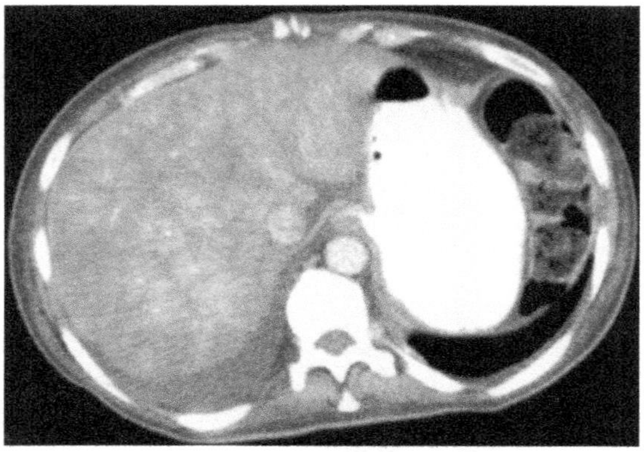

FIGURE 6-48. Axial contrast-enhanced CT in a 49-year-old man with passive venous congestion (nutmeg liver). There is also ascites.

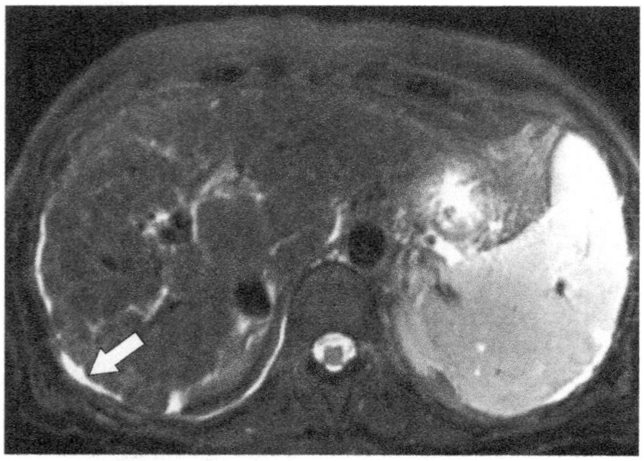

FIGURE 6-47. Axial T2-weighted fat-saturated MRI in a 72-year-old woman with cirrhotic features of an irregular liver, splenomegaly, and slight ascites (*arrow*) resulting from primary biliary cirrhosis.

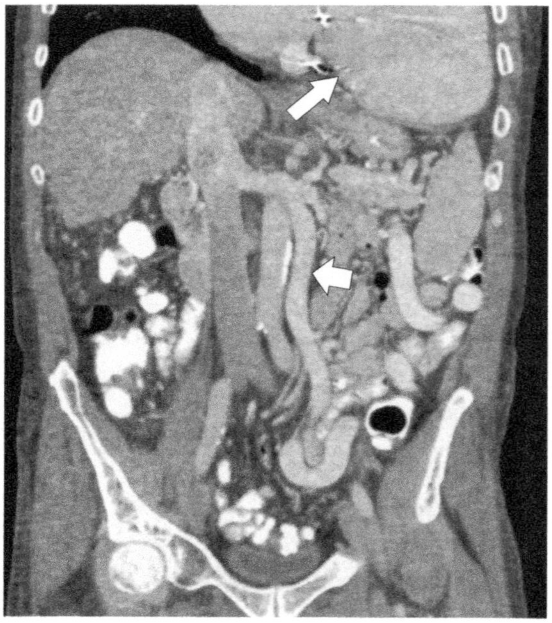

FIGURE 6-49. Coronal contrast-enhanced CT in a 67-year-old with cardiac cirrhosis and an enlarged heart (*arrow*), cirrhotic liver, and multiple mesenteric venous collaterals (*small arrow*) caused by portal venous hypertension.

newer chemotherapeutic agents are delivering better outcomes for patients with metastatic disease, these patients are tending to live longer and chemotherapeutic-induced cirrhosis is being observed more often (Fig. 6-46).

Primary Biliary Cirrhosis

The cause of primary biliary cirrhosis (PBC) is unknown but is most likely autoimmune. The course is chronic destruction of bile canaliculi and subsequent cholestasis, inflammation, fibrosis, scarring, and finally cirrhosis (Fig. 6-47). PBC is far more common in women (9:1), who usually have elevated antimitochondrial and antinuclear antibody levels. It is also associated with other autoimmune hepatic and nonhepatic diseases, including primary sclerosing cholangitis, autoimmune hepatitis, scleroderma, and rheumatoid arthritis, among others.

Primary biliary cirrhosis is difficult to differentiate from other forms of cirrhosis at imaging, but the diagnosis is suggested by clinical history in a female patient. Regenerative nodules are prominent features of the disease, and fibrosis may be less evident. Lymphadenopathy is more common in PBC than in other forms of cirrhosis, but HCC occurs less frequently. Portal hypertension tends to occur early.

Passive Venous Congestion and Cardiac Cirrhosis

Passive venous congestion and cardiac cirrhosis are secondary to right-sided heart failure from any cause (congestive failure, cardiomyopathy, constrictive pericarditis, valve disease), resulting in increased suprahepatic IVC pressure, which is transmitted into the hepatic venous system. Lower pressures and milder disease can be observed on contrast-enhanced CT as early arterial filling of the IVC and hepatic veins owing to right atrial reflux. The PVP shows a characteristic diffuse heterogeneous parenchymal mottled or mosaic enhancement pattern (Fig. 6-48), also known as a "nutmeg-appearing" liver. This can be differentiated from Budd-Chiari syndrome by IVC and hepatic venous dilatation rather than attenuation or obliteration.

As the chronic heart failure worsens, hepatic venous pressure ultimately leads to cirrhosis and portal hypertension and appears similar to Budd-Chiari syndrome. Aside from the specific imaging features of each disease, the effect on the portal vein is the same, namely an increase in pressure, which is classified as a hepatic wedge pressure >10 mm Hg. The imaging findings include gastroesophageal and splenic varices, splenorenal varices, recannulization of the portal vein, and numerous other smaller collaterals. If the disease is severe, splenomegaly and ascites develop (Fig. 6-49).

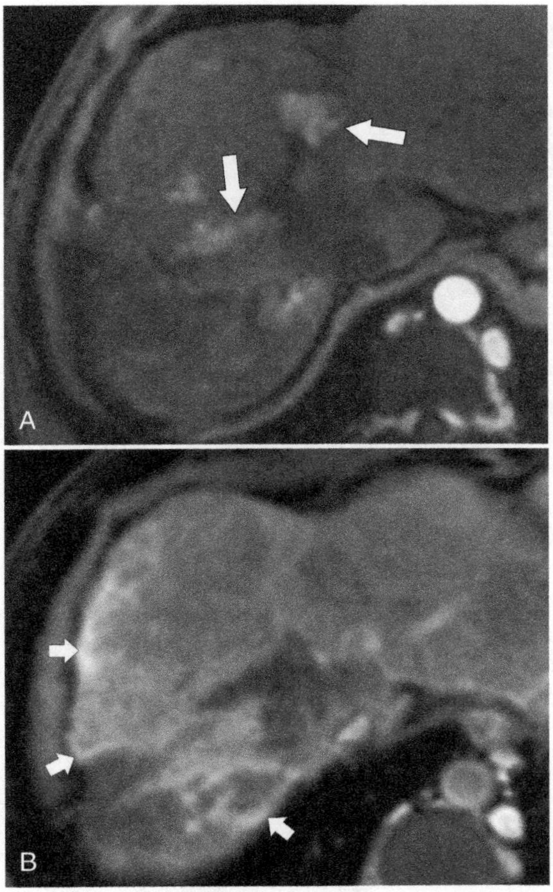

FIGURE 6-50. Axial arterial (A) and PVP (B) postcontrast fat-saturated MRI in a 43-year-old woman with Budd-Chiari syndrome. There is early central arterial enhancement (*arrows*) and late peripheral enhancement (*small arrows*) (flip-flop effect).

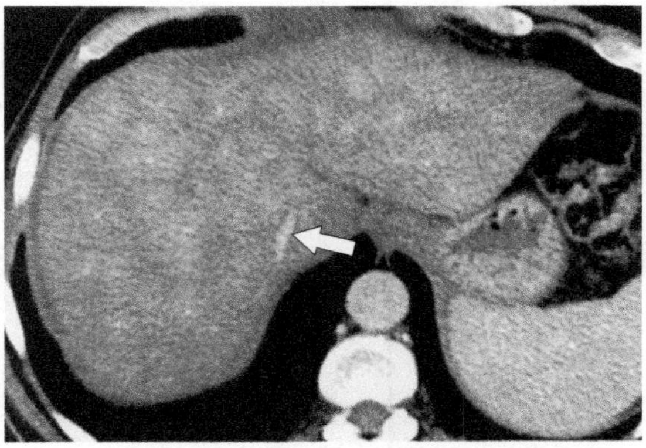

FIGURE 6-51. Axial contrast-enhanced CT in a 41-year-old woman with Budd-Chiari syndrome and a mosaic enhancement pattern to the liver. Note the attenuated IVC (*arrow*).

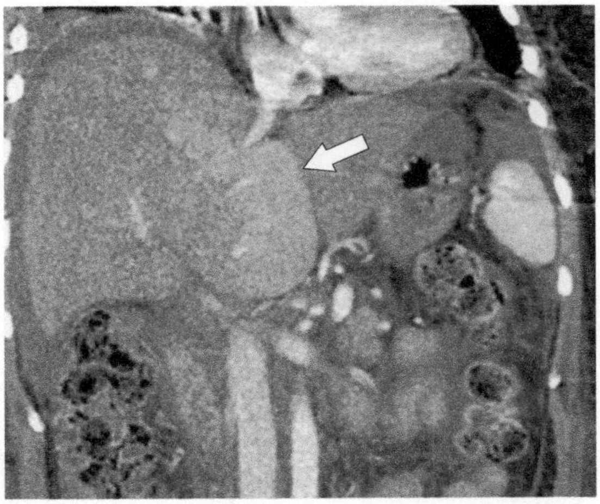

FIGURE 6-52. Coronal contrast-enhanced CT in a 49-year-old woman with Budd-Chiari cirrhosis and characteristic enlargement of the caudate lobe (*arrow*). There is also abdominal ascites.

Budd-Chiari Syndrome

Budd-Chiari syndrome consists of abdominal pain, hepatomegaly, and ascites secondary to lobar or segmental hepatic venous occlusion. A primary form is due to outflow obstruction, mainly idiopathic, but can also be secondary to congenital venous webs, trauma, and infections, especially tuberculosis (TB). Secondary forms are usually thrombotic, either at the hepatic venous outflow or within the hepatic central hepatic veins as a result of external venous compression by adjacent hepatic tumors, chemotherapy or radiation, or hypercoagulable states.

Presentation may be acute or chronic depending on the cause. Acute presentation may be fulminant with hepatomegaly and hepatic failure. On noncontrast CT the liver is enlarged and the hepatic veins are attenuated and hyperdense secondary to the thrombus. There are usually associated splenomegaly and ascites. Contrast-enhanced CT demonstrates a characteristic "flip-flop" enhancement pattern with early central liver enhancement (particularly in the caudate lobe and region surrounding the IVC) and decreased peripheral enhancement that reverses on the late PVP with peripheral enhancement and central relative lack of enhancement (Fig. 6-50) as a result of portal and sinusoidal stasis. Parenchymal enhancement in both acute and chronic presentations can also mimic the imaging findings of passive venous congestion (Fig. 6-51), with a diffusely heterogeneous "nutmeg" or mosaic-type pattern of parenchymal enhancement. Other features of chronic presentation include hepatic atrophy, sometimes with imaging appearances of cirrhosis (irregular contour, regenerative nodules), and usually hypertrophy of the caudate lobe (Fig. 6-52). The intrahepatic IVC and hepatic veins are attenuated and barely visible. Intrahepatic arterioportal shunting is frequently present.

Venoocclusive Disease

Venoocclusive disease usually results from the toxic effects on hepatic sinusoidal endothelium of high-dose chemotherapy, particularly when used with stem cell transplantation, when it is also known as sinusoidal obstruction syndrome. Less often, it occurs after ingestion of some plant alkaloids. The hepatic venules become occluded from inflammation and fibrosis. The clinical effect from the increased intrahepatic sinusoidal pressure leads to portal venous hypertension with hepatomegaly, portal hypertension, varices, splenomegaly, and ascites (Fig. 6-53).

Amyloidosis

Amyloid proteins, particularly monoclonal immunoglobulin light chains (AL-type) from primary systemic amyloidosis, accumulate within multiple organs (many within the abdomen and pelvis). Diffuse hepatic and splenic protein deposition causes hepatosplenomegaly (Fig. 6-54).

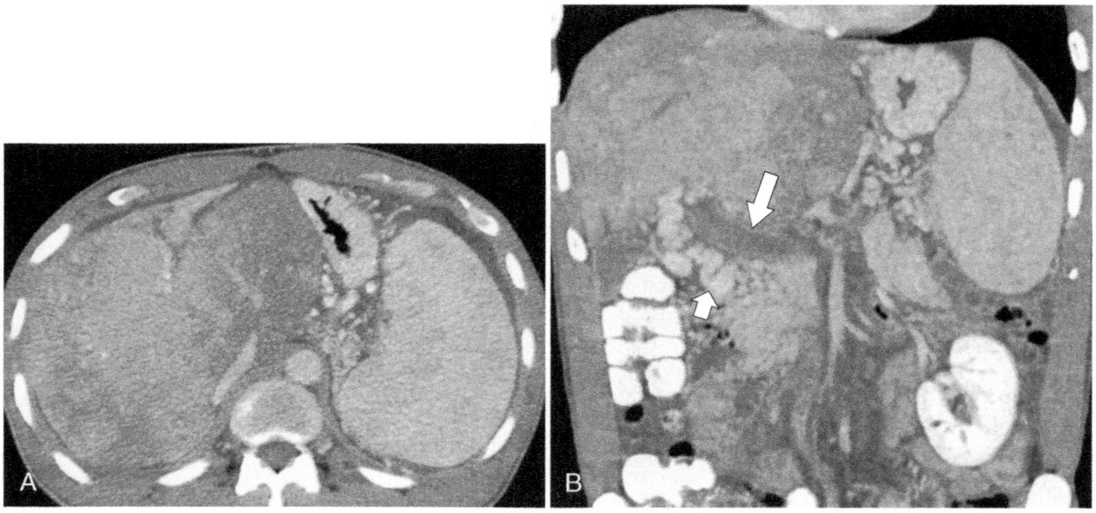

FIGURE 6-53. Axial (**A**) and coronal (**B**) contrast-enhanced CT in a 50-year-old man with venoocclusive disease. Hepatomegaly, heterogeneous hepatic enhancement, portal vein thrombus (*arrow*) leading to cavernous transformation of the portal vein (*small arrow*), and splenomegaly are present.

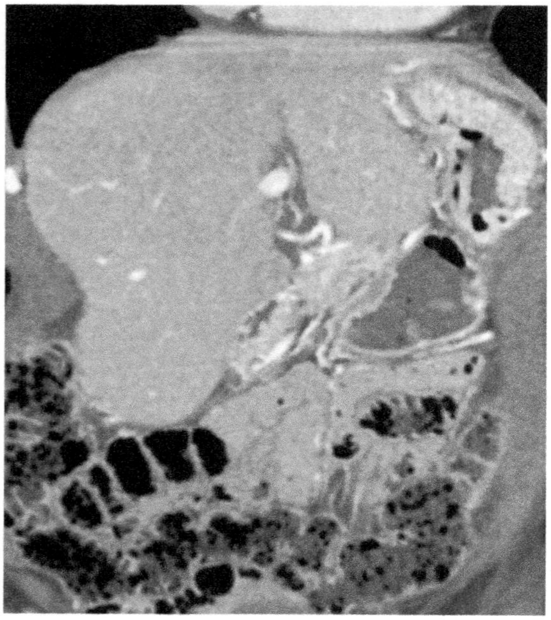

FIGURE 6-54. Coronal contrast-enhanced CT in a 77-year-old woman with primary systemic amyloidosis and hepatomegaly.

Sarcoidosis

Sarcoidosis, a multisystemic disease of unknown cause, produces noncaseating granulomatous disease that primarily affects lymph nodes and the lungs but also the eyes, skin, liver, and spleen. Hepatic involvement can lead to diffuse hepatosplenomegaly, which otherwise appears homogeneous at cross-sectional imaging (Fig. 6-55). Multiple small sarcoid nodules can also be present, but these are more common in the spleen.

Granulomatosis with Polyangiitis (Wegener Granulomatosis)

A group of multisystem vasculitic disorders includes Churg-Strauss* syndrome, which affects mainly small vessels (microscopic

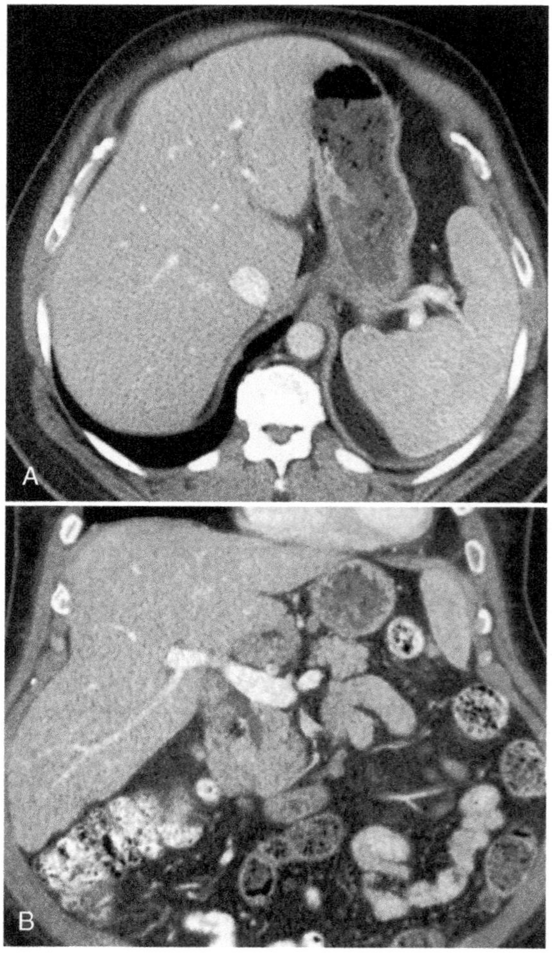

FIGURE 6-55. Axial (**A**) and coronal (**B**) contrast-enhanced CT in a 50-year-old man with hepatosplenic sarcoidosis. Imaging demonstrates moderate hepatosplenomegaly.

*Jacob Churg (1910-2005), American pathologist; Lotte Strauss (1913-1985), American pathologist.

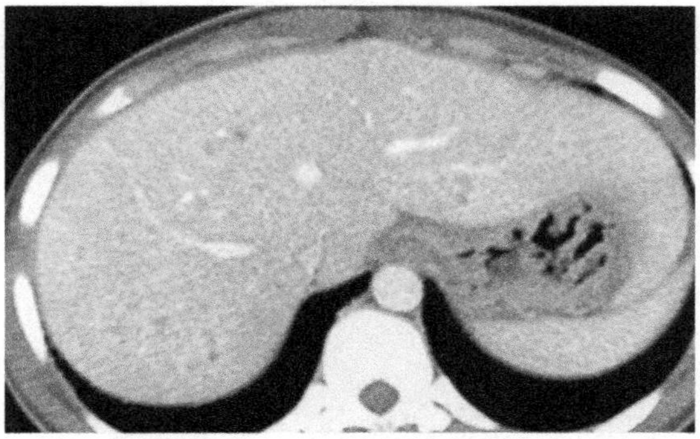

FIGURE 6-56. Axial contrast-enhanced CT in a 44-year-old man with granulomatosis with angiitis (Wegener type). There are numerous small nonspecific hypodense hepatic granulomatous lesions.

Box 6-5. Solitary Liver Lesions

BENIGN
Cyst
Hemangioma
Hamartoma
THIDS and THADS
Infections—abscess
Regenerating nodule
FNH
Adenoma
Peliosis
Epithelioid hemangioendothelioma
Lipoma
Fibroma
Focal fat
Biliary anomalies: Caroli, cystadenoma, hamartoma, biloma, peribiliary cysts
Adrenal/pancreatic heterotopic tissue

MALIGNANT
Metastasis
Dysplastic nodules (premalignant)
HCC
Fibrolamellar HCC
Cholangiocarcinoma
Angiosarcoma
Lymphoma
Biliary cyst adenocarcinoma
Hepatoblastoma

FNH, Focal nodular hyperplasia; *HCC*, hepatocellular carcinoma; *THADS*, transient hepatic attenuation differences; *THIDS*, transient hepatic intensity differences.

angiitis), and Wegener† granulomatosis, which involves larger vessels. They mainly affect the renal, pulmonary, and nasal regions, predominantly inducing local tissue necrosis, but in their acute forms they can also cause granulomatous hepatic and splenic involvement, seen as multiple hypodense lesions (Fig. 6-56) that are difficult to differentiate from other infiltrative diseases (metabolic, neoplastic, and infective).

FOCAL LIVER LESIONS

Focal liver lesions may be solitary or multiple and have numerous causes (Boxes 6-5 and 6-6). The detection of focal liver lesions is common in clinical practice now that cross-sectional imaging techniques are routinely used in the workup, diagnosis, and follow-up of many diseases. In a patient without a known history of malignancy, most prove benign. Many can be characterized at the time of the initial imaging examination; others require more dedicated imaging protocols to evaluate and characterize the mass. Lesion stability, either when compared with prior imaging or when observed at follow-up imaging, usually signifies benignity. The approach to lesion characterization therefore first depends on clinical history, age of the patient, and availability of prior imaging studies. There are a number of specific characteristic imaging features for both benign and malignant lesions, especially if dedicated imaging protocols are used. These will be discussed in turn.

Box 6-6. Multiple Liver Lesions

BENIGN
Cysts
Hemangioma
Focal fat
Infections (especially fungal)
Regenerating nodules
Adenoma
FNH
Epithelioid hemangioendothelioma
Peliosis
Caroli disease

MALIGNANT
Metastases
Multifocal HCC

FNH, Focal nodular hyperplasia; *HCC*, hepatocellular carcinoma.

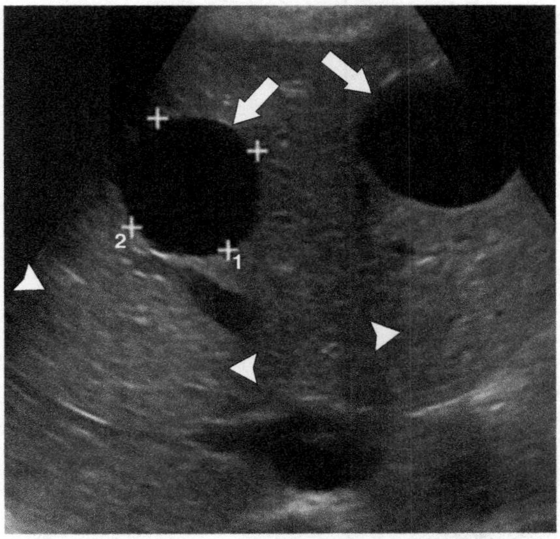

FIGURE 6-57. Sagittal US and noncontrast CT in an 87-year-old man with simple hepatic cysts (*arrows*). On US they are smooth walled and anechoic, with posterior acoustic shadowing (*arrowheads*).

Simple Hepatic Cysts

Simple hepatic cysts are the most common incidental hepatic lesions and are present in a large portion of the population. They usually gradually develop in adulthood as serous-filled simple cysts but less commonly can be congenital as a result of abnormal development of bile ducts. They are usually readily characterized by most imaging techniques. US demonstrates smooth-walled, anechoic, interior, and linear posterior acoustic shadowing (Fig. 6-57). Noncontrast CT demonstrates a uniform, smooth-walled,

†Friedrich Wegener (1907-1990), German pathologist.

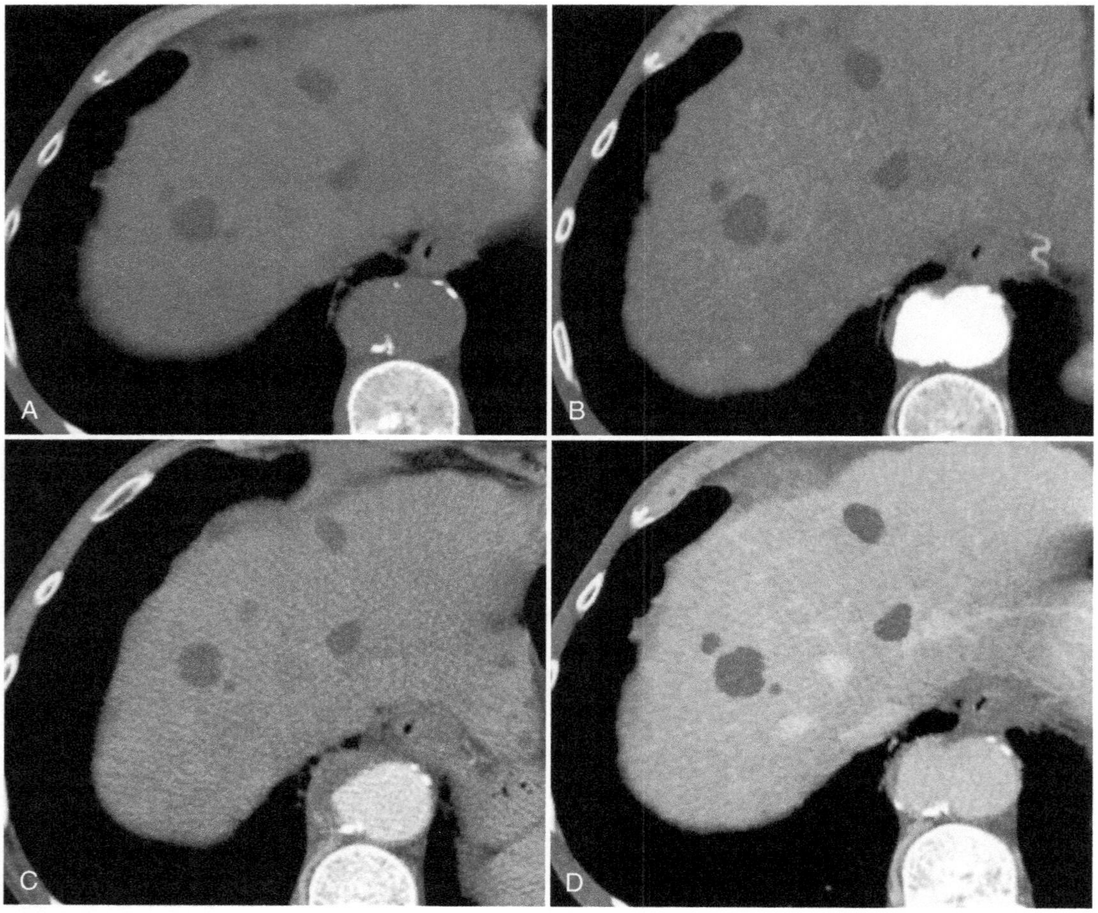

FIGURE 6-58. Axial noncontrast (**A**) and arterial (**B**), PVP (**C**), and delayed (**D**) contrast-enhanced CT in a 70-year-old man with multiple hepatic cysts. The cysts have a water density <10 HU and demonstrate no enhancement in any phase.

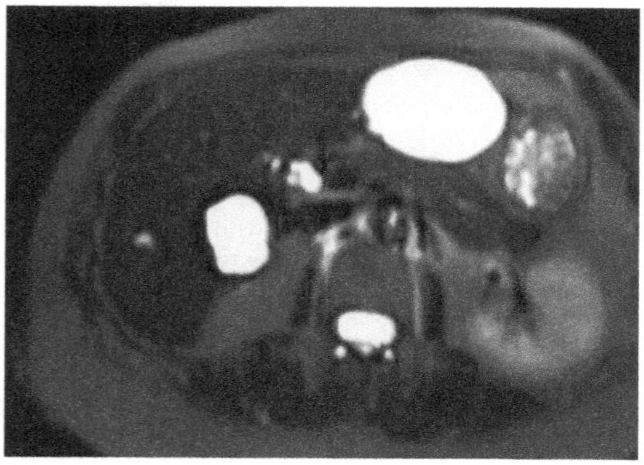

FIGURE 6-59. Axial T2-weighted MRI with several T2 hyperintense liver cysts in both the left and right lobes.

homogeneous, low-density mass, with typical densities of <10 Hounsfield Units (HU), that generally does not enhance after administration of IV contrast medium (Fig. 6-58). Slight enhancement may occur (similar to simple renal cysts), but generally <10 HU. On MRI, simple cysts are represented by low T1 and high T2 signal (Fig. 6-59). Cysts are often multiple, but numerous cysts are more likely associated with polycystic kidney disease (Fig. 6-16).

On occasion, simple cysts can be confused with other diagnoses. Biliary cystadenomas can appear cystic on cross-sectional imaging (Fig. 6-60), but they are usually large and contain internal septa. Biliary hamartomas appear cystic, but they are usually small and numerous (Fig. 6-61). Some metastases are predominantly cystic

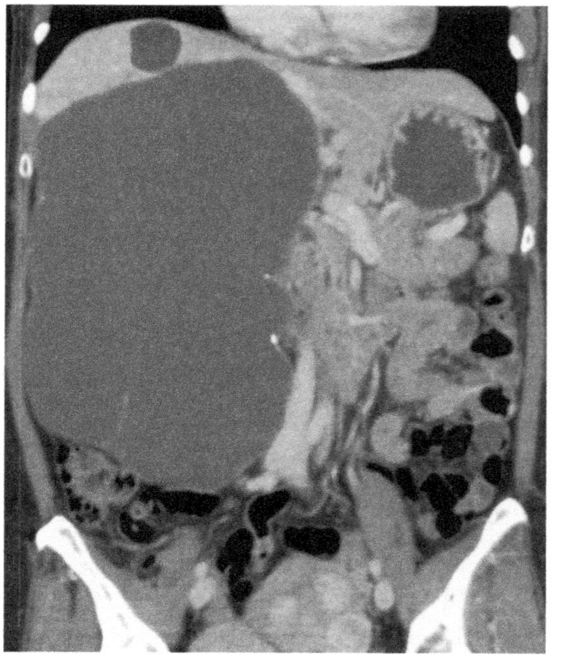

FIGURE 6-60. Coronal contrast-enhanced CT in a 57-year-old man with a large cystic mass caused by biliary cystadenoma. Simple hepatic cysts are unlikely to reach such size. There is a further smaller cystadenoma in the dome of the liver.

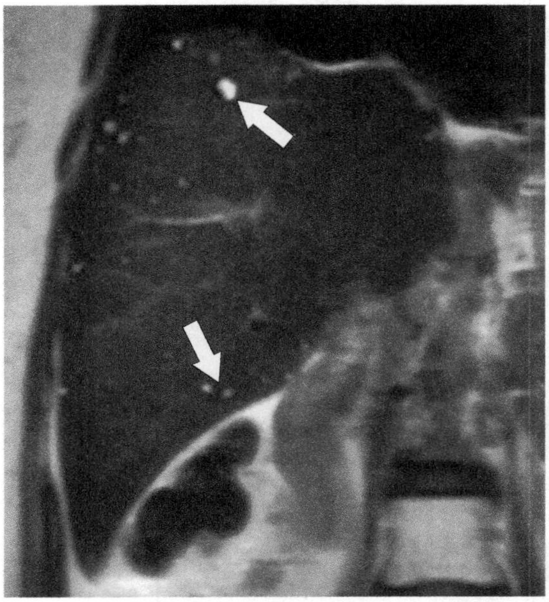

FIGURE 6-61. Coronal T2-weighted MRI in a 44-year-old woman with multiple small biliary cystic lesions (*arrows*) caused by biliary hamartoma.

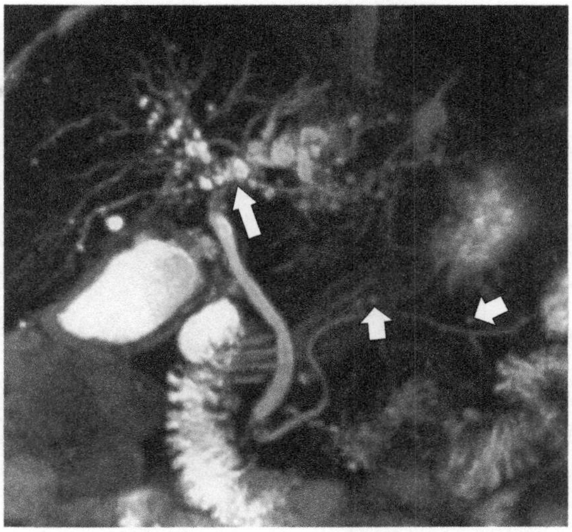

FIGURE 6-63. MRCP in a 70-year-old man with multiple small peribiliary T2 bright cysts (*arrow*) caused by peribiliary cystic disease. There are several small associated side-branch intraductal papillary neoplasms (*small arrows*).

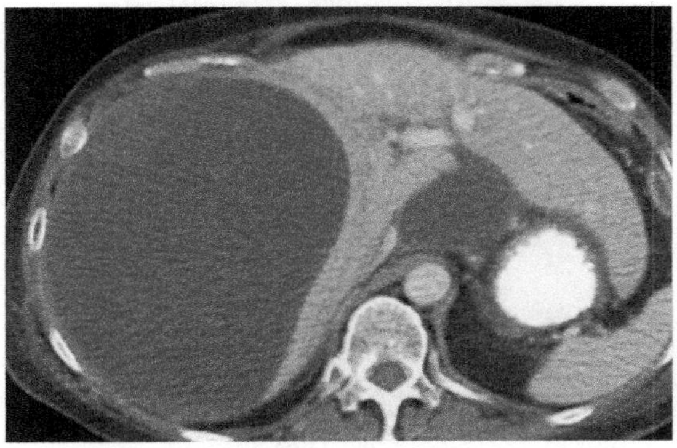

FIGURE 6-62. Contrast-enhanced CT in a 64-year-old woman with large cystic ovarian metastases that appear similar to simple cysts, yet are capsular metastases compressing the liver.

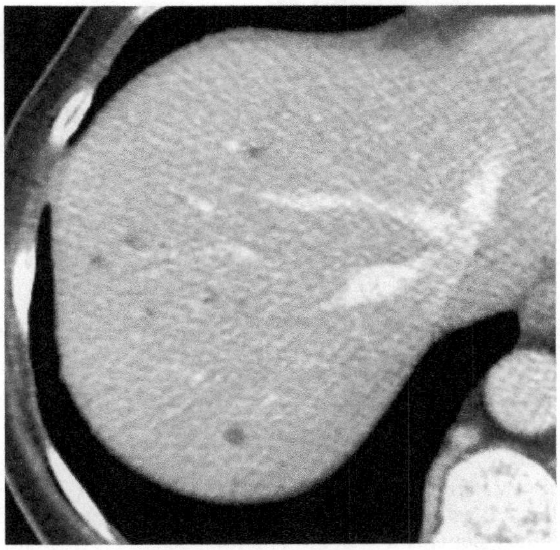

FIGURE 6-64. Axial contrast-enhanced CT in a 42-year-old woman with multiple tiny hepatic hypodensities caused by biliary hamartoma.

(particularly GI stromal tumors, ovarian cancer, and mucinous colon cancer), so knowledge of the underlying primary malignancy should alert the radiologist to consider metastases rather than cysts in these circumstances (Fig. 6-62). Less commonly, necrotic metastases and infectious cystic lesions (*Echinococcus*, amebic, fungal) can appear cyst like. An obstructed intrahepatic gallbladder and biloma can also appear cystic.

Peribiliary Cysts

Peribiliary cysts are uncommon but associated with cirrhosis and portal vein thrombosis. They represent focal dilatation of periductal glands that become obstructed through an inflammatory process. They are recognized at imaging as multiple small, hypodense, cyst-like lesions on noncontrast CT, but are best seen with T2-weighted MRI as multiple high T2 signal cysts (Fig. 6-63).

Biliary Hamartoma (von Meyenberg Complex)

Biliary hamartomas, also known as von Meyenberg* complex, are rare benign hepatic tumors that occur as a congenital anomaly in which malformation of the bile ducts results in multiple biliary cystic lesions. They are also associated with polycystic liver disease. Usually the lesions are asymptomatic and of no concern, being detected incidentally by cross-sectional imaging. At imaging they appear as multiple, small (usually <1.5 cm), cystic lesions identified on US, CT, or MRI (Figs. 6-61 and 6-64). US therefore shows multiple, diffuse, small anechoic lesions, although some may demonstrate mixed echogenicity because they have solid components (fibrous stroma). On CT, the density similarly depends on the proportion of cystic versus solid components and therefore ranges from water to soft tissue density. A hallmark, however, is the large number and small size of cyst-like lesions. On contrast-enhanced CT the solid elements may enhance, but cystic areas do not. MRI can show similar features, with low signal on T1-weighted imaging, bright T2 signal for cystic lesions, and intermediate signal for the more solid components (Fig. 6-61).

*Hans von Meyenburg (1887-1971), Swiss pathologist.

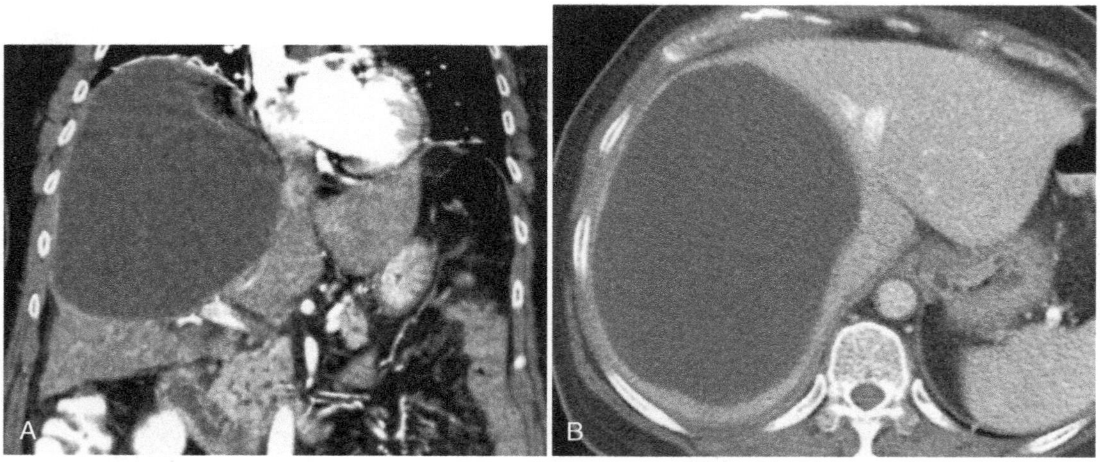

FIGURE 6-65. Axial (A) and coronal (B) contrast-enhanced CT in a 61-year-old man with a large right hepatic biliary cystadenoma.

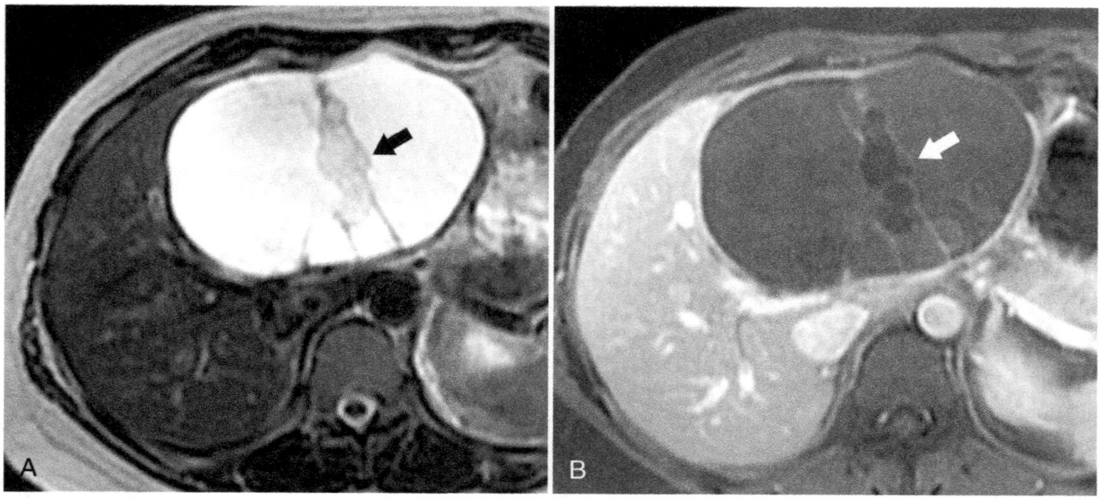

FIGURE 6-66. Axial T2-weighted (A) and postcontrast (B) MRI in a 36-year-old woman with a complex cystic 9-cm biliary cystadenoma. Note internal septa (*arrows*).

Biliary Cystadenoma (see Chapter 8)

Biliary cystadenomas are rare cystic tumors, most common in middle-aged women, derived from biliary endothelium, and usually solitary, sometimes septated, and large (Fig. 6-65), although they can be multiple (Fig. 6-60). They are usually benign and may contain ovarian stroma, but they have premalignant potential with a risk of degeneration into biliary cystadenocarcinoma. Under these circumstances they can be difficult to differentiate from cystic metastases, infected cysts (hydatid or echinococcal), or even resolving hematomas or bilomas.

At US, a large, usually multiseptated, cyst will be observed, sometimes with wall calcification. The diagnosis is best suggested with contrast-enhanced CT or MRI, which demonstrates a large multiseptated cyst with a well-defined wall that can calcify. The cyst at MRI may be of variable signal on both T1- and T2-weighted imaging, depending on the serous or mucoid nature of the cyst contents (Fig. 6-66). Malignant degeneration is suggested by enhancing septa and masses within the cyst.

Type V Choledochal Cyst (Caroli Disease) (see Chapter 8)

Caroli disease usually presents in young adulthood with complications of multiple cyst-like cavernous bile duct dilatations resulting from an autosomal-recessive disorder. Caroli syndrome is further complicated by congenital hepatic fibrosis and portal hypertension and presents in childhood. The intrahepatic dilated ducts are readily recognizable by CT or MRI (Fig. 6-67). A characteristic CT appearance is the central dot sign, representing enhancing portal tracts within the dilated bile duct (Fig. 6-67).

Hemangioma

The hemangioma is the second most common benign hepatic tumor after the hepatic cyst (approximately 5% of population). Hemangiomas are more common in females (and in pregnancy) and can be single or multiple. Usually hemangiomas are asymptomatic and of no significance (unless they are confused with metastases in a patient with cancer), but they can be symptomatic and bleed when very large (giant hemangioma). They can be differentiated into small capillary (usually seen in children), larger cavernous (the most common), hyalinized or sclerosed, or very large giant hemangiomas. Atypical forms are not infrequently recognized, but this is sometimes the result of suboptimal imaging rather than true idiosyncratic characteristics.

The characterization of hemangiomas is one of the most common diagnostic dilemmas facing abdominal radiologists, since they must be differentiated from malignant hepatic lesions, most commonly metastases. Fortunately, the a priori chance that a liver lesion is malignant in a patient with no history of malignancy

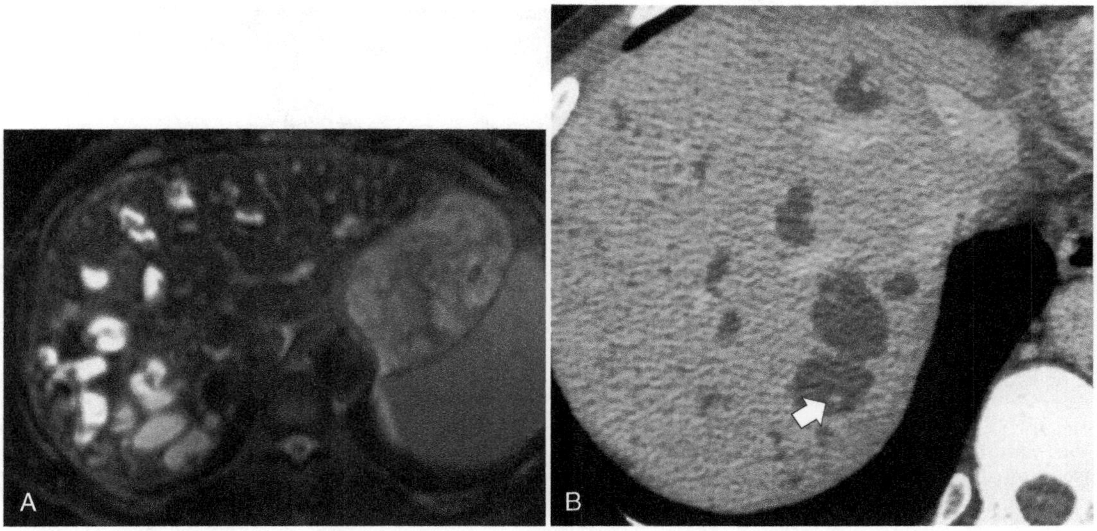

FIGURE 6-67. Axial T2-weighted fat-saturated MRI (A) and axial contrast-enhanced CT (B) in a 39-year-old woman with type V choledochal cyst (Caroli disease), multiple T2 bright ectatic bile ducts, and a CT central dot sign (*small arrow*).

TABLE 6-5 Imaging Features of Hemangioma

Imaging Modality	Features
US	Mostly hyperechoic (sometimes hypoechoic in fatty liver) Color Doppler may demonstrate peripheral vessels Posterior acoustic enhancement
CT	Hypodense on NCCT May or may not demonstrate enhancement on AP Characteristic nodular or globular peripheral on PVP Progressive centripetal enhancement of the lesion Almost complete enhancement on delayed images (larger lesions may have persistent central hypodensity
MRI	Low TI signal, very high (similar to CSF) T2 signal Postgadolinium features similar to CT (as above)
Nuclear medicine	SPECT with ^{99m}Tc-labeled RBC Rarely performed Increased activity on blood pool images at 1-2 hours

AP, Arterial phase; *CSF*, cerebrospinal fluid; *CT*, computed tomography; *MRI*, magnetic resonance imaging; *NCCT*, noncontrast CT scan; *PVP*, portal venous phase; *RBC*, red blood cell; *SPECT*, single-photon emission computed tomography; *US*, ultrasound.

strongly favors benign disease, especially if the patient is young. Under these circumstances, even if an incidentally detected enhancing liver lesion (particularly if solitary and small) does not show the classic imaging features of a hemangioma, it is still unlikely to be malignant. Therefore, for lesions that do not demonstrate the classic imaging features, the need to definitively characterize the lesion depends on the patient's age, the presence of underlying malignancy, the patient's or physician's request, or other suspect features by imaging. In practice, however, most radiologists would probably recommend further corroborative tests (MRI is the most specific) if the imaging features are not diagnostic at CT or US, even in the absence of malignancy.

All methods can show characteristic imaging features (Table 6-5). Even US, which is generally less sensitive than CT or MRI for evaluating most hepatic lesions, has characteristic features, that, with the appropriate patient and operator, should be sufficient to allow the radiologist to definitively diagnose the lesion. US shows a well-defined hyperechoic lesion with posterior acoustic through-transmission (Fig. 6-68). However, because contrast-enhanced MRI is both more sensitive and specific for the detection and characterization of hemangiomas and has no ionizing radiation, it is the method of choice, even though it is more expensive and less widely available. However, CT, being complementary to MRI in many respects, demonstrates similar findings after the administration of IV contrast material.

The classic CT findings of capillary hemangiomas are small, intense, arterial-phase flash-filling lesions (Fig. 6-69). They can have a very similar appearance to other small arterially enhancing lesions with both benign and malignant etiologies, including FNH (Fig. 6-70), adenoma (Fig. 6-71), dysplastic nodules (Fig. 6-40), HCC (Fig. 6-72), and hypervascular metastases (Fig. 6-73).

In comparison with capillary hemangiomas, cavernous hemangiomas are larger (1 to 5 cm), more common, and more characteristic at imaging. They are discrete hypodense masses on noncontrast CT (Fig. 6-74), although some may be relatively isodense to the liver because of their vascular nature. After administration of IV contrast material, hemangiomas demonstrate a highly characteristic peripheral nodular (sometimes called puddling) late arterial or early PVP enhancement, which with sequential imaging (late portal venous to equilibrium phase) gradually enhances toward the center of the lesion, referred to as the lesion "filling in" with contrast material (Fig. 6-74). Ultimately, in the late equilibrium phase, there is complete (or almost complete) opacification of the mass (particularly if small), which usually is slightly hyperdense compared with the surrounding parenchyma (Fig. 6-74). MRI findings follow the same pattern after contrast medium administration, and the diagnosis is further confirmed by low-signal intensity on T1-weighted imaging and high-signal (similar to water) T2-weighted signal (Fig. 6-75). Hepatobiliary agent imaging is thought to be slightly less sensitive than imaging with conventional MRI extracellular contrast agents because the vascular concentration of gadolinium is less within these agents. They are therefore not used as the first-line contrast agent in the follow-up of a suspected hemangioma that was inconclusively characterized on a prior imaging study (US or CT). However, close observation of the images should identify some peripheral nodular enhancement. Because hemangiomas have no hepatocyte function, they are hypointense relative to normal liver on delayed hepatobiliary agent imaging (Fig. 6-76). Furthermore,

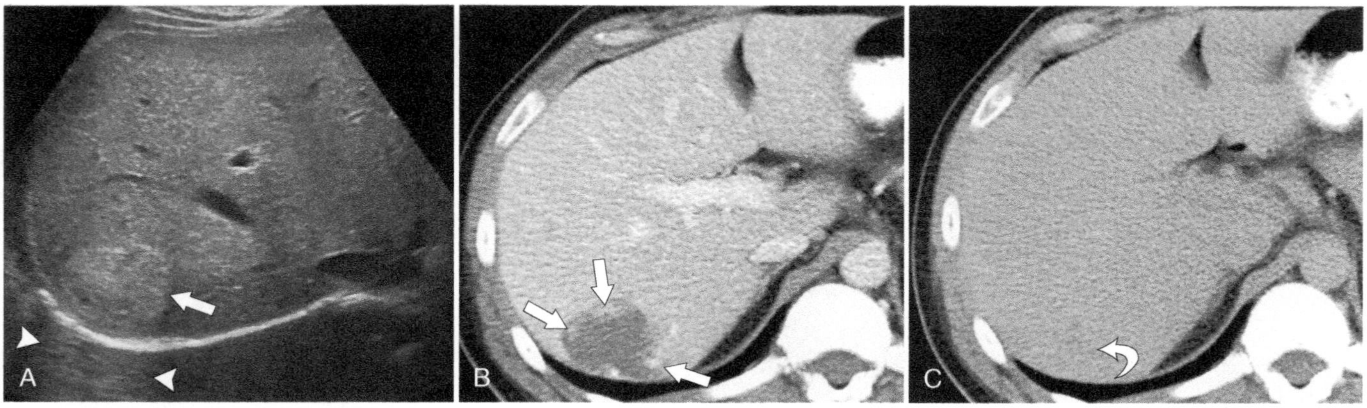

FIGURE 6-68. Sagittal US (**A**) and PVP (**B**) and delayed (**C**) contrast-enhanced CT in a 46-year-old woman with a cavernous hemangioma. It is hyperechoic at US (*arrow*) with through-transmission (*arrowheads*). At PVP CT, there is peripheral nodular enhancement (*arrows*) and the lesion is almost isodense to the liver in the delayed phase because of contrast fill-in (*curved arrow*).

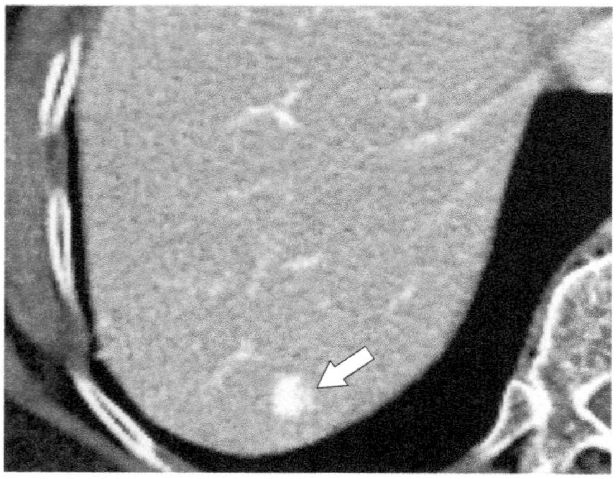

FIGURE 6-69. Axial arterial-phase contrast-enhanced CT in a 33-year-old man with a 1.5-cm hypervascular lesion (*arrow*) in segment VII as a result of a "flash-filling" capillary hemangioma.

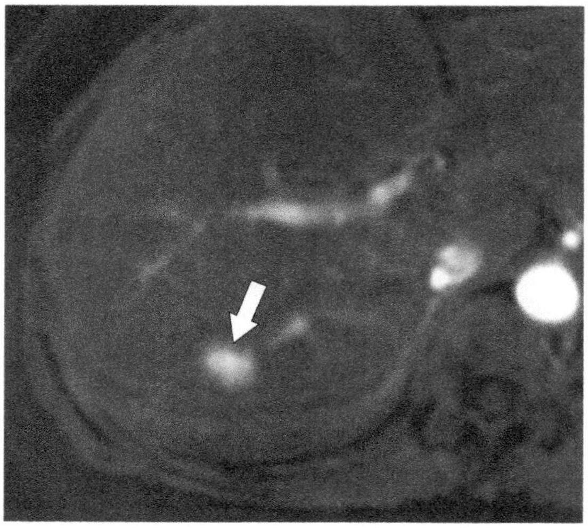

FIGURE 6-71. Axial arterial-phase contrast-enhanced MRI in a 36-year-old woman with a 1.5-cm segment VII hypervascular lesion (*arrow*) resulting from hepatic adenoma.

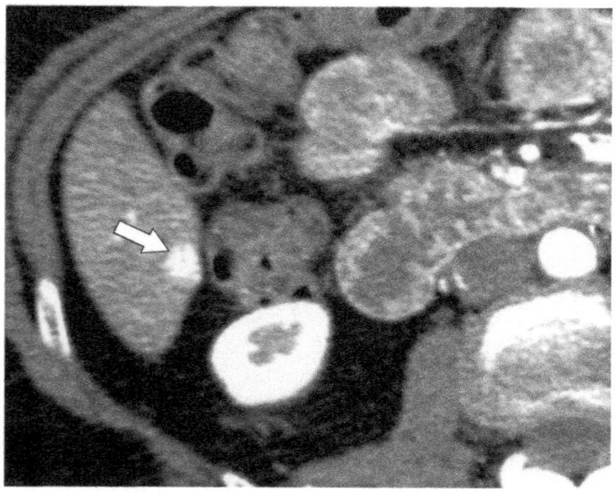

FIGURE 6-70. Arterial-phase contrast-enhanced CT in a 41-year-old woman with a 1.5-cm hypervascular segment VI lesion (*arrow*) resulting from focal nodular hyperplasia.

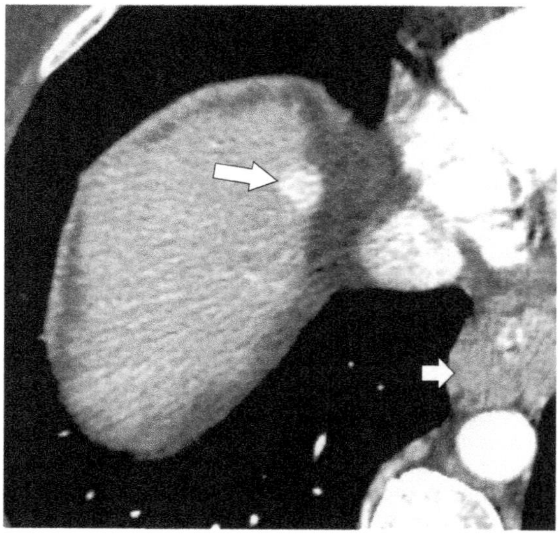

FIGURE 6-72. Axial arterial-phase contrast-enhanced CT in a 57-year-old man with a 1-cm segment VIII hypervascular mass (*arrow*) that represents hepatocellular carcinoma. Associated esophageal varices are present (*small arrow*).

diffusion-weighted imaging may be unhelpful in the characterization of hemangiomas. Often they show increased DWI signal, the reverse of what one would expect for a benign lesion. This is probably best explained by the slow-flowing blood within these lesions. Protons, therefore, do not travel far between the initial DWI and subsequent rephasing pulse, which therefore appear restricted. However, they are usually bright on the ADC maps, which serve to confirm the benign nature of the mass (Fig. 6-77).

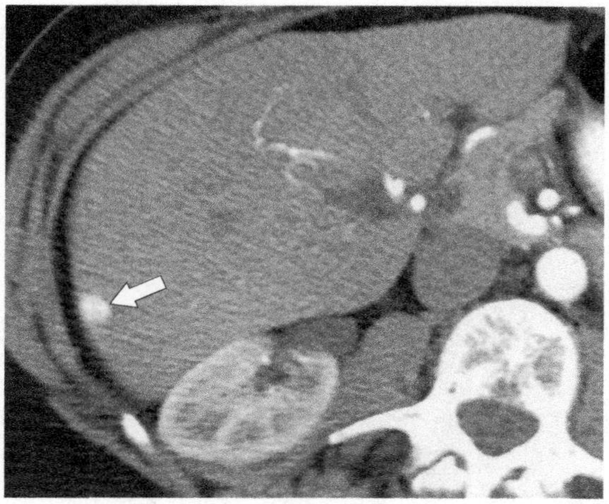

FIGURE 6-73. Axial arterial-phase contrast-enhanced CT in a 71-year-old man with a 1-cm hypervascular mass (*arrow*) that is a carcinoid metastasis.

Giant hemangiomas (>10 cm) usually demonstrate peripheral nodular enhancement but typically do not fully "fill in" on delayed imaging (Fig. 6-78). Many demonstrate a central scar that does not enhance (Fig. 6-79), which can be confused with some hepatocellular and fibrolamellar carcinomas. Their T2 signal characteristics are typically not as bright as smaller hemangiomas but should still be significantly brighter than malignant lesions. The central scar is typically hyperintense (Fig. 6-79).

Given the frequency of hemangiomas in the population, it is not surprising that a number demonstrate atypical imaging patterns on a particular imaging method and that further characterization with another method may be required. For instance, the peripheral enhancement may not be classically nodular at contrast-enhanced CT or MRI, or the signal characteristics on T2-weighted MRI may not be sufficiently high to diagnose hemangioma confidently. More than one imaging method may therefore be required. When using multiple methods, it is important to evaluate all the imaging characteristics of the hemangioma from all the images acquired. One method may demonstrate one or two of the classic features of a hemangioma, but another might show other features. By collating all the imaging findings from the different tests, it should be possible to make a definitive diagnosis in the majority of cases. Sometimes three methods may be required to make the formal

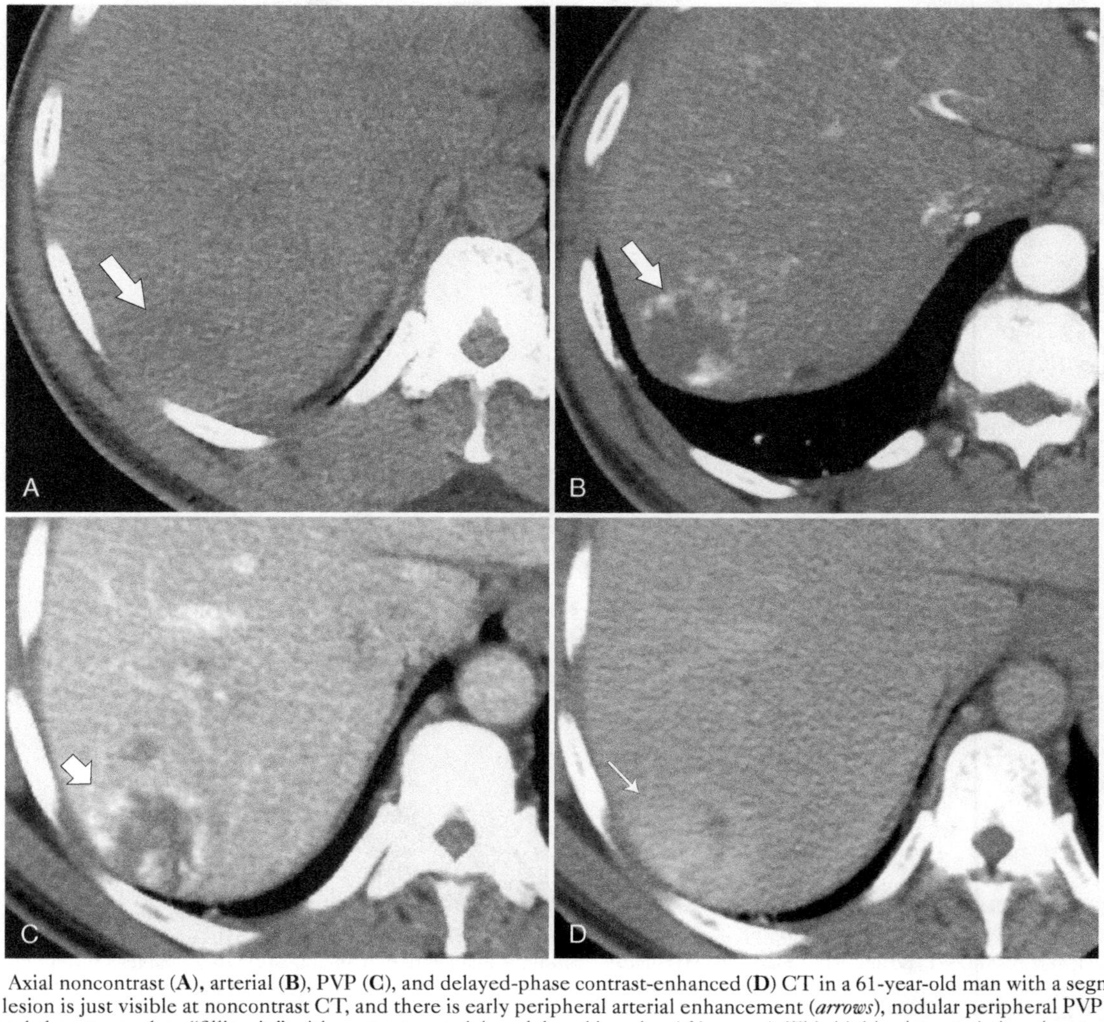

FIGURE 6-74. Axial noncontrast (**A**), arterial (**B**), PVP (**C**), and delayed-phase contrast-enhanced (**D**) CT in a 61-year-old man with a segment VII hemangioma. The lesion is just visible at noncontrast CT, and there is early peripheral arterial enhancement (*arrows*), nodular peripheral PVP enhancement (*small arrow*), and almost complete "filling-in" with contrast material on delayed imaging (*thin arrow*). This highly characteristic enhancement pattern is diagnostic for hemangioma.

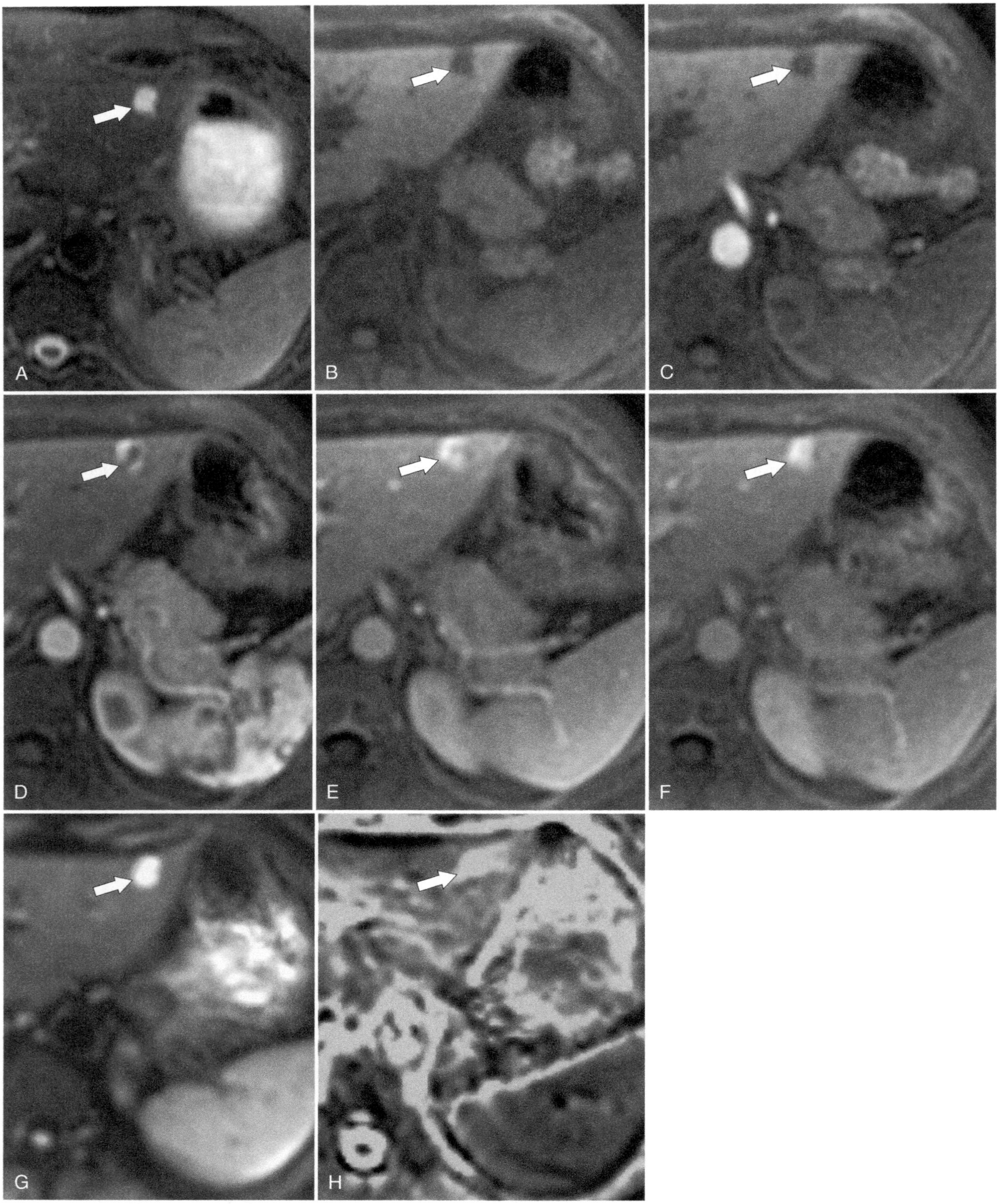

FIGURE 6-75. Axial T2-weighted (**A**), T1-weighted fat-saturated precontrast (**B**), arterial (**C**), PVP (**D**), early delayed-contrast (**E**) and late delayed-contrast (**F**) MRI, and B500 DWI (**G**) and ADC map MRI (**H**) in a 70-year-old woman with hemangioma (*arrows*). The lesion is intensely T2 bright, T1 dark before contrast material, which progressively fills in from the periphery on subsequent imaging. The lesion is bright on both B500 and ADC maps.

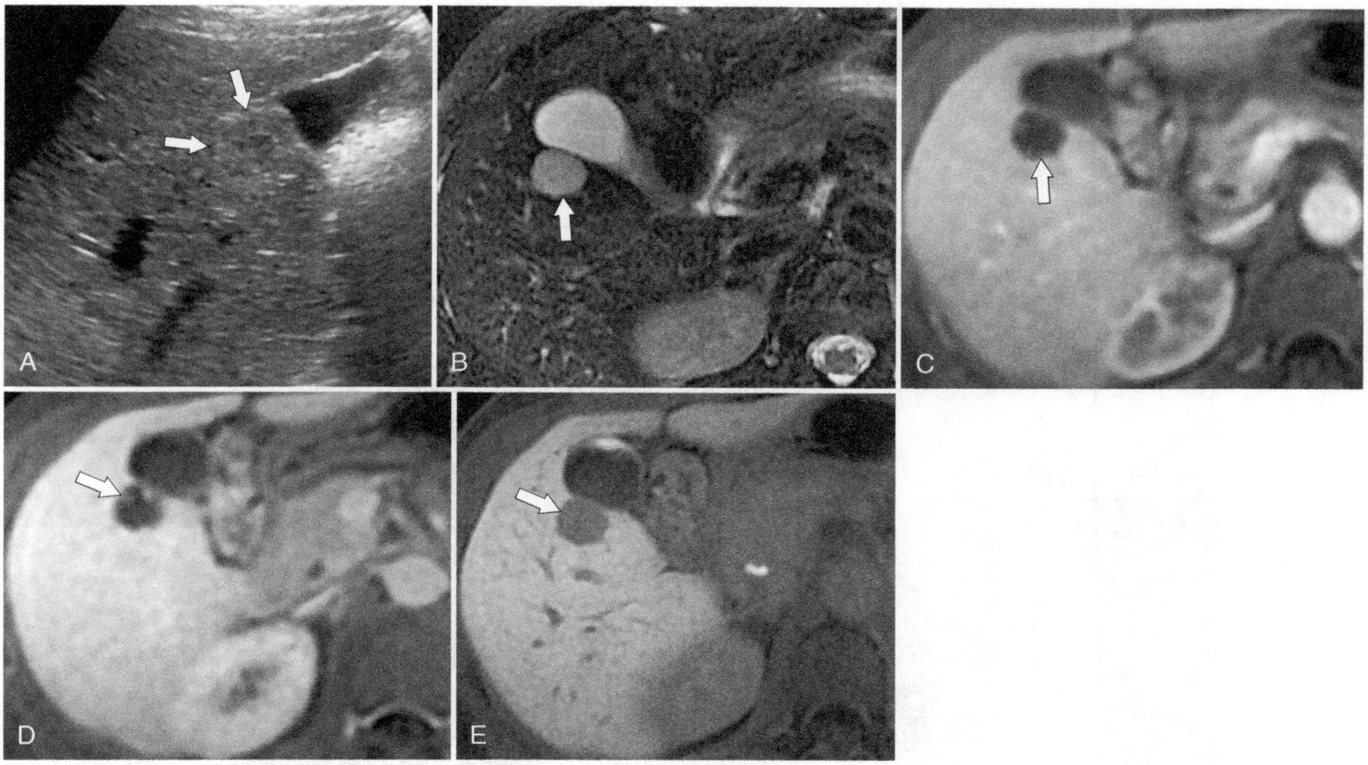

FIGURE 6-76. Sagittal US (**A**), T2 (**B**), PVP (**C**), delayed (**D**), and 20-minute delayed (**E**) T1-weighted fat-saturated hepatobiliary agent imaging of a hemangioma (*arrows*). The lesion is of intermediate echotexture at US and therefore required further characterization. The lesion is T2 bright, consistent with hemangioma, but demonstrates poor peripheral enhancement (*arrows*). At 20-minute delayed imaging, the lesion demonstrates no hepatocyte function (*arrow*, **E**).

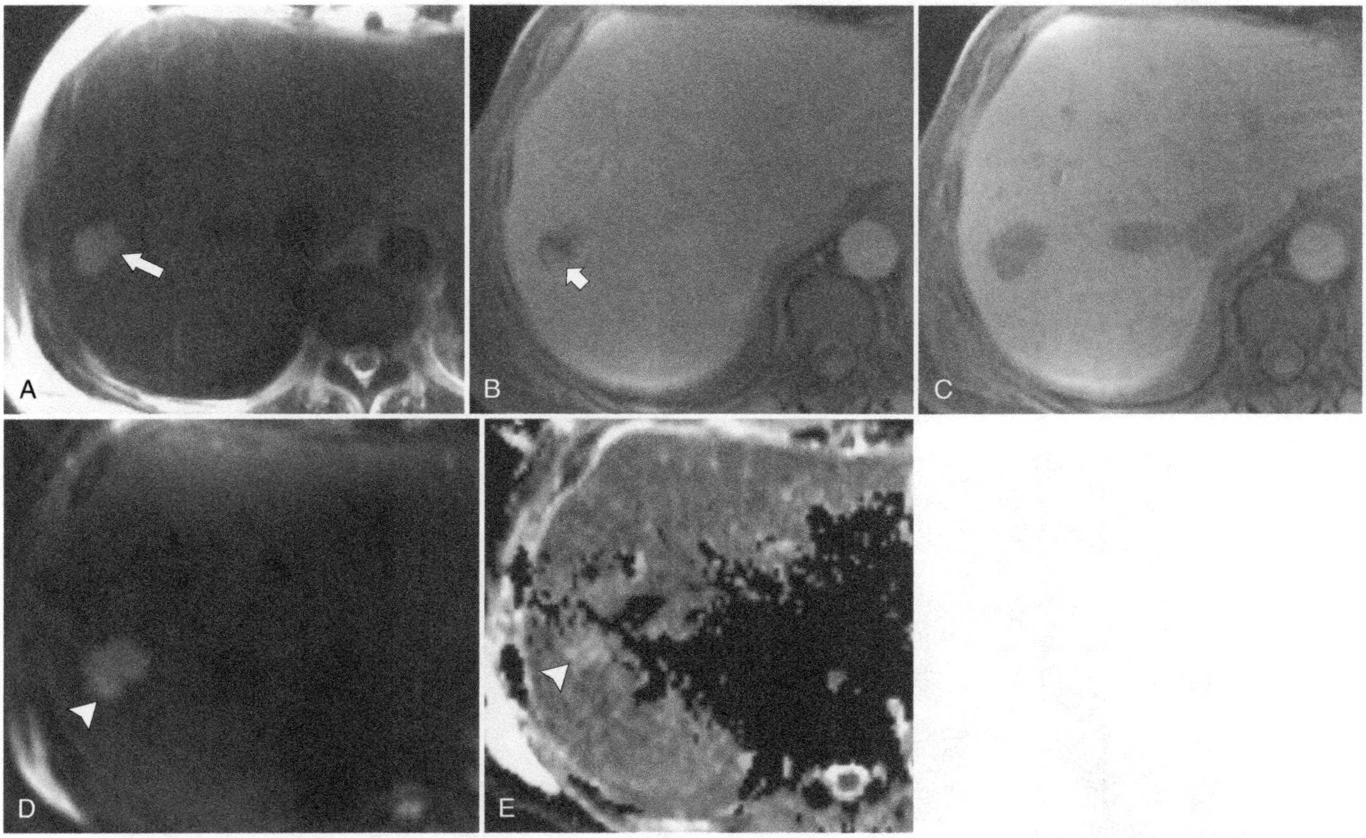

FIGURE 6-77. Axial T2-weighted (**A**), PVP (**B**), delayed-hepatobiliary agent T1-weighted fat-saturated (**C**), B100 DWI (**D**) and ADC map (**E**) MRI imaging in a 43-year-old woman with hemangioma. The lesion (*arrow*) is T2 bright and demonstrates subtle peripheral nodular enhancement (*small arrow*) but no hepatocyte activity at 20-minute delayed imaging. The lesion is bright at B100 DWI and on ADC maps (*arrowheads*).

diagnosis. For instance, steatotic livers at US can alter the usual lesion echo characteristics because the liver parenchyma is relatively echogenic compared with that of normal. Therefore hemangiomas may appear hypoechoic relative to the hyperechoic background liver rather than the normal situation, which is the converse (Fig. 6-80). Further imaging with CT may not demonstrate all the classic features of hemangioma (Fig. 6-81), and an MRI might ultimately be required to demonstrate all the classic features (Fig. 6-82). As previously discussed, however, it should be remembered that the a priori chance that these atypical lesions are malignant in a patient without malignant disease is very small. In general, the use of multiple methods to fully characterize atypical lesions is reserved for the patient who has an underlying malignancy, and metastatic liver disease must be excluded before a decision of which therapy to offer the patient.

Sclerosing hemangiomas are particularly challenging because they may not enhance at all (since the vascular spaces are sclerosed) and at MRI the features may be of intermediate signal on T2-weighted imaging, suggesting the lesion may be malignant (Fig. 6-83). The diagnosis may ultimately require percutaneous biopsy, particularly if definitive characterization is required in a patient with an extrahepatic malignancy to rule out metastatic disease. Although biopsy of a hemangioma should be avoided when possible, percutaneous biopsy with thin aspirate needles is

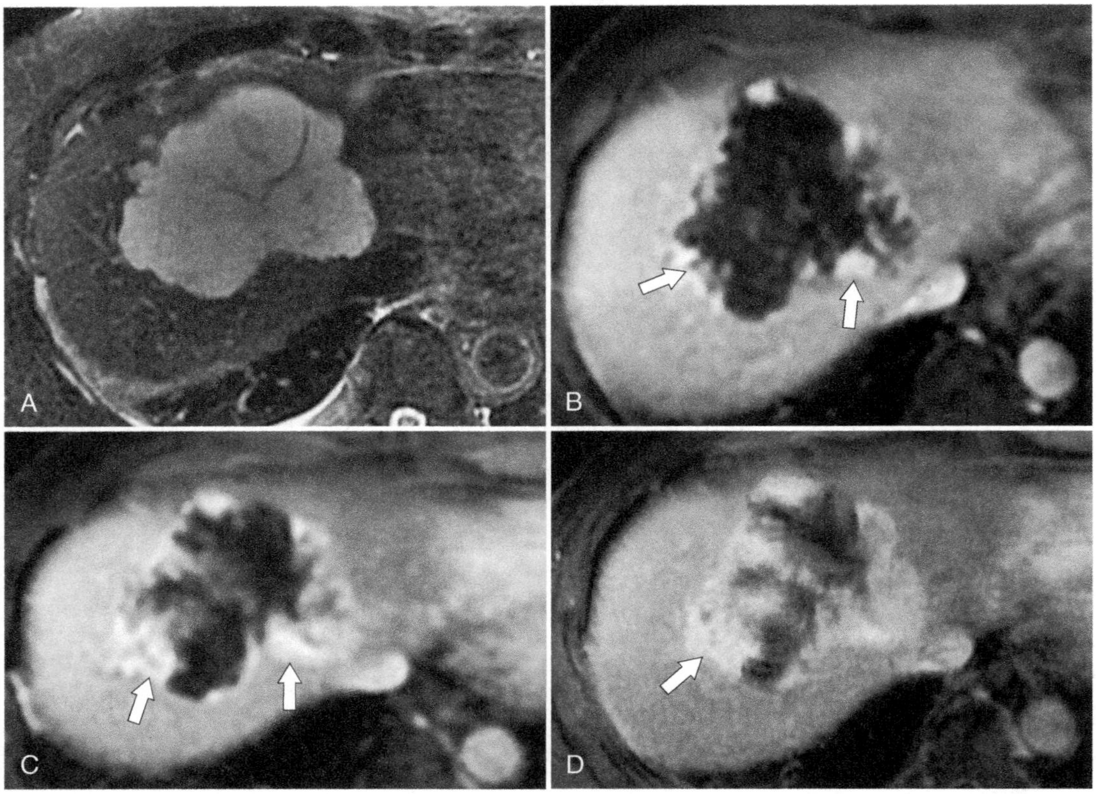

FIGURE 6-78. Axial T2 (**A**), postcontrast arterial (**B**), PVP (**C**), and delayed T1-weighted (**D**) fat-saturated MRI in a 35-year-old man and a giant hemangioma. The lesion is relatively T2 bright and demonstrates typical peripheral nodular enhancement (*arrows*) that steadily "fills in" from arterial to delayed-phase imaging but not completely.

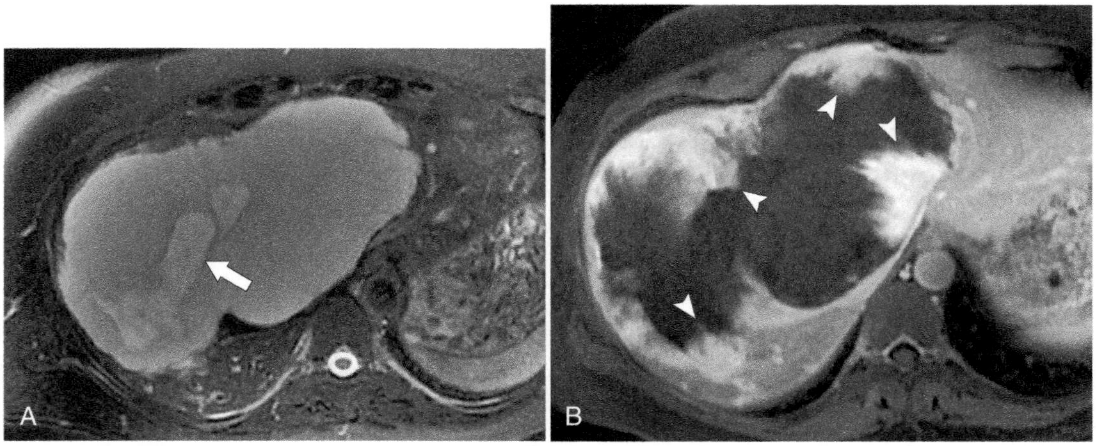

FIGURE 6-79. Axial T2-weighted (**A**) and delayed postcontrast T1-weighted (**B**) fat-saturated MRI in a 50-year-old woman with a giant hemangioma with peripheral nodular enhancement (*arrowheads*) and a T2 bright, nonenhancing scar (*arrow*).

generally safe. Larger, core biopsy needles should be avoided if a hemangioma is being considered.

Peliosis

Peliosis in Greek means "dusky" or "purple," reflecting the color of the liver in this condition. It is an uncommon lesion caused by sinusoidal dilatation and multiple blood-filled spaces (1 mm to several centimeters) in the hepatic parenchyma, but can also occur in the spleen, lymph nodes, and other organs. It is often idiopathic but is associated with a variety of disparate causes, including drugs (including the oral contraceptive pill), infections (including HIV, in which it is called bacillary peliosis), and malignancy. Its pathophysiology is poorly understood but may be related to hepatic outflow obstruction at the sinusoidal level. Peliosis is usually self-limiting after the causal agent (e.g., drugs) is removed.

On noncontrast CT, a hypodense lesion (or lesions) is identified, which may contain areas of higher attenuation because of internal hemorrhage. Lesions typically demonstrate centrifugal progression of globular-like enhancement (the opposite of hemangiomas) (Fig. 6-84), although less commonly lesions can display the reverse (such as hemangiomas) and can be slightly hyperattenuating on delayed-phase imaging. On MRI, lesions can demonstrate a variety of signal intensities on T1- and T2-weighted imaging depending on the concentration of blood products.

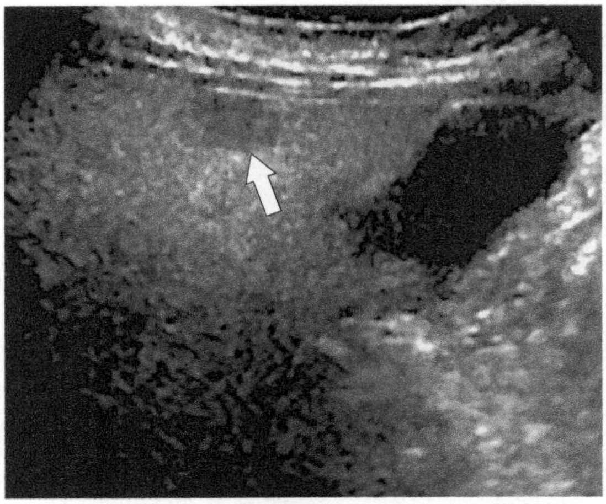

FIGURE 6-80. Sagittal US in a 52-year-old woman with breast cancer and hepatic steatosis and hemangioma. US demonstrates a hypoechoic lesion (*arrow*) surrounded by an echogenic steatotic liver.

Focal Nodular Hyperplasia

The third most common benign liver mass (after cyst and hemangioma) is FNH, and it is usually asymptomatic. Its significance is that it is detected incidentally at cross-sectional imaging performed for other reasons (usually CT) and requires differentiation from other hypervascular liver lesions, including adenoma, HCC, and metastases, with which it has some similar imaging characteristics. Its pathogenesis is not clear but may be a response to vascular injury. It is far more common in women (approximately 9:1) and usually seen in the third and fourth decades of life. Lesions are multiple in approximately 25% of patients. Differentiation between classic (approximately 80%) and nonclassic (20%) FNH is made at the histological level. The hallmark of FNH is the central scar, representing abnormal vascular structures and fibrous connective tissue, although other lesions (adenoma, hemangioma, some metastases, fibrolamellar HCC, and some other HCCs) may show similar features.

Imaging features can be diagnostic, particularly with MRI (Table 6-6). On US the lesion is often isoechoic (Fig. 6-85), but some demonstrate a hyperechoic halo surrounding the lesion. The central scar, if large, can be seen as hypoechoic. Color Doppler might be helpful if it demonstrates a "spoke-wheel" appearance of a central vessel feeding smaller vessels that course out to the periphery to drain into veins at the margins of the lesion. Most lesions, however, are detected with CT, which can be diagnostic if classic imaging findings are present. On noncontrast CT the lesion typically has smooth, lobulated margins and is slightly hypodense to isodense, but enhances avidly in the arterial phase (Figs. 6-70 and 6-86). However, it may return to being isodense, or even hypodense, during the PVP (Fig. 6-86). The central scar, if large, is generally hypodense in the arterial phase but gradually enhances such that on delayed imaging it is hyperdense (Fig. 6-86), which is a highly characteristic and diagnostic feature of FNH. Not all central scars, however, are hyperdense on delayed imaging (Fig. 6-87).

MRI is the most specific test, and if the lesion is detected by US and further characterization is required, MRI is indicated in preference to CT. On T1-weighted imaging the mass is typically isointense or hypointense. FNH can be difficult to visualize with T2-weighted imaging because it is mildly hyperintense or isointense (Fig. 6-88). This is in contradistinction to HCC and

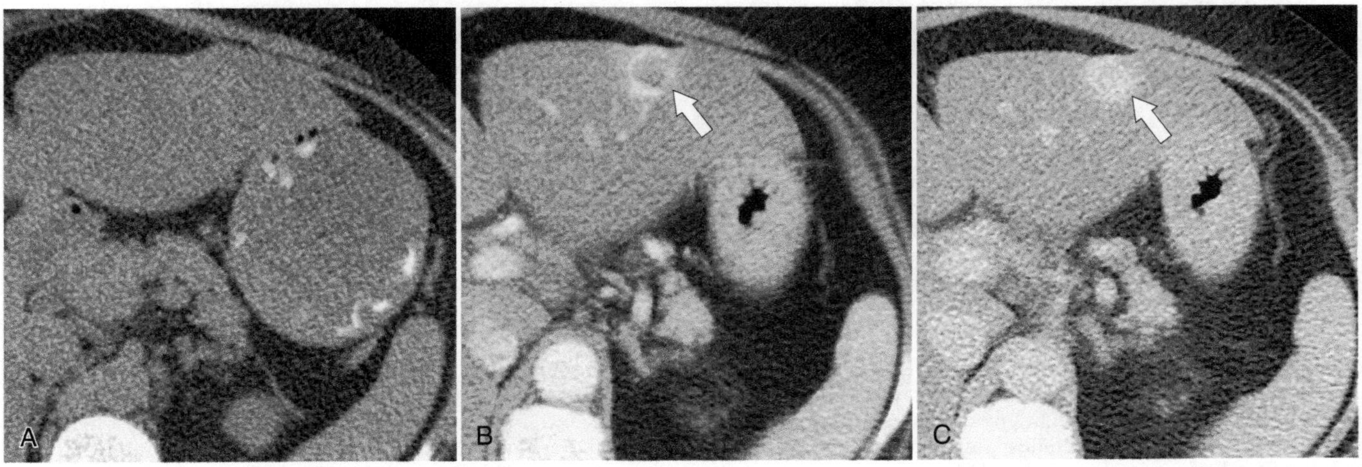

FIGURE 6-81. Noncontrast (**A**), PVP (**B**), and delayed (**C**) contrast-enhanced CT with steatotic liver and hemangioma. Because the steatotic liver is hypodense, the hemangioma cannot be clearly identified. Enhancement at PVP is circumferential but not nodular (*arrows*). Delayed contrast enhancement, however, confirms hemangioma with complete "fill-in" of contrast medium.

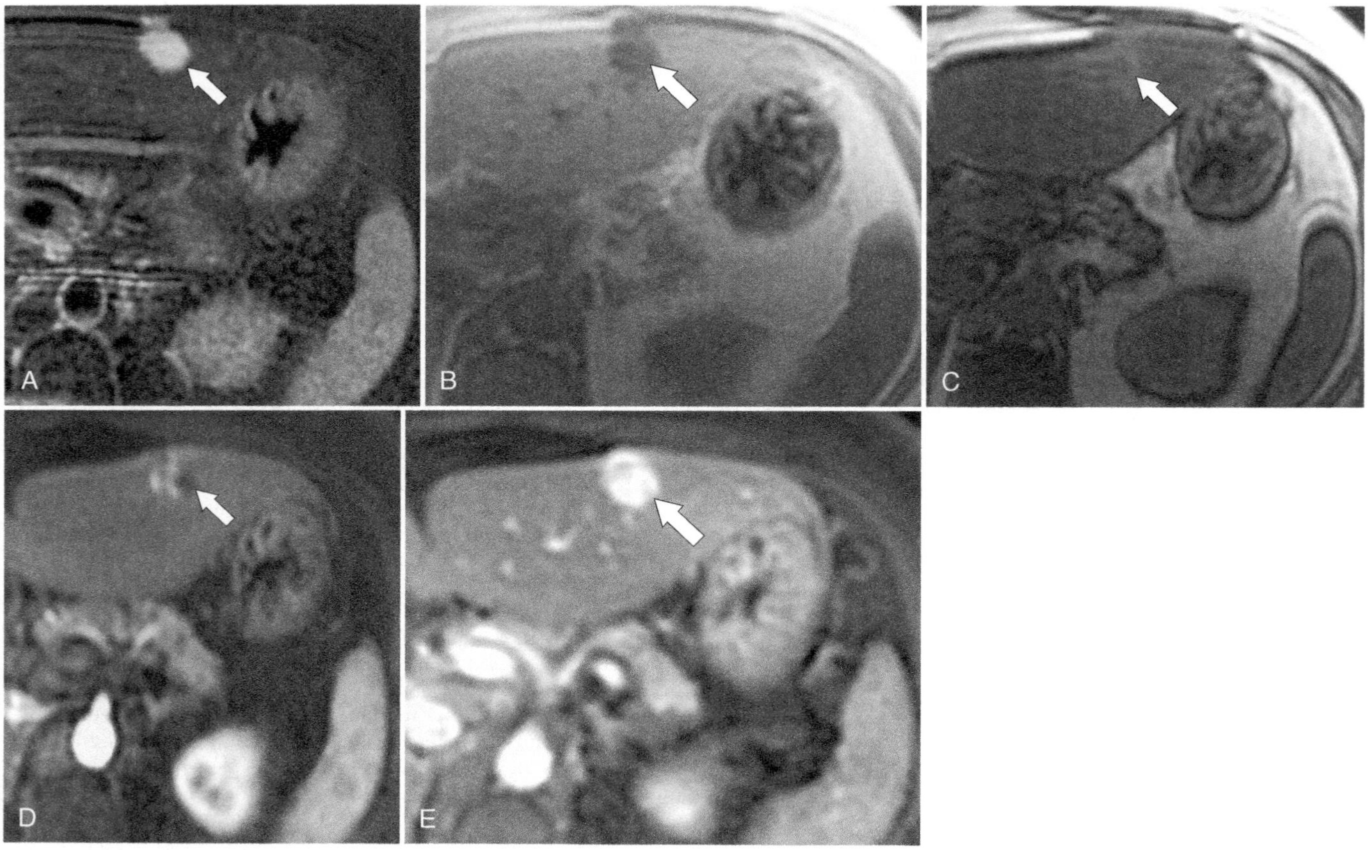

FIGURE 6-82. T2, in-phase (**A**), out-of-phase (**B**), T2-weighted (**C**), PVP (**D**), and delayed-phase (**E**) contrast-enhanced MRI (same patient as in Fig. 6-81) with a steatotic liver and hemangioma. The lesion (*arrows*) is better seen on in-phase MRI because of the T1 bright steatotic liver that loses signal on out-of-phase images, reducing the contrast differences between liver parenchyma and the hemangioma. The lesion is T2 bright, characteristic of hemangioma, and demonstrates peripheral nodular enhancement at PVP and almost complete contrast "fill-in" at delayed imaging.

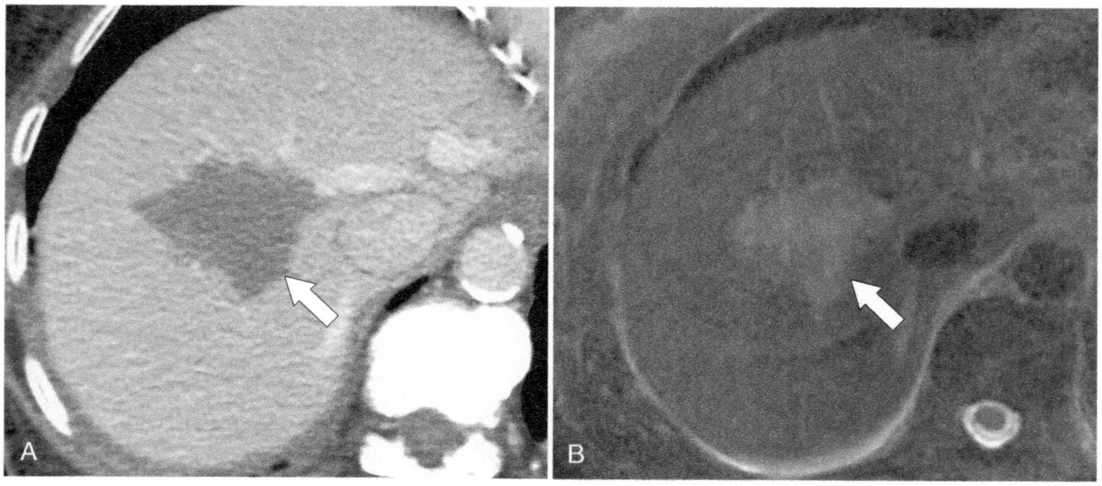

FIGURE 6-83. Axial contrast-enhanced CT (**A**) and T2-weighted fat-saturated MRI (**B**) in an 81-year-old woman with a sharply marginated, nonenhancing, mass at CT, which is mildly hyperintense on T2-weighted imaging, (*arrows*) caused by a sclerosed hemangioma.

metastases, which tend to have intermediate T2 signal. After administration of extracellular contrast agents, the lesion, in similarity to contrast-enhanced CT, briefly enhances intensely in the arterial phase but rapidly becomes isointense in the PVP. The scar usually enhances in later phases (Fig. 6-88).

Hepatobiliary imaging can be helpful and diagnostic and is the contrast agent of choice when attempting to characterize suspected FNH because most FNH lesions retain hepatocyte function. These are similarly hypervascular at hepatobiliary imaging and enhance intensely on dynamic arterial-phase imaging, which may partially wash out in the PVP and be relatively isointense to the liver. At delayed imaging, however, the lesion is again hyperintense because its hepatocytic function leads to marked retention of contrast agent (Fig. 6-89). The central scar may enhance on

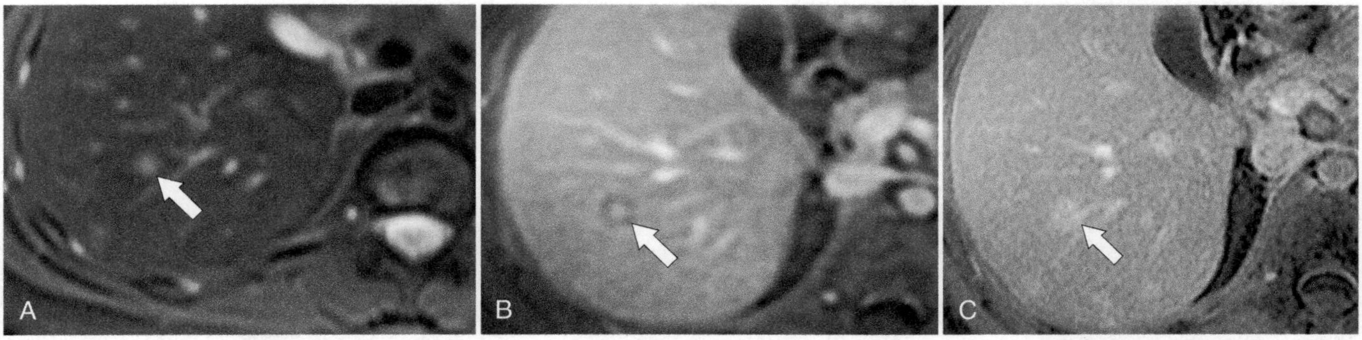

FIGURE 6-84. Axial fat-saturated T2 (**A**), PVP (**B**), and delayed postcontrast (**C**) T1-weighted MRI in a 17-year-old male adolescent with peliosis. The lesion is of intermediate T2 signal and enhances from the center of the lesion outward (*arrows*).

TABLE 6-6 Distinguishing Features of FNH, Adenoma, Fibrolamellar HCC, and HCC

	FNH	Adenoma	Fibrolamellar HCC	HCC
Sex	Female	Female	Both	Both
Age	Young	Young	Young	Usually older
Multiple	++	+	–	+
Calcification	+/–	+	++	+
AP	+++ and uniform	+++ and heterogeneous	++ and heterogeneous	+++ and usually uniform
PVP	+/–	+/–	+/–	+/–
Delayed	Iso to liver	Iso to liver	?	Washout
Hepatobiliary agents	+++	–	–	–
RES uptake	++	++		–
Scar	++	–	++	–
Scar enhancement	++	n/a	–	n/a

AP, Arterial phase; *FNH*, focal nodular hyperplasia; *HCC*, hepatocellular carcinoma; *PVP*, portal venous phase; *RES*, reticuloendothelial system.

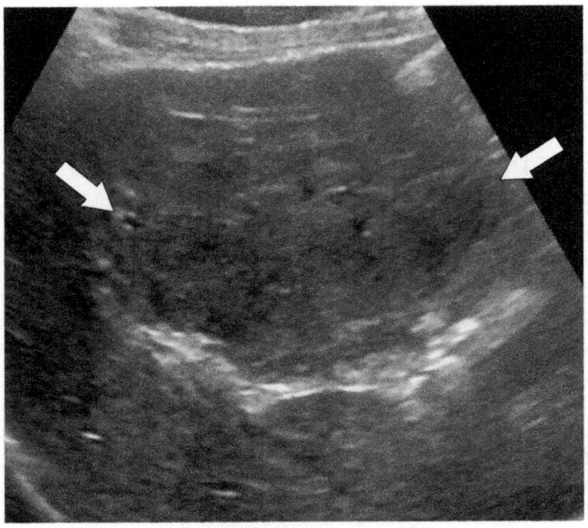

FIGURE 6-85. Sagittal US in a 38-year-old woman demonstrates an isoechoic 7-cm mass (*arrows*) in the left lobe caused by focal nodular hyperplasia.

arterial-phase imaging but typically does not enhance on delayed imaging. Some well-differentiated HCCs also retain hepatocyte function, and therefore enhancing lesions in the delayed hepatobiliary phase should not always be assumed to be FNH. However, patients with HCC usually have cirrhosis, and on delayed imaging (after intense arterial phase enhancement), there is usually marked washout of contrast material from the lesion when both extracellular and hepatobiliary gadolinium-based contrast agents are used. Fibrolamellar HCC can be even more difficult to differentiate from FNH because it often also retains hepatocyte function and has a central scar. However, delayed hepatobiliary enhancement is less homogeneous, and the central scar fails to enhance during arterial-phase imaging. Fibrolamellar HCC typically demonstrates higher T2-weighted signal than FNH, which, as discussed, is usually isointense or only mildly hyperintense relative to the normal liver.

Hepatic Adenoma

This tumor has some similar imaging features to those of FNH, hypervascular metastases, and HCC, so its characterization is important. It is far less common than FNH but is also more common in women, partly because it is detected far more frequently in patients taking the oral contraceptive pill. Pregnancy is known to exacerbate its growth (sometimes to a point of rupture), and it is also associated with anabolic steroid use. Multiple adenomas or adenomatosis is recognized more frequently than multiple FNH lesions and is also recognized in glycogen storage disease, type 1 (von Gierke disease). The adenomas are composed of sheets of hepatocytes with increased amounts of glycogen and lipid. The latter finding is important because the presence of fat within the lesion helps differentiate it from FNH, although some HCCs also contain fat. Hepatic adenomas often contain a pseudocapsule, which is also not recognized in FNH (Table 6-5). Very rarely, an adenoma (particularly if large) undergoes malignant

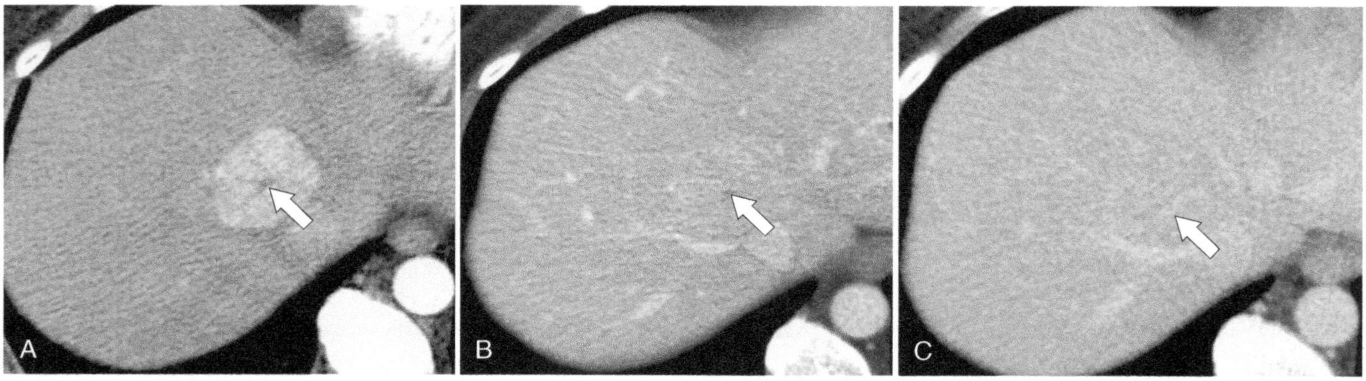

FIGURE 6-86. Axial arterial (**A**), PVP (**B**), and delayed-phase (**C**) contrast-enhanced CT in a 39-year-old woman with FNH. The lesion is hypervascular at arterial phase but then isodense on PVP and delayed imaging. A central scar (*arrows*) is seen on arterial phase and just visible on delayed imaging.

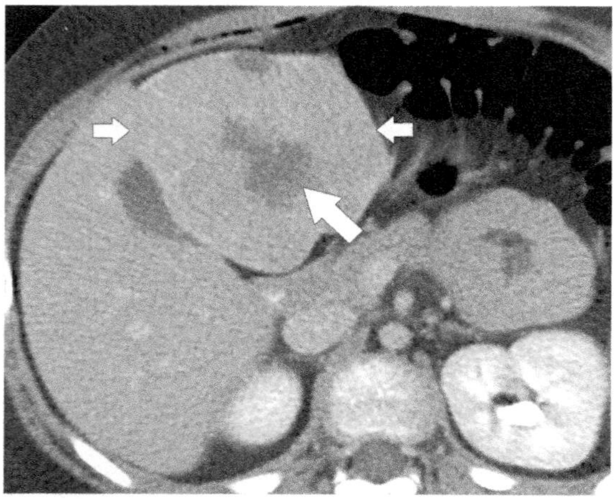

FIGURE 6-87. Axial delayed contrast-enhanced CT in a 37-year-old woman with FNH (*small arrows*). The central scar (*arrow*) remains hypodense on delayed imaging.

transformation to HCC. Large adenomas are therefore removed because of the risk of rupture and the remote risk of malignant degeneration.

On US, an adenoma is usually echogenic (and therefore easier to recognize than FNH), primarily because of its fat content, although appearances can be heterogeneous. On noncontrast CT, the lesion may be slightly hypodense, again because of the presence of fat. Adenomas are, however, prone to hemorrhage, and therefore foci on increased density may be observed. Macroscopic fat and calcification are seen in 10% to 20%. On contrast-enhanced CT the lesion enhances intensely in the arterial phase, although often less than that observed with FNH. During the PVP the lesion can be hypodense or isodense or remain hyperdense to the liver parenchyma (Fig. 6-90). A pseudocapsule may be identified, but no central scar.

MRI, similar to the imaging evaluation of FNH, is more specific for characterization of adenomas. At T1-weighted imaging, most lesions are isointense or hypointense, but they can be heterogeneous with fat (Fig. 6-91) and sometimes recent hemorrhage (Fig. 6-92). T2-weighted imaging may also demonstrate a combination of mixed signal intensities because of the variable proportion of fat, blood, calcification, and tumor. Similar to contrast-enhanced CT, the lesion enhances intensely on contrast-enhanced MRI but less homogeneously than FNH. During the PVP the lesion may remain mildly hyperintense, and a pseudocapsule is usually seen on delayed imaging (Fig. 6-92).

Hepatobiliary agents help to differentiate adenomas from FNH. Being hypervascular, adenomas also enhance avidly during arterial-phase imaging, but although they retain variable hepatocyte function, the excretion of hepatobiliary agents into the biliary system is impaired and so enhancement within the lesion is variable. If enhancement is present, it is poor and heterogeneous (Fig. 6-91). Frequently there is little or no retention of hepatobiliary contrast agent at delayed imaging (Fig. 6-93). The diagnosis is usually made in the correct clinical setting (e.g., young woman taking the oral contraceptive pill), combined with characteristic MRI or CT findings. Detection of fat is a highly characteristic finding, although fat can be seen in some HCCs. However, these tumors usually occur in patients with cirrhosis, and there is intense contrast washout on PVP and delayed imaging with gadolinium extracellular and hepatobiliary agents (Table 6-5).

Solitary Necrotic Nodule

Solitary necrotic nodules are poorly understood, rare, benign, small, solitary, hepatic lesions of uncertain cause that on pathological analysis have a necrotic center surrounded by a hyalinized fibrotic capsule. They are usually located close to the liver capsule, particularly in the right hepatic lobe. They are hypoechoic on US (although some calcify and so can be hyperechoic) and on CT are hypodense (unless calcified) and do not enhance. With MRI they are hypointense on both T1- and T2-weighted images and do not enhance.

Hepatic Inflammatory Pseudotumor

Hepatic inflammatory pseudotumor is a rare benign mass whose cause is unknown, although it may develop from an autoimmune disorder, usually associated with elevations of IgG4. In addition, there is some association with gastrointestinal tract malignancies. Inflammatory pseudotumors have also been described in the lung. On contrast-enhanced CT, the pseudotumor appears as an enhancing mass of variable size (may be several centimeters) and can be confused with other malignant lesions (Fig. 6-94). However, the enhancement is usually in the PVP and delayed phase, helping to distinguish the lesion from HCC and metastases, although differentiation from peripheral cholangiocarcinoma can be challenging. On MRI the lesion is typically hypointense on T1-weighted imaging and mildly hyperintense on T2-weighted imaging, again serving to confuse this benign lesion with other malignant lesions. Diagnosis is usually made with percutaneous biopsy.

Intrahepatic Spleen

Splenic tissue can implant throughout the abdomen after splenic trauma. This rarely occurs within the liver and is usually associated with liver laceration, allowing the splenic tissue to embed itself within the liver parenchyma (Fig. 6-95). The diagnosis can

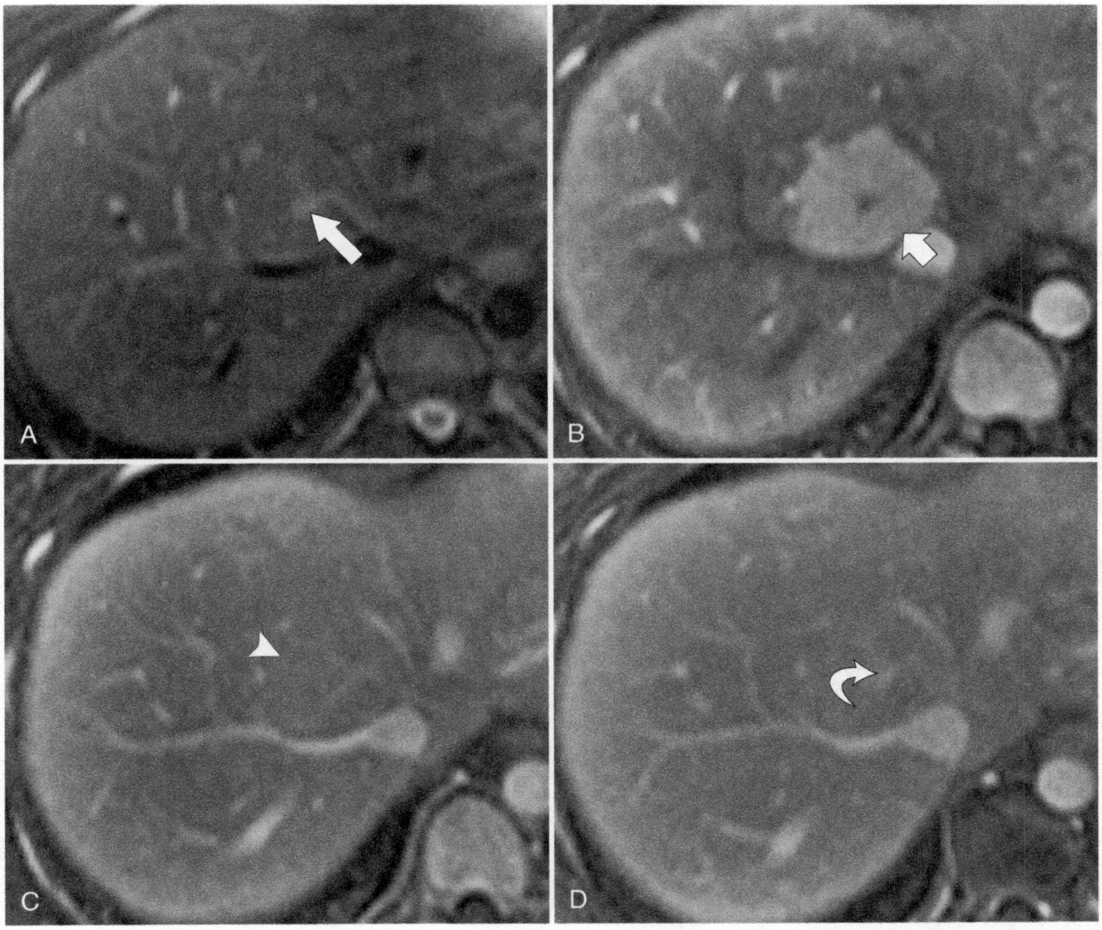

FIGURE 6-88. Axial T2 (**A**), T1-weighted arterial (**B**), PVP (**C**), and delayed fat-saturated contrast-enhanced (**D**) MRI (same patient as in Fig. 6-86). The lesion is isointense at T2, although a small T2 bright central scar is observed (*arrow*). The lesion avidly enhances on arterial phase (*small arrow*) but then becomes isointense of PVP (*arrowhead*) and delayed imaging, although the central scar has enhanced at delayed imaging (*curved arrow*).

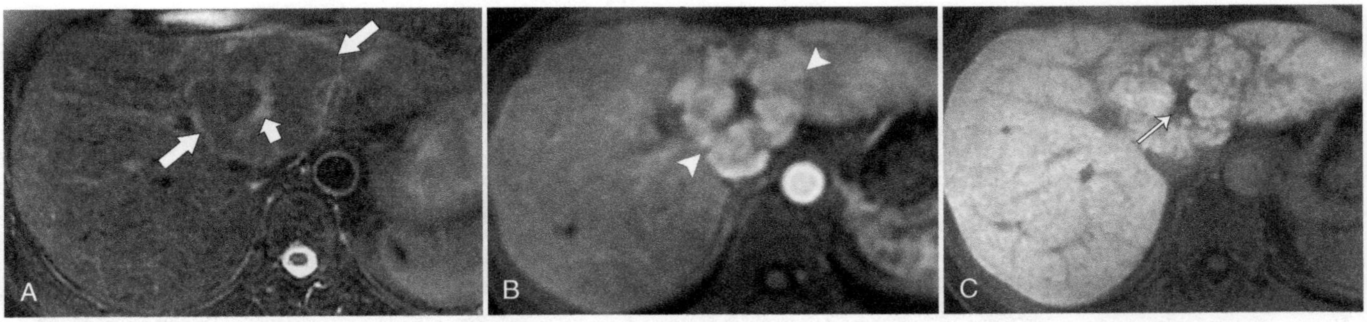

FIGURE 6-89. Axial T2 (**A**) and T1 fat-saturated arterial (**B**) and 20-minute delayed (**C**) phase hepatobiliary agent MRI in a 28-year-old woman. The lesion is T2 isointense (*arrows*) but with a bright central scar (*small arrow*) that enhances avidly in the arterial phase (*arrowheads*) and retains contrast in the 20-minute delayed hepatobiliary phase (*arrows*), diagnostic of FNH. The central scar is hypointense on delayed imaging (*thin arrow*).

be challenging, as it may be unsuspected, although there is usually evidence of prior splenic trauma or surgery. The lesion may be confirmed by ^{99m}Tc sulfur colloid imaging, with the splenic tissue absorbing the radioisotope (see Chapter 7). Otherwise, biopsy may be required for a definitive diagnosis.

MALIGNANT LIVER LESIONS

Hepatic Metastases

The liver is a frequent repository for metastatic disease; approximately 30% of patients with nonhepatic primary disease will ultimately develop liver metastases. Numerous malignancies from almost all anatomical locations can metastasize to the liver, but the most common are colon, stomach, pancreatic, breast, and lung cancer. Given that the presence of hepatic metastases affects disease staging and prognosis of the primary disease, both detection and characterization of detected hepatic lesions by cross-sectional imaging are mandatory in patients with a known malignancy. Although newer cross-sectional imaging methods offer thin-section, high-resolution imaging, both MRI and CT have limitations, particularly size limitations in that they are unable to detect or characterize submillimeter lesions, although newer imaging with hepatobiliary agents can detect lesions as small as 1 mm. Prior imaging can be critical in this regard because any new lesion, even if small, is likely to be metastatic (Fig. 6-96). Every attempt should be made therefore to evaluate prior images, even if they have been obtained at an outside institution, because they could obviate the need for further imaging workup. When these lesions have increased to a detectable size, particularly if multiple, it may already be too late for appropriate therapies to offer a chance of longer term survival (Fig. 6-97). Detecting a single lesion in the left lobe but missing the 2-mm lesion in the right lobe means that potentially unnecessary surgery may be performed for curative intent, since the presence of lesions in both lobes usually means that curative surgery is inappropriate. More recent functional and molecular imaging techniques, which can detect disease far earlier than conventional morphological tests (conventional CT and MRI), offer the opportunity to detect disease very early (Fig. 6-97).

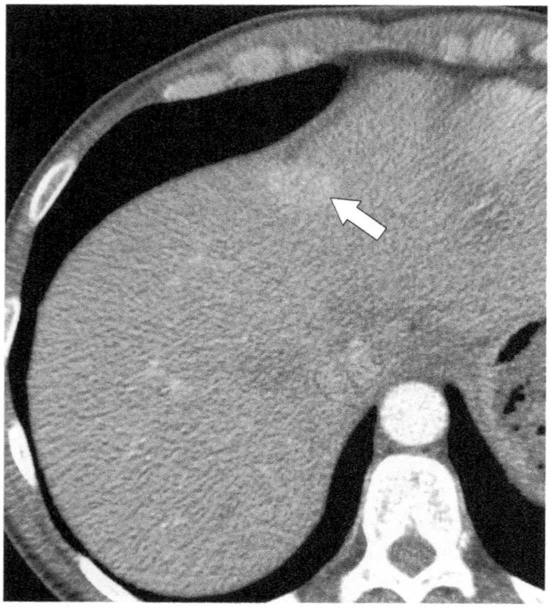

FIGURE 6-90. Axial arterial-phase CT in a 47-year-old woman with a 2-cm subtly enhancing hepatic adenoma (*arrow*).

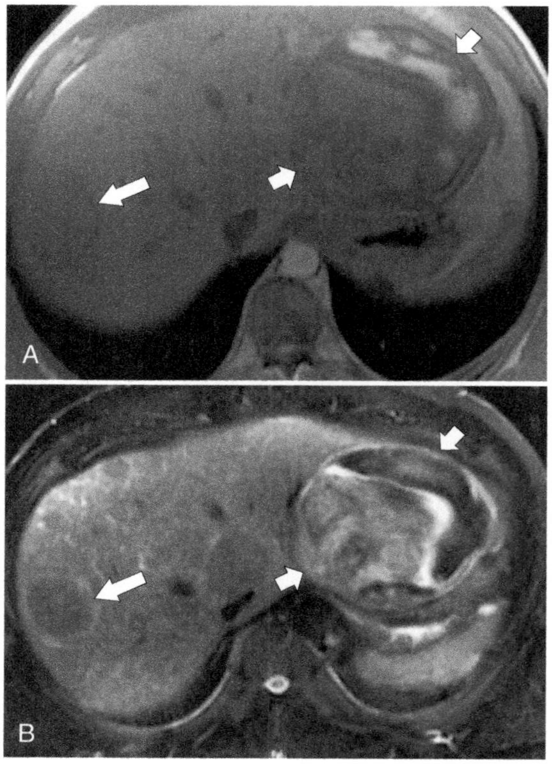

FIGURE 6-92. Axial T1- (**A**) and T2-weighted (**B**) MRI images in a 39-year-old man on self-medicated steroids demonstrate multiple right lobe T1 isointense and T2 hypointense adenomas (*arrows*) but a larger mixed signal hemorrhagic mass in the left lobe (*small arrows*) due to spontaneous hemorrhage.

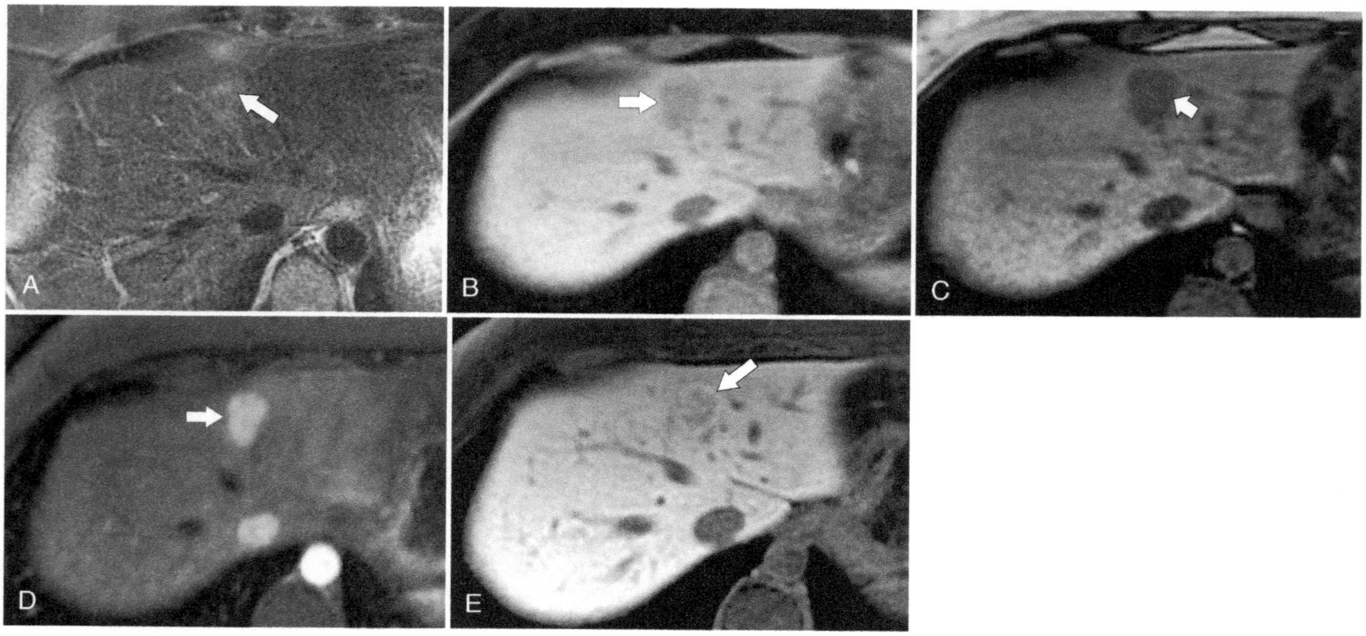

FIGURE 6-91. Axial T2-weighted (**A**), in-phase (**B**), out-of-phase (**C**), arterial (**D**), and 20-minute delayed (**E**) hepatobiliary contrast MRI study in a 50-year-old woman with adenoma. The lesion demonstrates mild T2 hyperintensity (*arrows*) and fat as shown by signal drop-off on out-of-phase images (*small arrow*). It avidly enhances during arterial-phase imaging, and demonstrates a capsule and slight internal retention of hepatobiliary agent at 20 minutes. These features are diagnostic of adenoma.

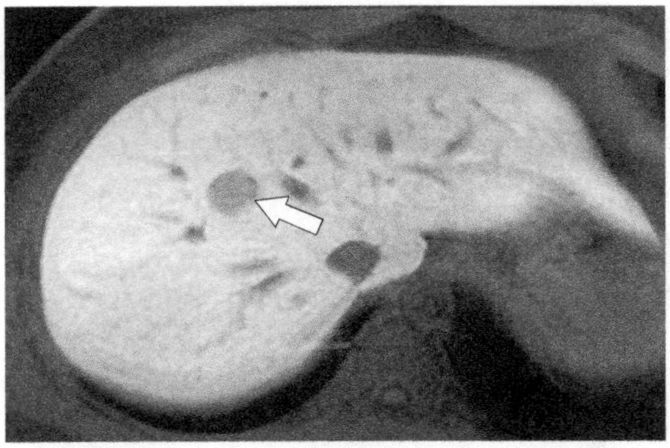

FIGURE 6-93. Axial delayed postcontrast hepatobiliary agent MRI in a 34-year-old woman with a 2-cm hypointense nonhepatocytic lesion (*arrow*), due to an adenoma.

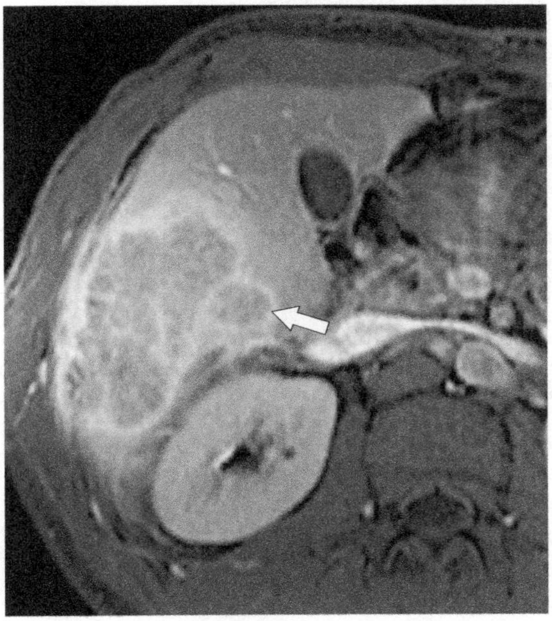

FIGURE 6-94. Axial postcontrast T1-weighted fat-saturated MRI in a 34-year-old woman with a complex heterogeneous segment VI mass (*arrow*) representing an IgG4 pseudotumor.

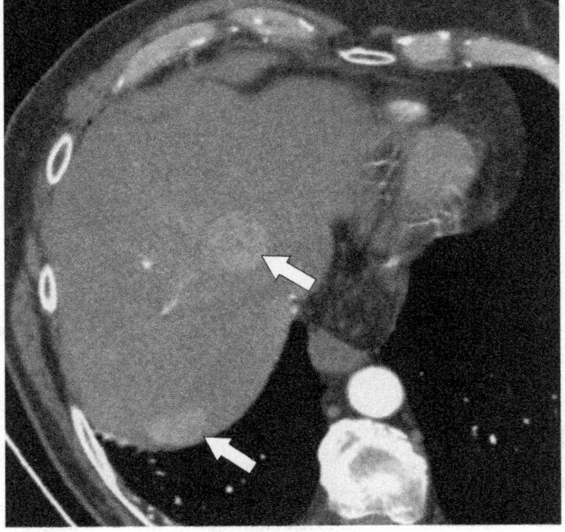

FIGURE 6-95. Axial contrast-enhanced CT in a 38-year-old man with two enhancing liver lesions (*arrows*) due to intrahepatic splenic tissue.

Because US is a less sensitive imaging tool than CT and MRI for evaluating liver lesions, its use is not recommended to screen for metastatic disease. It is too operator and patient dependent to be consistently reliable. If US is performed, however, metastatic lesions are usually hypoechoic, and a "bull's eye" pattern (hypoechoic margin) is characteristic (Fig. 6-98). Some metastases can be hyperechoic, including gastrointestinal tumors and HCC. Calcified metastases (e.g., mucinous malignancies) are also hyperechoic with posterior shadowing, in keeping with other US findings of calcification.

Given its speed and cost, contrast-enhanced CT is the method of choice to evaluate for the presence of hepatic metastases, although MRI is generally more sensitive for lesion detection and specific for lesion characterization. Multidetector scanners with the timing of imaging tailored to maximal metastatic or hepatic parenchymal enhancement are highly effective for the detection

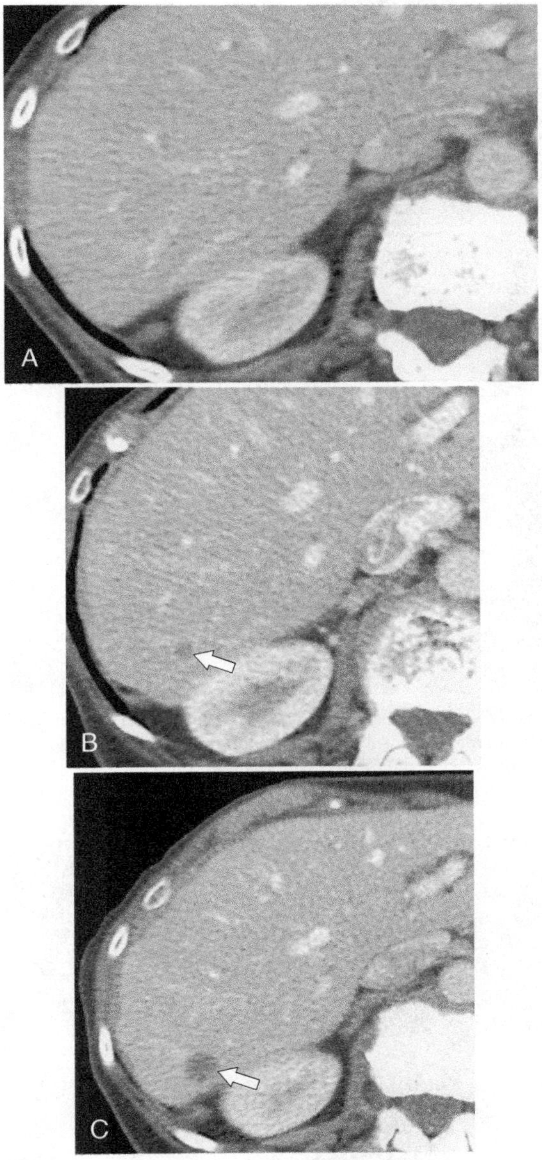

FIGURE 6-96. Axial contrast-enhanced CT in a 66-year-old woman with a breast cancer metastasis evolving on serial imaging. Initial imaging (**A**) demonstrates no lesion. Six-month follow-up CT demonstrates a 7-mm hypodense new lesion (**B**) in segment VII of the liver (*arrow*), which, although highly suspect for a new metastasis, is too small to fully characterize. Four months later (**C**), a follow-up CT demonstrated an increase in the size of the lesion (*arrow*) proving metastatic disease.

of most lesions >5 mm. Some metastatic lesions follow the same enhancement pattern as their "parent" primary malignancy and enhance predominantly in the arterial phase (Box 6-7). The knowledge that the patient has one of these underlying malignancies necessitates both arterial and PVP imaging because many of these lesions, particularly if small, can be detected only during the arterial phase (Figs. 6-3 and 6-99). Hepatic metastases, which

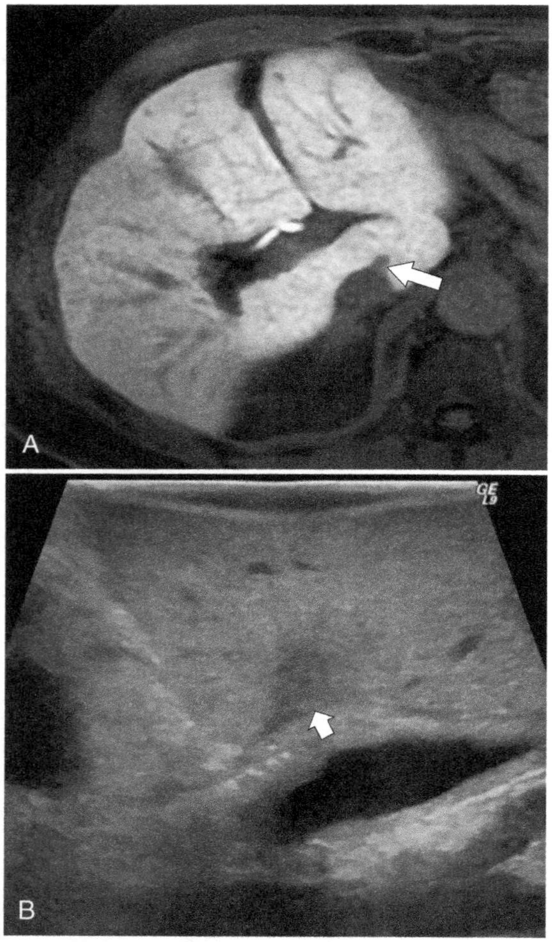

FIGURE 6-97. Axial delayed postcontrast hepatobiliary agent MRI (**A**) in a 69-year-old man with a small caudate lobe metastasis (*arrow*), confirmed at intraoperative US (**B**) (*small arrow*).

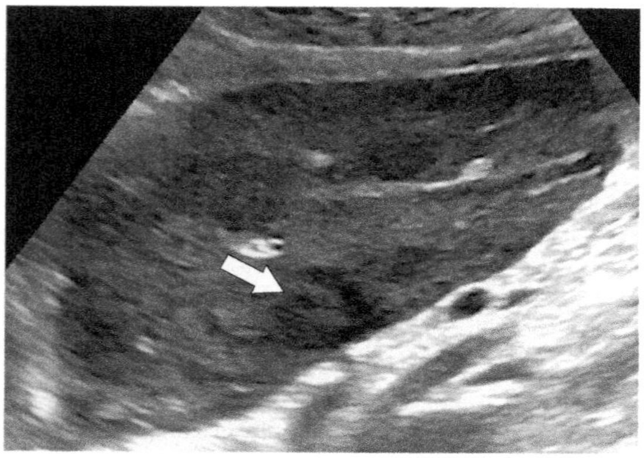

FIGURE 6-98. Sagittal US in a 59-year-old woman with predominantly hypoechoic breast cancer metastases (*arrow*) with "bull's-eye" appearances.

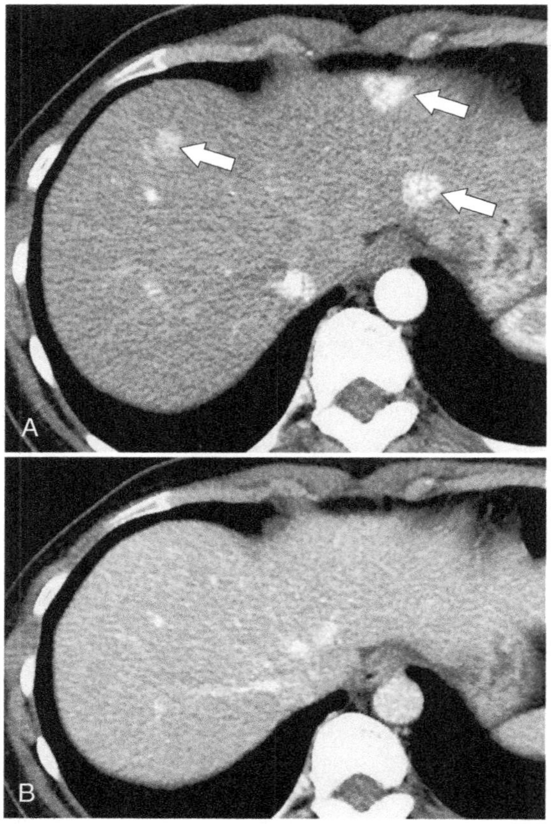

FIGURE 6-99. Axial arterial (**A**) and PVP (**B**) contrast-enhanced CT in a 42-year-old woman with metastatic pancreatic neuroendocrine tumor. The hypervascular lesions (*arrows*) are identified only during the arterial phase.

Box 6-7. Hypervascular Hepatic Metastases

Neuroendocrine (from any site)
Renal
Melanoma
Sarcoma
Thyroid
Hepatocellular carcinoma
Choriocarcinoma
Some breast metastases

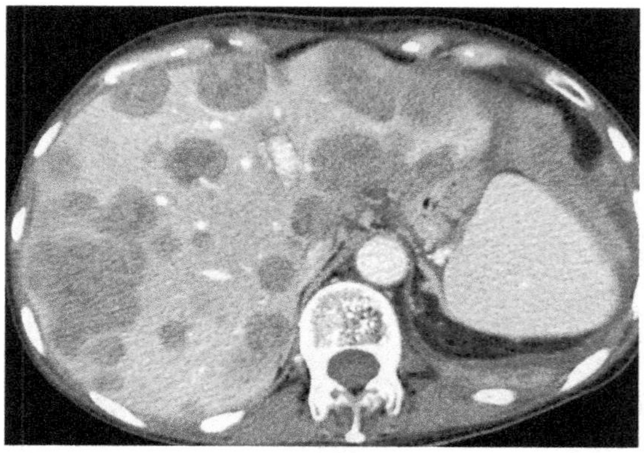

FIGURE 6-100. Axial PVP contrast-enhanced CT in a 66-year-old woman with multiple metastases from colon cancer.

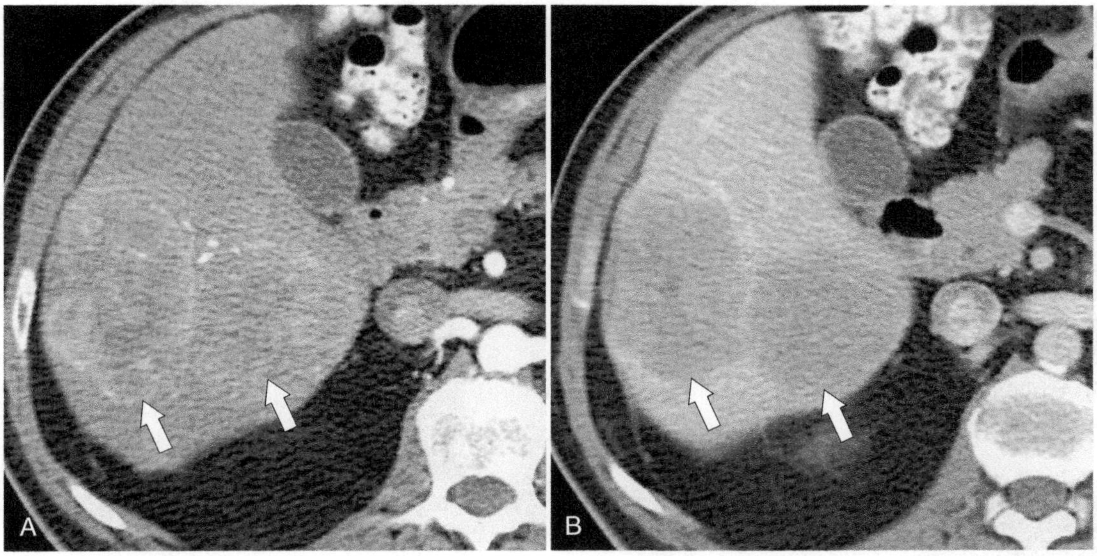

FIGURE 6-101. Axial arterial (**A**) and PVP (**B**) CT in a 77-year-old man with two segment VI liver lesions demonstrating subtle peripheral hypervascular enhancement (*arrows*) that is not as evident in the PVP.

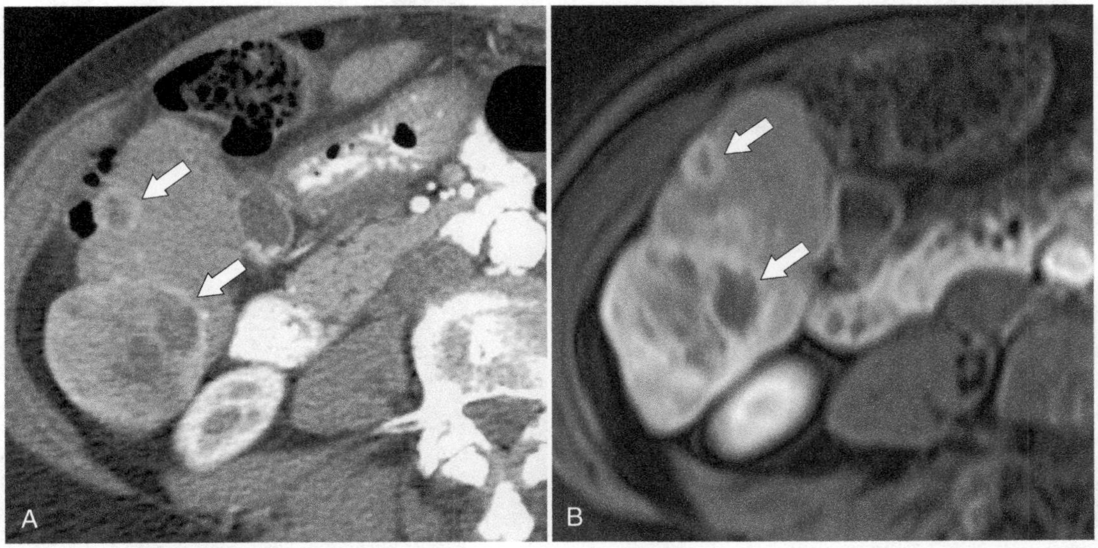

FIGURE 6-102. Axial contrast-enhanced CT (**A**) and T1-weighted fat-saturated MRI (**B**) in a 73-old-woman with heterogeneous metastases (*arrows*) from gastric cancer.

are not generally hypervascular and are often multiple, are best imaged in the PVP when the normal liver parenchyma is maximally enhanced (Fig. 6-100). Many metastatic lesions do, however, show some peripheral subtle irregular enhancement in the arterial phase, which represents peripheral hypervascular tumor neovascularization, the actively growing part of the tumor (Fig. 6-101). Lesions are also often highly heterogeneous at contrast-enhanced CT, with areas of variable enhancement (Fig. 6-102) and other areas of necrosis (Fig. 6-103). On the whole, however, lesion detection is determined by optimal hepatic parenchymal enhancement in the PVP, rendering the relatively hypovascular metastasis more conspicuous. If very large, the bulk of the lesion may appear necrotic (Fig. 6-103) and even cystic. Some lesions are purely cystic, such as those from ovarian cancer, gastrointestinal stromal tumors, and mucinous gastrointestinal tumors (Fig. 6-104). Even other metastases that are usually noncystic (e.g., melanoma) can rarely appear predominantly cystic (Fig. 6-105). These lesions can sometimes be difficult to differentiate from simple cysts. Some metastases can calcify, particularly those from mucinous gastrointestinal tumors (Fig. 6-106), and others are fatty (teratoma, liposarcoma) (Fig. 6-107). Still others can be capsular, scalloping the hepatic surface, as is most commonly observed in metastases from ovarian cancer (Fig. 6-108). The most specific imaging feature of hepatic metastases, however, is either central or peripheral washout on portal venous or delayed contrast-enhanced CT, representing washout of contrast material from the central component of the metastasis (Fig. 6-109). If this sign is visualized, the lesion is almost certainly metastatic.

On MRI, metastatic lesions, similar to most other malignant hepatic lesions, are mildly hyperintense on T2-weighted imaging and hypointense on T1-weighted imaging (Fig. 6-110). Extracellular contrast agents (e.g., gadolinium chelates) demonstrate enhancement characteristics similar to those on CT (Fig. 6-111). If the lesions are small, they may be difficult to visualize on T2-weighted imaging and identified only after the administration of IV contrast-enhanced material (Fig. 6-111). Melanoma metastases characteristically demonstrate high precontrast T1-weighted signal because melanin shortens T1 values (Fig. 6-112).

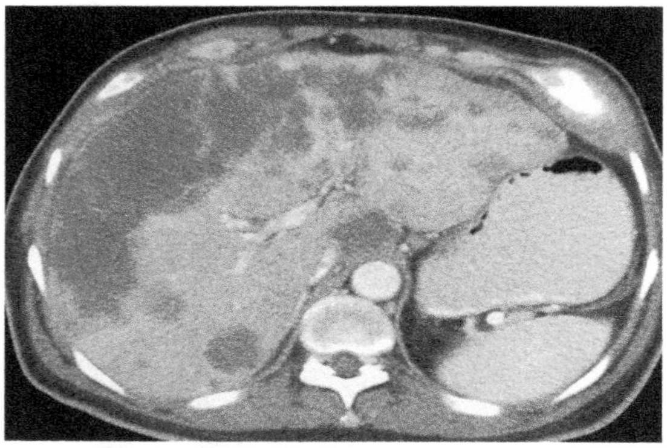

FIGURE 6-103. Axial PVP CT in 65-year-old man with hypodense predominantly necrotic metastases from rectal cancer.

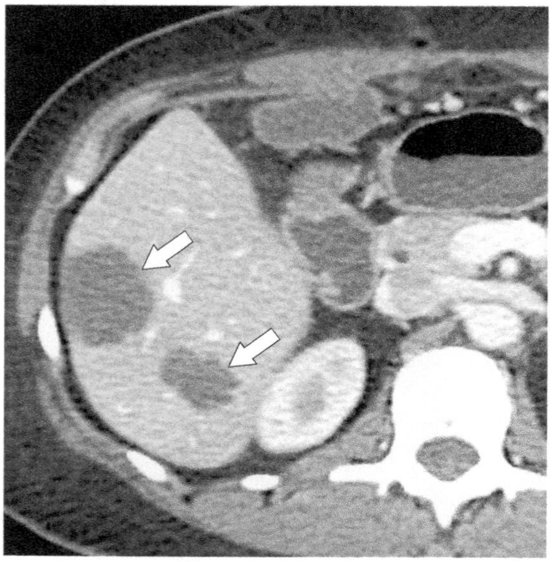

FIGURE 6-104. Axial PVP CT in a 71-year-old woman with cystic gastric colon metastases (*arrows*).

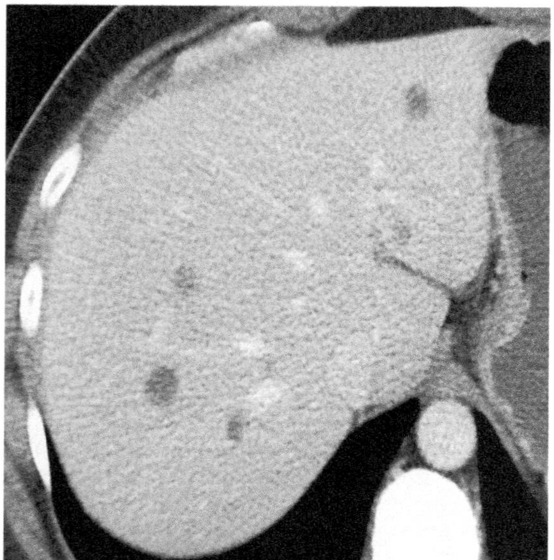

FIGURE 6-105. Axial PVP CT in a 49-year-old woman with multiple, small, hypodense, cystic-appearing metastases caused by melanoma.

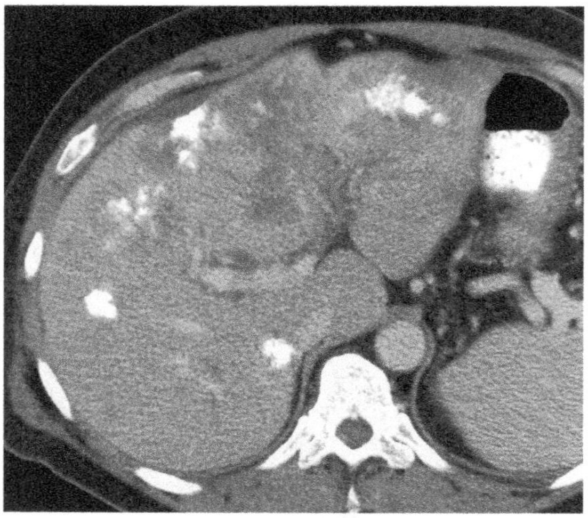

FIGURE 6-106. Axial PVP contrast-enhanced CT in a 46-year-old man with calcified mucinous metastases from colon cancer.

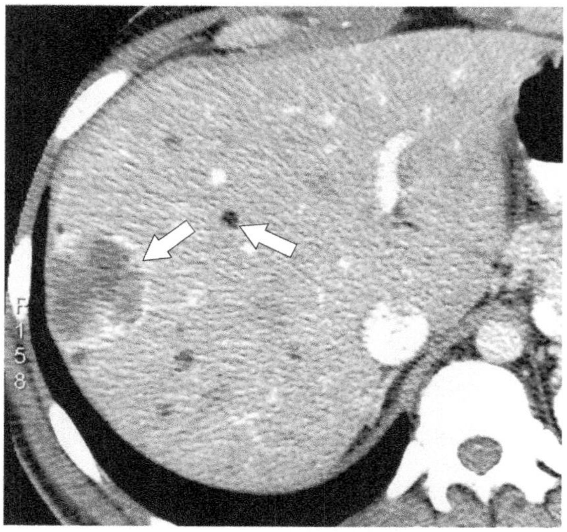

FIGURE 6-107. Axial contrast-enhanced CT in a 19-year-old woman with metastatic thoracic teratoma and fatty metastases (*arrows*).

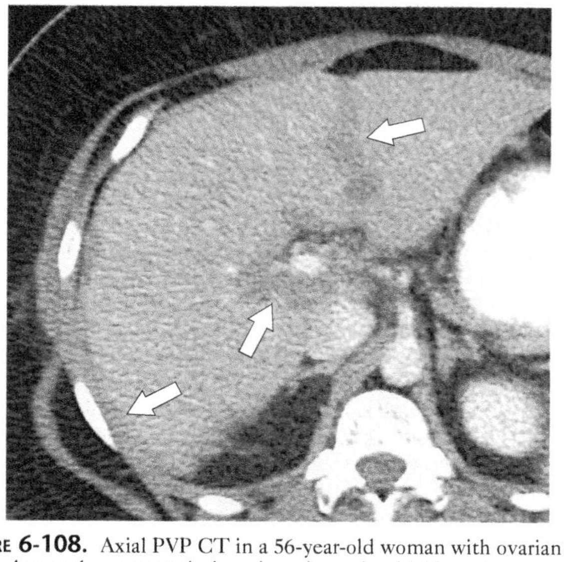

FIGURE 6-108. Axial PVP CT in a 56-year-old woman with ovarian cancer and capsular metastatic invasion along the falciform ligament, the porta hepatis, and segment VII surface (*arrows*).

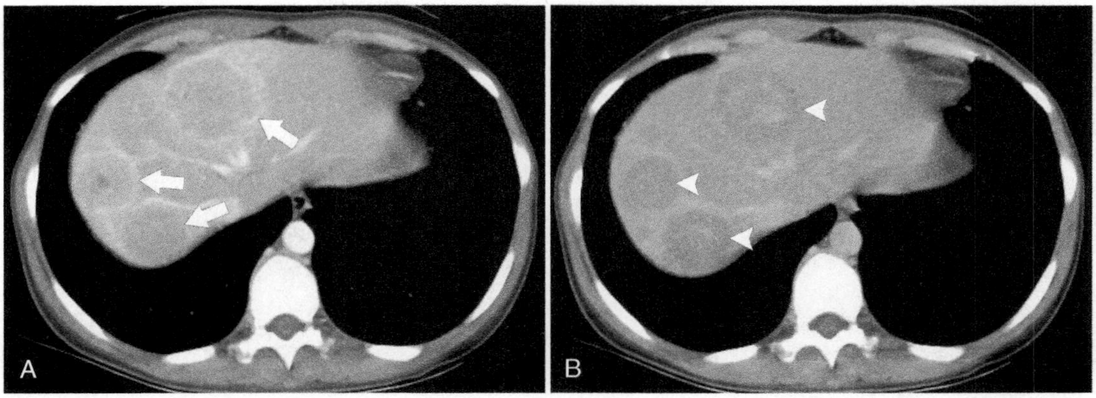

FIGURE 6-109. Axial PVP (**A**) and delayed (**B**) contrast-enhanced CT in a 29-year-old woman with metastatic carcinoid (*arrows*) and peripheral washout (*arrowheads*) on delayed imaging, highly specific for metastatic disease.

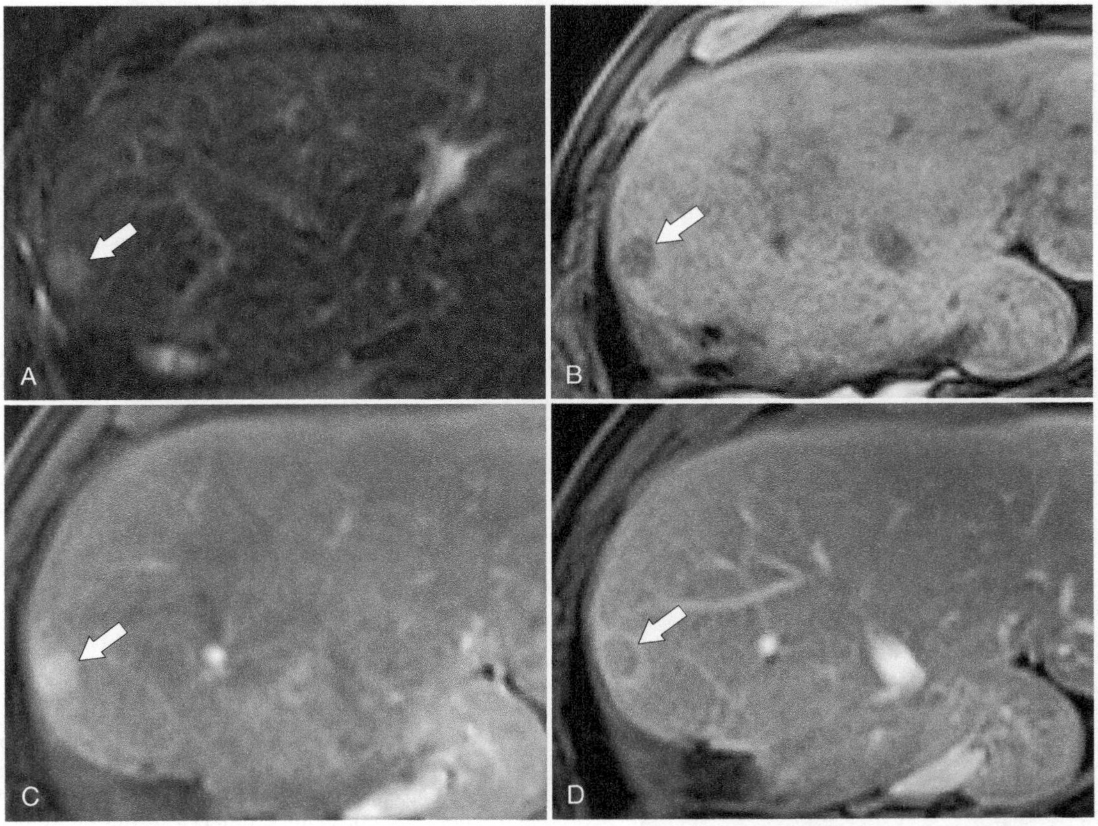

FIGURE 6-110. Axial T2 (**A**), T1-weighted precontrast (**B**) and postcontrast (**C**) PVP and delayed (**D**) fat-saturated MRI T1 in a 44-year-old man with metastatic melanoma. There is a 1.5-cm T2 intermediate signal metastasis (*arrows*) in segment VIII of the liver that is hypointense on precontrast T1-weighted images. After contrast administration, the lesion enhances but demonstrates washout on delayed imaging, highly characteristic of metastatic disease.

Diffusion-weighted imaging has become a routine additional pulse sequence in the evaluation of focal liver lesions because it offers some increased sensitivity for lesion detectability and generally increased specificity for lesion characterization. Given the frequency of metastatic disease in clinical practice, it is not surprising that not all lesions demonstrate the classic imaging findings as described. This pulse sequence adds little time to the overall MRI protocol yet can give greater confidence for lesion characterization, particularly for atypical lesions. Malignant lesions are generally diffusion restricted and demonstrate low DWI signal and moderate to high ADC map signal (Fig. 6-113). Some benign lesions (hemangioma and abscess) sometimes demonstrate restricted diffusion, but these lesions generally demonstrate low signal on ADC maps, distinguishing them from malignant disease.

Hepatobiliary contrast agents have offered the opportunity to increase liver lesion detection and characterization. The liver can be imaged dynamically (during the extracellular phase), demonstrating findings similar to those with conventional gadolinium chelates, albeit usually with less signal intensity because of the lower dose of administered gadolinium. However, after normal hepatobiliary uptake on delayed imaging, metastases (which have little or no hepatocyte function) are hypointense and clearly outlined by normally enhancing hepatic parenchyma (Fig. 6-114). Often this technique demonstrates additional small lesions

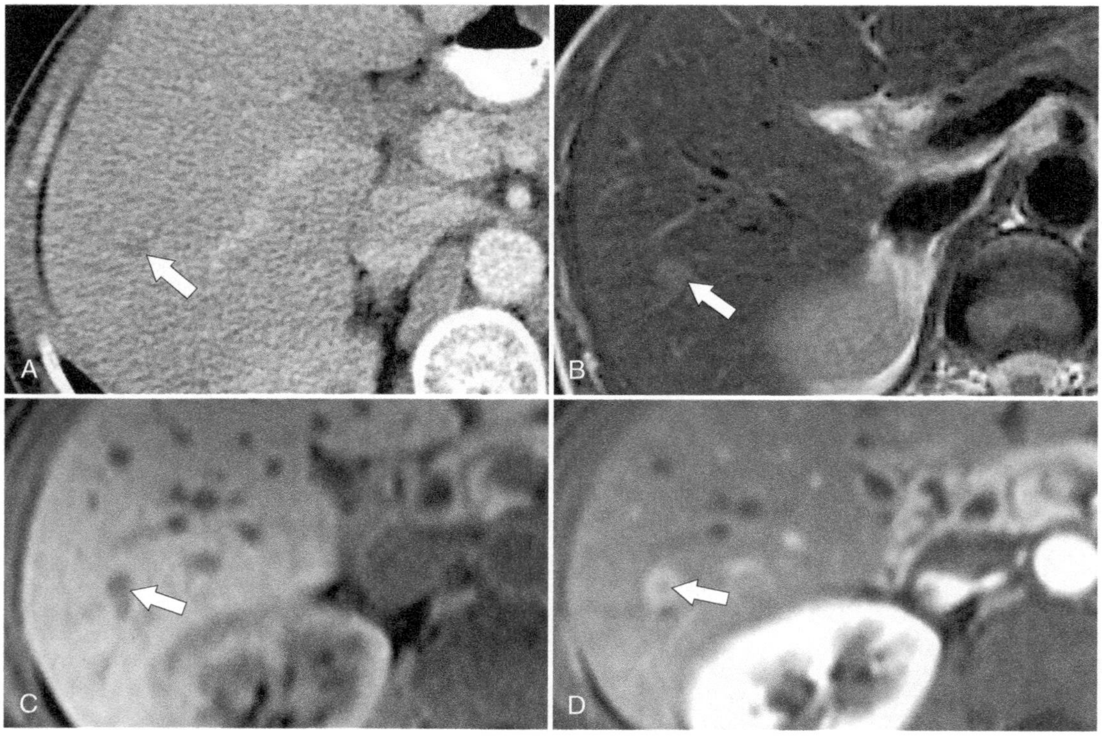

FIGURE 6-111. Axial contrast-enhanced CT (**A**) and T2- (**B**) and T1-weighted pre- (**C**) and post-contrast-enhanced (**D**) MRI in a 67-year-old man with metastatic lung cancer (*arrows*). The lesion in segment VII (*arrows*) is barely visible at CT, T1-, and T2-weighted precontrast MRI but is clearly seen after IV contrast administration.

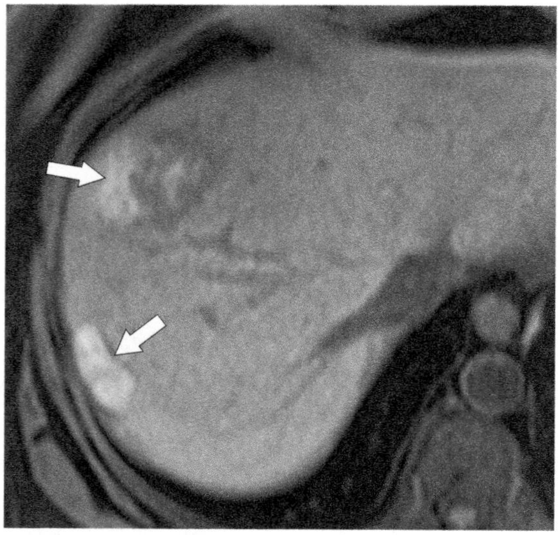

FIGURE 6-112. Axial precontrast T1-weighted MRI in a 61-year-old man with melanoma metastases that are characteristically bright (*arrows*).

hitherto unsuspected with other imaging protocols, which is critical for hepatic surgeons contemplating lesion or lobar curative resection (Fig. 6-114). Identification of lesions in both lobes of the liver often precludes curative surgery. Given the expense and morbidity of such surgery, it seems prudent to evaluate patients with hepatobiliary contrast agents before embarking on surgery. The most sensitive method, however, particularly for patients being considered for surgical resection of hepatic metastasis, is intraoperative US (Fig. 6-115), which is usually performed at the time of surgery to evaluate for any metastatic disease that might have been missed on prior imaging and could preclude curative surgery.

PET imaging, especially with PET/CT, has proved a useful tool for staging of malignant disease, particularly cancers of the colon or lung, lymphoma, melanoma, and several other diseases. Given the relative spatial resolution limitations of PET, contrast-enhanced CT performed as part of the same investigation with image fusion has shown greater accuracy for detecting and characterizing metastatic lesions, including in the liver. Lesions demonstrate variable increased activity, depending on the malignant nature and differentiation of the tumor (Fig. 6-116). Given the accuracy of multidetector CT and MRI, however, PET imaging is usually performed not to evaluate a patient solely for liver metastases, but rather to evaluate metastatic disease throughout the chest and abdomen.

Hepatocellular Carcinoma

Hepatocellular carcinoma (HCC) is the most common primary malignant hepatic tumor and mostly (up to 90%) arises in patients with underlying cirrhosis (see earlier in chapter). Noncirrhotic causes include toxins (aflatoxin and possibly androgens and Thorotrast) or genetic defects, including hemochromatosis, Wilson disease (both of which can cause HCC with or without cirrhosis), and tyrosinosis. More recently, obesity and type II diabetes mellitus have been associated with an increased risk of developing HCC as a result of chronic steatohepatitis. It is for these reasons that steatohepatitis, currently an epidemic, is being managed far more aggressively (with weight loss and effective diabetic treatment) than in the past.

In patients with cirrhosis there is a well-recognized pathway from regenerative nodule formation to dysplasia and ultimately carcinoma. Considering that cirrhosis is a common disease and the development of HCC is a major risk factor, periodic screening for the development of HCC is warranted, particularly because small, early lesions are potentially curable. Screening is usually performed with US, although given that the liver has a diffuse heterogeneous appearance on US, small HCCs can be difficult to detect. The rationales for persisting with US (rather than the more sensitive MRI or CT tests) are the expense

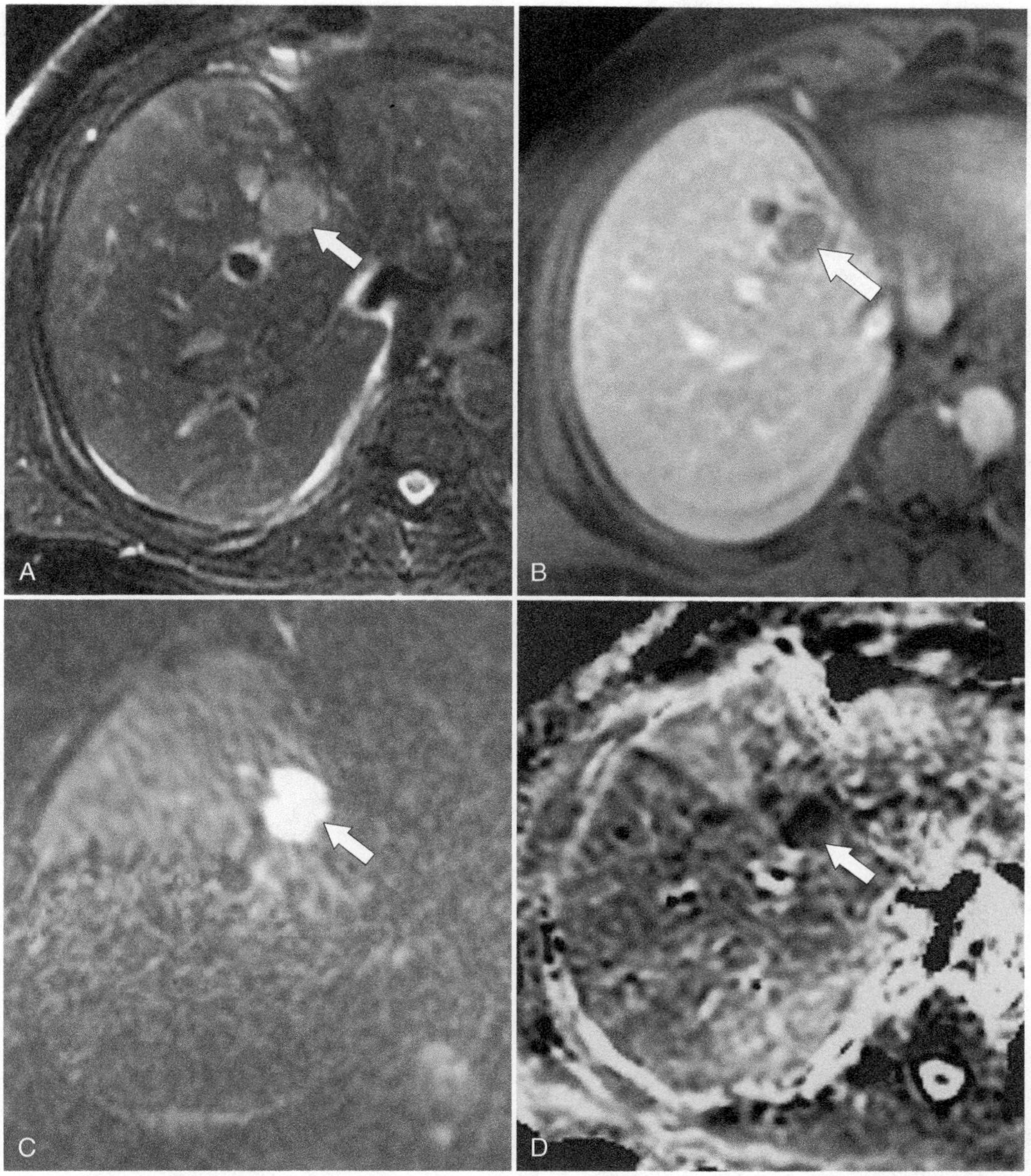

FIGURE 6-113. Axial T2 (**A**), postcontrast T1-weighted fat-saturated MRI (**B**) and B 600 DWI (**C**) and ADC (**D**) maps in a 45-year-old woman with a hepatic metastasis (*arrows*) from cervical cancer. The metastasis has characteristic malignant T2 and postcontrast characteristics and demonstrates restricted diffusion on DWI and ADC maps.

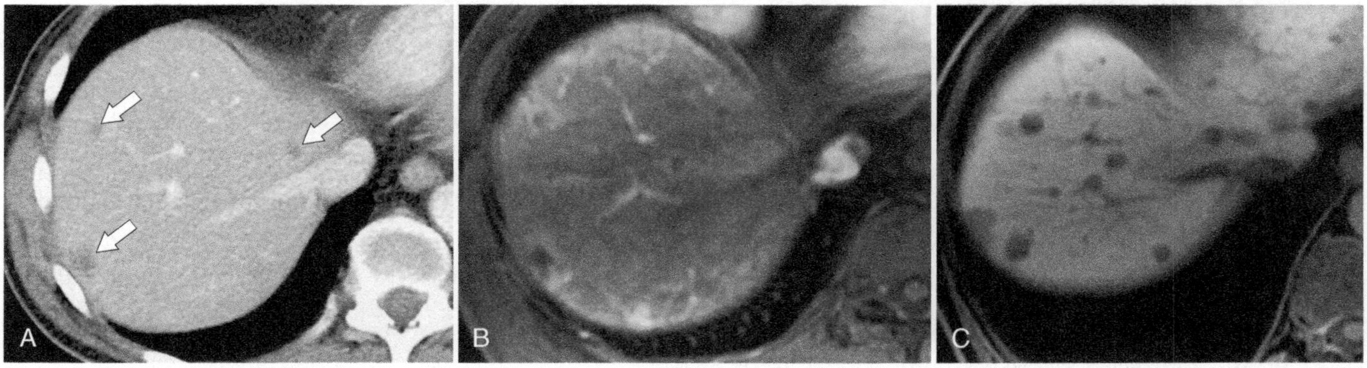

FIGURE 6-114. Axial PVP post-contrast-enhanced CT (**A**) and MRI (**B**) and 20-minute delayed hepatobiliary agent MRI (**C**) in a 61-year-old man with metastatic colon cancer. Only three lesions are identified at CT (*arrows*), several more during PVP MRI, but numerous hypointense lesions at delayed postcontrast imaging.

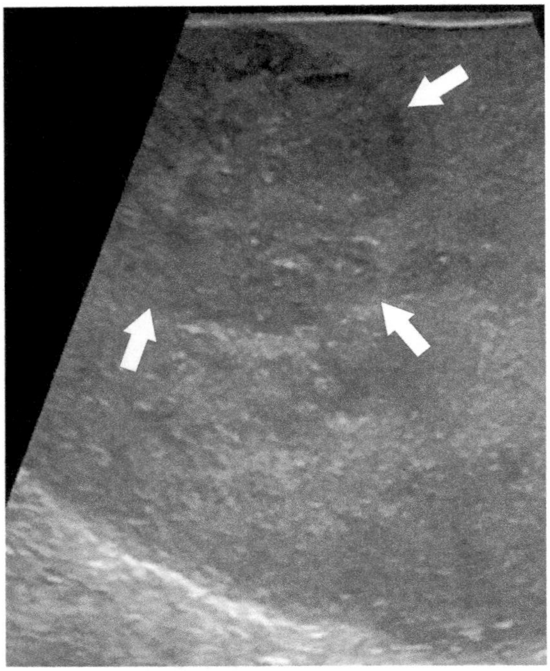

Figure 6-115. Intraoperative US in a 58-year-old man with a hypoechoic heterogeneous liver metastasis (*arrows*).

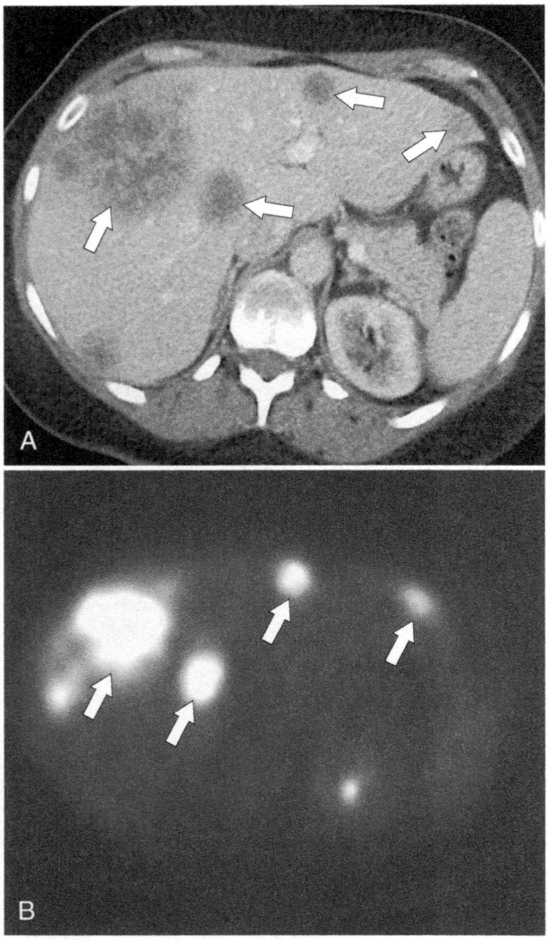

Figure 6-116. Axial contrast-enhanced CT (**A**) and PET (**B**) in a 50-year-old with metastatic colon cancer. There are multiple CT hypodense lesions that are PET avid (*arrows*). There is normal activity in the left renal pelvis.

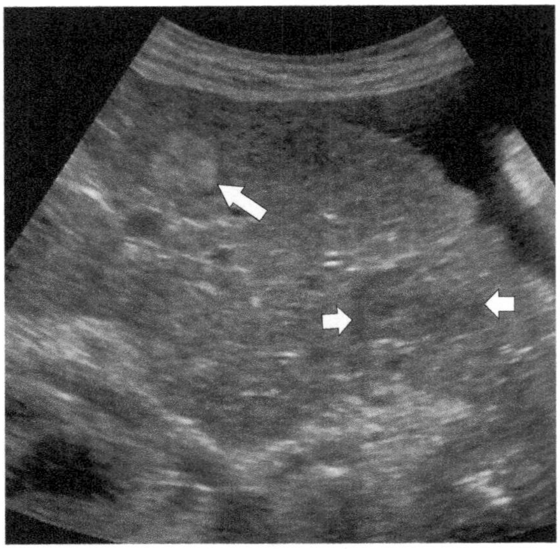

Figure 6-117. US in a 56-year-old man with cirrhosis and a hyperechoic (*arrow*) and hypoechoic HCC in the left lobe of the liver (*small arrows*).

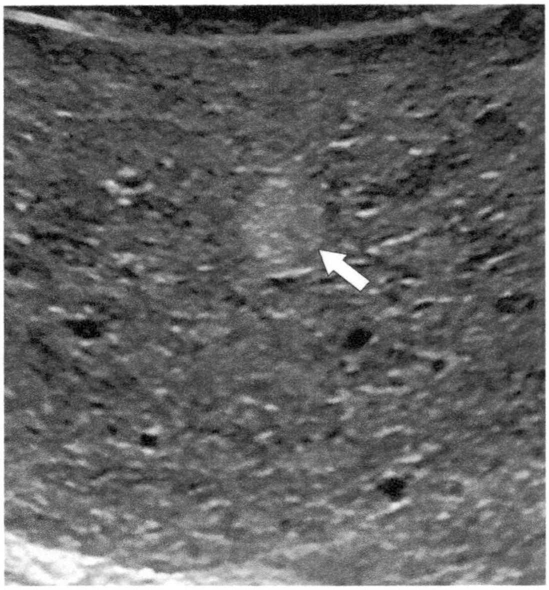

Figure 6-118. Intraoperative US in a 75-year-old man with a 1-cm hyperechoic liver mass (*arrow*) representing HCC.

and availability of CT and MRI and the potential for cure of most HCCs up to 3 cm (the size at which they can usually be detected by US). Lesions are suspected when a focal hypoechoic (or hyperechoic because some contain fat) mass is identified (Fig. 6-117). However, contrast-enhancing computed tomography (CECT) and contrast-enhanced magnetic resonance imaging (CEMRI) are well recognized to be far more sensitive and specific for detecting HCC, unless intraoperative US is to be performed (Fig. 6-118).

On cross-sectional imaging lesions appear either nodular or diffuse, and on noncontrast CT fat and calcification may be identified (Fig. 6-119). On contrast-enhanced CT the lesions typically enhance avidly in the arterial phase, especially if poorly differentiated, and many (particularly small lesions) are isodense in the PVP and may be encapsulated (Fig. 6-120). The differentiation from a dysplastic nodule can be difficult, although dysplastic nodules are generally smaller, and MRI may help distinguish

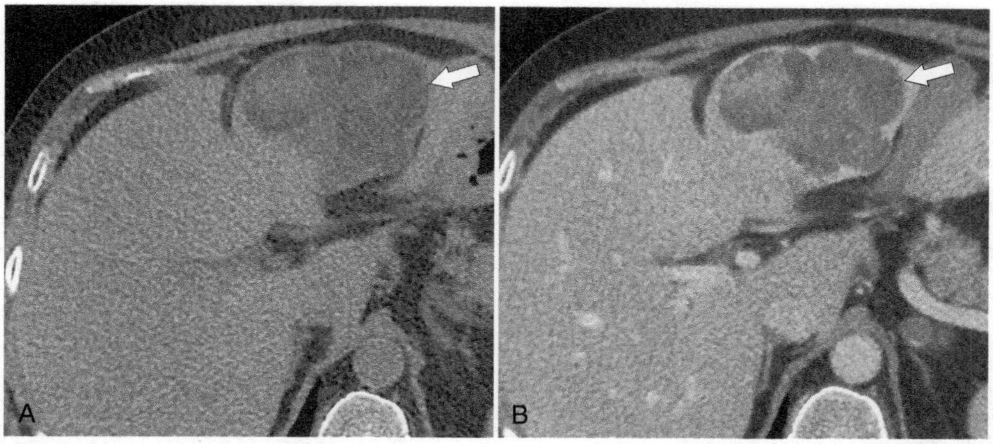

FIGURE 6-119. A and B, Axial non-contrast-enhanced CT in a 56-year-old woman with a left lobe HCC that has large hypodense fat elements (*arrows*).

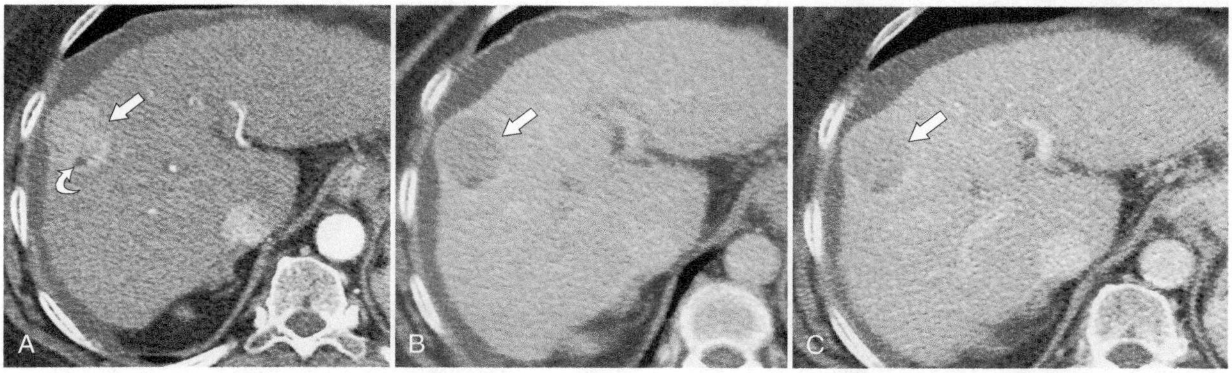

FIGURE 6-120. Axial arterial (A), PVP (B), and delayed (C) contrast-enhanced CT in a 79-year-old woman with a cirrhotic liver and a segment V HCC (*arrows*) that demonstrates arterial enhancement, a capsule at PVP, and contrast washout on delayed imaging. There is a focus on intratumoral fat (*curved arrow*) and abdominal ascites.

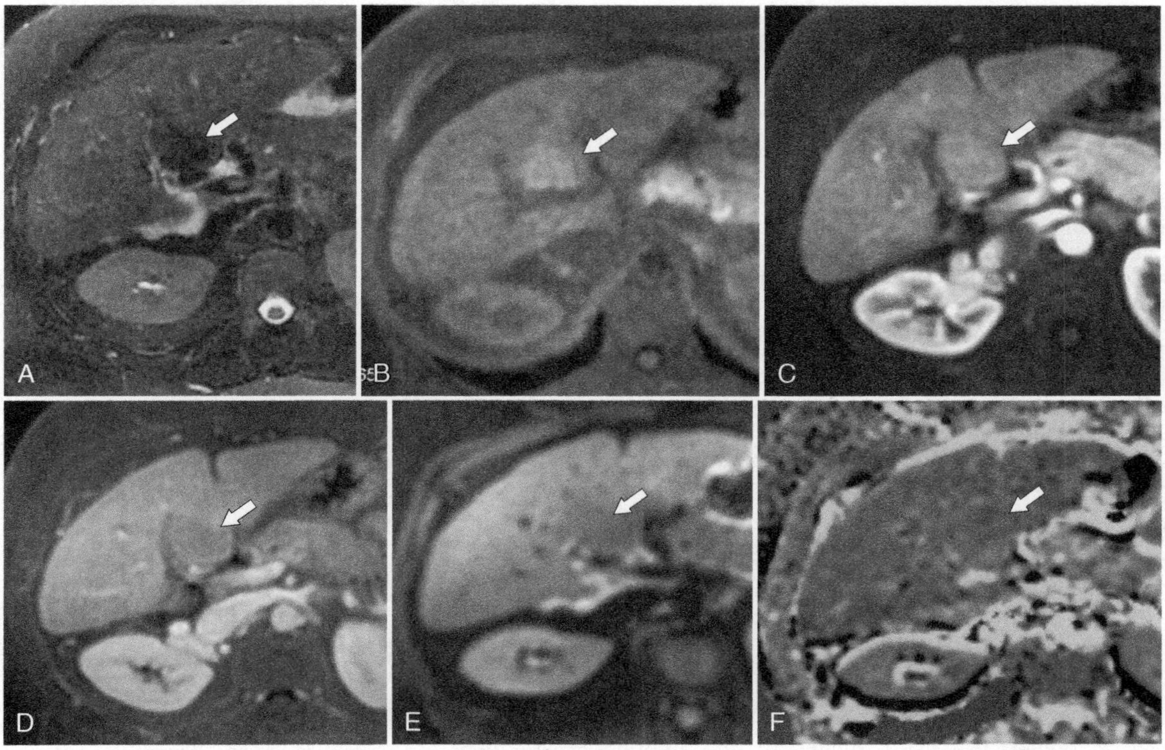

FIGURE 6-121. Axial fat-saturated T2-weighted (A), fat-saturated T1-weighted (B), AP (C), PVP (D), and hepatobiliary postcontrast MRI, and B500 DWI (E) and ADC maps (F) in a 63-year-old woman with a dysplastic nodule (*arrows*) that has low T2 signal, unlike an HCC, which would show moderate to high T2 signal. It does not demonstrate hepatocyte activity on delayed hepatobiliary agent imaging.

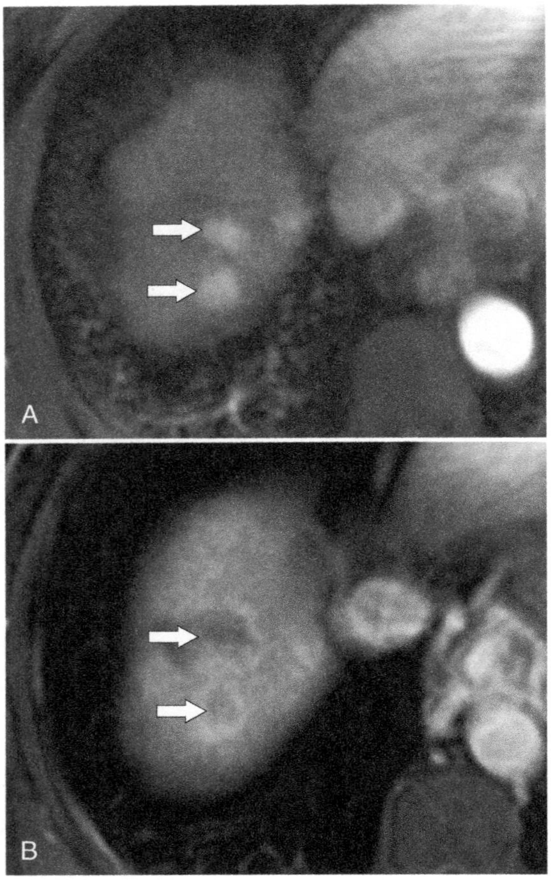

Figure 6-122. Axial arterial (**A**) and delayed (**B**) post-contrast-enhanced MRI in a 54-year-old with two foci of HCC that washed out on delayed imaging (*arrows*).

between the two (Fig. 6-121). A highly characteristic feature of HCC is delayed contrast washout from the lesion (Fig. 6-122), which helps differentiate HCC from benign lesions. On MRI the lesions may have variable T1-weighted appearances, but they are usually hyperintense on T2-weighted imaging. Degeneration of a dysplastic nodule is suggested by an area of increased T2 signal within a region of low T2 signal (dysplastic nodules are usually hypointense on T2-weighted imaging) (Fig. 6-123). Contrast-enhanced MRI shows brisk, intense enhancement with delayed washout, again characteristic of HCC (Fig. 6-122). More diffuse or metastatic lesions are generally easier to diagnose, given their multifocal nature, particularly when observed in a patient with cirrhosis (Fig. 6-124). Larger tumors may invade the portal vein and can be differentiated from nontumorous thrombus by subtle enhancement within the thrombus (Fig. 6-125). Larger lesions may also demonstrate a central scar and therefore need to be differentiated from other lesions with a central scar, including hemangioma, FNH, fibrolamellar HCC, and some metastases (Fig. 6-126). Differentiation from other hepatic tumors (FNH) is also aided by the use of hepatobiliary contrast agents, although some well-differentiated HCCs retain hepatocellular function. Poorly differentiated tumors, however, do not retain hepatocellular function and therefore are hypointense on delayed postcontrast imaging (Fig. 6-127), similar to metastatic disease.

Fibrolamellar Hepatocellular Carcinoma

Fibrolamellar hepatocellular carcinoma occurs in noncirrhotic livers, typically in younger patients. Histologically they are quite different from HCC, usually less aggressive, and potentially curable. Their imaging features have some similarity to those of

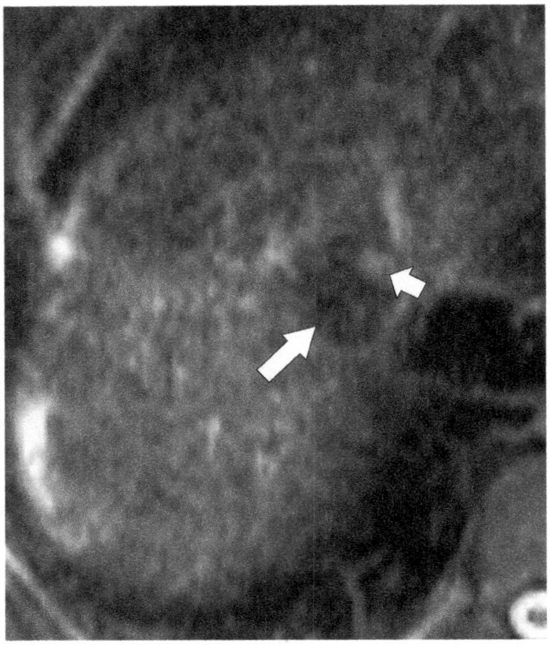

Figure 6-123. Axial T2-weighted MRI in a 66-year-old man with a predominantly hypointense dysplastic nodule (*arrow*), with an area of T2 increased signal resulting from malignant degeneration to HCC (*small arrow*).

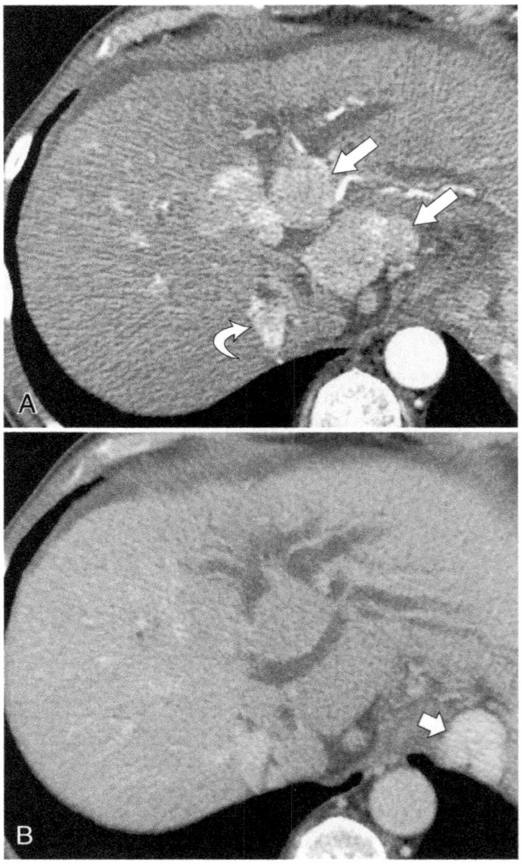

Figure 6-124. Axial arterial (**A**) and delayed (**B**) contrast-enhanced CT in a 57-year-old with cirrhosis with a multifocal enhancing HCC (*arrows*) that washes out on delayed imaging. There are ascites and esophageal varices (*small arrow*), as well as enhancing tumor thrombus in the IVC (*curved arrow*). The main hepatic mass also causes biliary obstruction.

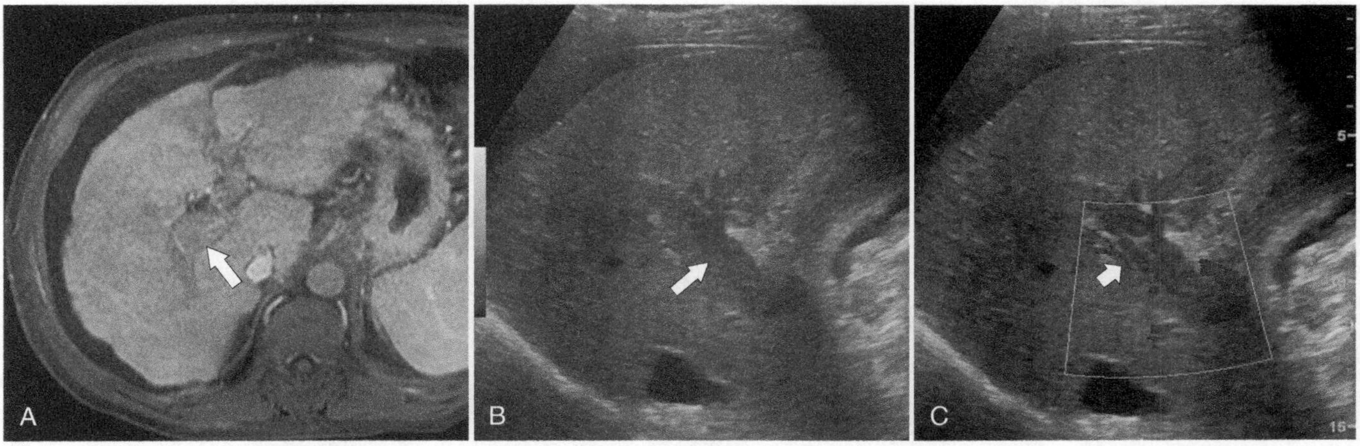

FIGURE 6-125. Axial T1-weighted fat-saturated postcontrast MRI (A) and US (B) of the portahepatic region in a 68-year-old man with metastasis of HCC to the portal vein (*arrows*). The tumor thrombus expands the vein and demonstrates increased vascular flow on Doppler (*small arrow*). *See ExpertConsult.com for color image.*

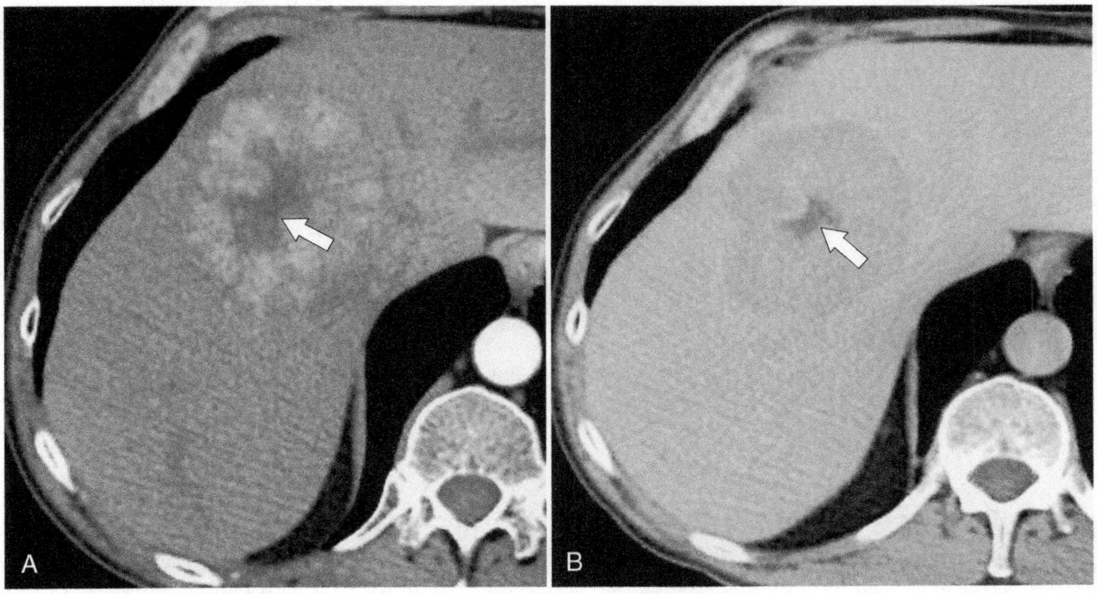

FIGURE 6-126. Axial arterial-phase (A) and delayed (B) contrast-enhanced CT in a 49-year-old man with a 5-cm hypervascular HCC that washes out on delayed imaging and contains a central scar (*arrows*).

FNH, hepatic adenoma, and HCC (Table 6-5) and less commonly to hemangiomas, metastases, and cholangiocarcinomas. They are usually discovered when they enlarge and the patient is evaluated because of abdominal pain. On contrast-enhanced CT an often large lobulated mass enhances avidly in the arterial phase, with washout in the PVP (Fig. 6-128). Characteristically, fibrolamellar hepatocellular carcinoma, like FNH, often demonstrates a central hypoattenuating scar (which can calcify), with several hypoattenuating septa radiating out from the center (Fig. 6-129). Satellite lesions are recognized but uncommon. Some have hepatocellular function and may absorb hepatobiliary contrast agents, at least partially so, although the majority do not. They also demonstrate restricted diffusion at DWI (Fig. 6-130).

Peripheral Cholangiocarcinoma (see Chapter 8)

The histology of peripheral cholangiocarcinoma is the same as for cholangiocarcinoma (most are adenocarcinoma) associated with the gallbladder or bile ducts. Peripheral cholangiocarcinoma represents tumor arising in more peripheral intrahepatic bile ducts. The mass tends to grow in an infiltrative pattern, alongside the bile ducts (periductal) or within the ducts (intraductal). Its diagnosis should be considered for any large, irregular, heterogeneous mass with capsular retraction that demonstrates gradual centripetal enhancement, particularly when there is delayed enhancement (Fig. 6-131). It should easily be distinguishable from hemangioma, which demonstrates some similar enhancing features, because cholangiocarcinoma enhancement is mild to moderate and the mass is heterogeneous and irregular. At MRI the lesion is heterogeneous and predominantly hypointense on T1-weighted imaging and shows peripheral hyperintensity on T2-weighted imaging with less signal toward the center of the lesion. Lesions enhance in a similar fashion to contrast-enhanced CT with initial peripheral enhancement and then show mild centripetal enhancement on subsequent imaging and noticeable enhancement on delayed imaging.

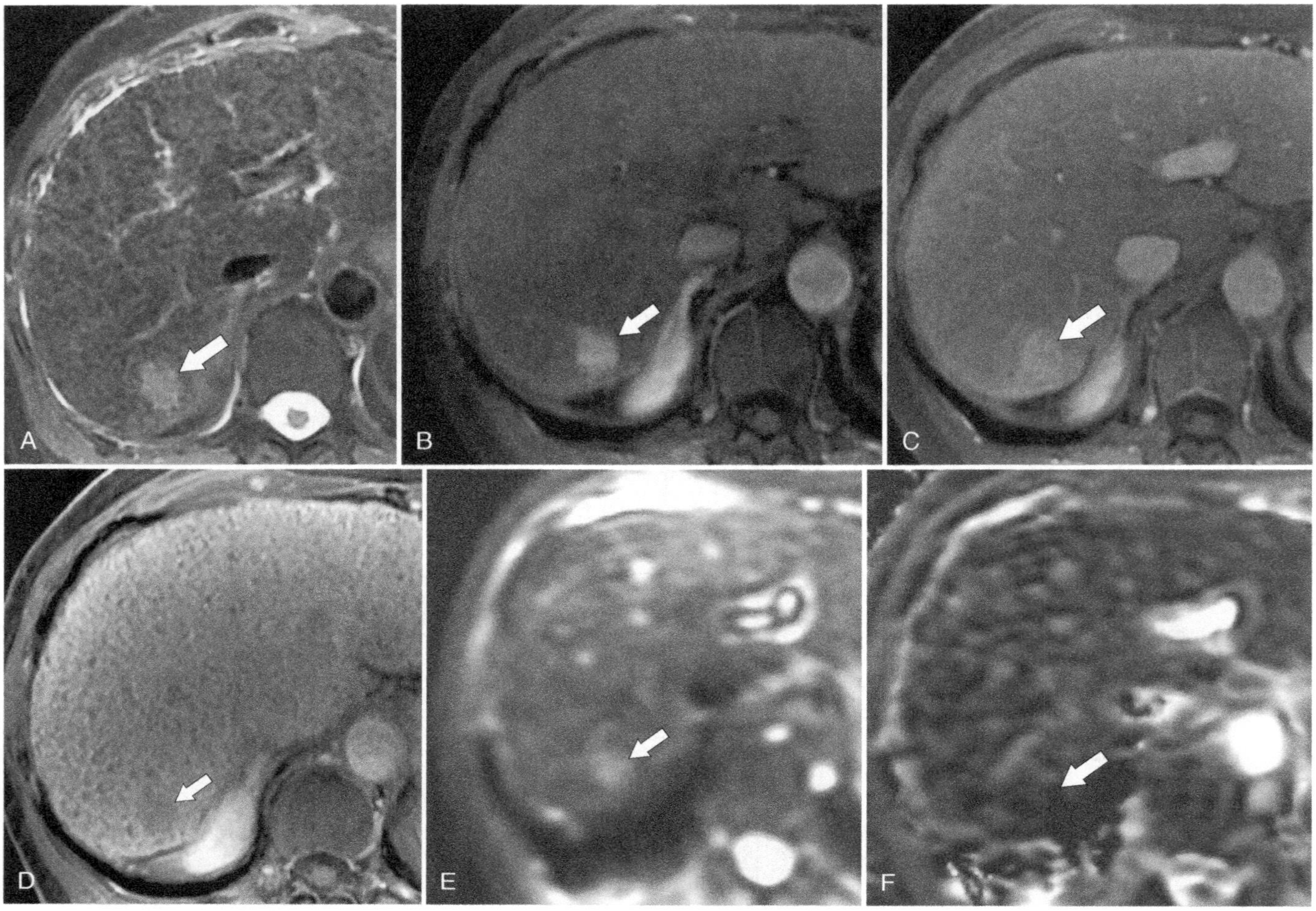

FIGURE 6-127. Axial T2-weighted (**A**), T1-weighted arterial (**B**), PVP (**C**), and delayed (**D**) postcontrast hepatobiliary agent MRI and DWI (**E**) and ADC map (**F**) in a 57-year-old man with HCC. The lesion (*arrows*) is of intermediate T2 signal, avidly enhances at arterial phase, less so on PVP, and has no hepatocyte activity on 20-minute delayed imaging. The lesion is bright on B100 DWI and dark on ADC map.

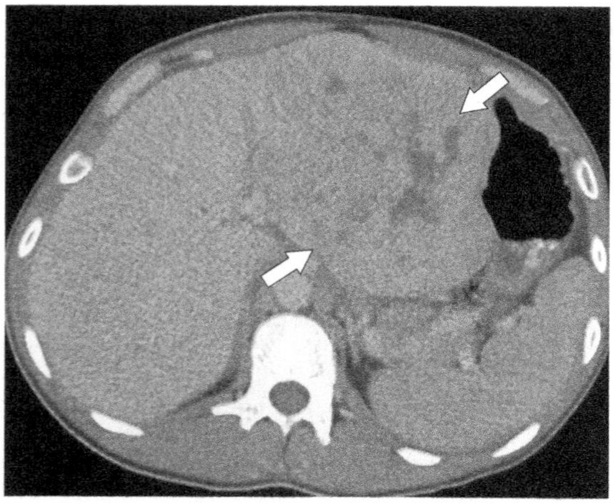

FIGURE 6-128. Axial contrast-enhanced CT (with a relatively poor contrast bolus) in a 30-year-old man with a fibrolamellar HCC. A large complex and heterogeneous mass replaces the left lobe of the liver (*arrows*) with a central scar.

Hepatic Lymphoma

Hepatic lymphoma can be primary or more commonly metastatic. When involved with Hodgkin disease, hepatic lymphoma generally signifies a poorer prognosis. The primary form is rare but is more common in HIV-infected patients or other immunosuppressed states. Lesions can be single or multiple and vary from small to very large (>15 cm). There are no particular distinguishing features on cross-sectional imaging. On PVP imaging at contrast-enhanced CT or MRI, the lesions are generally heterogeneous, similar to other malignant lesions, although they tend to enhance to a lesser degree (Fig. 6-132). The diagnosis can sometimes be inferred from a relatively smooth but lobular border with peripheral enhancement (Fig. 6-132). The diagnosis should be considered in the appropriate clinical setting, particularly for solitary hepatic lesions.

Posttransplant Lymphoproliferative Disorder (see Chapter 4)

In posttransplant lymphoproliferative disorder (PTLD), hepatic involvement is usually in the form of solitary hypodense lesions with relatively poor enhancement after IV contrast administration. Unlike more common forms of lymphoma, they are more likely to obstruct the biliary system if it is invaded by the mass.

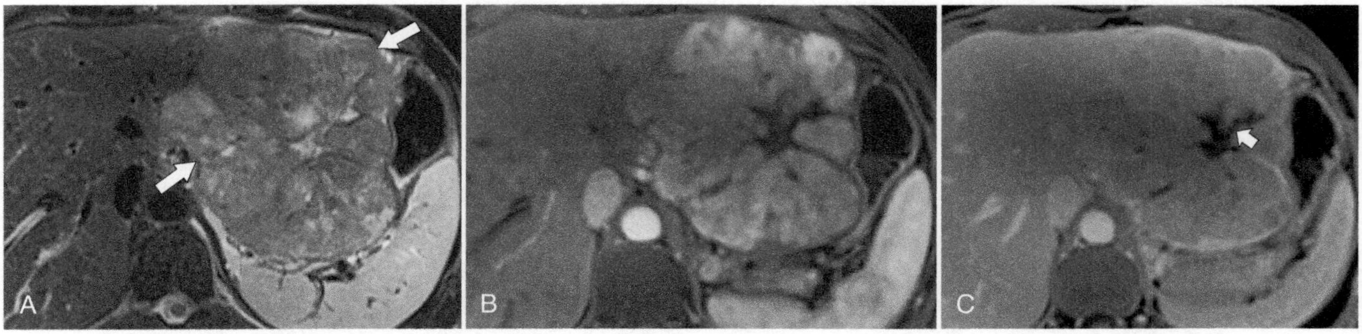

FIGURE 6-129. Axial T2 (**A**), arterial (**B**), and PVP (**C**) T1-weighted post-contrast fat-saturated MRI in a 31-year-old man with fibrolamellar HCC. A large heterogeneous T2 mass (*arrows*), which has replaced the left lobe of the liver, avidly enhances on arterial and PVP CT. A T2 bright, nonenhancing central scar radiates out from the center (*small arrow*).

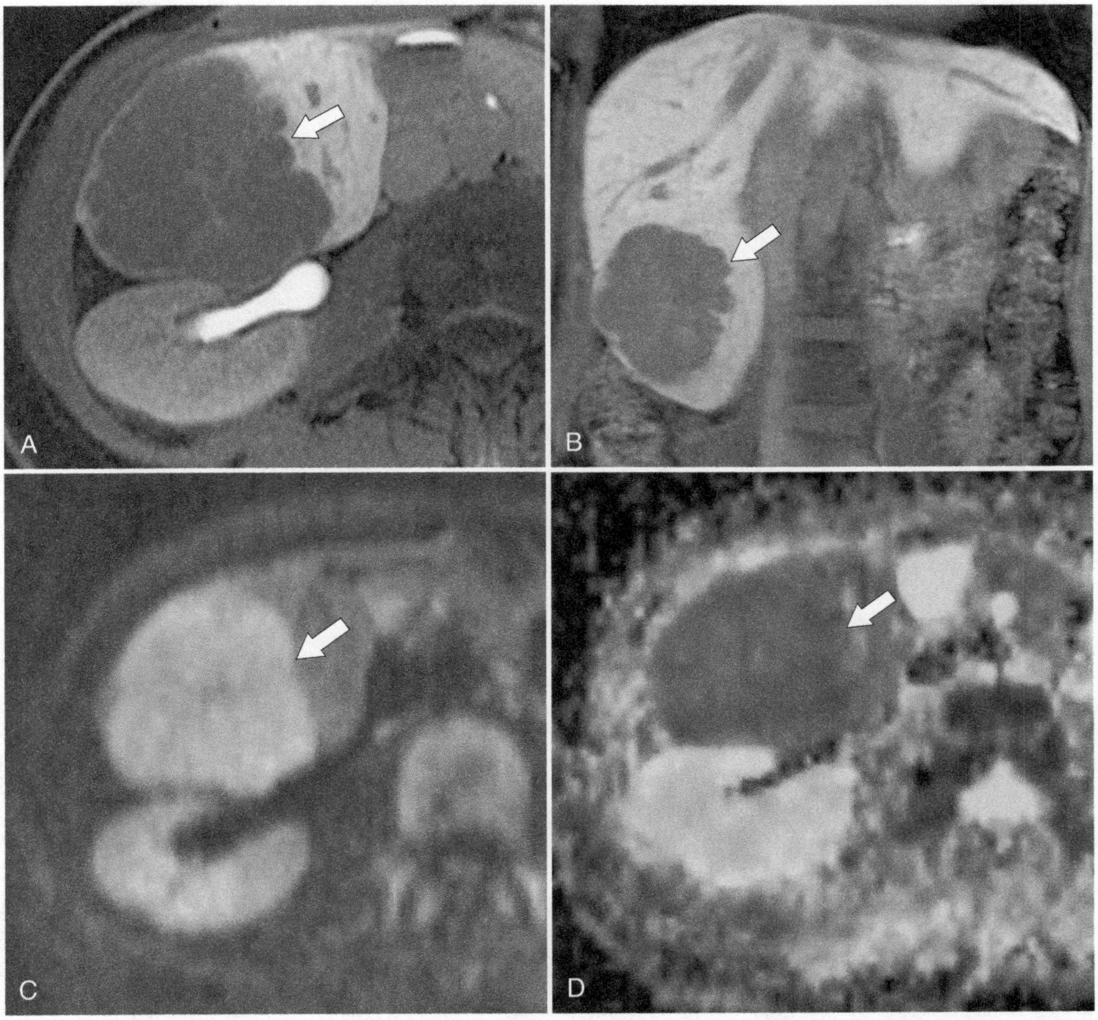

FIGURE 6-130. Axial (**A**) and coronal (**B**) 20-minute delayed postcontrast hepatobiliary agent imaging and B 600 DWI (**C**) and ADC maps (**D**) in a 36-year-old woman with fibrolamellar HCC (*arrows*). The lesion has no hepatocyte function and therefore is hypointense on delayed imaging. There is restricted diffusion with bright DWI signal and a dark ADC map.

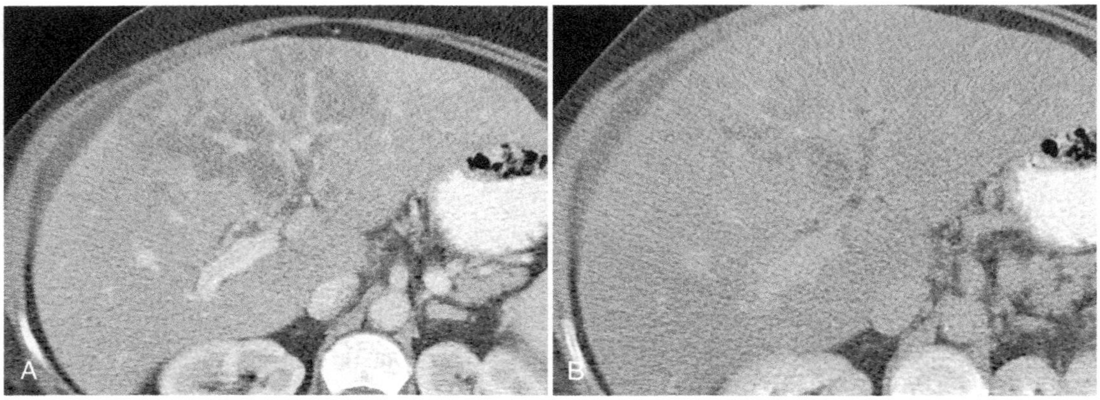

FIGURE 6-131. Axial PVP (**A**) and delayed (**B**) PVP contrast-enhanced CT in a 60-year-old woman with peripheral cholangiocarcinoma. A heterogeneous mass predominantly in segment IV of the liver mostly "fills in" on delayed imaging.

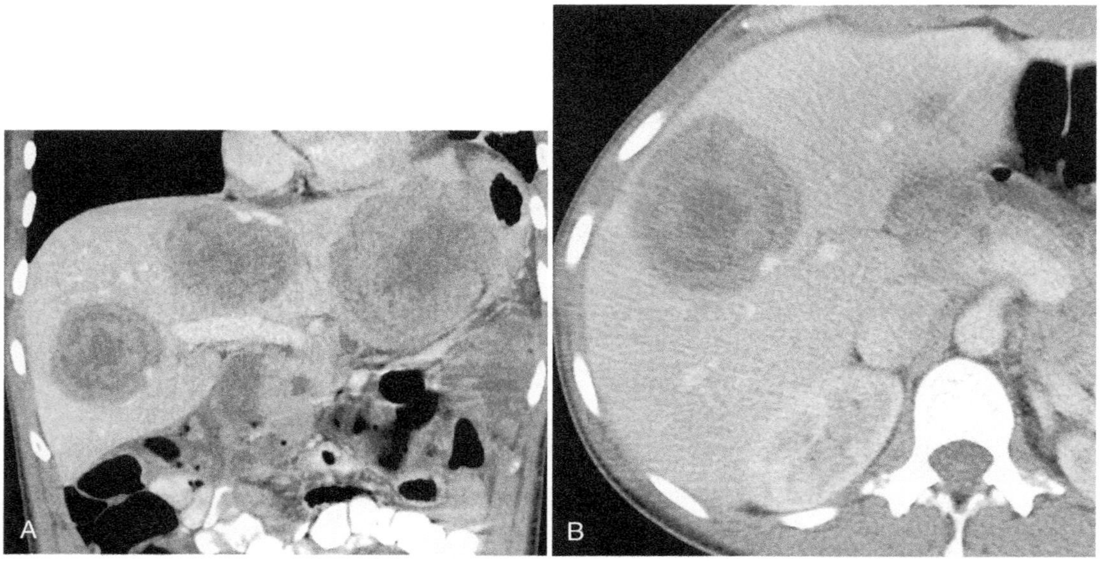

FIGURE 6-132. Coronal (**A**) and axial (**B**) contrast-enhanced CT in a 63-year-old man with several lesions representing primary hepatic non-Hodgkin lymphoma. The concentric peripheral washout is highly characteristic for malignant disease.

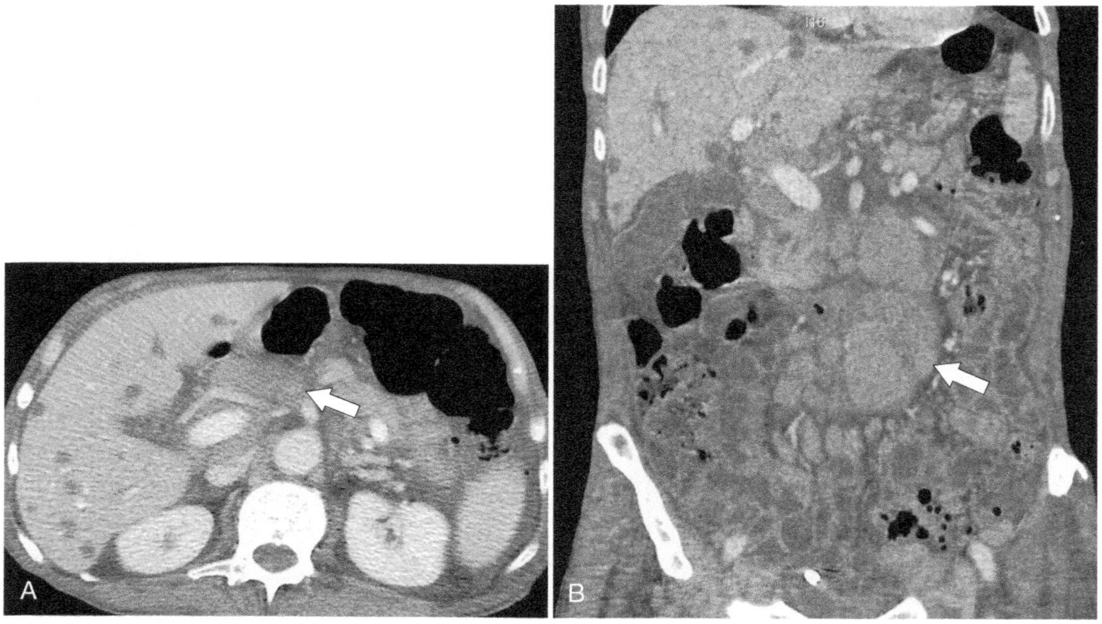

FIGURE 6-133. Axial (**A**) and coronal (**B**) contrast-enhanced CT in an 81-year-old man with multiple low-density hepatic lesions owing to acute lymphocytic leukemia. There is also marked mesenteric lymphadenopathy (*arrows*).

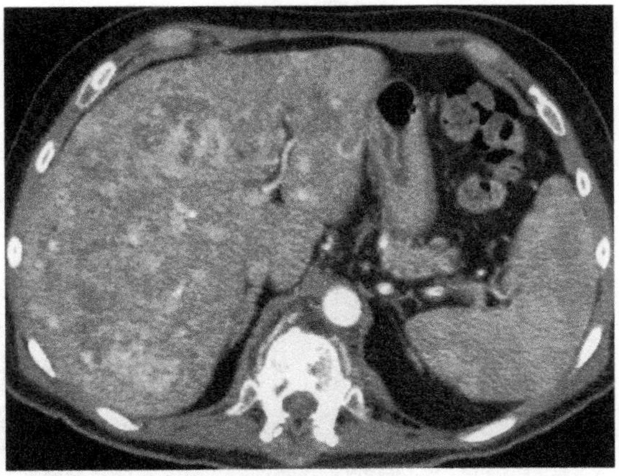

FIGURE 6-134. Arterial-phase contrast-enhanced CT in a 72-year-old man with angiosarcoma with a larger heterogeneous vascular mass almost completely replacing the right lobe. Smaller hypervascular metastases are also present in the left lobe.

Splenic manifestation of PTLD includes solitary nonspecific hypodense masses or, more usually, multiple, small, hypodense lesions.

Leukemia

Hepatic leukemic infiltration more commonly causes diffuse hepatomegaly (and often splenomegaly), but multiple, small, discrete neoplastic lesions are sometimes observed (Fig. 6-133).

Angiosarcoma

Angiosarcoma is a rare aggressive endothelial malignancy originating from mesenchymal cells. Predisposing risk factors include Thorotrast (radioactive alpha emitters), arsenic, hemochromatosis, neurofibromatosis, postradiation, and vinyl chloride. At cross-sectional imaging, the mass is highly heterogeneous, with, as its name suggests, areas of intense enhancement resulting from its vascularity (Fig. 6-134), particularly peripherally. Small angiosarcoma lesions can sometimes be confused with a hemangioma because the enhancement may be delayed.

Hepatoblastoma

The hepatoblastoma is the most common type of hepatic malignancy occurring in a younger population, usually children; most patients present before the age of 3 years. Presentation is usually accompanied by pain and an abdominal mass, which therefore is quite large at presentation. As with HCC, the alpha-fetoprotein level is often elevated. The disease is associated with familial adenomatous polyposis and Beckwith-Wiedemann* syndrome. At imaging there is usually a large heterogeneous mass, sometimes with areas of scattered calcification (Fig. 6-135).

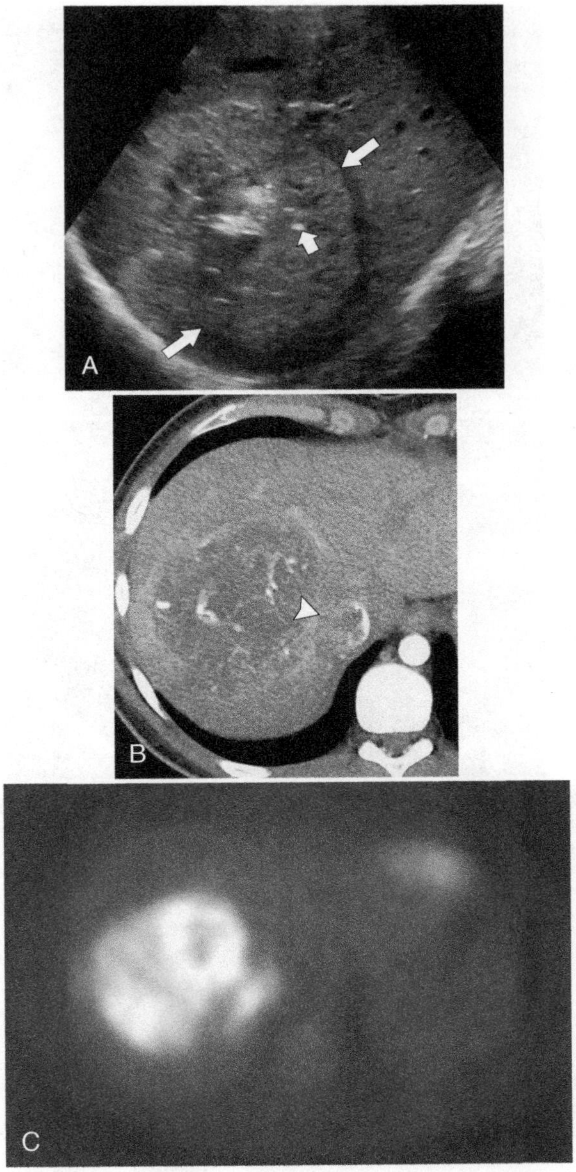

FIGURE 6-135. Sagittal US (**A**), axial arterial-phase contrast-enhanced CT (**B**), and PET (**C**) in a 20-year-old man with hepatoblastoma (*arrows*). Fine scattered calcification is present (*small arrow*). On CT the lesion demonstrates heterogeneous enhancement. There is an IVC tumor thrombus (*arrowhead*), and the lesion demonstrates marked FDG uptake at PET.

Hemangioendothelioma

Hemangioendothelioma is a disease seen in children; in adults it is known as epithelioid hemangioendothelioma. They are two distinct diseases. The former is the most common benign vascular tumor of childhood, and most patients present in the first 6 months of life, sometimes with heart failure because of marked arteriovenous shunting. Lesions are usually single, complex, and heterogeneous, demonstrating peripheral enhancement, often with evidence of arteriovenous shunting, so much so that the aorta may be attenuated below the origin of the celiac axis because of large-volume shunting to the hepatic tumor. Most lesions regress after 12 to 18 months, and no treatment is required.

Epithelioid hemangioendothelioma is a rare adult hepatic tumor, most common in middle-aged women, and is associated with the oral contraceptive pill and previous exposure to vinyl chloride. This is a highly aggressive and invasive tumor. At cross-sectional imaging, the diagnosis can be inferred from its frequent multinodular findings, mostly peripherally located, which can cause hepatic capsular retraction (owing to tumor fibrosis) with compensatory hypertrophy of the other normal liver segments. Some lesions can calcify. At contrast-enhanced CT, there is typically a thin, outer, nonenhancing rim, within which is an enhancing rind of tumor and nonenhancing inner regions. This feature may also be shown with CT and MRI (Fig. 6-136).

*John Bruce Beckwith (1933), American pathologist; Hans-Rudolph Wiedemann (1915-2006), German pediatrician.

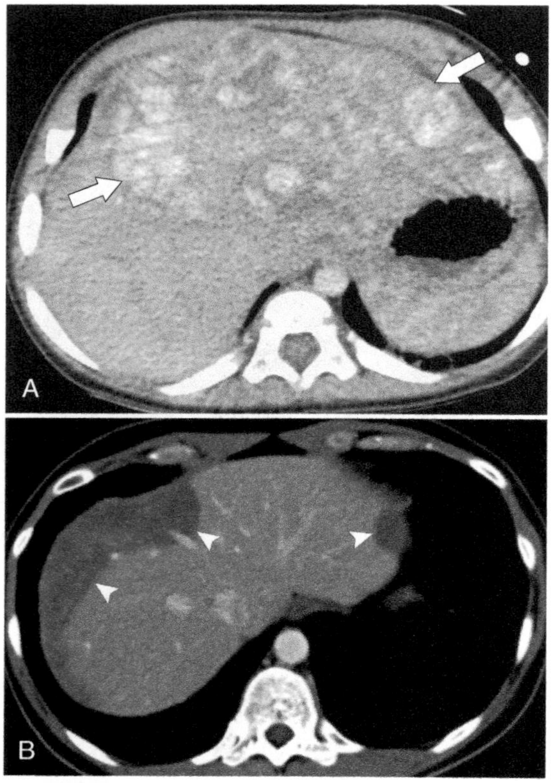

FIGURE 6-136. **A,** Axial contrast-enhanced CT in a 2-year-old boy with a large hypervascular hepatic hemangioendothelioma (*arrows*). **B,** Axial contrast-enhanced CT in a 55-year-old woman with a peripherally based mass representing epithelioid hemangioendothelioma (*arrowheads*).

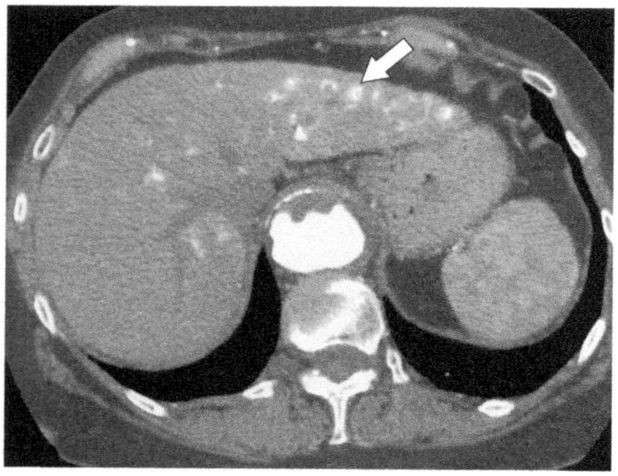

FIGURE 6-137. Arterial-phase CT in a 75-year-old man being investigated for aortic aneurysm demonstrates subtle left lobe arterial hyperattenuation (*arrow*) caused by transient hepatic attenuation defects from benign hepatic arterial portal shunting. These disappeared in the PVP.

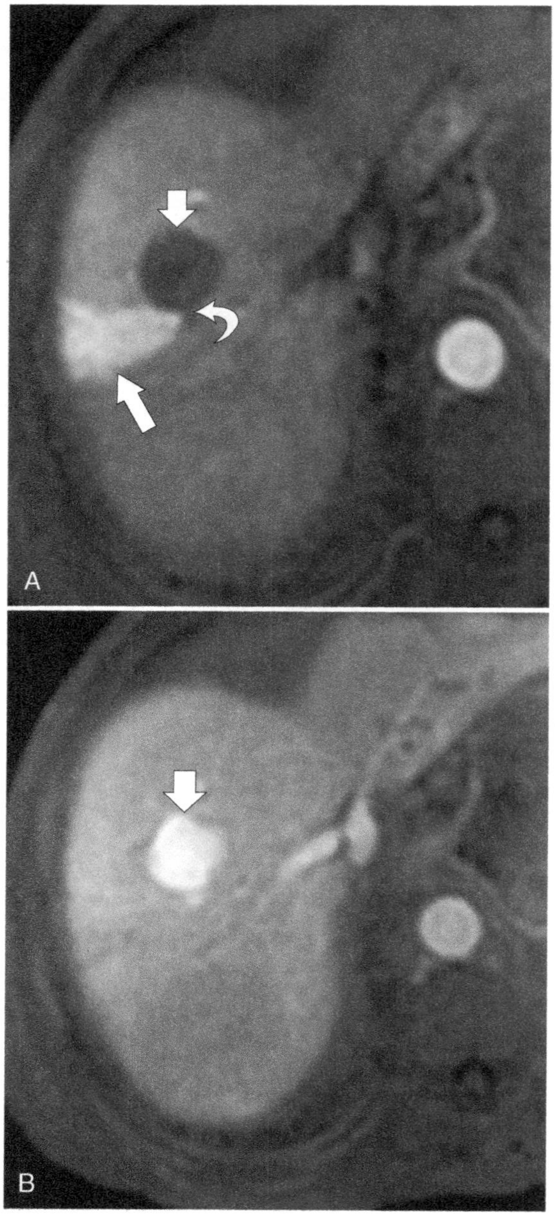

FIGURE 6-138. Axial arterial (**A**) and PVP (**B**) T1-weighted fat-saturated contrast-enhanced MRI in a 56-year-old man with an arterial peripheral wedge-shaped enhancement (*arrow*) that is transient (not seen on PVP). This is caused by a 3-cm portal hepatic vein shunt (*small arrows*) from a previous liver biopsy that compresses the portal vessels (*curved arrow*) to that hepatic segment outlined by the transient arterial shunt.

VASCULAR ANOMALIES

Transient Hepatic Attenuation and Intensity Differences

Transient hepatic attenuation differences (THADs) refer to CT (Fig. 6-137), and transient hepatic intensity differences (THIDs) to MRI (Fig. 6-138). These are brief (hence transient), typically peripheral, wedge-shaped or straight-lined arterial-phase blushes of enhancement seen at contrast-enhanced CT or MRI that disappear during the PVP. They can be observed within a whole lobe, a lobar segment, a segment, or a subcapsular region. They are caused by a number of mechanisms, including arterioportal shunts secondary to variety of nontumoral and tumoral causes, such as cirrhosis, trauma, hemangioma, cholangiocarcinoma, and HCC. Another cause is a reduction in portal venous inflow, either by a mass (tumor, abscess) or by portal or hepatic vein occlusion (Fig. 6-139). Under these circumstances the restricted portal venous flow is compensated for by increased arterial inflow, best seen beyond the compressive abnormality.

Arterioportal Shunts

Arterioportal shunts are caused by an abnormal direct communication between hepatic arteries and portal venous radicals. Therefore, on contrast-enhanced CT, there is early hepatic

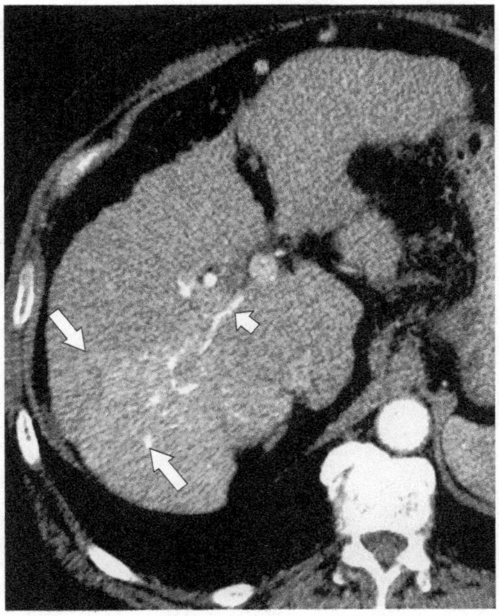

FIGURE 6-139. Axial arterial-phase contrast-enhanced CT in a 56-year-old man with cirrhosis and right portal vein thrombosis and a hyperdense wedge-shaped area on the right hepatic lobe (*arrows*) and prominent right hepatic artery (*small arrow*) resulting from arterial shunting.

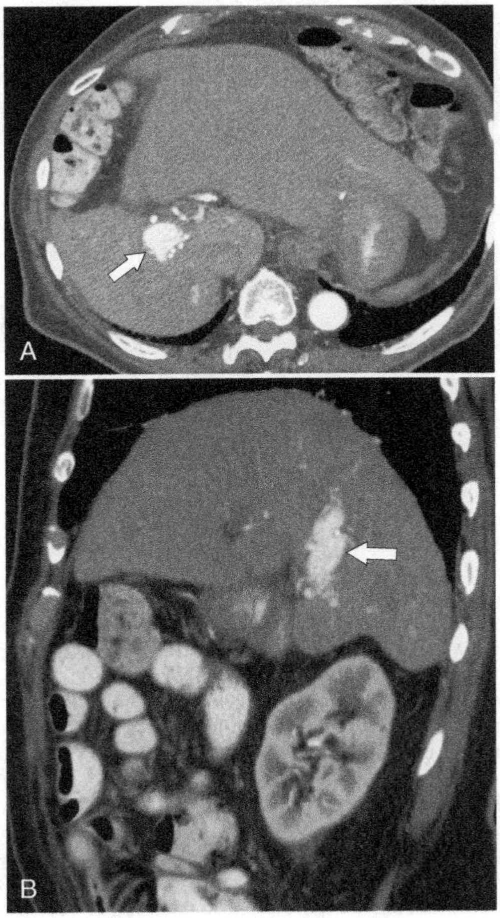

FIGURE 6-140. Axial (**A**) and sagittal (**B**) contrast-enhanced CT in a 76-year-old man with prior hepatic surgery and now with an arteriovenous fistula with early right portal vein enhancement (*arrows*).

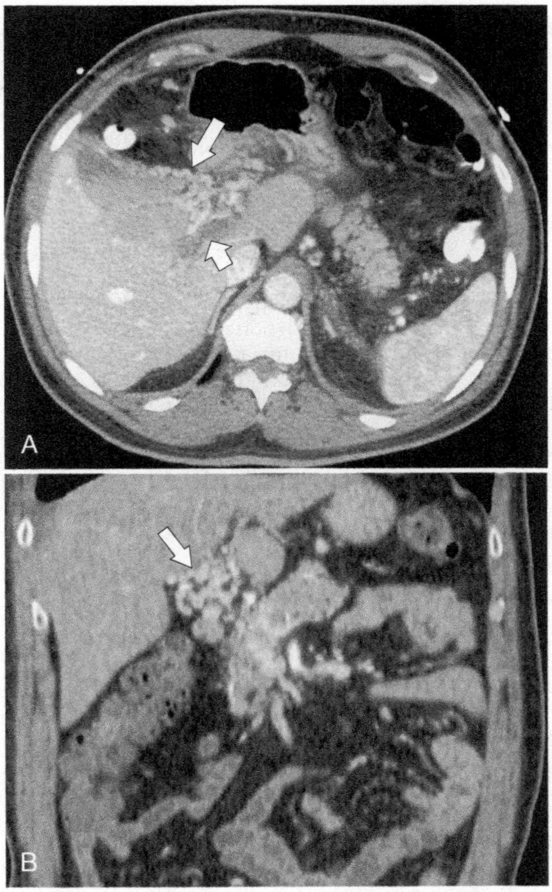

FIGURE 6-141. Axial (**A**) and coronal (**B**) CT in a 66-year-old man with PVP thrombosis (*short arrow*) and cavernous transformation of the portal vein (*arrows*).

enhancement of the portal venous area in question, typically wedge shaped. Most often, this is caused by cirrhosis and is trans-sinusoidal. This phenomenon can also unmask the presence of a small, as yet unrecognized metastasis that has created an arterioportal shunt and a wedge-shaped hypervascular area beyond it. HCCs frequently cause arterioportal shunting either within the primary tumor or as a result of treatment with radiofrequency ablation. Transplexal shunting is caused by arterial blood shunting to peribiliary venous plexuses and is typically seen in the perihilar region. This is less common and occurs with cirrhosis and portal vein obstruction. Hepatic arterial blood is abnormally diverted directly into the portal venous system at the level of the main vessels, sinusoids, or peribiliary venules. Causes are posttraumatic (particularly after interventional imaging procedures) or spontaneous in cirrhosis, but shunts can also be secondary to benign (hemangioma) and malignant (HCC) hepatic tumors (Fig. 6-140).

Evidence that a shunt is present at contrast-enhanced CT or MRI can be visualized as early (arterial phase) portal venous opacification, either of the larger portal veins or as isolated segmental or subsegmental enhancement. The latter is usually identified by a small, rounded, or oval blush, which is evidence of early portal opacification, not dilated arterial structures. Other features include a peripheral wedge-shaped area of enhancement (as in THIDs as high-pressure arterial blood is pumped into the segmental or subsegmental portal structures). Most shunts are not visible and are isodense by the time of portal venous scanning. Shunts in the setting of cirrhosis can be hard to differentiate from small HCCs, and close interval follow-up is indicated to exclude an enlarging tumor.

Hereditary Hemorrhagic Telangiectasia (Osler-Weber-Rendu Disease)

Hereditary hemorrhagic telangiectasia, or Osler-Weber-Rendu* disease, is an autosomal-dominant genetic defect resulting in excessive angiogenesis and the development of multiple telangiectasia of the skin, mucous membranes, and gastrointestinal tract with arteriovenous malformations in the lungs, liver, and brain. Hepatic arteriovenous malformations may be accompanied by portal venous shunting, which can lead to high-output cardiac failure.

Imaging with contrast-enhanced CT demonstrates an enlarged hepatic artery and branches with portal and hepatic venous dilatation caused by the multiple shunts (arteriovenous and telangiectasia), which cause early portal and hepatic venous opacification. The liver has a mosaic enhancement pattern (also seen in passive congestion and Budd-Chiari syndrome). Telangiectasia is recognized as small peripheral hyperattenuating blushes in the arterial phase (similar to some THIDs). Sometimes larger confluent vascular masses are identified. These findings along with a pertinent history and examination are usually diagnostic for the disease.

Portal Venous Occlusion

Portal venous occlusion is usually chronic in onset, mainly as a sequela of thrombosis secondary to venous stasis in cirrhosis. The thrombosis can also result from chronic local inflammatory conditions (e.g., pancreatitis). More acute onset is caused by thrombophlebitis from seeding of infected material (e.g., diverticulitis, appendicitis), hypercoagulable states, or invasion of the portal vein by tumor thrombus (e.g., HCC, pancreatic carcinoma). Segmental thrombosis is also common with localized intrahepatic tumors (e.g., cholangiocarcinoma, HCC, and metastases) (Fig. 6-125).

The imaging findings reflect whether the etiology is acute or chronic. At contrast-enhanced CT, the chronic form demonstrates portal vein occlusion, variceal dilatation of upstream (proximal) mesenteric veins, and formation of multiple portosystemic collaterals. Numerous periportal venous collaterals can also develop, permitting mesenteric venous return to bypass the occluded main portal vein, termed "cavernous transformation of the portal vein" (Fig. 6-141). Acute thrombosis on contrast-enhanced CT demonstrates a nonenhancing thrombus within the portal vein (Fig. 6-142), although tumor thrombus, particularly from HCC, may itself enhance and expand the portal vein. The diminished hepatic blood supply is compensated for by an increase in arterial blood (often with a visibly enlarged hepatic artery), which is recognized by high-attenuation enhancing parenchyma in the affected regions on the arterial phase as a result of the arterioportal shunting, which equilibrates on the PVP (Fig. 6-139). These findings can also be seen with contrast-enhanced MRI. Acute thrombus is typically high signal on both T1- and T2-weighted images. US can be the most useful imaging investigation, particularly in the acute phase, showing a hypoechoic defect in the portal vein with no flow at color Doppler, unless there is evidence of flow within a tumor thrombus (Fig. 6-143).

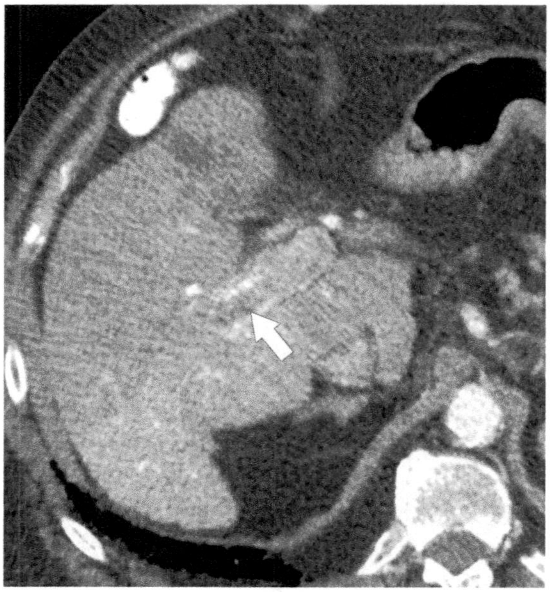

FIGURE 6-142. Axial contrast-enhanced CT in a 78-year-old with cirrhosis and acute portal vein thrombus (*arrow*).

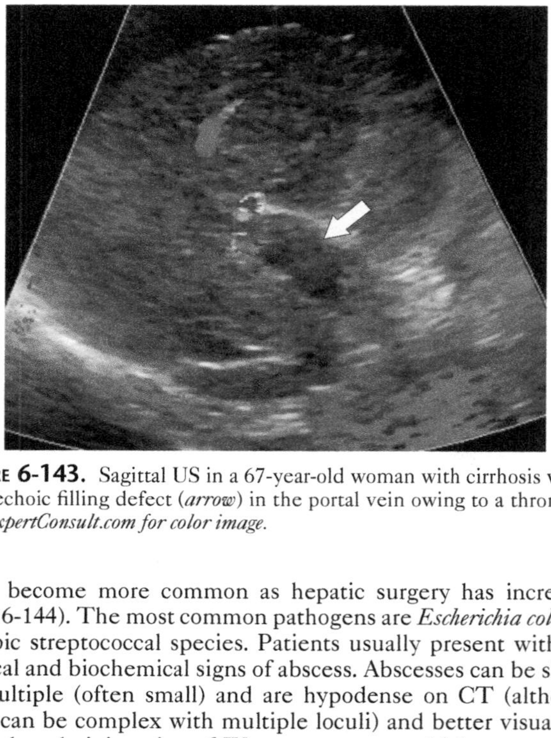

FIGURE 6-143. Sagittal US in a 67-year-old woman with cirrhosis with a hypoechoic filling defect (*arrow*) in the portal vein owing to a thrombus. *See ExpertConsult.com for color image.*

HEPATIC ABSCESS

Bacterial Abcess

Most hepatic abscesses are pyogenic and typically seed from the gastrointestinal tract (diverticulitis, appendicitis, inflammatory bowel disease) or biliary radicals (ascending cholangitis). Other causes include arterial seeding from bacterial endocarditis (or other chronic infective causes) and postoperative infections, which have become more common as hepatic surgery has increased (Fig. 6-144). The most common pathogens are *Escherichia coli* and aerobic streptococcal species. Patients usually present with the clinical and biochemical signs of abscess. Abscesses can be single or multiple (often small) and are hypodense on CT (although they can be complex with multiple loculi) and better visualized after the administration of IV contrast agent, which may resolve a thick, irregular, often enhancing wall (Fig. 6-145). They range from multiple small lesions, which are less common (Fig. 6-146), to lesions that can replace a whole lobe (Fig. 6-147). Gas within the collection is highly indicative of its infected nature because of gas-forming organisms (Fig. 6-148). Multiple septa are common and are better appreciated on US or MRI, but usually reflect multiple, small, coalescing lesions (Fig. 6-149). The surrounding hepatic parenchyma may enhance heterogeneously because of the adjacent inflammatory abscesses. On MRI the abscesses are usually hyperintense at T2-weighted imaging, often with associated periinflammatory increased T2 signal (Fig. 6-150). The lesions do not usually enhance, although rim enhancement, similar to that seen with CT, is observed.

*William Osler (1849-1919), Canadian physician; Frederick P. Weber (1863-1962), German physician; Henri J.L.M. Rendu (1844-1902), French physician.

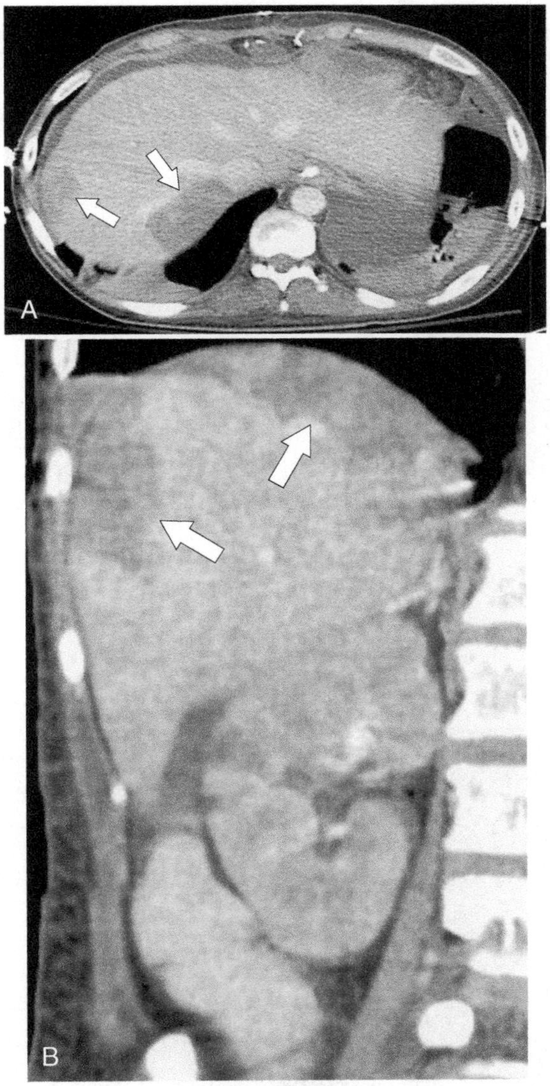

FIGURE 6-144. Axial (**A**) and coronal (**B**) contrast-enhanced CT in a 76-year-old with bacterial endocarditis and multiple hepatic septic emboli (*arrows*).

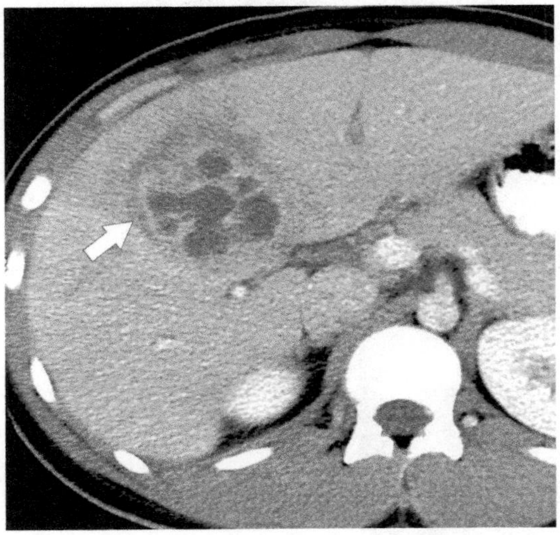

FIGURE 6-145. Axial contrast-enhanced CT in a 19-year-old man with a complex hypodense mass in segment V because of bacterial abscess. Peripheral hypodense areas (*arrow*) are commonly identified secondary to the associated hepatic inflammatory response.

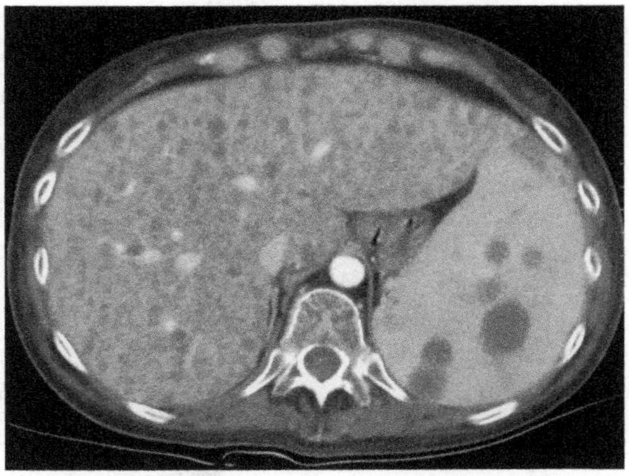

FIGURE 6-146. Axial contrast-enhanced CT in a 27-year-old with *Bartonella* infection (cat-scratch disease) of the liver and spleen as evidenced by muliple low-density abscesses in the liver and spleen.

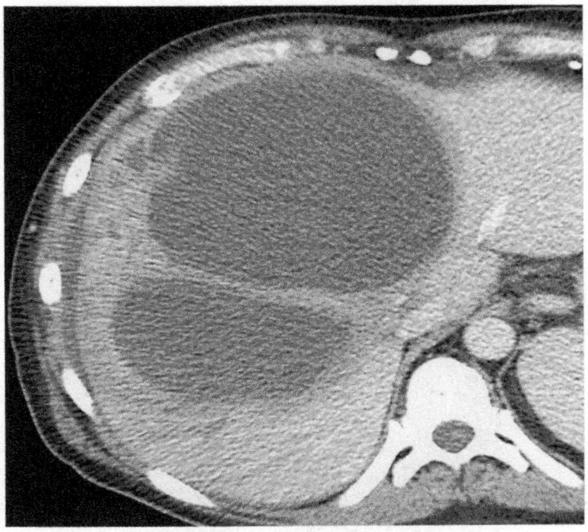

FIGURE 6-147. Axial contrast-enhanced CT in a 73-year-old man with a large, thick-walled loculated hepatic abscess.

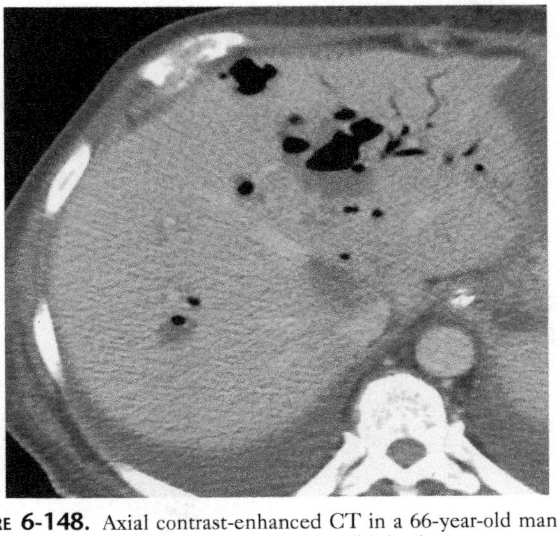

FIGURE 6-148. Axial contrast-enhanced CT in a 66-year-old man with multiple hepatic gas-fluid levels owing to multiple abscesses.

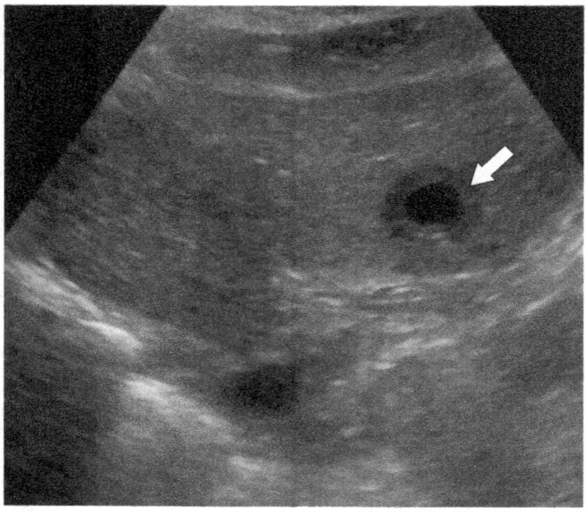

FIGURE 6-149. Transverse US in a 77-year-old female with a left lobe liver abscess (*arrow*). Hypoechoic pus is surrounded by a rind of infected liver.

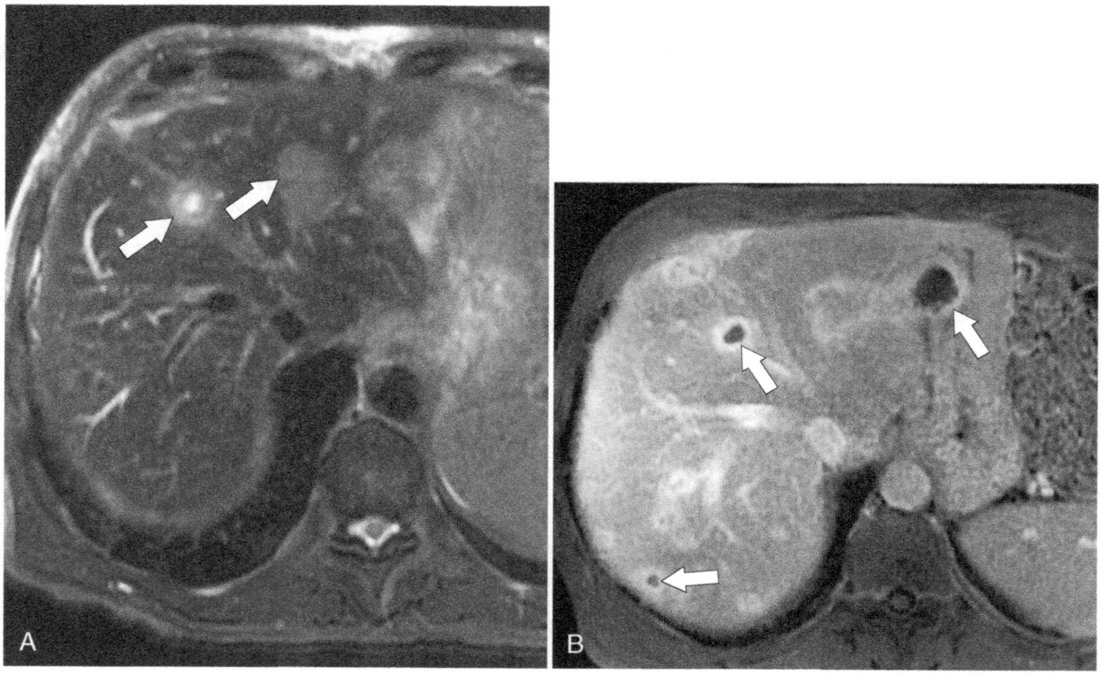

FIGURE 6-150. Axial T2-weighted (**A**) and postcontrast T1-weighted fat-saturated (**B**) MRI in a 66-year-old with multiple liver abscesses (*arrows*) caused by actinomycetes. T2 signal and wall enhancement are variable at CT.

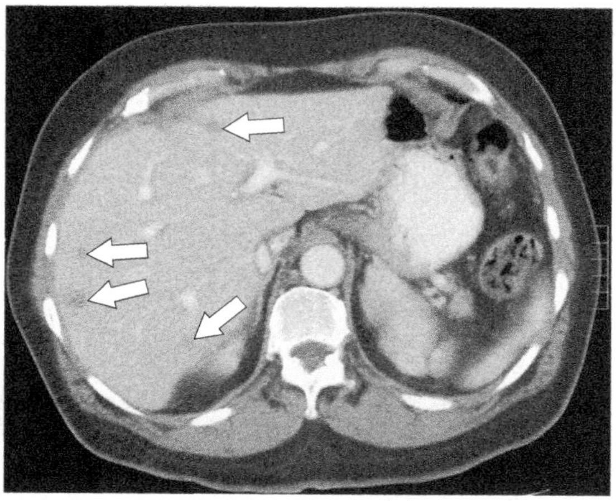

FIGURE 6-151. Axial CT in a 56-year-old man with several hypodense liver lesions (*arrows*) caused by candidal abscesses.

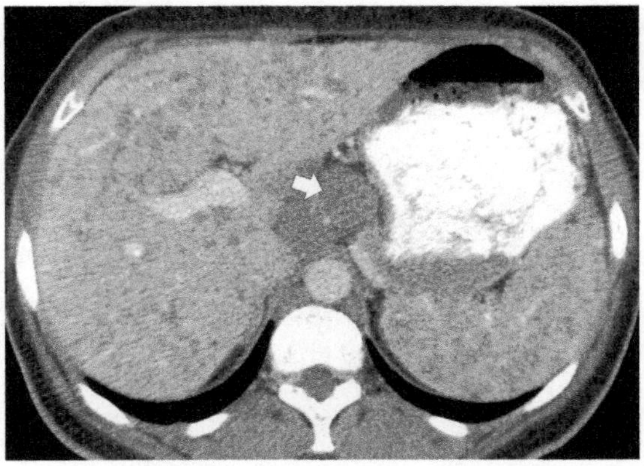

FIGURE 6-152. Axial contrast-enhanced CT in a 23-year-old man with diffuse hepatosplenic TB and retroperitoneal lymphadenopathy (*small arrow*).

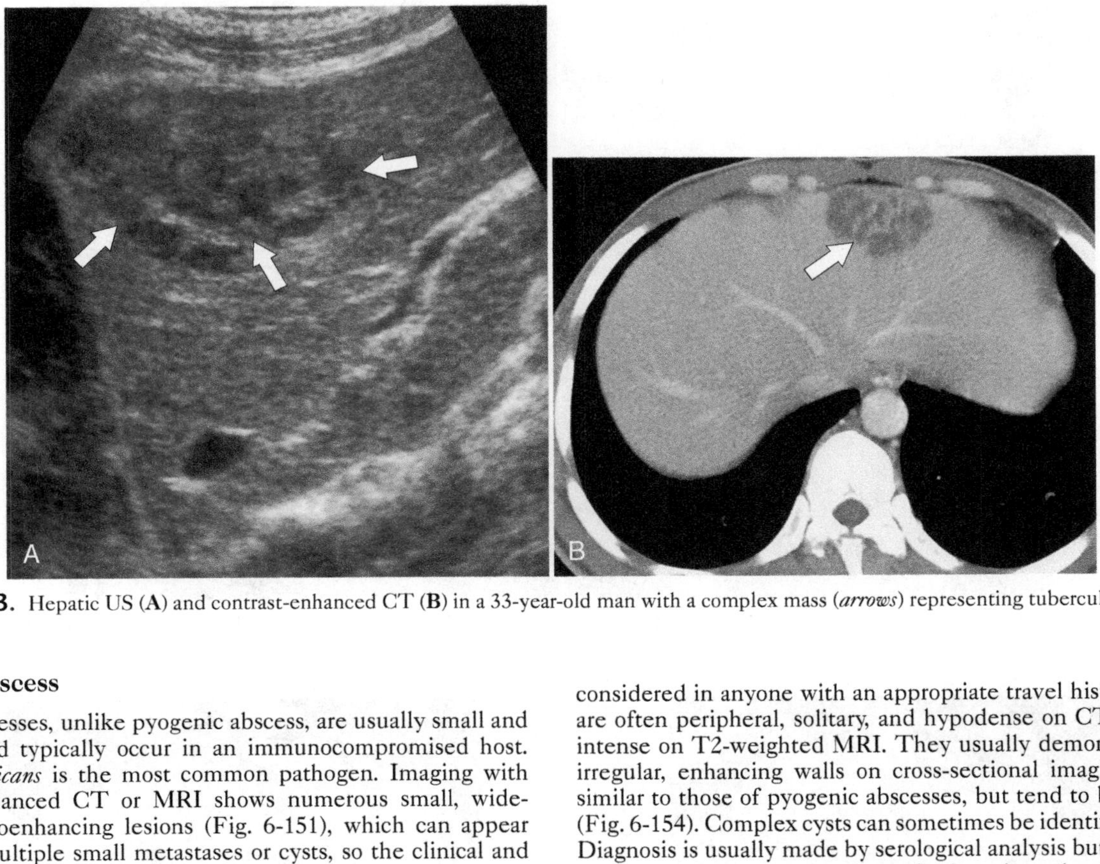

FIGURE 6-153. Hepatic US (**A**) and contrast-enhanced CT (**B**) in a 33-year-old man with a complex mass (*arrows*) representing tuberculous infection.

Fungal Abscess

Fungal abscesses, unlike pyogenic abscess, are usually small and multiple and typically occur in an immunocompromised host. *Candida albicans* is the most common pathogen. Imaging with contrast-enhanced CT or MRI shows numerous small, widespread, hypoenhancing lesions (Fig. 6-151), which can appear similar to multiple small metastases or cysts, so the clinical and laboratory findings are the key to the diagnosis.

Tuberculosis

With acute tuberculous hepatic infection (as in the spleen), numerous scattered hypoenhancing lesions (similar to fungal infection) are typically seen (Fig. 6-152). Diagnosis can be difficult because TB may be unsuspected unless there is overt evidence of the disease elsewhere. Less commonly the infection produces a solitary tuberculous abscess (Fig. 6-153).

Amebic Abscess

The organism *Entamoeba histolytica* typically seeds to the liver from the colon after cyst ingestion from contaminated water, with release of trophozoites into the mesenteric venous system. Abscess formation can be single or multiple and should be considered in anyone with an appropriate travel history. Lesions are often peripheral, solitary, and hypodense on CT and hyperintense on T2-weighted MRI. They usually demonstrate thick, irregular, enhancing walls on cross-sectional imaging, not dissimilar to those of pyogenic abscesses, but tend to be unilocular (Fig. 6-154). Complex cysts can sometimes be identified with US. Diagnosis is usually made by serological analysis but less often is based on culture after needle aspiration, since the diagnosis will not have been considered.

Echinococcus (Hydatid)

Echinococcus granulosus infection results from the dog tapeworm and is endemic in cattle-rearing areas, with the human acting as an intermediate host. *Echinococcus multilocularis* is acquired from rat tapeworms and is less common. The tapeworm embryos can disseminate throughout the human body after penetrating the small intestine. Patients usually present with long-standing infection. In the liver, infection is typically cystic and multilocular (Fig. 6-155), with calcified walls, depending on the longevity of infection (Fig. 6-156). Circumferential wall calcification usually indicates nonactive infection. A highly characteristic feature is "daughter cysts," which are cysts, predominantly located peripherally, within a larger "mother" cyst (Fig. 6-155). Another highly

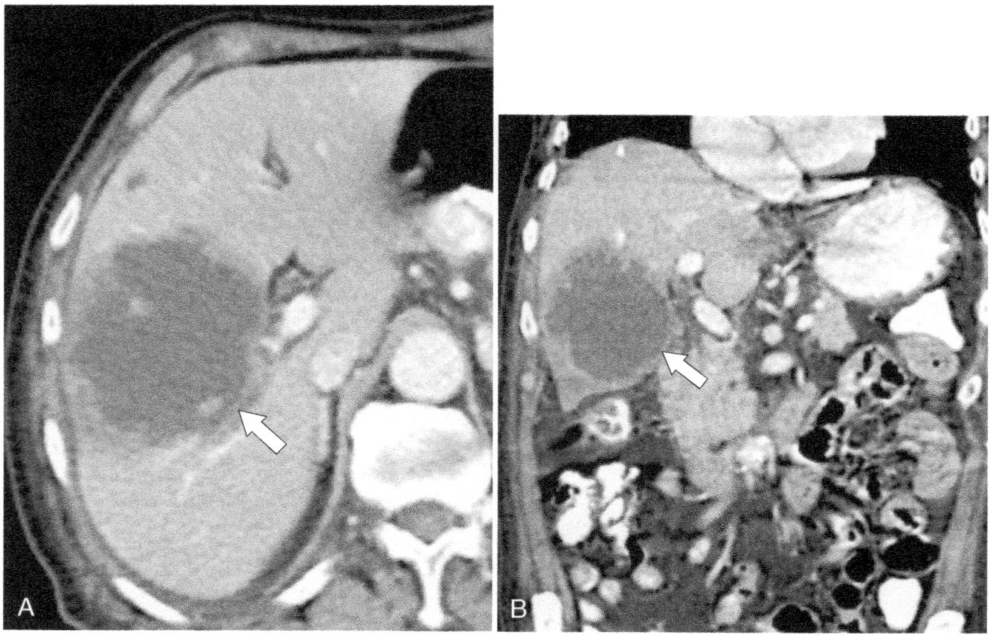

FIGURE 6-154. Axial (**A**) and coronal (**B**) contrast-enhanced CT in a 51-year-old man with amebic liver abscess (*arrows*).

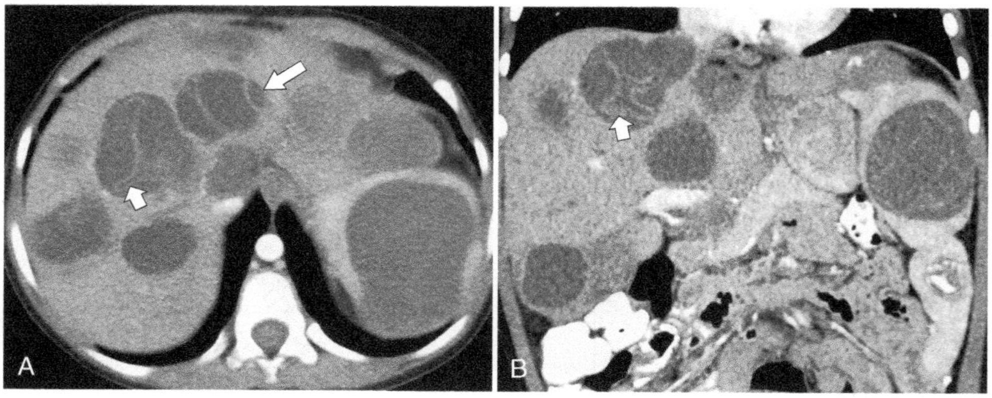

FIGURE 6-155. Axial (**A**) and coronal (**B**) contrast-enhanced CT in a 7-year-old boy with hydatid disease of the liver and spleen with daughter cysts (*arrow*) and a "drooping lily" sign (*small arrows*).

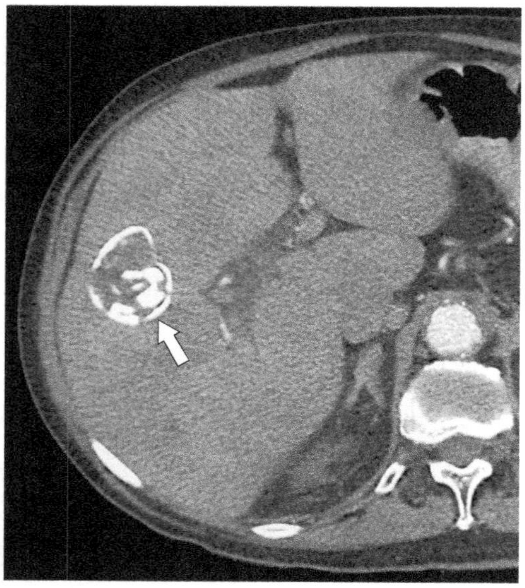

FIGURE 6-156. Axial contrast-enhanced CT in a 67-year-old woman with a calcified mass due to prior hydatid infection and cyst "death" (*arrow*).

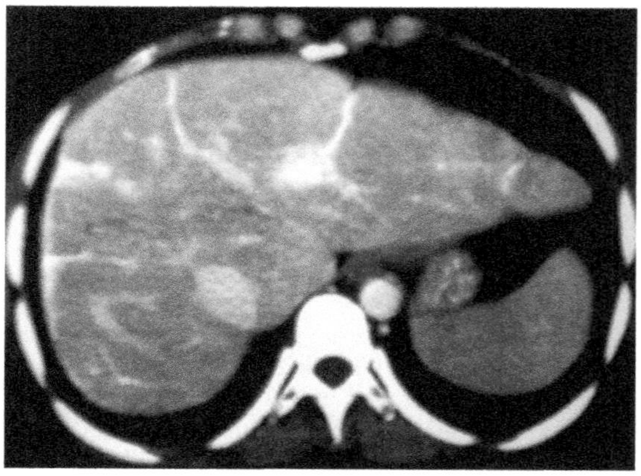

FIGURE 6-157. Axial contrast-enhanced CT in a 19-year-old man with a fibrotic "turtle-backed" liver as a result of chronic schistosomiasis.

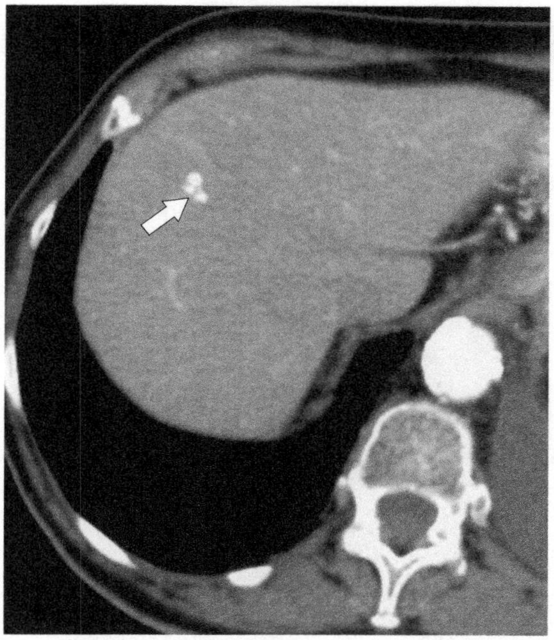

FIGURE 6-158. Axial contrast-enhanced CT with intrahepatic calcification (granuloma) owing to prior TB infection (*arrow*).

characteristic feature is the "water lily" sign, representing the walls of a dead or dying cyst (Fig. 6-155) that collapses within the larger cystic complex. The cyst wall may enhance, similar to other infected abscesses.

The major risk from hepatic hydatid cyst infection is rupture, which can be fatal if into the lungs or peritoneum. Percutaneous aspiration, however, is not contraindicated unless the wall is calcified because of difficulty penetrating the cyst wall. Rarely, hydatid cysts are large enough to cause obstructive jaundice. The diagnosis is readily made with an accompanying history and serological testing. Similar to that of amebic abscess, the diagnosis may not be made until an aspirate is cultured or analyzed microscopically. Treatment is with antiparasitic medication and aspiration for smaller lesions or catheter placement for larger lesions.

Hepatic Schistosomiasis

Of the three main schistosomal species (*Schistosoma hematobium, S. japonicum,* and *S. mansoni*), *S. mansoni* is most likely to infect the liver. The life cycle involves an intermediate freshwater snail host (asexual reproductive stage) and humans as the definitive host for sexual reproduction. Eggs excreted by humans release miracidia that infest the intermediate host, a freshwater snail, where they evolve into cercariae, which are released back into the water. These penetrate the skin of human bathers and are transported to the lungs and heart, then to the mesenteric venous system, and finally come to reside in periportal venules. Host immune response can result in parasitic death with granulomatous formation and subsequent fibrosis, resulting in cirrhosis (particularly centrally) and portal hypertension. Because the disease is endemic in countries with endemic hepatitis B and C, the two diseases often exacerbate the complications of each other, and the complications of cirrhosis are more profound and develop earlier.

The imaging findings are periportal edema and fibrosis, mainly at the porta hepatis, but as with other cirrhoses the liver is generally irregular in shape. Capsular and hepatic septal calcification can be identified, characteristic of schistosomal infection, and there may be linear hyperdense strands of fibrotic tissue, giving a so-called turtle-backed appearance (Fig. 6-157). Secondary effects of portal hypertension are common (mesenteric varices, splenomegaly, and ascites).

Box 6-8. Hepatic Calcifications

Granulomatous disease (TB, sarcoid)
Metastatic disease: mucinous tumors (ovarian, colon, stomach, appendiceal), osteosarcoma
HCC
Abscess
Parasitic disease
Cyst
Hemangioma
Hematoma

TB, Tuberculosis; *HCC*, hepatocellular carcinoma.

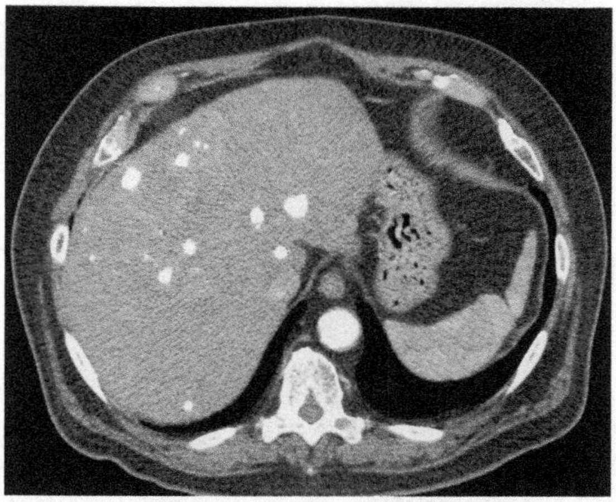

FIGURE 6-159. Axial contrast-enhanced CT in a 50-year-old man with multiple calcified osteosarcoma metastases in the liver.

HEPATIC CALCIFICATIONS (BOX 6-8)

Calcified granulomas from TB are common worldwide but rarer outside endemic countries (Fig. 6-158). In the United States, histoplasmosis is more common and even endemic in some areas. Typically, caseating granulomas heal with small, punctate areas of calcification, sometimes throughout the liver (and also spleen). The calcification in TB is often coarser than that seen with histoplasmosis. Sarcoidosis, a noncaseating granulomatous disease, can also develop multiple, small, punctate, calcified areas within the hepatic parenchyma. Other infections that can lead to hepatic calcification include wall calcification in treated abscess (e.g., pyogenic, amebic, and hydatid disease).

Malignant calcification within the liver is usually secondary to mucinous metastatic disease (e.g., from the colon, ovary, or pancreas) (Fig. 6-105). Very rarely, osteosarcoma can metastasize and calcify within the liver (Fig. 6-159). Hepatic calcification also occurs in primary liver tumors. HCC calcification is uncommon but definitely recognized and is observed far more often (up to 30%) in fibrolamellar HCC (Fig. 6-160). Rarer hepatic primary tumors, including hemangioendotheliomas, hamartomas, and hepatoblastomas, can also calcify (Fig. 6-135). Hamartoma, a rare hepatic benign tumor, can demonstrate calcification (Fig. 6-161). Very rarely, benign large hemangiomas also calcify.

Hematomas, particularly if subcapsular, are prone to calcification. Other capsular calcification can occur with diffuse peritonitis (particularly meconium peritonitis).

Rarely identified in the West, the parasite *Armillifer armillatus* can invade the liver and result in multiple, small, comma-shaped calcifications when healed.

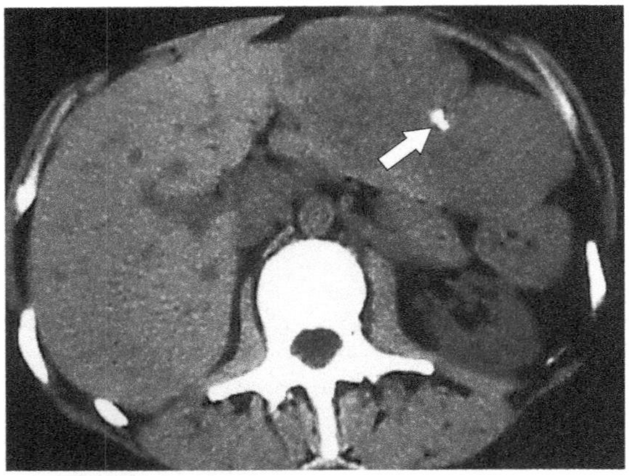

FIGURE 6-160. Axial noncontrast CT in a 35-year-old woman with central scar calcification (*arrow*) in a fibrolamellar HCC.

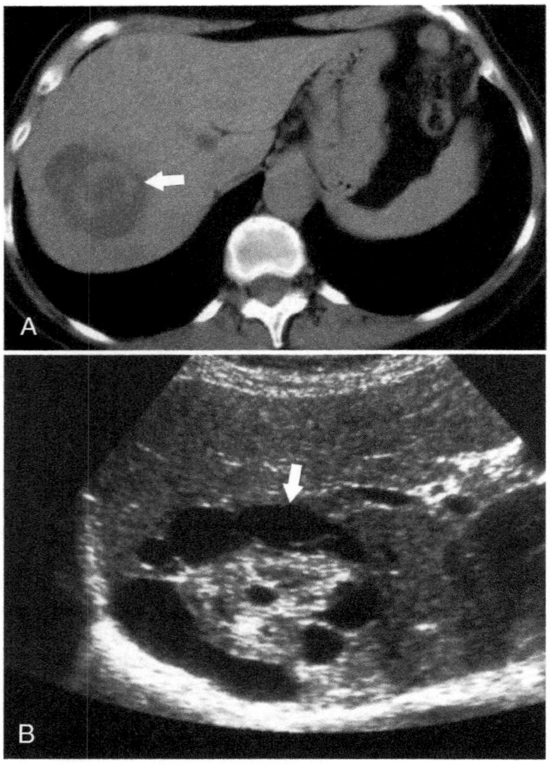

FIGURE 6-161. Axial non-contrast-enhanced CT (**A**) and US (**B**) in a 48-year-old man with a hepatic hamartoma (*arrows*).

THOROTRAST

Thorotrast was a widely used angiographic contrast agent that was withdrawn from the market in the 1950s because of its alpha-emitting properties. After intravenous administration it distributed throughout many tissues, particularly the liver and spleen. The biological half-life is approximately 22 years, so residual Thorotrast exposed patients to lifelong radiation and the risk of carcinogenesis, particularly angiosarcoma, cholangiocarcinoma, and leukemia. Its appearance at imaging is characteristic, with diffuse hyperdense splenic and hepatic material on CT (Fig. 6-162).

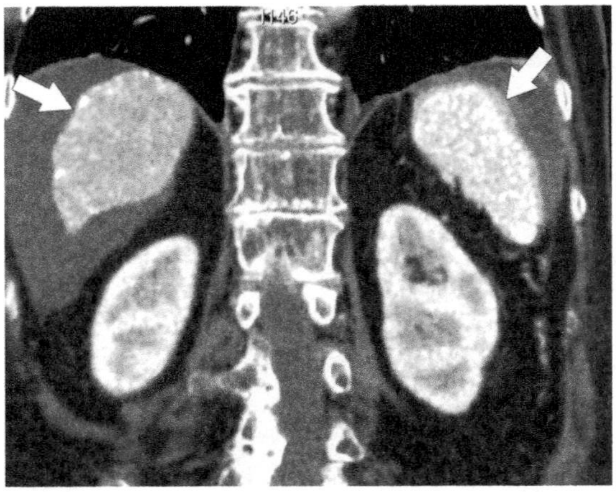

FIGURE 6-162. Coronal contrast-enhanced CT with diffuse hyperattenuation in the liver and spleen resulting from prior Thorotrast administration (*arrows*).

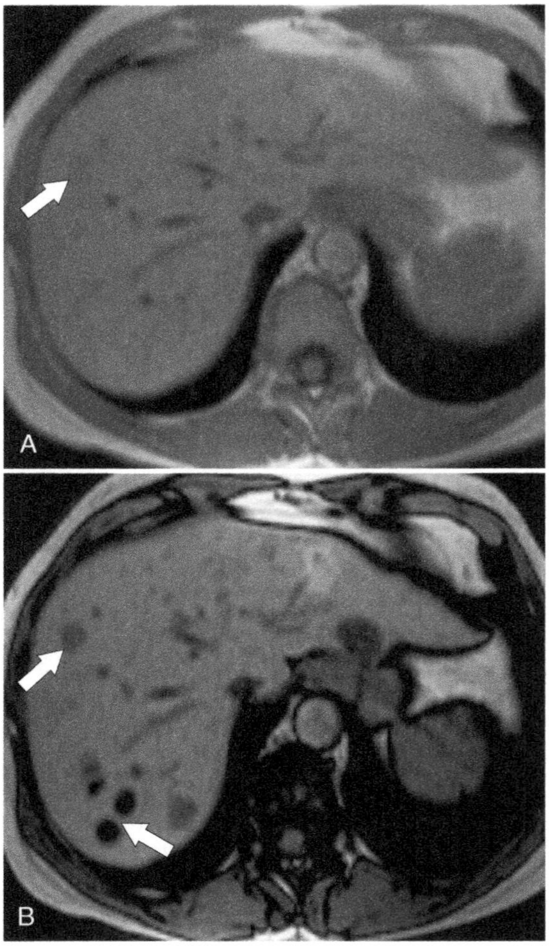

FIGURE 6-163. Axial in-phase (**A**) and out-of-phase (**B**) MRI in a 35-year-old with multiple adenomas (*arrows*) that contain fat (signal drop-off on out-of-phase MRI).

Box 6-9. Hepatic Lesions Containing Macroscopic Fat

BENIGN
Adenoma
Angiomyolipoma
Adrenal rest
Teratoma
Lipoma
Langerhans cell histiocytosis
Extramedullary hematopoiesis
Pseudolipoma of Glisson capsule
Omentum (postoperative packing)

MALIGNANT
Hepatocellular carcinoma
Fibrolamellar carcinoma
Metastases (liposarcoma, teratoma, renal cell)
Primary liposarcoma

FAT-CONTAINING LIVER LESIONS

Given that the characterization of hepatic tumors is generally required regardless of whether the patient has an underlying primary malignancy, the presence and distribution of macroscopic fat within the lesion help to minimize the differential diagnosis (Box 6-9). The presence of fat can be detected with US or CT, but the most specific imaging test is fat suppression MRI, particularly for smaller lesions. Ideally, CT is performed with and without contrast administration because subtle fatty areas might be overlooked with contrast-enhanced CT only.

Benign Fatty Lesions

Focal Fat

Focal fat is described earlier in this chapter.

Hepatic Adenoma (see earlier in this chapter)

Hepatic adenomatous cells may contain fat, which can be intracellular or intercellular. It can sometimes be recognized macroscopically, although recognition is reported to be <10% with CT but up to 77% with MRI, which is more sensitive for the detection of smaller concentrations of fat (Fig. 6-163). The detection of macroscopic fat is useful in distinguishing adenoma from FNH, which rarely contains fat.

Angiomyolipoma

Hepatic angiomyolipoma (AML) is histologically similar to the more common renal AML but is much rarer and less commonly associated with tuberous sclerosis. The appearance of AMLs on cross-sectional imaging depends on the proportion of lipomatous, angiomatous, and myelomatous tissue (Fig. 6-164). The angiomyomatous components tend to be on the periphery, which enhances intensely and generally for a longer period than HCC, with which AML is sometimes confused. The fat component also enhances because it is well vascularized, unlike HCCs that also contain macroscopic fat. However, up to 50% of hepatic AMLs do not contain macroscopic fat, making them even harder to differentiate from other hepatic tumors.

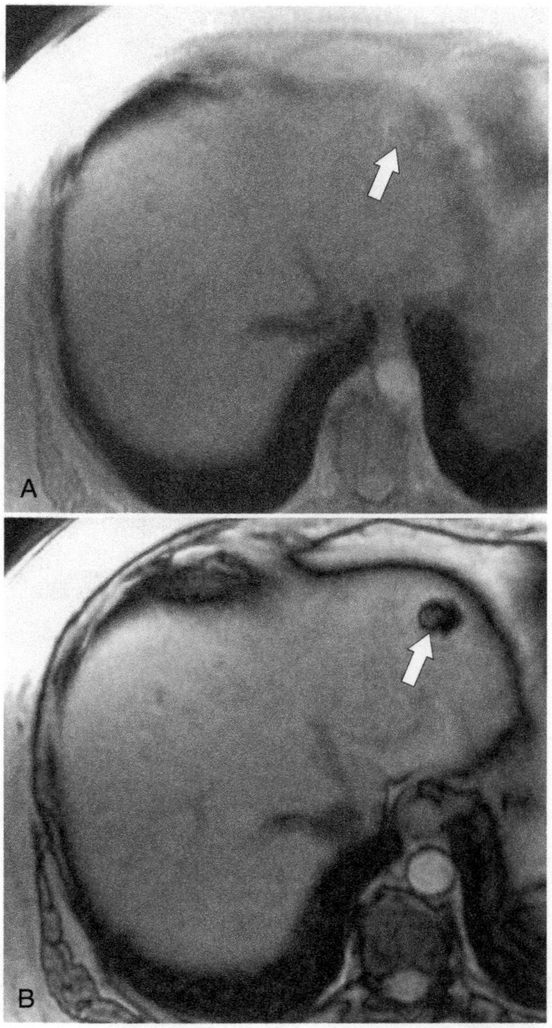

FIGURE 6-164. Axial in-phase (**A**) and out-of-phase (**B**) MRI in a 55-year-old woman with signal drop-off on out-of-phase imaging in a hepatic AML (*arrows*).

Adrenal Rest

The adrenal rest is a rare phenomenon in which ectopic adrenocortical cells collect in an extraadrenal location and can be hormonally functional. Its appearance can be difficult to distinguish from fat-containing adenoma, HCC, and angiomyelolipoma because it shows patchy areas of macroscopic fat within the lesion and areas of soft tissue enhancement. The diagnosis will probably be made only at biopsy, although the clue to the diagnosis may be inferred from the clinical findings if the lesion is hyperfunctioning.

Hepatic Teratoma

Even though rare in the liver, teratomas are usually secondary to extrahepatic teratomas that are enveloped by the liver rather than true primary liver lesions. As with teratomas elsewhere, the lesion can contain a variety of tissues, including calcification, fat, hair, teeth, and proteinaceous material (Fig. 6-107). As in the pelvis, the lesion shows a fat/fluid level that is highly suggestive of a teratoma.

Lipoma

A rare fatty tumor within the liver, lipoma is readily recognized on CT by its uniform fat content, lack of enhancement on contrast-enhanced CT and MRI, and signal loss with MRI fat-suppression techniques (Fig. 6-165).

Langerhans Cell Histiocytosis

Hepatic involvement in Langerhans* cell histiocytosis is uncommon, and most patients have extensive disease elsewhere. Most lesions are of soft tissue density, but some contain xanthomatous components, the lipomatous macroscopic nature of which can be recognized with US, CT, and MRI.

*Paul Langerhans (1847-1888), German pathologist.

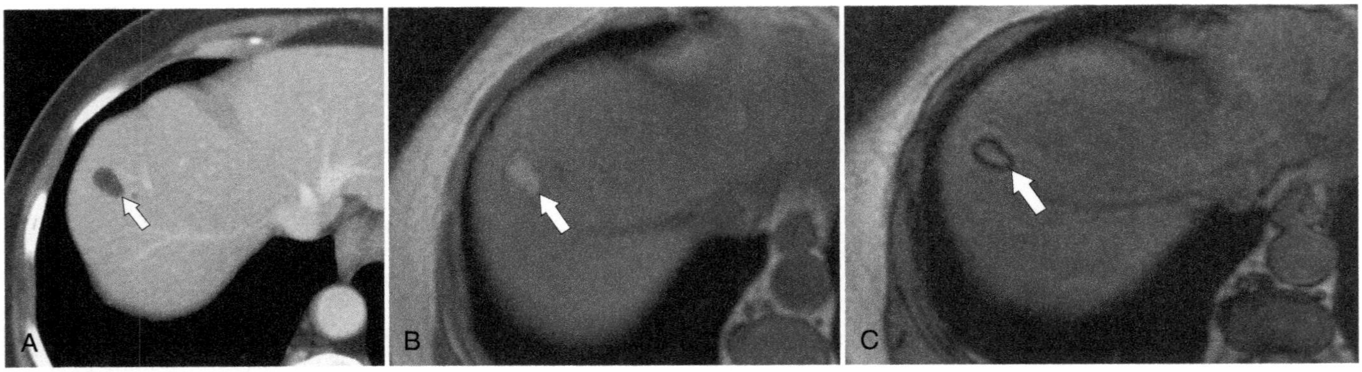

FIGURE 6-165. Axial postcontrast CT (**A**) and in-phase (**B**) and out-of-phase (**C**) MRI in a 57-year-old woman with a segment VIII lipoma. The lesion is of fat density at CT and bright on in-phase MRI, and demonstrates a chemical shift artifact on out-of-phase MRI (*arrows*).

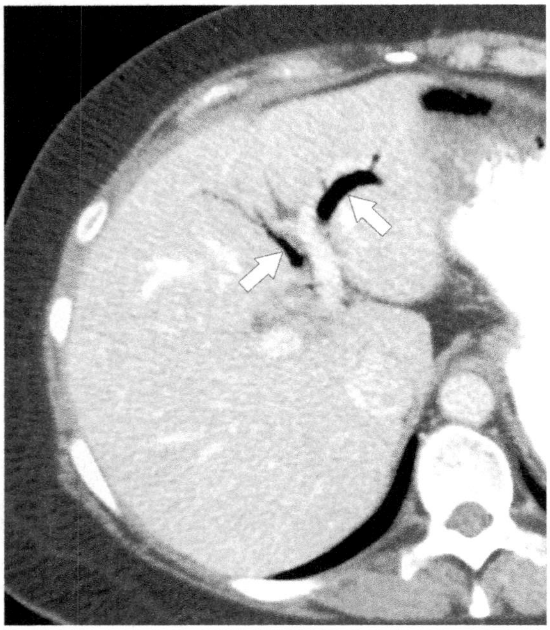

FIGURE 6-166. Axial contrast-enhanced CT in a 59-year-old woman with biliary gas (*arrows*), centered more centrally than portal venous gas.

Pseudolipoma of Glisson Capsule

Pseudolipoma of the Glisson† capsule is more commonly known as hepatic pseudolipoma and is not a true hepatic lesion. Rather, it occurs when the liver envelops degenerated peritoneal fat, most likely detached epiploic appendix.

Lipopeliosis

Peliosis (see earlier in this chapter) is caused by dilated blood-filled sinusoids in the liver. Lipopeliosis, however, is peliosis in a steatotic liver, in which fatty necrosis fills the dilated liver sinusoids.

Extramedullary Hematopoiesis

Usually extramedullary hematopoiesis involves the liver and spleen diffusely, but rarely it is focal and mass like, sometimes with macroscopic fat. When in the liver, extramedullary hematopoiesis may be confused with HCC.

†Francis Glisson (1599-1677), British anatomist and physician.

Box 6-10. Intrahepatic Gas

Intraductal biliary gas (common after surgery or ERCP, rarely cholangitis)
Portal venous gas
Abscess
Emphysematous cholecystitis

ERCP, Endoscopic retrograde cholangiopancreatography.

Postoperative Packing

Sometimes omentum is used to pack the space of a resected hepatic tumor or a larger cystic lesion (e.g., hydatid cyst) that has been drained. The correct diagnosis is made with adjacent surgical clips as evidence of prior surgery.

Malignant Fatty Lesions

Hepatocellular Carcinoma

Hepatocellular carcinoma develops in a cirrhotic liver, which usually presents as a hypervascular mass (see earlier in this chapter), but irregular and patchy fatty change caused by fatty metamorphosis can be observed in up to 35% of patients (Fig. 6-119). The diagnosis of HCC rather than other fat-containing lesions is suspected because of its presence in a cirrhotic liver and intense arterial enhancement characteristics. Fibrolamellar carcinoma (see earlier in this chapter) sometimes contains patches of macroscopic fat, although less commonly than HCC.

Liposarcoma

Most hepatic liposarcomas are metastatic, but primary hepatic liposarcoma has been reported. Its appearance is similar to liposarcoma elsewhere, with a large, predominantly lipomatous mass and multiple septa interspersed with enhancing soft tissue components.

Metastatic Disease

Liposarcoma uncommonly metastasizes to the liver, and the diagnosis is usually evident because of the retroperitoneal or extremity primary malignancy. Very rarely, renal cell cancer contains macroscopic fat. Metastatic teratomas, when they metastasize to the liver, may also demonstrate fatty lesions (Fig. 6-107).

INTRAHEPATIC GAS

The presence of intrahepatic gas is either benign and of little concern or the harbinger of a fatal outcome for the patient (Box 6-10).

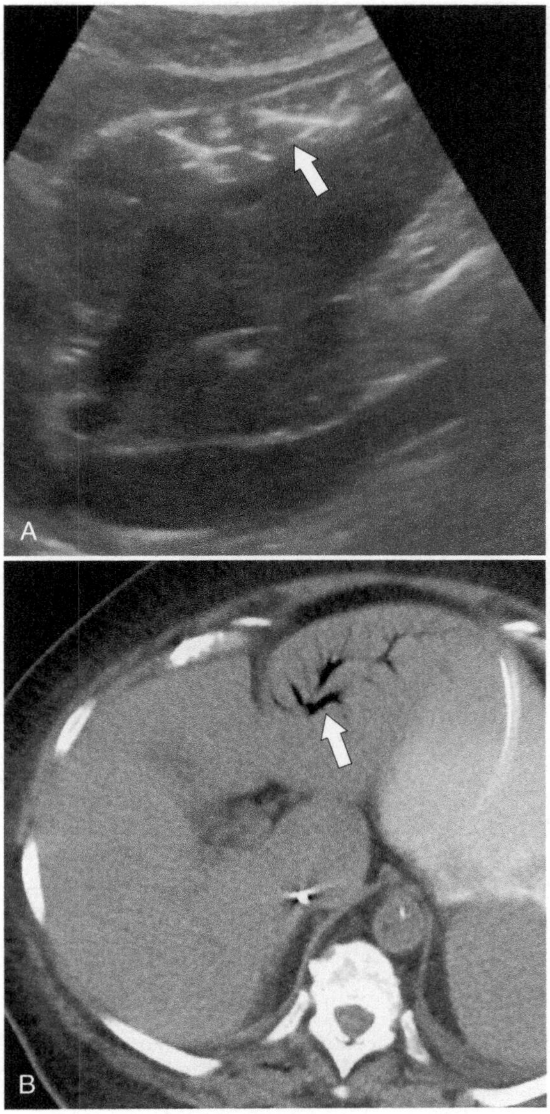

FIGURE 6-167. Sagittal US (**A**) and axial noncontrast CT (**B**) in a 67-year-old patient with portal venous gas. At US, there is echogenic nondependent shadowing, and the gas is in the most nondependent lobe at CT (*arrows*).

Portal Venous Gas

The finding of portal venous gas on plain radiograph, US, or CT rarely represents an innocent condition (unless the patient has had recent gastrointestinal surgery or endoscopic investigation). Usually the finding is a secondary sign of more serious disease elsewhere and denotes violation of the small and large bowel mucosal barrier by instrumentation, ischemia, infection, or perforation. Alternatively, gas may originate from gas-forming organisms in infected thrombophlebitis in the mesenteric tributaries, usually itself a manifestation of bacterial seeding from the large bowel.

In general, the diagnosis of portal venous gas should be straightforward. It should be distinguished from intrahepatic biliary gas, which is almost always benign and more central in location, since it is present mainly in the larger left and right main biliary radicals (Fig. 6-166). Gas, being nondependent, rises to the most superior location, and in the supine position the left biliary radicals are generally more anterior than those in the right, so biliary gas is more commonly identified in the left lobe. Furthermore, bile flows toward the hepatic hilum, keeping the gas relatively central

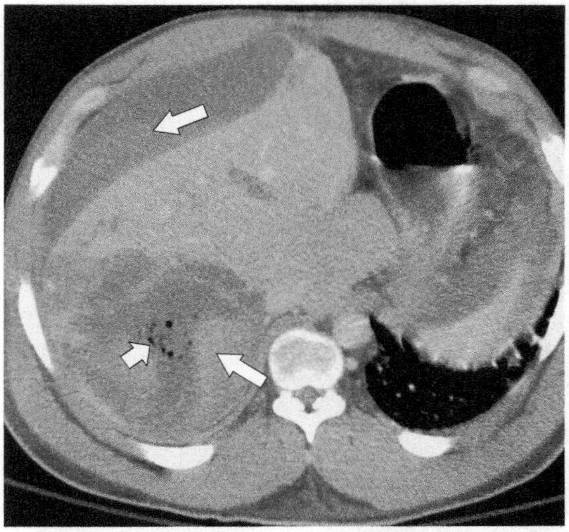

FIGURE 6-168. Axial contrast-enhanced CT in a 31-year-old man with right hepatic gas (*small arrow*) due to infarction secondary from embolization of a bleeding hepatic adenoma. There is also hepatic hemorrhage and hemorrhagic ascites (*arrows*).

(i.e., downstream to flowing bile). Conversely, portal venous gas follows the centrifugal flow of venous blood away to the periphery of the liver. Gas is located in the most nondependent location and is therefore most commonly present in the peripheral right and left lobes (Fig. 6-167).

Hepatic Infarction

Because of the dual hepatic blood supply, hepatic parenchymal necrosis is uncommon and usually requires disruption of both portal and arterial blood supply. Causes are usually iatrogenic (surgery, interventional imaging procedures) or traumatic. Patients undergoing liver transplant are particularly susceptible. Other causes include hypercoagulable states, vasculitis, or infections. On noncontrast CT, there is a hypoattenuating, usually wedge-shaped defect, although more central, rounded, low-density regions are also recognized. As necrosis progresses, gas formation can be seen within the affected regions. On contrast-enhanced CT, the infarcted regions are generally geographical in appearance and either fail to enhance or demonstrate patchy enhancement because of formation of collaterals (Fig. 6-168).

HEPATIC TRAUMA

In addition to iatrogenic causes (particularly interventional imaging procedures), hepatic trauma is most commonly a result of blunt trauma from motor vehicle injury and secondarily from penetrating injuries (knife wound or gunshot). CT is the preferred imaging method, particularly because other organs can be assessed simultaneously. A laceration without significant hemorrhage is identified as a linear, hypodense, hepatic lesion (Fig. 6-169). Areas of acute hemorrhage are identified as hyperdense regions on noncontrast CT and may even be hyperdense on contrast-enhanced CT if clotted, often in a subcapsular location (Fig. 6-170). There may be hemoperitoneum, the appearance of which varies from simple fluid to frank blood depending on the stage of bleeding. The degree of hemorrhage within and outside of the liver is generally more profound with hepatic laceration, which itself can be seen as a fracture within the hepatic parenchyma (Fig. 6-171). Areas of hepatic infarction are recognized as wedge-shaped hypodense defects. Pseudoaneurysm can be either an acute or a chronic complication.

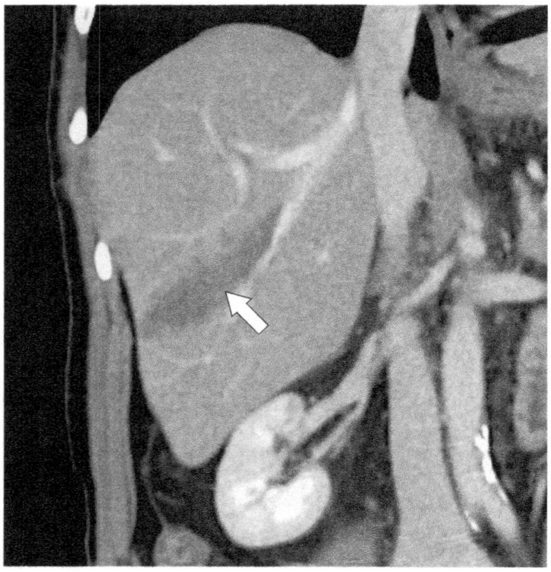

FIGURE 6-169. Coronal contrast-enhanced CT in a 27-year-old woman with a linear hypodense defect caused by a liver laceration (*arrow*).

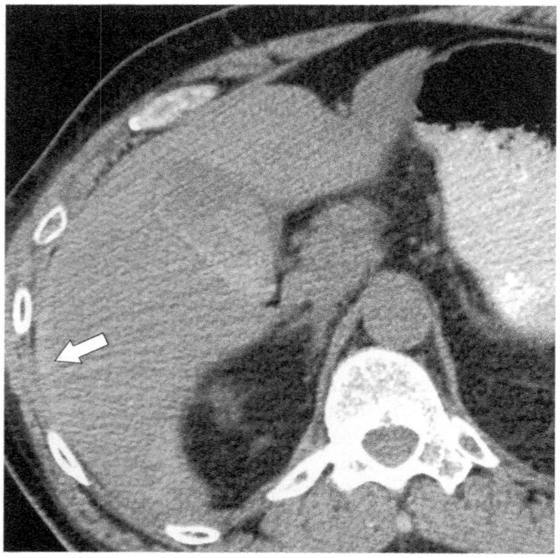

FIGURE 6-170. Axial noncontrast CT in a 55-year-old man with recent trauma and liver laceration and a sliver of hyperdense acute blood surrounding the liver margin (*arrow*).

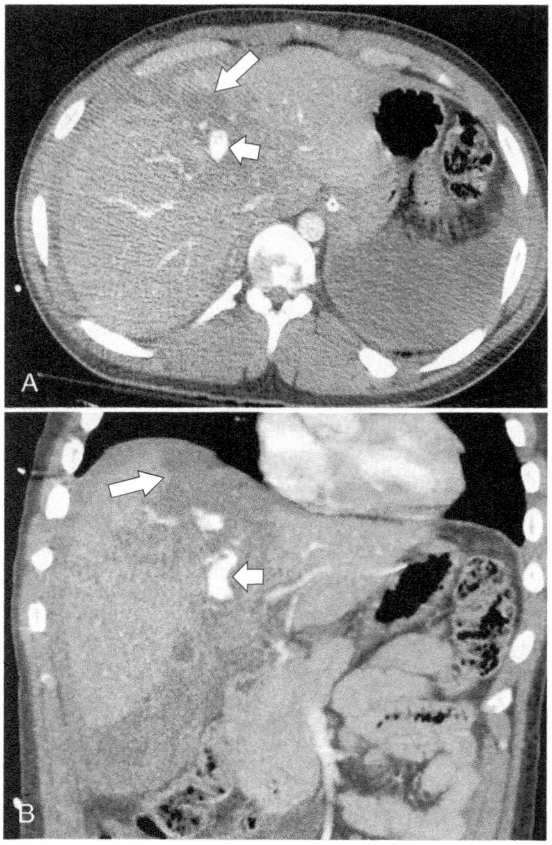

FIGURE 6-171. Axial (**A**) and coronal (**B**) contrast-enhanced CT in a 30-year-old man after a motor vehicle injury, which demonstrates a fractured liver (*arrows*), hemorrhage, and pseudoaneurysm formation (*small arrows*).

POSTOPERATIVE LIVER

Liver Transplant

The most common procedure is the orthotopic liver transplant, in which an allograft from a cadaveric donor wholly or partly replaces the diseased liver, or in the case of living donor allografts, the right lobe is given to adult recipients and the left lobe to child recipients. The procedures are understandably complex, involving anastomoses of biliary and vascular structures. Imaging plays a crucial postoperative role in evaluating both the normal state and postoperative complications.

Deteriorating liver function requires early imaging, usually with US to exclude a mechanical cause (refer to Box 6-11 and Table 6-7), in particular whether there is normal main, right, and left hepatic arterial flow. This is usually best evaluated by Doppler US to document absent flow (occlusion) or reduced flow (high-grade stenosis, hepatic edema, hypotension). Normal US findings include a low-resistance waveform best evaluated by the semiquantitative resistive index (RI), with normal values ranging from 0.5 to 0.7. Normal portal venous waveform is of continuous hepatopetal flow, whereas hepatic venous waveforms are phasic and secondary to variations in cardiac pulsations. Hepatic arterial occlusion (usually complete thrombosis) shows no flow or a tardus-parvus pattern with arterial collateral formation (RI <0.5 and acceleration time >80 msec) (Fig. 6-172). Hepatic arterial stenosis shows a prolonged systemic acceleration Doppler waveform and an RI of <0.5. At the site of anastomosis there is increased peak velocity of >2 m/s.

Portal vein complications are less common than those of the hepatic artery and include thrombosis and stenosis, best evaluated by US, which may demonstrate an intraluminal filling defect (thrombus) or no Doppler flow or both. Other complications, including evidence of hepatic infarction, bile leak, hemorrhage, and abscess, are usually diagnosed with CT. Biliary strictures or leaks can be confirmed by contrast medium injection via the T-tube placed perioperatively or by endoscopic retrograde cholangiopancreatography and, less commonly, transhepatic cholangiography. Biliary strictures can be caused by anastomotic or secondary rejection, ischemia, infection, or recurrent sclerosing cholangitis (in patients with that underlying disease). Other rare complications include recurrent HCC or PTLD. The latter occurs in approximately 5% of patients within the first year after liver transplantation. It is precipitated by aggressive immunosuppression that causes unregulated B-cell proliferation (often associated with Epstein-Barr virus) and development of B-cell lymphoma.

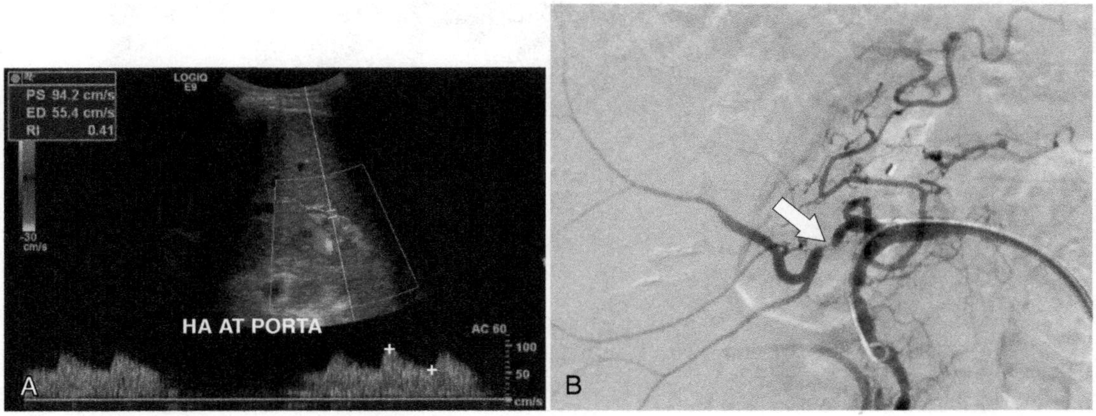

FIGURE 6-172. Color Doppler (**A**) and digital subtraction angiogram (**B**) of the hepatic artery demonstrating increased hepatic arterial velocity (94 cm/s) and elevated diastolic flow (55 cm/s) with low resistive index because of a hepatic arterial stricture (*arrow*). *See ExpertConsult.com for color image.*

BOX 6-11. Normal Postoperative Liver

Right pleural effusion
Periportal portal tract edema (lucency around portal tracts)
Hepatic artery resistive index 0.5-0.7
Anastomotic flow velocity < 0.3 m/s
Biliary anastomosis: may show mild narrowing
Normal parenchymal enhancement

TABLE 6-7 Complications Following Liver Transplant

Vascular	Arterial: Decreased RI (<0.5) Anastomotic narrowing: turbulent flow at anastomosis (flow velocity >0.3 m/s) Thrombosis: no arterial flow Pseudoaneurysm Arteriovenous fistula Hemorrhage Infarction
	Venous: Anastomotic stenosis (turbulent flow) Arteriovenous fistula IVC anastomotic stenosis
Biliary	Bile leak (anastomosis, intrahepatic ducts) Anastomotic stricture/obstruction Biliary necrosis (usually secondary to arterial occlusion) Stone formation
Infectious	Abscess

IVC, Inferior vena cava; *RI*, resistance index.

Liver Resection

Hepatic lobe resection is becoming more commonplace because of greater familiarity with and advances in techniques, with a mortality of less than 5% when performed by an experienced operator. Large volumes of the liver can be removed because compensatory hypertrophy rapidly develops in the remaining liver lobes. Indications for resection in benign disease include lesions that are symptomatic (pain from larger lesions) or at risk of hemorrhage (i.e., giant hemangioma and adenoma) or difficulty in excluding malignant disease. Resection is commonly performed for primary malignant lesions, especially HCC. Increasingly, patients are being offered surgery for removal of metastatic

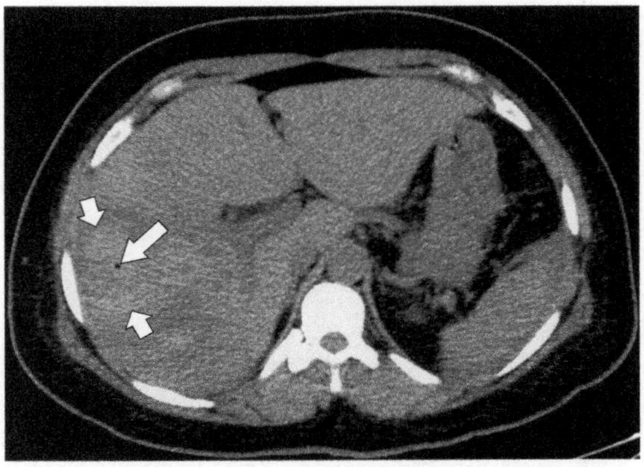

FIGURE 6-173. Axial noncontrast CT in a 33-year-old woman with a hepatic hematoma after a recent percutaneous biopsy. Hyperdense blood (*small arrows*) and a small focus of gas (*arrow*) are the result of the biopsy.

lesions, particularly colorectal metastases (providing they are few in number, usually three or fewer, and their location within the liver is amenable for removal) (Fig. 6-173). Patients are often first treated with chemotherapy to reduce the tumor burden.

Lobar removal is based on knowledge of the Couinaud segmental anatomy (see earlier in this chapter). Classic lobar resections include right lobectomy (segments V to VIII), extended right lobectomy (or right trisegmentectomy, segments IV to VIII), left lobectomy (segments II to IV), extended left lobectomy (or left trisegmentectomy, segments II to V and VIII), and left lateral segmentectomy (segments II and III). Because of advances in technique, individual lobar resections are now also performed.

Complications of hepatic lobe resection are similar to those of hepatic surgery in general, including hemorrhage, infection, biliary complications, and acute hepatic dysfunction (Fig. 6-173).

INTERVENTIONAL PROCEDURES

Percutaneous Biopsy

Percutaneous biopsy is usually performed for the tissue diagnosis of focal liver lesions or diffuse parenchymal disease. It is generally a safe procedure with low morbidity, but complications are well recognized, partly because of the frequency with which the procedure is performed. Immediate complications include hemorrhage (particularly in patients with bleeding disorders, a common associated finding in liver disease) that is usually self-limiting and intrahepatic but can be subscapular and sometimes intraperitoneal (Fig. 6-174). As with any percutaneous procedure, infection

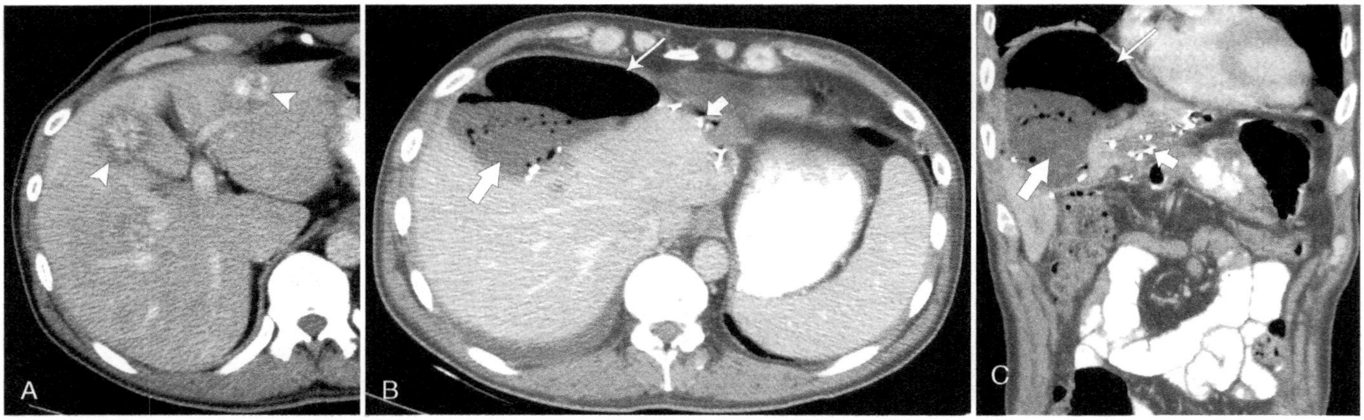

FIGURE 6-174. Preoperative axial (**A**) and postoperative left hepatectomy axial (**B**) and coronal (**C**) contrast-enhanced CT in a 64-year-old woman. Preoperative CT demonstrates two partially calcified mucinous colonic metastases in the left lobe (*arrowheads*). Subsequent resection by left hepatectomy (*small arrows*) resulted in a postoperative abscess (*arrows*) with subphrenic gas (*thin arrows*).

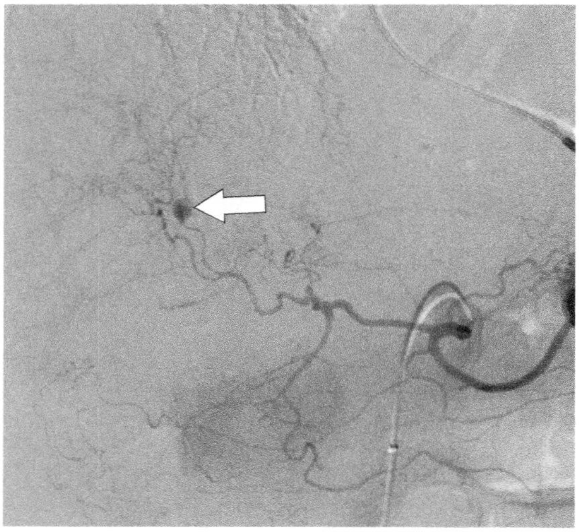

FIGURE 6-175. DSA of a 65-year-old man with a pseudoaneurysm (*arrow*) of the hepatic artery after percutaneous biopsy.

is possible, but very uncommon. Puncture of adjacent structures, including the lung (pneumothorax) and gallbladder (bile leak), is well recognized. Longer term complications include arteriovenous fistula, pseudoaneurysm formation (Fig. 6-175), and, occasionally, tumor seeding along the percutaneous tract after biopsy of malignant liver lesions.

Catheter Placement

Hepatic complications are more commonly associated with percutaneous catheter placement than with biopsy, mainly because of their size. These include arterial injury with hemorrhage or arteriovenous malformation, bile duct injury, and pneumothorax (transpleural catheter placement).

Transarterial Chemoembolization

Transarterial chemoembolization (TACE) uses selective arterial catheter placement for administration of large local doses of chemotherapeutic agents for inoperable focal malignant liver lesions, both primary and secondary. Complications include infarction and necrosis of normal liver, infection, and arteriovenous shunts (Figs. 6-168 and 176).

Radiofrequency Ablation

Radiofrequency ablation is a percutaneous imaging technique for the treatment of inoperable HCCs and metastatic disease that

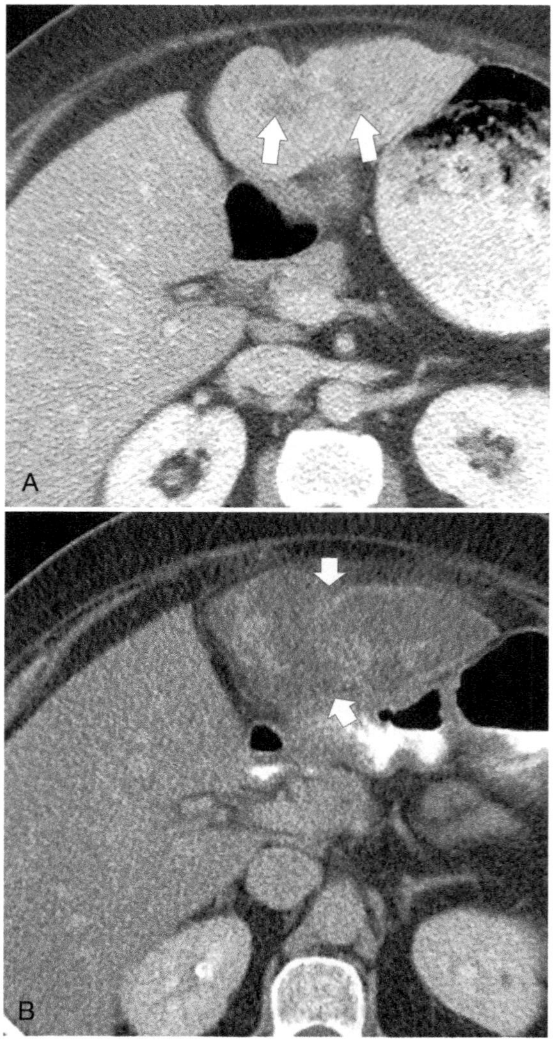

FIGURE 6-176. Contrast-enhanced CT in a 63-year-old man with colon cancer and a left lobe liver metastasis (**A**) (*large arrows*). After chemoembolization (**B**), there is almost complete infarction of the left lobe (*small arrows*).

induces tumor death by coagulable necrosis (Fig. 6-177). Complications are those associated with any percutaneous interventional hepatic procedure, including hemorrhage, infection, bile leak, and arteriovenous fistula formation. Dedicated follow-up imaging, either CT or MRI, is required to evaluate for tumor recurrence (Fig. 6-178). Both noncontrast and contrast-enhanced imaging is required to evaluate for any area of subtle enhancement (usually at the periphery of the lesion), which usually signifies tumor recurrence. This can be inferred from increased signal at T2-weighted imaging. Successful imaging follow-up should show a treatment region that is hypodense (or hypointense on both T1- and T2-weighted imaging), although it may be hyperdense in the immediate postprocedure period because of hemorrhage.

Transhepatic Intrahepatic Portosystemic Shunt

The transhepatic intrahepatic portosystemic shunt (TIPS or TIPPS) is an interventional imaging procedure used to treat portal hypertension. In this procedure a fistula is created between the portal and hepatic veins by use of a balloon-expandable metallic stent (Fig. 6-179). In addition to complications of

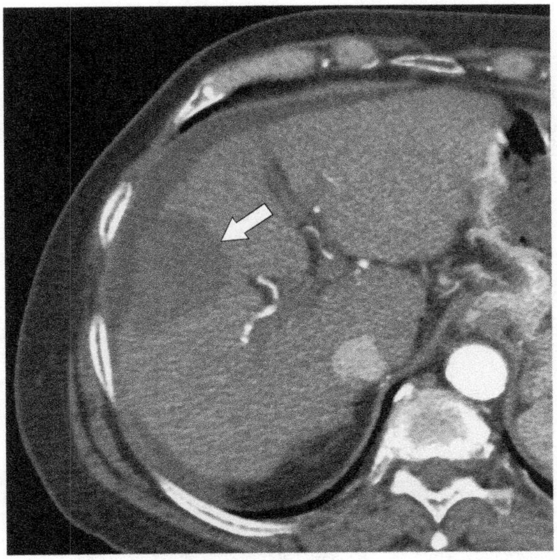

FIGURE 6-177. Axial arterial-phase CT in a 66-year-old man with a hypodense region after prior radiofrequency ablation (*arrow*) for hepatocellular carcinoma. There is no abnormal enhancement and therefore no evidence of recurrence.

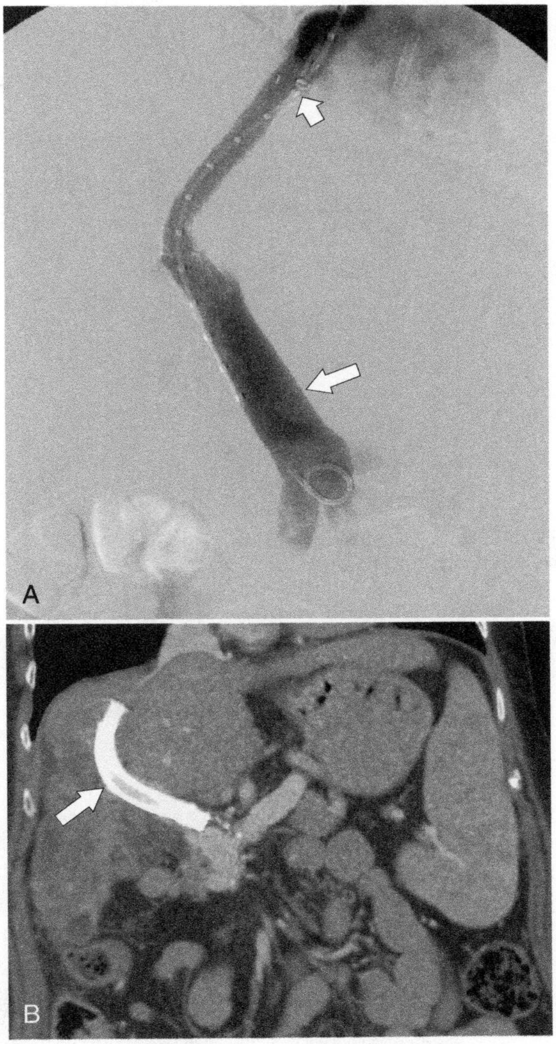

FIGURE 6-179. Digital subtraction angiographic view (**A**) of normal TIPPS with iatrogenic fistula between the portal vein (*arrows*) and hepatic vein (*short arrow*). Coronal contrast-enhanced CT (**B**) demonstrates the metallic stent (*arrow*).

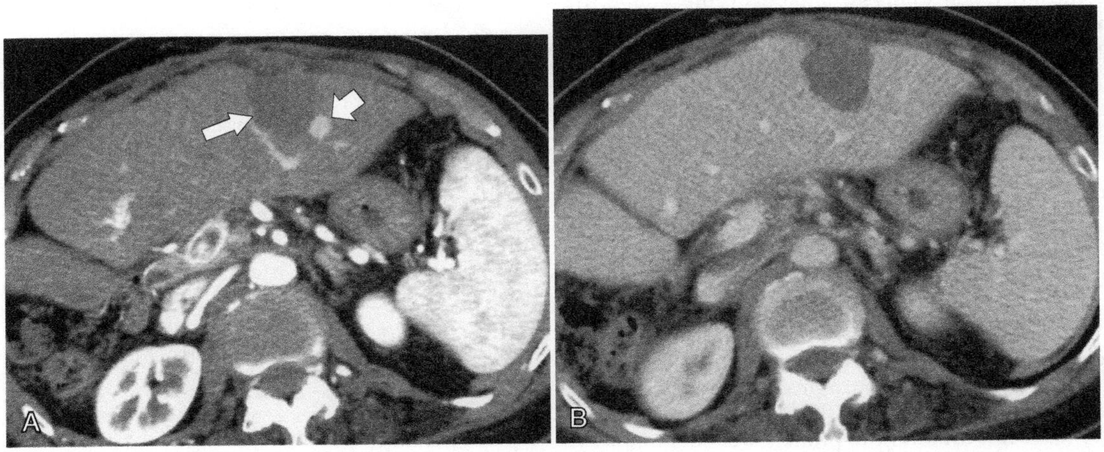

FIGURE 6-178. Arterial (**A**) and PVP (**B**) CT in a 56-year-old man who previously had radiofrequency ablation for HCC (*arrow*) and now has a new arterially enhancing recurrence (*small arrow*). The lesion is not identified at PVP.

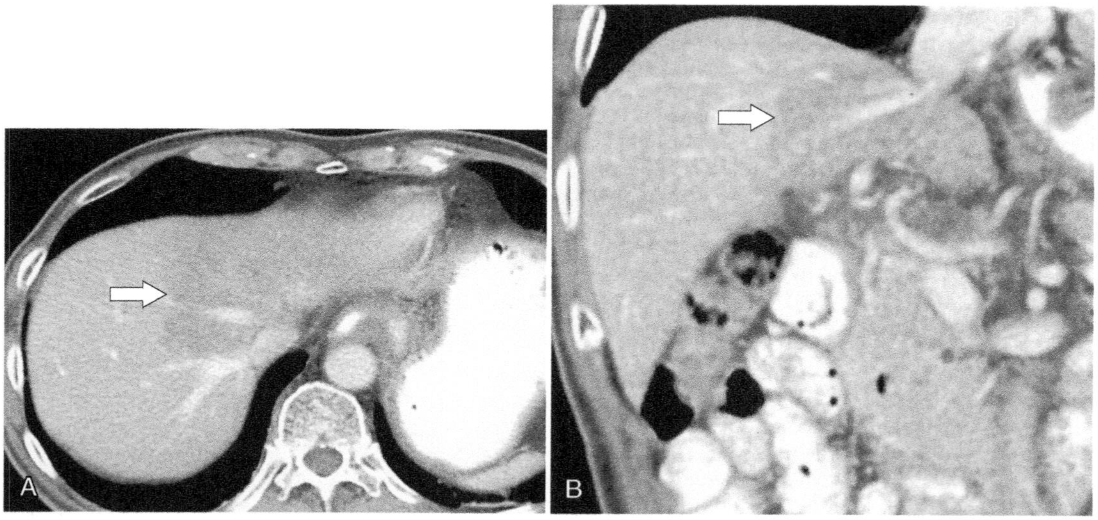

FIGURE 6-180. Axial (**A**) and coronal (**B**) contrast-enhanced CT in a 70-year-old man with a linear hypodense appearance of the liver (*arrows*) secondary to previous mediastinal radiation.

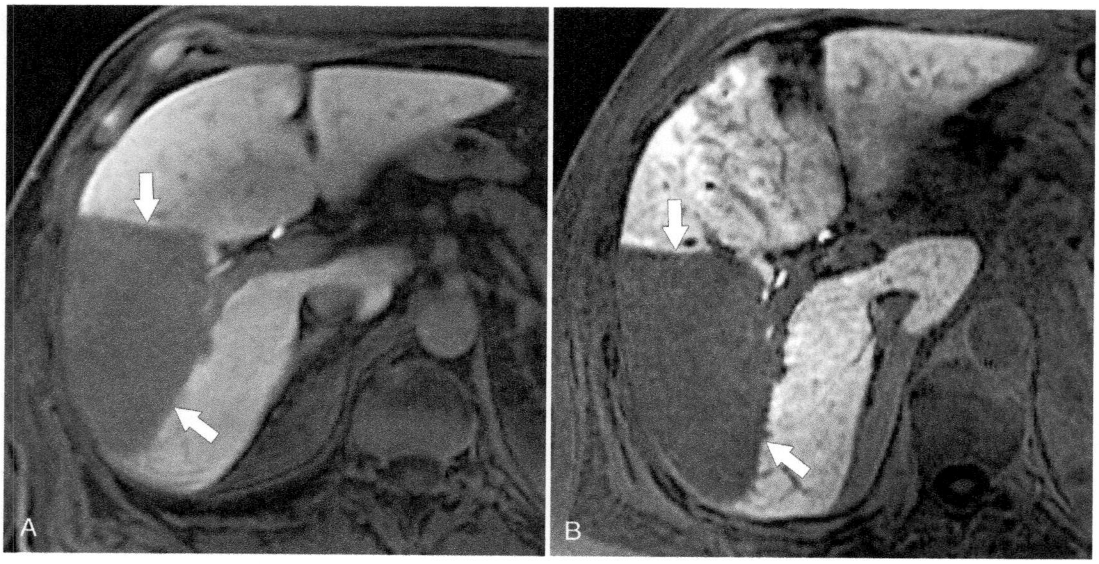

FIGURE 6-181. **A** and **B**, Axial delayed post–hepatobiliary agent contrast-enhanced MRI of the liver in a 53-year-old woman with a hepatic defect following proton beam therapy (*arrows*).

hemorrhage and infarction from the immediate procedure, the most common complication is stenosis from intimal fibroplasia in the hepatic vein. The direction of blood flow is best evaluated by Doppler US. Normal venous flow is hepatofugal, but in obstruction or stenosis the flow is slow (peak velocity <35 cm/s), absent, or hepatopetal or there may be increased flow at the point of anastomosis (>50 cm/s).

Hepatic Radiation

Given the size of the liver in the upper abdomen, it is not surprising that this organ is often in the radiation field in the treatment of upper abdominal malignancies, most often in combination with chemotherapy (chemoradiation) before curative surgical resection is attempted. If the liver is within the radiation field, it may show acute radiation changes as a discrete area of hypoattenuation at CT, typically with linear margins corresponding to the margins of the radiation field (Fig. 6-180). More recently, proton beam therapy has been used for the primary treatment of some hepatic malignancies, which leaves characteristic wedge-shaped defects within the irradiated field (Fig. 6-181).

SUGGESTED READINGS

Abikhzer G et al: Altered hepatic metabolic activity in patients with hepatic steatosis on FDG PET/CT. AJR 196:176-180, 2011.

Acunas B et al: Hydatid cyst of the liver: identification of detached cyst lining on CT scans obtained after cyst puncture. AJR 156:751-752, 1991.

Agnello F et al: High-b-value diffusion-weighted MR imaging of benign hepatocellular lesions: quantitative and qualitative analysis. Radiology 262(2):511-519, 2012.

Ahrar K et al: Percutaneous radiofrequency ablation of renal tumors: technique, complications, and outcomes. J Vasc Interv Radiol 16(5):679-688, 2005.

Asayama Y et al: Delayed-phase dynamic CT enhancement as a prognostic factor for mass-forming intrahepatic cholangiocarcinoma. Radiology 238(1):150-155, 2006.

Bahl M et al: Liver steatosis: investigation of opposed-phase T1-weighted liver MR signal intensity loss and visceral fat measurement as biomarkers. Radiology 249(1):160-166, 2008.

Bargellini I et al: Hepatocellular carcinoma: CT for tumor response after transarterial chemoembolization in patients exceeding Milan criteria—selection parameter for liver transplantation. Radiology 255(1):289-300, 2010.

Basaran C et al: Fat-containing lesions of the liver: cross-sectional imaging findings with emphasis on MRI. AJR 184(4):1103-1110, 2005.

Beaty SD et al: Teaching file: incidental hepatic mass. AJR 190:S62-S64, 2008.

Berrocal T et al: Pediatric liver transplantation: a pictorial essay of early and late complications. Radiographics 26(4):1187-1209, 2006.

Bhargava P et al: Imaging of orthotopic liver transplantation: review. AJR 196:WS15-WS25, 2011.
Bhargava P et al: Imaging of orthotopic liver transplantation: self-assessment module. AJR 196:S35-S38, 2011.
Bilaj F et al: MR imaging findings in autoimmune hepatitis: correlation with clinical staging. Radiology 236(3):896-902, 2005.
Blachar A et al: Primary biliary cirrhosis: clinical, pathologic, and helical CT findings in 53 patients. Radiology 220(2):329-336, 2001.
Bonkovsky HL et al: Hepatic iron concentration: noninvasive estimation by means of MR imaging techniques. Radiology 212(1):227-234, 1999.
Boonsirikamchai P et al: CT findings of response and recurrence, independent of change in tumor size, in colorectal liver metastasis treated with bevacizumab. AJR 197:W1060-W1066, 2011.
Brancatelli G et al: Benign regenerative nodules in Budd-Chiari syndrome and other vascular disorders of the liver: radiologic-pathologic and clinical correlation. Radiographics 22(4):847-862, 2002.
Brancatelli G et al: Fibropolycystic liver disease: CT and MR imaging findings. Radiographics 25(3):659-670, 2005.
Brancatelli G et al: Focal confluent fibrosis in cirrhotic liver: natural history studied with serial CT. AJR 192(5):1341-1347, 2009.
Brancatelli G et al: Focal nodular hyperplasia: CT findings with emphasis on multiphasic helical CT in 78 patients. Radiology 219(1):61-68, 2001.
Brancatelli G et al: Large regenerative nodules in Budd-Chiari syndrome and other vascular disorders of the liver: CT and MR imaging findings with clinicopathologic correlation. AJR 178(4):877-883, 2002.
Buetow PC et al: Focal nodular hyperplasia of the liver: radiologic-pathologic correlation. Radiographics 16(2):369-388, 1996.
Buetow PC et al: Malignant vascular tumors of the liver: radiologic-pathologic correlation. Radiographics 14(1):153-166, 1994. quiz 167-168.
Caiado AH et al: Complications of liver transplantation: multimodality imaging approach. Radiographics 27(5):1401-1417, 2007.
Catalano OA et al: Differentiation of malignant thrombus from bland thrombus of the portal vein in patients with hepatocellular carcinoma: application of diffusion-weighted MR imaging. Radiology 254(1):154-162, 2010.
Chen WP et al: Spectrum of transient hepatic attenuation differences in biphasic helical CT. AJR 172(2):419-424, 1999.
Choi SH et al: Hepatic arterial injuries in 3110 patients following percutaneous transhepatic biliary drainage. Radiology 261(3):969-975, 2011.
Chung GE et al: Transarterial chemoembolization can be safely performed in patients with hepatocellular carcinoma invading the main portal vein and may improve the overall survival. Radiology 258(2):627-634, 2011.
Chung JJ et al: Nonhypervascular hypoattenuating nodules depicted on either portal or equilibrium phase multiphasic CT images in the cirrhotic liver. AJR 191(1):207-214, 2008.
Colagrande S et al: Transient hepatic attenuation differences and focal liver lesions: sump effect due to primary arterial hyperperfusion. J Comput Assist Tomogr 33(2):259-265, 2009.
Czermak BV et al: Echinococcosis of the liver. Abdom Imaging 33(2):133-143, 2008.
Di Martino M et al: Intraindividual comparison of gadoxetate disodium-enhanced MR imaging and 64-section multidetector CT in the detection of hepatocellular carcinoma in patients with cirrhosis. Radiology 256(3):806-816, 2010.
Donadon M et al: Intraoperative ultrasound of the liver. AJR 198:W398, 2012.
Doyle DJ et al: Clinical observations: imaging features of sclerosed hemangioma. AJR 189:67-72, 2007.
Ebied O et al: Hepatocellular-cholangiocarcinoma: helical computed tomography findings in 30 patients. J Comput Assist Tomogr 27(2):117-124, 2003.
Faria SC et al: Hepatic adenoma. AJR 182:1520, 2004.
Ferlicot S et al: MRI of atypical focal nodular hyperplasia of the liver: radiology-pathology correlation. AJR 182:1227-1231, 2004.
Furata A et al: Hepatic enhancement in multiphasic contrast-enhanced MDCT. AJR 183:157-162, 2004.
Gaba RC et al: Comprehensive review of TIPS technical complications and how to avoid them. AJR 196:675-685, 2011.
Gastrointestinal imaging. AJR 198, 2012. 198_5_Supplement_E130.
Gervais DA et al: Percutaneous tumor ablation for hepatocellular carcinoma. AJR 197:789-794, 2011.
Glatard A-S et al: Obliterative portal venopathy: findings at CT imaging. Radiology, April 2, 2012. 111785; Published online.
Goshima S et al: Hepatic hemangioma and metastasis: differentiation with gadoxetate disodium-enhanced 3-T MRI. AJR 195:941-946, 2010.
Grazioli L et al: Accurate differentiation of focal nodular hyperplasia from hepatic adenoma at gadobenate dimeglumine-enhanced MR imaging: prospective study. Radiology 236(1):166-177, 2005.
Grazioli L et al: Focal nodular hyperplasia: morphologic and functional information from MR imaging with gadobenate dimeglumine. Radiology 221(3):731-739, 2001.
Grazioli L et al: Hepatic adenomas: imaging and pathologic findings. Radiographics 21(4):877-892, 2001. discussion 892-894.
Grazioli L et al: Hepatocellular adenoma and focal nodular hyperplasia: value of gadoxetic acid-enhanced MR imaging in differential diagnosis. Radiology 262(2):520-529, 2012.
Grazioli L et al: Liver adenomatosis: clinical, histopathologic, and imaging findings in 15 patients. Radiology 216(2):395-402, 2000.
Gryspeerdt S et al: Evaluation of hepatic perfusion disorders with double-phase spiral CT. Radiographics 17(2):337-348, 1997.
Gwon D II et al: Hepatocellular carcinoma associated with membranous obstruction of the inferior vena cava: incidence, characteristics, and risk factors and clinical efficacy of TACE. Radiology 254(2):617-626, 2010.
Hamer OW et al: Imaging features of perivascular fatty infiltration of the liver: initial observations. Radiology 237(1):159-169, 2005.
Han JK et al: Hilar cholangiocarcinoma: thin-section spiral CT findings with cholangiographic correlation. Radiographics 17:1475-1485, 1997.
Hanna RF et al: Cirrhosis-associated hepatocellular nodules: correlation of histopathologic and MR imaging features. Radiographics 28(3):747-769, 2008.
Hanna RF et al: Double-contrast MRI for accurate staging of hepatocellular carcinoma in patients with cirrhosis. AJR 190(1):47-57, 2008.
Hashimoto A et al: Safety and optimal management of hepatic arterial infusion chemotherapy after pancreatectomy for pancreatobiliary cancer. AJR 198:923-930, 2012.
Hirooka M et al: Splenic elasticity measured with real-time tissue elastography is a marker of portal hypertension. Radiology 261(3):960-968, 2011.
Hussain HK et al: T2-weighted MR imaging in the assessment of cirrhotic liver. Radiology 230(3):637-644, 2004.
Hussain HK et al: T2-weighted MR imaging in the assessment of cirrhotic liver. Radiology 230(3):637-644, 2004.
Hussain SM et al: Benign versus malignant hepatic nodules: MR imaging findings with pathologic correlation. Radiographics 22(5):1023-1036, 2002. discussion 1037-1039.
Hussain SM et al: Cirrhosis and lesion characterization at MR imaging. Radiographics 29(6):1637-1652, 2009.
Hussain SM et al: Focal nodular hyperplasia: findings at state-of-the-art MR imaging, US, CT, and pathologic analysis. Radiographics 24(1):3-17, 2004.
Iannaccone R et al: Hepatocellular carcinoma in patients with nonalcoholic fatty liver disease: helical CT and MR imaging findings with clinical-pathologic comparison. Radiology 243(2):422-430, 2007.
Iannaccone R et al: Peliosis hepatis: spectrum of imaging findings. AJR 187:W43-W52, 2006.
Ichikawa T et al: Fibrolamellar hepatocellular carcinoma: imaging and pathologic findings in 31 recent cases. Radiology 213(2):352-361, 1999.
Itai Y et al: Blood flow and liver imaging. Radiology 202(2):306-314, 1997.
Ito K et al: Hepatocellular carcinoma: association with increased iron deposition in the cirrhotic liver at MR imaging. Radiology 212(1):235-240, 1999.
Jha P et al: Radiologic mimics of cirrhosis. AJR 194:993-999, 2010.
Jhaveri KS et al: Association of hepatic hemangiomatosis with giant cavernous hemangioma in the adult population: prevalence, imaging appearance, and relevance. AJR 196:809-815, 2011.
Joe E et al: Feasibility and accuracy of dual-source dual-energy CT for noninvasive determination of hepatic iron accumulation. Radiology 262(1):126-135, 2012.
Kamel IR et al: Comprehensive analysis of hypervascular liver lesions using 16-MDCT and advanced image processing. AJR 183:443-452, 2004.
Kamel IR et al: Pictorial essay: focal nodular hyperplasia: lesion evaluation using 16-MDCT and 3D CT angiography. AJR 186:1587-1596, 2006.
Khosa F et al: Pattern of the month: hypervascular liver lesions on MRI. AJR 197:W204-W220, 2011.
Kim HC et al: Preoperative evaluation of hepatocellular carcinoma: combined use of CT with arterial portography and hepatic arteriography. AJR 180:1593-1599, 2003.
Kim HJ et al: Isolated perihepatic tuberculosis: imaging findings. Clin Radiol 64(2):184-189, 2009.
Kim JE et al: Hypervascular hepatocellular carcinoma 1 cm or smaller in patients with chronic liver disease: characterization with gadoxetic acid-enhanced MRI that includes diffusion-weighted imaging. AJR 196:W758-W765, 2011.
Kim MJ et al: Hepatic iron deposition on magnetic resonance imaging: correlation with inflammatory activity. J Comput Assist Tomogr 26(6):988-993, 2002.
Kim MJ et al: Technical essentials of hepatic Doppler sonography. Curr Probl Diagn Radiol 38(2):53-60, 2009.
Kim SH et al: Focal peliosis hepatic as a mimicker of hepatic tumors: radiological-pathological correlation. J Comput Assist Tomogr 31(1):79-85, 2007.
Kim Y-s et al: Recurrence of hepatocellular carcinoma after liver transplantation: patterns and prognostic factors based on clinical and radiologic features. AJR 189:352-358, 2007.
Koizumi J et al: Computed tomography during arterial portography under temporary balloon occlusion of the hepatic artery: evaluation of pseudolesions caused by arterio-portal venous shunts. Abdom Imaging 25(6):583-586, 2000.
Lee KH et al: Triple phase MDCT of heptocellular carcinoma. AJR 182:643-649, 2004.
Lee YH et al: Focal nodular hyperplasia-like nodules in alcoholic liver cirrhosis: radiologic-pathologic correlation. AJR 188:W459-W463, 2007.
Lencioni R et al: Early-stage hepatocellular carcinoma in patients with cirrhosis: long-term results of percutaneous image-guided radiofrequency ablation. Radiology 234(3):961-967, 2005.
Lewandowski RJ et al: Chemoembolization for hepatocellular carcinoma: comprehensive imaging and survival analysis in a 172-patient cohort. Radiology 255(3):955-965, 2010.
Lewin M et al: Liver adenomatosis: classification of MR imaging features and comparison with pathologic findings. Radiology 241(2):433-440, 2006.
Lim JH: Cholangiocarcinoma: morphologic classification according to growth pattern and imaging findings. AJR 181(3):819-827, 2003.
Liu CH et al: Imaging of focal hepatic lesions: self-assessment module. AJR 190:S65-S68, 2008.
Lonergan GJ et al: Autosomal recessive polycystic kidney disease: radiologic-pathologic correlation. Radiographics 20(3):837-855, 2000.

Lu DS et al: Radiofrequency ablation of hepatocellular carcinoma: treatment success as defined by histologic examination of the explanted liver. Radiology 234(3):954-960, 2005.

Maetani Y et al: MR imaging of intrahepatic cholangiocarcinoma with pathologic correlation. AJR 176(6):1499-1507, 2001.

Malayeri AA et al: Principles and applications of diffusion-weighted imaging in cancer detection, staging, and treatment follow-up. Radiographics 31(6):1773-1791, 2011.

Matsui O et al: Benign and malignant nodules in cirrhotic livers: distinction based on blood supply. Radiology 178:493-497, 1991.

Miraglia R et al: Interventional radiology procedures in pediatric patients with complications after liver transplantation. Radiographics 29(2):567-584, 2009.

Morgan DE et al: Polycystic liver disease: multimodality imaging for complications and transplant evaluation. Radiographics 26(6):1655-1668, 2006. quiz 1655.

Mortele KJ et al: Cystic focal liver lesions in the adult: differential CT and MR imaging features. Radiographics 21(4):895-910, 2001.

Mortele KJ et al: The infected liver: radiologic-pathologic correlation. Radiographics 24(4):937-955, 2004.

Motosugi U et al: Imaging of small hepatic metastases of colorectal carcinoma: how to use superparamagnetic iron oxide-enhanced magnetic resonance imaging in the multidetector-row computed tom+ography age? J Comput Assist Tomogr 33(2):266-272, 2009.

Mullan CP et al: Can Doppler sonography discern between hemodynamically significant and insignificant portal vein stenosis after adult liver transplantation? AJR 195:1438-1443, 2010.

Murakami T et al: Liver necrosis and regeneration after fulminant hepatitis: pathologic correlation with CT and MR findings. Radiology 198(1):239-242, 1996.

Nomura R et al: Clinical observations: development of hepatic steatosis after pancreatoduodenectomy. AJR 189:1484-1488, 2007.

Oei T et al: Radiofrequency ablation of liver tumors: a new cause of benign portal venous gas. Radiology 237(2):709-717, 2005.

Pandharipande PV et al: Perfusion imaging of the liver: current challenges and future goals. Radiology 234(3):661-673, 2005.

Park SH et al: Macrovesicular hepatic steatosis in living liver donors: use of CT for quantitative and qualitative assessment. Radiology 239(1):105-112, 2006.

Park S-Y et al: Radiofrequency ablation of hepatic metastases after curative resection of extrahepatic cholangiocarcinoma. AJR 197:W1129-W1134, 2011.

Patten RM et al: CT detection of hepatic and splenic injuries: usefulness of liver window settings. AJR 175(4):1107-1110, 2000.

Peterson MS et al: Hepatic angiosarcoma: findings on multiphasic contrast-enhanced helical CT do not mimic hepatic hemangioma. AJR 175(1):165-170, 2000.

Pickhardt PJ et al: Original research: visceral adiposity and hepatic steatosis at abdominal CT: association with the metabolic syndrome. AJR 198:1100-1107, 2012.

Poletti PA et al: CT criteria for management of blunt liver trauma: correlation with angiographic and surgical findings. Radiology 216(2):418-427, 2000.

Prasad SR et al: Fat-containing lesions of the liver: radiologic-pathologic correlation. Radiographics 25(2):321-331, 2005.

Purysko AS et al: Characteristics and distinguishing features of hepatocellular adenoma and focal nodular hyperplasia on gadoxetate disodium–enhanced MRI. AJR 198:115-123, 2012.

Qayyum A et al: CT of benign hypervascular liver nodules in autoimmune hepatitis. AJR 183(6):1573-1576, 2004.

Ringe KI et al: Gadoxetate disodium-enhanced MRI of the liver: part 1, protocol optimization and lesion appearance in the noncirrhotic liver. AJR 195:13-28, July 2010.

Ross AG et al: Schistosomiasis. N Engl J Med 346(16):1212-1220, 2002.

Rossi S et al: Contrast-enhanced ultrasonography and spiral computed tomography in the detection and characterization of portal vein thrombosis complicating hepatocellular carcinoma. Eur Radiol 18(8):1749-1756, 2008.

Rossi S et al: Percutaneous radio-frequency thermal ablation of nonresectable hepatocellular carcinoma after occlusion of tumor blood supply. Radiology 217(1):119-126, 2000.

Rossi S et al: Percutaneous RF interstitial thermal ablation in the treatment of hepatic cancer. AJR 167(3):759-768, 1996.

Ruppert-Kohlmayr AJ et al: Focal nodular hyperplasia and hepatocellular adenoma of the liver: differentiation with multiphasic helical CT. AJR 176:1493-1498, 2001.

Sacks A et al: Value of PET/CT in the management of primary hepatobiliary tumors, part 2. AJR 197:W260-W265, 2011.

Sacks A et al: Value of PET/CT in the management of liver metastases, part 1. AJR 197:W256-W259, 2011.

Sandrasegaran K et al: Distinguishing gelatin bioabsorbable sponge and postoperative abdominal abscess on CT. AJR 184(2):475-480, 2005.

Sandrasegaran K et al: Hepatic peliosis (bacillary angiomatosis) in AIDS: CT findings. Abdom Imaging 30(6):738-740, 2005.

Sauter A et al: Imaging findings in immunosuppressed patients with Epstein Barr virus–related B cell malignant lymphoma. AJR 194:W141-W149, 2010.

Savastano S et al: Pseudotumoral appearance of peliosis hepatic. AJR 185(2):558-559, 2005.

Shah PA et al: Hepatic gas: widening spectrum of causes detected at CT and US in the interventional era. Radiographics 31(5):1403-1141, 2011.

Shah RP et al: Review: arterially directed therapies for hepatocellular carcinoma. AJR 197:W590-W602, 2011.

Sharma P et al: Liver and spleen stiffness in patients with extrahepatic portal vein obstruction. Radiology 111046; Published online. April 20, 2012.

Siegelman ES et al: Abdominal iron deposition: metabolism, MR findings, and clinical importance. Radiology 199:13-22, 1996.

Simon CJ et al: Pulmonary radiofrequency ablation: long-term safety and efficacy in 153 patients. Radiology 243(1):268-275, 2007.

Smith MT et al: Best cases from the AFIP: fibrolamellar hepatocellular carcinoma. Radiographics 28(2):609-613, 2008.

Sneag DB et al: Extrahepatic spread of hepatocellular carcinoma: spectrum of imaging findings. AJR 197:W658-W664, 2011.

Sondag MJ et al: Case 179: Hereditary hemochromatosis. Radiology 262(3):1037-1041, 2012.

Soyer P et al: Detection of hypovascular hepatic metastases at triple-phase helical CT: sensitivity of phases and comparison with surgical and histopathologic findings. Radiology 231:413-420, 2004.

Stankovic Z et al: Normal and altered three-dimensional portal venous hemodynamics in patients with liver cirrhosis. Radiology 262(3):862-873, 2012.

Stewart BG et al: Imaging and percutaneous treatment of secondarily infected hepatic infarctions. AJR 190(3):601-607, 2008.

Sueyoshi E et al: Vascular complications of hepatic artery after transcatheter arterial chemoembolization in patients with hepatocellular carcinoma. AJR 195:245-251, 2010.

Suh YJ et al: Differentiation of hepatic hyperintense lesions seen on gadoxetic acid–enhanced hepatobiliary phase MRI. AJR 197:W44-W52, 2011.

Tamada T et al: Hepatic hemangiomas: evaluation of enhancement patterns at dynamic MRI with gadoxetate disodium. AJR 196:824-830, 2011.

Taouli B: Diffusion-weighted MR imaging for liver lesion characterization: a critical look. Radiology 262(2):378-380, 2012.

Taouli B et al: Diffusion weighted MR imaging of the liver. Radiology 254(1):47-66, 2010.

Tohme-Noun C et al: Multiple biliary hamartomas: magnetic resonance features with histopathologic correlation. Eur Radiol 18(3):493-499, 2008.

Torabi M et al: CT of nonneoplastic hepatic vascular and perfusion disorders. Radiographics 28(7):1967-1982, 2008.

Torrisi JM et al: CT findings of chemotherapy-induced toxicity: what radiologists need to know about the clinical and radiologic manifestations of chemotherapy toxicity. Radiology 258(1):41-56, 2011.

Umeoka S et al: Pictorial review of tuberous sclerosis in various organs. Radiographics 28(7):e32, 2008.

van Aalten SM et al: Hepatocellular adenomas: correlation of MR imaging findings with pathologic subtype classification. Radiology 261(1):172-181, 2011.

Vandermeer FQ et al: Imaging of whole-organ pancreas transplants. Radiographics 32(2):411-435, 2012.

Vilgrain V et al: Hepatic nodules in Budd-Chiari syndrome: imaging features. Radiology 210(2):443-450, 1999.

Vilgrain V et al: Prevalence of hepatic hemangioma in patients with focal nodular hyperplasia: MR imaging analysis. Radiology 229(1):75-79, 2003.

Wagnetz U et al: Intraoperative ultrasound of the liver in primary and secondary hepatic malignancies: comparison with preoperative 1.5-T MRI and 64-MDCT. AJR 196:562-568, 2011.

Wah TM et al: Image-guided percutaneous radiofrequency ablation and incidence of post-radiofrequency ablation syndrome: prospective survey. Radiology 237(3):1097-1102, 2005.

Wai-Kit L et al: Imaging assessment of congenital and acquired abnormalities of the portal venous system. Radiographics 31(4):905-926, 2011.

Walser EM et al: Extrahepatic portal biliopathy: proposed etiology on the basis of anatomic and clinical features. Radiology 258(1):146-153, 2011.

Wang SL et al: Treatment of hepatic venous outflow obstruction after piggyback liver transplantation. Radiology 236(1):352-359, 2005.

Ward J et al: Colorectal hepatic metastases: detection with SPIO-enhanced breath-hold MR imaging—comparison of optimized sequences. Radiology 228:709-718, 2003.

Wilcox DM et al: MR imaging of a hemorrhagic hepatic cyst in a patient with polycystic liver disease. J Comput Assist Tomogr 9(1):183-185, 1985.

Willatt JM et al: MR Imaging of hepatocellular carcinoma in the cirrhotic liver: challenges and controversies. Radiology 247(2):311-330, 2008.

Yamada A et al: Quantitative evaluation of liver function with use of gadoxetate disodium–enhanced MR imaging. Radiology 260(3):727-733, 2011.

Yao DC et al: Using contrast-enhanced helical CT to visualize arterial extravasation after blunt abdominal trauma: incidence and organ distribution. AJR 178(1):17-20, 2002.

Yoon W et al: CT in blunt liver trauma. Radiographics 25:87-104, 2005.

Yoshimitsu K et al: Pseudolesions of the liver possibly caused by focal rib compression: analysis based on hemodynamic change. AJR 172(3):645-649, 1999.

Yoshimitsu K et al: Unusual hemodynamics and pseudolesions of the noncirrhotic liver at CT. Radiographics 21:S81-S96, Spec No 2001.

Young ST et al: Appearance of oxidized cellulose (Surgicel) on postoperative CT scans: similarity to postoperative abscess. AJR 160(2):275-277, 1993.

Zeitoun D et al: Congenital hepatic fibrosis: CT findings in 18 adults. Radiology 231(1):109-116, 2004.

Zhang YJ et al: Hepatocellular carcinoma treated with radiofrequency ablation with or without ethanol injection: a prospective randomized trial. Radiology 244(2):599-607, 2007.

CHAPTER 7

Spleen

The spleen is part of the mononuclear phagocytic system (formally known as reticuloendothelial) and the largest lymphatic organ. Its red pulp is responsible for red blood cell and platelet metabolism and acts as a monocyte reservation. Its white pulp is critical to the immune response, producing antibodies and removing antibody-laden bacteria (humoral immune response), as well as producing macrophages and lymphocytes (cell-mediated immune response). Therefore splenic infiltration by disease or absence of the spleen can render the patient susceptible to various infections, particularly bacterial and protozoal. It also functions as a red blood cell reservoir in case of blood loss.

Because spleen size varies by individual, splenomegaly can be difficult to determine and small increases in size may not be readily appreciated. Prior cross-sectional imaging can help distinguish whether the spleen is changing in size. It is typically 11 to 12 cm in long axis, usually measured by ultrasound (US). Its transverse dimension is rarely measured but is typically 7 to 8 cm in width and 4 to 5 cm in breadth. Splenomegaly is classified as >14 cm in length (longitudinal axis). Rarely, the spleen is absent (asplenia) or is composed of multiple smaller splenunculi (termed polysplenia and particularly associated with congenital cardiovascular anomalies). Also rarely, the splenic mesentery is abnormally long, so depending on the length of the mesentery, the spleen may be positioned outside its usual left upper quadrant position in the abdomen.

The spleen is best imaged using contrast-enhanced computed tomography (CT) or magnetic resonance imaging (MRI), although because it is adjacent to the abdominal surface, it is amenable to sonographic evaluation. Usually on plain radiography the spleen is only identified unless it is calcified or significantly enlarged (Fig. 7-1). Splenic tissue can also be imaged with technetium 99m (^{99m}Tc) labeled sulfur colloid, which is rapidly sequestered by the mononuclear phagocytic system (including in the liver and bone marrow). The vascularity of the red pulp creates a variable enhancement pattern, particularly in the arterial phase, and should not be mistaken for splenic disease. Any difficulty is usually resolved by imaging during the portal venous phase (PVP) when the spleen is homogeneously enhanced (Fig. 7-2).

Being highly vascular, the spleen is susceptible to many bloodborne pathogens, particularly metastatic and infectious disease, either as discrete lesions or as diffuse infiltration of the whole organ with or without splenomegaly. Differentiation between benign and malignant splenic lesions, either single or multiple, may ultimately require positron emission tomography (PET) or preferably PET/CT or even percutaneous biopsy, a relatively safe procedure when performed by experienced interventionalists.

SPLENIC DISORDERS

Congenital Disorders

Accessory Spleen

Typically the spleen is a single organ, but it is not uncommon for smaller amounts of splenic tissue (splenule or accessory spleen) to surround the main body, particularly close to the pancreatic tail. Usually these are single, but sometimes a few are present. Splenules are characteristically rounded, smooth-walled masses, most often 1 to 2 cm (but can be larger), that are located in the proximity of the spleen (usually the splenic hilum). They typically demonstrate a similar density to the spleen, whether on contrast-enhanced or noncontrast imaging (Fig. 7-3), which usually differentiates them from lymphadenopathy or peritoneal and omental masses.

Asplenia and Polysplenia Syndromes

Asplenia and polysplenia syndromes belong to a spectrum of heterotaxic syndromes referring to abnormal positioning of the internal organs. Situs solitus refers to the normal position, and situs inversus to the mirror image. When the position of the organs is between the two (or ambiguous), it is referred to as situs ambiguus. There are two primary classifications of situs ambiguus, which depend on the cardiac atrial morphology. If both atria have right-sided morphologies, it is known as right isomerism or asplenic syndrome (the spleen is absent). Conversely, if both atria have left atrial morphologies, this is known as left isomerism or polysplenism (multiple small splenic masses). However, the features and positioning of the abdominal organs in situs ambiguus are inconsistent, and precise definition of the type is often difficult.

Right isomerism (asplenia) usually presents in infancy with numerous other congenital anomalies, such as imperforate anus, Hirschsprung* disease, and annular pancreas. It is often fatal. Left isomerism (polysplenia) can be fatal, but not usually as early as right isomerism. Patients with left isomerism are prone to biliary obstruction, esophageal and duodenal atresia, and biliary atresia, as well as other anomalies.

On CT, right isomerism is identified with asplenia, a centrally located liver, the aorta and inferior vena cava on the same side (usually the right), both lungs trilobed, and bilateral morphological right atria. Left isomerism is characterized by multiple splenic

*Harald Hirschsprung (1830-1916), Danish physician.

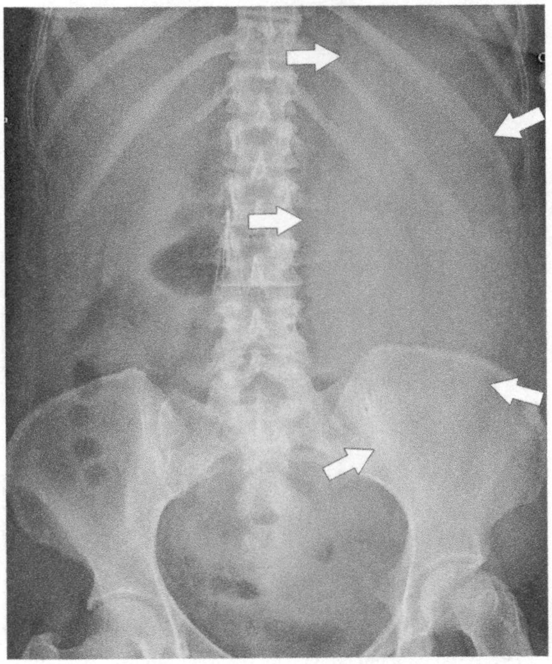

FIGURE 7-1. Plain abdominal radiograph in a 37-year-old woman with leukemic splenic infilration and splenomegaly (*arrows*).

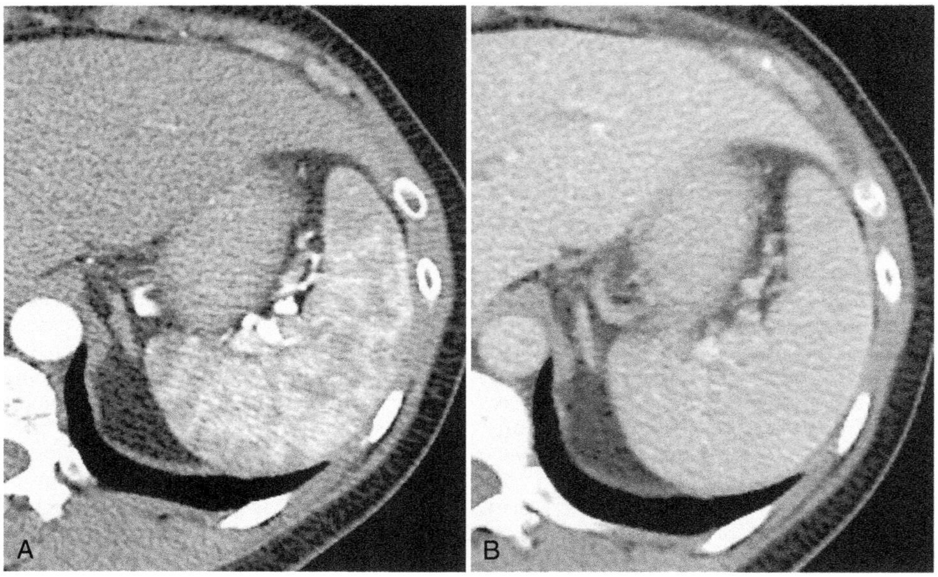

FIGURE 7-2. Axial arterial and PVP CT in a 36-year-old woman demonstrating marked irregular arterial enhancment (**A**) becoming uniform during the PVP (**B**).

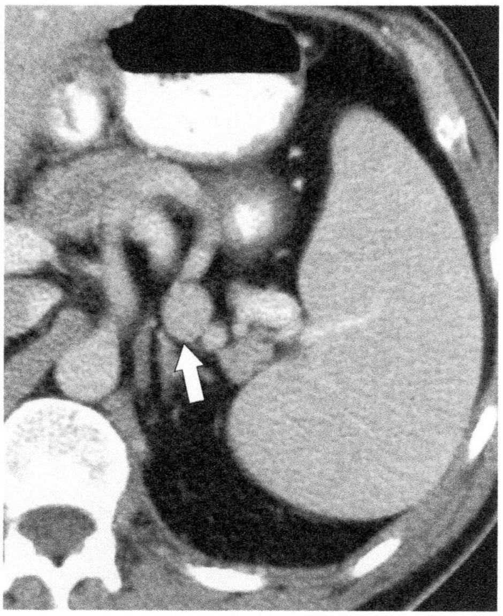

FIGURE 7-3. Axial contrast-enhanced CT in a 45-year-old woman with a splenule (accessory splenic tissue) (*arrow*).

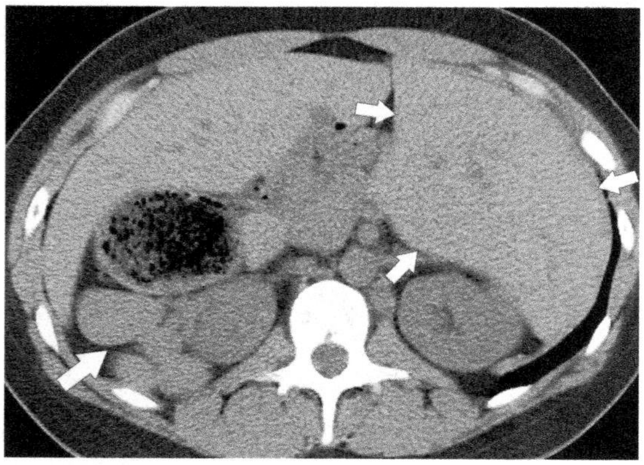

FIGURE 7-4. Axial noncontrast CT in a 26-year-old man with polysplenia (*large arrow*). The liver is predominantly on the left (*small arrows*) with splenic tissue on the right.

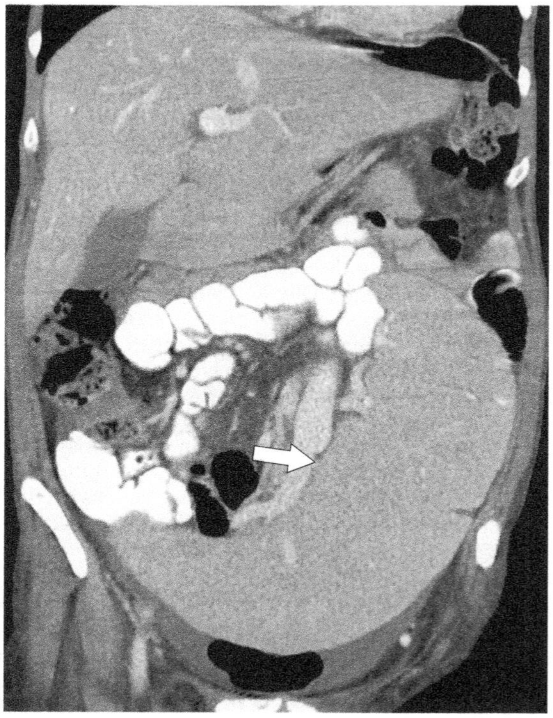

FIGURE 7-5. Coronal contrast-enhanced CT in a 57-year-old woman with splenomegaly caused by polycythemia rubra vera and a "wandering" spleen in the left lower quadrant (*arrow*).

nodules, intrahepatic inferior vena cava interruption with azygous or hemiazygous continuation of the inferior vena cava, bilobed lungs, and bilateral left-sided atria (Fig. 7-4).

Wandering Spleen

The so-called wandering spleen is caused by an abnormal congenital development of the lienorenal ligament, resulting in a long splenic vascular pedicle that allows the spleen the "freedom to wander" within the peritoneum. Given that it is on a long pedicle, its position within the abdomen or pelvis can vary from one scan to another (Fig. 7-5). For similar reasons, it is susceptible to torsion.

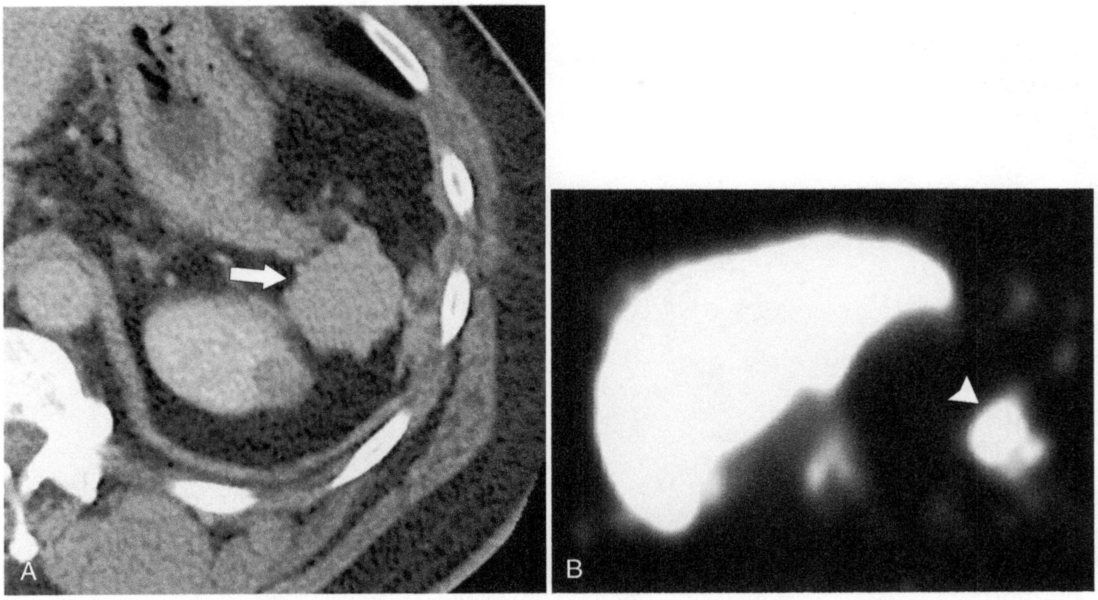

FIGURE 7-6. Axial contrast-enhanced CT (**A**) in a 47-year-old woman with prior splenectomy and now a 3-cm left upper quadrant mass (*arrow*), proved to be splenic tissue on ^{99m}Tc sulfur colloid scan (**B**; *arrowhead*). There is also normal hepatic uptake.

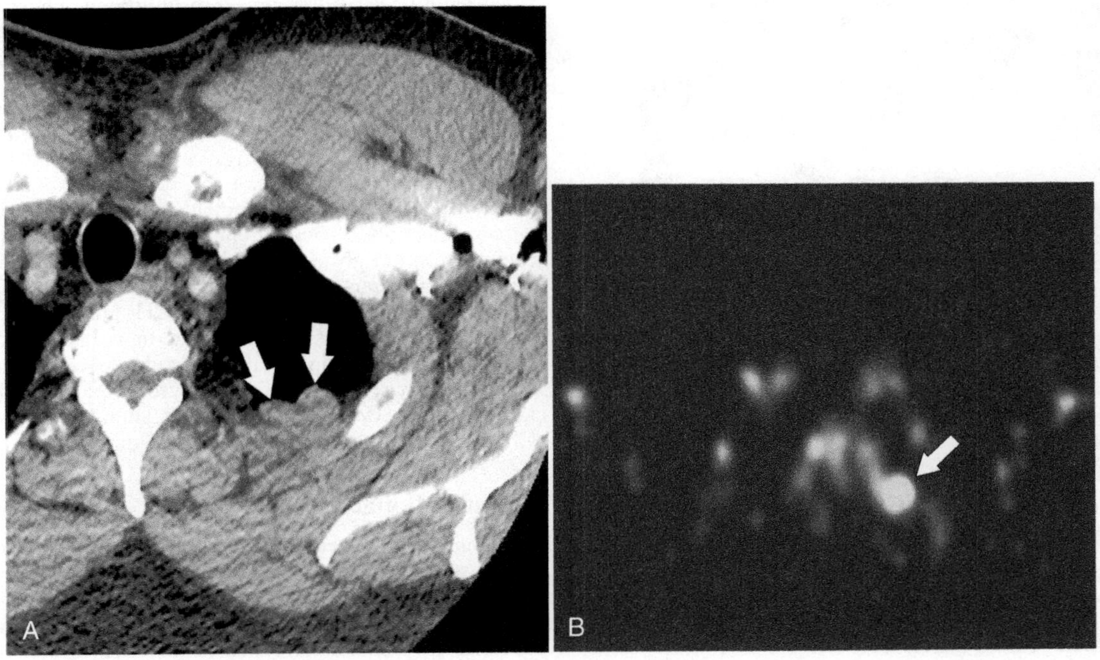

FIGURE 7-7. Axial contrast-enhanced CT (**A**) in the same patient as in Figure 7-6 with a 2-cm pleural-based left upper lobe mass (*arrows*) demonstrating splenic activity at ^{99m}Tc sulfur colloid imaging (**B**).

SPLENOSIS AND RESIDUAL SPLENIC TISSUE

Splenosis is usually secondary to blunt splenic trauma, in which either the whole or parts of the shattered spleen distribute splenic tissue throughout the abdomen and pelvis. The chest may be involved if the diaphragm is breached, and sometimes other organs are affected if they also underwent traumatic laceration. Similarly, splenic remnants can remain after splenectomy (Fig. 7-6). These nodules, which are often multiple, must be differentiated from other abdominal masses, although their smooth-walled, homogeneous, and rounded appearance and their enhancement characteristics, similar to those of the spleen, should be a clue to the diagnosis. The diagnosis may ultimately require ^{99m}Tc-labeled red blood cells or sulfur colloid tests to confirm the splenic nature of the mass, whether in the abdomen (Fig. 7-6) or in the mediastinum (Fig. 7-7).

SPLENOMEGALY

Splenomegaly is defined as splenic enlargement and should not be confused with hypersplenism (see later in the chapter), which is caused by splenic functional abnormalities in distinction to simple splenic enlargement. There are numerous disparate causes of an enlarged spleen (Box 7-1), usually defined on US as >13 cm in long axis or >500 cm^3 volume, although these measurements are relative given the size and morphology of the individual.

Box 7-1. **Causes of Splenomegaly**

VASCULAR CONGESTION
Portal hypertension
Sickle cell disease
Hereditary spherocytosis
Thalassemia
Right heart failure

MALIGNANCY
Lymphoma
Leukemia
Metastases
Myelofibrosis
Multiple myeloma

HEMATOLOGICAL
Polycythemia rubra vera
Trauma (hemorrhage)

INFECTIOUS
Infectious mononucleosis
Leptospirosis
Brucellosis
Malaria
Leishmaniasis
Acute tuberculosis and histoplasmosis
Typhoid
Fungal infection
Schistosomiasis
HIV-related
Multiple splenic infected emboli (endocarditis)

STORAGE
Gaucher disease
Niemann-Pick disease
Mucopolysaccharidosis
Langerhans cell histiocytoses
Amyloidosis

AUTOIMMUNE
Rheumatoid arthritis (Felty syndrome)
Sjögren syndrome
Systemic lupus erythematosus
Idiopathic thrombocytopenia purpura
Autoimmune hemolytic anemia

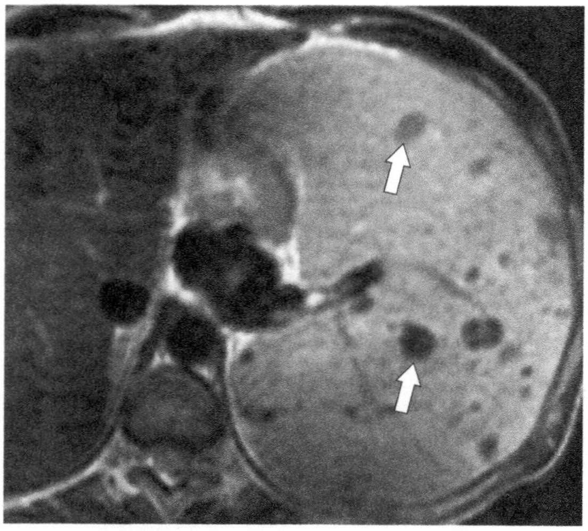

FIGURE 7-8. Axial T2-weighted MRI in a 46-year-old man with Gaucher disease and multiple splenic gaucheromas (*arrows*).

Congenital Splenomegaly

Hematological Abnormalities

Hematological genetic abnormalities usually result in splenomegaly because the continuously produced defective red blood cells are sequestered in a steadily increasing spleen. These include thalassemia, early sickle cell disease (in the later stages, the spleen infarcts and becomes small), hereditary spherocystosis, and elliptocytosis.

Depositional Metabolic Disease

Gaucher* disease is the most common lysosomal storage disease caused by a genetic defect (autosomal recessive) in the enzyme glucosylceramidase, resulting in glucosylceramide accumulation, predominantly in tissues abundant in mononuclear leukocytes (macrophages), namely the spleen, lungs, kidneys, liver, brain, and bone marrow. There are types I, II, and III, and patients with types I and III usually survive into adulthood. These may present with hepatosplenomegaly (Fig. 7-8) as the unmetabolized lipids steadily accumulate within the spleen, or they may be deposited as complex focal masses known as gaucheromas.

Niemann-Pick* disease is a lysosomal storage disorder in which sphingomyelin accumulates (owing to lack of sphingomyelinase) in the liver, spleen, brain, lungs, and bone marrow.

Mucopolysaccharidoses are a group of lysosomal storage disorders caused by deficiency of lysosomal enzyme activity (the subclassification is dependent on the missing enzyme) with accumulation of glycosaminoglycans, which are deposited in the peripheral nervous cysts, eyes, liver, and spleen.

Langerhans† cell histiocytoses (LCH) are a group of disorders with excessive deposition of Langerhans histiocytic cells. The systemic manifestations involve multiple organs and include splenomegaly. Subtypes (now all referred to as LCH) were known as histiocytosis X, eosinophilic granuloma, Hand-Schüller-Christian* disease, and Letterer-Siwe† disease.

Vascular Congestion

The most common cause of splenomegaly is portal hypertension as a result of liver cirrhosis, although any cause of portal hypertension can lead to splenomegaly, including right-sided heart failure, hepatic fibrosis, Budd-Chiari syndrome, portal or splenic vascular thrombosis, and occlusion. The findings are readily appreciated with CT, particularly when signs of liver cirrhosis are obvious. Splenic venous enlargement and tortuosity are caused by the chronically raised venous pressure, and collaterals commonly form, particularly around the splenic hilum (Fig. 7-9). At MRI, multiple small T1 and T2 hypointense lesions, known at Gamna-Gandy* bodies, can be observed, which represent areas of hemosiderosis, probably from prior microhemorrhages induced by the vascular congestive process (Fig. 7-10).

*Phillippe Gaucher (1854-1918), French dermatologist.

*Albert Niemann (1880-1921), German pediatrician; Ludwig Pick (1868-1935), German physician.

†Paul Langerhans (1847-1888), German pathologist.

*Alfred Hand (1868-1949), US pediatrician; Artur Schüller (1822-1884), Austrian physician; Henry A. Christian (1876-1951), American internist.

†Eric Letterer (1895-1982), German pathologist; Sture A. Siwe (1897-1966), Swedish pediatrician.

*Carlos Gamna (1866-1950), Italian physician; Charles Gandy (1872-1943), French physician.

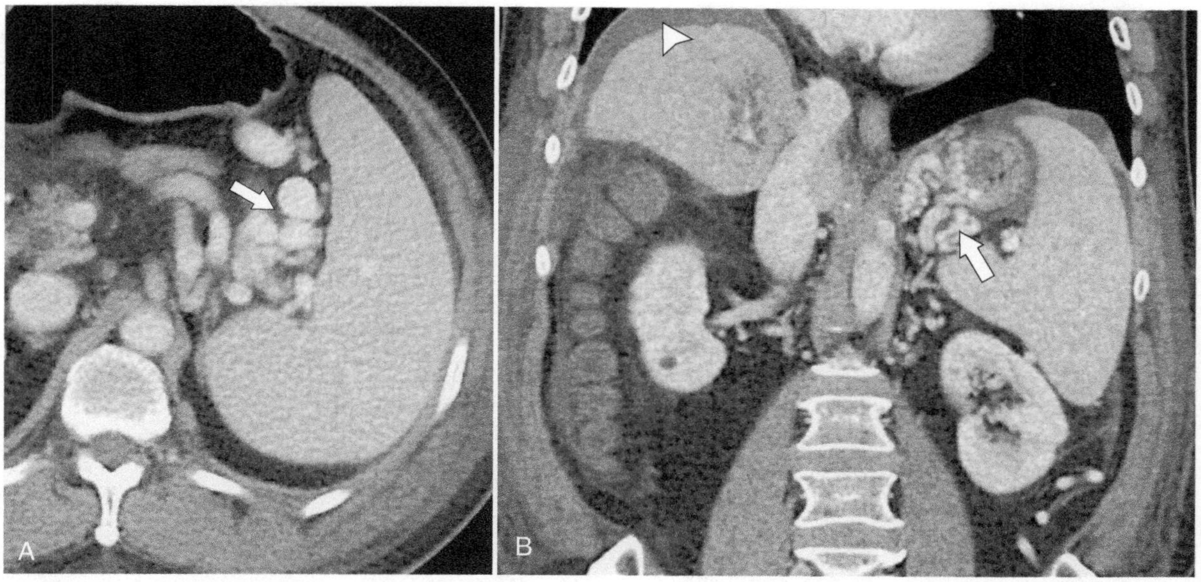

FIGURE 7-9. Axial (**A**) and coronal (**B**) contrast-enhanced CT in a 57-year-old man with cirrhosis, ascites (*arrowhead*), splenic varices (*arrows*), and splenomegaly.

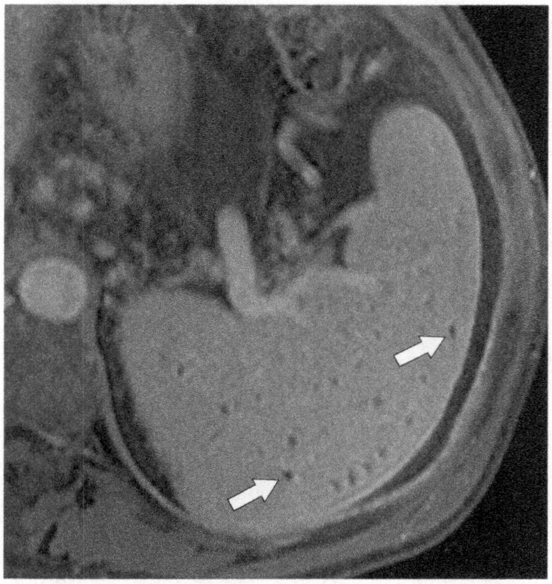

FIGURE 7-10. Axial T1-weighted fat-saturated postcontrast MRI in a 44-year-old man with cirrhosis and multiple hypointense foci in the spleen (*arrows*) caused by Gamna-Gandy bodies.

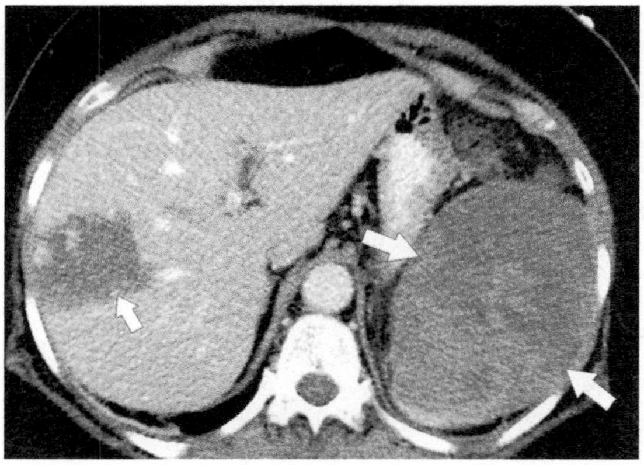

FIGURE 7-11. Axial contrast-enhanced CT in a 66-year-old woman with almost complete splenic replacement by a primary lymphomatous mass (*arrows*). There is an incidental hemangioma in the liver (*small arrow*).

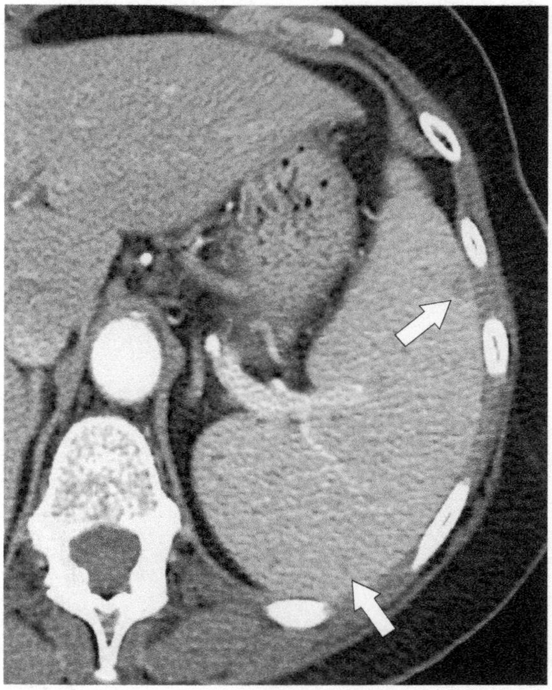

FIGURE 7-12. Axial contrast-enhanced CT in a 75-year-old woman with multiple tiny splenic lesions (*arrows*) caused by small lymphocytic lymphoma.

Lymphoma

Lymphoma is the most common malignant tumor of the spleen and frequently a site of both Hodgkin† (30%) and non-Hodgkin disease (30%). Secondary or metastatic involvement from lymphoma elsewhere is more common than isolated primary splenic lymphoma. For staging purposes, splenomegaly is considered nodal in Hodgkin disease and extranodal in non-Hodgkin disease (see "Lymphoma Staging," Chapter 4).

At imaging, the disease may be a solitary mass (Fig. 7-11), a few or multiple small (Fig. 7-12) or larger (Fig. 7-13) masses, or diffuse

†Alan Lloyd Hodgkin (1914-1998), British physiologist.

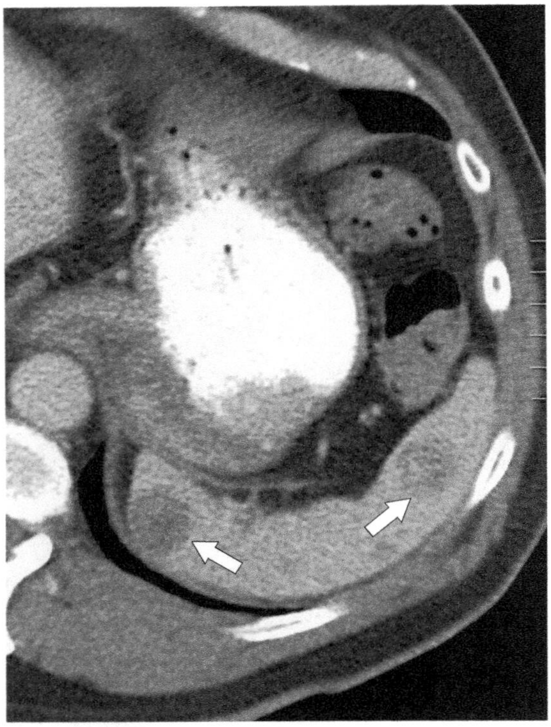

FIGURE 7-13. Axial contrast-enhanced CT in a 51-year-old woman with multiple hypodense splenic lesions (*arrows*) caused by B-cell lymphoma.

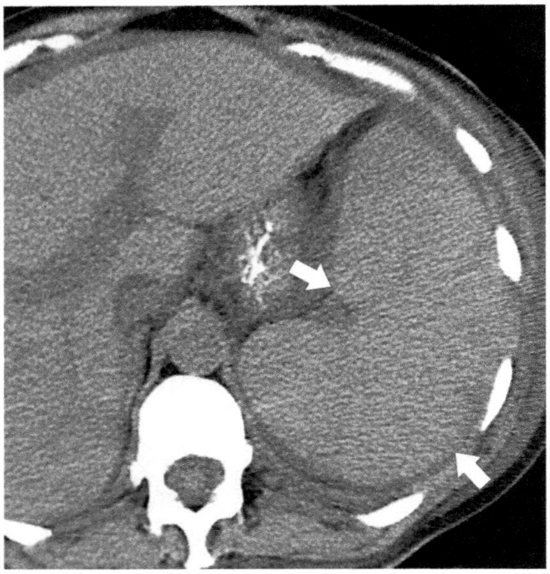

FIGURE 7-14. Axial noncontrast CT in a 37-year-old man with splenomegaly (*arrows*) caused by diffuse infiltration with Epstein-Barr virus–induced lymphoma. There is associated ascites.

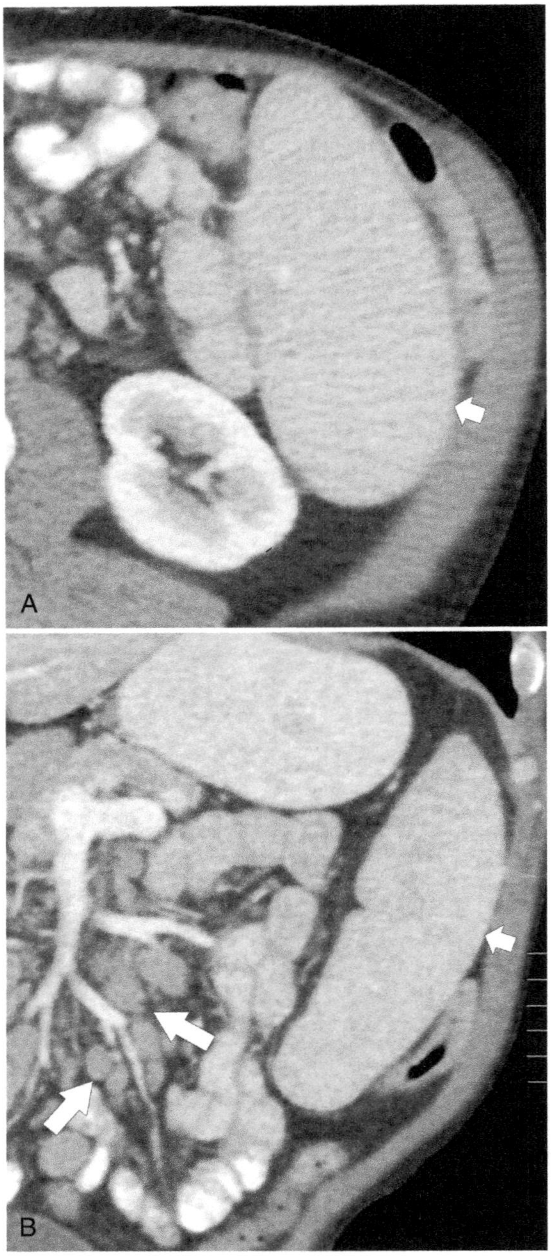

FIGURE 7-15. Axial (**A**) and coronal (**B**) contrast-enhanced CT in a 66-year-old woman demonstrating homogeneous splenomegaly (*short arrows*) caused by non-Hodgkin lymphoma. There is diffuse intraabdominal adenopathy (*arrows*).

splenic involvement (Fig. 7-14). These are mostly hypodense on contrast-enhanced CT, but larger lesions can demonstrate some necrotic or cystic areas. There is usually evidence of extrasplenic lymphoma, particularly mesenteric or retroperitoneal adenopathy (Fig. 7-15). The splenic CT findings are relatively nonspecific, since other infectious or infiltrative disease (Box 7-1) can give similar appearances.

Leukemia

Most leukemias involve the spleen, although this is less common with acute lymphoblastic leukemia. The disease typically affects the spleen uniformly as an infiltrative process of malignant leukemic cells. Splenomegaly can reach massive sizes, particularly with chronic leukemias (especially chronic myelocytic leukemia) (Fig. 7-16). At imaging, the spleen appears uniformly and homogeneously enlarged. With massive splenomegaly the spleen may demonstrate some heterogeneous regions because of either tumor deposits or areas of splenic infarction (wedge shaped or rounded), since some anatomy of the speen is arterially compromised owing to its massive size (Fig. 7-16).

Myeloproliferative Disease

Myeloproliferative disease is a group of bone marrow disorders, including chronic myelogenous leukemia, myelofibrosis (Fig. 7-17), polycythemia rubra vera (Fig. 7-18) (overproduction of red blood cells), and essential thrombocythemia (platelet overproduction).

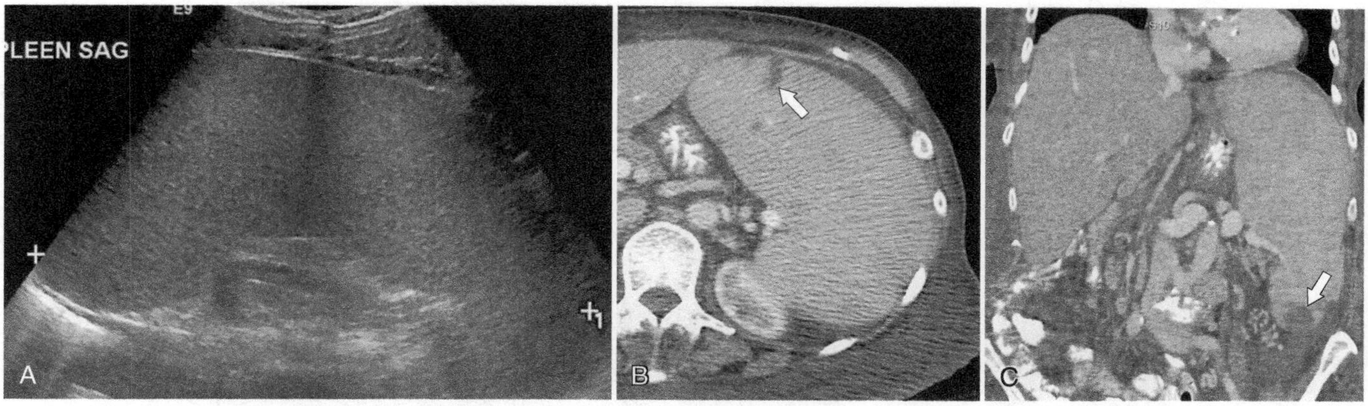

FIGURE 7-16. Sagittal US (**A**), axial (**B**), and coronal (**C**) contrast-enhanced CT in a 76-year-old woman with splenomegaly resulting from chronic lymphocytic leukemia. On US the spleen measures 21 cm in length. CT demonstrates small associated peripheral splenic infarctions (*arrows*).

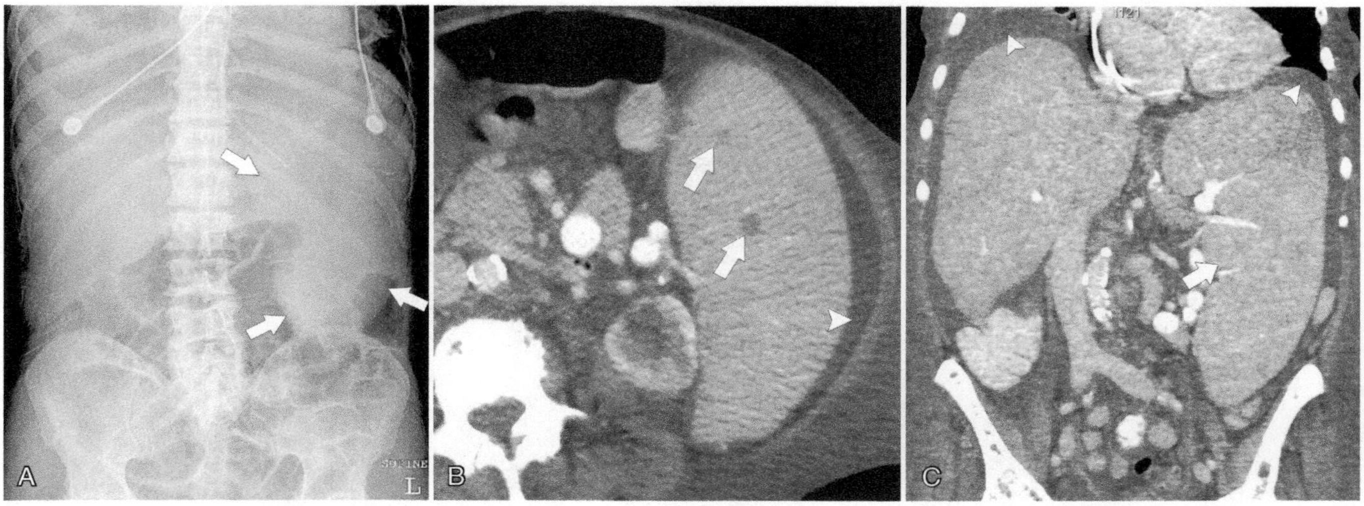

FIGURE 7-17. Plain frontal abdominal radiograph (**A**) in a 77-year-old woman with myelofibrosis and massive splenomegaly (*arrows*). Axial (**B**) and coronal (**C**) contrast-enhanced CT demonstrates splenomegaly and several small hypodense splenic tumors (*small arrow*). There is associated ascites.

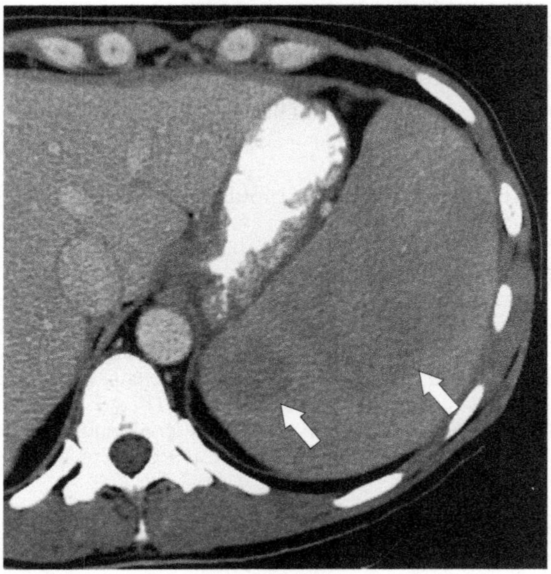

FIGURE 7-18. Axial contrast-enhanced CT in a 58-year-old man with polycythemia rubra vera with splenomegaly and ill-defined splenic hypodensities (*arrows*) caused by extramedullary hematopoiesis.

They may evolve into a myelodysplastic syndrome and acute myeloid leukemia. Splenomegaly is due either to sequestration of the overproduced cell lines, which can also cause vascular occlusion and infarction, ultimately reducing the splenic size, or to extramedullary hemopoiesis as a result of the infiltrative marrow disorder or infiltration with malignant leukemic cells.

Splenic Metastases

Hematogenous metastases are common because of the rich splenic vascular supply and are observed in numerous malignancies, but particularly melanoma, breast cancer, and lung cancer. There is often a history of malignant disease, which helps to differentiate single or multiple splenic lesions from other neoplastic, infectious, or infiltrative causes. Should metastatic disease cause splenomegaly, it is usually because of mass effect from single or, more often, multiple lesions rather than homogeneous enlargement (Fig. 7-19).

Infectious Splenomegaly

Parasites

Many infectious diseases cause splenomegaly (and often hepatosplenomegaly), particularly parasitic diseases that sometimes cause massive enlargement (especially leishmaniasis, schistosomiasis, and malaria). Splenomegaly can be secondary to the

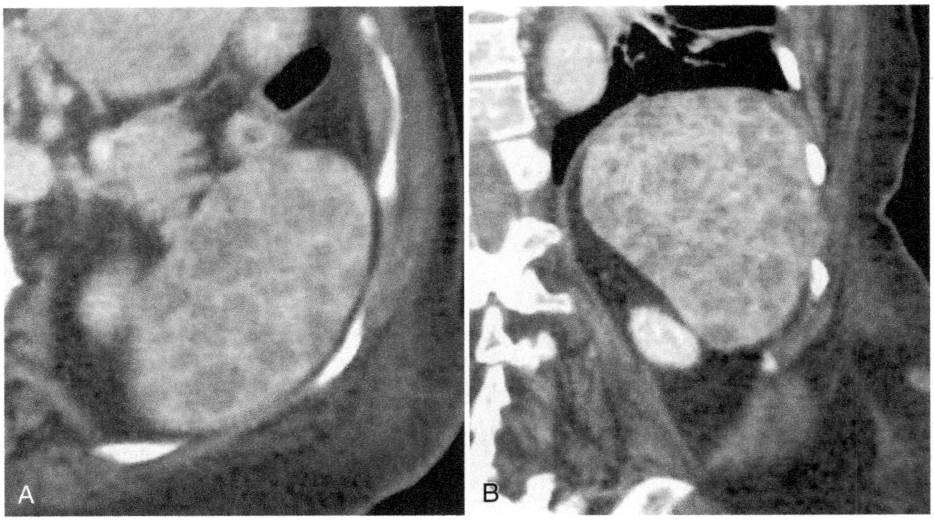

FIGURE 7-19. Axial (**A**) and coronal (**B**) contrast-enhanced CT in a 74-year-old man with lung cancer demonstrating splenomegaly and numerous hypodense splenic metastases.

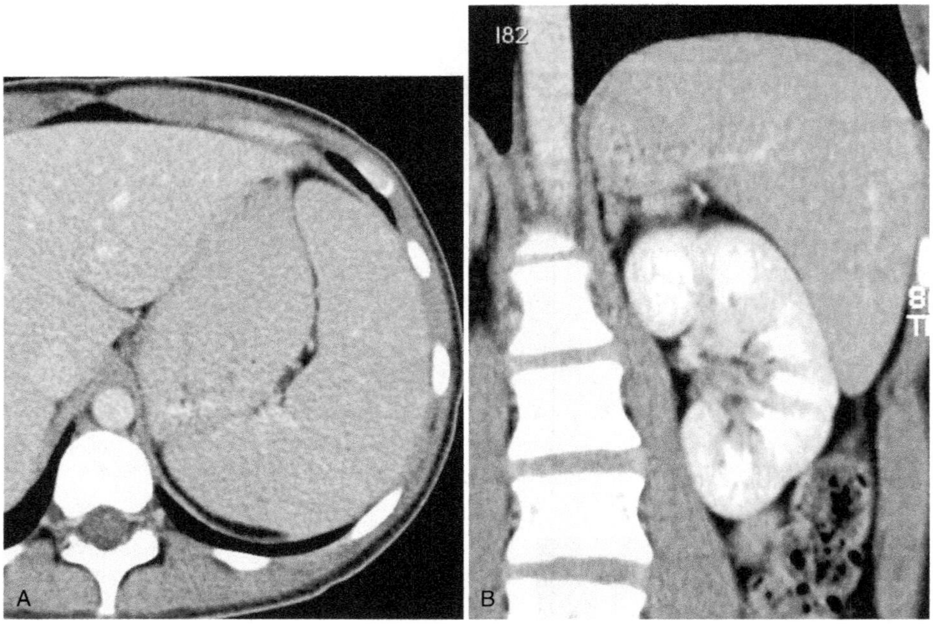

FIGURE 7-20. Axial (**A**) and coronal (**B**) contrast-enhanced CT in a 28-year-old woman with splenomegaly resulting from chronic malarial infection. By CT, the splenomegaly cannot be differentiated from many other causes of splenomegaly.

sequestration of parasitic agents or, as in malaria, an immunoglobulin M (IgM) response from repeated infections with splenic lymphocytic infiltration, also known as tropical splenomegaly syndrome (Fig. 7-20).

Viral Splenic Infection

Similar to other infective agents, viral splenic infection is usually associated with hepatomegaly (see Chapter 6). It can be part of a generalized acute viral hepatitis (hepatitis A through E, human immunodeficiency virus [HIV]) or infectious mononucleosis, but can also be seen in cytomegalovirus and rubella infection. Infectious mononucleosis is secondary to infection with the Epstein-Barr* virus (a herpes virus), and there is characteristic preferential splenic enlargement, which is at particular risk of spontaneous rupture, especially following contact sport injuries (Fig. 7-21).

Bacterial Splenic Infection

A number of bacterial infections can cause diffuse splenomegaly, particularly brucellosis, leptospirosis, and typhoid fever. *Mycobacterium tuberculosis* and histoplasmosis often cause diffuse hepatosplenomegaly in the acute phase and are usually associated with concomitant multiple, hypodense lesions (Fig. 7-22). Repeated embolic assault, particularly from bacterial endocarditis, can cause splenomegaly, including splenic abscess (Fig. 7-23).

Depositional Disease

Amyloidosis (see Chapter 4)

Splenomegaly is usually secondary to primary systemic amyloidosis (AL-type) with accumulation of monoclonal immunoglobulin light chains within the spleen and multiple other organs.

---

*Michael A. Epstein (1921-), British pathologist and virologist; Yvonne Barr (1932-), British virologist.

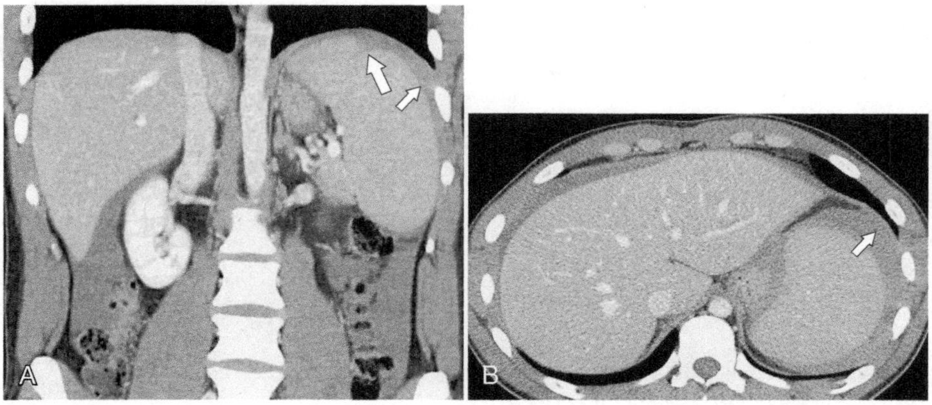

FIGURE 7-21. Coronal (**A**) and axial (**B**) contrast-enhanced CT in a 24-year-old woman with infectious mononucleosis and splenomegaly, splenic rupture (*large arrow*), and intraabdominal hemorrhage (*small arrows*).

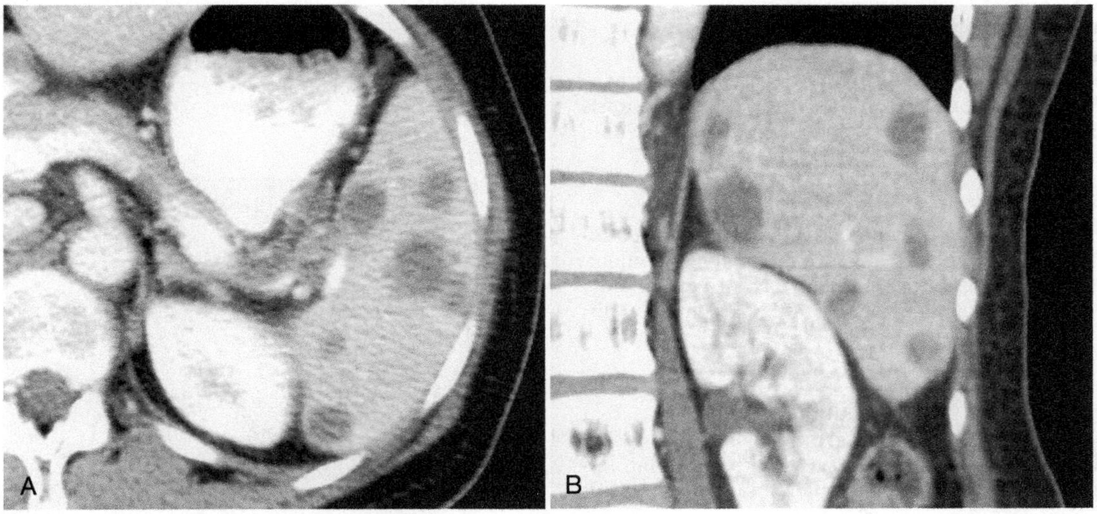

FIGURE 7-22. Axial (**A**) and coronal (**B**) contrast-enhanced CT in a 53-year-old man with tuberculosis and mild splenomegaly and multiple hypodense tuberculous splenic lesions.

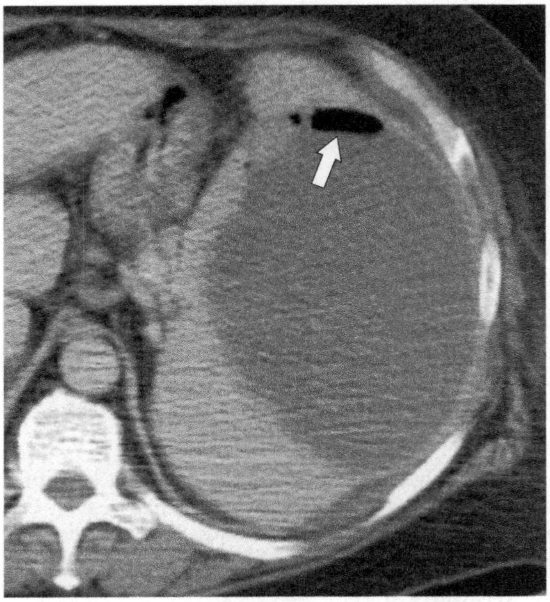

FIGURE 7-23. Axial contrast-enhanced CT in a 66-year-old man with splenomegaly and a 10-cm splenic abscess with air/fluid level (*arrow*) caused by gas-forming organisms.

Hypersplenism

Hypersplenism is a pancytopenia (erythrocytes, platelets, and granulocytes) to a variable degree caused by an enlarged spleen that is responsible for their premature destruction. Hypersplenism results from splenomegaly from almost any cause (Box 7-2), but not all cases of splenomegaly cause hypersplenism. Hypersplenism may or may not be associated with increased bone marrow activity as a counter to the pancytopenia.

Autoimmune Disease

Many autoimmune conditions can cause splenomegaly (Box 7-1).

Autoimmune Hemolytic Anemia

As its name suggests, autoimmune hemolytic anemia is an autoimmune reaction to red blood cells. The primary disease is idiopathic, whereas secondary disease can be caused by a number of lymphoproliferative or autoimmune disorders (systemic lupus erythematosus, ulcerative colitis, rheumatoid arthritis, and scleroderma). The damaged red blood cells are sequestered in the spleen, leading to splenomegaly.

Idiopathic Thrombocytopenic Purpura

Idiopathic thrombocytopenic purpura (ITP) is an autoimmune disorder in which antibody production against platelets leads to thrombocytopenia and hypersplenism as the defective platelets

Box 7-2. Causes of Small Spleen

Congenital (Fanconi syndrome)
Sickle cell anemia
Essential thrombocytopenia
Irradiation
Thorotrast
Wegener granulomatosis

are sequestered in the spleen. The disease may be asymptomatic but often causes purpura or bleeding diathesis.

Systemic Lupus Erythematosus

Systemic lupus erythematosus is a systemic autoimmune disease with repeated episodes of vasculitis and inflammatory disease. In the acute phase, this can result in hepatosplenomegaly, although it more commonly causes glomerulonephritis, dermatological rashes, arthritis, and neuropsychiatric disorders.

Granulomatosis with Polyangiitis (Wegener Granulomatosis)

A multisystemic vasculitis, usually requiring lifelong immunosuppressive therapy, Wegener* granulomatosis (granulomatosis with polyangiitis) can cause repeated splenic infarctions leading ultimately to a "shrunken" spleen (Fig. 7-24).

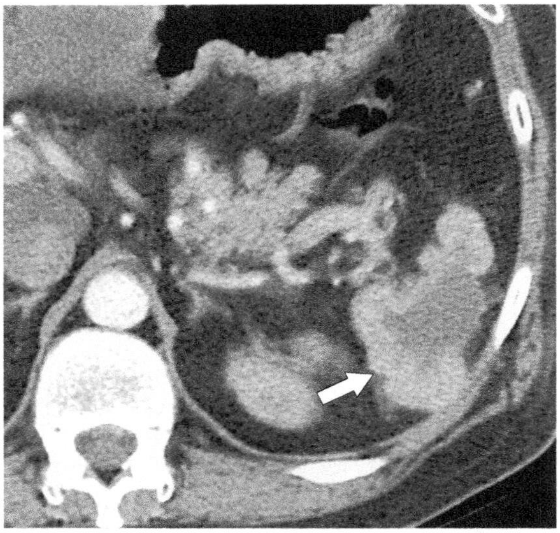

FIGURE 7-24. Axial contrast-enhanced CT in a 41-year-old man with Wegener granulomatosis and a shrunken heterogeneous spleen (*arrow*) as a result of multiple infarctions.

Felty Syndrome

Splenomegaly is part of Felty* syndrome with associated neutropenia (secondary to splenic sequestration from granulocytic abnormalities) and rheumatoid arthritis. The spleen can be markedly enlarged. Anemia and thrombocytopenia often accompany this syndrome.

Sjögren Syndrome

Sjögren† syndrome is a systemic autoimmune disease that predominantly affects the exocrine glands (parotid and salivary glands). However, it is often associated with other autoimmune connective tissue disorders, and splenomegaly may result (Fig. 7-25).

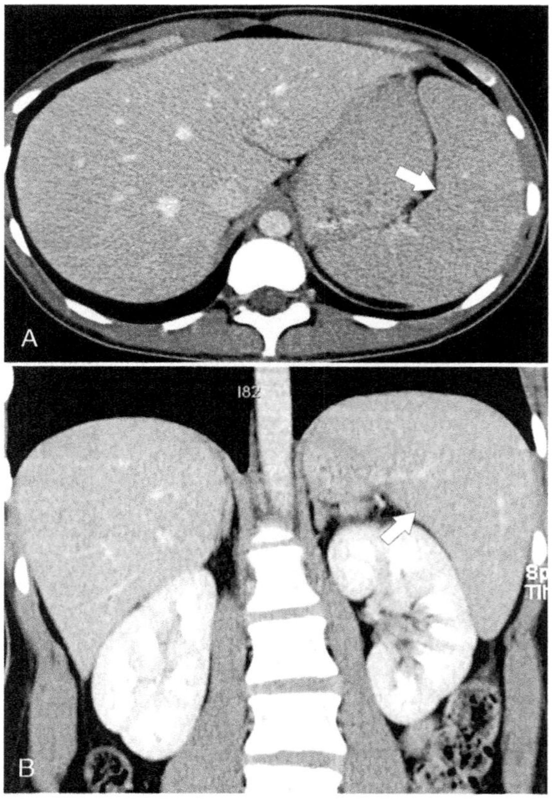

FIGURE 7-25. Axial (**A**) and coronal (**B**) contrast-enhanced CT in a 28-year-old woman with Sjögren syndrome and spelnomegaly (*arrows*).

SMALL OR SHRUNKEN SPLEEN (BOX 7-2)

Congenital (Fanconi Syndrome)

A small spleen as a congenital condition is very uncommon but has been described in Fanconi‡ syndrome, a disease of the proximal renal tubules with loss of bicarbonate renal tubular acidosis and phosphate and rickets formation. Causes of Fanconi syndrome include cystinosis and Wilson* disease, among others.

Sickle Cell Disease

Although the spleen is commonly enlarged in the more acute phases of sickle cell disease, the repetitive splenic infarctions ultimately lead to a small, often fibrotic spleen that is effectively nonfunctioning, such that it is frequently termed an autosplenectomy (Fig. 7-26). The small residual mass may calcify (Fig. 7-27).

Essential Thrombocythemia (Thrombocytosis)

Essential thrombocythemia, or thrombocytosis, is a myeloproliferative disease with overproduction of platelets by megakaryocytes in the bone marrow. Initially splenomegaly occurs, but ultimately numerous splenic infarcts caused by platelet aggregates can lead to a small spleen, as in sickle cell disease.

Splenic Irradiation

Radiation change that produces endarteritis obliterans and chronic multiple small splenic infarctions results in hyposplenism.

*Friedrich Wegener (1907-1990), German pathologist.
*Augustus R. Felty (1895-1964), U.S. internal medicine physician.
†Henrick Sjögren (1899-1986), Swedish ophthalmologist.
‡Guido Fanconi (1892-1979), Swiss pediatrician.
*Samuel A.K. Wilson (1878-1937), British neurologist.

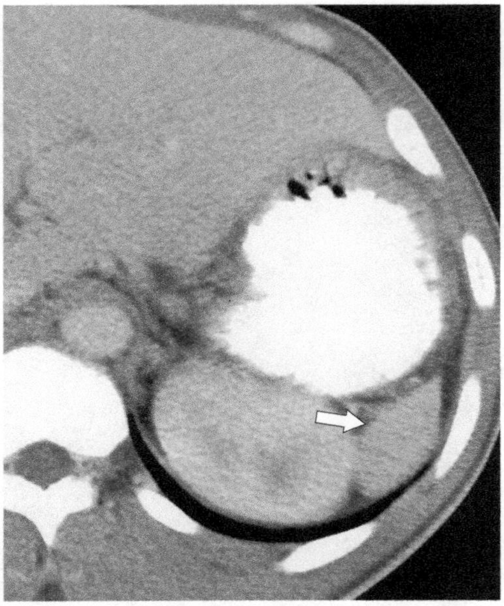

FIGURE 7-26. Axial contrast-enhanced CT in a 39-year-old woman with sickle cell disease and a small spleen (*arrow*) resulting from repeated thrombotic episodes.

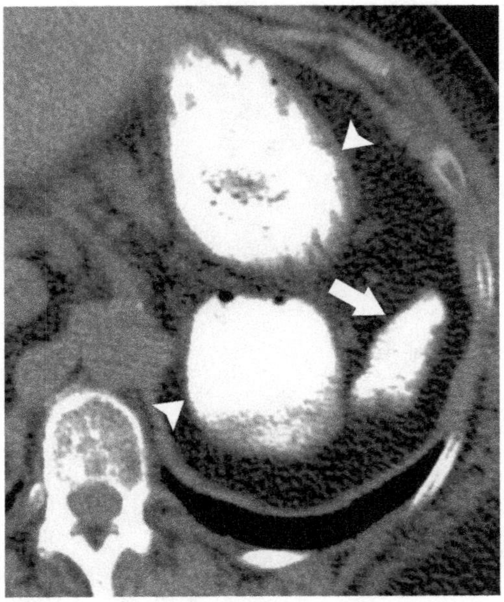

FIGURE 7-27. Axial noncontrast CT in a 44-year-old woman with sickle cell disease and a small calcified "shrunken" spleen (*arrow*). The stomach is filled with oral contrast material (*arrowheads*).

Thorotrast

The presence of Thorotrast is now rarely identified because its use as an intravascular angiographic contrast agent was terminated in the 1950s following the discovery that its alpha-emitting particles could lead to malignancies (mainly splenic angiosarcoma). It was readily sequestered by the mononuclear phagocytic system, mainly the liver and spleen, resulting in hyperdense organs (particularly the spleen). Thorotrast in the spleen sets up a chronic reactive process, ultimately leading to fibrosis and splenic contraction (Fig. 7-28).

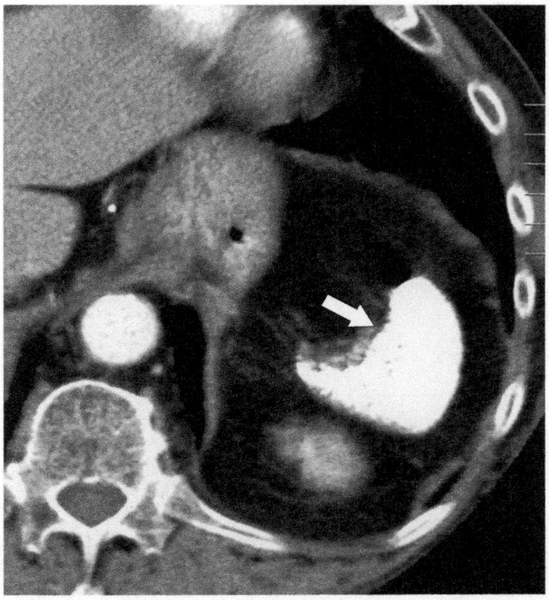

FIGURE 7-28. Axial contrast-enhanced CT in a 79-year-old man with previous Thorotrast contrast agent administration and a hyperdense spleen (*arrow*), representing sequestered Thorotrast.

TABLE 7-1 Benign Splenic Lesions

Type	Etiology	Single	Multiple
Cyst	Pseudocyst	++	+
	Epithelioid	++	+
Infection	Bacterial abscess	++	+
	Fungal	+	+++
	Mycobacterial	+	+++
	Parasitic	+	+
	Yeast	+	+++
Infarction	Infarction	+	+
	Hematoma	+	+
Neoplasm	Hemangioma	++	+
	Hamartoma	++	+
	Littoral cell angioma	+	++
	Lymphangioma	++	+
	SANT	+	–
	PEComa	+	–
	Inflammatory pseudotumor	+	–
	Epithelioid granuloma	+	–
	Chondroma	+	–
	Myxoma	+	–
	Osteoma	+	–
Infiltrative	Granuloma (sarcoid)	+	++
	Gaucher disease	+	++

PEComa, Perivascular epitheliod cell tumor; *SANT*, sclerosing angiomatoid nodular transformation.

SPLENIC MASS LESIONS

Splenic mass lesions can be classified as either single or multiple, benign (Table 7-1) or malignant (Table 7-2) lesions. Benign and malignant primary splenic lesions tend to be single, whereas metastatic and infectious lesions are multiple.

Benign Splenic Lesions

Gaucher Disease

Gaucher disease types 1 and 3 can survive into adulthood and usually lead to hepatosplenomegaly caused by accumulation of

TABLE 7-2 Malignant Splenic Lesions

Etiology	Single	Multiple
Lymphoma	+	+
Metastasis	+	+
Angiosarcoma	++	+
Hemangiosarcoma	++	+
Hemangiopericytoma	++	–
Kaposi sarcoma	+	++
Fibrosarcoma	+	–
Leiomyosarcoma	+	–

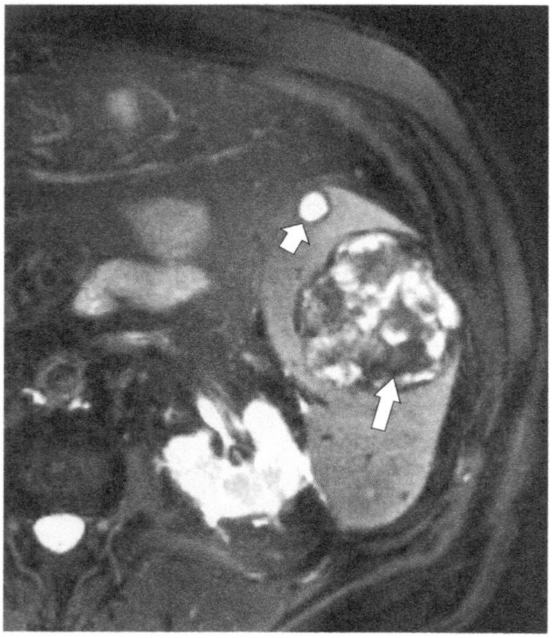

FIGURE 7-29. Axial T2 fat-saturated MRI in a 77-year-old with Gaucher disease demonstrating a complex splenic mass consistent with "gaucheroma" (*large arrow*). There is an incidental simple splenic cyst in the anterior spleen (*small arrow*).

glucocerebroside. The unmetabolized lipids may accumulate as discrete focal hepatic or splenic masses known as gaucheromas (Fig. 7-29).

Splenic Cysts

The majority of splenic cysts are thought to be pseudocysts and probably posttraumatic because they have no epithelial lining (Fig. 7-30). True epidermoid cysts are less common, lined by epithelial tissue, and most likely congenital (Fig. 7-31). The walls of both types can calcify. They are not usually associated with cystic disease elsewhere (kidney, liver, pancreas). On imaging they are generally simple and are uniformly hypodense on CT or uniformly sonolucent on US (Fig. 7-31). On MRI they demonstrate typical cystic features of low T1-weighted and high T2-weighted signal. Occasionally they are complicated by secondary infection or hemorrhage.

Splenic Infections

Most infective splenic lesions are multiple rather than solitary, although isolated splenic lesions are sometimes found.

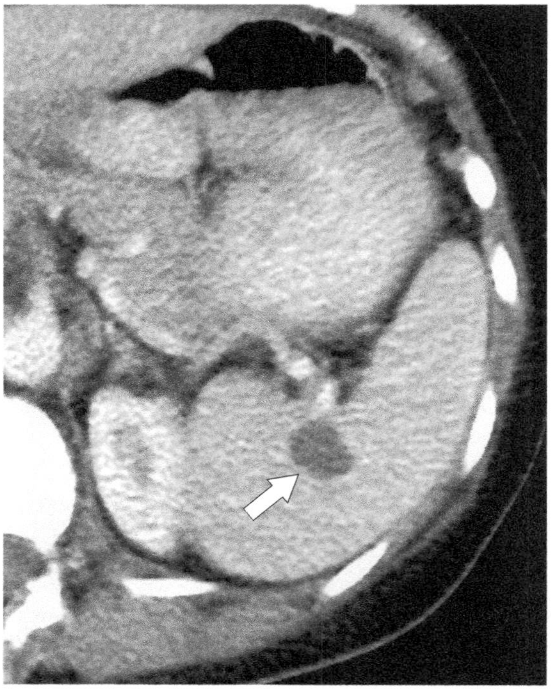

FIGURE 7-30. Axial contrast-enhanced CT in a 66-year-old woman with a 1.8-cm simple splenic cyst (*arrow*).

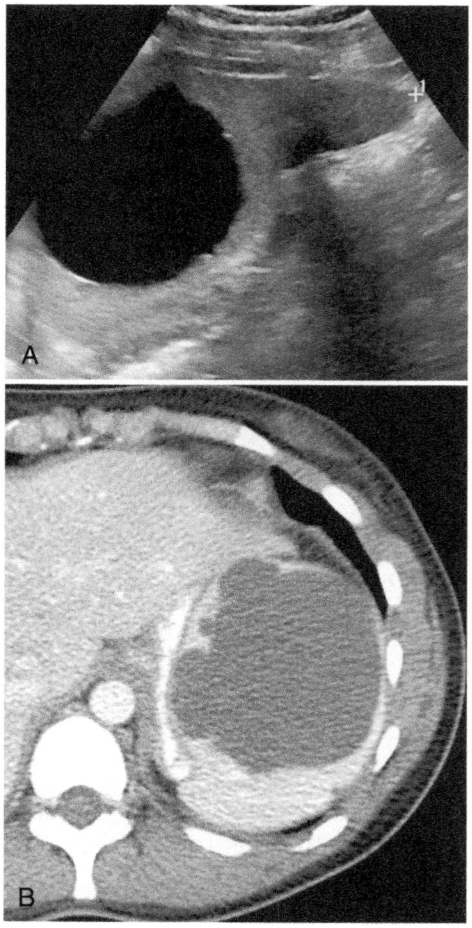

FIGURE 7-31. Sagittal US (**A**) and axial contrast-enhanced CT (**B**) in a 28-year-old woman with a sonolucent 7-cm lesion that is uniformly hypodense at CT and represents a splenic epidermoid cyst.

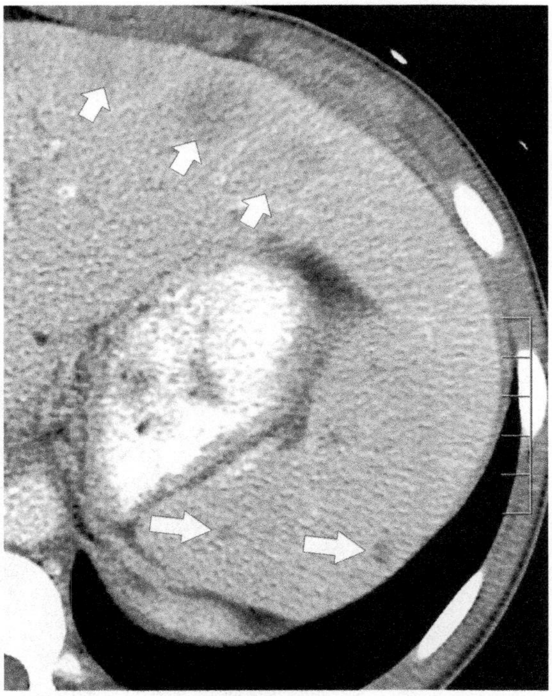

FIGURE 7-32. Axial contrast-enhanced CT in a 17-year-old man with *Bartonella* sp. infection, or "cat-scratch fever," demonstrating multiple splenic and hepatic hypodense bacterial lesions (*arrows*). There are also subtle hepatic lesions (*small arrows*).

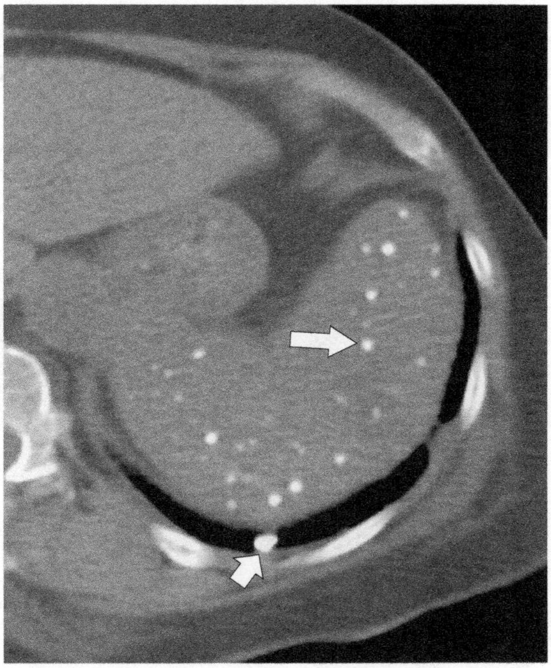

FIGURE 7-34. Axial noncontrast CT in a 55-year-old man with previous histoplasmosis and multiple calcified splenic granulomata (*arrow*). An associated calcified granuloma is in the right lower lobe (*short arrow*).

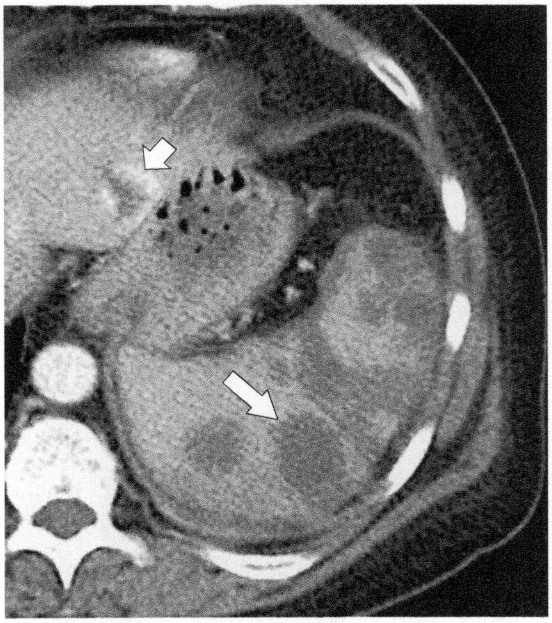

FIGURE 7-33. Axial contrast-enhanced CT demonstrating multiple hypodense fungal splenic masses (*long arrow*) in a 28-year-old woman taking high-dose steroids. There is an incidental liver hemangioma (*short arrow*).

Bacterial Abscess

Pyogenic abscesses may be single (Fig. 7-22) but are more often multiple (Fig. 7-33). They can be unilocular or multilocular and present with the expected symptoms of fever, pain, and elevated white blood cell count. They are often caused by septic emboli, particularly endocarditis. On CT they are nonenhancing, complex, low-density masses (Figs. 7-22 and 7-32).

Fungal Abscess

Fungal (*Candida, Cryptococcus,* and *Aspergillus* spp.) splenic abscesses may be single but are usually multiple (Fig. 7-33) and often smaller than pyogenic abscesses. A history of immunosuppression strongly suggests the diagnosis. Histoplasmosis often heals by calcification (Fig. 7-34).

Mycobacterial Infection

Tuberculous infection is rarely limited to the spleen. Patients are often immunocompromised. The splenic findings are nonspecific, with single or multiple low-density lesions that can be large (Fig. 7-21) or small (Fig. 7-35) on CT imaging. Similar to tuberculosis elsewhere, the infection often heals by calcification. *Mycobacterium avium-intracellulare* infection gives a similar appearance but is usually confined to patients with AIDS.

Parasitic Disease

Hydatid (*Echinococcus granulosus*) disease of the spleen is rare and usually occurs in association with hepatic disease. The splenic disease, like that of the liver, is much more likely to originate in countries where animal husbandry is common. The CT features are similar to those in the liver and include single or multiple irregular low-density cysts, some with daughter cysts, and a thick wall. The "drooping lily" sign of a collapsing cyst wall from cyst death is also recognized (Fig. 7-36).

Yeast Infections

Infection with *Pneumocystis jirovecii* (previously known as *Pneumocystis carinii* and misclassified as a protozoan) usually occurs in patients with AIDS and may infiltrate both the liver and spleen and is commonly associated with pneumocystis pneumonia. CT imaging features demonstrate multiple low-density lesions, but these are nonspecific findings. Yeast infection differs from fungal disease as it may demonstrate calcification in some lesions. Lesions also tend to be larger than those seen in other splenic infective diseases (Fig. 7-37).

Splenic Infarct

Splenic infarcts are the most common cause of solitary or multiple splenic defects and should therefore always be considered in the differential dignosis for any discrete splenic lesion (Box 7-3). Most demonstrate peripheral wedge-shaped hypoattenuating defects at CT (Fig. 7-38), best visualized after the administration of intravenous contrast material. Many splenic infarcts, however, do not demonstrate the classic peripheral wedge-shaped defect and are more irregular or even rounded in shape, both at the periphery and within the spleen (Figs. 7-13 and 7-39).

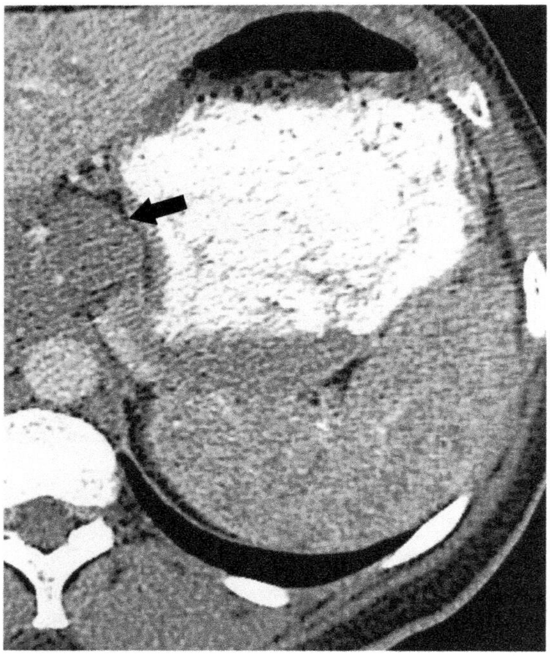

Figure 7-35. Axial contrast-enhanced CT in a 49-year-old man with numerous small hepatic and splenic hypodense lesions caused by tuberculosis. There is associated intraabdominal adenopathy (*arrow*).

Sarcoidosis

Granulomatous splenic infiltration can occur with sarcoidosis, recognized as numerous, smaller, hypodense lesions (Fig. 7-40). PET imaging can determine the degree of splenic sarcoid as either diffuse or isolated (Fig. 7-41).

Epithelioid Granuloma

Epithelioid granuloma is a very rare, sometimes large, granulomatous mass with or without necrosis. It is caused by various systemic intraabdominal diseases involving multiple organs (Fig. 7-42).

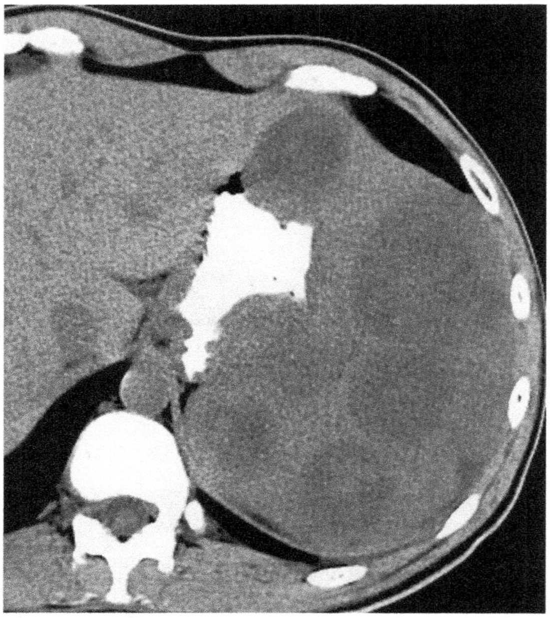

Figure 7-37. Axial noncontrast CT in a 38-year-old man with AIDS and multiple low-density splenic lesions caused by *Pneumocystis jirovecii* infection.

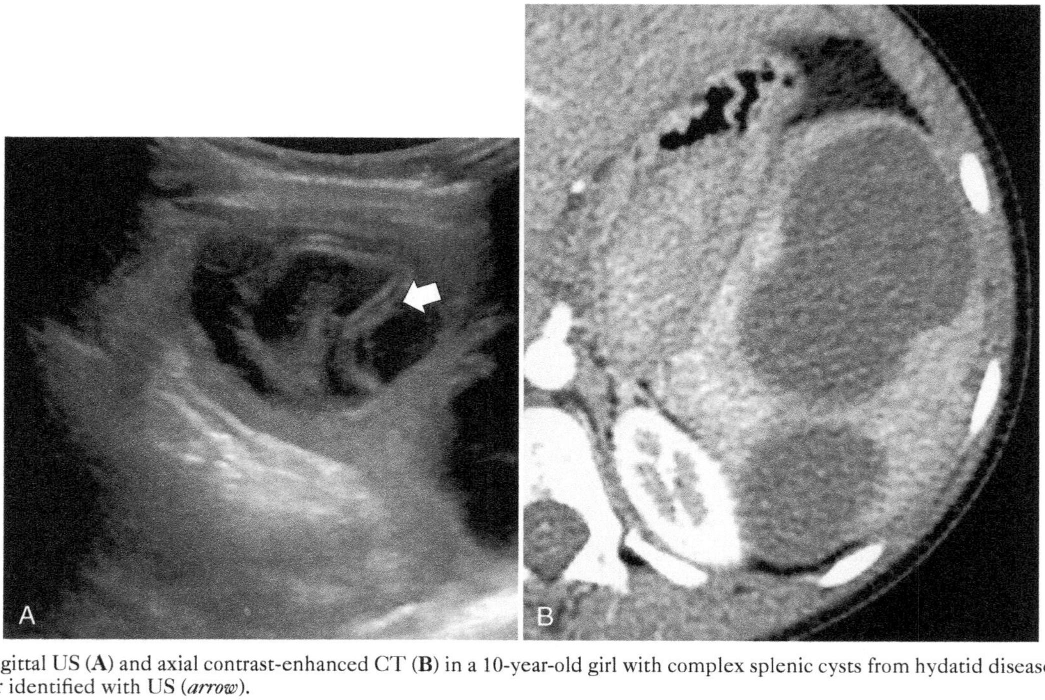

Figure 7-36. Sagittal US (**A**) and axial contrast-enhanced CT (**B**) in a 10-year-old girl with complex splenic cysts from hydatid disease. The "drooping lily" sign is better identified with US (*arrow*).

Box 7-3. Causes of Splenic Infarct

EMBOLIC
Infectious endocarditis
Atheroma
Valve vegetations, atrial fibrillation
Mitral stenosis

TUMOR
Lymphoma (hematogenous)
Leukemia
Pancreatic (local invasion)

INFLAMMATORY
Pancreatitis
Connective tissue diseases

THROMBOTIC
Sickle cell disease
Polycythemia rubra vera
Hypercoagulable states (diffuse intravascular dissemination, malignancy)

HYPERSPLENISM
Any cause (refer to Box 7-1)

MECHANICAL
Splenic torsion (i.e., wandering spleen)
Splenic trauma

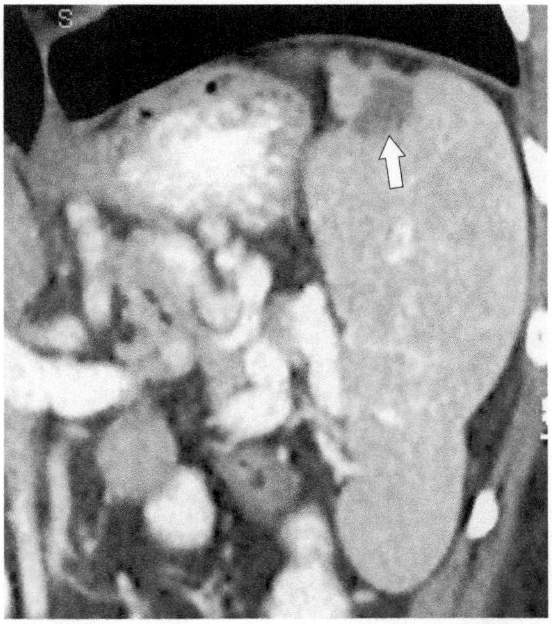

FIGURE 7-39. Coronal contrast-enhanced CT in a 43-year-old woman with a partially rounded hypodense splenic lesion (*arrow*) caused by an infarct. There is also splenomegaly.

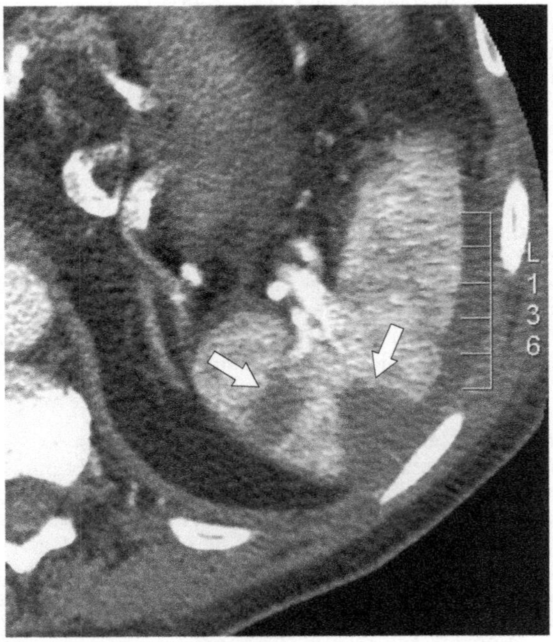

FIGURE 7-38. Axial contrast-enhanced CT in an 83-year-old woman with peripheral hypoattenuating nonenhancing splenic defects (*arrows*) caused by infarcts.

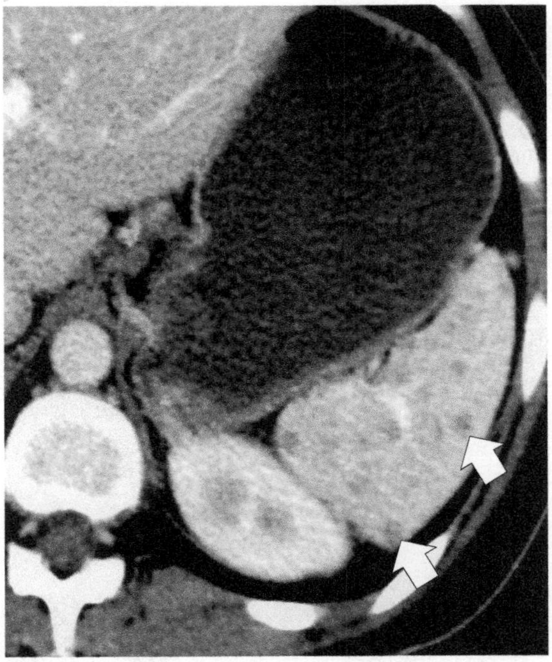

FIGURE 7-40. Axial contrast-enhanced CT in a 34-year-old woman with multiple splenic granulomas (*arrows*) from sarcoidosis.

Splenic Hemangioma

Although uncommonly seen by imaging, hemangioma is the most common benign splenic tumor and has been noted in up to 14% of autopsy studies. The sonographic appearances are variable, sometimes hyperechoic (Fig. 7-43), like hepatic hemangiomas but in other cases complex and of mixed echogenicity (Fig. 7-44). The tumors can be solid or cystic, heterogeneous or homogeneous. They can uncommonly calcify. On contrast-enhanced cross-sectional imaging they demonstrate less reliable appearances, and so, unlike hemangiomas in the liver, many are difficult to characterize. For instance, they may demonstrate peripheral enhancement after the administration of IV contrast medium that progressively fills in toward the center (Fig. 7-44), but these appearances are unpredictable. At MRI, they may or may not show hyperintense T2 signal and their enhancement is similar to that observed with CT. The major differential diagnosis is with splenic hamartoma, whose enhancement characteristics can be identical.

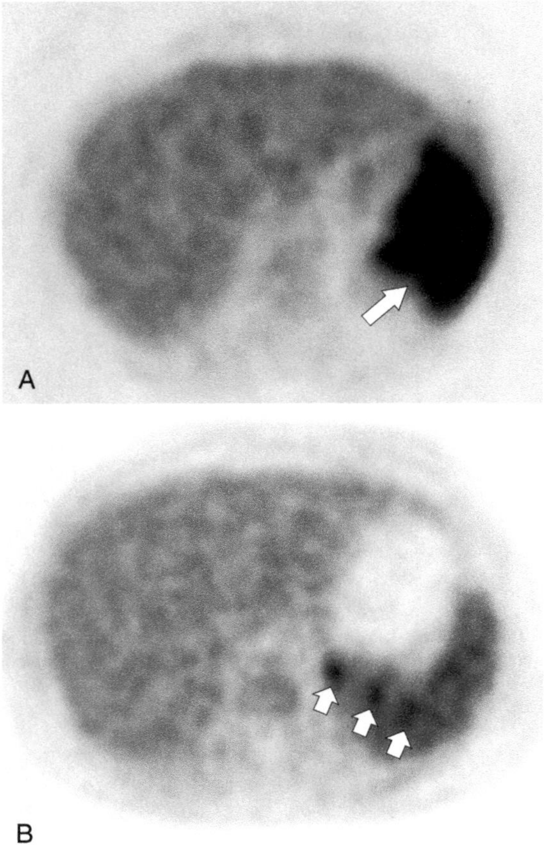

FIGURE 7-41. PET imaging in two patients with splenic sarcoid, one with diffuse and marked FDG uptake (**A**, *arrow*), the other with discrete subtle areas of uptake (**B**, *small arrows*).

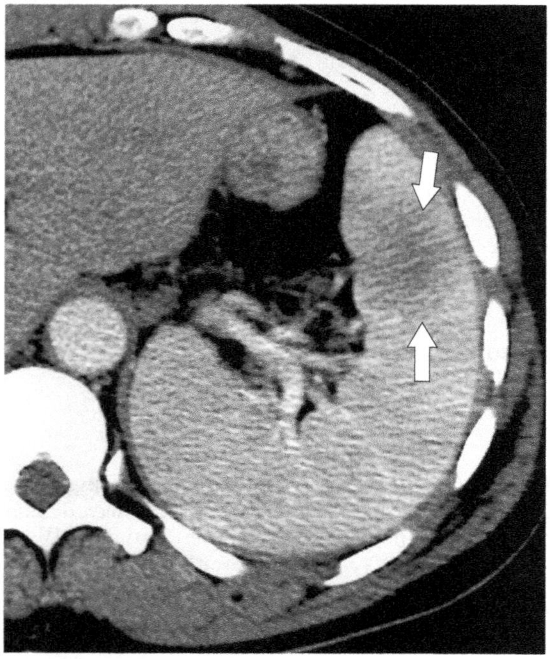

FIGURE 7-42. Axial contrast-enhanced CT in a 39-year-old man with an ill-defined, 3.5-cm splenic mass (*arrows*) due to an epithelioid granuloma.

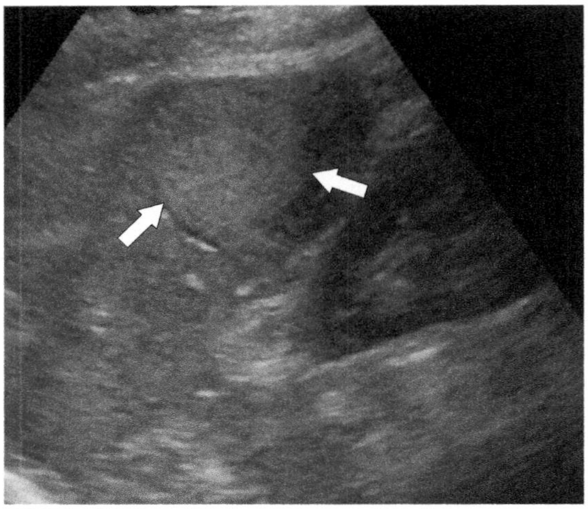

FIGURE 7-43. Sagittal US in a 36-year-old woman with a 3.5-cm hyperechoic splenic mass (*arrows*) representing a hemangioma.

Splenic Hamartoma

Hamartomas are uncommon vascular tumors of the spleen that are usually an incidental finding. They are generally hyperechoic on US and can be difficult to visualize. On CT they appear similar to hemangiomas, although the enhancement tends to be more heterogeneous with variable filling-in toward the center on delayed images (Fig. 7-45). They can therefore be difficult or impossible to differentiate from hemangiomas by imaging. On MRI they are often isointense on T1-weighted imaging and slightly hyperintense on T2-weighted images (Fig. 7-45). As with CT, they generally show peripheral nodular enhancement and variable centripetal filling-in of contrast material. Similar to hemangiomas, they can also show areas of calcification.

Splenic Lymphangioma

Splenic lymphangiomas are rare and classically of low density at CT, sometimes cyst like, with thin walls and sharp margins, often in a subcapsular location. The walls may demonstrate curvilinear calcifications. Fine internal septa are frequently seen (Fig. 7-46) and are better identified after the administration of IV contrast agent or with MRI.

Littoral Cell Angioma

Littoral cell angiomas are rare benign vascular splenic tumors arising from littoral cells in the red pulp sinuses. They can be as large as 6 to 8 cm and are often multiple. They appear hypodense on noncontrast CT imaging and demonstrate irregular enhancement after administration of IV contrast material (Fig. 7-47). They may become relatively isodense with the spleen on delayed imaging, which makes differentiation from splenic hamartomas and hemangiomas difficult because they can show similar features. Usually the diagnosis can be made only by percutaneous biopsy or splenectomy.

Sclerosing Angiomatoid Nodular Transformation

Sclerosing angiomatoid nodular transformation (SANT) is a rare benign vascular tumor composed of multiple red pulp nodules made from endothelial cells interspersed with fibrous bands, sometimes with a central scar. At imaging, unless the scar is identified, there are no particular identifying features. The tumors are typically hypodense but may demonstrate some peripheral enhancement and, like hemangiomas and hamartomas, can become isodense with the spleen on delayed imaging (Fig. 7-48).

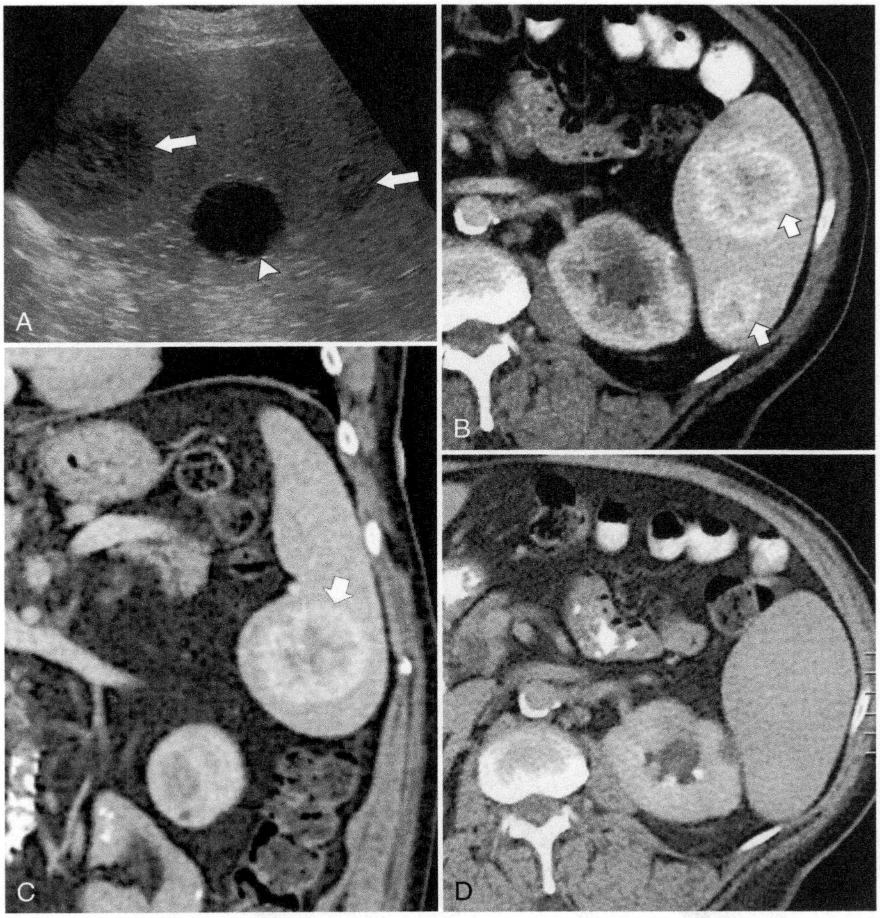

FIGURE 7-44. Sagittal US (**A**), axial (**B, D**), and coronal (**C**) contrast-enhanced CT in a 70-year-old man with splenic hemangiomas. US demonstrates hypoechoic splenic lesions (*arrows*), and CT demonstrates heterogeneous but predominantly peripherally enhancing lesions (*small arrows*). The lesions show complete contrast "fill-in" on delayed images such that they are barely perceptible against the normal parenchyma. There is an incidental renal cyst (*arrowhead*).

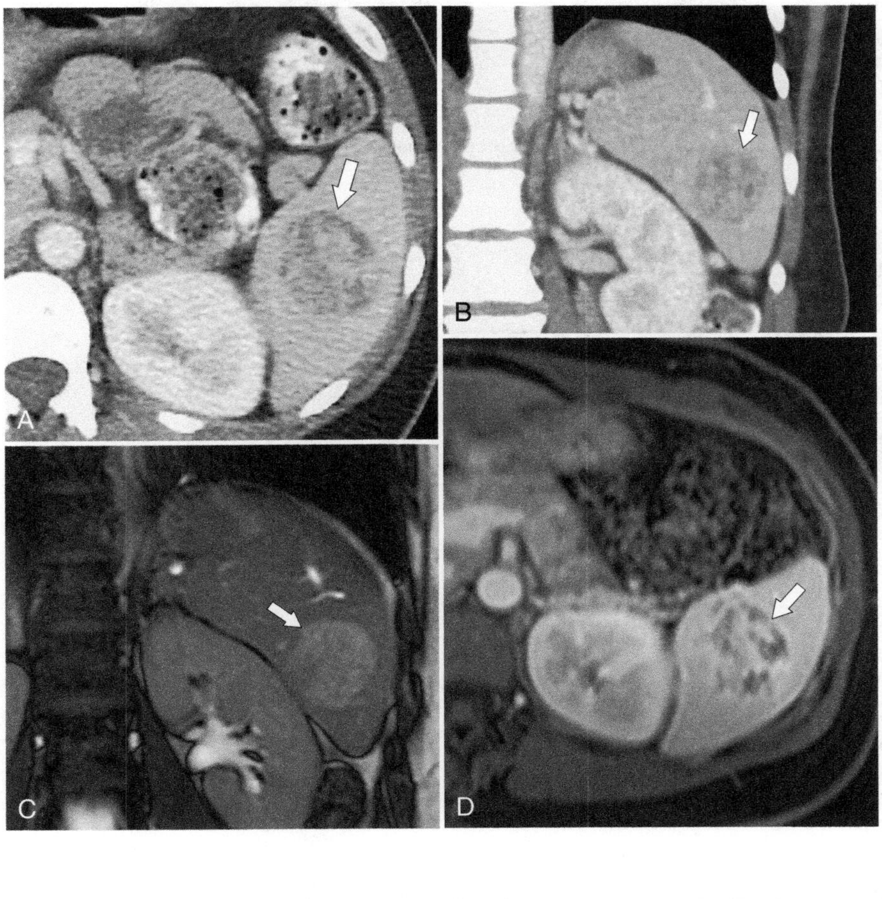

FIGURE 7-45. Axial (**A**) and coronal (**B**) contrast-enhanced CT and coronal T2-weighted (**C**) and postcontrast fat-saturated T1-weighted (**D**) MRI in a 45-year-old woman with a slightly T2 hyperintense and heterogeneously enhancing 5-cm splenic mass (*arrows*). The appearance was similar to a hemangioma but proved to be a hamartoma.

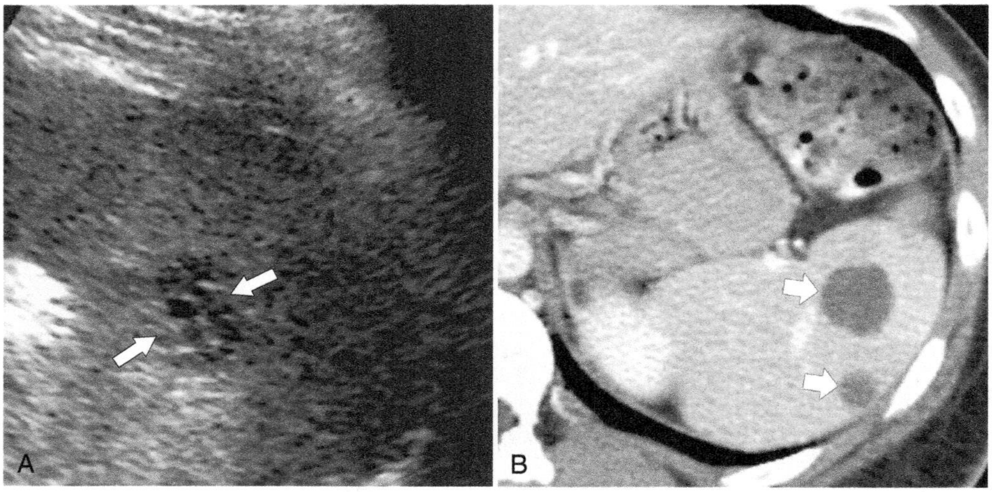

Figure 7-46. Sagittal US (**A**) and axial (**B**) contrast-enhanced CT in a 38-year-old woman with splenic lymphangioma. US demonstrates an ill-defined, small, complex, cyst-like structure (*arrows*) with internal septa. CT demonstrates low-density complex cysts with the septa barely visible (*small arrows*).

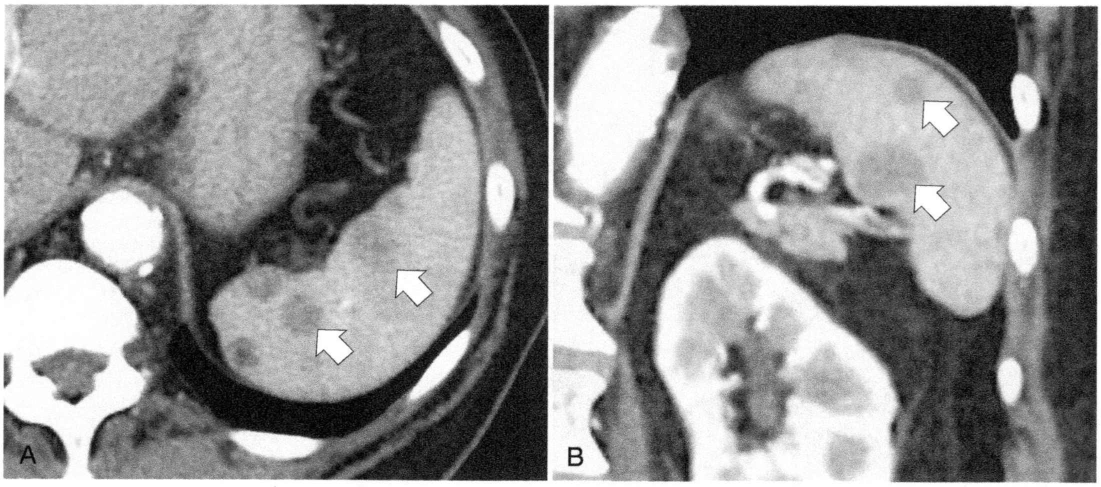

Figure 7-47. Axial (**A**) and coronal (**B**) contrast-enhanced CT in a 66-year-old woman with multiple hypodense splenic lesions (*arrows*) that proved to be littoral cell angiomas.

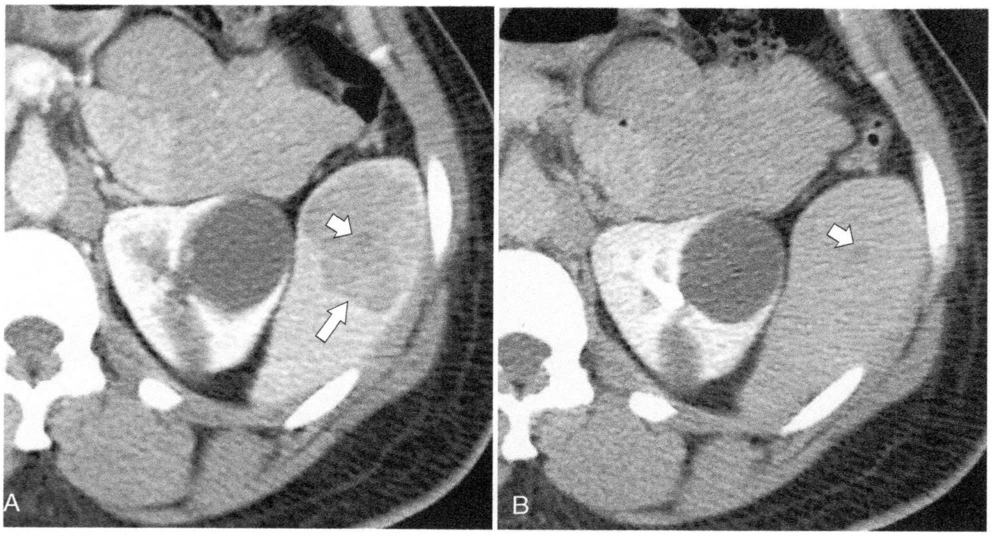

Figure 7-48. Axial portal venous phase (**A**) and delayed (**B**) contrast-enhanced CT in a 48-year-old woman with a 4-cm heterogeneously enhancing mass (*arrows*) representing a sclerosing angiomatoid nodular transformation (SANT) that is almost isodense with the spleen on delayed imaging. There is a small central nonenhancing scar (*small arrows*).

Perivascular Epithelioid Cell Tumor

The perivascular epithelioid cell tumor (PEComa; clear cell "sugar" tumor) is a very rare benign lesion, far more common in women, that more commonly occurs in the lung. It has been described anywhere in the abdomen. It is a mesenchymal neoplasm related to angiomyolipoma and lymphangiomyomatosis, both of which are more common in tuberous sclerosis. Contrast-enhanced CT demonstrates diffuse heterogeneity with some areas of intense enhancement and other areas with little or no enhancement (Fig. 7-49).

Inflammatory Pseudotumor

Inflammatory pseudotumors, also known as inflammatory myofibroblastic tumors, are rare benign tumors that contain inflammatory cells (lymphocytes, plasma cells, and eosinophils) and can occur within any organ in the body. The pathogenesis is uncertain. At imaging they typically demonstrate enhancement (Fig. 7-50), but it is not possible to differentiate them from other benign or malignant splenic lesions. Biopsy or surgical removal is required for diagnosis.

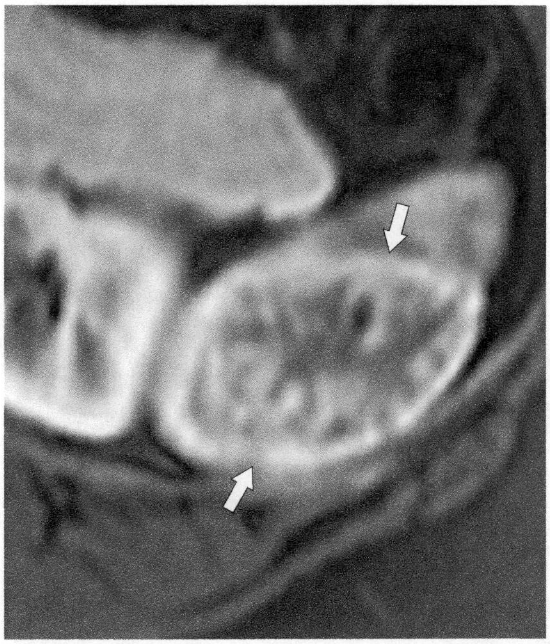

FIGURE 7-50. Axial T1-weighted fat-saturated contrast-enhanced MRI in a 44-year-old man with a rounded heterogeneously enhancing splenic mass (*arrows*) that proved to be an inflammatory pseudotumor.

Malignant Splenic Lesions

Lymphoma (see also Chapter 4)

Lymphomatous splenic involvement is the most common malignancy to affect the spleen. In addition to diffuse splenomegaly described earlier in this chapter, lymphoma can present with focal or multiple discrete masses (Figs. 7-10 and 7-11), often indistinguishable from other splenic diseases. The lymphoma is usually secondary to non-Hodgkin or Hodgkin lymphoma elsewhere, but when primary, it is commonly associated with AIDS.

Metastases

Splenic metastases are less common than hepatic metastases, but given the vascularity of the spleen, it is a relatively common site for hematogenous spread of metastatic disease. The most common splenic metastases are from breast, lung, stomach, and ovarian cancer and from melanoma. They may be single (Fig. 7-51), or multifocal, solid or cystic (Fig. 7-52), They are typically

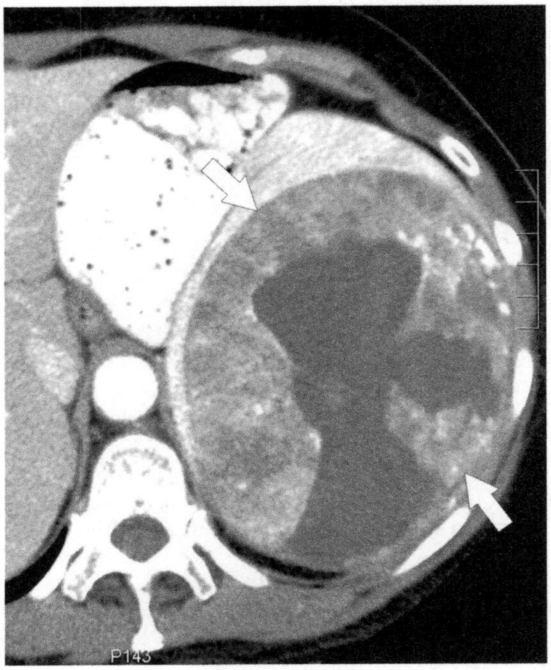

FIGURE 7-49. Axial contrast-enhanced CT in a 70-year-old woman with a complex heterogeneous mass (*arrows*) in the spleen that is a PEComa ("sugar" tumor).

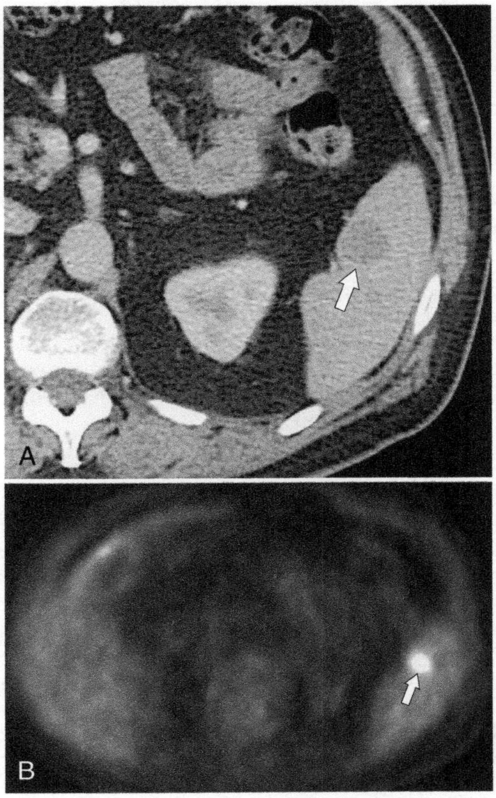

FIGURE 7-51. **A** and **B**, Axial contrast-enhanced PET/CT in a 48-year-old man with splenic metastases from melanoma (*arrows*). This solitary lesion cannot be differentiated from many other benign splenic lesions by CT alone.

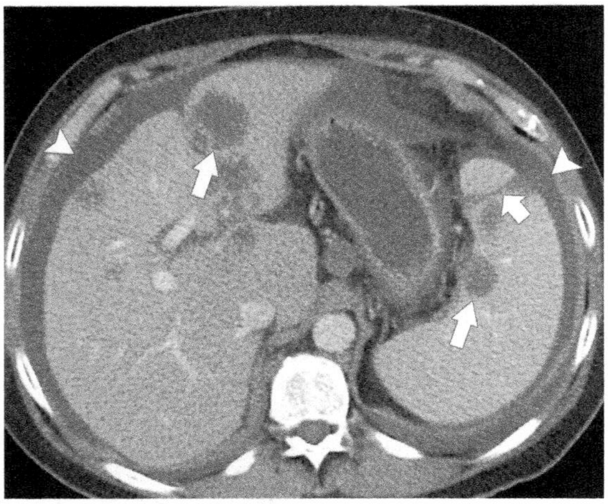

FIGURE 7-52. Axial contrast-enhanced CT in a 60-year-old man with lung cancer and multiple cystic-appearing splenic and hepatic metastases (*arrows*). Abdominal ascites (*arrowheads*) and a splenic infarct (*small arrow*) are also present.

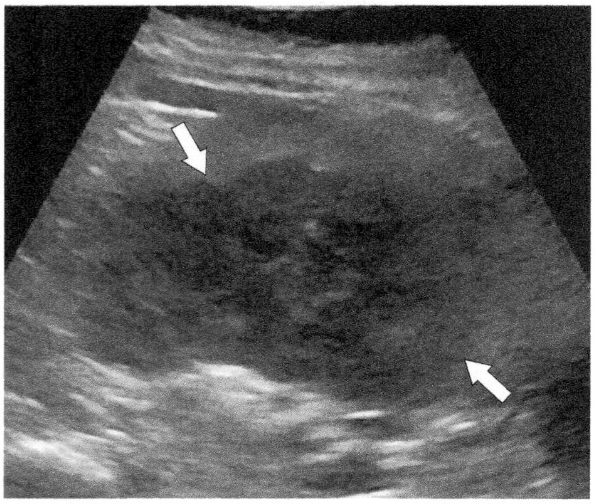

FIGURE 7-53. Sagittal US in a 71-year-old woman with a 7-cm hypoechoic splenic metastasis (*arrows*) from breast carcinoma.

hypoechoic on US (Fig. 7-53) and hypodense on CT and are difficult to differentiate from other solitary or multiple splenic lesions. If disease has spread to the spleen by the peritoneal route (e.g., gastric and ovarian cancer), the lesions may be capsular (Fig. 7-54). Other tumors (e.g., pancreas, colon, stomach) may invade the spleen by direct invasion (Fig. 7-55).

Angiosarcoma

Angiosarcoma is the second most common primary splenic malignant tumor after lymphoma. A rare, aggressive tumor associated with a poor prognosis, angiosarcoma is sometimes associated with prior Thorotrast use because of its alpha-emitting properties. As its name suggests, angiosarcoma is highly vascular in appearance and metastasizes early. Contrast-enhanced CT imaging often demonstrates splenomegaly with a heterogeneous hypervascular mass, which can be either focal or diffuse. Not all tumors avidly enhance, however (Fig. 7-56). The tumor may demonstrate increased density before contrast enhancement because of its highly vascular nature. There is often tumoral calcification.

Kaposi Sarcoma

Induced virally (human herpes virus 8), Kaposi sarcoma is often associated with AIDS and typically presents with cutaneous lesions, but it can be present anywhere in the mediastinum and abdomen. Kaposi sarcoma is rare in the spleen but can present there as either a single mass or multiple masses (Fig. 7-57).

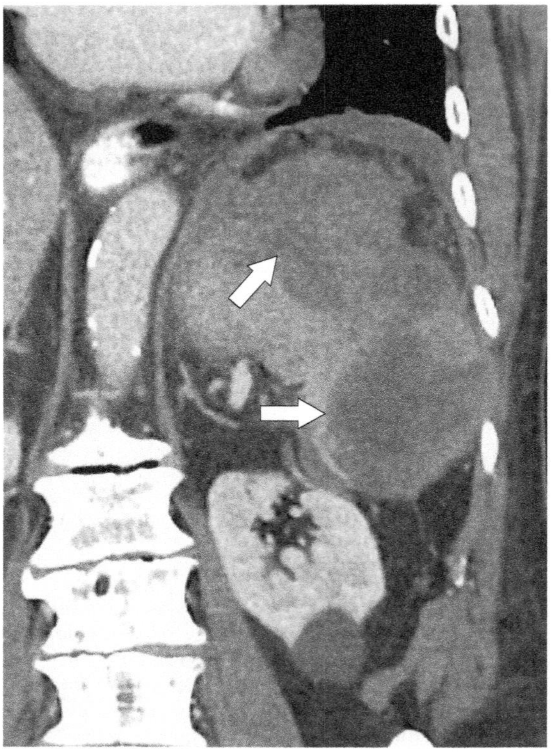

FIGURE 7-54. Coronal contrast-enhanced CT in a 49-year-old woman with splenic capsular invasion (*arrows*) from ovarian cancer.

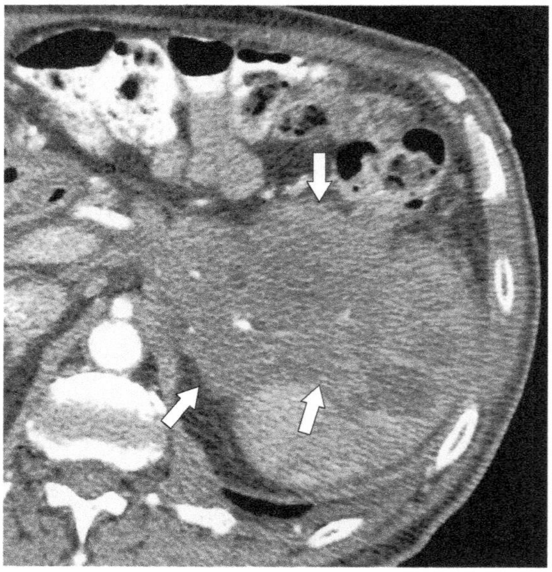

FIGURE 7-55. Axial contrast-enhanced CT in a 68-year-old man demonstrating a large pancreatic tail adenocarcinoma with direct invasion into the spleen (*arrows*).

Very Rare Splenic Neoplasms

Very rare splenic neoplasms include epithelioid tumors, hemangioendothelioma, hemangiopericytoma (Fig. 7-58), malignant fibrous histiocytoma, follicular dendritic cell tumor (Fig. 7-59), fibrosarcoma, and leiomyosarcoma. They are usually focal, heterogeneous, hypervascular, splenic masses on contrast-enhanced CT, and tissue diagnosis is usually made by splenectomy or percutaneous biopsy.

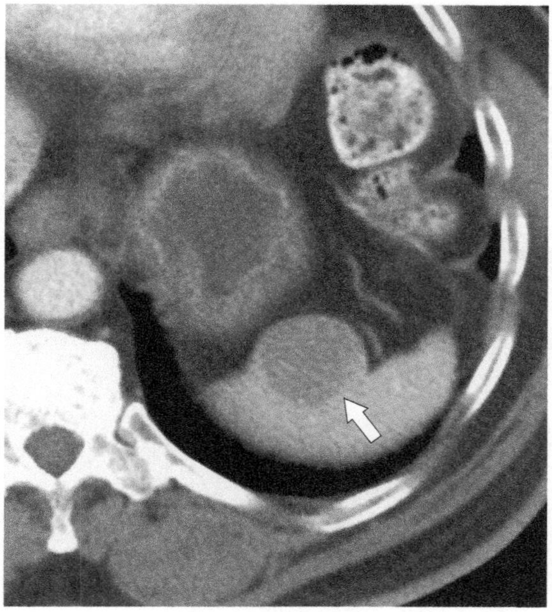

FIGURE 7-56. Axial contrast-enhanced CT in a 55-year-old man with a 3-cm splenic mass (*arrow*) that has relatively poor enhancement and proved to be angiosarcoma at surgery.

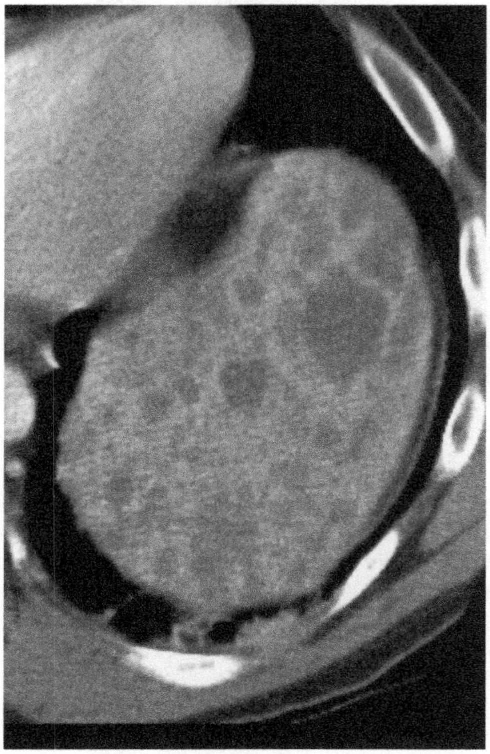

FIGURE 7-57. Axial contrast-enhanced CT in a 33-year-old man with HIV infection and multiple splenic masses caused by Kaposi sarcoma.

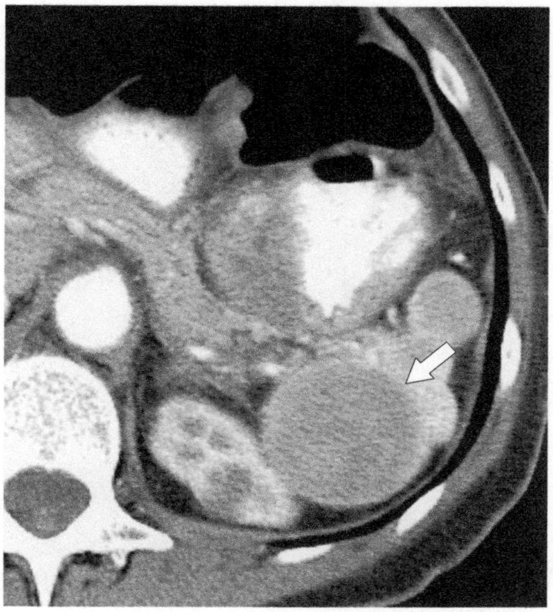

FIGURE 7-58. Axial contrast-enhanced CT in a 55-year-old man with a solid poorly enhancing splenic mass (*arrow*) representing hemangiopericytoma.

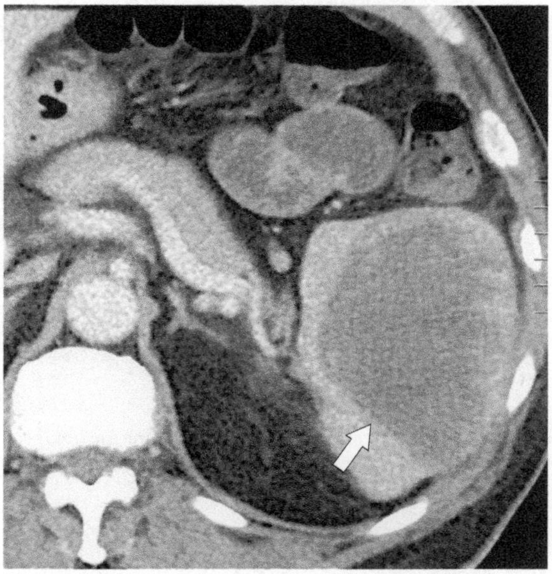

FIGURE 7-59. Axial contrast-enhanced CT in a 75-year-old man with follicular dendritic cell tumor (*arrow*). The mass is heterogeneous at CT and cannot be differentiated from other malignant splenic lesions by CT alone.

SPLENIC TRAUMA

Usually occurring as blunt trauma (e.g., motor vehicle crash injuries) rather than penetrating injuries (e.g., gunshot or knife injuries), splenic trauma may also be caused by spontaneous rupture from marked splenomegaly (e.g., in infectious mononucleosis) (Fig. 7-20). The diagnosis is usually based on the appropriate history, signs of left upper quadrant pain, and contrast-enhanced CT, which demonstrates a low-attenuation splenic laceration that fails to "fill in" with IV contrast medium on delayed imaging. The laceration may be severe enough to cause splenic fracture (Fig. 7-60) or a contained laceration (Fig. 7-61), both of which can cause severe hemorrhage. There may be active extravasation as evidenced by a high-density focus (similar in attenuation to the aorta), with surrounding, slightly lower density hemorrhage (but still hyperdense relative to the spleen and surrounding tissues) (Fig. 7-62). Hemorrhage may be within the spleen, in a subcapsular region, or freely into the peritoneum. With severe trauma there may be splenic avulsion, with little or no enhancement within the spleen but diffuse hemorrhage from the ruptured splenic artery.

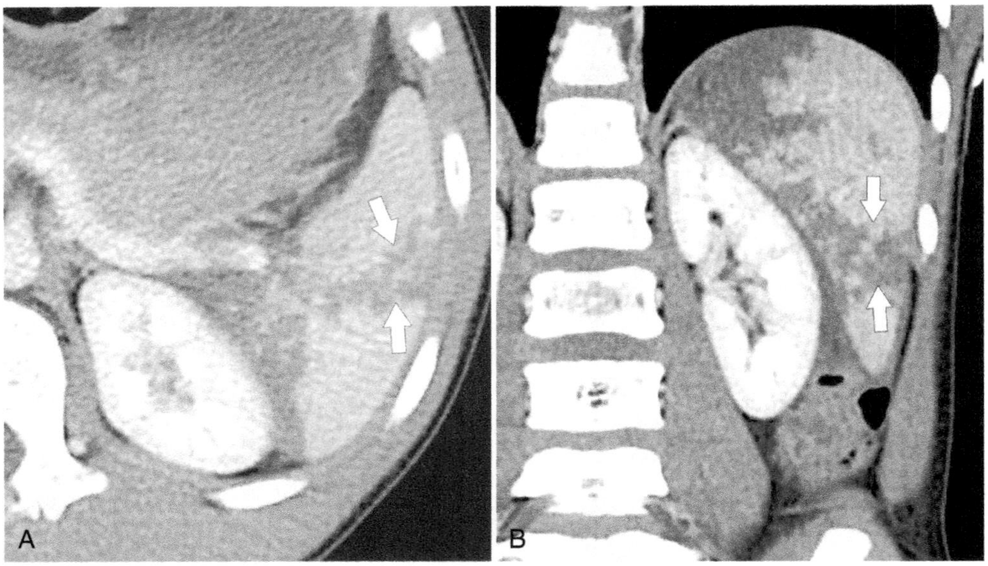

FIGURE 7-60. Axial (**A**) and coronal (**B**) contrast-enhanced CT in a 24-year-man who has a motor vehicle injury with splenic fracture (*arrows*) and perisplenic hemorrhage.

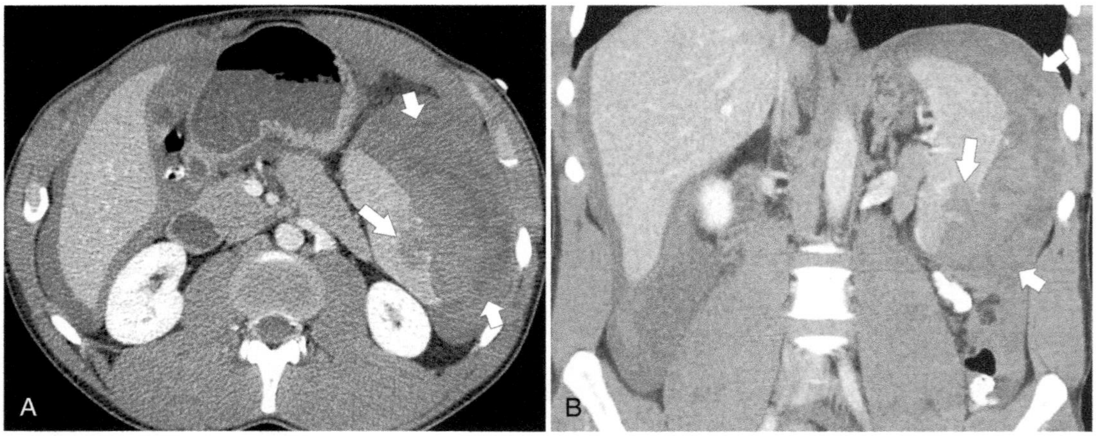

FIGURE 7-61. Axial (**A**) and coronal (**B**) contrast-enhanced CT in a 23-year-old man with splenic trauma incurred during a hockey game. An inferior splenic laceration (*arrows*) and extensive perisplenic hyperdense blood and peritoneal hemorrhage (*small arrows*) can be seen.

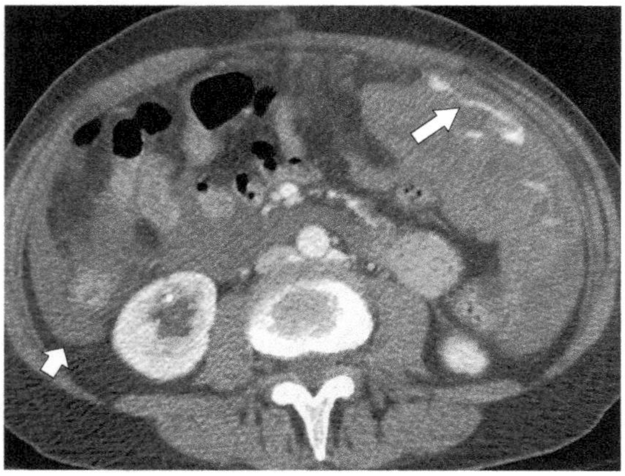

FIGURE 7-62. Axial contrast-enhanced CT in a 56-year-old woman after a motor vehicle injury with splenic trauma and active arterial extravasation (*large arrow*) and abdominal hemorrhage (*small arrow*).

SPLENIC CALCIFICATION

Splenic calcification most commonly results from prior infection, tuberculosis, histoplasmosis (Fig. 7-34), or hydatid disease (Fig. 7-63 and Box 7-4). Repeated splenic infarctions from sickle cell disease often create either a completely (Fig. 7-26) or partially calcified spleen (Fig. 7-64). Some vasculitic diseases may heal with diffuse splenic calcification (Fig. 7-65).

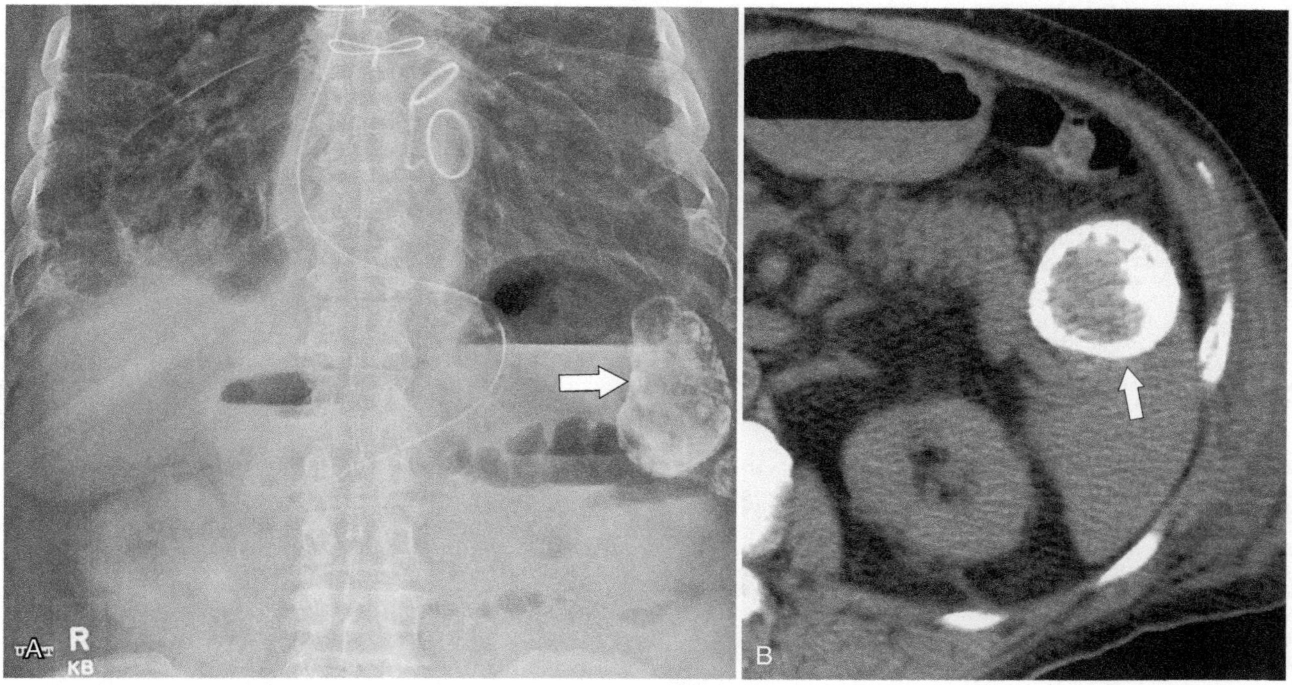

FIGURE 7-63. Plain upper abdominal radiograph (**A**) and axial noncontrast CT (**B**) in a 64-year-old man with a calcified splenic mass (*arrows*) resulting from prior treated splenic echinococcal infection.

***Box 7-4.* Splenic Calcification**

Vascular calcification
Tuberculosis
Histoplasmosis
Hydatid disease
Sickle cell disease
Vasculitis (SLE)
Prior hemorrhage

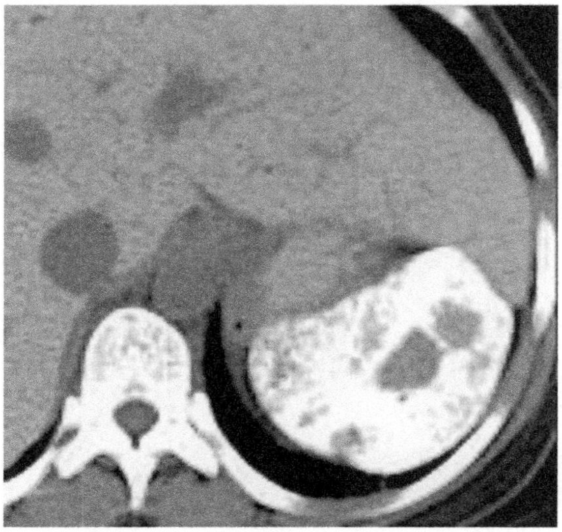

FIGURE 7-64. Axial noncontrast CT in a 38-year-old woman with irregular splenic calcification caused by sickle cell disease.

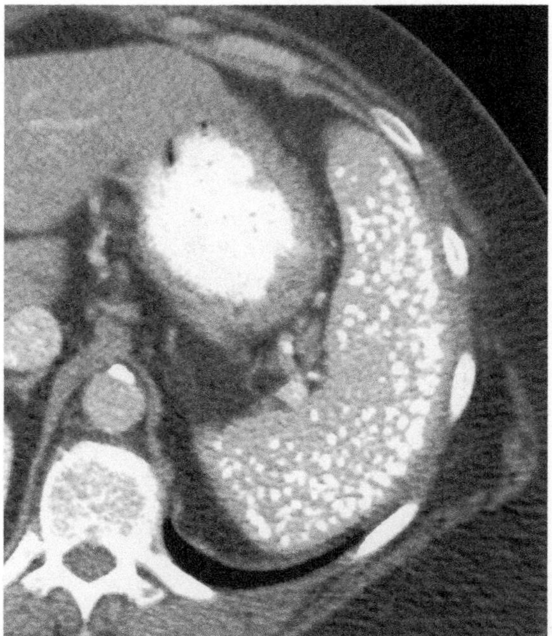

FIGURE 7-65. Axial contrast-enhanced CT in a 56-year-old woman with systemic lupus erythematosus and multiple splenic calcifications.

Suggested Readings

Andrews MW: Ultrasound of the spleen. World J Surg 24(2):183-187, 2000.

Anis M et al: Imaging of abdominal lymphoma. Radiol Clin North Am 46(2): 265-285, viii-ix. 2008.

Bensinger TA et al: Thorotrast-induced reticuloendothelial blockage in man. Am J Med 51:663-668, 1971.

Bessoud B et al: Nonoperative management of traumatic splenic injuries: is there a role for proximal splenic artery embolization? AJR 186:779-785, 2006.

Brancatelli G et al: Case 80: splenosis. Radiology 234(3):728-732, 2005.

Brancatelli G et al: Fibropolycystic liver disease: CT and MR imaging findings. Radiographics 25(3):659-670, 2005.

Chua SC et al: Iimaging features of primary extranodal lymphomas. Clin Radiol 64(6):574-588, 2009.

Dachman AH et al: Nonparasitic splenic cysts: a report of 52 cases with radiologic-pathologic correlation. AJR 147:537-542, 1986.

de Jong PA et al: CT and ^{18}F-FDG PET for noninvasive detection of splenic involvement in patients with malignant lymphoma. AJR 192:745-753, 2009.

Doody O et al: Blunt trauma to the spleen: ultrasonographic findings. Clin Radiol 60(9):968-976, 2005.

Elsayes KM et al: MR imaging of the spleen: spectrum of abnormalities. Radiographics 25(4):967-982, 2005.

Freeman JL et al: CT of congenital and acquired abnormalities of the spleen. Radiographics 13(3):597-610, 1993.

Fulcher AS et al: Abdominal manifestations of situs anomalies in adults. Radiographics 22(6):1439-1456, 2002.

Harris GN et al: Accessory spleen causing a mass in the tail of the pancreas: MR imaging findings. AJR 163(5):1120-1121, 1994.

Lee WK et al: Abdominal manifestations of extranodal lymphoma: spectrum of imaging findings. AJR 191(1):198-206, 2008.

Leite NP et al: Cross-sectional imaging of extranodal involvement in abdomino-pelvic lymphoproliferative malignancies. Radiographics 27(6):1613-1634, 2007.

Levy AD et al: Littoral cell angioma of the spleen: CT features with clinicopathologic comparison. Radiology 230(2):485-490, 2004.

Luna A et al: MRI of focal splenic lesions without and with dynamic gadolinium enhancement. AJR 186:1533-1547, 2006.

Marmery H et al: Optimization of selection for nonoperative management of blunt splenic injury: comparison of MDCT grading systems. AJR 189:1421-1427, 2007.

Mortele KJ et al: CT features of the accessory spleen. AJR 183(6):1653-1657, 2004.

Nunweiler CG et al: The imaging features of nontuberculous mycobacterial immune reconstitution syndrome. J Comput Assist Tomogr 33(2):242-246, 2009.

Paterson A et al: A pattern-oriented approach to splenic imaging in infants and children. Radiographics 19(6):1465-1485, 1999.

Radin DR et al: Visceral and nodal calcification in patients with AIDS-related *Pneumocystis carinii* infection. AJR 154:27-31, 1990.

Rezai P et al: Splenic volume model constructed from standardized one-dimensional MDCT measurements. AJR 196:367-372, 2011.

Singh AK et al: Image-guided percutaneous splenic interventions. Radiographics 32(2):523-534, 2012.

Thanos L et al: Percutaneous CT-guided drainage of splenic abscess. AJR 179(3):629-632, 2002.

Thompson WM et al: Angiosarcoma of the spleen: imaging characteristics in 12 patients. Radiology 235(1):106-115, 2005.

Thorelius L: Emergency real-time contrast-enhanced ultrasonography for detection of solid organ injuries. Eur Radiol 17(Suppl 6):F107-F111, 2007.

Urrutia M et al: Cystic masses of the spleen: radiologic-pathologic correlation. Radiographics 16(1):107-129, 1996.

CHAPTER 8

Gallbladder

The biliary tree develops embryologically along the course of the portal venous anatomy and is defined proximally by right and left intrahepatic biliary ducts, which join to form the common hepatic duct. A side appendage, the gallbladder, is attached to the common hepatic duct by the cystic duct to form the common bile duct (CBD), which traverses the pancreas to join the main pancreatic duct and drain into the duodenum at the ampulla of Vater.* The gallbladder usually lies distinct from the liver within the gallbladder fossa, mostly in an anteroinferior location to the liver, although some gallbladders are totally intrahepatic. A normal gallbladder fold (or septation) known as a Phrygian cap† is often demonstrated toward the gallbladder fundus (Fig. 8-1).

Biliary anatomy has numerous variants, particularly the insertion of the cystic duct into the common hepatic duct. They are a variety of aberrant ducts, perhaps the best known being the duct of Luschka,‡ knowledge of which is critical to prevent surgical transection at cholecystectomy (Fig. 8-2). Less commonly, congenital gallbladder anomalies arise, including duplicated gallbladder or gallbladder agenesis. Gallbladder agenesis is present in approximately 1 per 10,000 individuals. Its only significance is that it is almost always unsuspected and patients with right upper quadrant pain are sometimes inappropriately diagnosed with chronic cholecystitis. They are then referred for cholecystectomy, upon which the gallbladder cannot be identified. This may confound the radiologist and surgeon, who thought they had definitive sonographic finding of a contracted gallbladder full of stones. Rather, the hyperechoic structure in the region of the gallbladder represented gas within the duodenal lumen. Occasionally the gallbladder has a long mesentery and is therefore at risk of torsion with consequent gangrene and perforation.

Oral cholecystography, once the mainstay of gallbladder imaging, is no longer used because of its variable gallbladder opacification and because it caused relatively frequent allergic reactions. More recently, however, it has been used in conjunction with multidetector computed tomography (CT) to evaluate biliary tree disease, but its use is not widespread. Ultrasonography (US) has largely replaced oral cholecystograph and is the primary imaging method for the gallbladder given its superficial location and fluid-filled nature. US detects most gallstones in patients who are prepared appropriately and is useful for the evaluation of acute and chronic cholecystitis. It can also detect very small (<5 mm) anomalies, including polyps and cholesterosis. US is also useful for evaluating the intrahepatic and extrahepatic biliary system, particularly if distended. US may detect CBD stones, but more distal stones may prove challenging because of overlying bowel gas that attenuates the sound waves. Subtle biliary dilatation can be observed, and the CBD caliber is readily identified in most patients where the duct crosses the hepatic artery (Fig. 8-3). Normal measurements depend on the age of the patient and any prior cholecystectomy. The CBD typically measures 2 to 3 mm in younger patients, increasing to 4 to 6 mm in the elderly. A CBD greater than 7 mm is considered dilated in the elderly unless there has been prior cholecystectomy, in which case the duct can measure up to 10 mm normally.

CT is less useful than US, although thin-section multidetector CT with multiplanar reformatting can sometimes prove clinically useful. Many gallstones demonstrate variable calcific concentrations, and CT detects only 50% to 70% of gallstones and even fewer CBD stones. Its main use is to evaluate for biliary malignancies (gallbladder carcinoma and intrahepatic cholangiocarcinoma). Common hepatic duct and CBD cholangiocarcinomas are often small and difficult to identify by CT, but their presence can be inferred when they occlude the duct, resulting in biliary obstruction.

Imaging of the biliary system with magnetic resonance cholangiopancreatography (MRCP) has improved dramatically with fast fat-suppressed two- or three-dimensional T2-weighted sequences. Bile is hyperintense on these sequences and is readily differentiated from surrounding anatomy. Images are evaluated either coronally as a composite three-dimensional image or on individual axial maximum intensity projections. This is often useful when evaluating more subtle pancreaticobiliary abnormalities, particularly of the distal pancreatic or bile duct. Although MRCP in its own right is indicated for detection and characterization of pancreaticobiliary disease, the indication for MRCP is often as a replacement for failed endoscopic retrograde cholangiopancreatography (ERCP), either because of absolute or relative contraindications or because of procedure failure. ERCP has better fine-detail resolution, particularly for small intrahepatic or aberrant bile ducts. Furthermore, ERCP offers the opportunity for therapeutic intervention. However, when ERCP is to be avoided for whatever reason, MRCP is an effective screening tool to evaluate for ductal stone disease, choledochal cysts, and intrahepatic ductal anomalies (sclerosing cholangitis, peribiliary cysts).

CHOLEDOCHAL CYST

All of the five different forms of choledochal cyst represent variations of congenital cystic dilatation of the bile ducts (Fig. 8-4 and Table 8-1). Their significance is that patients are at increased risk of developing cholangiocarcinoma. Type I is by far the most common (Fig. 8-5), representing approximately 80% to 90% of all forms. Choledochal cysts usually present in childhood, although type IV is just as common in adulthood. There are numerous associated anomalies, including gallbladder agenesis or duplication, biliary atresia, polycystic liver disease and fibrosis (hepatic fibrocystic disease), and annular pancreas. Patients may be asymptomatic, although most present in childhood with secondary signs of cholangitis and jaundice, with or without intraductal stone formation.

Caroli* disease is a congenital disease with two forms, a simple autosomal-dominant type and a complex autosomal-recessive type, but is also classified as a type V choledochal cyst. The simple variety, which usually presents in young adulthood, has isolated ectatic cavernous intrahepatic bile ducts, whereas the complex

*Abraham Vater (1684-1751), German anatomist.
†Phrygian cap: refers to the hats worn by residents in the ancient city in central Anatolia.
‡Hubert von Luschka (1820-1875), German anatomist.

*Jacques Caroli (1902-1979), French gastroenterologist.

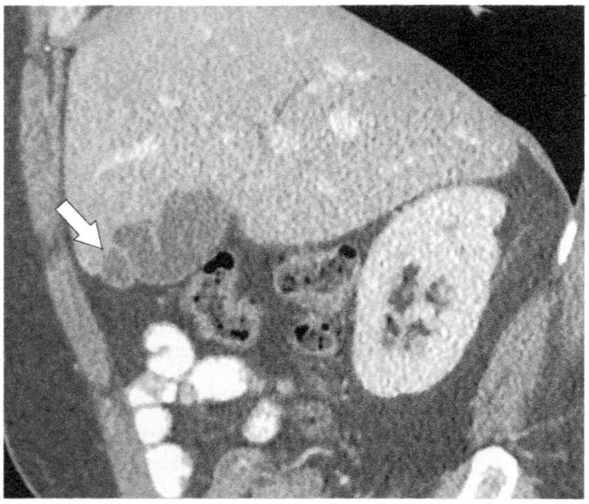

FIGURE 8-1. Sagittal contrast-enhanced CT in a 47-year-old man with "Phrygian cap" appearance of the gallbladder fundus (*arrow*).

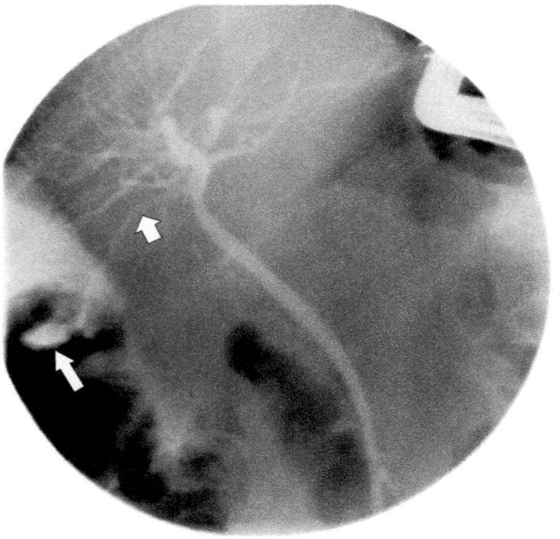

FIGURE 8-2. ERCP in a 43-year-old woman with recent cholecystectomy and a current bile leak (*arrow*) from an aberrant duct of Luschka (*small arrow*).

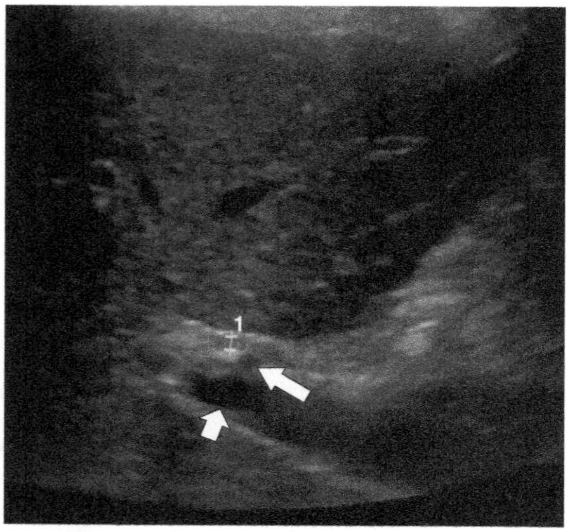

FIGURE 8-3. US of a normal common bile duct (*between +s*) at the level of the hepatic artery (*large arrow*), which is anterior to the portal vein (*small arrow*).

variety forms part of a Caroli syndrome with ectatic ducts, congenital hepatic fibrosis, and portal hypertension, which usually presents in childhood. The complex form is also associated with autosomal-recessive polycystic kidney disease, medullary sponge kidney, and biliary hamartomas. The defective biliary anatomy is best visualized by ERCP (Fig. 8-6), which shows marked and irregular segmental biliary cavernous ectasia. However, all cross-sectional imaging techniques can identify these findings. A characteristic feature at contrast-enhanced CT is the "central dot" sign, representing enhancing portal tracts within the grossly dilated bile ducts (Fig. 8-5).

GALLSTONES AND GALLBLADDER SLUDGE

Stone formation is secondary to biliary material concretions within the gallbladder, but depending on their size, stones can pass into the cystic or bile ducts, pancreatic duct, or duodenum. Stones may be single (sometimes large) or multiple and when granular are referred to as pseudoliths or, more commonly, gallbladder sludge. Cholesterol makes up approximately 80% of the composition in most stones (75% to 80%). Pigment stones are less common (approximately 20%) and are composed mainly of bilirubin and calcium salts (80%), the remainder being cholesterol. Mixed stones are less common and are composed of between 20% and 80% cholesterol and a mixture of calcium and phosphate salts and bilirubin. A number of predisposing factors are associated with gallstone formation, including obesity, diabetes mellitus, cirrhosis, hemolytic anemias (pigment stones), small bowel malabsorption abnormalities (ulcerative colitis, Crohn disease, and small bowel resection), and hyperthyroidism.

Gallstones are commonly identified at imaging and are usually asymptomatic. Most gallstones are not sufficiently calcified to be visible on plain radiographs, but some mixed (owing to their calcium concentration) stones are visible in the right upper quadrant (Fig. 8-7). US is the investigation of choice but needs adequate patient preparation, which requires the patient to fast for up to 8 hours to ensure gallbladder distention (the gallbladder usually contracts on feeding). Almost all gallstones can then be identified. They are hyperechoic, rounded structures with strong acoustic shadowing (Fig. 8-8). Their presence can be confirmed by placing the patient in the decubitus position, which should cause the stone to drop into the most dependent part of the gallbladder (Fig. 8-8). Stones impacted in the gallbladder neck (or occasionally adherent to the gallbladder wall) may not move, however. Gallstones can be difficult to identify definitively in patients with a contracted gallbladder from chronic cholecystitis. A large stone in a chronically contracted gallbladder can be almost impossible to differentiate from a gas-filled duodenum, which also demonstrates marked hyperechogenicity (Figs. 8-9 and 8-10). Under these circumstances a definitive diagnosis of gallstones can be made only by the presence of the sonographic wall-echo-shadow (WES) sign. In this sign the wall represents the gallbladder wall, the echo the superficial acoustic reflective surface of the gallstone, and the shadow the attenuated sound (or shadow) beyond the gallstone surface (Fig. 8-10). However, between the gallbladder wall and the echogenic stone surface, a sliver of radiolucent bile must be observed to document gallstones definitively and exclude duodenal gas. Without the presence of the WES sign in these circumstances, exclusion of duodenal gas can be made by requesting that the patient swallow water and immediately performing repeat imaging with the patient in the right lateral decubitus position. Swirling ingested gas and water should be observed, confirming the location of the duodenum.

Gallbladder sludge is less commonly observed than gallstones but more commonly recognized in the fasting state, particularly in acutely ill hospitalized patients because fasting and multiple cholestatic medications cause gallbladder stasis, which encourages the deposition of biliary particulate material (calcium bilirubinate or cholesterol crystals). Most patients are asymptomatic. At US the sludge is recognized as a layering, nonshadowing, and slightly

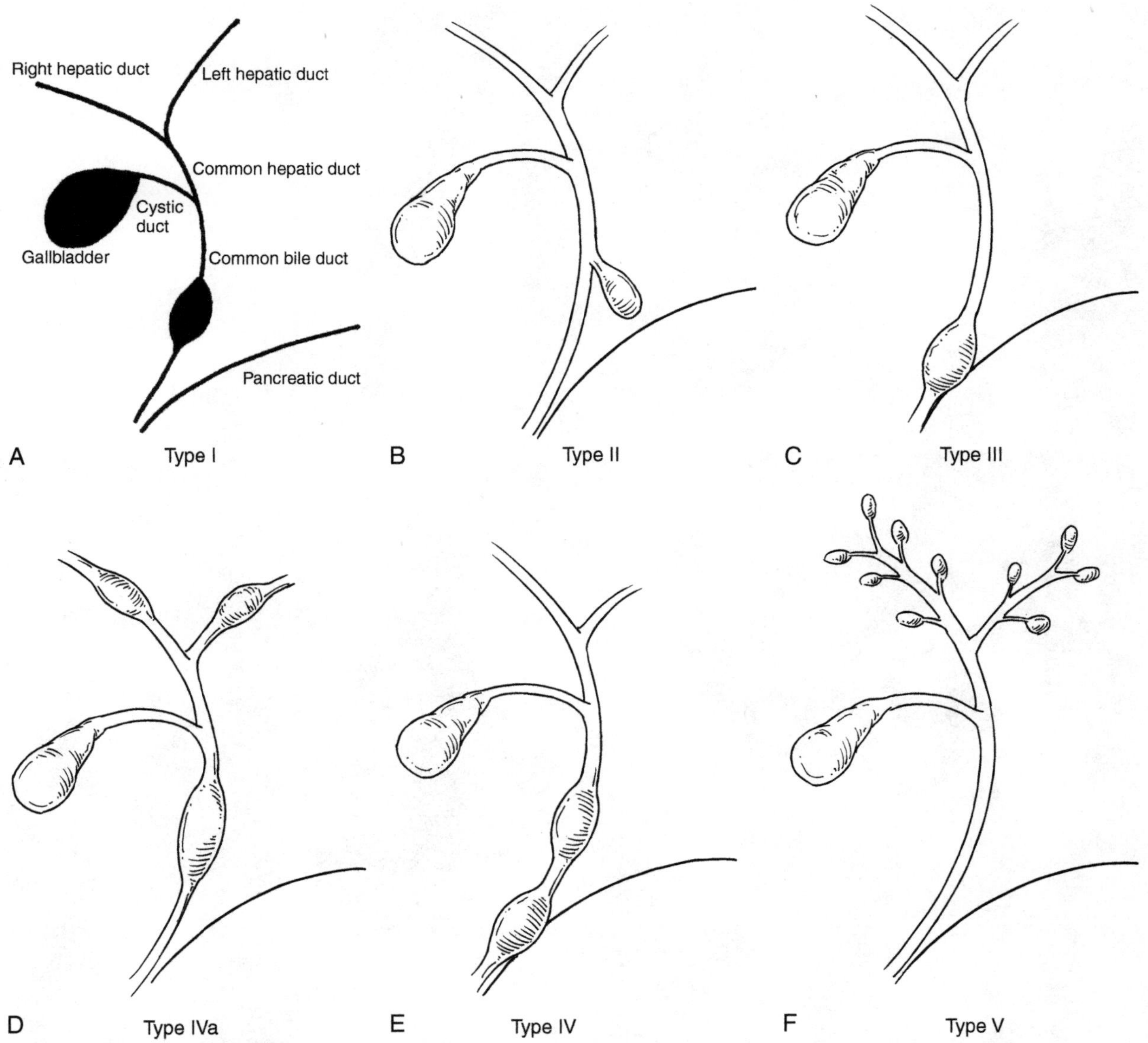

FIGURE 8-4. **A** through **F**, Schematic representation of types I through V choledochal cysts (choledochoceles).

TABLE 8-1 Classification of Choledochal Cysts (see Figs. 8-5 and 8-6)

Type I	Fusiform dilatation of all or part of CBD (i.e., extrahepatic)
Type II	CBD diverticulum (extrahepatic)
Type III	Choledochocele (dilatation at junction of CBD and pancreatic duct)
Type IVa	Fusiform intrahepatic and extrahepatic duct dilatation
Type IVb	Combination of Types I and III
Type V	Caroli disease (cystic dilatation of intrahepatic ducts)

CBD, Common bile duct.

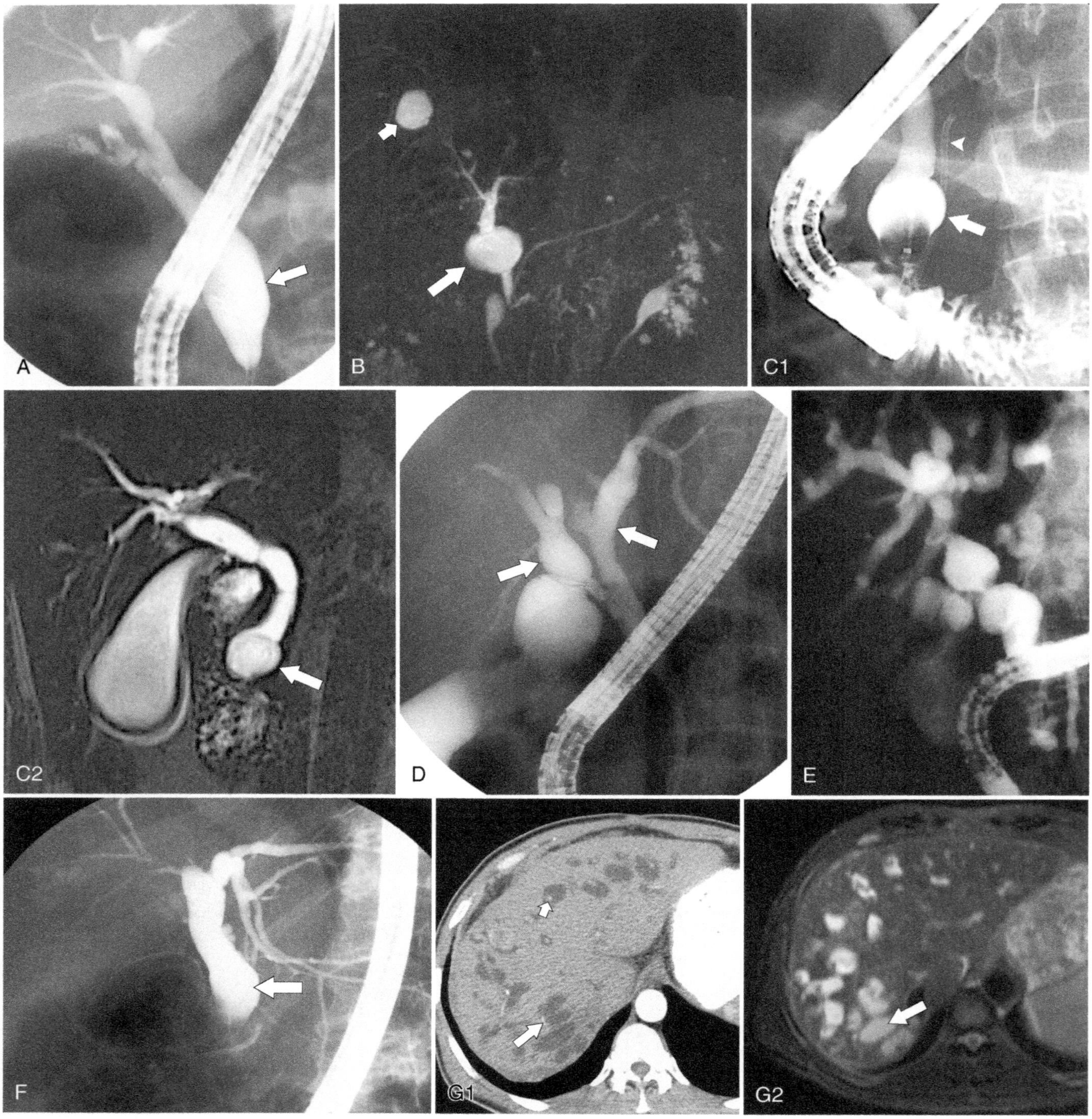

FIGURE 8-5. Choledochoceles types I through V. **A**, Type I ERCP demonstrates fusiform dilatation of the distal CBD (*arrow*). **B**, MRCP in a 36-year-old man with a type II choledochal cyst (*arrow*). There is an incidental liver cyst (*small arrow*). **C1** and **C2**, Type III MRCP and ERCP in a 40-year-old man with choledochocele (*arrows*). A pancreatic stent (*arrowhead*) is present. **D**, ERCP in a 47-year-old woman with fusiform intrahepatic duct dilatation (*arrows*) caused by a type IVa choledochal cyst. **E**, ERCP in a 39-year-old woman with a type IVa choledochal cyst. **F**, Type IVb choledochal cyst. ERCP in a 56-year-old man with fusiform dilatation (*arrow*) of the CBD and choledochocele of the distal duct. **G1** and **G2**, Type V choledochal cyst. Axial contrast-enhanced CT and T2-weighted MRI in a 40-year-old with Caroli disease with abundant dilated intrahepatic biliary ducts (*arrows*) and a central dot sign (*small arrow*) typical of this disease.

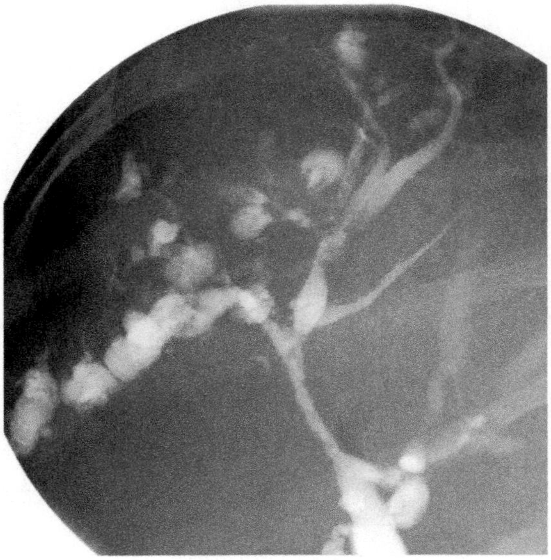

FIGURE 8-6. ERCP in a 63-year-old woman with Caroli disease and multiple cystic intrahepatic ducts.

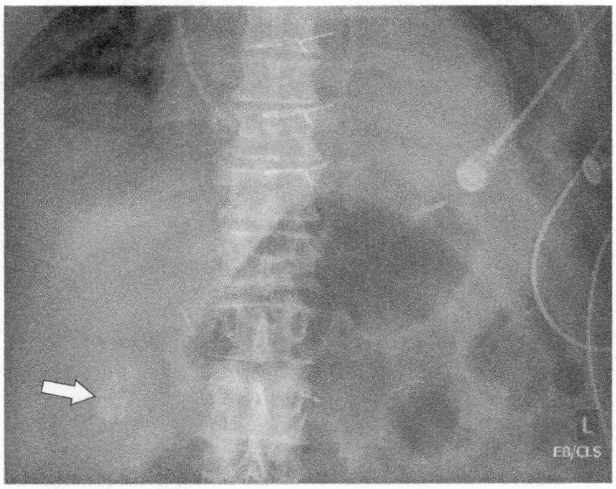

FIGURE 8-7. Plain abdominal radiograph in a 75-year-old man with calcified gallstones in the right upper quadrant (*arrow*).

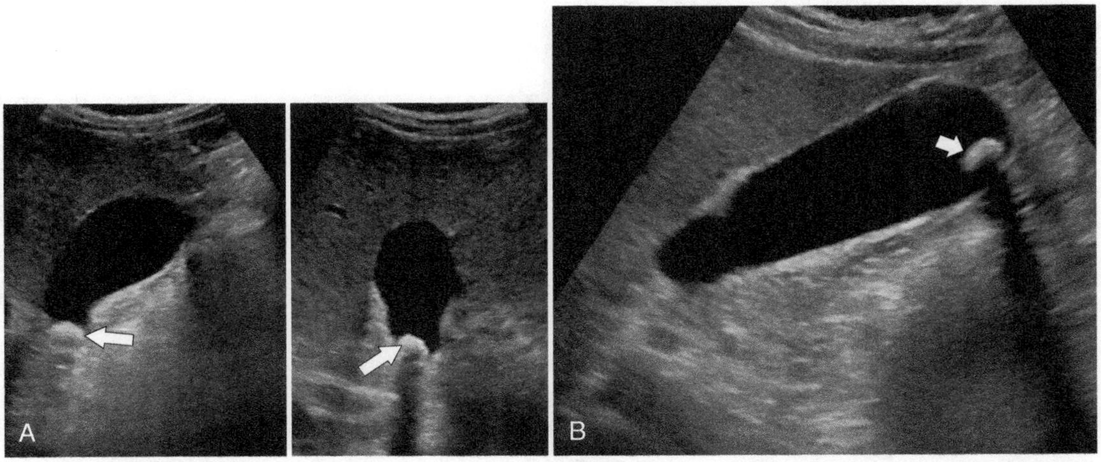

FIGURE 8-8. **A** and **B**, Sagittal, transverse, and lateral decubitus US in a 47-year-old woman with a hyperechoic gallstone in the gallbladder neck with strong posterior acoustic shadowing (*large arrows*) that moves in the decubitus position to the gallbladder fundus (*small arrow*).

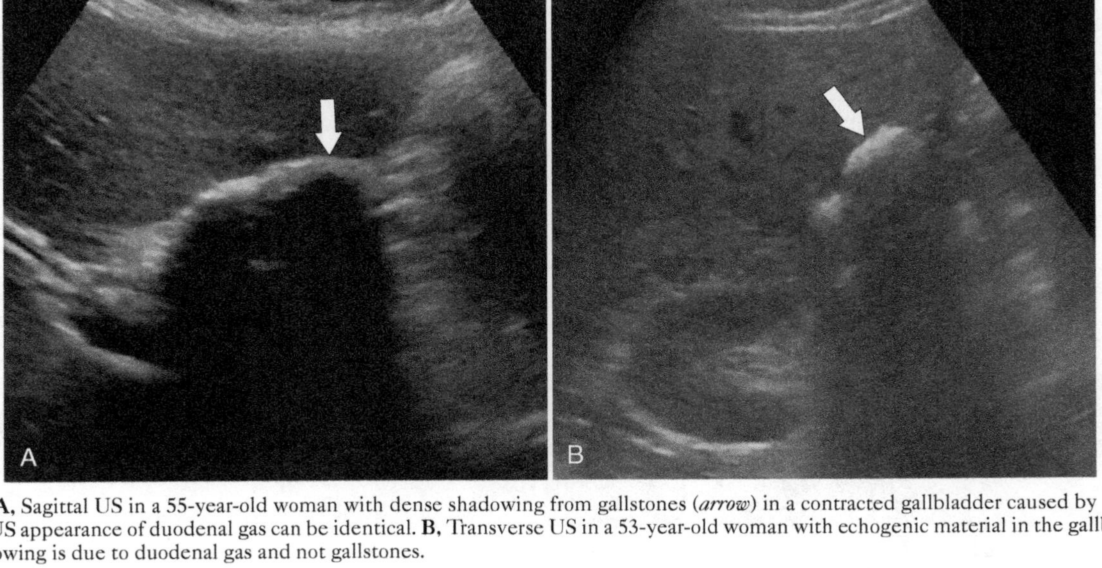

FIGURE 8-9. **A**, Sagittal US in a 55-year-old woman with dense shadowing from gallstones (*arrow*) in a contracted gallbladder caused by chronic cholecystitis. The US appearance of duodenal gas can be identical. **B**, Transverse US in a 53-year-old woman with echogenic material in the gallbladder region (*arrow*). Shadowing is due to duodenal gas and not gallstones.

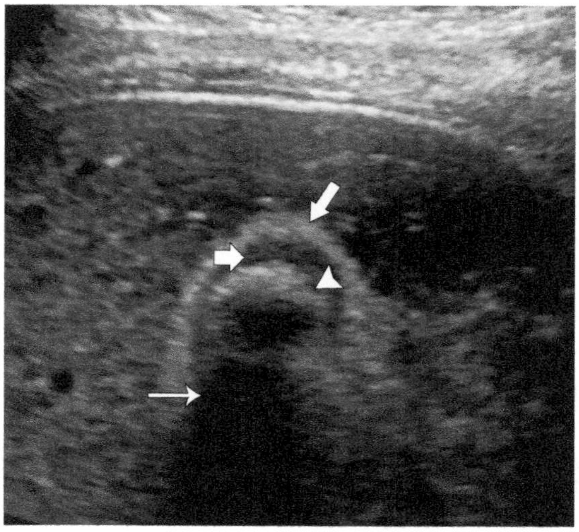

FIGURE 8-10. Transverse US in a 27-year-old woman with a hyperechoic gallbladder wall (*long arrow*), sonolucent bile (*short arrow*), hyperechoic stone (*arrowhead*), and posterior acoustic shadow (*thin arrow*), which constitute the WES sign.

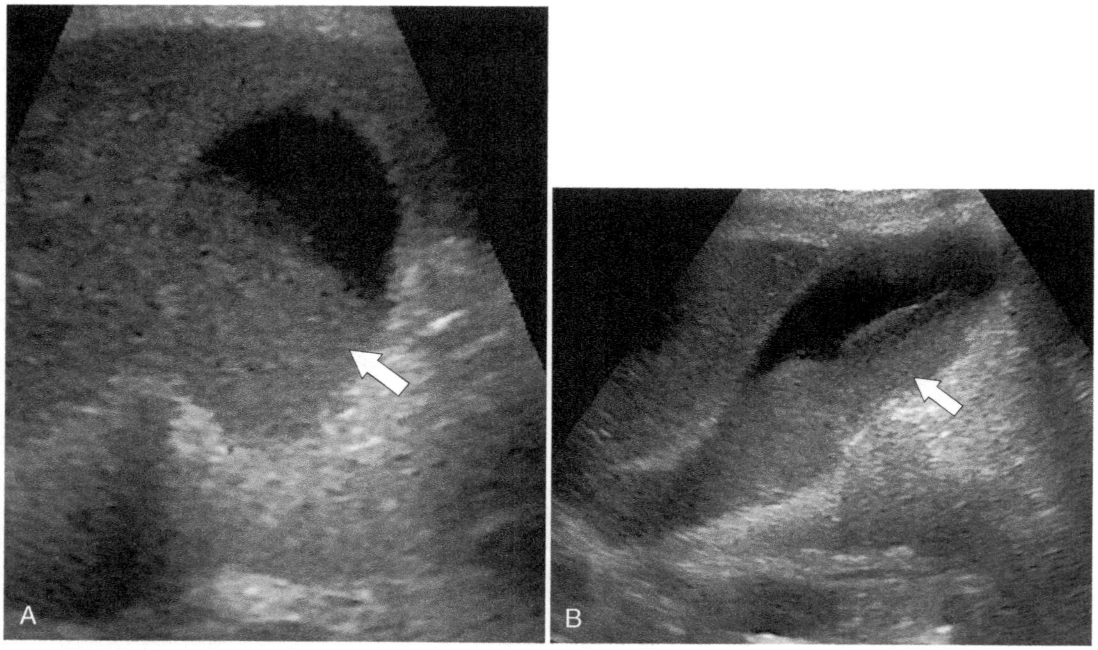

FIGURE 8-11. **A** and **B**, Sagittal and transverse US in a 55-year-old man with layering gallbladder sludge (*arrows*).

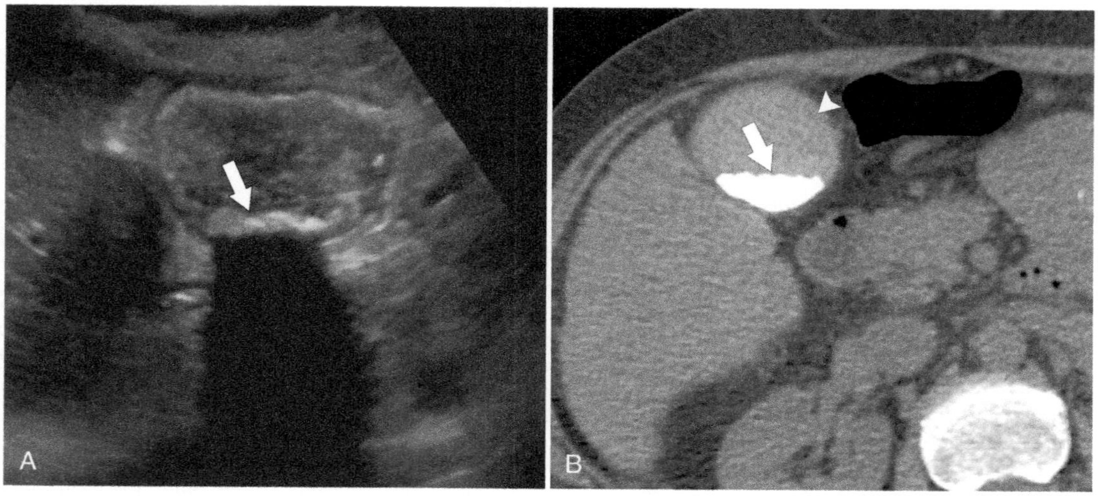

FIGURE 8-12. Transverse US (**A**) and axial noncontrast (**B**) in a 64-year-old woman with multiple hyperdense dependent small layering stones (*arrows*) and sludge, which fill the gallbladder. The sludge is slightly hyperdense at CT (*arrowhead*).

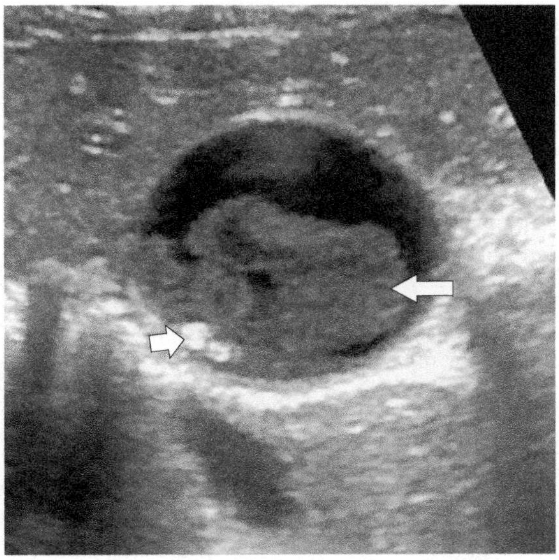

FIGURE 8-13. Gallstones and sludge. Transverse US images on the gallbladder in a 29-year-old woman with sickle cell disease, a tumefactive sludge ball (*large arrow*), and pigment stones, which do not shadow (*small arrow*).

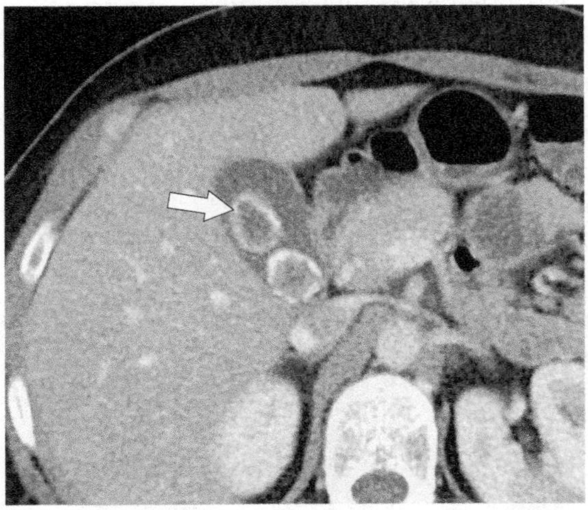

FIGURE 8-14. Axial contrast-enhanced CT in a 31-year-old woman with typical CT appearances of cholesterol gallstones (*arrow*).

hyperechoic material (Fig. 8-11), and at CT it is often slightly hyperdense (Fig. 8-12). Occasionally the sludge coalesces to a more mass-like form, known as tumefactive sludge (Fig. 8-13), which is sometimes mistaken for a gallbladder neoplasm, but the tumefactive mass is often accompanied by mobile sludge. Furthermore, the tumefactive sludge may itself move, and there is no color Doppler* flow within the sludge unlike tumors that frequently demonstrate some vascularity.

Approximately 80% of gallstones are incidentally detected at CT performed for other reasons. Pure cholesterol stones are hypodense (owing to their lipid content) and isodense to normal bile. The internal architecture can sometimes be appreciated as uniformly dense from predominantly calcified material, laminated from alternating cholesterol and calcified elements (Fig. 8-14), or stellate (also known as the Mercedes-Benz† sign), caused mainly by nitrogen gas trapped within the stone matrices (Fig. 8-15). The

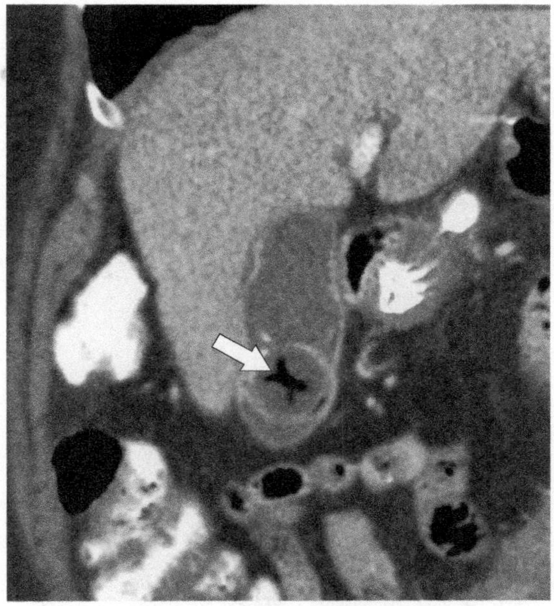

FIGURE 8-15. Coronal contrast-enhanced CT in a 61-year-old man with a stellate gallstone with internal nitrogen gas (*arrow*).

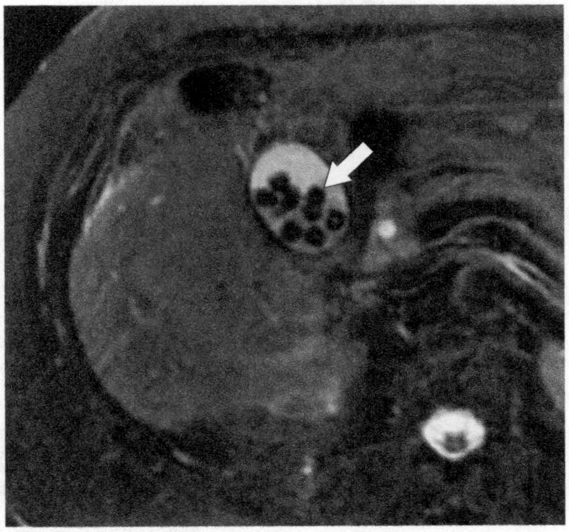

FIGURE 8-16. Axial fat-saturated T2-weighted image in a 44-year-old woman with multiple hypointense gallstones (*arrow*) surrounded by hyperintense bile.

routine use of CT is not warranted for detection of gallstones but is for some of their complicating features, including cholecystitis, perforation, carcinoma formation, pancreatitis, and ascending cholangitis from cholelithiasis. Gallstones are generally well identified by T2-weighted MRI because of the superior contrast characteristics of high-signal bile and low-signal stones (Fig. 8-16).

CHOLEDOCHOLITHIASIS

Choledocholithiasis is defined as the presence of gallstones within the biliary tree and outside the gallbladder, mostly in the CBD. The stones are usually secondary to the passage of smaller gallstones through the cystic duct into the CBD, where they can move up and down the duct freely or become lodged at the ampulla of Vater. However, primary bile or hepatic duct stone formation is recognized when there is excessive biliary material production (e.g., pigment stone formation in hemolytic anemia) or

*Christian Doppler (1803-1853), Austrian mathematician and physicist.
†Mercédès Adrienne Manuela Ramona Jellinek (1889-1929), daughter of Austrian automobile entrepreneur Emil Jellinek; Karl Freidrich Benz (1844-1929), German engine designer.

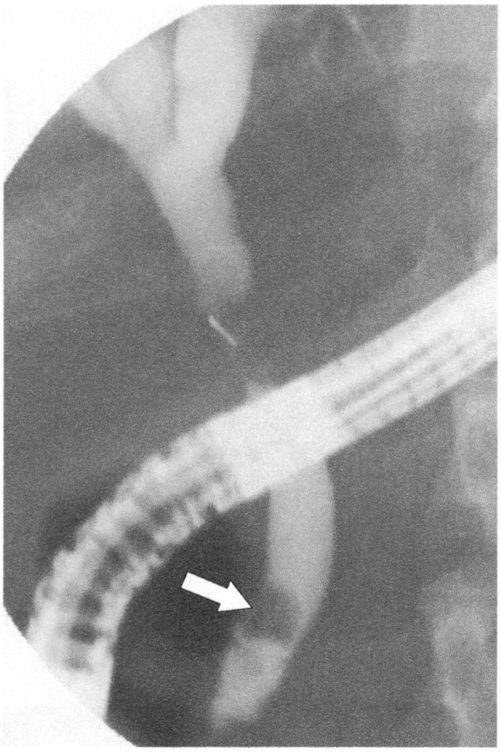

FIGURE 8-17. ERCP in a 49-year-old man with a radiolucent stone (*arrow*) in the lower duct.

biliary stasis conditions (congenital ductal anomalies, sphincter of Oddi* malfunction), foreign body material (e.g., suture material), or parasitic infections (*Ascaris lumbricoides, Clonorchis sinensis*). Small stones pass spontaneously, but unlike gallstones, CBD stones are symptomatic and patients may present with obstructive jaundice, fever, pain, or pancreatitis.

The most sensitive imaging test for CBD stone detection is the injection of water-soluble contrast material into the CBD via either ERCP (Fig. 8-17) or T-tube cholangiography, in which the opacified ducts outline a radiolucent stone. Confusion with an air bubble is usually resolved by placing the patient in the Trendelenburg* position (stones are dependent, and gas is nondependent). The stones are less readily identified by US because of normal overlying duodenal bowel gas and other anatomical structures. However, good US technique can identify many stones as hyperechoic shadowing structures within the hypoechoic lumen of the gallbladder. Obstructing stones should also distend the CBD, which then acts as a guide for detection of the offending impacted stone more distally, even if the stone itself is not clearly identified (Fig. 8-18). The absence of posterior acoustic shadowing should not deter the diagnosis, since approximately 10% of CBD stones do not shadow (Fig. 8-19). Most CBD stones are difficult to identify with CT, partly because biliary stones are less conspicuous on CT but also because smaller stones may not be resolved adequately (Fig. 8-20). Denser stones may be identified, particularly if impacting with a distended bile duct above the stone (Figs. 8-18 and 8-21). The absence of a stone at CT does

*Ruggero Oddi (1864-1913), Italian surgeon.
*Friedrich Trendelenburg (1802-1872), German surgeon.

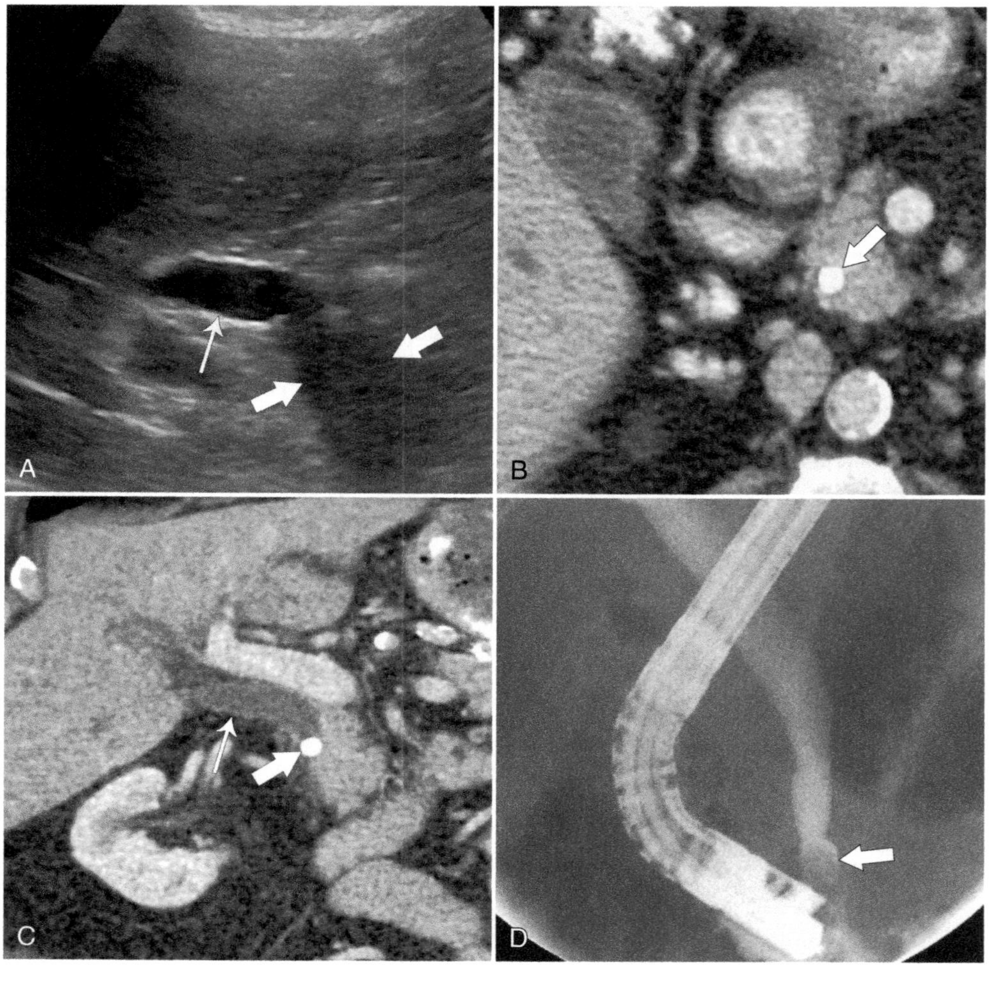

FIGURE 8-18. Sagittal right upper quadrant US (**A**), axial (**B**), and coronal (**C**) contrast-enhanced CT and ERCP (**D**) in a 66-year-old man with biliary dilatation due to common duct stone (*thin arrows*). The stone is not identified on US, but there is strong acoustic shadowing (*larger arrows in* **A**) implying a common duct stone. Secondary biliary dilatation and strong acoustic shadows from the impacted stone are identified with CT and ERCP (*arrows*).

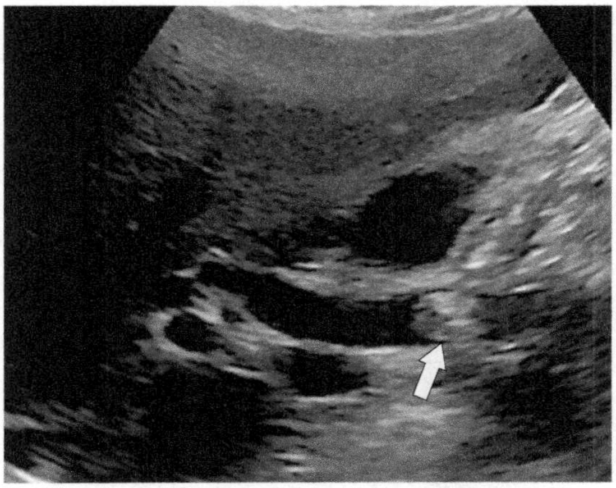

FIGURE 8-19. Sagittal US in a 49-year-old woman with bile duct dilatation caused by a stone in the lower duct (*arrow*).

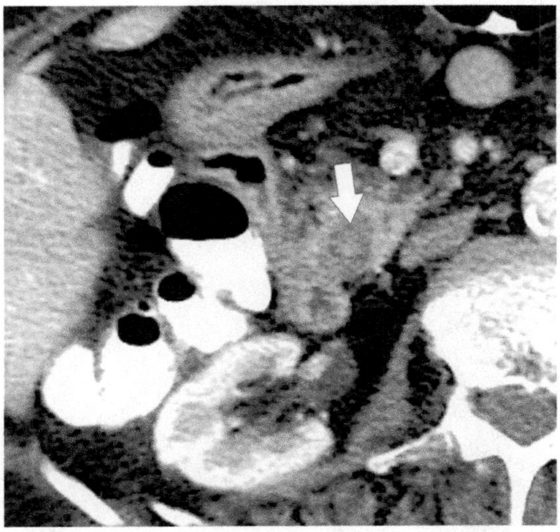

FIGURE 8-20. Axial contrast-enhanced CT in a 77-year-old man with gout and a urate stone in the lower bile duct. The stone is only just visible by CT (*arrow*).

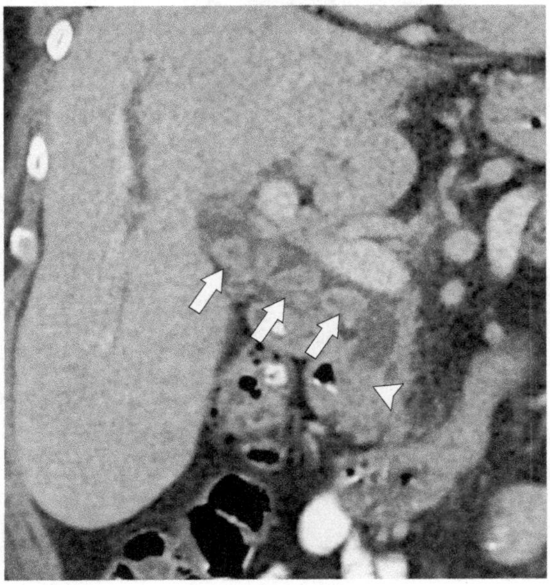

FIGURE 8-21. Coronal contrast-enhanced CT in a 70-year-old man with several CBD stones (*arrows*), one of which obstructs the lower duct (*arrowhead*), causing intrahepatic ductal dilatation.

not exclude choledocholithiasis. However, T2-weighted MRI sequences, particularly MRCP, are far more sensitive, detecting approximately 90% of stones because normal bile has intensely bright T2 signal (similar to water), which permits the visualization of even small bile duct stones (Fig. 8-22). This is therefore the noninvasive investigation of choice should US prove unhelpful and is often preferable to ERCP, an invasive procedure.

Gallstones may reside outside the gallbladder or biliary tree, either because not all gallstones were removed during cholecystectomy (so-called dropped gallstone) or because of gallbladder perforation resulting from chronic cholecystitis. In the former, the gallstones can be located anywhere in the peritoneal cavity (Fig. 8-23), but their visualization will depend, as in the gallbladder, on their calcium content. Some dropped stones therefore will not be visualized, but often they create a peritoneal or retroperitoneal (depending on where they drop) inflammatory reaction, which should not be confused with a mesenteric neoplasm (Fig. 8-24).

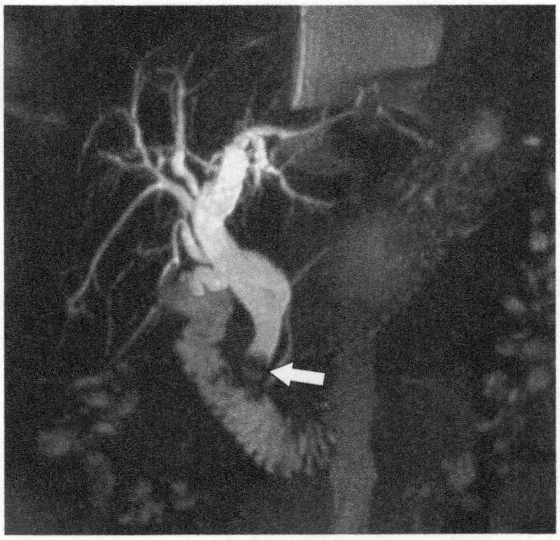

FIGURE 8-22. MRCP in a 59-year-old woman with CBD and intrahepatic duct dilatation caused by an impacted stone at the ampulla of Vater (*arrow*).

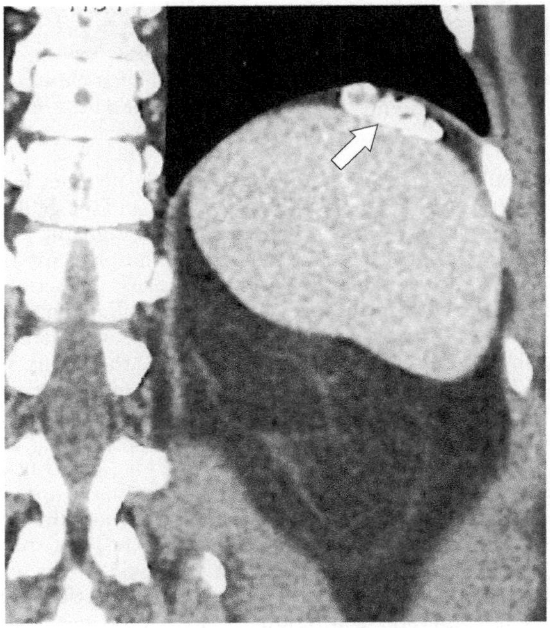

FIGURE 8-23. Coronal contrast-enhanced CT in a 54-year-old man with left subphrenic gallstones (*arrow*) due to "dropped" stones.

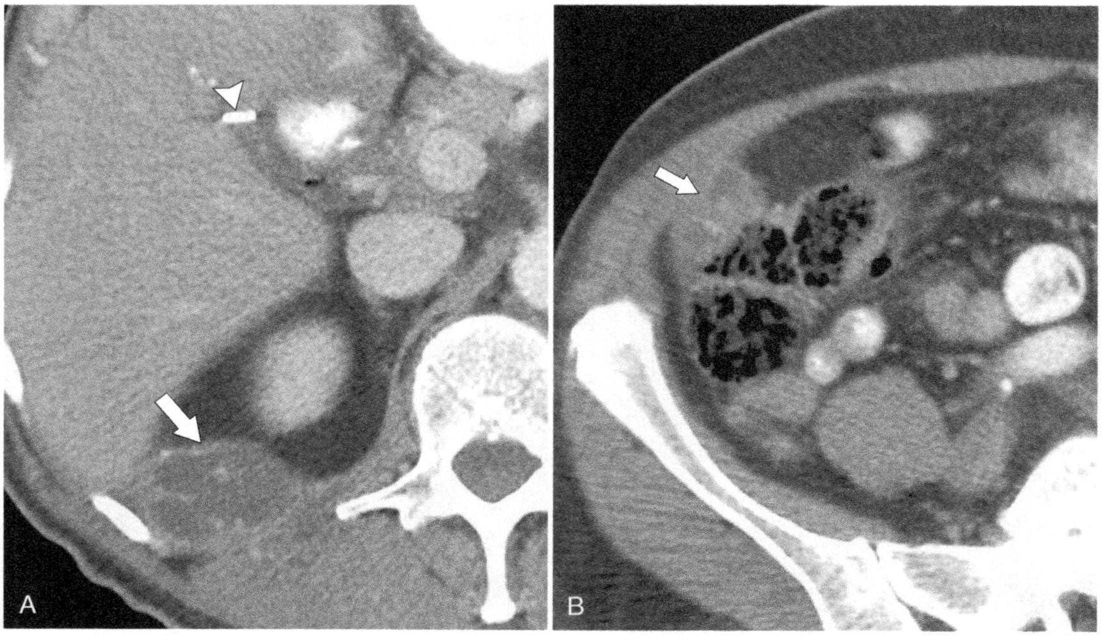

FIGURE 8-24. A and B, Axial contrast-enhanced CT in a 71-year-old man with abdominal pain and two abscesses (*arrows*) secondary to "dropped" gallstones. Note prior cholecystectomy clips (*arrowhead*).

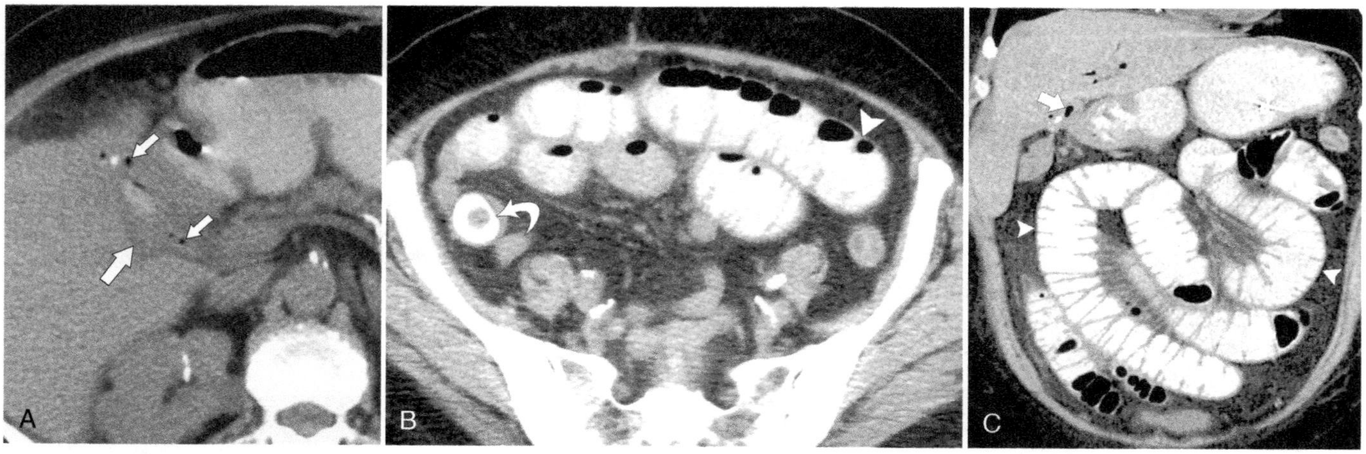

FIGURE 8-25. Axial (A and B) and coronal (C) contrast-enhanced CT in a 77-year-old woman with small bowel obstruction (*arrowheads*) caused by a gallstone ileus (*curved arrow*). Small inflammatory mass (*large arrow*) is due to a choleduodenal fistula with biliary gas (*small arrows*).

After gallbladder perforation the extruded gallstones can have an appearance similar to dropped gallstones, and the gallbladder itself will invariably appear contracted with signs of previous pericholecystic inflammation. Because of the proximity of the gallbladder to the duodenum, the inflammatory reaction from repeated bouts of cholecystitis may create a biliary enteric duodenal fistula as the gallstones erode into the intestinal lumen, with subsequent retrograde reflux of gas into the biliary system (Fig. 8-25). If small, they may be excreted through the rectum, but larger stones can become lodged in the distal ileum, particularly at its narrowest point, the ileocecal valve. This can cause small bowel obstruction called gallstone ileus (Fig. 8-25). Larger stones may obstruct the small bowel more proximally (Fig. 8-26). Alternatively, the gallstone may erode directly into the colon and be excreted through the rectum, since the colon is more distensible, although in rare cases gallstones are sufficiently large to even cause large bowel obstruction. Erosion directly into the stomach, jejunum, and ileum has also been recognized.

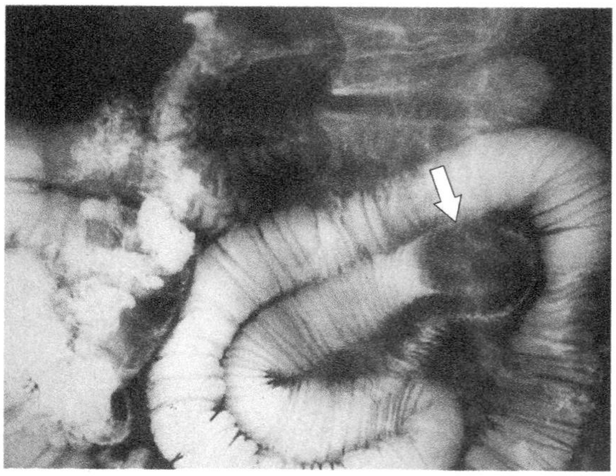

FIGURE 8-26. SBFT in a 56-year-old woman with a large obstructing jejunal gallstone (*arrow*).

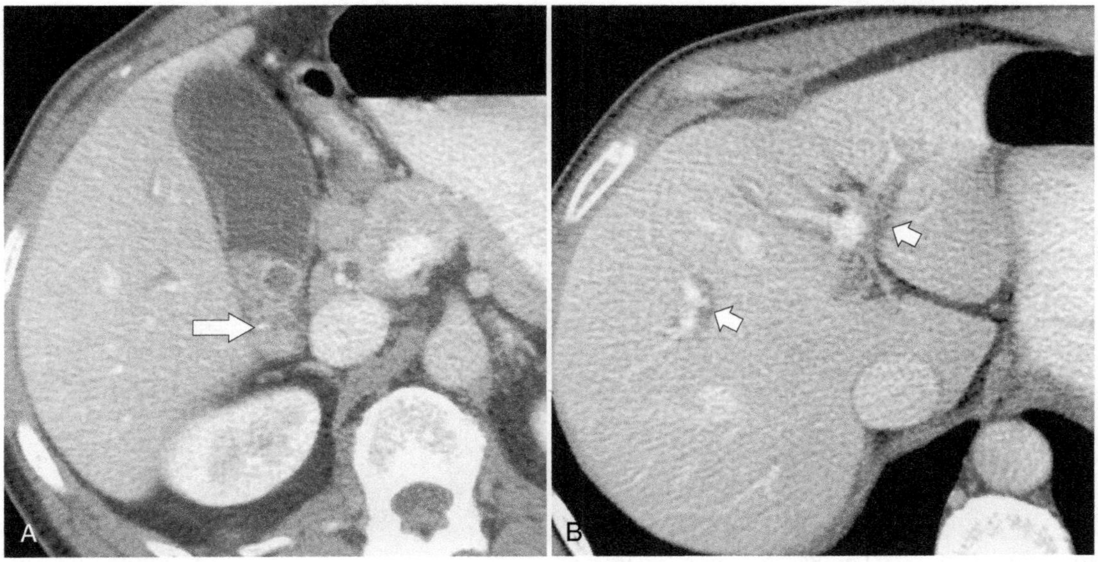

FIGURE 8-27. **A** and **B**, Axial contrast-enhanced CT in a 57-year-old man with multiple gallstones in the gallbladder neck (*large arrow*) causing gallbladder distention and intrahepatic duct dilatation (*small arrows*) owing to Mirizzi syndrome.

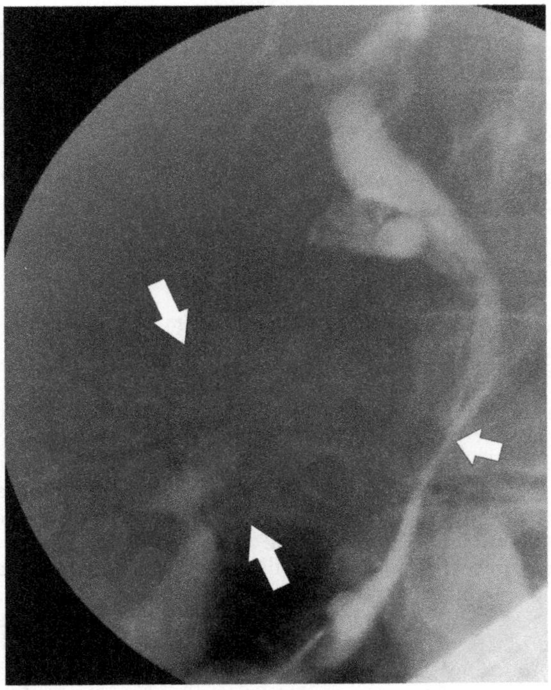

FIGURE 8-28. ERCP in a 49-year-old man with multiple gallstones (*large arrows*) and bile duct stricture (*small arrow*) caused by Mirizzi syndrome.

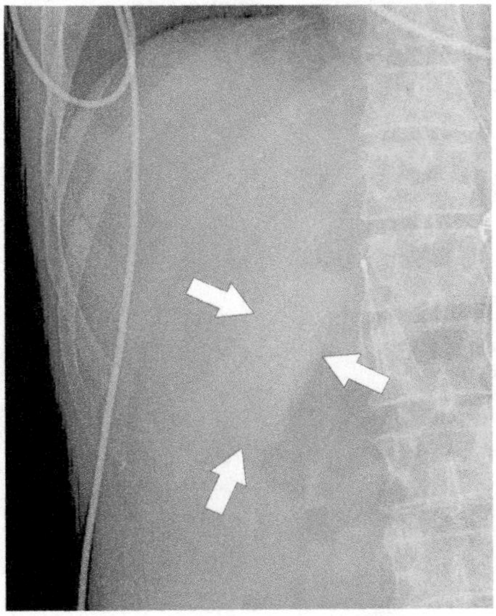

FIGURE 8-29. Plain abdominal radiograph of a 66-year-old man with a subtly dense gallbladder (*arrows*) caused by milk of calcium bile. There is an inferior vena cava filter in situ.

MIRIZZI SYNDROME

Mirizzi* syndrome is a rare complication of gallstone disease in which a large gallstone (usually within a chronically diseased gallbladder) becomes impacted in the cystic duct or gallbladder neck. The stone and the associated inflammatory reaction of the cystic duct then produce mass effect and impinge on the CBD to form a stricture and cause obstructive jaundice. Intrahepatic duct biliary dilatation can be identified on US, CT (Fig. 8-27), or MRI. The impacted stone is more likely to be identified with US or MRI than with CT, although gallbladder distention may or may not be identified because of the often associated chronic cholecystitis. Imaging with ERCP can be helpful, demonstrating a smooth tapering of the CBD, the region of cystic duct insertion, and intrahepatic duct obstruction (Fig. 8-28).

MILK OF CALCIUM BILE

Milk of calcium bile is caused by biliary stasis, which is usually secondary to chronic cystic duct obstruction. Calcium carbonate in static bile increases in concentration and then precipitates, which can then be identified radiographically (Fig. 8-29) or by CT (Fig. 8-30) as either diffuse or layering (Fig. 8-31) radiopacities within the gallbladder. It can be confused with a post-ERCP contrast-filled gallbladder, although this will be unusual (the gallbladder rarely fills with contrast medium injected at ERCP).

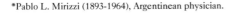

*Pablo L. Mirizzi (1893-1964), Argentinean physician.

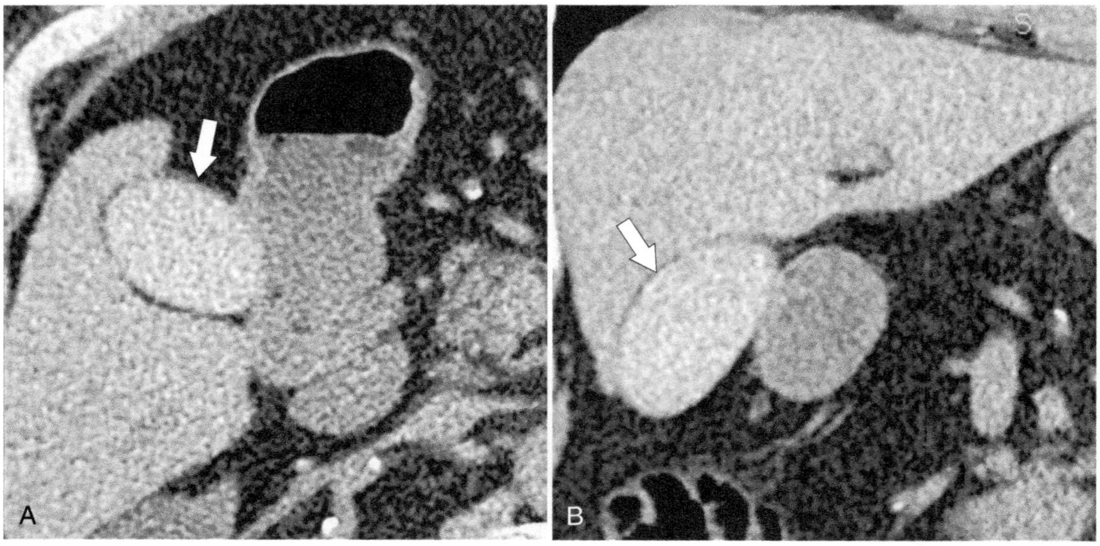

FIGURE 8-30. Axial (**A**) and coronal (**B**) contrast-enhanced CT in a 70-year-old man with dense bile caused by milk of calcium bile (*arrows*).

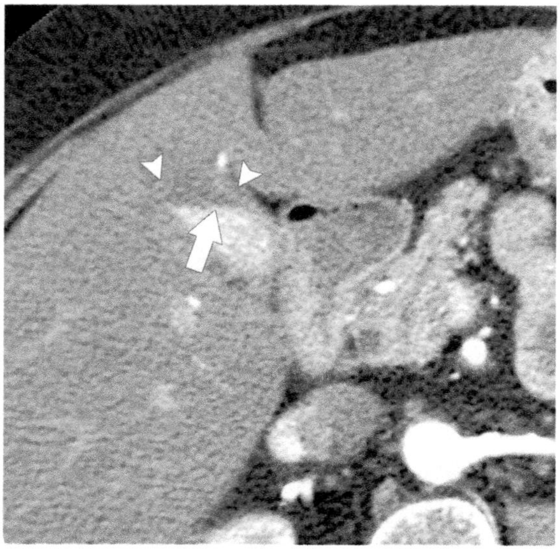

FIGURE 8-31. Axial contrast-enhanced CT in a 57-year-old woman demonstrates dense layering bile (*arrow*) within the gallbladder (*arrowheads*) resulting from milk of calcium bile.

VICARIOUS EXCRETION OF CONTRAST MATERIAL

The vicarious excretion of contrast material can have an imaging appearance similar to milk of calcium bile, with the bile uniformly increased in contrast (at plain radiography or CT) because of the biliary excretion of injected or ingested iodinated contrast material. The condition is usually observed in patients with renal failure who fail to excrete the circulating contrast medium; hence, the medium is "vicariously" excreted into bile instead. It is usually observed with CT (Fig. 8-32) because the concentration of contrast medium is generally insufficient to be observed on plain radiography unless the patient received iodinated contrast material in the presence of severe renal failure. Although generally unnecessary, it can be differentiated from milk of calcium bile by repeat imaging a few days later, allowing sufficient time for the biliary contrast medium to have cleared (Fig. 8-32).

PORCELAIN GALLBLADDER

Porcelain gallbladder is one of the sequelae of chronic cholecystitis. The chronically inflamed gallbladder wall steadily calcifies, sometimes sufficiently to be identified on plain radiography (Fig. 8-33), although most will be identified with US or CT, which will demonstrate curvilinear wall calcification (Fig. 8-34). On US the gallbladder is usually obscured by the calcific wall (Fig. 8-34) and may be confused with a gallbladder full of gallstones. Up to 30% of patients with porcelain gallbladder, left untreated by cholecystectomy, can develop gallbladder carcinoma. Consequently, patients are referred for prophylactic cholecystectomy.

INFLAMMATORY BILIARY DISEASES

Cholecystitis

Cholecystitis is a common cause of morbidity among the general population because of the prevalence of gallstones. It may present for the first time acutely or with chronic clinical symptoms. Less commonly (approximately 5%), acute cholecystitis is acalculous (see later in the chapter). Gallbladder inflammatory change typically results from obstruction of the gallbladder by a stone lodged within the cystic duct. Biliary stasis follows with continued mucosal biliary secretion, which distends the lumen and then thickens or inspissates and becomes secondarily infected, usually by *Escherichia coli* and *Bacteroides* spp. Symptoms may initially be intermittent and self-limiting, but the ensuing infections ultimately produce symptoms and signs of acute bacterial infection. The gallbladder wall becomes hyperemic, inflamed, and thickened. Treatment is usually antibiotics and interval cholecystectomy, although in severe infection, gallbladder perforation and peritonitis occur, requiring immediate surgery.

Imaging is highly sensitive and specific for the detection of acute cholecystitis, and most patients are referred for US. Classic sonographic features include a distended gallbladder, thickened gallbladder wall (>3 mm), intramural gallbladder wall lucencies (representing wall edema), gallstones (often a gallstone impacted in the gallbladder neck), and a Murphy* sign (Fig. 8-35). The Murphy sign is usually elicited by US and is maximal tenderness when the abdomen is compressed precisely over the distended gallbladder. If maximal pain is not directly over the gallbladder,

*John B. Murphy (1857-1916), American surgeon.

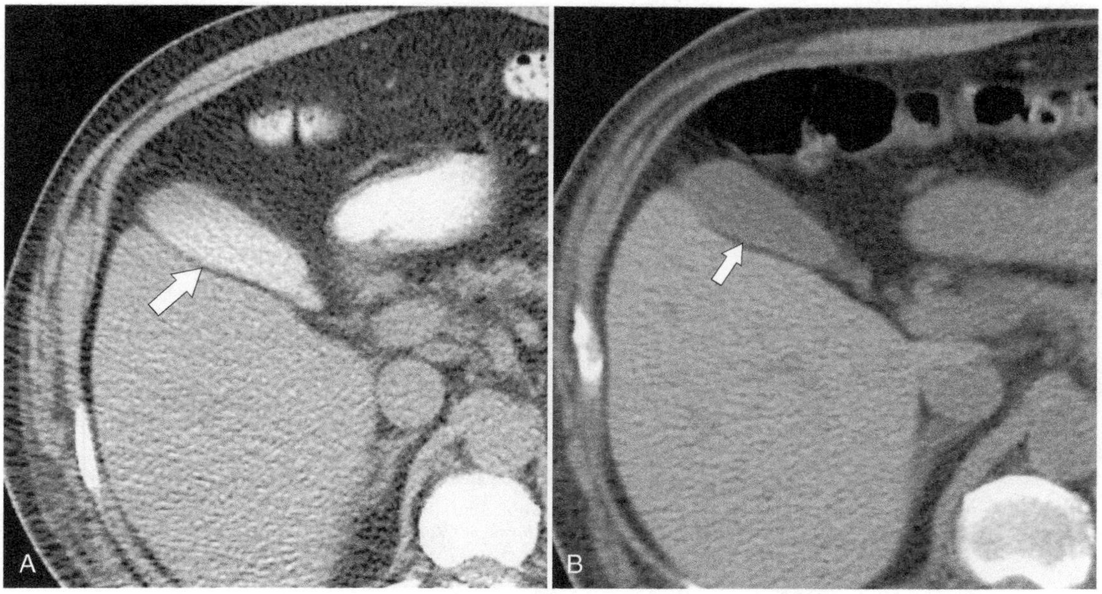

FIGURE 8-32. **A** and **B**, Axial noncontrast CT in a 51-year-old man with renal failure. There is dense bile caused by vicarious excretion of contrast material (*large arrow*) from a recent contrast angiographic study. Three weeks later (*small arrow*), the contrast medium has been excreted.

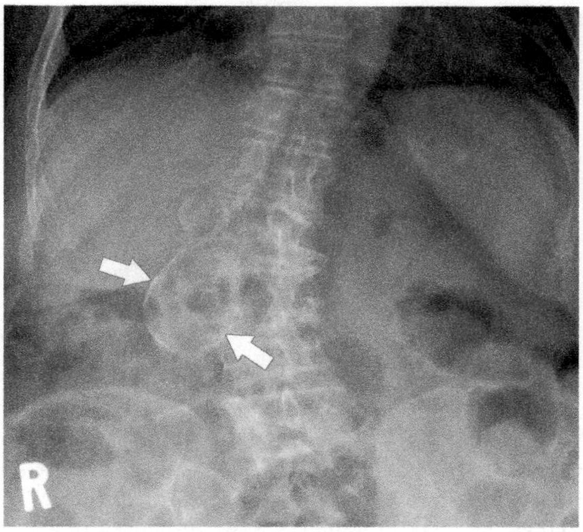

FIGURE 8-33. Plain abdominal radiograph in a 77-year-old woman with a porcelain gallbladder (*arrows*).

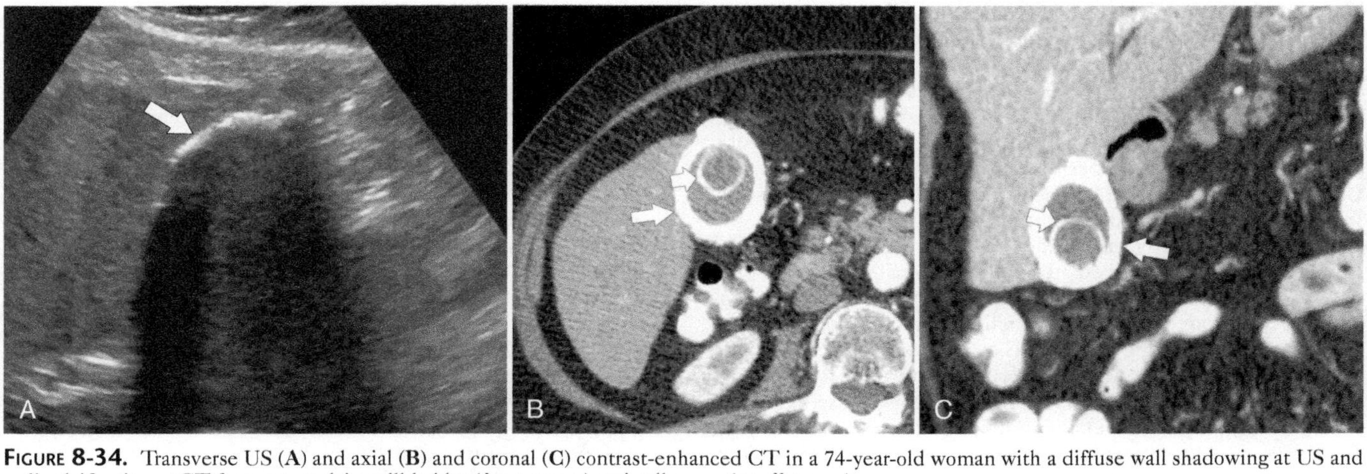

FIGURE 8-34. Transverse US (**A**) and axial (**B**) and coronal (**C**) contrast-enhanced CT in a 74-year-old woman with a diffuse wall shadowing at US and wall calcification at CT from a porcelain gallbladder (*large arrows*) and gallstones (*small arrows*).

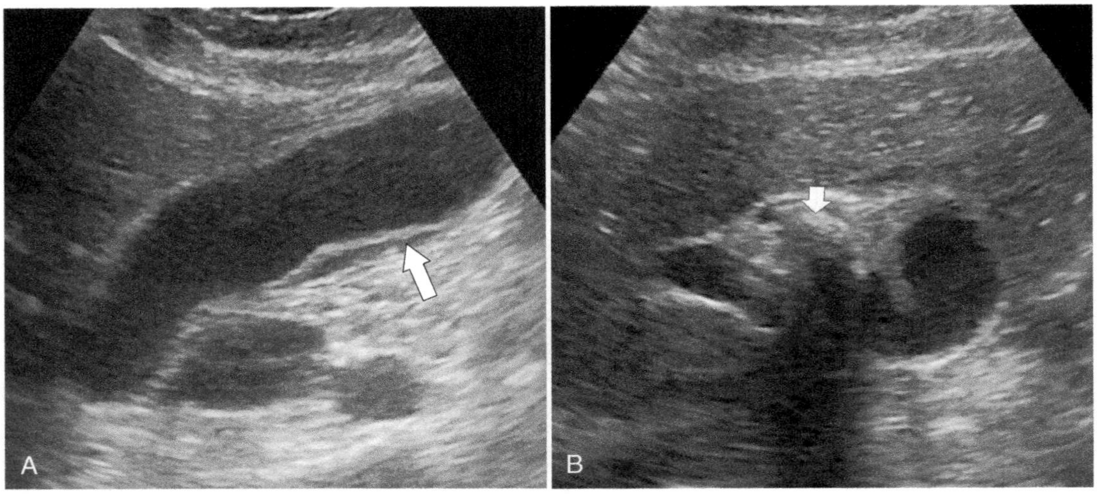

FIGURE 8-35. **A** and **B**, Sagittal US in a 29-year-old woman with a distended gallbladder, slight wall thickening, and intramural gallbladder lucencies (*long arrow*) caused by acute cholecystitis. There is an impacted stone at the gallbladder neck (*short arrow*). The patient had a positive sonographic Murphy sign.

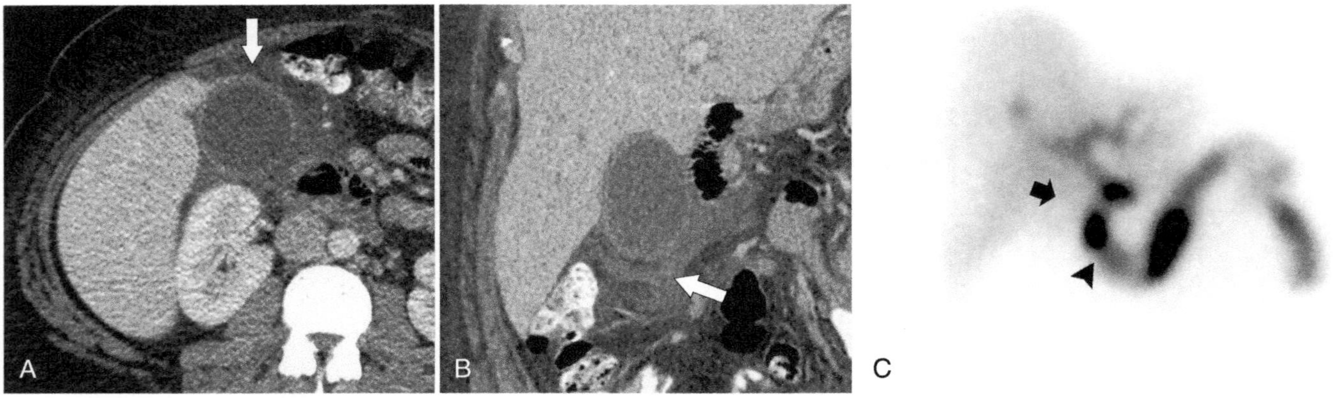

FIGURE 8-36. Axial (**A**) and coronal contrast-enhanced CT (**B**) and HIDA scan (**C**) in a 30-year-old man with an inflamed gallbladder. Pericholecystic edema (*large white arrows*) and wall thickening are due to acute cholecystitis. On HIDA scan there is no gallbladder filling (*small black arrow*) of Tc at 60 minutes because of an obstructed cystic duct. Isotope passes into the duodenum directly (*arrowhead*).

it is unlikely to be a Murphy sign and therefore not acute cholecystitis. However, since this test is often poorly performed, the sign is not necessarily elicited when acute cholecystitis is present.

Less commonly, patients are referred for CT because the clinical symptoms may not localize specifically to the gallbladder or the referring physician may not specifically suspect cholecystitis. Features on contrast-enhanced CT include a distended gallbladder with enhancement of a circumferentially thickened wall and pericholecystic inflammatory changes ("fat stranding") in the adjacent peritoneal fat (Fig. 8-36). Gallstones may or may not be identified, depending on their calcium content.

Nuclear scintigraphy with ^{99m}Tc hepatobiliary iminodiacetic acid (HIDA), now rarely performed because of the accuracy of US, has high specificity for the diagnosis of acute cholecystitis. Injected isotope is readily excreted into the biliary system, and a normally functioning gallbladder is usually identified at 1 hour. If no gallbladder is observed after 4 hours (because of cystic duct obstruction), a diagnosis of acute cholecystitis is made, assuming that there are accompanying clinical symptoms and signs (Fig. 8-36). Early in the injection (i.e., in the arterial phase), the hyperemic gallbladder wall may demonstrate increased activity and a "rim sign" may be observed, representing a crescentic band of isotope activity in the adjacent inflamed hepatic parenchyma, but this sign is less specific and rarely identified. MRI is rarely performed to evaluate for the diagnosis of acute cholecystitis but will demonstrate MR-equivalent findings to contrast-enhanced CT, with a distended gallbladder and a thickened enhancing wall, and most likely the offending gallstone will be identified. Pericholecystic inflammatory change will be manifest as increased T2 signal.

The complications of acute cholecystitis include gallbladder gangrene and perforation with pericholecystic abscess or gas in the gallbladder wall or lumen (Figs. 8-37 and 8-38). Once the gallbladder has been perforated, a positive Murphy sign is less likely because the gallbladder is no longer distended. The features of a perforated gallbladder are best imaged by CT, demonstrating the extent of pericholecystic abscess formation.

Chronic cholecystitis results from repetitive episodes of subacute cholecystitis caused by the presence of stones but usually is not sufficiently symptomatic to make the patient seek urgent medical care. The symptoms are mild to moderate intermittent pain in the right upper quadrant. There is sometimes biliary colic when the gallstone becomes temporarily impacted in the gallbladder neck, but not long enough to cause the sequelae of full-blown acute cholecystitis. The repetitive milder inflammatory episodes ultimately cause fibrosis, thickening, and contraction of the gallbladder, such that it becomes shrunken and compacted with stones (Figs. 8-9 and 8-10). At that point an increasing number of more painful episodes may develop, precipitating medical attention and subsequent cholecystectomy.

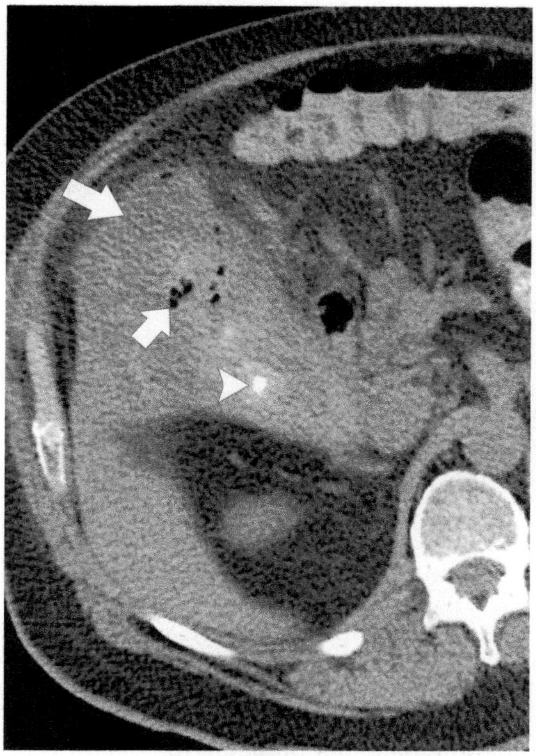

FIGURE 8-37. Axial noncontrast CT in a 77-year-old man with gangrenous cholecystitis with gallbladder perforation, pericholecytic abscess (*long arrow*), and intraluminal gas (*short arrow*). There is also a single gallstone that precipitated the infection (*arrowhead*).

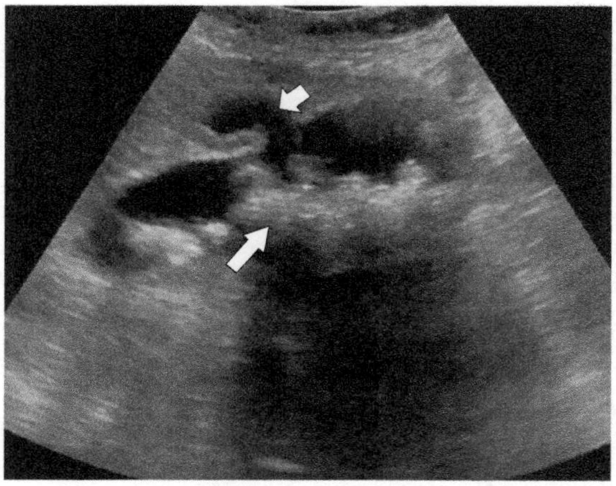

FIGURE 8-38. US in a 76-year-old woman with gallbladder perforation from acute cholecystitis. Numerous stones (*long arrow*) and a perforation are identified on US (*short arrow*).

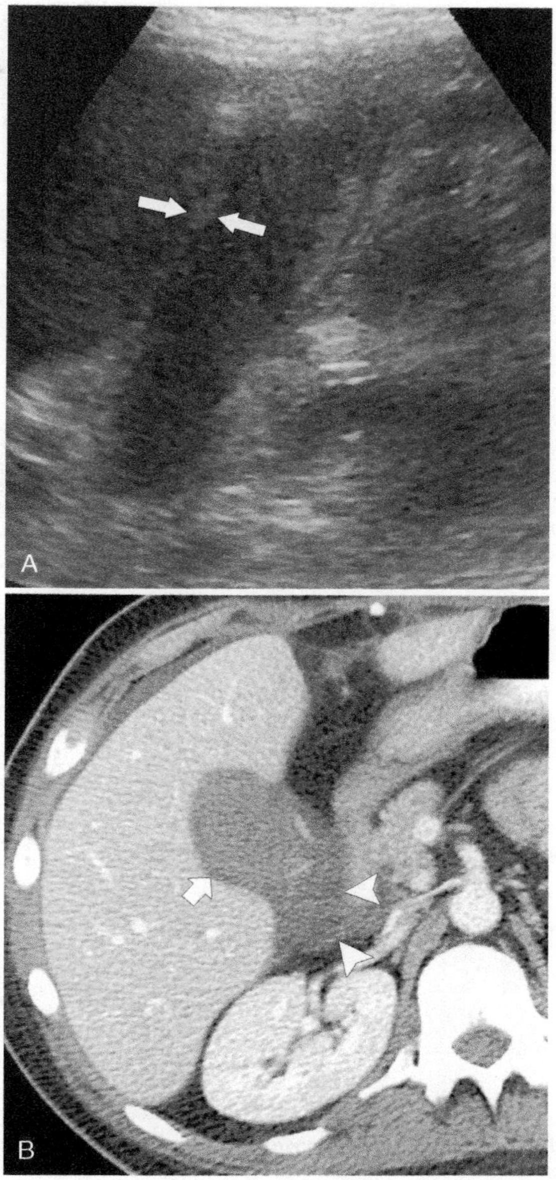

FIGURE 8-39. Sagittal US (**A**) and axial contrast-enhanced CT (**B**) in a 23-year-old man in the ICU with a distended gallbladder (*short arrow*) and pericholecystic edema (*arrowheads*) resulting from acute acalculous cholecystitis. The gallbladder wall (*long arrows*) measures 6 mm.

Acalculous Cholecystitis

Acalculous cholecystitis, a relatively unusual form of cholecystitis, demonstrates all the clinical and imaging features of cholecystitis except the presence of gallstones (Fig. 8-39). It is classically identified in patients after a prolonged stay in an intensive care unit (ICU) and less commonly in patients with diabetes mellitus, AIDS, vascular injury or insufficiency to the gallbladder, colitis, or postpartum state. The resulting gallbladder stasis (particularly after hyperalimentation or cholestatic drugs) can ultimately become secondarily infected, leading to cholecystitis. The diagnosis is often challenging because patients who stay in the ICU may not manifest classic clinical symptoms (pain is masked by narcotics, which in themselves are cholestatic). The diagnosis may be suspected only because of clinical features of sepsis and the knowledge by ICU physicians that these patients are at risk for acalculous cholecystitis. It has been demonstrated, however, that many of the sonographic features of cholecystitis in this group of patients can resolve spontaneously. Conversely, if acalculous cholecystitis is identified in the appropriate clinical setting, the gallbladder is often drained via percutaneous cholecystostomy, with culture of bile (typically milky white because of prolonged stasis) to exclude the gallbladder as the infectious source in a patient with a fever of unknown origin.

HIV-Induced Cholecystitis

Biliary abnormalities are relatively common in patients with AIDS. Cholestatic and cholecystitis-like findings on US include

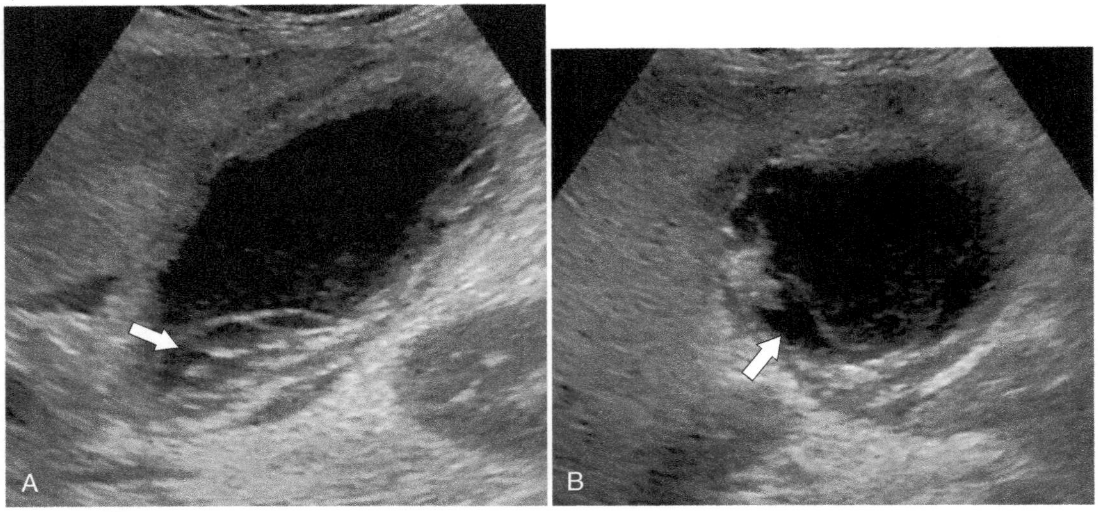

FIGURE 8-40. Sagittal US (**A**) and transverse US (**B**) in a 51-year-old man with HIV-associated cholecystitis, gallbladder wall thickening and intramural lucencies (*arrows*), and gallbladder distention.

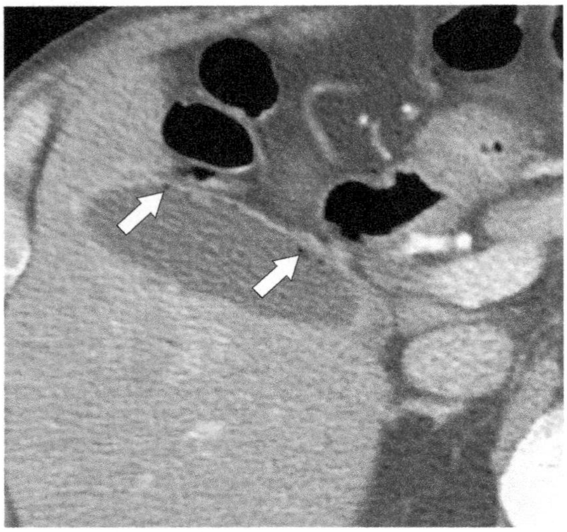

FIGURE 8-41. Axial contrast-enhanced CT in a 74-year-old man with diabetes mellitus with subtle gas in the gallbladder wall (*arrows*) from early emphysematous cholecystitis.

gallbladder wall thickening, pericholecystic lucencies, gallbladder dilatation, and sludge (Fig. 8-40).

Emphysematous Cholecystitis

Emphysematous cholecystitis is a rare presentation of acute cholecystitis and is caused by infection with gas-forming organisms, particularly *E. coli* and *Clostridium welchii.* It has similarities to emphysematous infections in other organs (kidney and bladder) in that it is much more commonly identified in patients with diabetes, who are particularly susceptible to these infections. It has a relatively high death rate. Patients with widespread atherosclerosis are also at risk (also common to patients with diabetes mellitus) because of relative ischemia. If severe, the gas may be identified on plain radiography, but the gas may obscure visualization of the gallbladder at US. CT is therefore the investigation of choice, readily identifying the inflamed gas-filled gallbladder wall (Fig. 8-41). Emphysematous cholecystitis should be differentiated from ascending cholangitis, which also is caused by gas-forming organisms that affect the gallbladder wall. In ascending cholangitis there is usually gas elsewhere in the biliary tree, whereas the gas in emphysematous cholecystitis is confined to the gallbladder.

Xanthogranulomatous Cholecystitis

Xanthogranulomatous cholecystitis, a rare form of chronic cholecystitis, is named for the yellow-gray material that results from its lipid-laden macrophages in the gallbladder wall. Most patients (usually those in the fifth to sixth decades) have associated gallstones, and the disease may be secondary to ulceration of the mucosa and extravasation of bile into the gallbladder wall, setting up an inflammatory response. The imaging findings are generally nonspecific and common to chronic cholecystitis in general, with gallstones or sludge and wall thickening, although the wall thickening may be asymmetrical. More characteristic features include hyperechoic nodules and bands within the gallbladder wall (Fig. 8-42), representing the lipid-laden xanthomatous material. On CT, there is mucosal enhancement and mural thickening, often asymmetrical, and the CT equivalent of lipid-laden macrophages within the wall, represented by hypodense intramural nodules (Fig. 8-42). The differentiation from cholangiocarcinoma can be difficult, and usually the diagnosis is made only after cholecystectomy.

OTHER BENIGN GALLBLADDER DISEASES

Gallbladder Hydrops

Gallbladder hydrops is also known as a mucocele of the gallbladder because of mucous or watery distention of the gallbladder. It results from obstruction, which sometimes is caused by a gallstone in the cystic duct or gallbladder neck but may also be from neoplastic disease. The gallbladder can distend markedly but remains sterile, although later infection and development of gallbladder empyema are common. Once empyema develops, the patient usually presents with pain and fever and a right upper quadrant mass may be palpated. At US, the gallbladder is markedly distended with echogenic material, usually with a markedly thickened wall (Fig. 8-43). When empyema ensues, gas formation can be identified with CT and US. A number of patients do not have a sonographic Murphy sign, which should not deter the diagnosis of gallbladder empyema. Patients are at significant risk of gallbladder perforation.

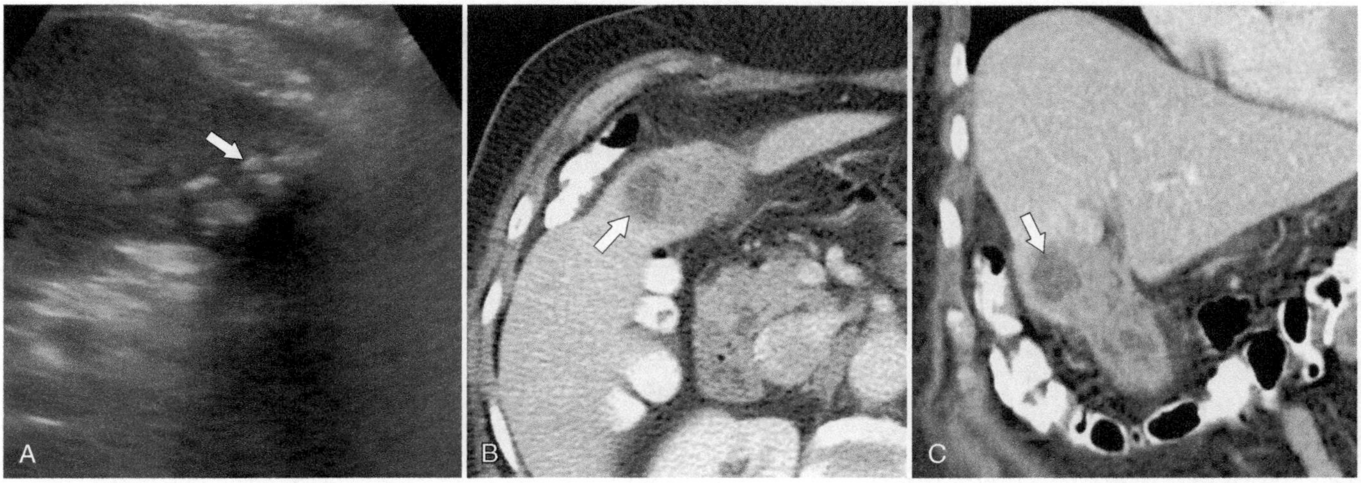

FIGURE 8-42. Sagittal US (**A**), axial (**B**), and coronal (**C**) contrast-enhanced CT in a 59-year-old woman with a heterogeneous material in the gallbladder and hypoechoic and hypodense lipid deposits in the gallbladder wall due to xanthogranulomatous cholecystitis (*arrows*).

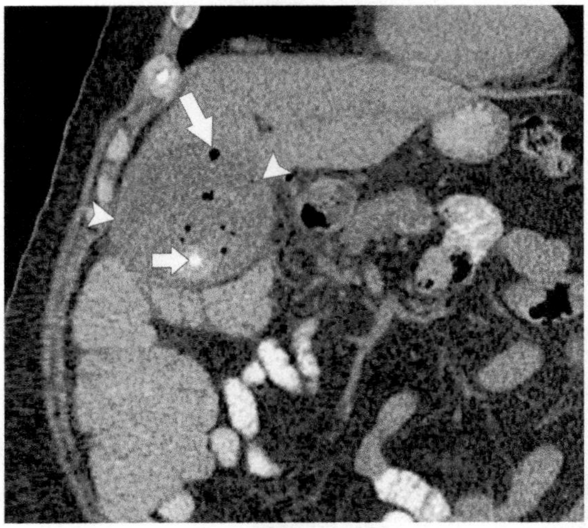

FIGURE 8-43. Coronal contrast-enhanced CT in a 57-year-old man with secondary infection (empyema) of a gallbladder hydrops (*arrowheads*) with intracystic gas (*long arrow*). There is an associated gallstone (*short arrow*).

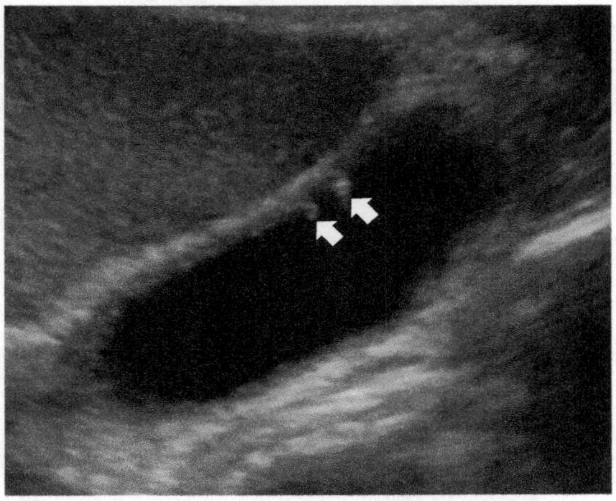

FIGURE 8-44. Sagittal US in a 50-year-old woman with two small filling defects (*arrows*) with ring-down artifacts caused by cholesterosis.

Hyperplastic Cholecystosis

Hyperplastic cholecystosis is a spectrum of benign inflammatory gallbladder changes, the cause of which is poorly understood. The disease is relatively common (approximately 3% to 5% of the population). Patients are frequently asymptomatic (although associated gallstones can occur in approximately 50% of patients), and usually hyperplastic cholecystosis is diagnosed only after cholecystectomy. However, it can present with intermittent right upper quadrant pain, usually in patients in the fifth decade. Hyperplastic cholecystosis has two predominant forms, adenomyomatosis and hyperplastic cholesterosis.

Adenomyomatosis, the more common form, is due to mucosal proliferation and hypertrophy of the muscularis in the gallbladder wall, which is sometimes marked. The gallbladder mucosa then invaginates the hypertrophied wall, forming Rokitansky-Aschoff* sinuses. These sinuses can be identified by US, especially in nonobese patients who have been appropriately fasted. The sinuses appear hypoechoic if filled with bile or hyperechoic if filled with sludge or small stones. A characteristic sonographic feature is a so-called comet tail ring-down artifact representing cholesterol crystals within the sinuses (Fig. 8-44), which may also be identified by CT or MRI. On T2-weighted images the Rokitansky-Aschoff sinuses are seen as small multiple cystic structures (sometimes referred to as a "pearl necklace" sign) within the gallbladder wall that may be filled with multiple small stones (a "rosary sign") at CT (Fig. 8-45). These findings can be diffuse, segmental, or localized. The diffuse form involves the whole gallbladder, the segmental form involves the proximal, middle, or distal gallbladder circumferentially, and the most common form, localized, involves only the fundus. The segmental form typically has waist-like narrowing of the affected gallbladder wall (Fig. 8-46). The fundal or localized form can present as simple mural thickening, but sometimes it is sufficient to appear mass-like and can be difficult to differentiate from gallbladder carcinoma, particularly because with both diseases the affected region may show increased activity on positron emission tomography.

Hyperplastic cholesterosis, sometimes referred to as a strawberry gallbladder because of multiple, small, bright-yellow fatty deposits, is caused by diffuse deposition of submucosal cholesterol/triglyceride-laden histiocytes. The accumulation of these fatty deposits causes mucosal polypoid enlargement, which sometimes can be recognized at US (Fig. 8-47).

*Karl Freiherr von Rokitansky (1804-1878), Austrian pathologist; Karl Albert Ludwig Aschoff (1866-1942), German pathologist.

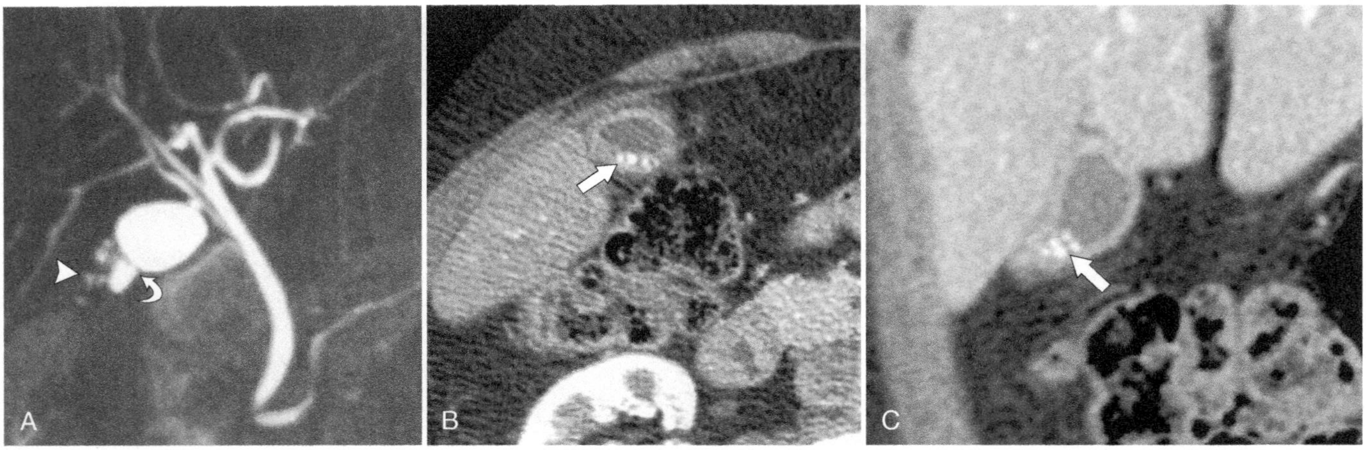

FIGURE 8-45. MRCP (**A**) and axial (**B**) and coronal (**C**) contrast-enhanced CT in a 58-year-old woman with adenomyomatosis and a CT "rosary sign" with several tiny stones (*arrows*) lodged within the Rokitansky-Aschoff sinuses and the "string of pearls" sign (*arrowhead*) and fundal constriction (*curved arrow*) at MRCP.

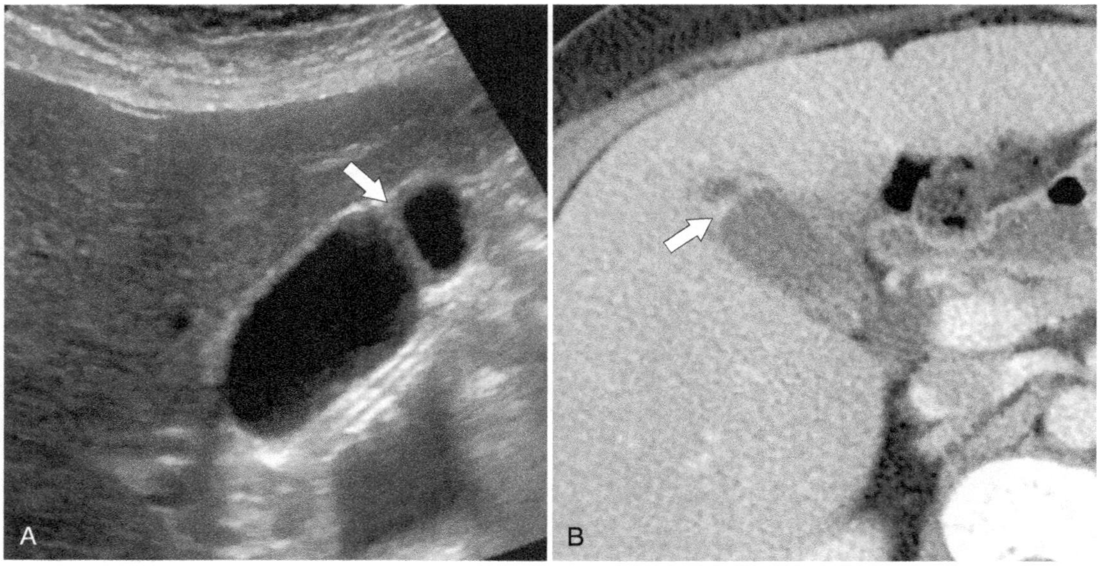

FIGURE 8-46. Sagittal US (**A**) and axial contrast-enhanced CT (**B**) in a 44-year-old woman with a fundal gallbladder constriction (*arrows*) caused by adenomyomatosis.

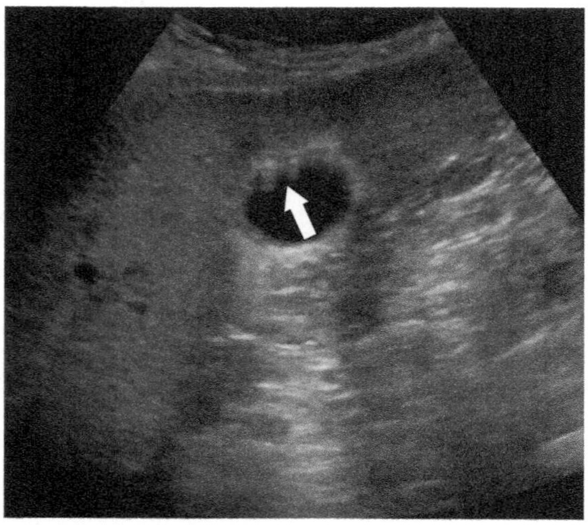

FIGURE 8-47. Transverse US in a 48-year-old woman with ring-down artifacts (*arrow*) in a "strawberry" gallbladder.

Primary Sclerosing Cholangitis

Primary sclerosing cholangitis (PSC) is a chronic disease of the extrahepatic and intrahepatic bile ducts that causes progressive and diffuse biliary duct inflammation and stricture formation, often termed either arborized (or "pruned tree") or bead like. Cholestasis ensues with the formation of multiple small segmental ectatic bile ducts. PSC is most likely autoimmune in origin because of the presence of numerous circulating autoantibodies and because up to 80% of patients also have ulcerative colitis. It is also, however, associated with Crohn disease and other autoimmune diseases, including autoimmune pancreatitis and thyroiditis. In most patients it appears before the age of 45 years, and the disease is usually unrelenting with progression through fibrosis and biliary cirrhosis, which may ultimately require liver transplantation, even though PSC is known to recur in the allograft. There is also an approximate 10% chance that cholangiocarcinoma will develop.

The diagnosis is best made with good biliary ductal opacification, and therefore ERCP (or transhepatic cholangiography) is the imaging method of choice (Fig. 8-48). Segmental strictures are found in the extrahepatic ducts but are most commonly observed

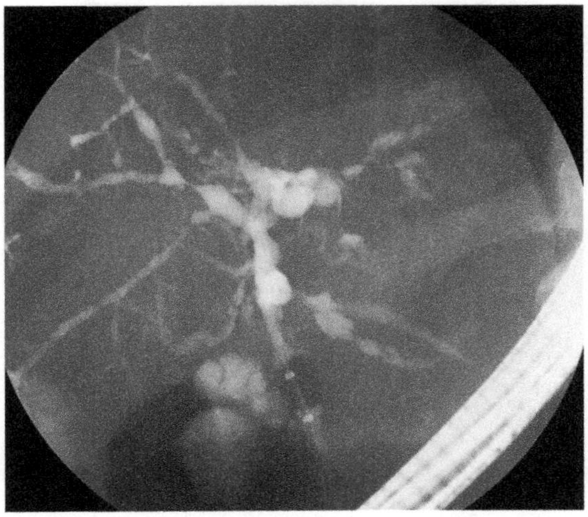

FIGURE 8-48. ERCP in a 73-year-old woman demonstrating diffuse intrahepatic duct irregularities with a bead-like appearance resulting from primary sclerosing cholangitis.

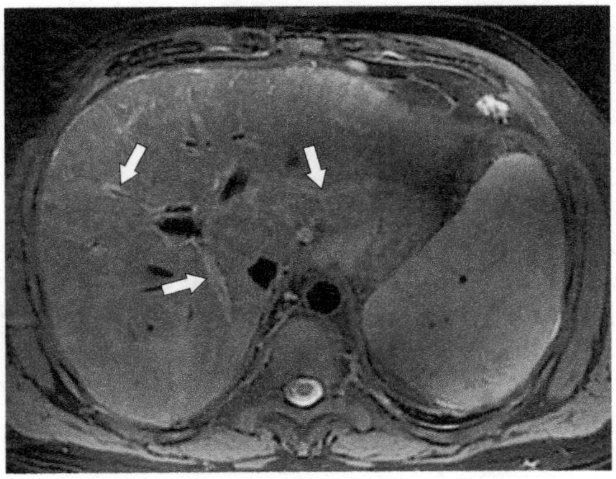

FIGURE 8-49. T2-weighted fat-saturated MRI in a 35-year-old man with primary biliary cirrhosis and high periductal T2 signal due to edema (*arrows*). There is associated splenomegaly.

in the right and left intrahepatic ducts as multiple short segmental strictures with intermittent focal ductal dilatation (Fig. 8-48). The fine, bead-like ductal abnormalities are generally not identified by CT, although focal bile lakes of ectatic ducts might be visualized. There is often evidence of periductal fibrosis, which is recognized by edematous tracking along the ducts that becomes broader and more confluent as fibrosis progresses and is observed particularly centrally (Fig. 8-49). Finally, as diffuse cirrhosis ensues, the liver has the typical cirrhotic appearances of a shrunken liver with distorted contour. As in other forms of cirrhosis, the caudate lobe is usually hypertrophied, but whereas in other forms the cause is preservation of vascular drainage, in PSC it is relative preservation of the caudate bile ducts. US is superior to CT for evaluating the ductal abnormalities, demonstrating wall thickening (caused by progressive inflammatory change), hypoechoic focal segmental strictures, and biliary ectasia. Echogenic portal triads correspond to fibrotic change. The gallbladder is not spared in this disease, so US may demonstrate segmental and asymmetrical wall thickening. The evolution of the disease is often monitored with MRI and MRCP, which clearly demonstrate the biliary ductal irregularity (Fig. 8-50), and high periductal T2-weighted signal implies edema and fibrosis. Identification of cholangiocarcinoma is suggested by the development of a mass (especially if it demonstrates delayed enhancement on contrast-enhanced CT or MRI) and upstream biliary dilatation.

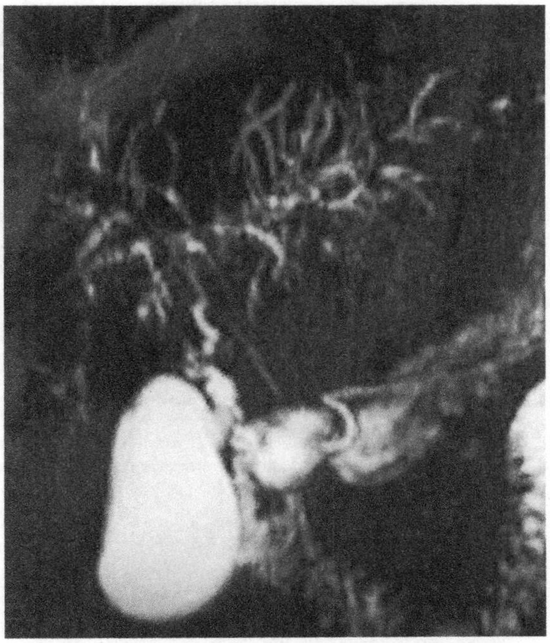

FIGURE 8-50. MRCP in a 33-year-old woman with diffusely irregular intrahepatic bile ducts caused by primary sclerosing cholangitis.

Infectious Cholangitis

Infectious cholangitis usually refers to an infection of the intrahepatic or extrahepatic biliary system, whereas gallbladder infection is termed cholecystitis. It is mostly bacterial in nature (often *E. coli*) and termed ascending cholangitis. Parasites (*Clonorchis sinensis* and *Ascaris lumbricoides*) are common infectious pathogens in many parts of the world. Other AIDS-related infections are responsible for AIDS-related cholangiopathy.

Ascending Cholangitis

Pyogenic cholangitis is usually associated with gallstones, and patients are particularly susceptible if these are associated with biliary obstruction (as can occur with other benign or malignant strictures). The infection can be devastating if not treated early. Patients present with pain, fever, and jaundice (Charcot* triad), and the infection can develop rapidly into bacteremia and overwhelming septicemia. In the correct clinical setting, US is often the imaging method of choice because it is rapidly available and is more sensitive than CT for the demonstration of intrahepatic and extrahepatic biliary duct dilatation, especially if mild (Fig. 8-51). Color Doppler is useful to differentiate normal portal venous strictures from dilated ducts, which are sometimes difficult to identify (Fig. 8-51). Once biliary dilatation has been confirmed, ERCP is usually performed to further define the anatomical site of obstruction and also to remove stones and perform sphincterotomy with or without stent placement, particularly for neoplastic forms of obstruction. Less commonly, transhepatic cholangiography and catheter drainage are performed, mainly for patients in whom ERCP is contraindicated or who have not responded to treatment (e.g., those who underwent prior upper gastrointestinal surgery) (Fig. 8-52).

AIDS-Related Cholangiopathy

Patients with AIDS-related immunosuppression are susceptible to multiple opportunistic infections, which can lead to repeated biliary inflammatory changes and ultimately strictures and obstruction. The

*Jean-Martin Charcot (1825-1893), French neurologist and pathologist.

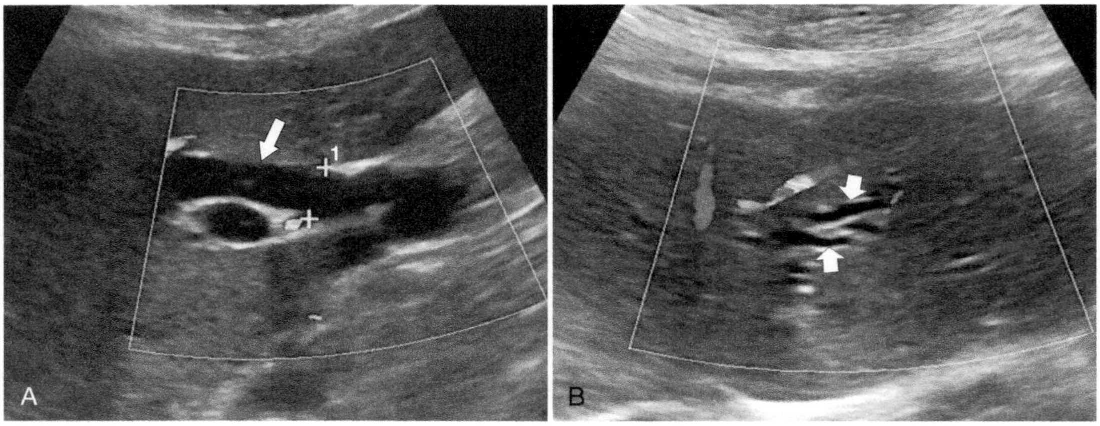

Figure 8-51. A and B, US in a 70-year-old man with ascending cholangitis caused by obstructive jaundice from pancreatic adenocarcinoma and a dilated CBD (16 mm) (*long arrow*) and intrahepatic ducts (*short arrows*).

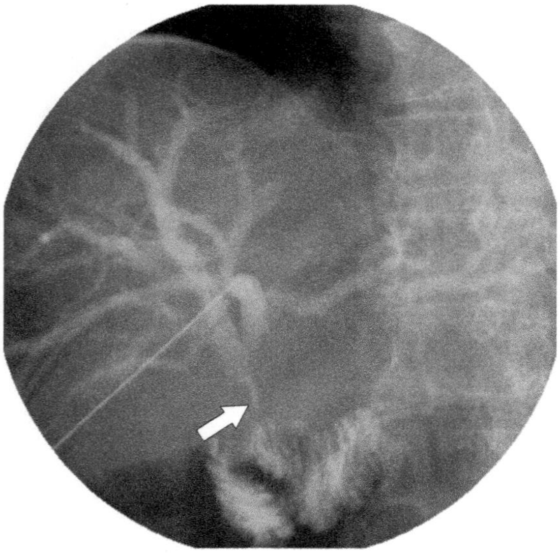

Figure 8-52. Transhepatic cholangiogram in a 46-year-old man with prior choledochojejunostomy that is strictured (*arrow*) with dilated intrahepatic ducts and ascending cholangitis.

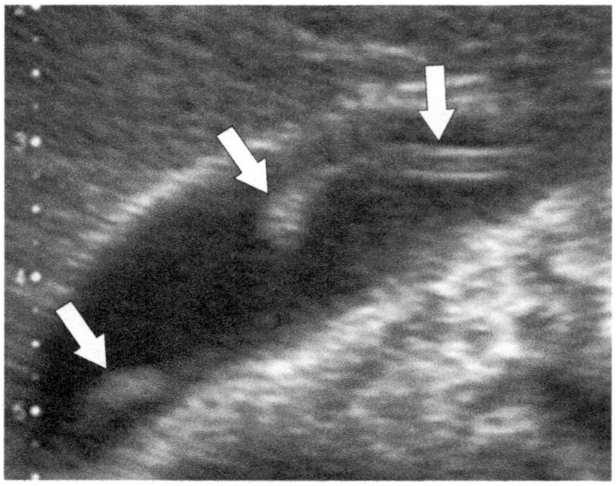

Figure 8-53. Sagittal US in a 43-year-old man with a tubular gallbladder filling defect (*arrows*) caused by *Ascaris* species worm.

most common opportunistic organism is *Cryptosporidium parvum*, but others include cytomegalovirus, microsporidia, and *Cyclospora*. Patients present with a Charcot* triad of fever, pain, and jaundice, and most already have a known diagnosis of AIDS. At imaging, both intrahepatic and extrahepatic duct dilatation is usually present, interspersed with multiple stricture formation not dissimilar to that in sclerosing cholangitis. The gallbladder is commonly thickened and often demonstrates irregular linear wall lucencies (Fig. 8-40). Evidence of opportunistic infection elsewhere in the abdomen (retroperitoneal adenopathy) or enteritis is often present.

Parasitic Cholangitis

Ascaris *Species Infection*

Ascaris lumbricoides is a parasitic nematode worm that typically grows to 20 to 30 inches long. These worms are highly prevalent in most developing countries, and patients are often infested with numerous worms. Given their thin tubular nature, they have a propensity to burrow into the lower CBD through the ampulla of Vater and may cause biliary and pancreatic duct obstruction, the latter leading to pancreatitis. Occasionally a worm manages to navigate up the bile duct and even into the gallbladder, where it can be identified by US or ERCP (Fig. 8-53).

Asiatic or Oriental Cholangitis

Oriental cholangiohepatitis, caused by *Clonorchis sinensis* (or Chinese liver fluke), is endemic in Southeast Asia and is responsible for Asiatic or oriental cholangitis, also known as recurrent pyogenic cholangitis. The fluke uses the fresh-water snail as an intermediate host in which cysts mature into cercariae, burrow their way out of the snail, and penetrate fish bodies. Humans who consume the fish become infected. The cercariae resist degradation in the small intestine and migrate to the biliary system, where they sexually reproduce and set up a biliary inflammatory response. The repeated infections lead to intrahepatic and extrahepatic duct inflammation (compounded by fluke volume and eggs), strictures, and stone formation, which are characteristic of this disease. The CT findings are characteristic in the appropriate clinical setting, with irregular and dilated ducts (Fig. 8-54), many of which are filled with stone material (Fig. 8-55). As with gallstones, the overall stone burden may not be evident on CT. Given that the stones are predominantly intrahepatic and many are in distal locations, they can prove almost impossible to remove and repeated cholangitic attacks occur. Cholangiocarcinoma is a complication of the disease and is common in regions where the disease is endemic (Fig. 8-54).

Chemotherapy-Induced Cholangitis

Chemotherapy-induced cholangitis is a complication of transarterial chemoembolization (TACE) with toxic chemotherapeutic

*Jean-Martin Charcot (1825-1893), French neurologist.

agents for treatment of malignant primary and secondary hepatic disease. The injected agents can cause an occlusive ischemic biliary injury and also damage the biliary tree via their direct toxic effects. The larger hepatic ducts are those usually affected and heal by fibrotic strictures, often multiple, which may extend into the distal intrahepatic ducts (i.e., those closer to the hepatic bifurcation). Peripheral (proximal) ducts are usually unaffected. Proximal biliary dilatation seen on cross-sectional MRI is evidence of stricturing. The actual stricture usually requires direct contrast visualization with ERCP or THC. Treatment is usually with balloon dilatation and ultimately liver transplant, providing the primary tumor has not metastasized.

Portal Biliopathy

In the presence of extrahepatic portal venous occlusion (which may also extend into the intrahepatic portal veins), multiple hepatopetal portal cavernous veins (or transformation) occur. These act as a means to divert mesenteric blood around the thrombosed portal vein from the peripancreatic region and into the liver. Depending on the acuity of the portal vein obstruction, the portal venous thrombus may or may not be identified, but there will be multiple serpiginous venous collaterals in and around the region of the thrombosed vessel. These dilated collaterals can impinge in the extrahepatic bile duct and cause biliary obstruction, usually mild, within the intrahepatic ducts (Fig. 8-56).

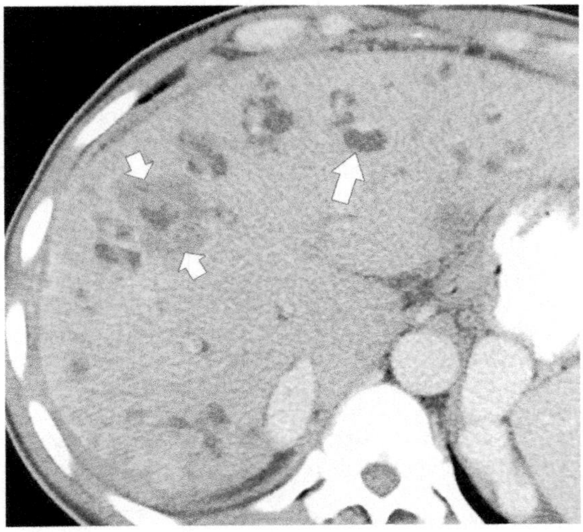

FIGURE 8-54. Axial contrast-enhanced CT in a 43-year-old woman with multiple dilated ducts caused by oriental cholangitis (*long arrow*). The patient subsequently developed cholangiocarcinoma (*short arrows*).

Gallbladder Wall Thickening

Thickening of the gallbladder wall is defined as a thickness greater than 3 mm. It is important to measure the thickness in transverse diameter; spurious recordings will be made if the wall is measured in oblique or tangential planes. A number of primary gallbladder diseases are responsible for gallbladder wall thickening (Box 8-1). Most causes have already been discussed in this chapter. Gallbladder carcinoma is discussed later in the chapter.

Secondary causes of gallbladder wall thickening are adjacent inflammation, hepatitis or pancreatitis (Fig. 8-57), or ascites from any cause (particularly right-sided heart failure and renal failure). The precise reason is poorly understood but is thought to be elevated portal venous pressure. The gallbladder wall thickening can be surprisingly alarming, particularly in hepatitis, and should not be confused with gallbladder gangrene or necrosis (Fig. 8-58). The wall at US is often multilayered with multiple intramural lucencies (Fig. 8-58). These features all resolve once the immediate inflammatory condition subsides, and cholecystectomy is not warranted.

Cystic Biliary Masses

Peribiliary Cysts

Peribiliary cysts are uncommon but are associated with cirrhosis and portal vein thrombosis. They represent focal dilatation of periductal glands that become obstructed owing to an inflammatory process. They are recognized at imaging as single or multiple small CT-hypodense or MRI-hyperintense cystic lesions along the length of the biliary tree and are sometimes confused with small simple cysts. They are better appreciated with T2-weighted MRI as multiple high-signal cysts (Fig. 8-59).

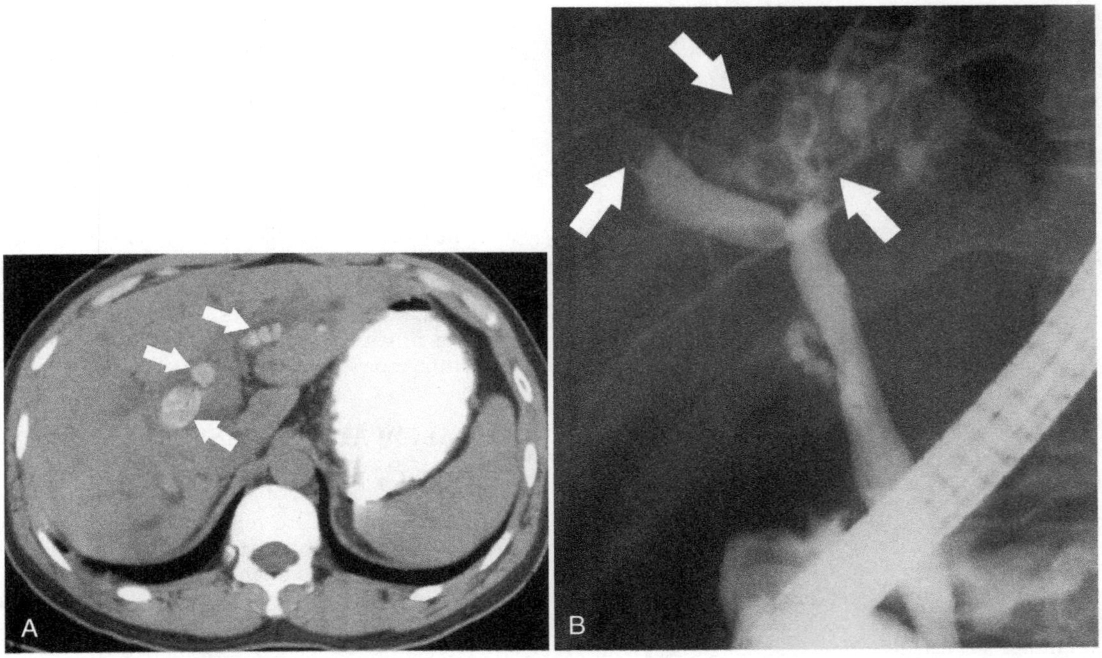

FIGURE 8-55. Axial non-contrast-enhanced CT (**A**) and ERCP (**B**) in a 28-year-old woman with multiple intrahepatic stones (*arrows*) caused by oriental cholangiohepatitis.

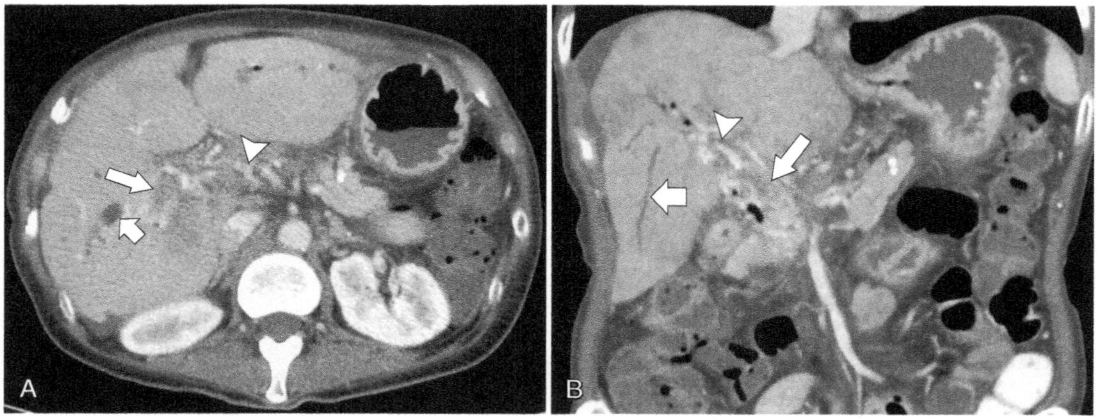

FIGURE 8-56. Axial (**A**) and coronal (**B**) contrast-enhanced CT in a 61-year-old woman with cirrhosis, portal vein occlusion (*large arrows*), and biliary dilatation (*small arrows*) caused by portal biliopathy (*arrowheads*).

Box 8-1. Gallbladder Wall Thickening

Acute and chronic cholecystitis (calculus and acalculous)
Emphysematous cholecystitis
Xanthogranulomatous cholecystitis
Adenomyomatosis
Porcelain gallbladder
Ascites (from any cause)
Hepatitis
Cirrhosis
Pancreatitis
HIV cholangiopathy
Gallbladder carcinoma

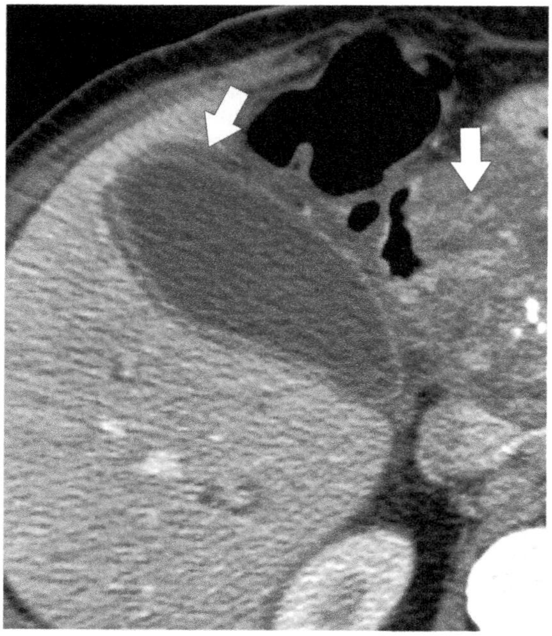

FIGURE 8-57. Axial contrast-enhanced CT in a 42-year-old man with gallbladder wall thickening (*left arrow*) caused by adjacent pancreatitis (*right arrow*).

Biliary Cystadenoma

Biliary cystadenomas are rare cystic tumors most commonly occurring in middle-aged women. They are derived from biliary endothelium and are usually solitary, although occasionally multiple, and often septated and large. They frequently contain ovarian stroma, a diagnostic feature at histological examination. They are usually benign, but some have a malignant potential with a risk of degeneration into biliary cystadenocarcinoma. The cysts are usually complex, which makes them difficult to differentiate from cystic metastases, infected cysts (hydatid or *Echinococcus*), resolving hematomas, or bilomas. The clinical history is therefore important because most biliary cystadenomas are detected incidentally.

On US a large multiseptated cyst is observed (Fig. 8-60), sometimes with wall calcification. The diagnosis is best suggested with contrast-enhanced CT or MRI, which demonstrates a large multiseptated cyst with a well-defined wall that can calcify. Malignant degeneration demonstrates enhancing septa and larger solid masses within the cyst. The cyst may be of variable signal on both T1- and T2-weighted MRI, depending on the serous or mucoid nature of the cyst contents.

Bile Duct Hamartomas

Bile duct hamartomas, also known as von Meyenburg* complexes, are rare benign hepatic tumors. A congenital anomaly with malformation of the bile ducts results in multiple biliary cystic lesions. Biliary hamartomas are either incidental or associated with polycystic liver disease, in which they are relatively common. They are usually asymptomatic and of no concern, being detected incidentally on US, CT, or MRI as multiple small (usually <1.5 cm) cystic lesions (Fig. 8-61). US demonstrates multiple, diffuse, small anechoic lesions, although some may display mixed echogenicity because they have solid components (fibrous stroma). On CT, the density similarly depends on the proportion of cystic versus solid components and therefore ranges from water to soft tissue density. A hallmark, however, is the large number and small size of cyst-like lesions, unlike simple hepatic cysts, which are generally not so numerous. On contrast-enhanced CT, the solid elements may enhance but cystic areas do not. MRI can demonstrate similar features, with low signal on T1-weighted imaging, bright T2 signal for cystic lesions, and intermediate signal for the more solid components.

GALLBLADDER MASSES

Gallbladder Polyps

Gallbladder polyps are relatively common and are small polypoid masses that project into the gallbladder lumen. They are most frequently adenomatous. When multiple they are associated with cholesterol deposits and therefore are part of

*Hans von Meyenburg (1887-1971), Swiss pathologist.

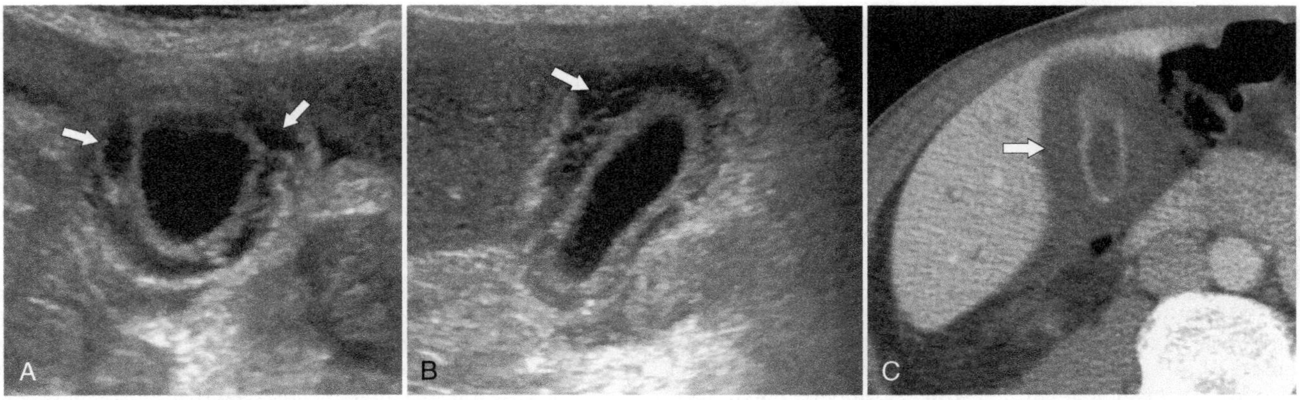

FIGURE 8-58. Transverse (**A**) and sagittal US (**B**) and axial CT (**C**) in a 61-year-old woman with a 7-mm gallbladder wall thickening and multiple wall lucencies (*arrows*) caused by hepatitis.

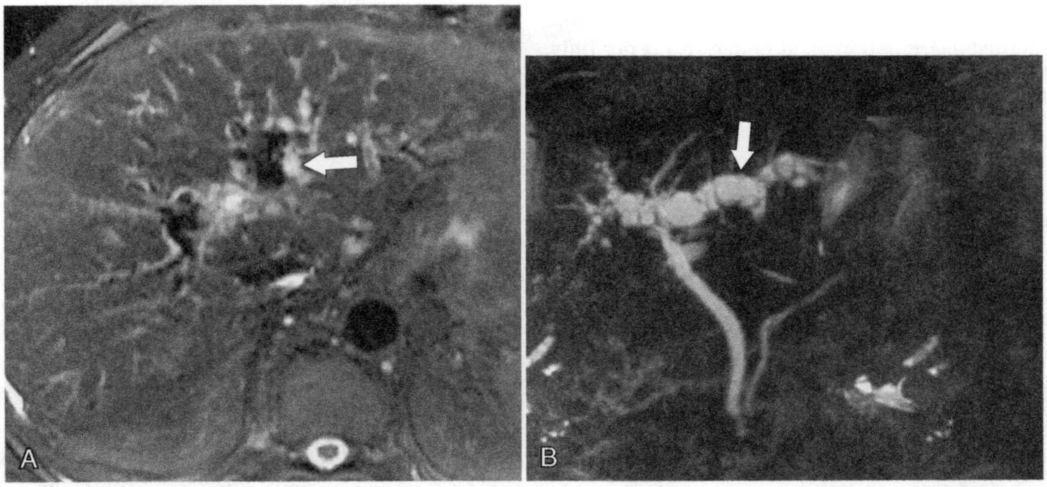

FIGURE 8-59. Axial fat-saturated T2-weighted MRI (**A**) and MRCP (**B**) in a 44-year-old man with multiple small T2 hyperintense peribiliary cysts (*arrows*).

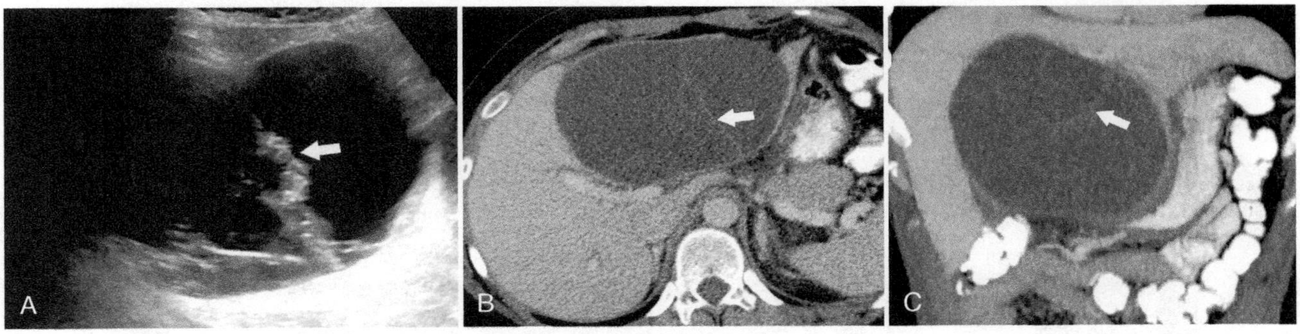

FIGURE 8-60. Sagittal US (**A**) and axial (**B**) and coronal (**C**) contrast-enhanced CT in a 36-year-old woman with a complex 9-cm intrahepatic cyst representing a biliary cystadenoma. Note internal septa (*arrows*).

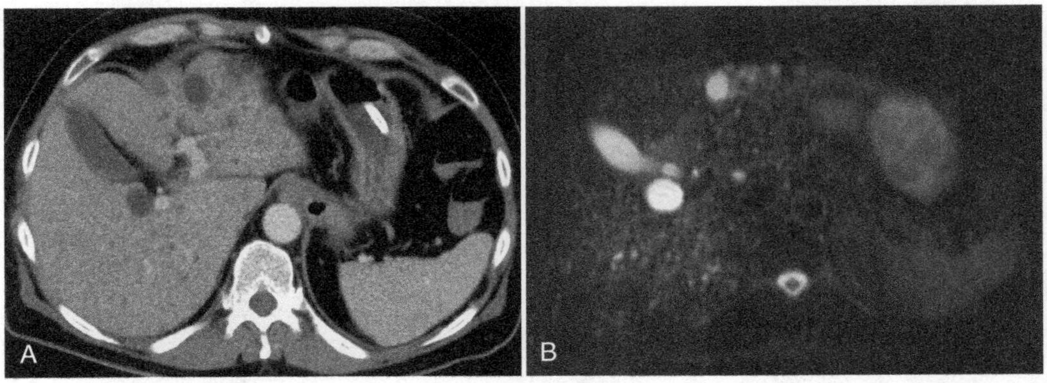

FIGURE 8-61. Axial contrast-enhanced CT (**A**) and T2-weighted MRI (**B**) in a 53-year-old man with multiple biliary hamartomas or von Meyenburg complexes that are low density at CT and high signal at MRI.

a spectrum of disease with hyperplastic cholecystosis and particularly cholesterolosis. Gallbladder polyps have also been recognized in Peutz-Jeghers (hamartomatous polyps) (see Chapter 4) and familial adenomatous polyposis (adenomatous polyps) (see Chapters 4 and 5). At US, they are recognized by a small intraluminal nonshadowing sessile mass, which helps to differentiate them from gallstones (Fig. 8-62). The presence of cholesterol is indicated by echogenicity within the polyp (without shadowing). Differentiation from tumefactive sludge is usually possible because sludge is typically mobile, larger, and irregular in contour. Furthermore, color Doppler flow can be observed in some larger polyps. If the polyp is sufficiently large (>5 mm), it can be identified with CT. Smaller polyps can be identified with T2-weighted MRI because of the superior contrast resolution between the high-signal bile and low-signal polyp.

Most polyps are asymptomatic and benign, but they are considered to have premalignant potential, although this is not fully substantiated. Polyps up to 1 cm are serially imaged to determine any increase in size that might indicate malignant transformation to cholangiocarcinoma. When polyps are larger than 1 cm (and especially if >1.5 cm), cholecystectomy is usually indicated to exclude cholangiocarcinoma (Fig. 8-63). Some surgeons remove polyps smaller than 1 cm because of this risk.

Biliary Intraductal Papillary Mucinous Neoplasm

Biliary intraductal papillary mucinous neoplasm (IPMN) causes both intrahepatic and extrahepatic biliary duct dilatation when mucin is secreted from papillary mucinous epithelial cells lining the ducts. Therefore a discrete mass may not be present. Biliary IPMN is far less commonly observed than IPMN of the pancreatic duct. Patients present with intermittent pain, fever, and jaundice. The diagnosis is suggested when ERCP demonstrates multiple intraluminal mucinous filling defects, with or without an associated mass. US, CT, and MRI usually show diffuse (and sometimes grossly enlarged) bile ducts filled with hypodense mucinous material (Fig. 8-64).

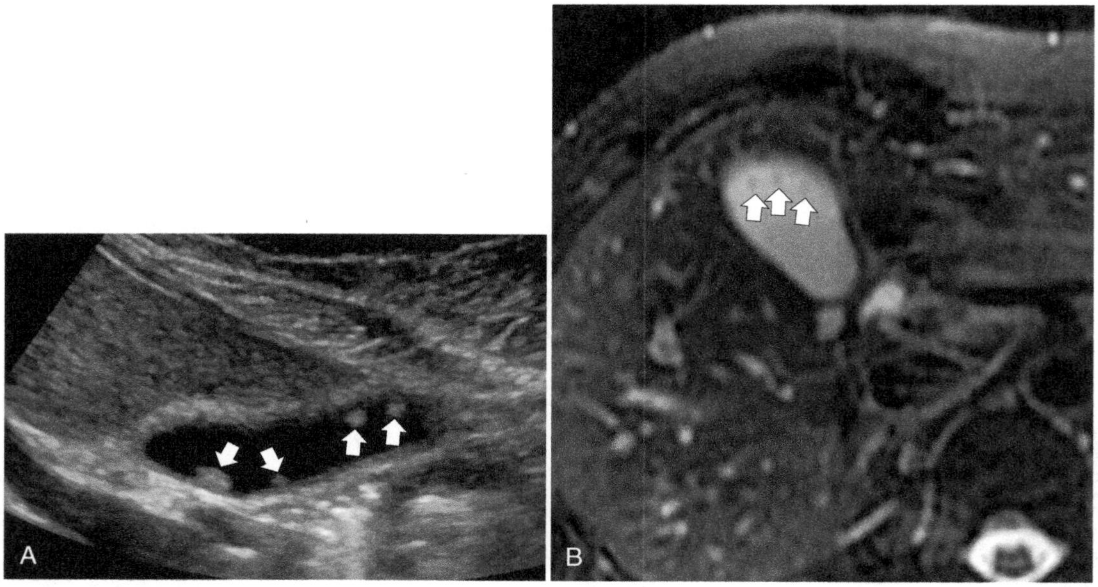

FIGURE 8-62. Sagittal US (**A**) and axial T2-weighted fat-saturated MRI (**B**) in a 49-year-old woman with several gallbladder polyps (*arrows*).

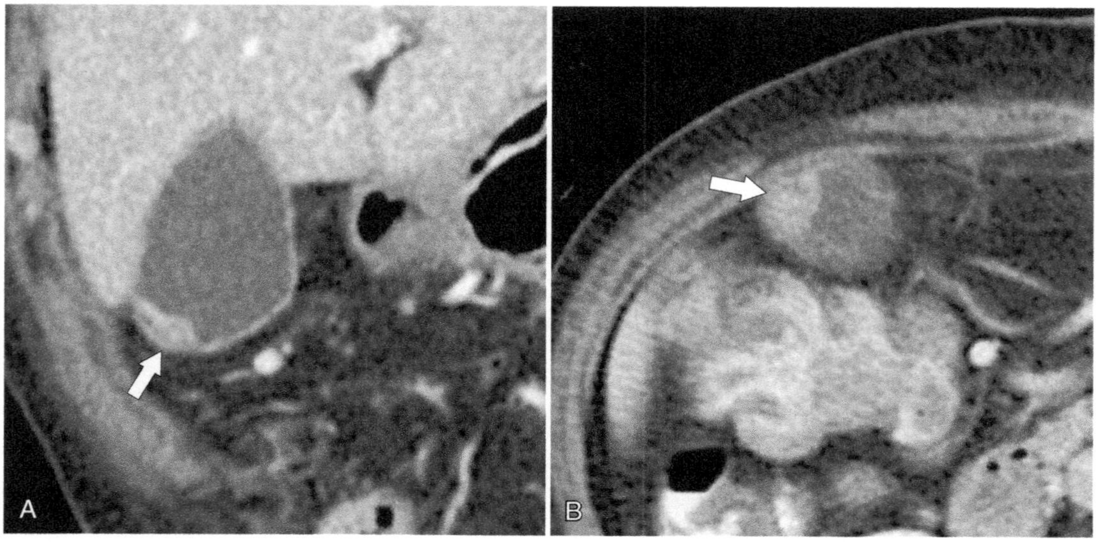

FIGURE 8-63. Coronal (**A**) and axial (**B**) contrast-enhanced CT in a 56-year-old woman with a small fundal polypoid mass (*arrows*) that was early gallbladder carcinoma at cholecystectomy.

Cholangiocarcinoma

Cholangiocarcinomas are rare tumors with an increased incidence in patients with primary sclerosing cholangitis, oriental cholangiohepatitis, chronic liver disease (especially cirrhosis), Caroli syndrome and other choledochal cysts, Thorotrast exposure, and Lynch syndrome. Tumors occur with equal frequency intrahepatically and extraheptically. Those originating at the biliary confluence are known as Klatskin* tumors. Tumors may be exophytic with a larger eccentric mass, polypoid with a smaller intraluminal mass, or infiltrative along the length of the duct. They are almost always ductal adenocarcinomas and invade the periductal tissues with a desmoplastic reaction, and this fibrotic reaction can make it difficult to diagnose the underlying malignancy.

Patients usually present in their sixth and seventh decades with pain and jaundice. The imaging method of choice is ERCP, particularly because many lesions produce little mass effect and are missed by CT. Furthermore, ERCP provides the opportunity to relieve any strictures, at least temporarily. After ductal injection, an irregular stricture should be identified with proximal or upstream biliary dilatation (Fig. 8-65). There may be a small (2- to 5-mm) intraductal papillary mass or a relatively long stricture as seen in the infiltrating type. On contrast-enhanced CT there is usually biliary dilatation but the mass is often not identified, although occasionally the tumor can be observed as subtle ductal enhancement along the affected duct (Fig. 8-66). A small mass in the region of the biliary bifurcation with converging obstructing ducts leading into the mass is highly suggestive of the diagnosis. Larger masses are easier to identify (Fig. 8-67). The mass is generally hypodense on noncontrast CT but often demonstrates peripheral enhancement in the arterial phase that gradually enhances toward the center, which remains hyperdense on delayed imaging, a characteristic feature (Fig. 8-67). This is caused by fibrous desmoplastic tissue that retains the contrast material for variable lengths of time. Imaging with MRCP can provide useful information about the stricture location and intrahepatic duct dilatation (Fig. 8-68). On contrast-enhanced MRI the tumor enhances similarly to that on CT (Fig. 8-69), with peripheral arterial enhancement that is retained on delayed imaging.

*Gerald Klatskin (1911-1986), American internal medicine physician.

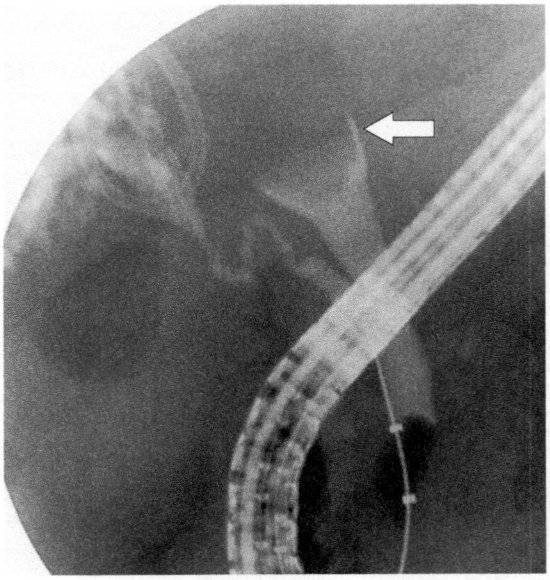

FIGURE 8-64. ERCP in a 56-year-old woman with a globular intraluminal CBD filling defect (*arrow*) caused by intraductal IPMN.

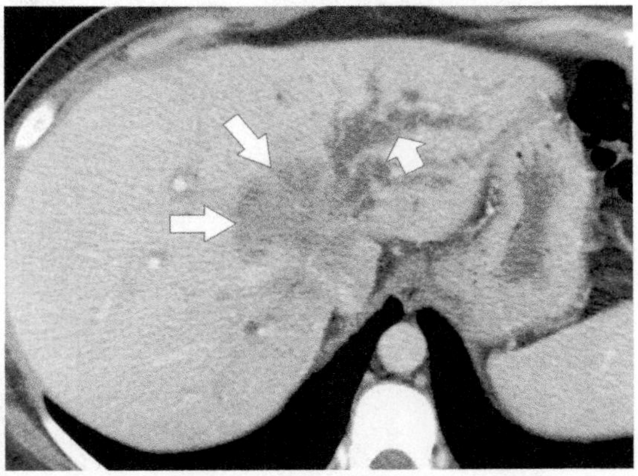

FIGURE 8-66. Axial contrast-enhanced CT in a 46-year-old man with a hilar cholangiocarcinoma (*long arrows*) that mainly obstructs the left-sided ducts (*short arrow*).

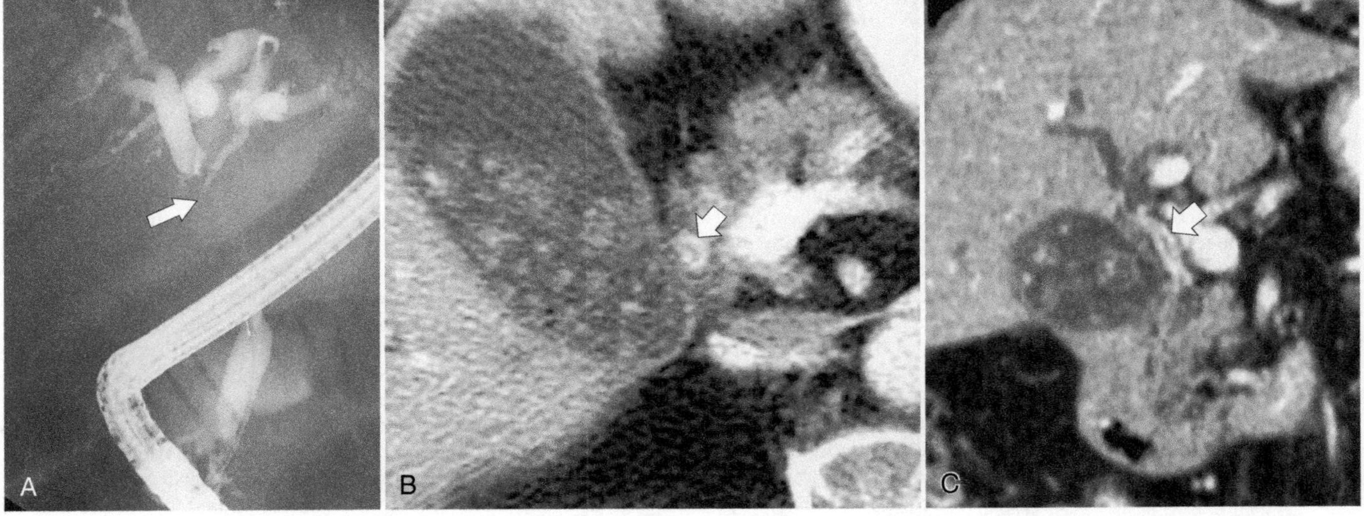

FIGURE 8-65. ERCP (**A**) and axial (**B**) and coronal (**C**) contrast-enhanced CT (**B** and **C**) in a 71-year-old man with a Klatskin tumor (*large arrow*) and intrahepatic duct dilatation. The tumor is just visible as an enhancing infiltrating mass along the length of the common hepatic duct (*small arrows*). Gallstones are present.

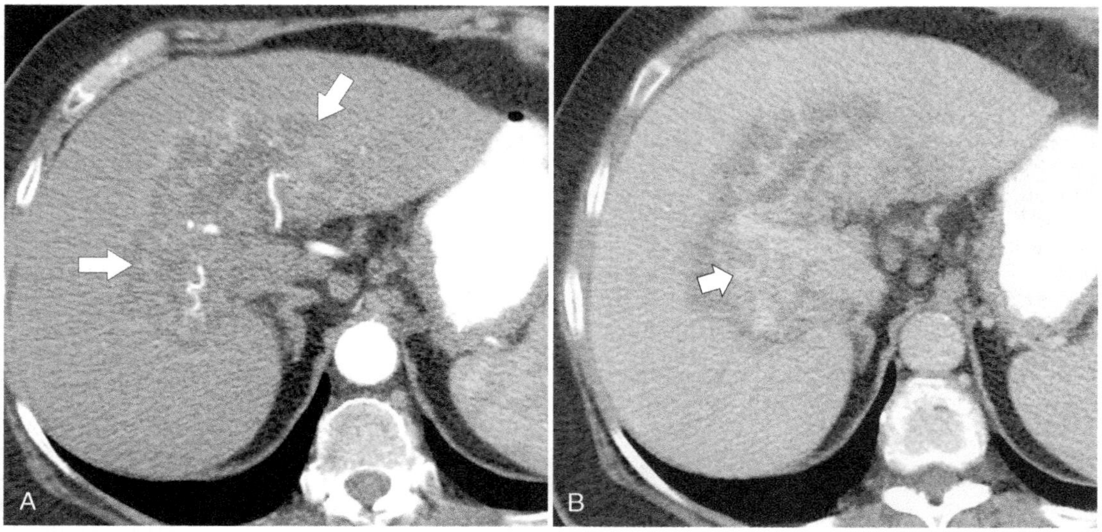

FIGURE 8-67. Axial arterial (**A**) and delayed (**B**) contrast-enhanced CT in a 77-year-old man with cholangiocarcinoma. A large hilar heterogeneous mass (*arrows*) demonstrates delayed enhancement (*short arrow*).

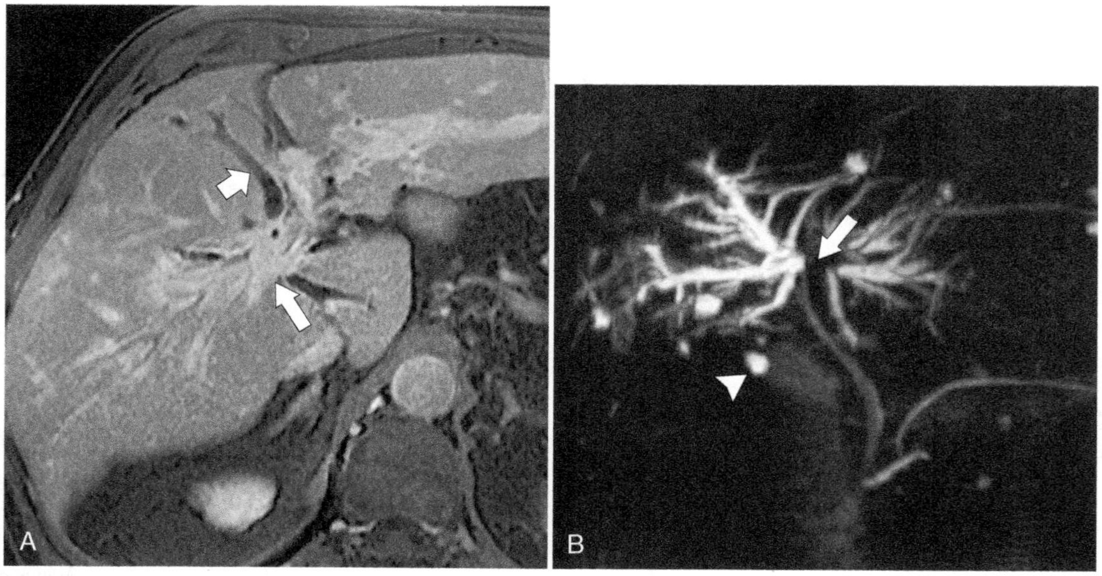

FIGURE 8-68. Axial postcontrast fat-saturated MRI (**A**) and MRCP (**B**) in a 63-year-old man with a Klatskin tumor (*arrows*) and dilated intrahepatic ducts (*small arrow*). There are several hepatic cysts (*arrowhead*).

Gallbladder Carcinoma

Gallbladder carcinoma (usually adenocarcinoma) is a rare malignancy. Patients present with pain, jaundice, and generalized symptoms of malignancy, particularly if it has metastasized, which it often has done by the time of presentation, primarily by local invasion of the liver. It has a strong association with gallstones, perhaps reflecting a chronic inflammatory contribution to development of neoplastic change. It is also recognized with increased frequency with porcelain gallbladder (Fig. 8-70) and is associated with gallbladder polyps, although this link is controversial.

Early in the course of disease a focal mass is confined to the gallbladder wall (Fig. 8-71), but at presentation the mass has often extended beyond the confines of the gallbladder, with an irregular soft-tissue mass infiltrating the liver and porta hepatis with or without associated adenopathy. The mass is usually hypovascular on contrast-enhanced CT and infiltrates the immediate region around the gallbladder fossa (Fig. 8-72).

Ampullary Carcinoma

Ampullary carcinoma is an adenocarcinoma arising from ductal epithelium in the region of the ampulla of Vater. The cause is unknown, but it is associated with polyposis and Gardner syndrome. The tumor is lobulated or infiltrating like other cholangiocarcinomas. Given its location, it leads to early bile and pancreatic duct dilatation ("double-duct" sign) and therefore mostly presents with jaundice. Its prognosis is also better than that of cholangiocarcinoma elsewhere, but the tumor may have metastasized to regional lymph nodes at the time of presentation. It is often not identified on cross-sectional imaging because of its small size but can appear hypodense on CT and similarly hypointense on contrast MRI. Evidence of an underlying mass is inferred from pancreatic and bile duct dilatation (Fig. 8-73). However, a dedicated contrast-enhanced CT using duodenal distention has a better chance than conventional CT of identifying the mass water (the patient drinks 500 mL immediately before imaging). Images are then reformatted into the coronal plane to

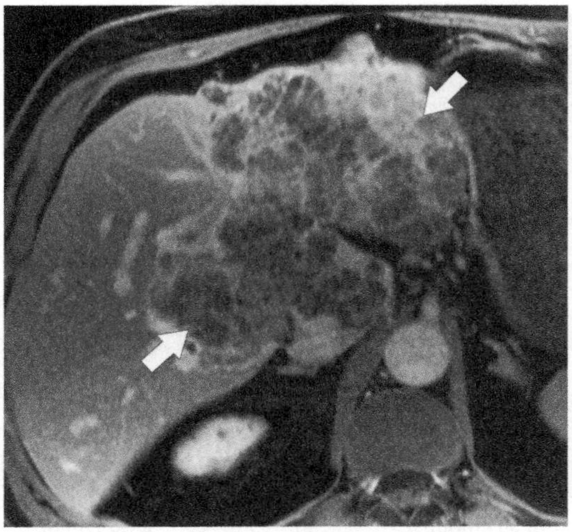

FIGURE 8-69. Axial postcontrast fat-saturated MRI in a 73-year-old woman with a large infiltrating heterogeneous cholangiocarcinoma (*arrows*).

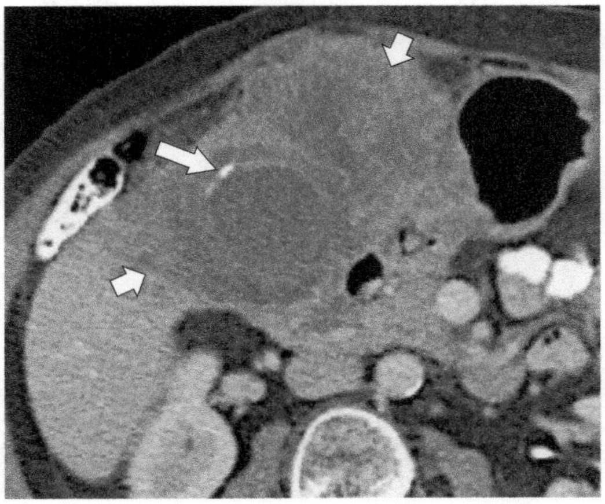

FIGURE 8-70. Contrast-enhanced CT in an 86-year-old woman with a partially calcified porcelain gallbladder (*large arrow*) and a large gallbladder carcinoma (*small arrows*).

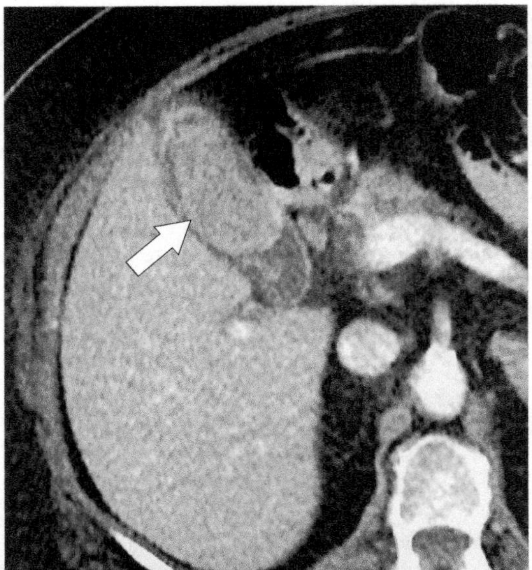

FIGURE 8-71. Axial contrast-enhanced CT in a 77-year-old man with a 4-cm gallbladder mass (*large arrow*) that represents a gallbladder carcinoma.

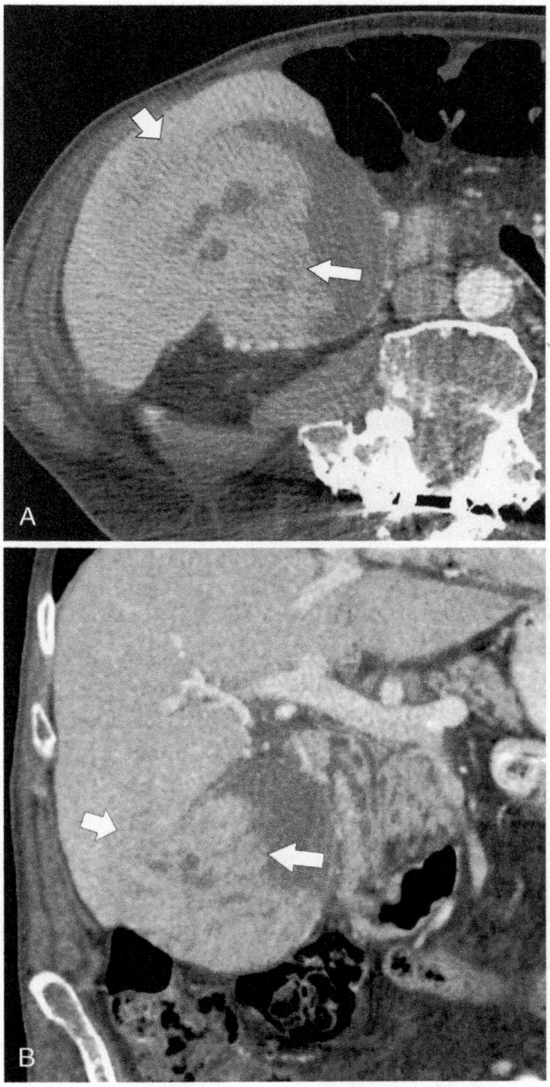

FIGURE 8-72. Axial (**A**) and coronal (**B**) contrast-enhanced CT in a 74-year-old man with gallbladder cholangiocarcinoma. A gallbladder-centered mass (*long arrows*) extends into segment VI of the liver (*short arrows*).

precisely define the location of the stricture and mass. In practice, once the patient presents with jaundice, ERCP is usually performed and directly visualizes a soft tissue mass at the ampulla.

Metastatic Disease

Gallbladder metastases are uncommon but are well recognized in melanoma (15% of patients with disseminated melanoma have gallbladder metastases). These patients can present with acute cholecystitis if an enlarging mass causes cystic duct obstruction. Other metastases are far less common and usually from lung cancer. The metastases are identified as an enhancing polypoid mass on contrast-enhanced CT or MRI. They also demonstrate increased color Doppler flow at US.

Common bile or hepatic duct obstruction occurs from either direct malignant extension or distant metastatic spread, usually lymphatic. Pancreatic head and uncinate adenocarcinomas often obstruct the pancreatic and CBD early, producing the "double-duct" sign (Fig. 8-74). Lymphatic metastatic disease is usually to lymph nodes at the porta hepatis, particularly from intestinal malignancies. Given the caliber of the bile duct at this point,

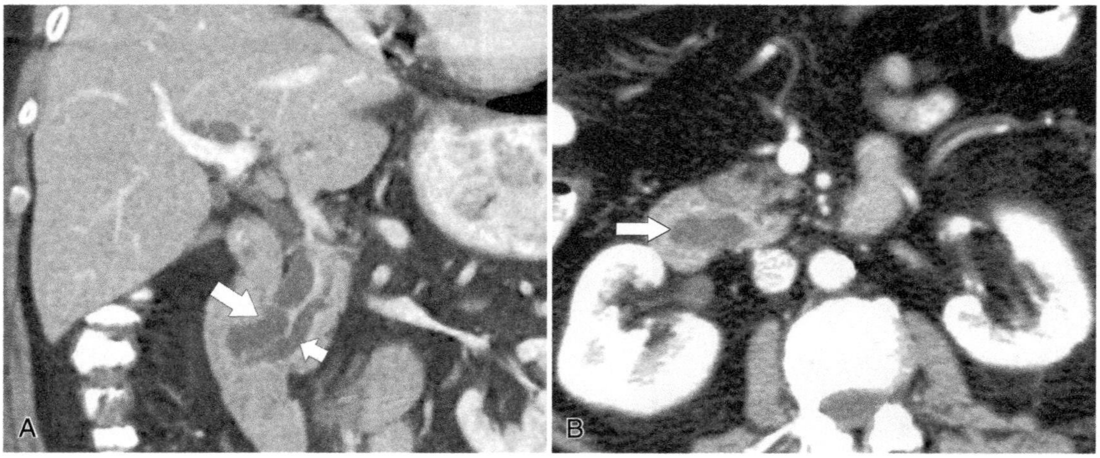

FIGURE 8-73. Coronal (A) and axial (B) contrast-enhanced CT in a 72-year-old woman with an ampullary tumor. The tumor cannot be visualized by CT but can be inferred from pancreatic (*small arrow*) and CBD dilatation (*large arrows*) proximal to the major papilla.

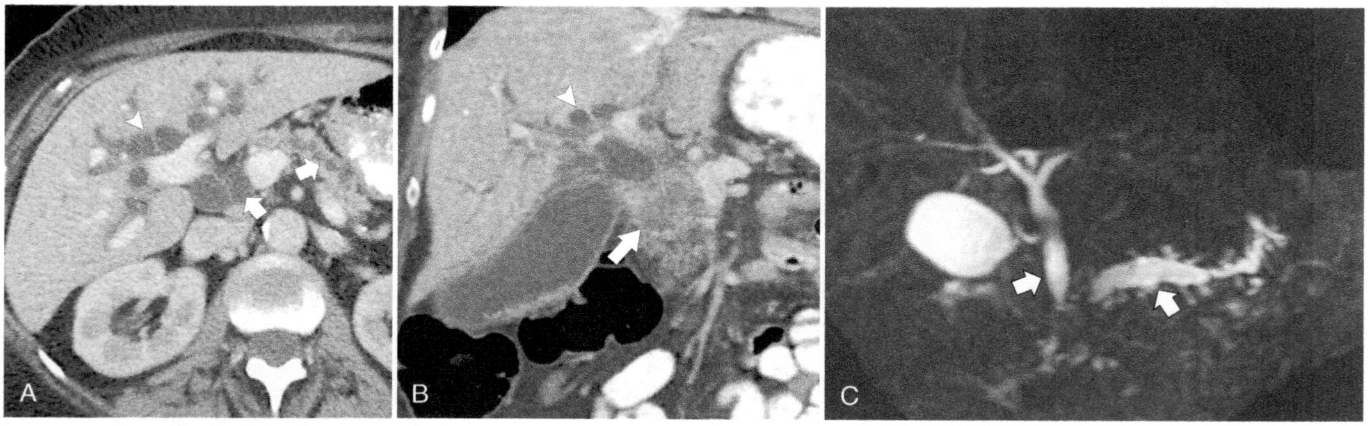

FIGURE 8-74. Axial (A) and coronal (B) contrast-enhanced CT and MRCP (C) in a 66-year-old woman with pancreatic adenocarcinoma (*large arrow*) obstructing both the pancreatic duct and the CBD (double-duct sign) (*small arrows*) that also results in intrahepatic duct dilatation (*arrowheads*).

even small nodes can impinge on and obstruct the duct. Because of their small size, they may not be identified with cross-sectional imaging but can be inferred from upstream biliary dilatation. They typically produce a smooth extrinsic tapering impression on the bile duct rather than the abrupt irregular strictures seen in cholangiocarcinoma (Fig. 8-75).

Gallbladder Lymphoma

Most lymphomatous biliary involvement is from metastatic spread from lymphoma elsewhere or as part of diffuse nodal disease throughout the abdomen. Primary gallbladder lymphoma is extremely rare and of the non-Hodgkin type. The gallbladder initially produces eccentric wall thickening, which develops into a larger, generally homogeneous mass. Before cholecystectomy is performed, it is generally not possible to distinguish lymphoma from other gallbladder malignancies, especially gallbladder adenocarcinoma.

AMPULLARY DYSFUNCTION

Ampullary dysfunction, also known as sphincter of Oddi dysfunction, is a difficult disease to diagnose and treat. It is seen in approximately 15% of patients after cholecystectomy, and patients report recurrent episodic abdominal pain. The cause is failure of the sphincter of Oddi to relax normally, causing temporary biliary dilatation until the spasm subsides. The diagnosis is usually one of exclusion, although it can be made using sphincter of Oddi manometry. MRCP performed at the time of sphincter spasm may show ductal distention (Fig. 8-76), but because the disease is transitory, the diagnosis may be missed. Further diagnostic steps involve challenging the sphincter after a fatty meal and imaging shortly afterward with US or preferably MRCP. A better noninvasive test is a secretin stimulation test (see Chapter 9). Injection of secretin causes excessive production of pancreatic exocrine digestive juices (primarily bicarbonate), which challenges the sphincter. This is best monitored by MCRP before and 1, 2, 5, and 10 minutes after secretin injection. The normal pancreatic and bile duct should demonstrate minimal ductal increase, which rapidly returns to normal. Sphincter dysfunction causes pancreatic and biliary sustained dilatation at the time of examination.

POSTOPERATIVE ANOMALIES

Intrahepatic Biliary Gas

Intrahepatic biliary gas is commonly observed after upper gastrointestinal surgery with choledochoenteric anastomoses. Intestinal gas (and sometimes fluid) passes into a patent bile duct and into intrahepatic ducts. This also commonly occurs after biliary sphincterotomy procedures. It can be differentiated from portal venous gas by being predominantly central and radiating from the hilum (Fig. 8-77). In contradistinction, portal venous gas is identified at the liver margins (Fig. 8-78). Far less commonly,

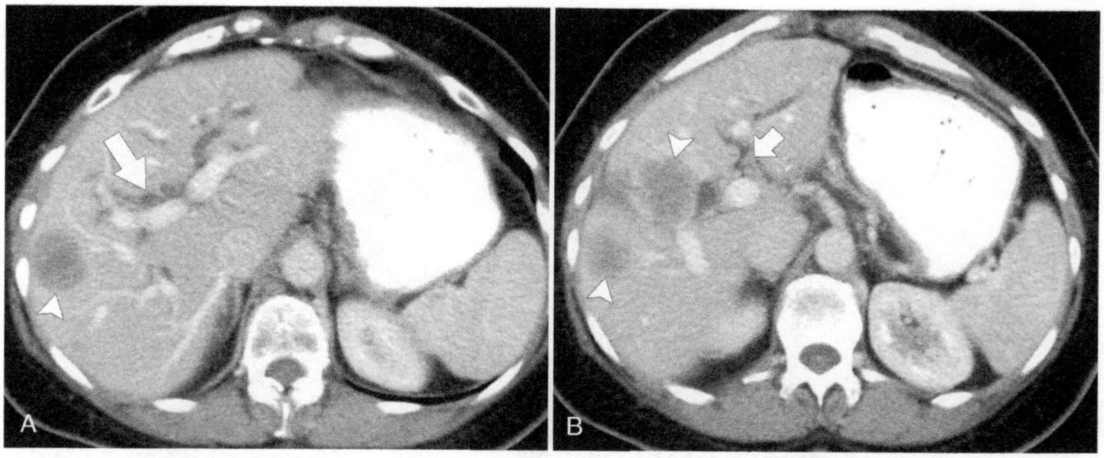

FIGURE 8-75. A and B, Contrast-enhanced CT in a 48-year-old woman with colon cancer and hepatic metastases (*arrowheads*). Biliary dilatation (*large arrow*) is due to small porta hepatic nodes (*small arrow* in B) obstructing the common hepatic duct.

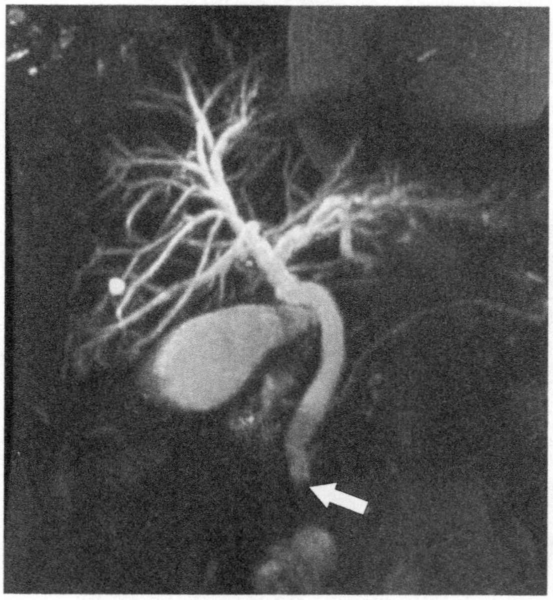

FIGURE 8-76. MRCP in a 74-year-old man. Dilatation of the CBD and intrahepatic ducts is due to ampullary stenosis (*arrow*).

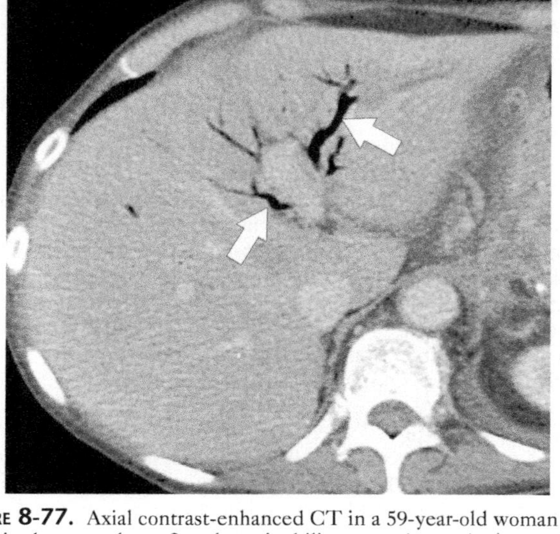

FIGURE 8-77. Axial contrast-enhanced CT in a 59-year-old woman after a Whipple procedure. Intrahepatic biliary gas (*arrows*) that radiates peripherally from the hepatic hilum is a normal finding.

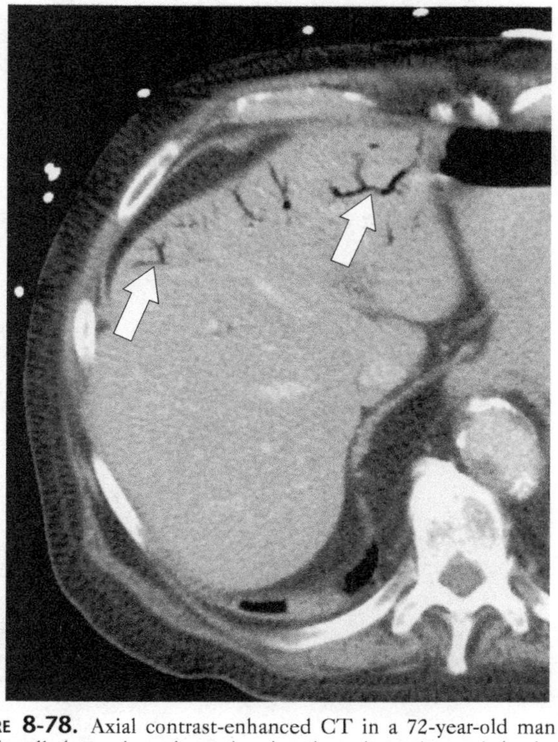

FIGURE 8-78. Axial contrast-enhanced CT in a 72-year-old man with peripherally located nondependent intrahepatic gas (*arrows*) that is portal venous in origin.

intrahepatic biliary gas is caused by gas-forming organisms, usually secondary to ascending cholangitis. The patient will almost certainly show signs of overwhelming sepsis.

Biloma

Bile leakage, either intrahepatically or extrahepatically, accumulates in loculated collections known as bilomas, with an attenuation on noncontrast CT similar to bile and therefore hypodense, close to water density. Leakage is usually iatrogenic from biliary surgery (cholecystectomy), percutaneous biopsy or catheter placement, perforation during ERCP, or radiation biliary necrosis after radiation treatment for cholangiocarcinoma (Fig. 8-79). Bilomas are also common after rupture from blunt or penetrating trauma. They usually are easily recognized on US, CT, and MRI as fluid-filled collections arising from the affected biliary structure (Fig. 8-80). Sometimes the cause of perihepatic fluid

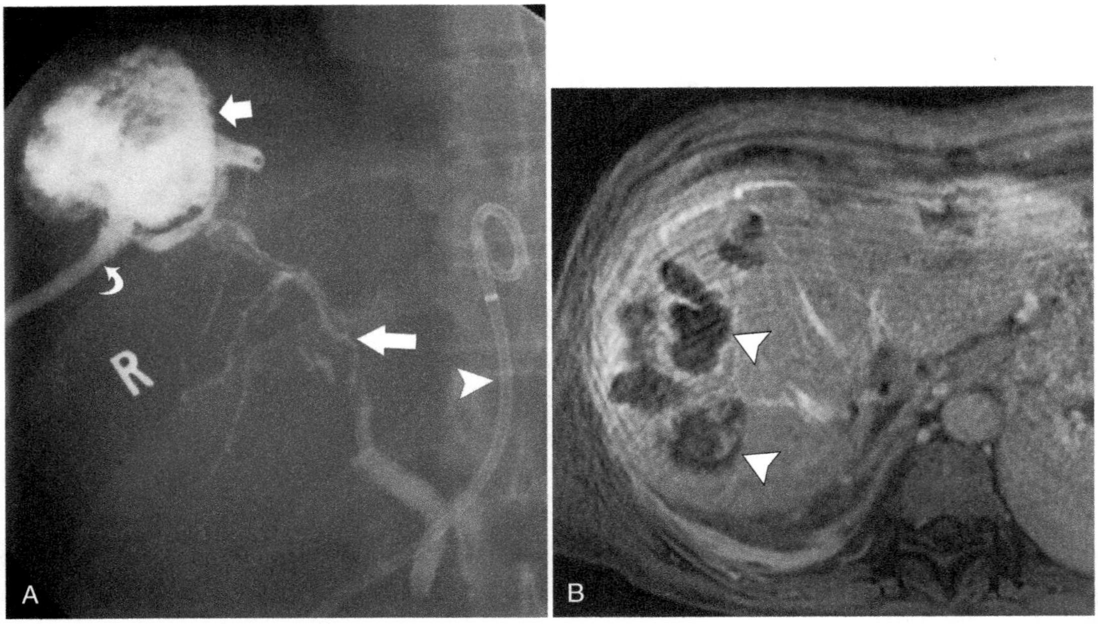

FIGURE 8-79. ERCP (**A**) and contrast-enhanced MRI (**B**) in a 57-year-old man with irregular intrahepatic ducts (*large arrow*) and a large biloma (*small arrow*) that drains externally via a biliary cutaneous fistula induced by previous percutaneous catheter drainage (*curved arrow*). There is a biliary drain in situ (*arrowhead*). Several other bilomas are also identified at MRI (*arrowheads*).

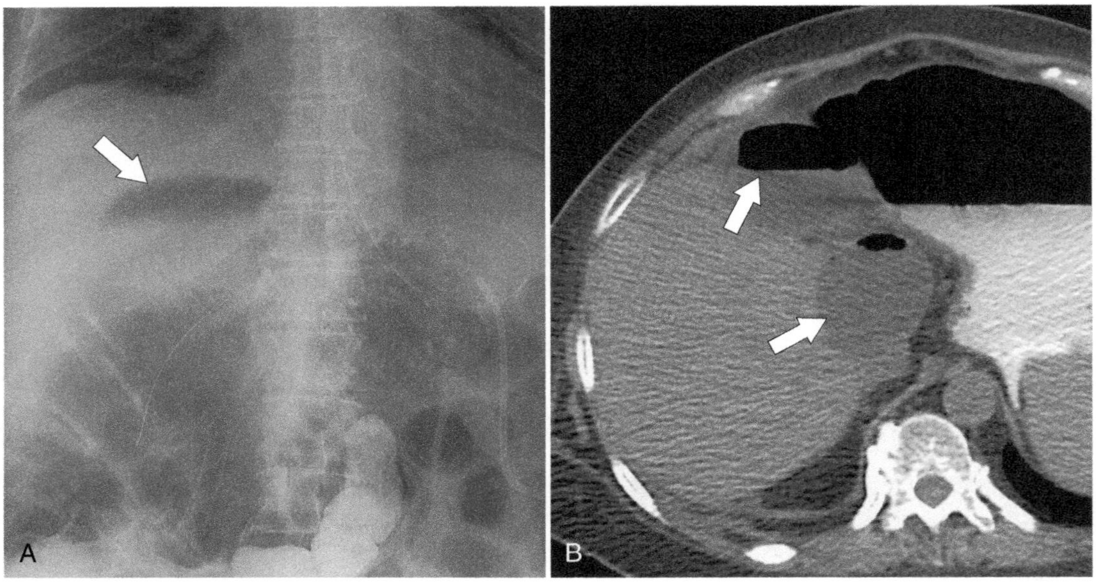

FIGURE 8-80. Plain abdominal radiograph (**A**) and axial noncontrast CT (**B**) in a 70-year-old man with a partially gas-filled biloma (*arrows*) as a result of a leak from recent biliary surgery.

collections is unclear, and imaging ^{99m}Tc HIDA can confirm the biliary nature of the fluid (Fig. 8-81). Leakage into the peritoneum causes severe peritonitis. Treatment is usually by percutaneous catheter drainage.

Biliary Traumatic Complications

Most biliary trauma is iatrogenic from bile duct or gallbladder surgery (open or laparoscopic and especially from liver transplantation), percutaneous catheter placement (Fig. 8-82) and biopsy, or complications from ERCP. Bile ducts can also become ischemic and undergo necrosis from radiation treatment, chemoembolization (TACE), or injury to the hepatic artery from hepatobiliary surgery (Fig. 8-79). Other injuries result from complete or partial rupture from blunt or penetrating trauma. These injuries may cause bile leakage (biloma), fistula (biliary-enteric fistula), and stricture formation, usually as a result of ischemia and healing fibrosis, or occasionally because of occlusion from inadvertent surgical suturing. Treatment for most complications is usually by temporizing biliary drainage and, if necessary, balloon dilatation or surgical repair of the offending stricture or defect. Cross-sectional imaging or nuclear scintigraphy may reveal evidence of biloma. Biliary strictures are best evaluated with ERCP but also may sometimes be observed on CT. Hemobilia, the presence of bloody bile, is usually caused by vascular injury, most commonly iatrogenic (e.g., percutaneous biliary catheter drainage that extravasates into the biliary tree). It is usually self-limiting but may require selective arterial catheterization and embolization if severe.

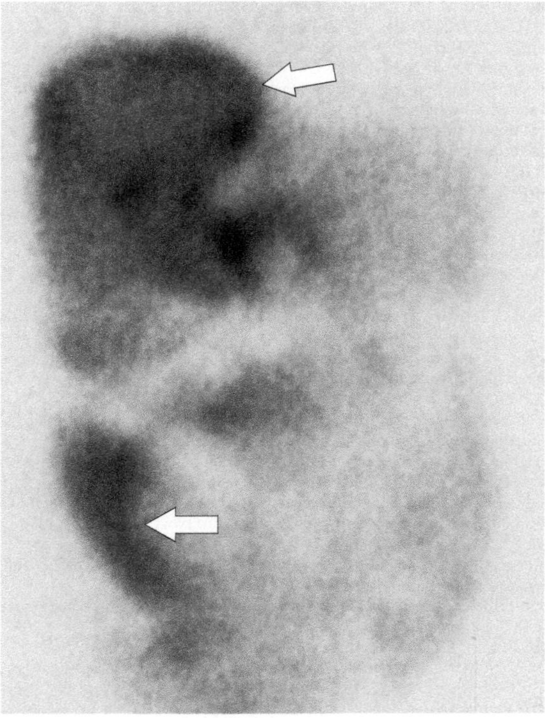

FIGURE 8-81. Technetium 99m HIDA imaging in a 67-year-old with fever and perihepatic and peritoneal fluid confirmed as biliary in origin (*arrows*).

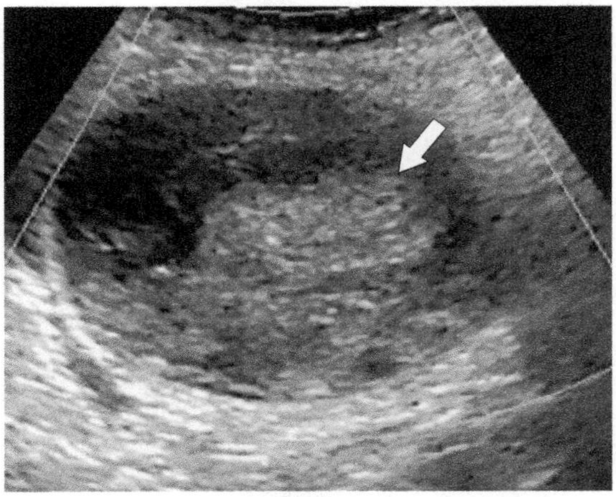

FIGURE 8-82. Transverse US in a 55-year-old man with recent percutaneous gallbladder placement. Irregular hyperechoic intraluminal mass (*arrow*) is due to gallbladder hemorrhage.

SUGGESTED READINGS

Ahualli J: The double duct sign. Radiology 244(1):314-315, 2007.
Altun E et al: Acute cholecystitis: MR findings and differentiation from chronic cholecystitis. Radiology 244(1):174-183, 2007; doi: 10.1148/radiol.2441060920.
Anderson SW et al: Accuracy of MDCT in the diagnosis of choledocholithiasis. AJR 187(1):174-180, 2006.
Anderson SW et al: Detection of biliary duct narrowing and choledocholithiasis: accuracy of portal venous phase multidetector CT. Radiology 247(2):418-427, 2008.
Arai K et al: Dynamic CT of acute cholangitis: early inhomogeneous enhancement of the liver. AJR 181(1):115-118, 2003.
Bader TR et al: MR imaging features of primary sclerosing cholangitis: patterns of cirrhosis in relationship to clinical severity of disease. Radiology 226(3):675-685, 2003.
Bennett GL et al: CT findings in acute gangrenous cholecystitis. AJR 178:275-281, 2002.
Bennett GL et al: Ultrasound and CT evaluation of emergent gallbladder pathology. Radiol Clin North Am 41(6):1203-1216, 2003.
Berk RN et al: Carcinoma in the porcelain gallbladder. Radiology 106:29-31, 1973.
Bilgin M et al: Hepatobiliary and pancreatic MRI and MRCP findings in patients with HIV infection. AJR 191(1):228-232, 2008.
Brancatelli G et al: Fibropolycystic liver disease: CT and MR imaging findings. Radiographics 25(3):659-670, 2005.
Bucceri AM et al: Common bile duct caliber following cholecystectomy: two-year sonographic survey. Abdom Imaging 19:251-258, 1994.
Catalano O et al: Complications of biliary and gastrointestinal stents: MDCT of the cancer patient. AJR 199:W187-W196, 2012; doi: 10.2214/AJR.11.7145.
Catalano OA et al: MR imaging of the gallbladder: a pictorial essay. Radiographics 28(1):135-155, 2008. quiz 324.
Chan WC et al: Gallstone detection at CT in vitro: effect of peak voltage setting. Radiology 241(2):546-553, 2006.
Chan YL et al: Choledocholithiasis: comparison of MR cholangiography and endoscopic retrograde cholangiography. Radiology 200:85-91, 1996.
Chavhan GB et al: Pediatric MR cholangiopancreatography: principles, techniques, and clinical applications. Radiographics 28(7):1951-1962, 2008.
Chen RC et al: Value of ultrasound measurement of gallbladder wall thickness in predicting laparoscopic operability prior to cholecystectomy. Clin Radiol 50: 570-578, 1995.
Choi E et al: Duplication of the extrahepatic bile duct with anomalous union of the pancreaticobiliary ductal system revealed by MR cholangiopancreatography. Br J Radiol 80(955):e150-154, 2007.
Choi JY et al: Hilar cholangiocarcinoma: role of preoperative imaging with sonography, MDCT, MRI, and direct cholangiography. AJR 191(5):1448-1457, 2008.
Chung YE et al: Varying appearances of cholangiocarcinoma: radiologic-pathologic correlation. Radiographics 29(3):683-700, 2009; doi: 10.1148/rg.293085729.
Corwin MT et al: Incidentally detected gallbladder polyps: is follow-up necessary? Long-term clinical and US analysis of 346 patients. Radiology 258(1):277-282, 2011; Published online August 9, 2010, doi: 10.1148/radiol.10100273.
Darge K et al: MR imaging of the abdomen and pelvis in infants, children, and adolescents. Radiology 261(1):12-29, 2011; doi: 10.1148/radiol.11101922.
Dave M et al: Primary sclerosing cholangitis: meta-analysis of diagnostic performance of MR cholangiopancreatography. Radiology 256:387-396, 2010.
Dohke M et al: Anomalies and anatomic variants of the biliary tree revealed by MR cholangiopancreatography. AJR 173(5):1251-1254, 1999.
Elsayes KM et al: Gastrointestinal manifestation of diabetes mellitus: spectrum of imaging findings. J Comput Assist Tomogr 33(1):86-89, 2009.
Fuks D et al: Acute cholecystitis: preoperative CT can help the surgeon consider conversion from laparoscopic to open cholecystectomy. Radiology 263(1):128-138, 2012; Published online February 13, 2012, doi: 10.1148/radiol.12110460.
Furlan A et al: Gallbladder carcinoma update: multimodality imaging evaluation, staging, and treatment options. AJR 191(5):1440-1447, 2008.
Ginat D et al: Incidence of cholangitis and sepsis associated with percutaneous transhepatic biliary drain cholangiography and exchange: a comparison between liver transplant and native liver patients. AJR 196:W73-W77, 2011; doi: 10.2214/AJR.09.3925.
Grand D et al: CT of the gallbladder: spectrum of disease. AJR 183:163-170, 2003.
Gupta RT et al: Dynamic MR imaging of the biliary system using hepatocyte-specific contrast agents. AJR 195:405-413, 2010; doi: 10.2214/AJR.09.3641.
Haller JO: Sonography of the biliary tract in infants and children. AJR 157: 1051-1058, 1991.
Han JK et al: Cholangiocarcinoma: pictorial essay of CT and cholangiographic findings. Radiographics 22(1):173-187, 2002.
Hashimoto M et al: Evaluation of biliary abnormalities with 64-channel multidetector CT. Radiographics 28(1):119-134, 2008; doi: 10.1148/rg.281075058.
Heffernan EJ et al: Recurrent pyogenic cholangitis: from imaging to intervention. AJR 192(1):W28-35, 2009.
Hoeffel C et al: Normal and pathologic features of the postoperative biliary tract at 3D MR cholangiopancreatography and MR imaging. Radiographics 26(6): 1603-1620, 2006; doi: 10.1148/rg.266055730.
Jutras JA: Hyperplastic cholecystoses. AJR 83:795-827, 1960.
Kiewiet JJS et al: A systematic review and meta-analysis of diagnostic performance of imaging in acute cholecystitis. Radiology, July 12, 2012; Published online. doi: 10.1148/radiol.12111561.
Kim JH et al: MR cholangiography in symptomatic gallstones: diagnostic accuracy according to clinical risk group. Radiology 224(2):410-416, 2002; Published online May 17, 2002, doi: 10.1148/radiol.2241011223.
Kim JH et al: CT findings of cholangiocarcinoma associated with recurrent pyogenic cholangitis. AJR 187:1571-1577, 2006; doi: 10.2214/AJR.05.0486.
Kim JY et al: Differentiation between biliary cystic neoplasms and simple cysts of the liver: accuracy of CT. AJR 195:1142-1148, 2010; doi: 10.2214/AJR.09.4026.
Kim JY et al: Spectrum of biliary and nonbiliary complications after lapatoscopic cholecystectomy: radiologic findings. AJR 191(3):783-789, 2008.
Kim OH et al: Imaging of the choledochal cyst. Radiographics 15:69-88, 1995.
Kim SJ et al: Peripheral mass–forming cholangiocarcinoma in cirrhotic liver. AJR 189:1428-1434, 2007; doi: 10.2214/AJR.07.2484.
Knowlton JQ et al: Imaging of biliary tract inflammation: an update. AJR 190(4):984-992, 2008.
Kumar A et al: Carcinoma of the gallbladder: CT findings in 50 patients. Abdom Imaging 19:304-310, 1994.
Lee WJ et al: Radiologic spectrum of cholangiocarcinoma: emphasis on unusual manifestations and differential diagnoses. Radiographics 21:S97-S116, 2001. Spec No.
Levy AD et al: Caroli's disease: radiologic spectrum with pathologic correlation. AJR 179(4):1053-1057, 2002.

Lim JH: Cholangiocarcinoma: morphologic classification according to growth pattern and imaging findings. AJR 181:819-827, 2003.
Lim JH et al: Intraductal papillary mucinous tumor of the bile ducts. Radiographics 24(1):53-66, 2004. discussion 66-67.
Lim JH et al: Parasitic diseases of the biliary tract. AJR 188(6):1596-1603, 2007.
Lim JH et al: Biliary parasitic diseases including clonorchiasis, opisthorchiasis and fascioliasis. Abdom Imaging 33(2):157-165, 2008.
Lim JH et al: Intraductal papillary mucinous tumors of the bile ducts. Radiographics 24:53-67, 2004.
Malet PF et al: Gallstone composition in relation to buoyancy at oral cholecystography. Radiology 177:167-169, 1990.
Mall JC et al: Caroli's disease associated with congenital hepatic fibrosis and renal tubular ectasia. Gastroenterology 66:1029-1035, 1974.
Martel JP et al: Melanoma of the gallbladder. Radiographics 29(1):291-296, 2009.
Menias CO et al: Mimics of cholangiocarcinoma: spectrum of disease. Radiographics 28(4):1115-1129, 2008; doi: 10.1148/rg.284075148.
Miller FH et al: Contrast-enhanced helical CT of choledocholithiasis. AJR 181:125-130, 2002.
Miller WJ et al: Imaging findings in Caroli's disease. AJR 165:333-340, 1995.
Mortelé KJ et al: Multimodality imaging of pancreatic and biliary congenital anomalies. Radiographics 26(3):715-731, 2006; doi: 10.1148/rg.263055164.
O'Connor OJ et al: Imaging of cholecystitis. AJR 196:W367-W374, 2011; doi: 10.2214/AJR.10.4340.
O'Connor OJ et al: Structured review: imaging of biliary tract disease. AJR 197:W551-W558, 2011; doi: 10.2214/AJR.10.4341.
Patel HT et al: MR cholangiopancreatography at 3.0 T. Radiographics 29:6, 2009; doi: 10.1148/rg.296095505. 1689-1706.
Reinhold C et al: MR cholangiopancreatography: potential clinical applications. Radiographics 16:309-331, 1996.
Rizzo RJ et al: Congenital abnormalities of the pancreas and biliary tree in adults, Radiographics 15:49-68, 1995.
Rybicki FJ: The WES sign. Radiology 214(3):881-882, 2000.
Sainani NI: Cholangiocarcinoma: current and novel imaging techniques. Radiographics 28(5):1263-1287, 2008.
Santiago I et al: Congenital cystic lesions of the biliary tree. AJR 198:825-835, 2012; doi: 10.2214/AJR.11.7294.
Savader SJ et al: Choledochal cysts: classification and cholangiographic appearance. AJR 156:327-331, 1991.
Schuster DM et al: Magnetic resonance cholangiography. Abdom Imaging 20: 353-361, 1995.
Shakespear JS et al: CT findings of acute cholecystitis and its complications. AJR 194:1523-1529, 2010; doi: 10.2214/AJR.09.3640.
Shanbhogue AKP et al: Benign biliary strictures: a current comprehensive clinical and imaging review. AJR 197:W295-W306, 2011; doi: 10.2214/AJR.10.6002.
Shanmugam V et al: Is magnetic resonance cholangiopancreatography the new gold standard in biliary imaging? Br J Radiol 78(934):888-893, 2005.
Sheng R et al: Cholangiographic features of biliary strictures after liver transplantation for primary sclerosing cholangitis: evidence of recurrent disease. AJR 166:1109-1116, 1996.
Shin SM et al: Biliary abnormalities associated with portal biliopathy: evaluation on MR cholangiography. AJR 188:W341-W347, 2007; doi: 10.2214/AJR.05.1649.
Silva AC et al: MR cholangiopancreatography: improved distention with intervenous morphine administration. Radiographics 24:677-687, 2004.
Silverthorn K: Sonographic follow-up of patients with gallbladder polyps. AJR 177:467, 2001.
Smith EA et al: Cross-sectional imaging of acute and chronic gallbladder inflammatory disease. AJR 192(1):188-196, 2009.
Sugita R et al: Periampullary tumors: high-spatial-resolution MR imaging and histopathologic findings in ampullary region specimens. Radiology 231(3):767-774, 2004.
Taourel P et al: Anatomic variants of the biliary tree: diagnosis with MR cholangiopancreatography. Radiology 199:521-527, 1996.
Valls C et al: Biliary complications after liver transplantation: diagnosis with MR cholangiopancreatography. AJR 184:812-820, 2005.
Vermani N et al: MR cholangiopancreatographic demonstration of biliary tract abnormalities in AIDS cholangiopathy: report of two cases. Clin Radiol 64(3): 335-338, 2009.
Ward J et al: Bile duct strictures after heptobiliary surgery: assessment with MR cholangiography. Radiology 231:101-108, 2004.
Weltman DI, Zeman RK: Acute diseases of the gallbladder and biliary ducts. Radiol Clin North Am 32:933-954, 1994.
Wiot JF, Felson B: Gas in the portal venous system. AJR 86:920-929, 1961.
Yeh BM et al: MR imaging and CT of the biliary tract. Radiographics 29:6, 2009; doi: 10.1148/rg.296095514. 1669-1688.
Yu J et al: Congenital anomalies and normal variants of the pancreaticobiliary tract and the pancreas in adults: part 1, biliary tract. AJR 187(6):1536-1543, 2006.
Yun EJ et al: Gallbladder carcinoma and chronic cholecystitis: differentiation with two-phase spiral CT. Abdom Imaging 29(1):102-108, 2003.

CHAPTER 9

Pancreas

The pancreas is an obliquely positioned retroperitoneal organ containing a tail, body, neck, head, and uncinate. It has a main duct (normal measurements, 2 to 3 mm in diameter) running the length of the pancreas from the tail proximally to the ampulla of Vater* distally. It has both endocrine and exocrine functions. As an endocrine organ, islets of Langerhans† within the pancreas secrete insulin, somatostatin, and glucagon. Exocrine function produces digestive enzymes necessary for food digestion. The size of the pancreas and the proportion of parenchymal fat vary considerably from one person to another, although it usually atrophies or undergoes a degree of fatty replacement in older patients.

Imaging of the pancreas typically requires contrast-enhanced computed tomography (CT), because although ultrasound (US) can be useful for detection of some pancreatic disease, the pancreas is often partially obscured by intraabdominal fat, depending on body habitus and intestinal gas. Magnetic resonance imaging (MRI) is indicated in specific instances, including allergy to iodinated contrast material, the detection of some hypervascular diseases, generation of three-dimensional ductal anatomical images, and evaluation of small cystic disease.

The development of multidetector thin-slice CT combined with arterial- or pancreatic-phase imaging offers the opportunity to increase detection and better characterize pancreatic disease, particularly adenocarcinoma. Some pancreatic diseases (e.g., neuroendocrine tumors) are highly vascular and preferentially enhance during the arterial phase (typically 20 to 25 seconds after administration of intravenous [IV] contrast medium) and sometimes only during this phase. Many small neuroendocrine tumors can be missed, even with optimized arterial-phase contrast-enhanced techniques, and as with image interpretation, close attention to a dedicated protocol is required so as not to miss subtle, small, usually hyperfunctioning neuroendocrine tumors. Conversely, most pancreatic adenocarcinomas enhance poorly, and their detection and delineation are best observed during pancreatic-phase imaging (typically 40 to 45 seconds after administration of IV contrast material), when the contrast between normal-enhancing pancreatic parenchyma and nonenhancing pancreatic adenocarcinoma is maximized (i.e., increased tumor conspicuity). Small adenocarcinomas, however, are notoriously difficult to detect by all imaging methods, except perhaps endoscopic or intraoperative US, and therefore pancreatic-phase CT may offer the only noninvasive hope of detecting tumors less than 2 cm. Furthermore, critical vascular structures (celiac axis, portal vein, and superior mesenteric artery and vein) that may be invaded or occluded by tumor are best evaluated during this phase, both because they are optimally enhanced at that time and because tumor conspicuity in relation to the pancreas and these vessels is maximized. During the portal venous phase (60 to 70 seconds after initiation of IV contrast administration), the normal pancreatic parenchyma may be less enhanced and the pancreatic tumor may have absorbed some IV contrast material, reducing the tumor conspicuity. Portal venous–phase imaging is performed predominantly to evaluate for distant metastases (liver, lung, and abdominal lymphadenopathy). Portal venous–phase imaging is also used in the evaluation of pancreatitis and other benign diseases.

Multiplanar image reconstructions add considerable value to the evaluation of pancreatic carcinoma. They can offer the surgeon and radiologist a better perspective of vascular tumor invasion or encasement, knowledge of which is necessary to stage the disease and decide on curative treatments.

*Abraham Vater (1684-1751), German anatomist.
†Paul Langerhans (1847-1888), German pathologist.

Because of the excellent contrast characteristics of T2-weighted imaging, pancreatic duct anomalies (either main duct or side branch) are best imaged noninvasively with magnetic resonance cholangiopancreatography (MRCP), although greater anatomical detail will require endoscopic retrograde cholangiopancreatography (ERCP) and, in some circumstances, therapeutic intervention (i.e., pancreatic stent).

CONGENITAL ANOMALIES

A brief understanding of pancreatic embryology is necessary to understand congenital pancreatic anomalies. The pancreas is formed by fusion of the ventral and dorsal buds of the embryonic foregut. The ventral bud is originally two buds that fuse early and form to the right of the developing duodenum, while the dorsal bud lies to the left (Fig. 9-1). The midgut (which includes the duodenum) then rotates clockwise, and the ventral bud rotates along with it and fuses with the dorsal pancreatic bud from behind. The fused pancreas now lies completely to the left of the duodenum. The dorsal duct (duct of Santorini*) from the original dorsal bud now drains the tail, body, and upper head and for a while drains into the minor papilla. The ventral duct (from the original ventral bud), also known as duct of Wirsung,† drains the lower head and uncinate into the major papilla along with the common bile duct. Normally, the ventral and proximal dorsal ducts fuse to form the main pancreatic duct, which drains into the major papilla (papilla of Vater). The remaining distal remnant of the dorsal duct usually regresses and drains into the accessory duct of Santorini.

Annular Pancreas

Annular pancreas is a rare anomaly resulting from abnormal or failed rotation of the ventral bud and/or rotation of the duodenum embryologically (Fig. 9-2) such that the bud fails to achieve its position to the left of the duodenum and instead forms a partial or complete ring of pancreatic tissue around the second part of the duodenum. It can also result when the bifid ventral ducts encircle the duodenum rather than fuse together. Many patients are asymptomatic, but annular pancreas can present early in childhood because it is commonly associated with other congenital atretic anomalies, including those of the esophagus, duodenum, and anus. Furthermore, the resulting ring can cause duodenal strictures, which if severe can be recognized in the neonate because of copious vomiting from duodenal obstruction, often requiring surgery to remove the stricture. Presentation in adults is usually after repeated episodes of epigastric pain, early satiety, and vomiting from subacute duodenal obstruction.

The diagnosis was formerly made with an upper gastrointestinal (GI) series, in which the second part of the duodenum appears strictured to a variable degree depending on the degree of the anomaly and associated with loss of the normal duodenal fold pattern (Fig. 9-3). Depending on the degree of stricture formation, the proximal duodenum may be distended or dilated. However, annular pancreas is now detected primarily by CT because of its increased use. The CT findings are characteristic of pancreatic tissue passing to the right and encircling the second part of the duodenum, which is sometimes better visualized on multiplanar imaging (Fig. 9-4). The diagnosis can also be made with ERCP that shows the ventral duct (Wirsung) completely encircling the

*Giovanni Domenico Santorini (1681-1737), Italian anatomist.
†Johann Georg Wirsung (1600-1643), German physician.

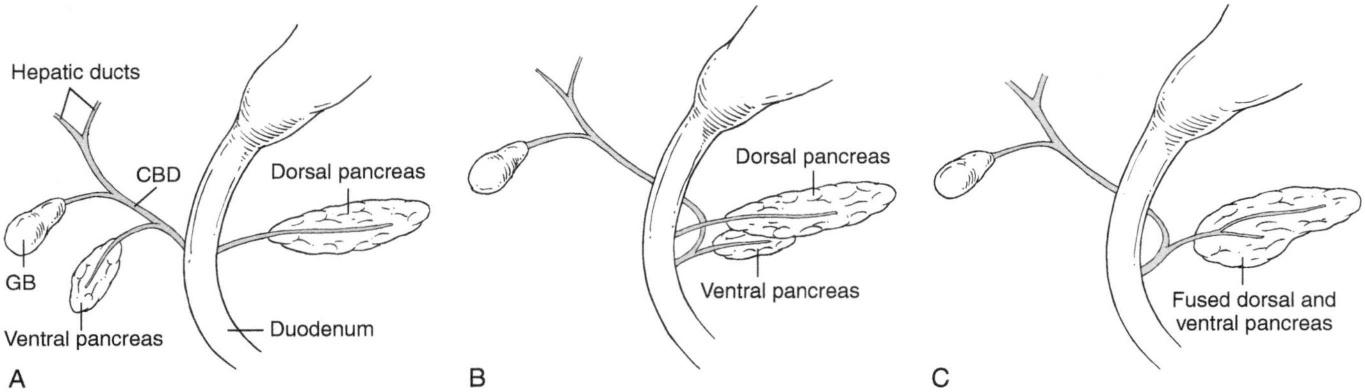

FIGURE 9-1. Schematic representation of embryological development of the pancreas. The ventral and dorsal buds are originally separate (**A**). The ventral pancreas then rotates clockwise to fuse with the dorsal pancreas (**B** and **C**).

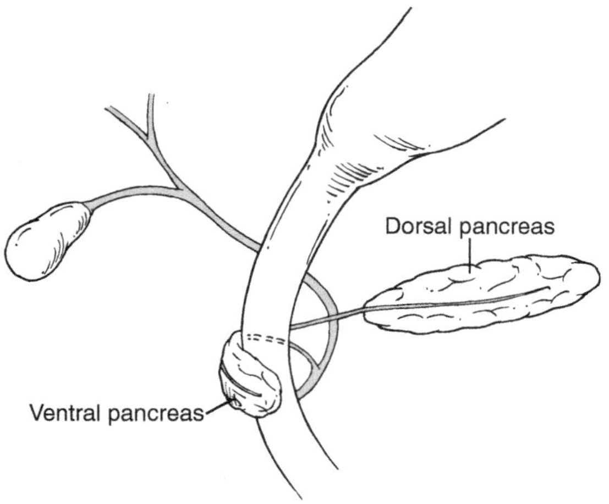

FIGURE 9-2. Schematic representation of an annular pancreas. The ventral pancreas rotates abnormally to variable degrees and either partially or whole envelops the second part of the duodenum.

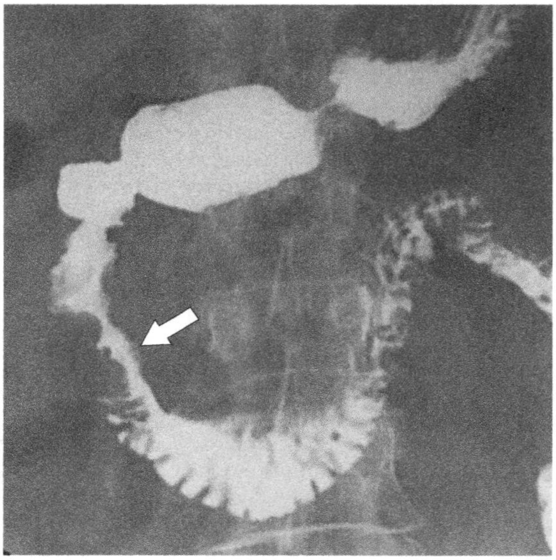

FIGURE 9-3. Upper GI series in a 44-year-old woman with narrowing of the second part of the duodenum (*arrow*) caused by an annular pancreas.

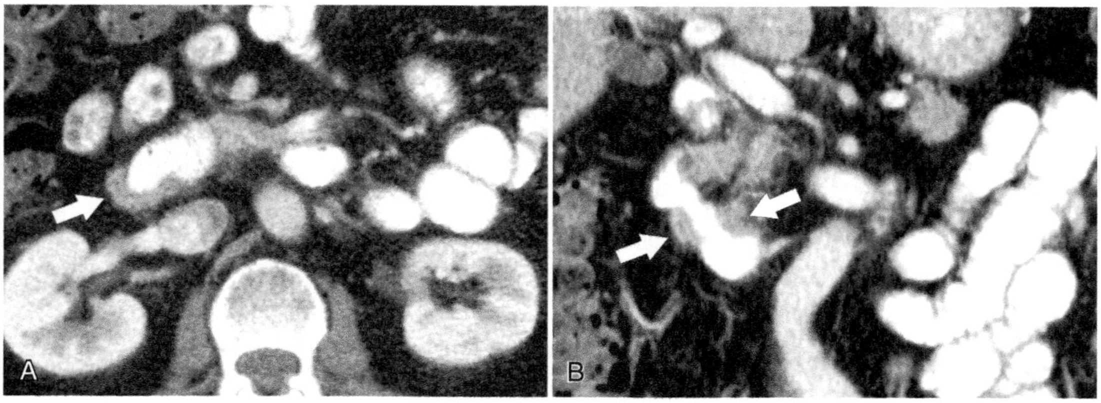

FIGURE 9-4. Axial (**A**) and coronal (**B**) CT in a 71-year-old man with an annular pancreas. A cuff of pancreatic tissue surrounds the second part of the duodenum (*arrows*).

duodenum. Annular pancreas is associated with an increased incidence of pancreatitis and peptic ulcer disease, both of which may be identified by CT.

Agenesis of the Dorsal Pancreas

Complete pancreatic agenesis, defined as absence of the neck, body, tail, duct of Santorini, and minor papilla, is extremely rare, particularly because many with this condition are stillborn or die of multiple other congenital anomalies as neonates. More commonly the agenesis is partial, with the neck, body, or tail missing (Figs. 9-5 and 9-6). Many patients are asymptomatic, but if present, symptoms include abdominal pain and an increased incidence of pancreatitis. Depending on the degree of agenesis, patients can also present with pancreatic insufficiency (diabetes mellitus and steatorrhea).

On imaging, pancreatic agenesis can be identified by a short pancreas, but the findings may be subtle. ERCP or MCRP, which will identify a ventral (Wirsung) duct but little or no accessory (Santorini) duct, confirms the diagnosis.

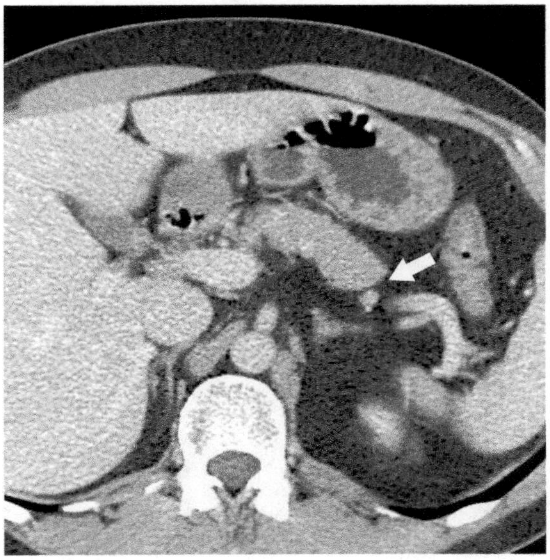

FIGURE 9-5. Axial contrast-enhanced CT in a 38-year-old woman with a congenitally short pancreas and missing tail (*arrow*).

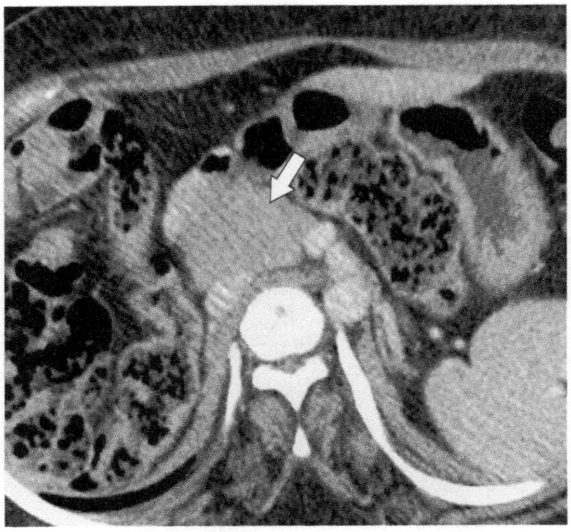

FIGURE 9-6. Axial contrast-enhanced CT in a 41-year-old woman with a pancreatic uncinate (*arrow*) but no body or tail because of partial agenesis.

Pancreas Divisum

Pancreas divisum is far more common than other pancreatic anomalies, with up to 10% of the population showing some variant, depending on the degree of ductal fusion anomalies. Essentially, despite normal rotation of the ventral bud, its duct (Wirsung) fails to fuse appropriately with the dorsal duct (Santorini), so a single pancreatic duct is not formed (Fig. 9-7). With complete lack of fusion, the dorsal duct now drains exclusively into the minor papilla, which remains patent, and the body and upper pancreatic head drain through the minor papilla. The ventral duct continues to drain into the major papilla, draining the uncinate and lower half of the pancreatic head.

Many patients are asymptomatic, but others have intermittent pain, which usually appears between 30 and 50 years of age and results from mild and occasionally severe pancreatitis, possibly because of the restricted drainage of the bulk of pancreatic fluid through the smaller minor papilla. Therefore pancreatitis, when present, is usually of the neck, body, and tail, although pancreatitis of the uncinate caused by reflux of bile into a short ventral duct can also occur.

The diagnosis of pancreas divisum can be challenging. At ERCP, injection of contrast material into the major papilla opacifies only the duct of Wirsung (Fig. 9-8). Ideally the minor papilla is also cannulated, but because of its small size, this sometimes fails. Should it prove successful, a long dorsal, noncommunicating duct is outlined. Imaging with MRCP, which demonstrates the anatomical anomaly in most patients noninvasively, may therefore be preferable (Fig. 9-9). Imaging with CT is less sensitive, and the anomaly is often missed unless the pancreatic ductal anatomy is closely scrutinized. The pancreatic head may be enlarged, and sometimes there is a subtle fatty cleft between the uncinate process and the remaining pancreas, but this is rarely observed and nonspecific. With thin-section and multiplanar imaging, the two distinct noncommunicating ducts can be observed (Fig. 9-10). Evidence of pancreatitis, a relatively common feature of pancreas divisum, may also be present (Fig. 9-10).

SECRETIN STIMULATION TEST

The secretin stimulation test is designed to determine any functional obstruction of the pancreatic duct. Secretin is a powerful hormonal stimulant for pancreatic bicarbonate production (required for duodenal neutralization of gastric acid). When injected, it causes a temporary increase in the production and therefore volume of pancreatic fluid, which should pass normally into the duodenum. Typically, in the healthy patient, after 0.4 μg/kg is injected, the duct dilates slightly (from a normal 1 to 3 mm to between 4 and 6 mm) but returns rapidly to normal. Conversely, the duct remains dilated for up to 30 minutes in the presence of a functional obstruction. Measurements are made using US or, more commonly, coronal MRCP (Fig. 9-11).

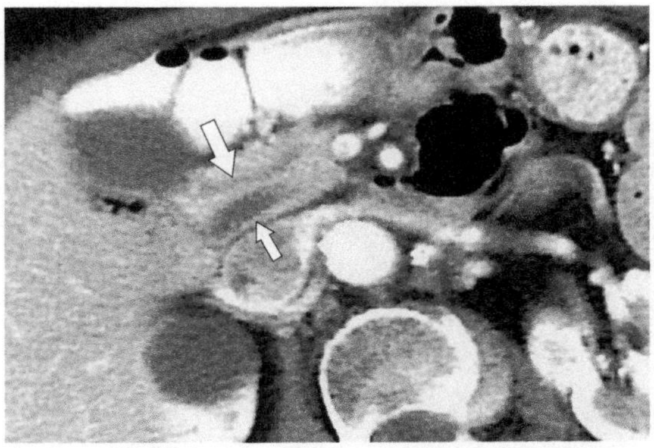

FIGURE 9-7. Axial and coronal contrast-enhanced CT in a 76-year-old man with pancreas divisum. The minor pancreatic duct (Santorini; *large arrow*) remains anterior to the bile duct and major pancreatic duct (Wirsung; *small arrow*).

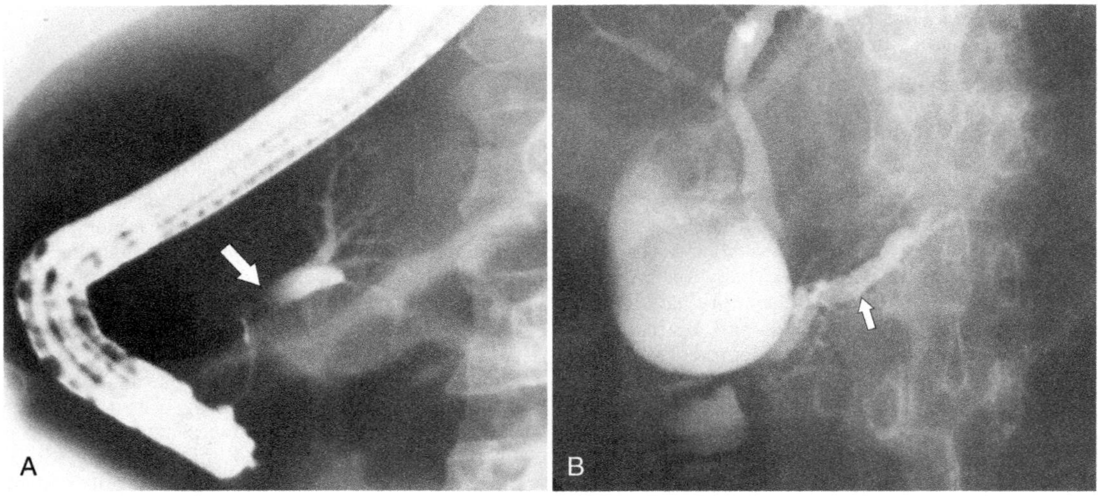

FIGURE 9-8. A and B, ERCP in a 53-year-old man with initial injection into the major duodenal papilla outlining only the duct of Wirsung (*arrow*). Subsequent cannulation of the minor papilla fills a dilated duct of Santorini (*small arrow*) owing to chronic pancreatitis resulting from pancreatic divisum. There are changes of chronic pancreatitis with a dilated irregular duct of Santorini.

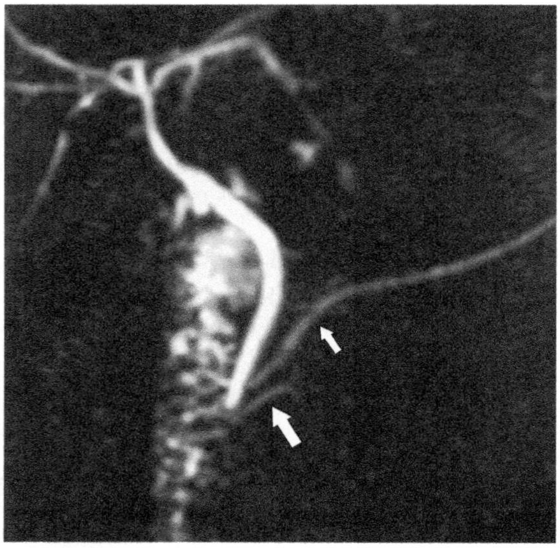

FIGURE 9-9. MRCP in a 43-year-old woman demonstrating drainage of the duct of Santorini (*small arrow*) via the minor papilla duct of Wirsung into the common bile duct and major papilla (*large arrow*).

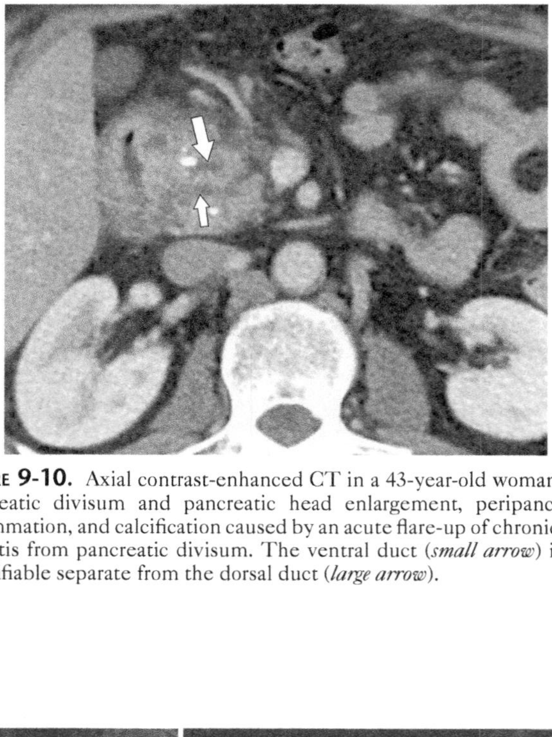

FIGURE 9-10. Axial contrast-enhanced CT in a 43-year-old woman with pancreatic divisum and pancreatic head enlargement, peripancreatic inflammation, and calcification caused by an acute flare-up of chronic pancreatitis from pancreatic divisum. The ventral duct (*small arrow*) is just identifiable separate from the dorsal duct (*large arrow*).

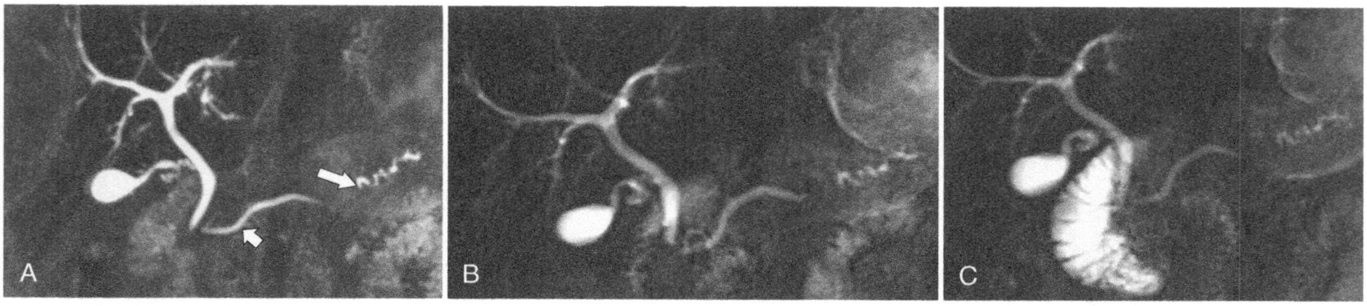

FIGURE 9-11. Secretin MRCP in a 63-year-old woman with papillary dysfunction. The pancreatic duct (*small arrow*) measured 3 mm at baseline (**A**), which increased to 5 mm at 5 minutes (**B**) and returned to 3 mm at 10 minutes (**C**). The distal duct is tortuous (*large arrow*) due to previous episodes of pancreatitis.

ECTOPIC PANCREAS

The true incidence of ectopic pancreas is unknown, but some figures put the incidence surprisingly at 10% of the population, although the condition is rarely seen in clinical practice. Ectopic pancreas is also known as pancreatic rest or aberrant pancreas. Small areas of pancreatic tissue come to "rest" in an ectopic position, usually in the distal gastric antrum along the greater curvature or near the pancreatic ampulla in the second portion of the duodenum. They can, however, be detected in more disparate locations, including other intestinal locations and even the pelvis, liver, and spleen.

Patients are usually asymptomatic, but ectopic pancreas can cause gastric or duodenal hemorrhage and, if large enough, biliary obstruction or even small bowel intussusception. Rests that are identified at imaging are usually in the expected location of the stomach or duodenum and found mostly with upper GI series because they are too small to be identified by cross-sectional imaging techniques (although they may be inferred from the presence of a small hypodense and cystic mass). The characteristic appearance is of a 1- to 2-cm submucosal mass, either round or eccentric in shape, sometimes lobular, with a central pit or depression that fills with contrast material in the dependent position.

FATTY PANCREATIC REPLACEMENT

Fatty pancreatic replacement can be a normal aging process as the pancreas becomes increasingly atrophic and fatty replaced (Fig. 9-12).

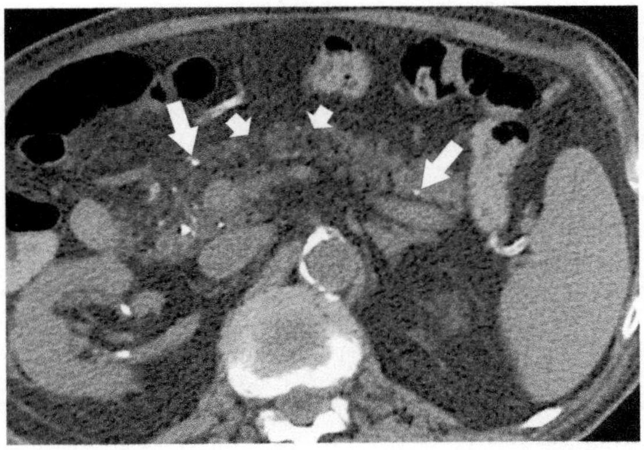

FIGURE 9-12. Axial noncontrast CT in a 79-year-old woman with an age-related atrophic fatty-replaced pancreas (*small arrows*) that has tiny punctate calcifications (*arrows*).

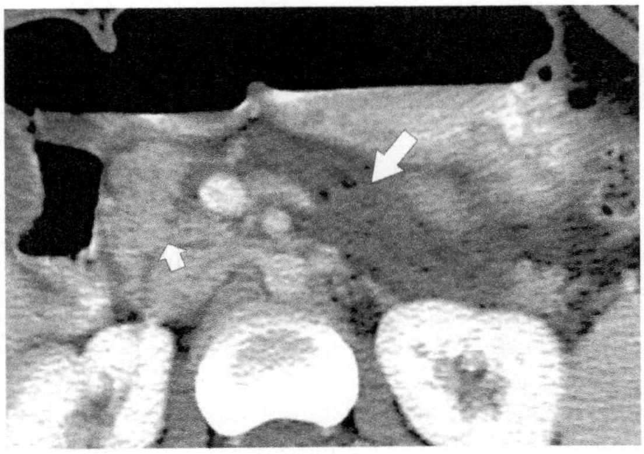

FIGURE 9-13. Axial contrast-enhanced CT in a 24-year-old woman with a partially fatty-replaced pancreas (*arrow*) resulting from cystic fibrosis. The pancreatic head and uncinate are normal (*small arrow*).

Cystic Fibrosis

Cystic fibrosis is an autosomal-recessive disease with a number of abdominal complications, including diffuse pancreatic insufficiency when severe. The pancreatic tissue becomes largely fatty replaced, sometimes with small cystic change. On US the fatty change is hyperechoic, but on CT the pancreas is partially replaced by fat (Fig. 9-13) or may not be seen at all, the fatty replacement merging into the surrounding retroperitoneal fat (Fig. 9-14). Other features may include small bowel dilatation and cecal thickening (see discussion in Chapters 4, on the small bowel, and 5, on the colon). The pancreas in cystic fibrosis can also become diffusely calcified or undergo cystosis (see later in the chapter).

Uneven Lipomatosis

Fatty pancreatic replacement can be either diffuse (Fig. 9-15) or focal, termed "uneven" (Fig. 9-16). It is of little clinical significance, except that it has been associated with pancreas divisum and can be confused with a pancreatic neoplasm. Fat-suppressed MRI can be helpful in distinguishing between the two.

Pancreatic Lipomatous Pseudohypertrophy

Pancreatic lipomatous pseudohypertrophy is of unknown but possibly congenital origin, causes pancreatic hypertrophy with

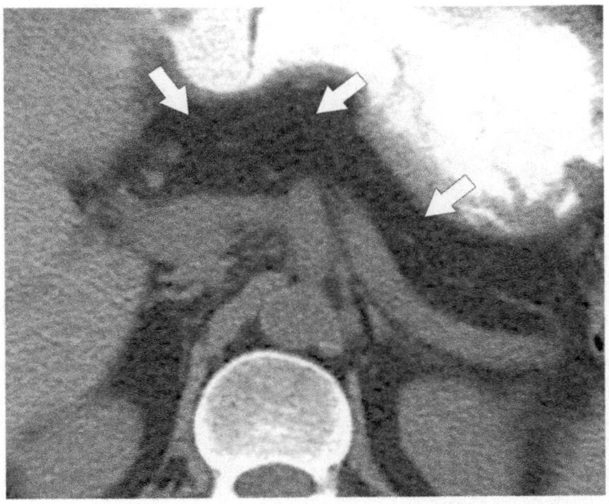

FIGURE 9-14. Axial noncontrast CT in a 39-year-old man with cystic fibrosis and complete pancreatic fatty replacement (*arrows*).

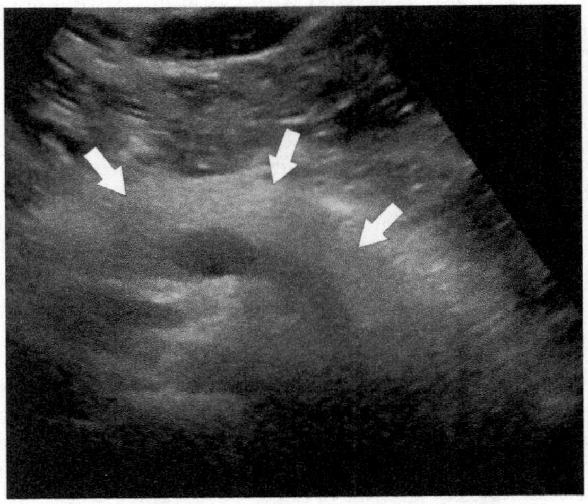

FIGURE 9-15. Transverse US of the pancreas in a 44-year-old woman with diffuse echogenicity (*arrows*) secondary to a fatty pancreas.

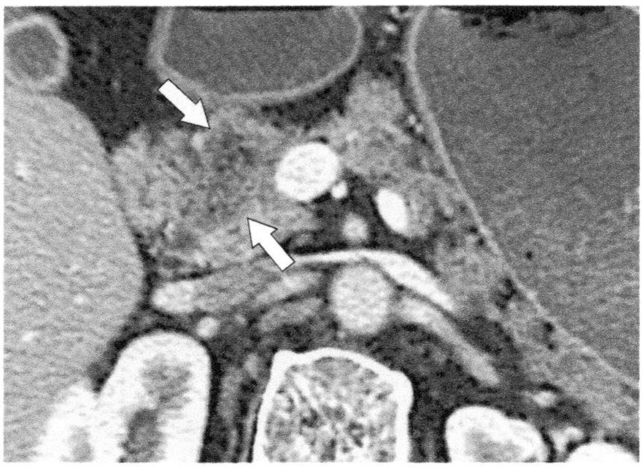

FIGURE 9-16. Axial contrast-enhanced CT in a 65-year-old man demonstrating a nondeforming hypodense anterior pancreatic head (*arrows*) consistent with uneven lipomatosis.

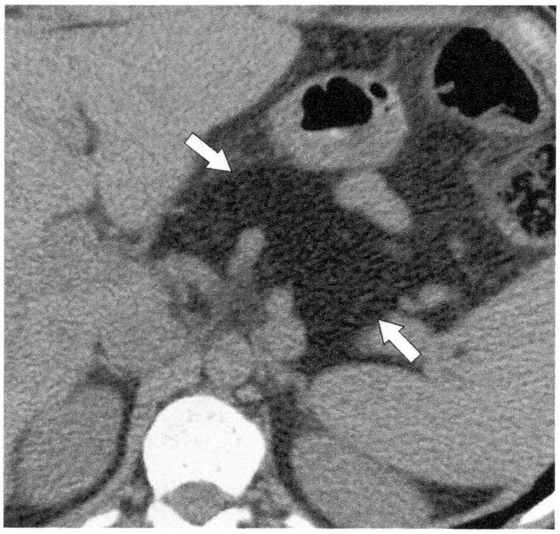

FIGURE 9-17. Axial noncontrast CT in a 28-year-old woman with cystic fibrosis and diffusely enlarged fatty pancreas (*arrows*) caused by pancreatic lipomatous pseudohypertrophy.

focal or diffuse fatty replacement, and is readily identified with CT or MRI (Fig. 9-17). It is, however, often associated with chronic liver disease (i.e., cirrhosis), which may therefore be contributory. It is also associated with cystic fibrosis but should be distinguished from diffuse pancreatic fatty replacement, which is also seen in cystic fibrosis but shows no pancreatic hypertrophy.

Pancreatic Lipoma

Lipomas are very rare in the pancreas, being much more common in the intestinal tract. In the pancreas, as elsewhere, lipomas are relatively straightforward to diagnose with CT because of their fat content, which is confined to the pancreas and is well circumscribed (Fig. 9-18).

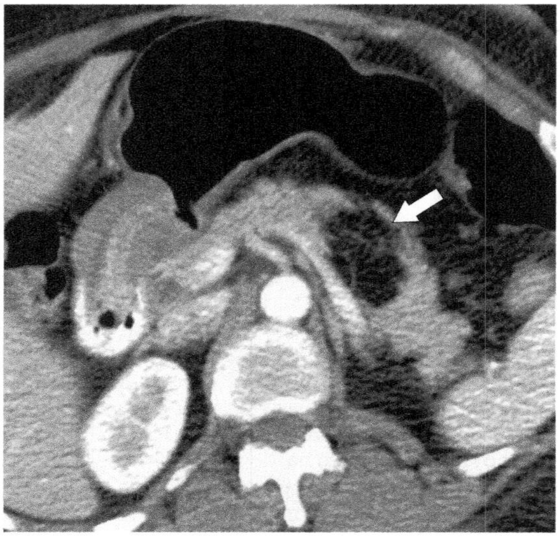

FIGURE 9-18. Axial contrast-enhanced CT in a 44-year-old woman with a 4-cm pancreatic hypodense fatty mass (*arrow*) that represents a pancreatic lipoma.

Box 9-1. Causes of Pancreatitis

Gallstones
Alcohol
Hyperparathyroidism
Hypercalcemia
Hypertriglyceridemia
Hypothermia
Pregnancy
Pancreas divisum
Viral infections: mumps
Pancreatic duct stones
Trauma
Postpump pancreatitis
Post-ERCP
Drugs: thiazide diuretics, sulfonamides, AIDS medication, valproic acid, azathioprine, statins
Hereditary pancreatitis (trypsinogen activation)
Porphyria

AIDS, Acquired immunodeficiency syndrome; *ERCP*, endoscopic retrograde cholangiopancreatography.

PANCREATITIS

Pancreatitis represents acute or chronic inflammation of the pancreas caused by release of pancreatic enzymes, mainly trypsin, into the pancreatic parenchyma rather than the duodenum. Pancreatitis has numerous precipitating factors (Box 9-1), but gallstones cause the majority of cases of acute pancreatitis, whereas alcohol is mainly responsible for chronic pancreatitis. The diagnosis is based on the clinical history, elevated serum amylase and lipase levels, and imaging. However, clinical symptoms and presentation vary widely and range from mild to severe. Patients with milder forms present with pain, vomiting, and abdominal tenderness, whereas those with severe forms present with shock, organ failure, and hemorrhage. The severe hemorrhagic clinical signs have been well recognized for more than a century. Grey Turner* sign is flank bruising, and Cullen† sign is periumbilical bruising, resulting from acute pancreatitis. Clinical severity is ranked by either Ranson or APACHE II criteria.

Many patients with pancreatitis have no imaging abnormalities. When pancreatitis is more severe, however, plain radiographs may demonstrate ileus, particularly a sentinel loop, representing a distended loop of small bowel immediately adjacent to the inflamed pancreas. A colon "cut-off" sign represents a distended transverse colon, with paucity of air from the splenic flexure distally because of colonic spasm (Fig. 9-19). Upper GI studies often demonstrate

*George Grey Turner (1877-1951), British surgeon.
†Thomas S. Cullen (1868-1953), Canadian-American gynecologist.

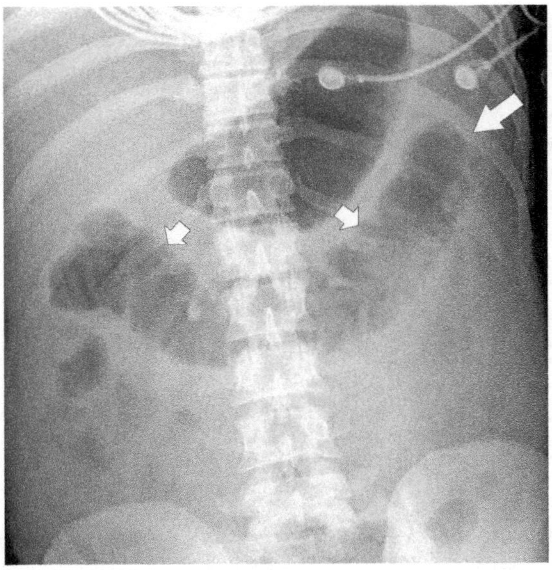

FIGURE 9-19. CT scout view in a 43-year-old man with distended transverse colon (*small arrows*) and a colon cut-off sign (*arrow*).

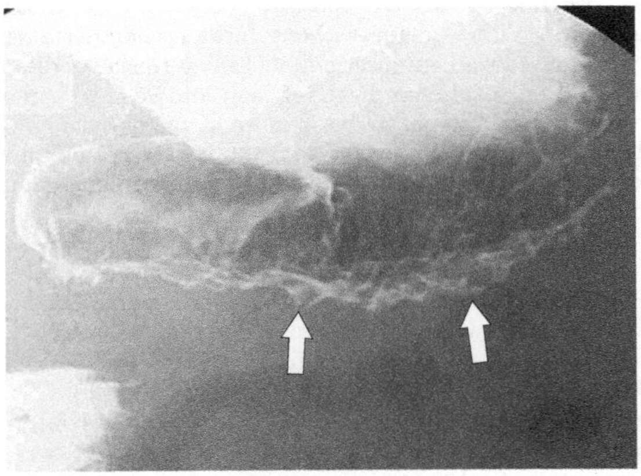

FIGURE 9-20. Upper GI series in a 66-year-old man with a "puckered" appearance to the greater curvature of the stomach (*arrows*) caused by inflammation from pancreatitis.

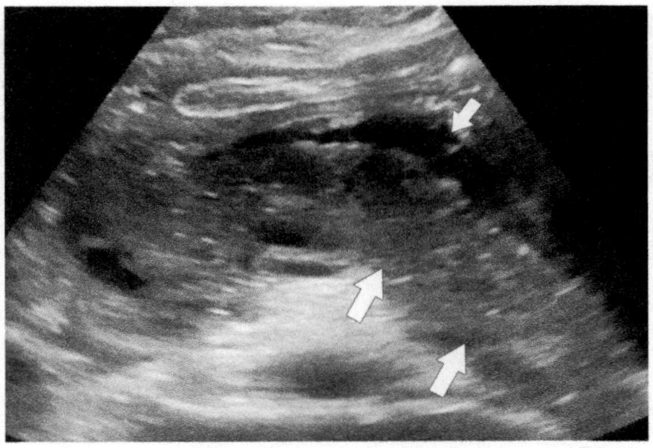

FIGURE 9-21. Transverse US in a 17-year-old male with acute pancreatitis, demonstrating an edematous, heterogeneously enlarged pancreas (*arrows*) with anterior peripancreatic fluid (*small arrow*).

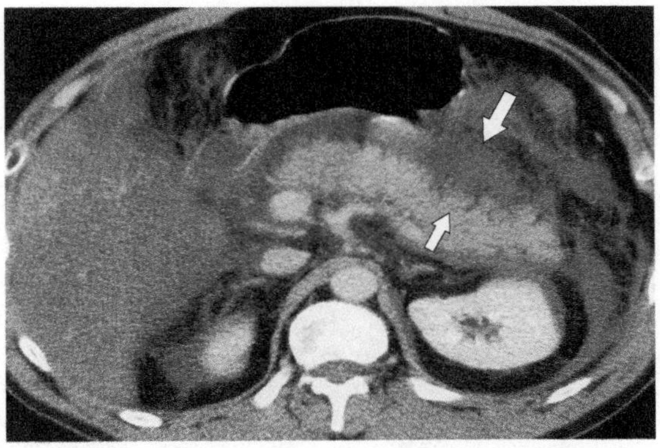

FIGURE 9-22. Axial contrast-enhanced CT in a 37-year-old man with hypertriglyceridemia-induced pancreatitis. The liver is markedly fatty, and pancreatic enlargement without necrosis (*small arrow*) and diffuse peripancreatic inflammation (*large arrow*) are present.

thickened and spiculated duodenal and gastric folds representing secondary edematous transmural enteric changes (Fig. 9-20). On US the pancreas can appear enlarged with a heterogeneous echo texture mixed with prominent hypoechoic regions (Fig. 9-21), although contrast-enhanced CT is usually performed to evaluate pancreatitis. Not all patients with clinical and biochemical pancreatitis have abnormal CT findings, although the majority of patients show abnormalities to a variable degree. The pancreas is typically enlarged, sometimes focally, with effacement of the normal indented pancreatic border combined with peripancreatic edematous changes (Fig. 9-22). The latter can be severe with widespread edema throughout the retroperitoneal space, producing single or multiple acute fluid collections (Fig. 9-23). Sometimes pancreatic adenocarcinoma has a similar appearance, and a useful CT sign is preservation of perivascular fat planes (unlike pancreatic adenocarcinoma, in which they are often obliterated), which strongly favors a benign diagnosis (Fig. 9-24). The reverse is not always true in that the peripancreatic inflammation in severe pancreatitis can sometimes obliterate this fat plane. Unless contraindicated, contrast-enhanced CT is administered to evaluate the vascular viability of the pancreatic parenchyma. Pancreatic necrosis is recognized by single or multiple focal hypodensities (or diffuse depending on the severity) surrounded by normally enhancing pancreas (Fig. 9-25). These hypodensities represent the hypovascularized or nonvascularized pancreatic parenchyma, which has been destroyed by the acute inflammatory process. Depending on the degree of pancreatic necrosis, it may be termed necrotizing pancreatitis if more than 50% of the gland is involved.

Documentation of pancreatic necrosis is critical because it places the patient in a much higher risk category than those with simple fluid collections. Necrotic areas can also become infected, which has an even higher mortality rate. Surgical debridement is the treatment of choice. Necrosis is usually associated with pancreatic and peripancreatic fluid collections (Figs. 9-23 through 9-25). There may be evidence of acute fluid collections in the retroperitoneum, which may also become infected and form an abscess. If contrast material is not administered, the pancreas is typically diffusely hypodense. MRI also demonstrates an enlarged gland with areas of necrosis that fail to enhance after IV administration of contrast medium. The terminology used in pancreatitis is defined in Table 9-1.

The severity of acute pancreatitis can be staged by contrast-enhanced CT (Table 9-2) and corresponds reasonably closely to the clinical course. When the percentage of gland necrosis is also included (0 to 30%, 30% to 50%, >50%), a CT severity index can be calculated, which corresponds even more closely to the clinical course (Table 9-3). However, the CT severity index does not always match the clinical course, and therefore its use in clinical practice is variable. The most important CT finding is pancreatic necrosis, which markedly increases morbidity and mortality rates associated with disease. Acute hemorrhagic pancreatitis is a particularly severe form of pancreatitis with, as its name suggests, hemorrhage within the pancreas (which might not be recognized

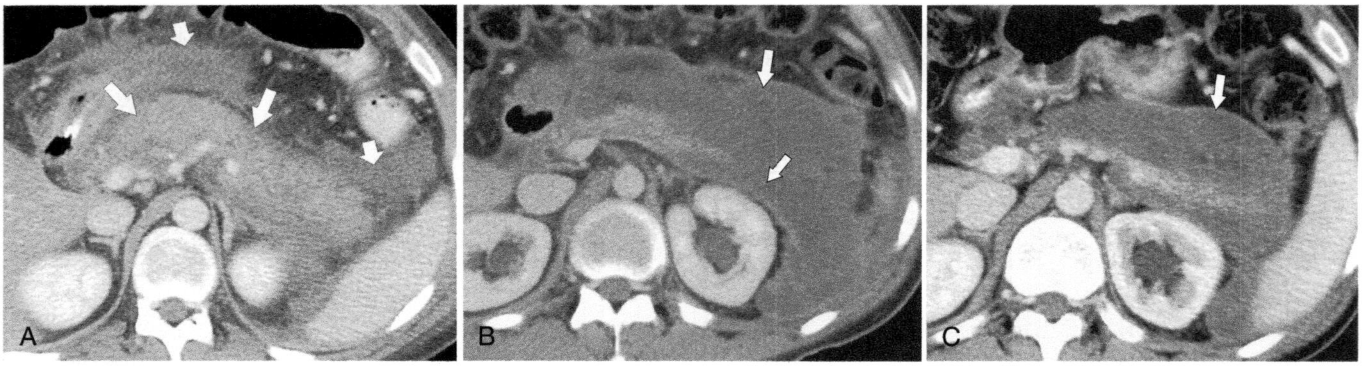

FIGURE 9-23. Axial contrast-enhanced CT in a 27-year-old man with acute pancreatitis demonstrating evolution of acute pancreatitis. **A,** Enlarged and inflamed pancreas (*arrows*) with diffuse peripancreatic inflammation (*small arrows*). **B,** Axial contrast-enhanced CT 1 month later demonstrating partial necrosis and partial loss of pancreatic tail (*small arrow*) and an organizing peripancreatic collection (*arrows*). **C,** Axial contrast-enhanced CT 2 months after **B,** demonstrating pancreatic body and tail of formation of a capsule (*arrow*) around the peripancreatic collection as a result of pseudocyst formation.

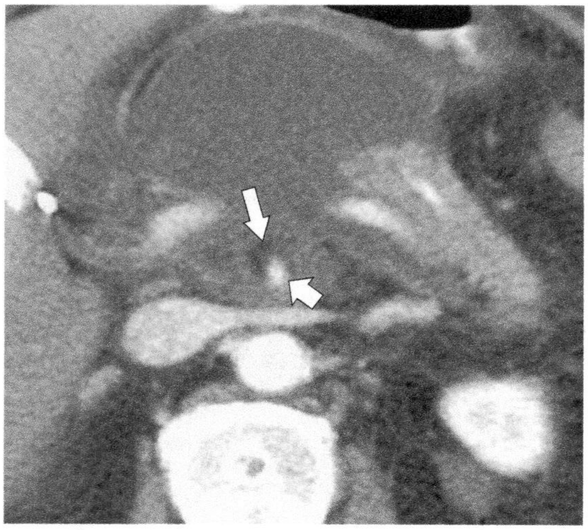

FIGURE 9-24. Axial contrast-enhanced CT in a 38-year-old man with acute pancreatitis and preservation of the fat plane (*large arrow*) surrounding the superior mesenteric artery (*small arrow*).

if IV contrast medium has been administered) along with diffuse pancreatic inflammation, enlargement, and necrosis. Splenic and portal vein thromboses (Fig. 9-26) and aneurysm formation, particularly of the splenic artery (Fig. 9-27), are other recognized complications of severe pancreatitis.

Mild or moderate pancreatitis usually involves pancreatic inflammation and enlargement that may or may not be focal (grades B and C). With more severe forms, peripancreatic fluid collections develop acutely, representing pancreatic fluid collections. Unlike chronic fluid collections (pseudocyst), they have no encapsulation or wall (Fig. 9-23). These collections can also occur within the pancreas or in other retroperitoneal locations. Many resolve spontaneously, but approximately 50% evolve into pseudocysts (see below).

Pancreatic Pseudocyst

Pancreatic pseudocyst is a complication of pancreatitis (usually acute but also chronic) and is defined as a well-circumscribed, rounded, and fibrous encapsulated pancreatic or peripancreatic fluid collection, rich in blood, necrotic material, and pancreatic enzymes. A pancreatic pseudocyst can be hard to differentiate from acute fluid collections, so the diagnosis is usually made by temporally relating the finding to the onset of symptoms. There is no radiological definition as to when an acute fluid collection becomes a pseudocyst, although the surgical definition is 6 weeks from the onset of symptoms. If ERCP is performed, a connection with the pancreatic duct is seen in up to 50% of patients.

Patients often have upper abdominal pain (radiating to the back) and, because pseudocysts can be quite large, a palpable mass. About 50% of pseudocysts resolve spontaneously with no treatment. Approximately 20% remain without further complications, but about 30% cause local complications, including erosion or dissection into adjacent organs, hemorrhage (erosion into vessels), aneurysm formation, rupture and peritonitis, and duodenal or biliary obstruction. Pseudocysts can also become infected and develop into pancreatic abscesses. These can be suitably drained percutaneously, unlike infected necrosis, which requires surgical debridement.

At imaging by CT, a rounded homogeneous hypodense and encapsulated mass is seen (acute fluid collections are not encapsulated) (Fig. 9-28). If the pseudocyst has become secondarily infected (with or without gas) or undergone hemorrhage, the contents of the mass may be heterogeneous. The fibrous rim usually shows fine enhancement on contrast-enhanced CT. MRI features match the CT findings, with hypointense contents on T1-weighted imaging and hyperintense contents on T2-weighted imaging (Fig. 9-29). Less commonly, US is performed, the results of which usually show the cyst filled with complex echoes because of the internal debris and blood.

Chronic Pancreatitis

Chronic pancreatitis, as its name suggests, is secondary to repeated bouts of acute pancreatitis, most often in unremitting alcoholics, although many of the causes of acute pancreatitis are also responsible for chronic pancreatitis (Box 9-1). The episodes of pancreatitis range from mild to severe, but the repeated injury to the pancreas ultimately takes its toll with irreversible parenchymal damage. Patients usually admit to episodes of acute pancreatitis and have recurrent or chronic abdominal pain, sometimes jaundice, and signs of pancreatic insufficiency (diabetes mellitus, steatorrhea) with malabsorption and weight loss. Serum amylase and lipase levels are typically elevated, although not usually to the degree seen in acute pancreatitis. The secretin stimulation test by ERCP has high sensitivity for the diagnosis but is not often performed, having been replaced by US or an MRCP technique (Fig. 9-11). Because of pancreatic dysfunction, pancreatic duct bicarbonate production is decreased.

In addition to the clinical features, the diagnosis is often made by cross-sectional imaging, although plain radiography may show diffuse pancreatic calcification (Fig. 9-30) and upper GI studies may show thickened duodenal folds and luminal narrowing. On CT there is usually diffuse dystrophic calcification (Fig. 9-31) within an atrophic gland and a dilated pancreatic duct, which

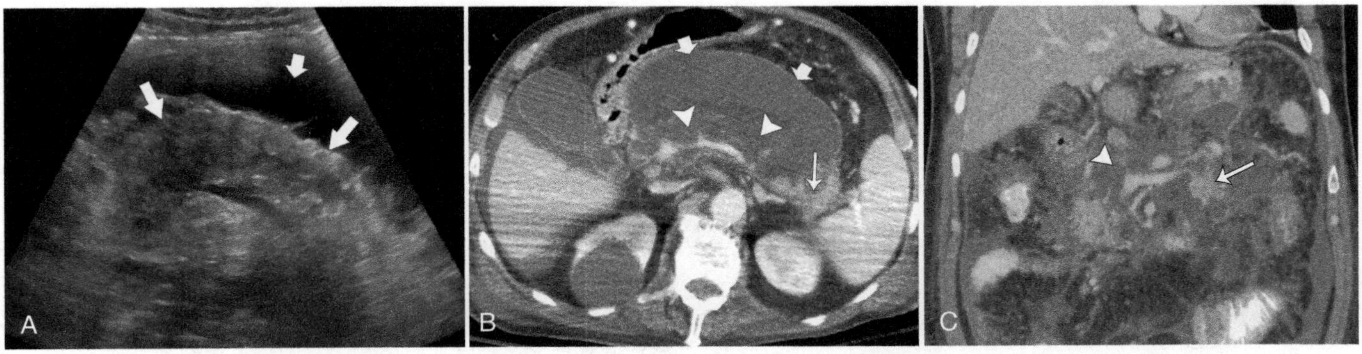

FIGURE 9-25. Transverse US (**A**) and axial (**B**) and coronal (**C**) contrast-enhanced CT in an 80-year-old man with acute pancreatitis. The pancreas is enlarged (*arrows*) and markedly heterogeneous at US with an anterior peripancreatic acute fluid collection (*small arrows*) confirmed by CT. CT also demonstrates almost complete pancreatic necrosis (*arrowheads*), except for the pancreatic tail (*thin arrows*), and a large peripancreatic acute fluid collection (*small arrows*).

TABLE 9-1 Definition of Findings in Pancreatitis

Pancreatic necrosis	Single or multiple nonenhancing intrapancreatic regions (necrotizing pancreatitis with >50% necrosis).
Exudative pancreatitis	Predominantly peripancreatic fluid collections with normally enhancing pancreas. It is synonymous with peripancreatic fat necrosis.
Acute fluid collection	Intrahepatic or extrahepatic fluid collections without defined wall in acute phase. Caused by inflammation or peripancreatic fat necrosis. May or may not be infected.
Pseudocyst	Fluid collection with defined fibrous capsule; develops 4-6 weeks after acute event. May or may not be infected.

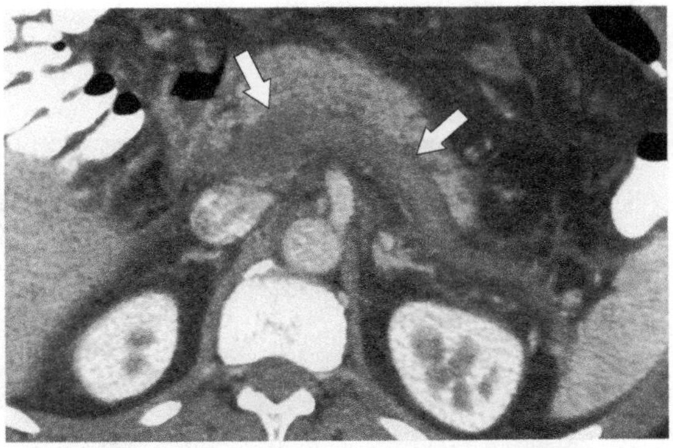

FIGURE 9-26. Axial contrast-enhanced CT in a 53-year-old woman with complete thrombosis of the splenic and superior mesenteric veins (*arrows*) secondary to acute pancreatitis.

TABLE 9-2 CT Staging of Pancreatitis

CT Grade		CT Grade Point
A	Normal pancreas	0
B	Gland enlargement (focal or diffuse) Heterogeneous gland attenuation (no necrosis) No peripancreatic inflammation	1
C	Peripancreatic inflammatory change Intrinsic pancreatic gland abnormalities	2
D	Small fluid collection	3
E	2 or more large fluid collections Gas in pancreas or retroperitoneum	4

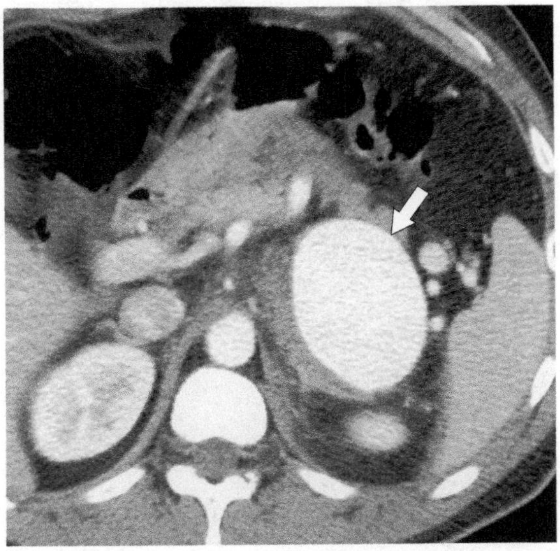

FIGURE 9-27. Axial contrast-enhanced CT in a 44-year-old woman with a 6-cm hyperenhancing left upper quadrant mass due to a splenic artery aneurysm (*arrow*) as a complication of acute pancreatitis.

TABLE 9-3 CT Severity Index

Index Point	Necrosis
0	None
2	0-30%
4	30%-50%
6	>50%

may also contain calcifications or stones. Pancreatic enhancement is variable depending on the degree of fibrosis. The chronic inflammatory change often causes splenic vein thrombosis and consequent splenic varices and splenomegaly. Sometimes intrapancreatic or extrapancreatic pseudocysts are observed. Findings at ERCP include a dilated irregular duct, sometimes beaded in both the main and side branches (Fig. 9-32), although the duct

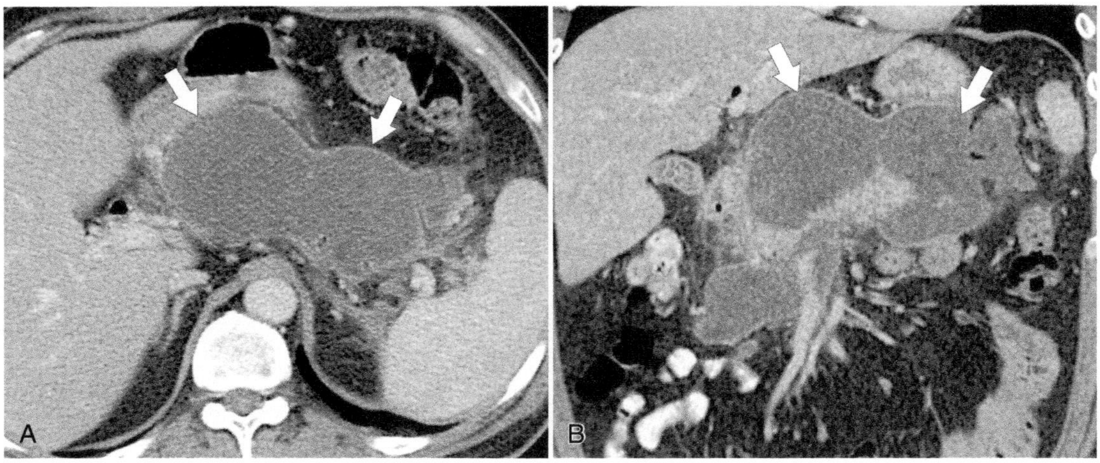

FIGURE 9-28. Axial (**A**) and coronal (**B**) contrast-enhanced CT in a 44-year-old woman with a 10-cm well-contained encapsulated fluid collection (*arrows*) representing a pancreatic pseudocyst.

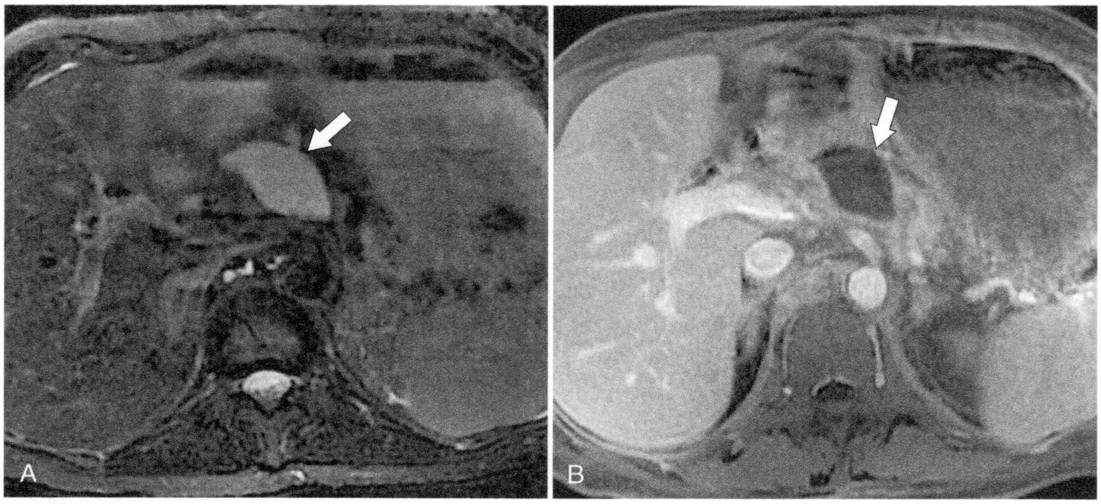

FIGURE 9-29. Axial T2-weighted (**A**) and coronal T1-weighted (**B**) fat-saturated postcontrast MRI in a 53-year-old man with a 5-cm pancreatic pseudocyst (*arrows*).

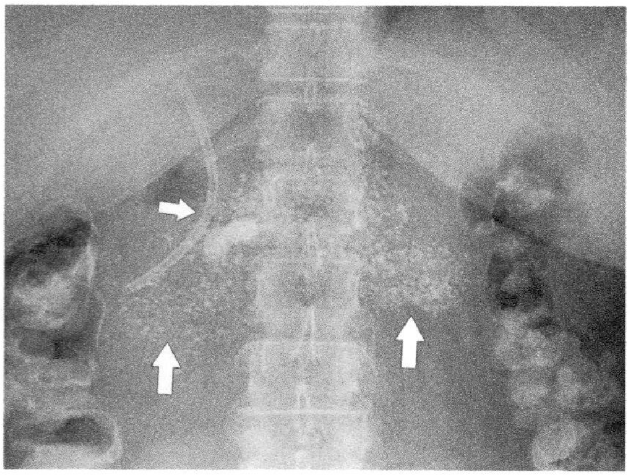

FIGURE 9-30. Plain abdominal radiograph and axial contrast-enhanced CT in a 47-year-old woman with chronic pancreatitis and diffuse pancreatic calcification (*arrows*). A plastic biliary stent (*small arrow*) is present because of an inflammatory biliary stricture.

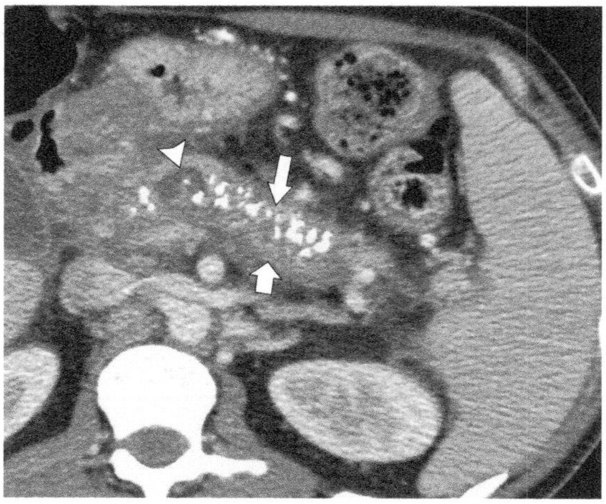

FIGURE 9-31. Axial contrast-enhanced CT in a 42-year-old man with an acute episode of chronic pancreatitis, demonstrating diffuse pancreatic calcification (*large arrow*), peripancreatic inflammatory changes (*small arrow*), and a focally enlarged pancreatic duct (*arrowhead*). Splenomegaly is caused by chronic splenic vein thrombosis.

can also be narrowed, usually tapered rather than abruptly constricted as is seen in pancreatic adenocarcinoma. Both the pancreatic duct and bile duct may be strictured in the head of the pancreas, giving a "double-duct" appearance in which there is proximal biliary and pancreatic duct dilatation to the stricture in the pancreatic head. This feature is far more commonly associated, however, with pancreatic carcinoma. Filling defects are usually secondary to pancreatic stones.

Autoimmune Pancreatitis

Autoimmune pancreatitis is a poorly understood entity that is also a form of chronic pancreatitis but with no discrete cause. Most patients have elevations of immunoglobulin 4 (IgG4) levels (a specific sign for the disease) and antinuclear antibody levels, which are associated with many other autoimmune diseases, hence the term autoimmune pancreatitis. The pancreas is filled with a lymphoplasmocytic infiltrate. Characteristically, the normal lobulated pancreatic external contour is effaced, producing a more tubular or sausage-shaped outline (Fig. 9-33). Usually the whole gland is affected, but the disease can be focal (Fig. 9-34). After IV contrast administration at CT, capsule-like enhancement that surrounds a low-density band or halo is demonstrated (Fig. 9-35). Peripancreatic adenopathy or inflammatory lesions elsewhere are sometimes observed (Fig. 9-36). The pancreatic duct, if evaluated with ERCP or MRCP, is typically irregularly narrowed and strictured, which may also affect the intrahepatic ducts and resemble primary sclerosing cholangitis.

Chronic Segmental Pancreatitis (Groove Pancreatitis)

Chronic segmental pancreatitis is a specific form of chronic pancreatitis confined to the pancreaticoduodenal groove (hence its common name "groove pancreatitis"), defined as the area between the head of the pancreas and the second portion of the duodenum. Its exact cause is unknown, but it is associated with excessive and chronic alcohol abuse (similar to chronic pancreatitis), minor papilla strictures (either congenital or caused by neoplasm), and chronic inflammation of the lower common bile duct resulting from prior surgery. Most patients present between 30 and 50 years of age with postprandial pain and vomiting and sometimes with weight loss and mild jaundice. In the correct clinical setting the imaging features at CT are highly suggestive, with separation between the head of the pancreas and the duodenal C-loop because of an intervening hypodense inflammatory mass (or hypointense on T1-weighted MRI) that is often associated with cystic change (Fig. 9-37).

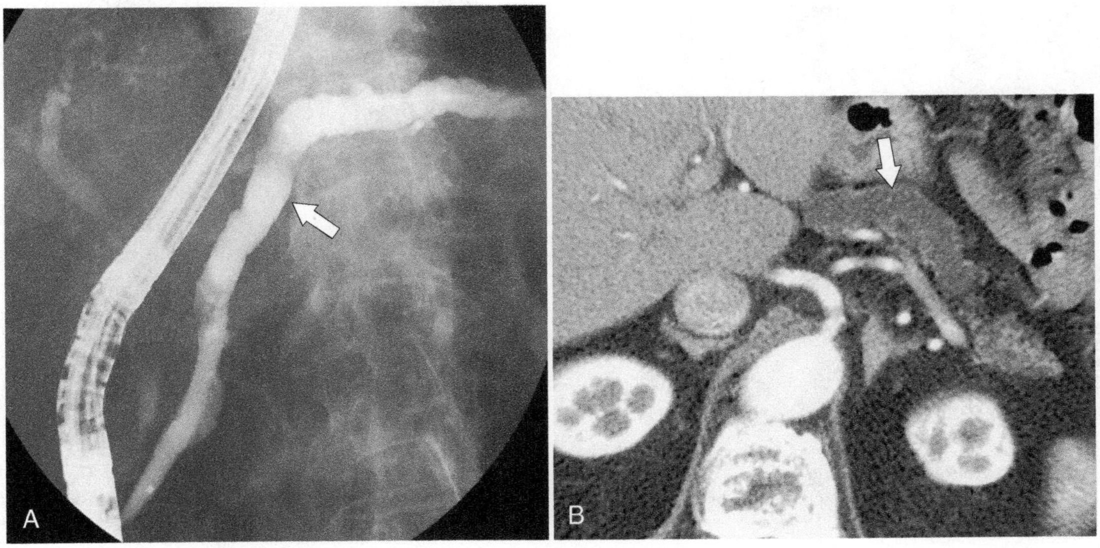

FIGURE 9-32. ERCP (**A**) and axial contrast-enhanced CT (**B**) in a 55-year-old man with a diffusely dilated and irregular pancreatic duct (*arrows*) from chronic pancreatitis.

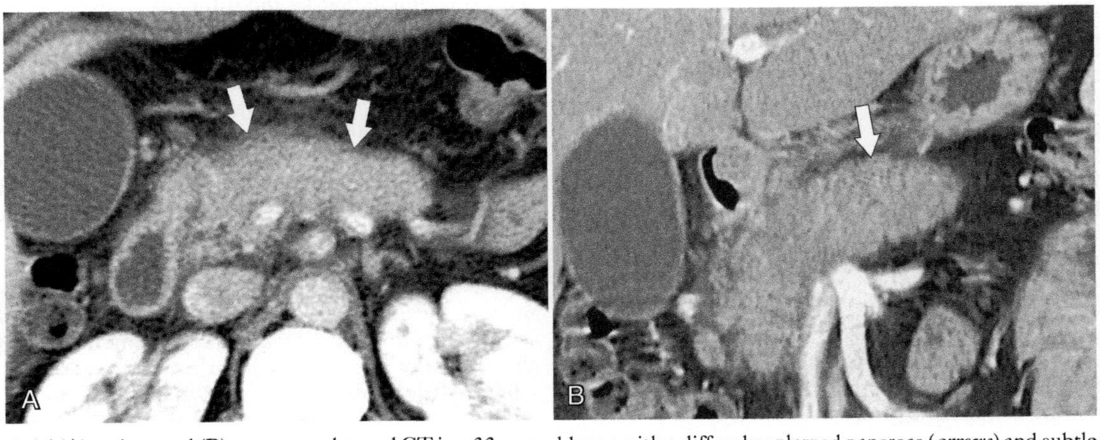

FIGURE 9-33. Axial (**A**) and coronal (**B**) contrast-enhanced CT in a 32-year-old man with a diffusely enlarged pancreas (*arrows*) and subtle peripancreatic inflammation caused by autoimmune pancreatitis. The pancreas is sometimes described as "sausage" shaped.

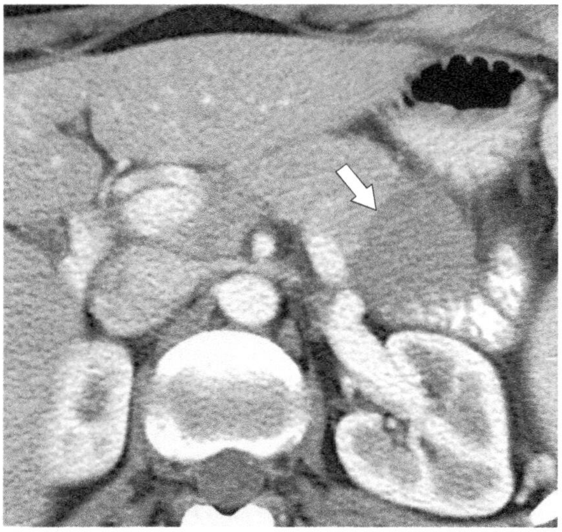

FIGURE 9-34. Axial contrast-enhanced CT in a 29-year-old woman with smooth enlargement of the pancreatic tail caused by autoimmune pancreatitis with a sharp margination from the normal pancreas (*arrow*).

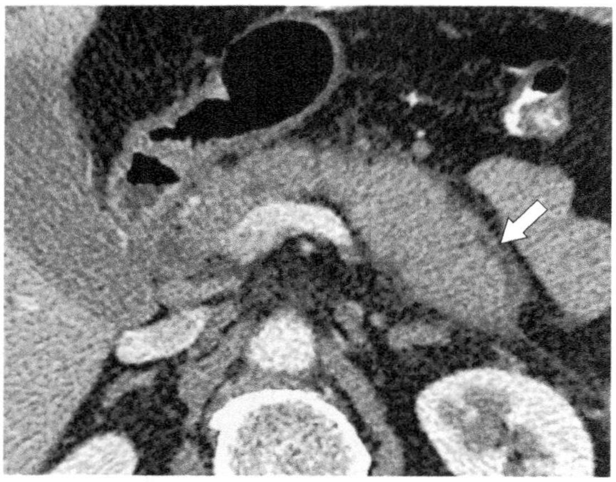

FIGURE 9-35. Axial contrast-enhanced CT in a 62-year-old man with raised IgG4 levels showing a smoothly enlarged body and tail of the pancreas with a peripancreatic halo (*arrow*) characteristic of autoimmune pancreatitis.

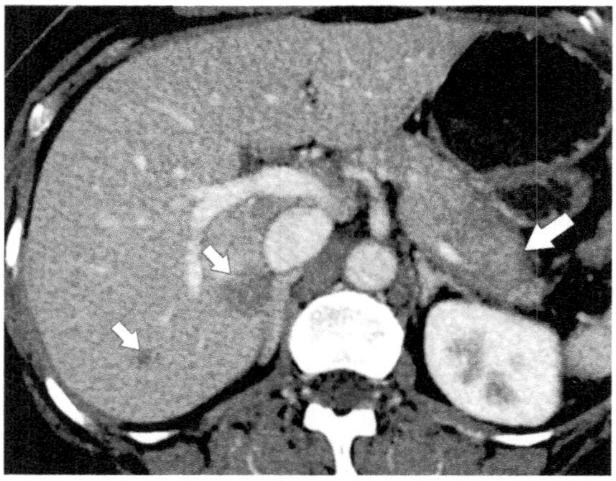

FIGURE 9-36. Axial contrast-enhanced CT in a 46-year-old woman with an enlarged and heterogeneous pancreatic body and tail (*large arrow*) and hypodense hepatic IgG4 inflammatory pseudotumors (*small arrows*) concomitant with autoimmune pancreatitis.

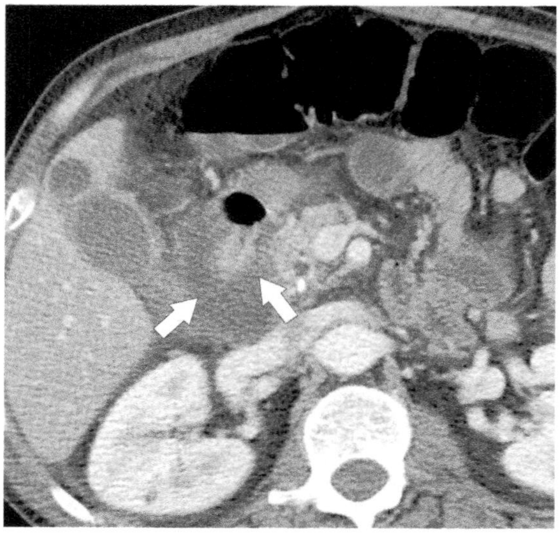

FIGURE 9-37. Axial contrast-enhanced CT in a 47-year-old woman with diffuse inflammation (*arrows*) in the duodenal pancreatic groove caused by "groove" pancreatitis.

SOLID PANCREATIC MASS LESIONS (BOX 9-2)

Pancreatic Adenocarcinoma

Pancreatic adenocarcinoma is the most common pancreatic neoplasm (90% of malignant pancreatic tumors) and the fourth most common cause of cancer death in the United States. Patients with this type of cancer still have a dismal prognosis (20% 5-year survival rate with surgery and 5% without). The tumor arises from the ductal epithelium of the exocrine pancreas, with two thirds in the head and the remainder in the body and tail. Patients are typically in their seventies and generally present with central abdominal or back pain, weight loss, and jaundice. The Courvoisier* sign is painless jaundice in the presence of a distended and palpable gallbladder secondary to biliary obstruction, an ominous sign. Rarer presentations include GI bleeding, diabetes mellitus, and pancreatitis. Pancreatic adenocarcinoma is staged according to the TNM classification (Table 9-4).

*Ludwig Georg Courvoisier (1843-1918), Swiss surgeon.

A primary reason for the grim prognosis is that most patients present late, when the tumor is already advanced and inoperable. This is compounded by the difficulty in detecting small lesions at imaging. Lesions less than 2 cm are notoriously difficult to detect, even with a dedicated pancreatic CT protocol. However, contrast-enhanced CT is still the initial imaging investigation of choice. The key to maximizing lesion detection and assessing resectability is pancreatic-phase scanning, which maximizes normal pancreatic parenchymal enhancement while the pancreatic tumor remains relatively unenhanced. This increase in tumor conspicuity is best evaluated with a 40- to 45-second scan delay after the initiation of IV contrast material. At that time, celiac and superior mesenteric arteries are well enhanced, so that local encasement by tumor can also be assessed (Fig. 9-38). Furthermore, sufficient delay for the mesenteric veins to be opacified has usually occurred, so any vascular encasement can be evaluated at the same time. Portal venous–phase scanning at 60 to 70 seconds adds additional diagnostic information about the mesenteric veins and, more important, about the presence of any potential hepatic metastases that were not optimally imaged during the earlier pancreatic-phase scanning.

Box 9-2. Solid Pancreatic Masses

MALIGNANT
Adenocarcinoma
PNET (islet cell, VIPoma, gastrinoma, glucagonoma)
Acinar cell carcinoma
Colloid carcinoma
Anaplastic carcinoma
Giant cell carcinoma
Small cell carcinoma
Pancreaticoblastoma
Lymphoma
Metastases
Sarcoma

BENIGN
PNET (islet cell, VIPoma, gastrinoma, glucagonoma)
SPEN
Intrapancreatic spleen
Lipoma

PNET, Pancreatic neuroendocrine tumor; *SPEN,* solid and papillary epithelial pancreatic neoplasm of the pancreas.

TABLE 9-4 TNM Classification of Pancreatic Adenocarcinoma

Primary Tumor (T)	
Tis	Carcinoma in situ
T1	Tumor ≤2 cm within pancreas
T2	Tumor >2 cm within pancreas
T3	Tumor beyond pancreas without SMA/SMV involvement
T4	Tumor involves SMA/SMV
Regional Lymph Nodes (N)	
N0	Absent
N1	Present
Distant Metastases (M)	
M0	Absent
M1	Present

Stage	T	N	M
0	Tis	N0	M0
IA	TI	N0	M0
IB	T2	N0	M0
IIA	T3	N0	M0
IIB	T1	N1	M0
	T2	N1	M0
	T3	N1	M0
III	T4	Any N	M0
IV	Any T	Any N	M1

SMA, Superior mesenteric artery; *SMV,* superior mesenteric vein.

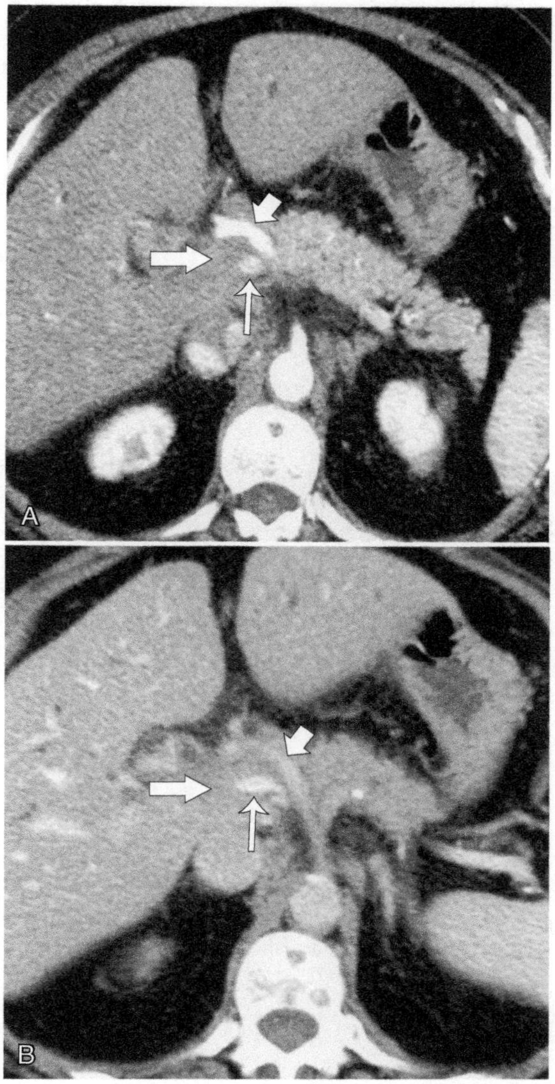

FIGURE 9-38. Axial pancreatic phase (**A**) and portal venous phase (**B**) contrast-enhanced CT in a 70-year-old woman with a pancreatic head adenocarcinoma. On pancreatic-phase imaging, the tumor (*large arrows*), celiac axis (*small arrows*), and superior mesenteric vein (*thin arrows*) are all visualized to better effect.

When a tumor is detected at contrast-enhanced CT, there may or may not be mass effect, depending on the size of the tumor. Lack of a pancreatic mass effect should not deter the diagnosis, but larger tumors will inevitably distort the normal pancreatic outline. Tumors are typically hypodense (particularly during the pancreatic phase) because of the central hypovascularity of the tumor (Fig. 9-38). As the tumor enlarges, recognition of hypodensity becomes easier, and large tumors may show frank necrosis (Fig. 9-39). As the mass grows in size, pancreatic duct dilatation becomes more evident, particularly if the tumor is in the head, resulting in upstream ductal dilatation (Fig. 9-40). Smaller tumors in the uncinate may cause little ductal dilatation because of their distance from the main pancreatic duct. Ultimately, the common bile duct may also become obstructed with large pancreatic head tumors (Fig. 9-41), which may progress to a "double-duct" sign when both the pancreatic and biliary ducts are dilated. This is best visualized by ERCP or MRCP (Fig. 9-42). The double-duct sign indicates that the likelihood of a pancreatic adenocarcinoma in the head of the pancreas is very high, even if the tumor is not visualized. Uncommonly, chronic pancreatitis can also cause a double-duct sign, but there should be other signs of chronic pancreatitis at CT and a prolonged clinical history. As the tumor extends beyond the pancreas, the peripancreatic fat becomes invaded or obliterated, which is recognized by increased (sometimes hazy) inflammatory change (i.e., stranding) (Fig. 9-43). Often the tumor causes local pancreatitis, further adding to the peripancreatic inflammation

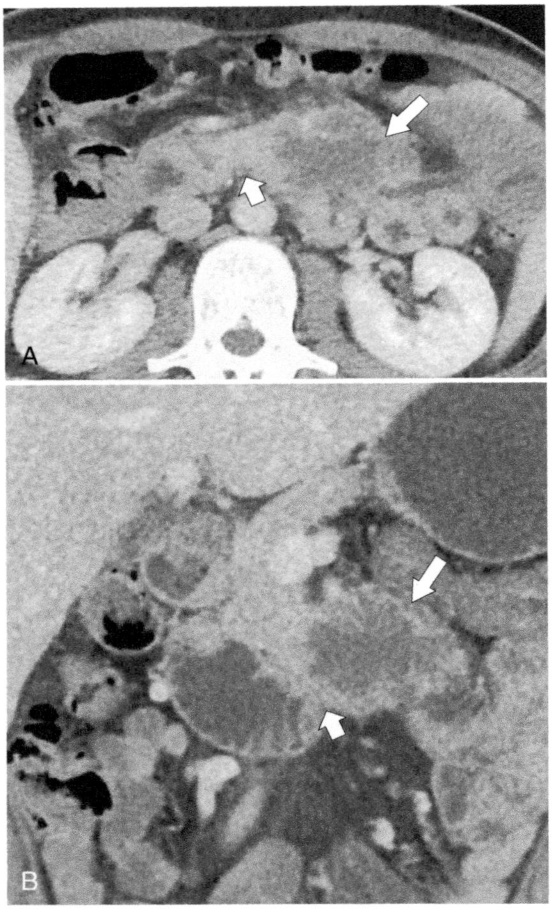

FIGURE 9-39. Axial (**A**) and coronal (**B**) contrast-enhanced CT in a 76-year-old man with a large pancreatic adenocarcinoma having a central hypodense necrotic area (*large arrows*). The tumor also obstructs the duodenum (*small arrows*).

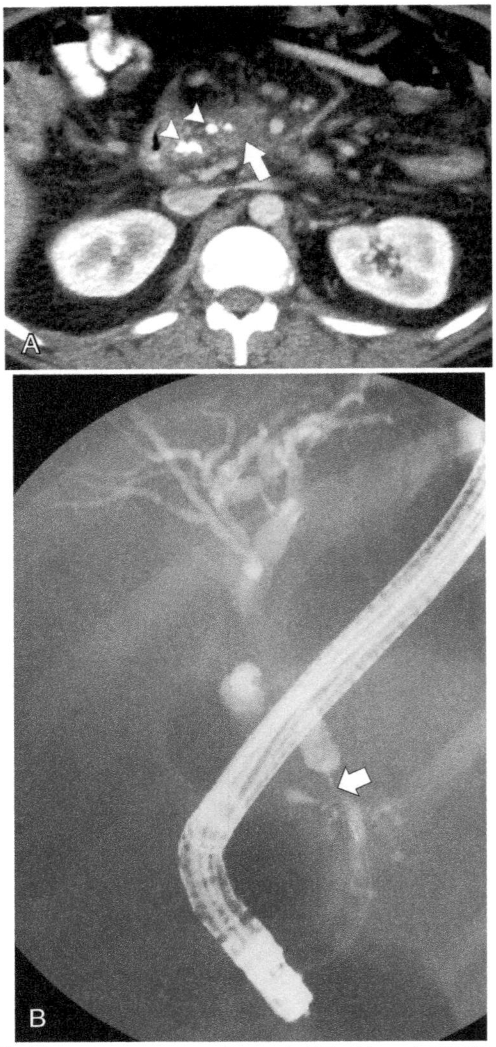

FIGURE 9-41. Axial contrast-enhanced CT (**A**) and ERCP (**B**) in a 53-year-old man with chronic pancreatitis and a new pancreatic head mass caused by adenocarcinoma (*large arrow*). A stricture is present in the lower bile duct (*small arrow*), as well as calcification (*arrowheads*).

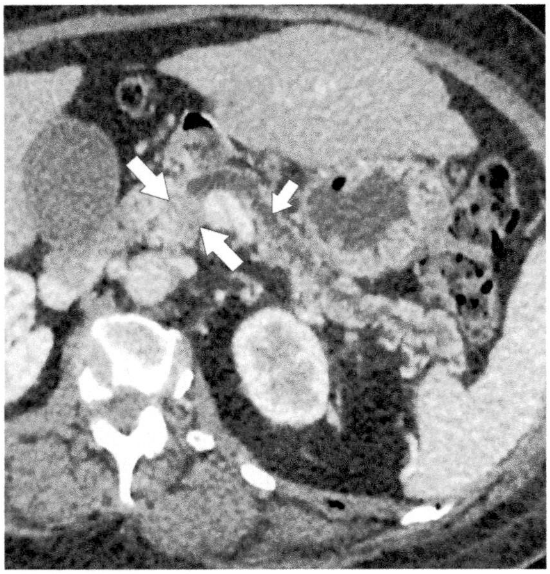

FIGURE 9-40. Axial reformatted contrast-enhanced CT in a 60-year-old man with a subtle 2-cm uncinate mass (*large arrow*) that obstructs the pancreatic duct (*small arrow*).

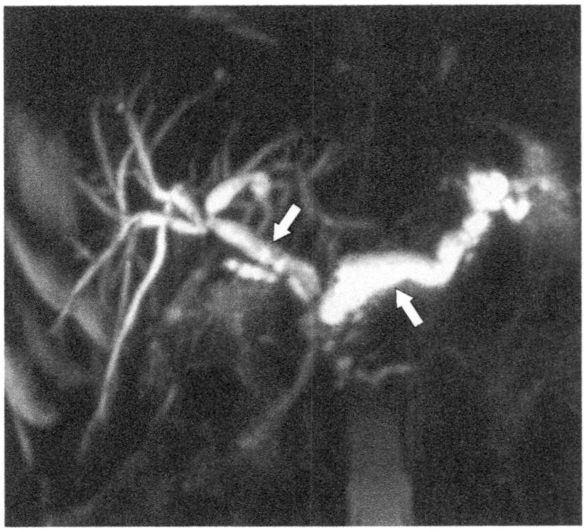

FIGURE 9-42. MRCP in a 61-year-old with dilated pancreatic and biliary ducts (double-duct sign) (*arrows*) resulting from an obstructing pancreatic adenocarcinoma.

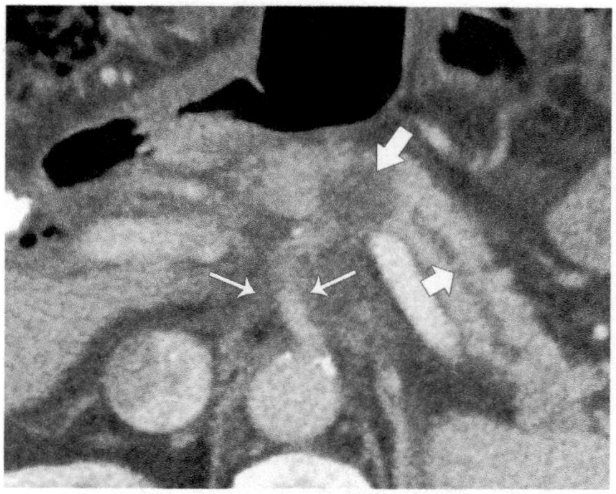

FIGURE 9-43. Axial pancreatic-phase contrast-enhanced CT in a 78-year-old man with an adenocarcinoma of the midpancreatic body (*large arrow*) with upstream pancreatic duct dilatation (*small arrow*) and peripancreatic extension of tumor. The tumor has extended to encase the celiac axis (*thin arrows*), rendering the patient inoperable.

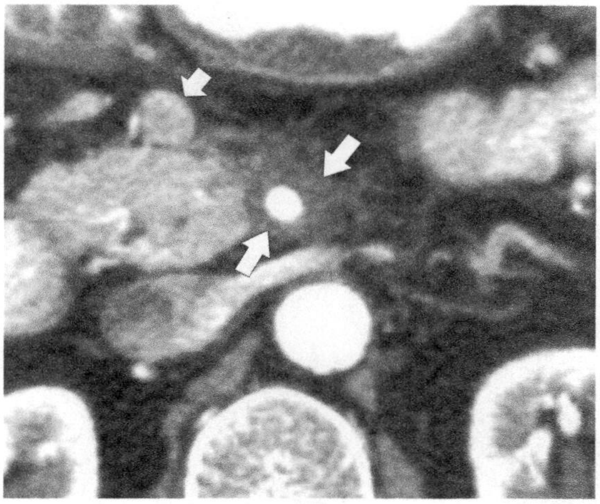

FIGURE 9-44. Axial pancreatic-phase contrast-enhanced CT in a 73-year-old woman with soft tissue encasement by pancreatic adenocarcinoma of the superior mesenteric artery (*arrows*), but the superior mesenteric vein is unaffected (*small arrow*). This patient was inoperable.

so that it is sometimes difficult to differentiate changes due to tumor from those due to pancreatitis. The local extension into the peripancreatic fat can abut and then surround key vascular structures, particularly the superior mesenteric artery (Fig. 9-44) or vein and sometimes both (Fig. 9-45). The superior mesenteric vein (SMV), however, is often compressed by tumor mass effect as it courses through the pancreas rather than becoming invaded and encased (Fig. 9-46). Multiplanar images can offer better depiction of the relationship of the tumor to the adjacent vessels (Fig. 9-47) and are often used to determine surgical resectability of the mass. Local invasion of splenic, celiac, and mesenteric vessels may preclude operability but will depend on the local surgical expertise. Tumors with more than 50% encasement of the SMV or portal vein (Figs. 9-46 through 9-48) are generally unresectable, although some surgeons are more aggressive and have shown some success with up to 75% circumferential encasement. Splenic vein invasion is not a contraindication to surgery. Celiac axis (celiac or hepatic artery or both) and superior mesenteric artery encasement greater than 25% is generally unresectable (Figs. 9-45 through 9-47). Splenic and gastroduodenal artery encasement is not a contraindication to surgery. Tumors with distant metastases, which are common in pancreatic cancer because of its late presentation, are unresectable. However, it is becoming increasingly apparent that some newer neoadjuvant therapies (e.g., FOLFIRINOX with or without radiation therapy) cause a dramatic reduction in tumor size and residual perivascular soft tissue changes now represent fibrosis rather than active tumor. Radiologists should therefore hesitate before assuming inoperability in these patients (Fig. 9-49). Contrast-enhanced CT has a high predictive value (close to 100%) for unresectability but only 75% to 80% for tumor resectability. Hence, when the CT features suggest unresectability, the radiologist is usually correct. The converse is not true, as a number of tumors deemed resectable by CT turn out not to be. Pancreatic positron emission tomography (PET)/CT does not usually add value to the diagnosis of the primary tumor because of variable fluorodeoxyglucose uptake (Fig. 9-50), but it can sometimes be useful to evaluate extrapancreatic disease, particularly regional adenopathy.

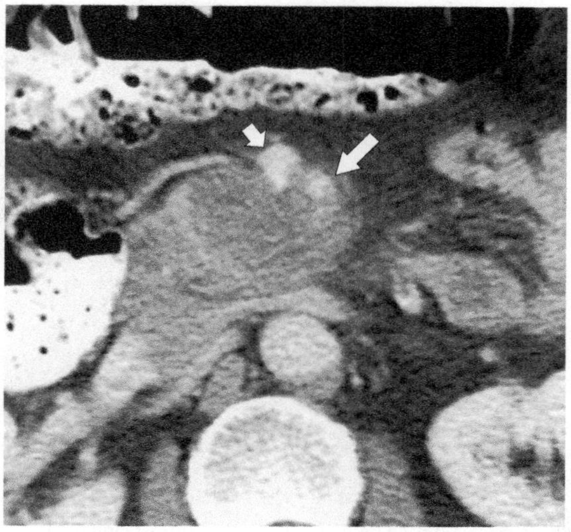

FIGURE 9-45. Axial contrast-enhanced CT in a 71-year-old with pancreatic adenocarcinoma and almost complete encasement of the superior mesenteric artery (*large arrow*) and approximately 50% of the superior mesenteric vein (*small arrow*), which has lost its normal ovoid shape. This patient proved inoperable.

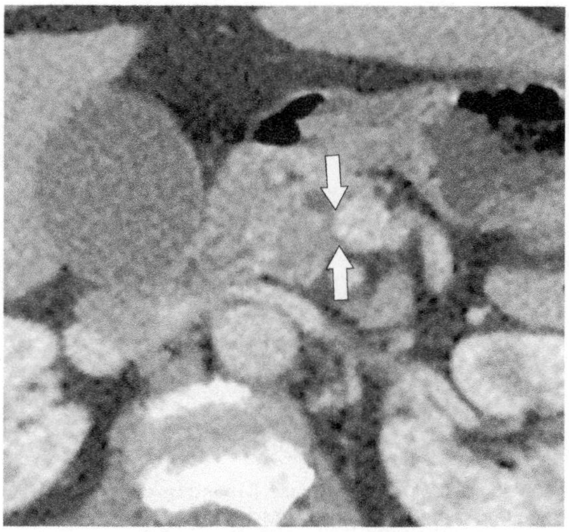

FIGURE 9-46. Axial pancreatic-phase contrast-enhanced images in a 66-year-old woman with a 1.5-cm subtle hypodense mass in the junction of the head and uncinate that abuts the superior mesenteric vein between the 6 and 11 o'clock positions with effacement of the normal fat plane (*arrows*) but preservation of vessel caliber. This patient was operable.

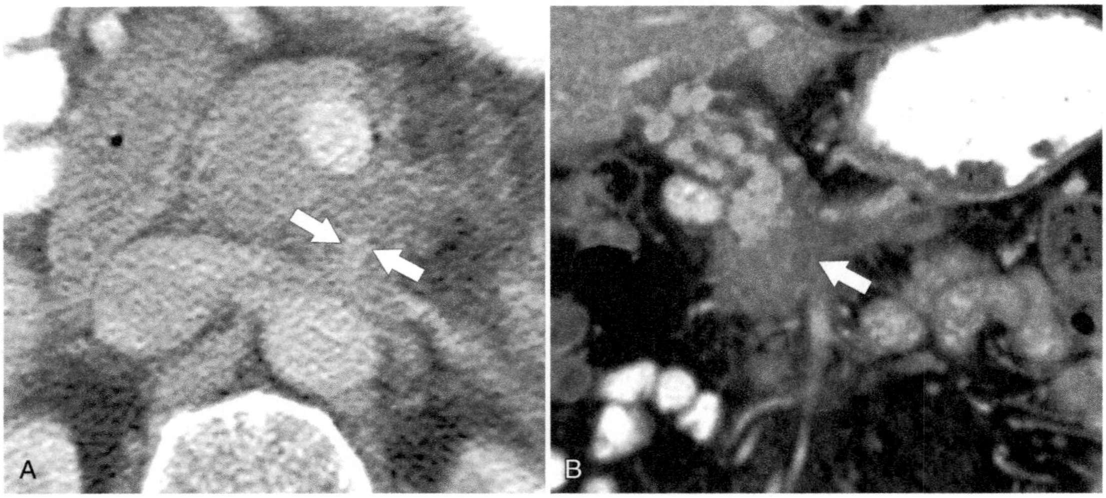

FIGURE 9-47. Axial (**A**) and coronal (**B**) contrast-enhanced CT in a 54-year-old man with inoperable pancreatic adenocarcinoma and complete encasement of the superior mesenteric artery (*arrows*).

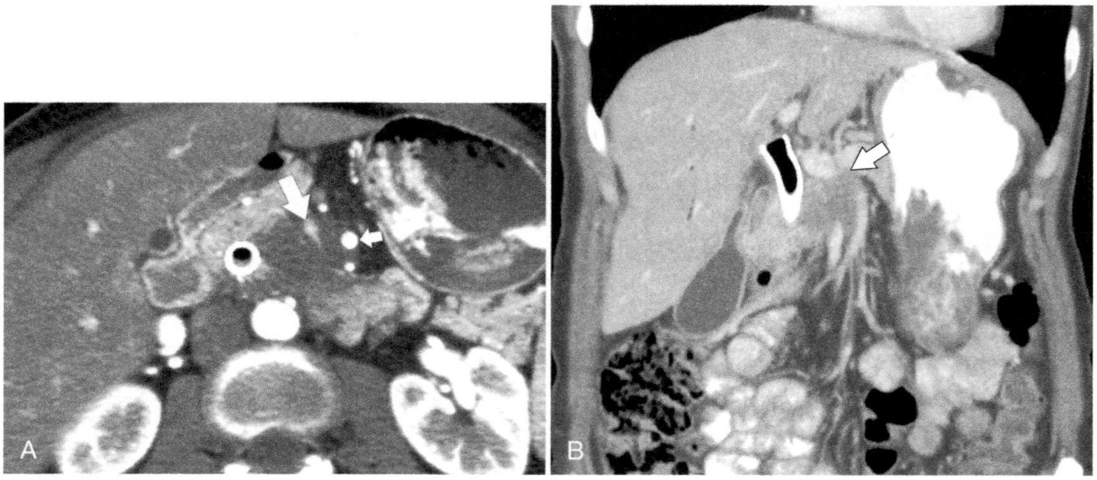

FIGURE 9-48. Axial (**A**) and coronal (**B**) contrast-enhanced CT in a 63-year-old woman with pancreatic adenocarcinoma showing complete encasement of the superior mesenteric vein (*arrows*).

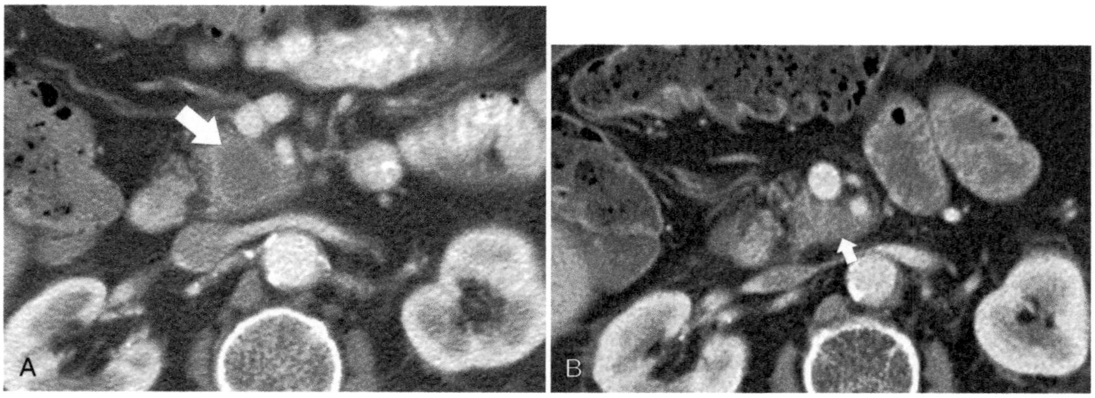

FIGURE 9-49. Axial contrast-enhanced CT in a 49-year-old woman with what was initially thought to be inoperable pancreatic cancer by imaging (**A**) as evidenced by encasement of the superior mesenteric artery (*large arrow*). After treatment with FOLFIRINOX (**B**), the mass has significantly reduced in size (*small arrow*). Even though there is some residual tissue around the superior mesenteric artery, this was proven to be fibrosis and no residual tumor at Whipple operation.

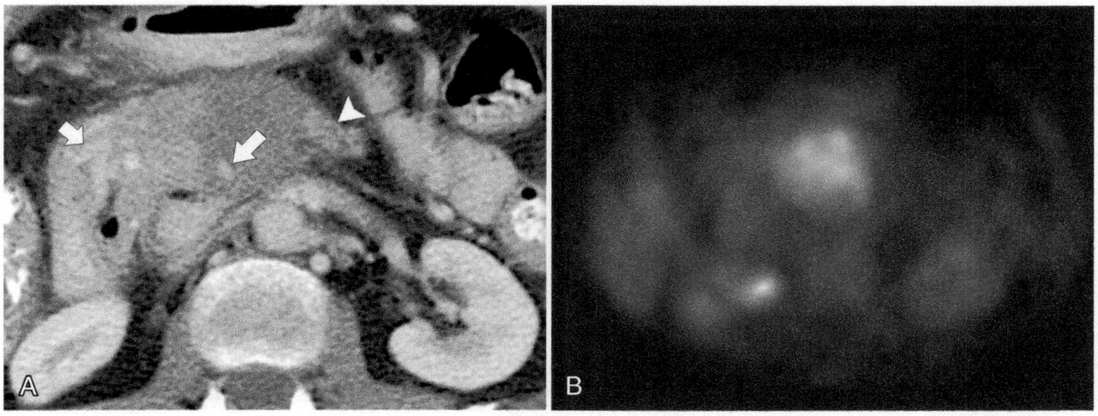

FIGURE 9-50. Axial contrast-enhanced CT (**A**) and PET (**B**) in a 63-year-old woman with pancreatic adenocarcinoma. A 5-cm hypodense mass in the body of the pancreas (*arrowheads*) completely surrounds the superior mesenteric artery (*large arrow*). There are also superior mesenteric vein occlusion and collateral formation (*small arrow*). PET shows increased fluorodeoxyglucose uptake in the pancreatic mass (*arrowhead*).

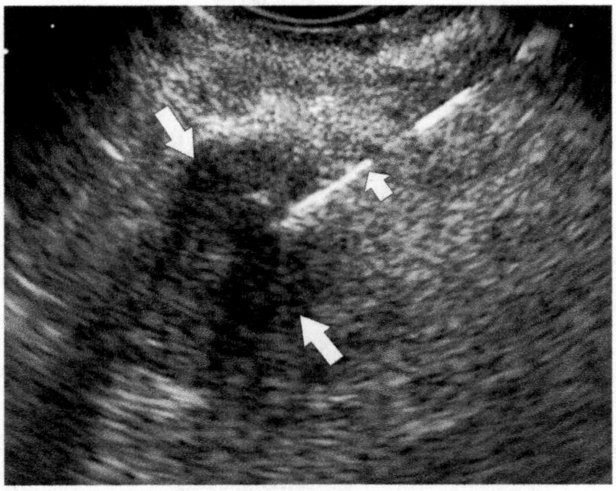

FIGURE 9-51. Endoscopic US in a 65-year-old woman with an ill-defined 2-cm hypoechoic mass (*arrows*) in the head of the pancreas that proved to be ductal adenocarcinoma at biopsy (*small arrow*).

Further extension of pancreatic tumor may involve local organs, including the stomach, small bowel, spleen, and even the kidneys. More regional extension frequently involves local lymphadenopathy, and further distant metastases often involve the liver and peritoneum and less frequently the lungs.

The tumor can be visualized with MRI, being hypointense on T1-weighted imaging, particularly with added fat suppression, which increases the contrast between the tumor and higher signal healthy pancreas. On contrast-enhanced MRI the pancreas and tumor show features similar to those with contrast-enhanced CT. Should these techniques fail to detect any lesion and with a high index of clinical suspicion, endoscopic US should detect most small tumors unrecognized on CT or MRI (Fig. 9-51). Furthermore, tissue sampling can be performed during the procedure. However, endoscopic US generally usually cannot detect distant metastases.

Pancreatic Neuroendocrine Tumor

Pancreatic neuroendocrine tumors (PNETs) are also known as islet cell tumors or amine precursor and uptake decarboxylation tumors. They can hypersecrete various hormones (insulin, glucagon, gastrin, and somtatostatin), producing unusual but classic clinical findings. The amine precursor and uptake decarboxylation cells are embryonic and migrate from the neural crest to the pancreas and also to the intestinal tract, thyroid, parathyroid, and adrenal gland. They are classified as either functioning (85% of all islet cell tumors) or nonfunctioning (15%) if no excessive hormones are produced. If hyperfunctioning, they may be part of a multiple endocrine neoplasia syndrome 1 (MEN 1), an autosomal-dominant disease associated with endocrine hyperplasia or neoplasia in disparate organs (Table 9-5). They can be benign or malignant (Table 9-6), although the most common type of tumor, insulinoma, is usually benign.

TABLE 9-5 MEN 1 (Wermer* Syndrome)

Organ	Tumor	Hormone	Frequency in Syndrome
Pancreas	Insulinoma (can be multiple)	Insulin	Approximately 50%
	Gastrinoma	Gastrin	Approximately 20%-40%
Pituitary		Adenocortico-tropic hormone	
Parathyroid		Calcitonin	

*Paul Wermer (1898-1975), American physician.

Insulinoma

Insulinomas are the most common islet cell tumors that are either functioning, producing insulin from hyperactivity of alpha cells, or nonfunctioning, without significant insulin elevation. Most tumors are small (<2 cm), isolated (70%), benign (90%), and hypervascular (70%). The resulting hyperinsulinemia leads to classic symptoms when florid, but milder forms can go clinically undetected for many years. Typical features are those of hypoglycemia with weakness, confusion, loss of consciousness, and even seizures. Because insulinomas are hypervascular, anyone suspected of having this tumor should undergo dedicated arterial-phase (rather than pancreatic-phase) multidetector CT pancreatic imaging. The lesion, particularly if small (as they frequently are), is often detected only during the arterial phase. Many are missed if the timing of the IV bolus is suboptimal. Classically, optimal CT scanning shows a small, uniform, hyperenhancing mass in the pancreas (Fig. 9-52), which rapidly washes out on portal venous–phase or later imaging, so much so that the sometime-lesion disappears. Dedicated contrast-enhanced MRI has slightly higher accuracy for islet cell tumor detection (especially with fat-saturated techniques) (Fig. 9-53), but if it is still not detected when there is a very high index of suspicion, selective angiography can delineate the hypervascular mass or excessive insulin at pancreatic venous sampling. Alternatively, endoscopic US has proved more accurate than either CT or MRI

TABLE 9-6 Features of Pancreatic Neuroendocrine Tumors

Type	Location	Cell Type	Hormone	Malignancy	Clinical Findings
Insulinoma	Pancreas	β	Insulin	10%	Hypoglycemia
Gastrinoma	Pancreas, duodenum, stomach	α-1	Gastrin	60%	Zollinger-Ellison syndrome
Glucagonoma	Pancreas	α-1	Glucagon	80%	Diabetes mellitus, necrolytic migratory erythema
VIPoma	Pancreas	δ-1	VIP	50%	WDHA syndrome
Somatostatinoma	Pancreas, chest, brain	δ	Somatostatin	60%-70%	Diarrhea, weight loss

WDHA, Watery diarrhea, hypokalemia, and achlorhydria.

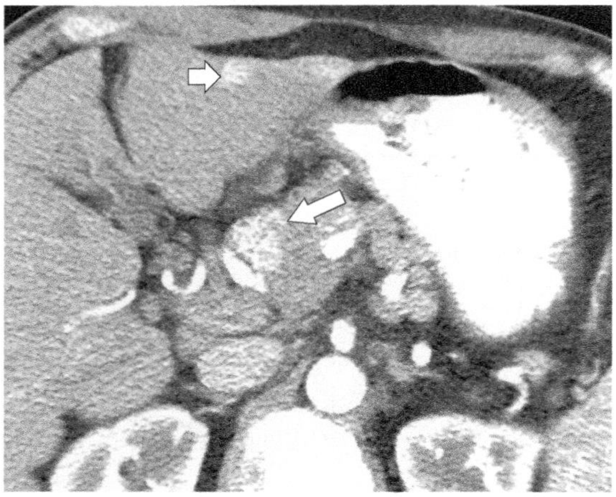

FIGURE 9-52. Axial arterial-phase contrast-enhanced CT in a 54-year-old man with a 2-cm enhancing mass in the pancreatic head (*large arrow*) that represents a functioning insulinoma. An additional hypervascular liver mass is in segment II of the liver (*small arrow*).

for the detection of small lesions (Fig. 9-54). Because lesions have high levels of somatostatin receptors, the somatostatin analogue indium-111 pentetreotide (octreotide) can help locate and characterize these pancreatic lesions (Fig. 9-55) as neuroendocrine in origin (insulinoma or otherwise). Ultimately, an exploratory laparotomy with intraoperative US may be required if the index of suspicion remains very high and noninvasive imaging tests fail to identify the mass (Fig. 9-56).

Not all islet cell tumors are hypervascular. Some are isodense or hypodense on CT imaging (even in the arterial phase) and may therefore occasionally be confused with adenocarcinoma. However, they tend to be more well circumscribed (Fig. 9-57) without peripancreatic extension unless very large with a late presentation. Others are heterogeneous and either partially cystic (Fig. 9-58) or almost completely cystic (Fig. 9-59).

Nonfunctioning insulinomas can be more sinister and indolent because they often present late owing to the lack of hormone production and early clinical signs. They are therefore usually larger at presentation with mass-like symptoms (pain, obstruction, and invasion of other organs) (Fig. 9-60). Because they are large, insulinomas are often necrotic, but the active periphery of the tumor can enhance avidly like other islet cell tumors. They can also be cystic in appearance, like functioning tumors, and calcification is present in 20% (Fig. 9-61). They are often metastatic (80% to 90%), either locally or distantly (hypervascular liver metastases), and consequently patients have a relatively poor 5-year survival rate (45%).

Gastrinoma

Gastrinomas are the second most common pancreatic neuroendocrine tumors and are associated with MEN1 in approximately 20% to 40% of patients. They arise from alpha-1 cells and typically reside in the pancreas but can be ectopic in the second part of the duodenum or stomach. They are often small, like insulinomas, but are more likely to be multiple (75%). Investigation of the patient is triggered by clinical symptoms (also known as Zollinger-Ellison* syndrome) that result from profuse ulceration of the gastric, duodenal, and even proximal jejunal mucosa because of gastrin hyperproductivity (Fig. 9-62). This peptide hormone normally stimulates gastric parietal cells to secrete hydrochloric acid, so with excessive hormonal production, profuse upper intestinal tract inflammation and ulceration ensue.

Because of their sometimes ectopic location outside the pancreas, gastrinomas are more frequently missed than insulinomas, and careful evaluation along the medial border of the second part of the duodenum is required. With optimal bolus timing and dedicated arterial multidetector CT, most tumors should be detected. Metastases are far more common (approximately 60% of gastrinomas) than with insulinomas (10%) (Fig. 9-63) and can also secrete gastrin, and palliative treatment involves gastrectomy or H_2-blocker therapy.

Glucagonoma

Glucagonomas are rarer than either insulinomas or gastrinomas and arise from alpha-2 islet cells. Even though they secrete glucagon, glucagonomas often present late and large, and up to 80% are metastatic to the liver or regional lymph nodes at the time of diagnosis. They are usually located in the body and tail of the pancreas (Fig. 9-64). Clinical findings are secondary to the elevated glucagon levels and include diabetes mellitus, anemia, weight loss, hypoaminoacidemia, and a characteristic necrolytic migratory erythema.

VIPoma

VIPomas secrete vasoactive intestinal polypeptide (VIP) from delta-1 islet cells, producing the WDHA (or WDHH) syndrome of watery diarrhea, hypokalemia, and achlorhydria and hypovolemia. Up to 50% are malignant, and most occur in the body and tail of the pancreas. Like other pancreatic neuroendocrine tumors at imaging, they are hypervascular and most likely to be detected during arterial-phase imaging (Fig. 9-65).

Somatostatinoma

Somatostatinomas are the rarest of the islet cell tumors, with excess somatostatin produced from delta islet cells. Most are malignant, cause diarrhea and weight loss, and can be confused with VIPomas. At imaging, they are also relatively large and hypervascular and

*Robert Milton Zollinger (1903-1992), American surgeon; Edwin H. Ellison (1918-1970), American surgeon.

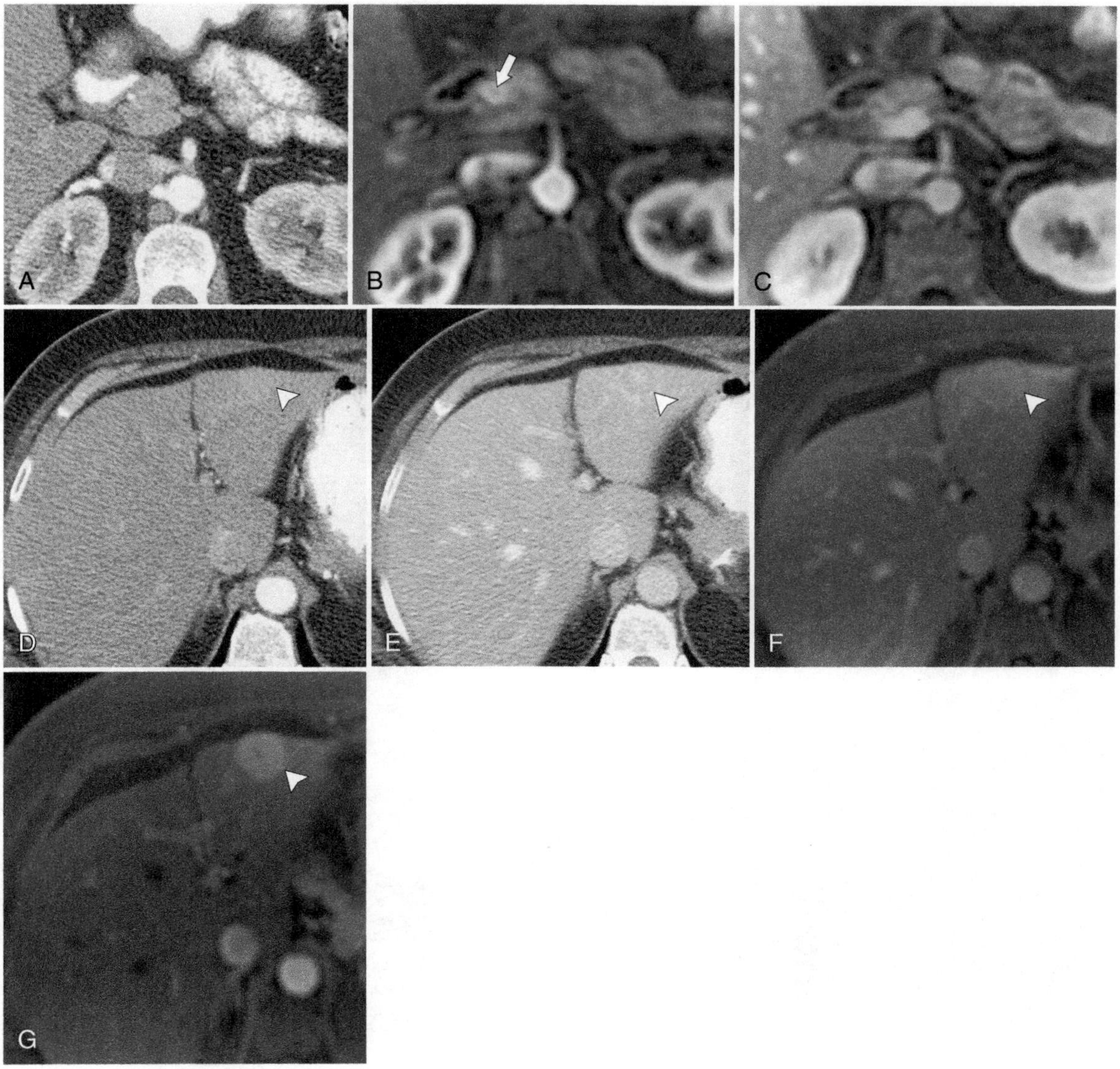

FIGURE 9-53. Axial arterial-phase CT (**A**) and T1-weighted fat-saturated arterial phase MRI (**B**) and portal venous–phase T1-weighted fat-saturated MRI (**C**) in a 50-year-old woman with a 1.2-cm pancreatic head neuroendocrine tumor (*arrow*) identified only on arterial-phase MRI (**B**). A segment II hepatic metastasis (*arrowheads*) is barely visible on arterial-phase CT (**D**) and portal venous–phase CT (**E**) and fat-saturated PVP MRI (**F**) but is clearly visible on arterial-phase T1-weighted fat-saturated MRI (**G**).

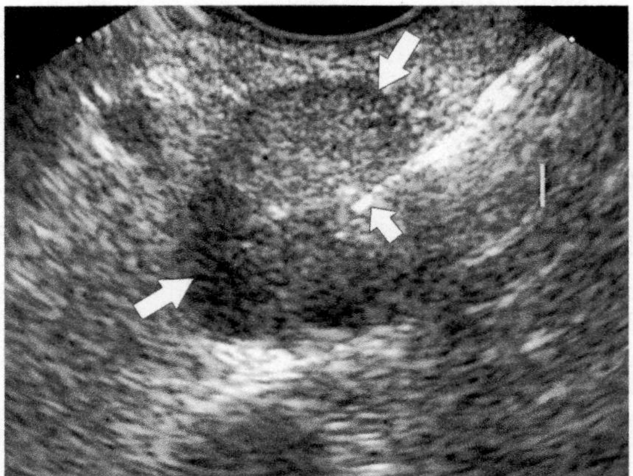

FIGURE 9-54. Endoscopic US in a 44-year-old woman with a normal CT and a 1.4-cm hypoechoic mass (*large arrows*) in the pancreatic tail that represents an insulinoma. A biopsy needle is inserted into the mass (*small arrow*).

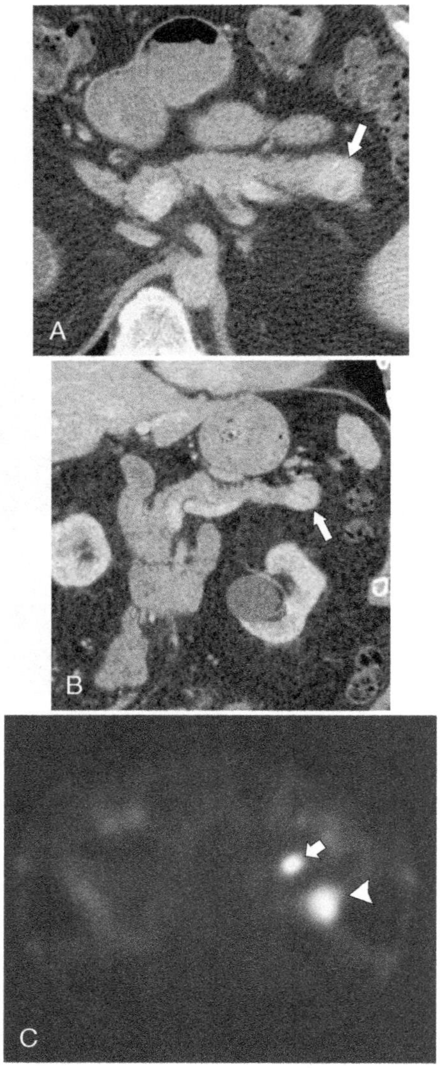

FIGURE 9-55. Axial (**A**) and coronal (**B**) contrast-enhanced CT and pentetreotide study (**C**) in a 66-year-old man with a 1.5-cm hypervascular neuroendocrine tumor in the pancreatic tail (*large arrows*). The lesion is hyperactive on pentetreotide imaging (*small arrow*). Other activity (*arrowhead*) is normal in the left kidney.

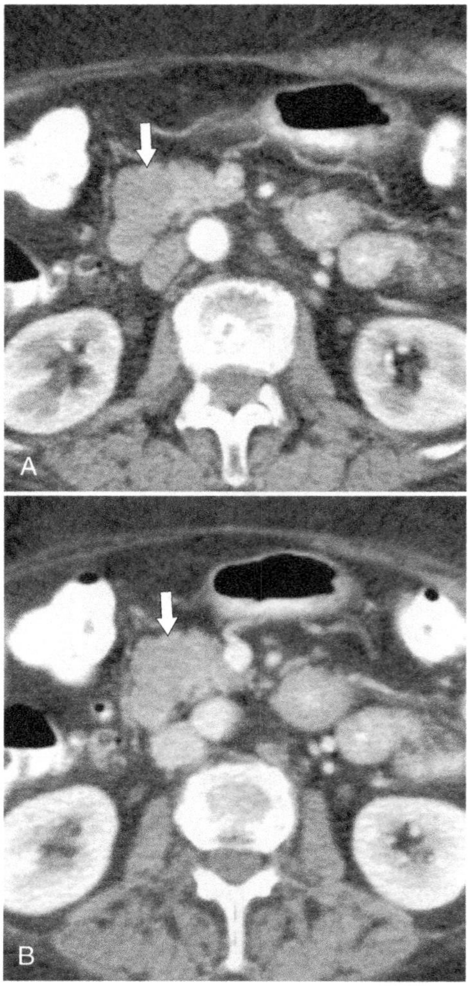

FIGURE 9-57. Axial contrast-enhanced CT in arterial (**A**) and portal venous (**B**) phases in a 55-year-old man with a proven neuroendocrine tumor in the pancreatic head (*arrows*). The 2.5-cm tumor enhances in neither phase.

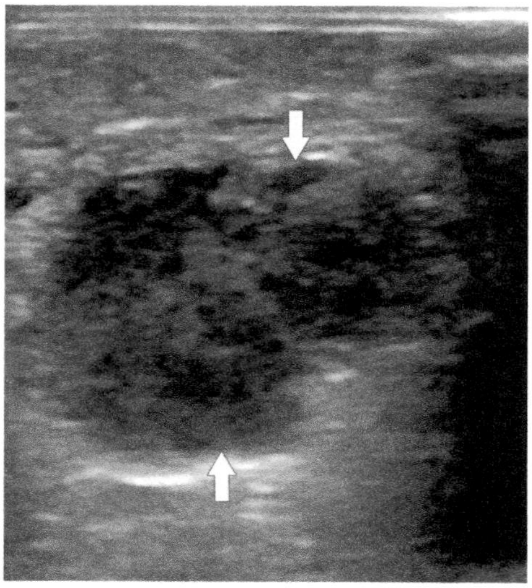

FIGURE 9-56. Intraoperative US in a 32-year-old woman with clinical signs of insulinoma. Contrast-enhanced CT was negative, but the hypoechoic tumor (*arrows*) was imaged perioperatively.

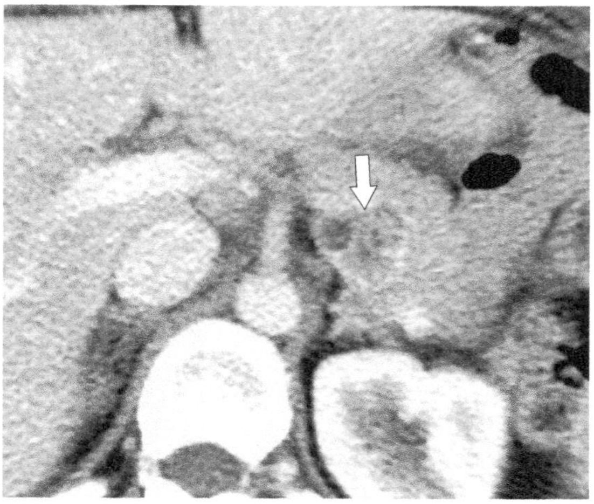

FIGURE 9-58. Axial contrast-enhanced CT in a 47-year-old woman showing a 2.5-cm complex partially cystic pancreatic neuroendocrine tumor in the body of the pancreas (*arrow*).

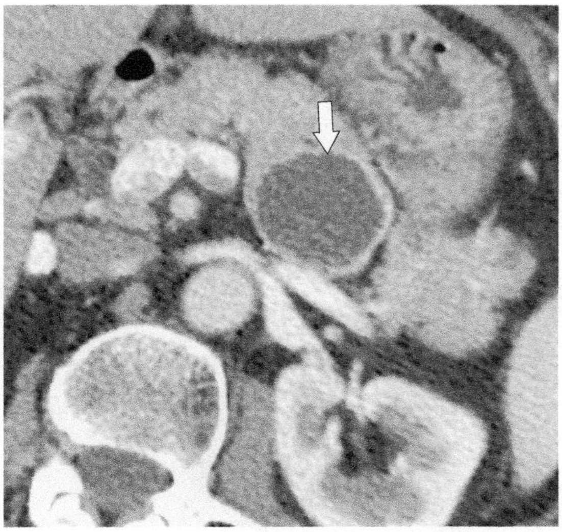

FIGURE 9-59. Axial contrast-enhanced CT in a 63-year-old woman with a 3.5-cystic insulinoma (*arrow*) in the pancreatic tail.

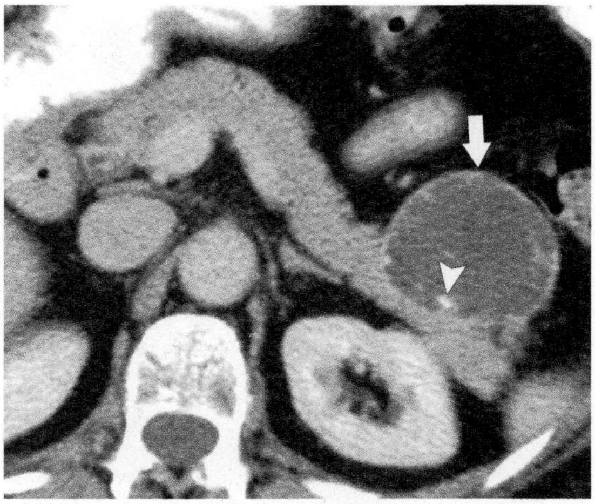

FIGURE 9-61. Axial contrast-enhanced CT in a 63-year-old woman with a 4.5-cm complex pancreatic tail mass (*arrow*) with partial calcification (*arrowhead*) that proved to be a cystic insulinoma tumor by pathological study.

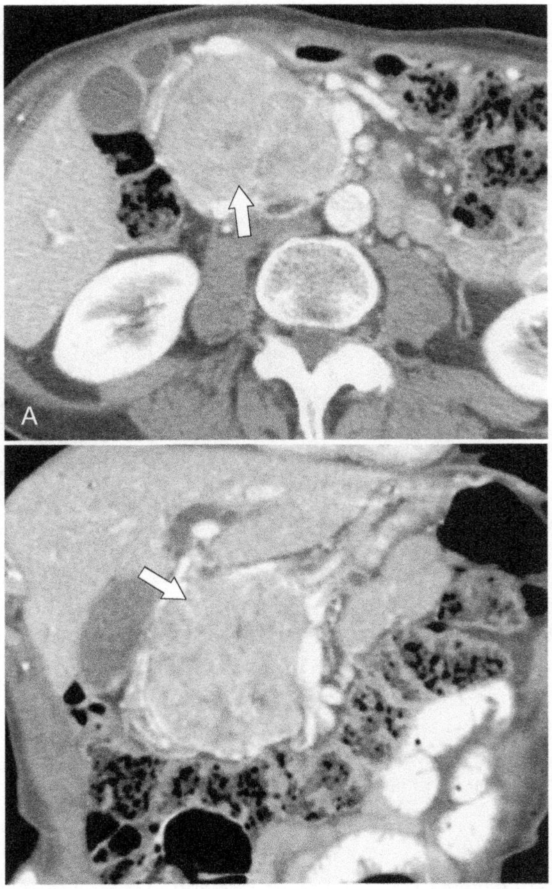

FIGURE 9-60. Axial (**A**) and coronal (**B**) contrast-enhanced CT in a 72-year-old man with a 9-cm complex pancreatic head mass (*arrows*) representing a nonfunctioning islet cell tumor. As the tumor was nonfunctioning, the patient presented late with abdominal pain.

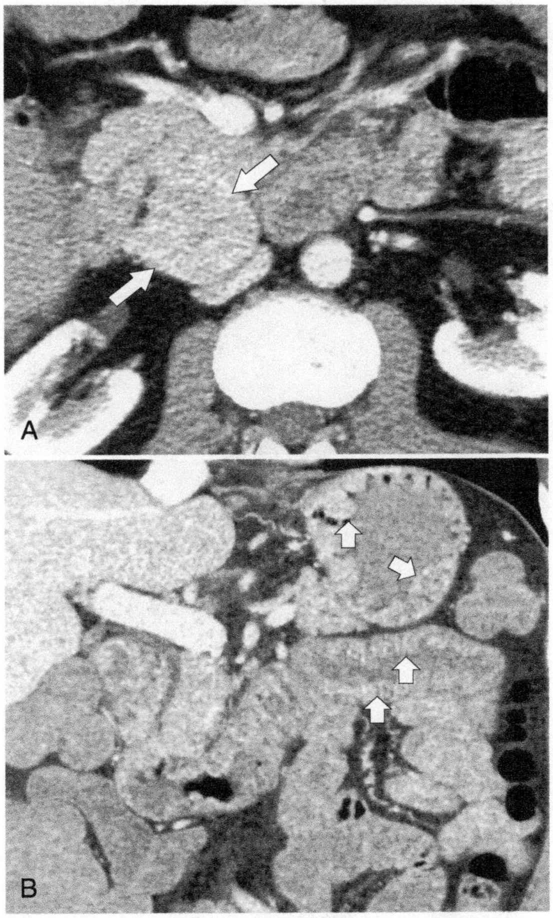

FIGURE 9-62. Axial (**A**) and coronal (**B**) contrast-enhanced CT in a 54-year-old man with a 4.5-cm hypervascular gastrinoma just posterior to the uncinate process (*large arrows*). Coronal images demonstrate marked gastric and small bowel mucosal thickening secondary to diffuse gastritis resulting from Zollinger-Ellison syndrome (*small arrows*).

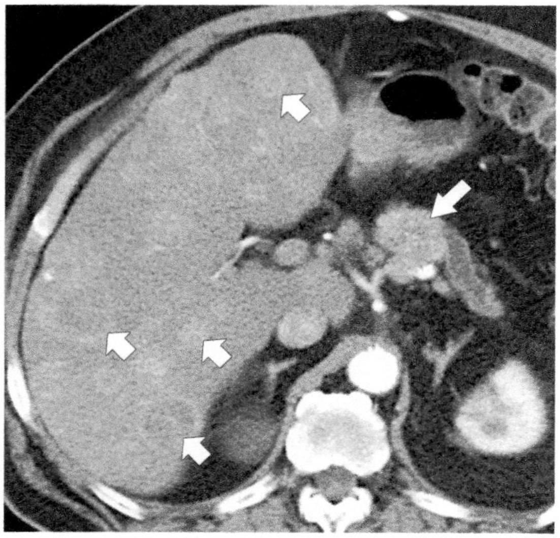

FIGURE 9-63. Axial arterial-phase contrast-enhanced CT in a 66-year-old man with a 2.5-cm pancreatic head gastrinoma (*arrow*) and an obstructed pancreatic duct. There are multiple subtle hepatic metastases (*small arrows*).

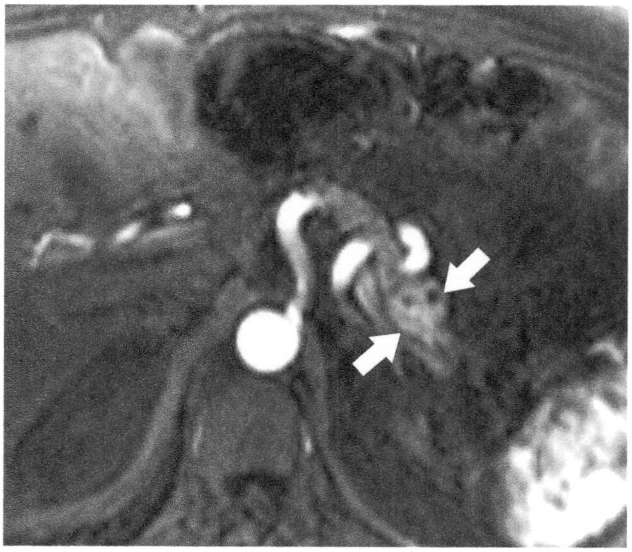

FIGURE 9-65. Axial T1-weighted fat-saturated postcontrast MRI in a 44-year-old woman with a 2-cm subtle and complex pancreatic tail mass (*arrows*) caused by a VIPoma.

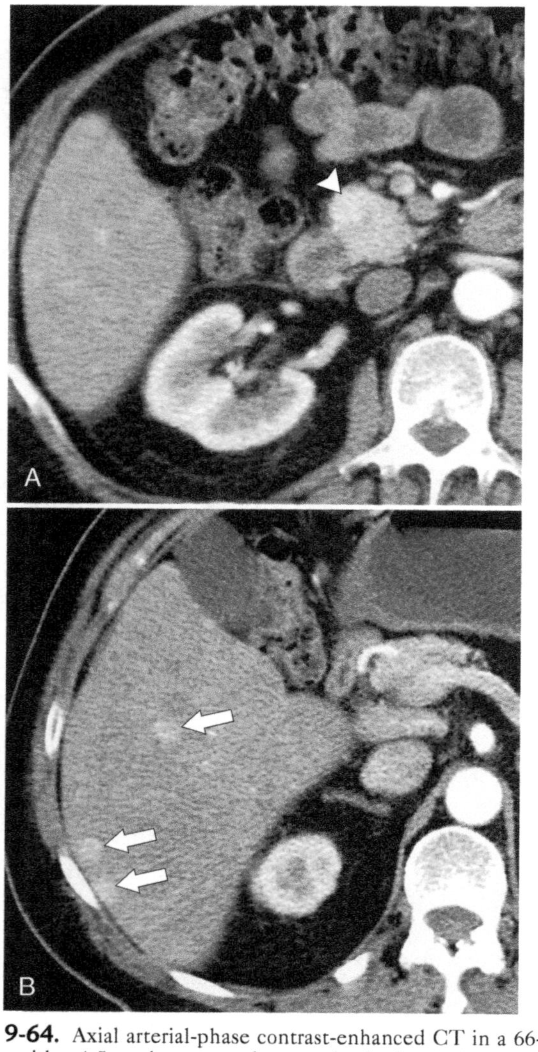

FIGURE 9-64. Axial arterial-phase contrast-enhanced CT in a 66-year-old man with a 1.5-cm hypervascular mass in the head of the pancreas (**A**; *arrowhead*) representing glucagonoma. Images of the liver during the same scan demonstrate three hypervascular metastases (**B**; *arrows*).

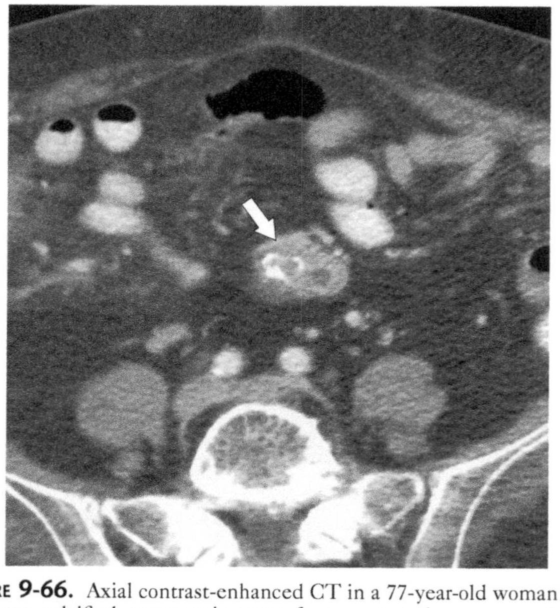

FIGURE 9-66. Axial contrast-enhanced CT in a 77-year-old woman with a 3.5-cm calcified mesenteric mass from metastatic somatostatinoma (*arrows*).

confined mostly to the pancreas. They can, however, occur in the chest and brain. Many have metastasized at the time of diagnosis, mainly to the liver and mesentery (Fig. 9-66).

Lymphoma

Primary pancreatic lymphoma is rare and usually non-Hodgkin. The pancreas is more commonly involved by direct invasion from extrapancreatic disease. When present, however, lymphoma presents with either an isolated relatively avascular homogeneous mass (Fig. 9-67) or diffuse pancreatic involvement with peripancreatic extension. As is common with lymphoma elsewhere, the tumor does not obliterate the immediate vasculature. Rather, vessels tend to course relatively normally through the tumor (Fig. 9-67). PET or PET/CT is useful to document response to treatment.

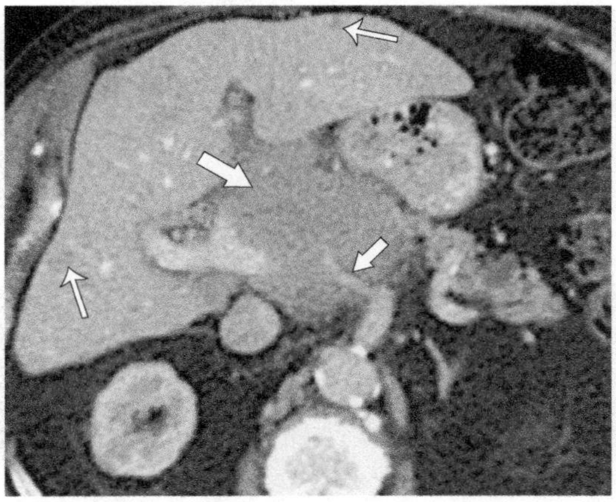

FIGURE 9-67. Axial contrast-enhanced CT in a 44-year-old man with pancreatic lymphoma and a large pancreatic head mass (*large arrow*). As with lymphoma elsewhere, vascular patency (hepatic artery) is preserved (*small arrow*). There are subtle liver metastases (*thin arrows*).

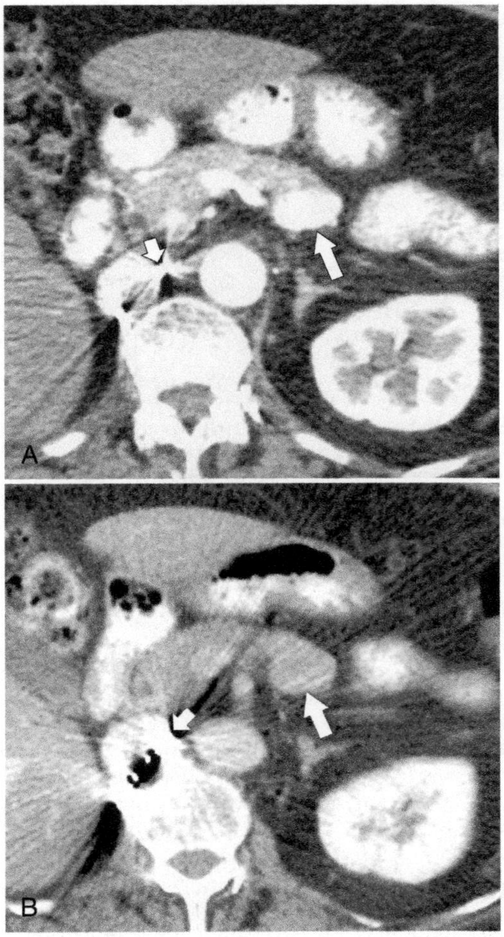

FIGURE 9-68. Axial arterial-phase contrast-enhanced CT (**A**) in a 70-year-old woman with a hypervascular renal cell metastasis (*large arrows*), poorly visualized on portal venous–phase images (**B**). Note surgical clips from prior right nephrectomy (*small arrows*).

Metastases

Local extension from adjacent malignancies (e.g., colon or stomach) is most common. When hematogenous, metastases can be either hypervascular (Fig. 9-68) or hypovascular (Fig. 9-69), depending on the primary tumor, and also multiple. Multiplicity may give a clue to the diagnosis because without a history of malignancy, these metastases could be confused with pancreatic neuroendocrine or pancreatic adenocarcinoma (Fig. 9-70). The most common primary malignancies are renal cell, lung, breast, colon, and melanoma. Renal cell metastases may occur many years after removal of the primary lesion.

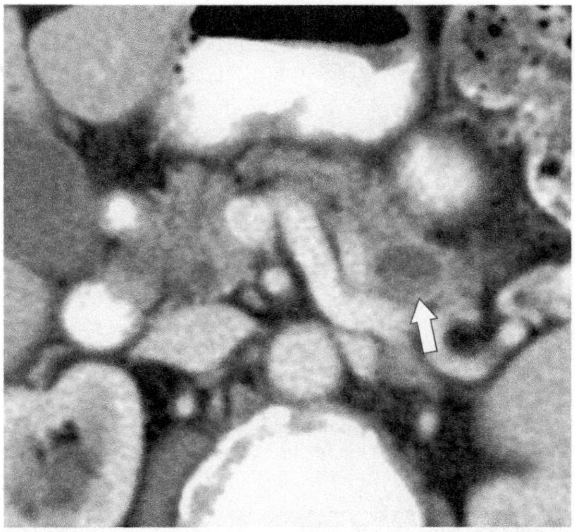

FIGURE 9-69. Axial contrast-enhanced CT in a 66-year-old woman with a 1.8-cm low-density cystic breast metastasis (*arrow*) in the pancreatic tail.

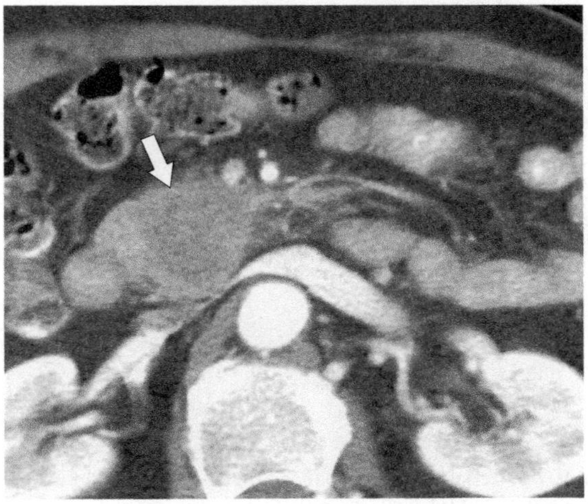

FIGURE 9-70. Axial contrast-enhanced CT in a 62-year-old man with a 3.8-cm hypodense lung metastasis in the pancreatic head and uncinate (*arrow*). This could be confused with a pancreatic adenocarcinoma.

Pancreaticoblastoma

Pancreaticoblastomas are rare tumors of early childhood but can rarely present in adults. They are usually indolent and slow growing and are therefore large at the time of initial presentation. They tend to be soft and gelatinous, so may not produce obstructive symptoms (i.e., ductal obstruction). Pancreaticoblastomas are associated with Beckwith-Wiedemann* syndrome, a spectrum usually seen in childhood with multiple congenital defects and increased incidence of malignancies. On contrast-enhanced CT, in addition to usually being large, pancreaticoblastomas show a multilobulated mass separated by enhancing septa (Fig. 9-71).

*John Bruce Beckwith (1933-), American pathologist; Hans Rudolf Wiedemann (1915-2006), German pediatrician.

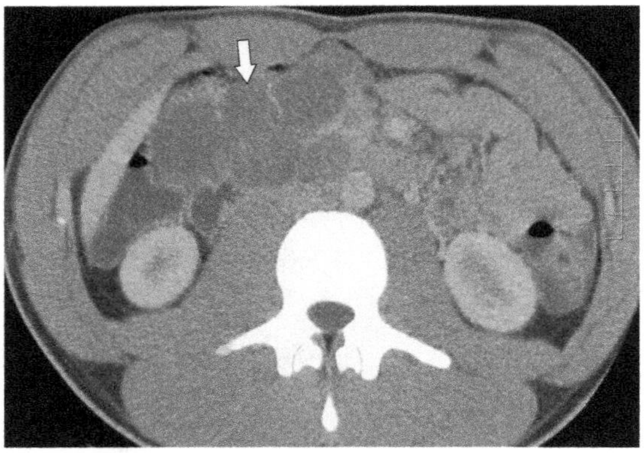

FIGURE 9-71. Axial contrast-enhanced CT in an 18-year-old man with a multilobulated pancreatic mass (*arrow*) caused by pancreaticoblastoma.

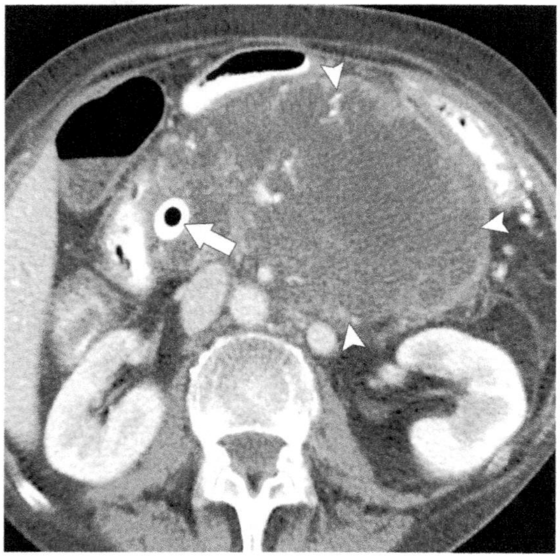

FIGURE 9-72. Axial contrast-enhanced CT in a 67-year-old woman with a large predominantly necrotic and cystic mass (*arrowheads*) caused by colloid carcinoma. There is a biliary metallic stent in situ (*arrow*).

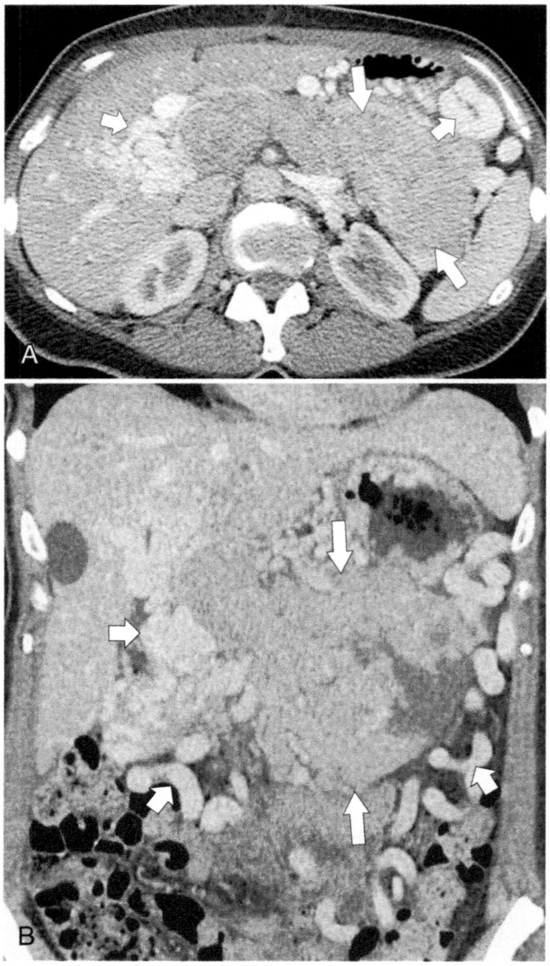

FIGURE 9-73. Axial (**A**) and coronal (**B**) contrast-enhanced CT in a 44-year-old woman with acinar cell carcinoma of the pancreas. There is a large heterogeneous pancreatic mass (*large arrows*) with multiple varices caused by splenic and portal vein thrombus (*small arrows*). There is an incidental hepatic cyst.

Colloid Carcinoma

Colloid carcinomas are rare pancreatic tumors that were previously classified as either adenocarcinoma or mucinous cystadenocarcinoma. Despite the usual large size of colloid carcinomas at presentation, patients with these tumors have a much better prognosis than do those with ductal adenocarcinoma. Even without surgical removal, patients can live for years. With contrast-enhanced CT, it can be understood why these tumors were confused with other tumors, because they often demonstrate large necrotic and cystic regions (Fig. 9-72).

Acinar Cell Carcinoma

Acinar cell carcinomas are very rare pancreatic neoplasms arising from acinar cells, which are usually responsible for exocrine enzyme production. Therefore they often oversecrete lipase, causing widespread fat necrosis, which may present clinically as subcutaneous nodules. Patients with these carcinomas have a slightly better prognosis than those with ductal adenocarcinomas. On contrast-enhanced CT the tumors have no distinguishing features and are often large and heterogeneous with areas of necrosis (Fig. 9-73). Occasionally they appear cystic and may be confused with other cystic pancreatic neoplasms.

Anaplastic Carcinoma

Anaplastic carcinomas are rare malignant pancreatic masses that are highly aggressive and readily metastasize to the liver and lungs. They are usually seen in the elderly and present in patients with a relatively short history of pain and general loss of well-being, particularly if they are metastatic. At imaging, the mass is usually found in the body and tail and is large and highly heterogeneous with areas of hypervascularity and necrosis.

Small Cell Carcinoma

Small cell carcinomas are rare pancreatic tumors that are usually large at presentation but generally less aggressive than anaplastic carcinomas. They respond relatively well to chemotherapy. Small cell carcinomas are usually found in the pancreatic head.

Giant Cell Carcinoma

Giant cell carcinoma is another type of rare malignant pancreatic tumor, characteristically presenting as a relatively large complex mass at presentation, but often appearing similar to mucinous neoplasms in that it can be exophytic and multicystic,

***Box 9-3.* Cystic Pancreatic Masses**

NEOPLASMS
Serous (microcystic)
  Mucinous
    Mucinous cystic neoplasm (macrocystic)
    IPMN
Cystic islet cell tumor (rare)
Necrotic large pancreatic adenocarcinoma
Necrotic metastases
SPEN
Cystic teratoma
Acinar cell carcinoma

INFLAMMATORY/INFECTIOUS
Pseudocyst
Abscess
Hydatid

SIMPLE CYSTS
Solitary (congenital)
Cystic fibrosis
von Hippel-Lindau disease
Adult polycystic kidney disease

IPMN, Intraductal papillary mucinous neoplasm; *SPEN*, solid and pseudopapillary neoplasm of the pancreas.

TABLE 9-7 Differentiation of Pancreatic Cystic Neoplasms

Characteristic	Serous Cystic Neoplasm	Mucinous Cystic Neoplasm	IPMN
Malignant potential	No	Yes	Yes
Age	>60 years	40-60 years	>60 years
Sex	F/M 1.5:1	F/M 8:1	M>F
Location	Head (70%)	Body and tail (95%)	Head/uncinate 55% Body/tail 10% Multiple/diffuse 35%
Ductal involvement	No	No	Main/side branch 70% Side branch only 30%
Size of cyst	<20 mm	>20 mm	Usually <20 mm
Number of cysts	>6	<6	Usually single (can be multiple)
Enhancement	Hypervascular	Hypovascular	Hypovascular
Calcification	40% amorphous	20% rim	Usually no, but possible when malignant
Cyst content	Glycogen	Mucin	Mucin

IPMN, Intraductal papillary mucinous neoplasms.

with multiple internal septa and calcification of the wall and septa. Giant cell carcinomas rarely metastasize, so the prognosis is usually good in these patients if the primary tumor is removed surgically.

CYSTIC PANCREATIC MASSES

Cystic Pancreatic Neoplasms

Approximately 90% of cystic pancreatic neoplasms are benign, with the remaining malignant 10% arising predominantly arising from mucinous tumors. Many lesions appear similar at imaging, however, and the challenge for the radiologist is to determine which lesions need to be monitored more closely than others. With modern imaging techniques, it is possible to differentiate many by their location, size, and internal architecture along with the sex and age of the patient (Box 9-3 and Table 9-7). However, some lesions can be identified only by endoscopic US and biopsy or complete surgical removal.

Simple Pancreatic Cysts

Simple pancreatic cysts are uncommon and may be congenital in origin, since they are more commonly seen in neonates. At imaging, they are usually thin walled and less than 2 cm, without septa, mural nodules, or thickening, and are therefore innocent (Fig. 9-74). They are usually single but can be multiple. Up to 10% of patients with adult polycystic kidney disease show simple pancreatic cysts, as do 50% of patients with von Hippel-Lindau* disease (Fig. 9-75). Pancreatic cysts can also be seen in patients with Beckwith-Wiedemann syndrome.

Pancreatic Enteric Duplication Cyst

Pancreatic enteric duplication cysts are rare and most commonly found in children. They are usually incidental but can present with complications of pancreatitis and therefore can be confused with pancreatic pseudocyst. They are, however, usually well circumscribed and cystic in appearance and tend to be larger than simple cysts (Fig. 9-76).

Pancreatic Cystosis

In patients with cystic fibrosis, the pancreas typically becomes fatty replaced (Figs. 9-13 and 9-14) or less commonly calcified. In some patients, however, pancreatic epithelial cysts develop because some exocrine function remains, but their ducts are blocked by the viscous inspissated secretions (Fig. 9-77). The older the individual is, the more likely these cysts are to develop.

Serous Microcystic Pancreatic Neoplasm

Serous microcystic pancreatic neoplasms are of uncertain cause but are considered benign. Their walls consist of cuboidal epithelium and secrete glycogenic-type material. They are more common in women (4:1) and in patients with von Hippel-Lindau disease. They are much less common than mucinous tumors and account for approximately 15% of cystic pancreatic neoplasms. They are difficult to differentiate from other cystic neoplasms, particularly when small, but as they enlarge, these neoplasms may show characteristic features (Table 9-7). They are usually discovered incidentally but if large can produce symptoms of bowel or biliary duct obstruction.

At imaging, the lesion is usually well circumscribed and positioned in the pancreatic head. Multiple small (<2 cm, often <1 cm) lace-like cysts are identified, giving them their well-known "honeycomb" and microcystic appearance (seen in approximately 90% of serous cystadenomas) (Fig. 9-78). Approximately 10% show larger cysts and are termed oligocystic or macrocystic (not to be confused with macrocystic mucinous cysts). The cyst walls may enhance and show a central scar, which can calcify, a useful differentiating feature from mucinous tumors (Fig. 9-79). The tumor typically does not cause

*Eugen von Hippel (1867-1939), German ophthalmologist; Arvid Vilhelm Lindau (1892-1958), Swedish pathologist.

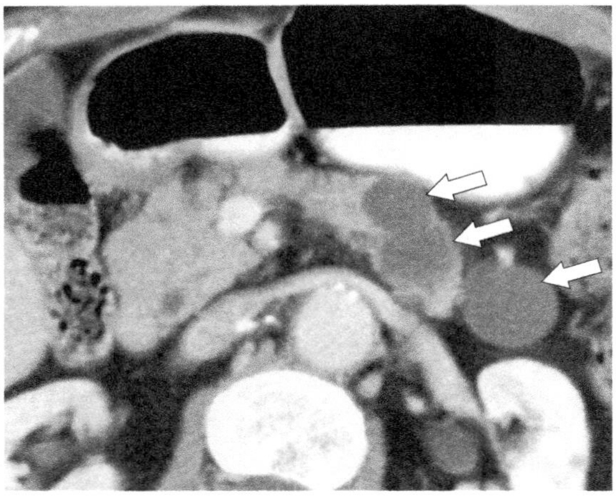

FIGURE 9-74. Axial contrast-enhanced CT in a 71-year-old woman with three smooth-walled simple pancreatic cysts (*arrows*).

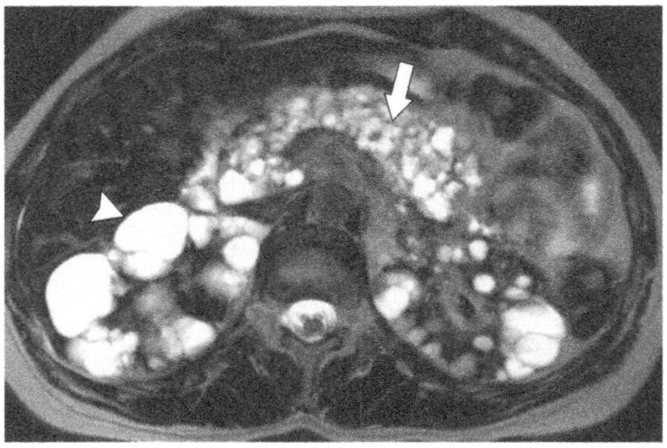

FIGURE 9-75. Axial T2-weighted MRI in a 32-year-old woman with von Hippel-Lindau disease. There are numerous simple pancreatic (*arrow*) and renal cysts (*arrowhead*).

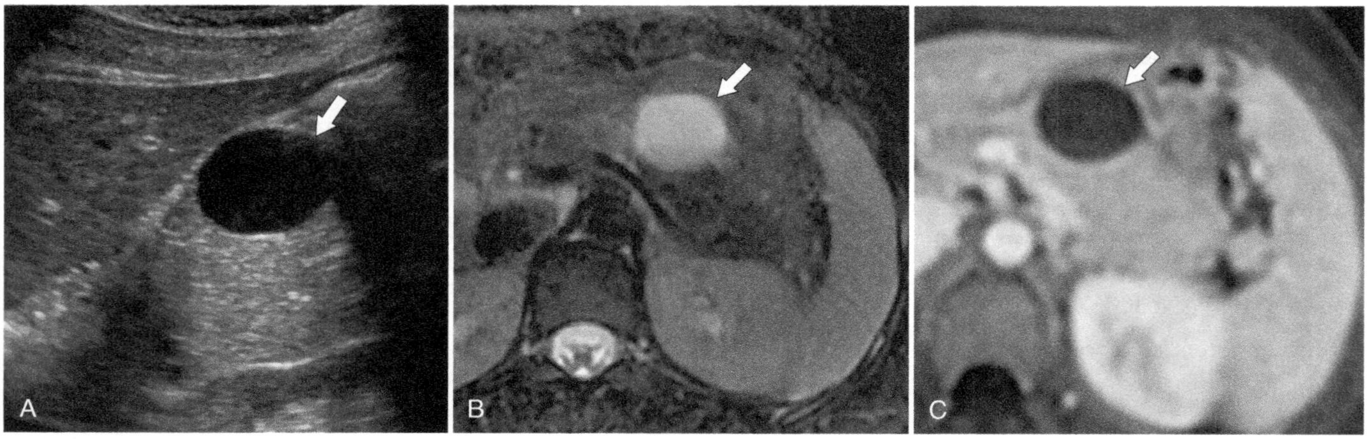

FIGURE 9-76. Transverse US (**A**) and T2-weighted (**B**) and postcontrast (**C**) MRI of the pancreatic body in a 24-year-old man demonstrating a uniform hypoechoic, nonenhancing, cystic, 3-cm mass (*arrows*) representing a pancreatic duplication cyst.

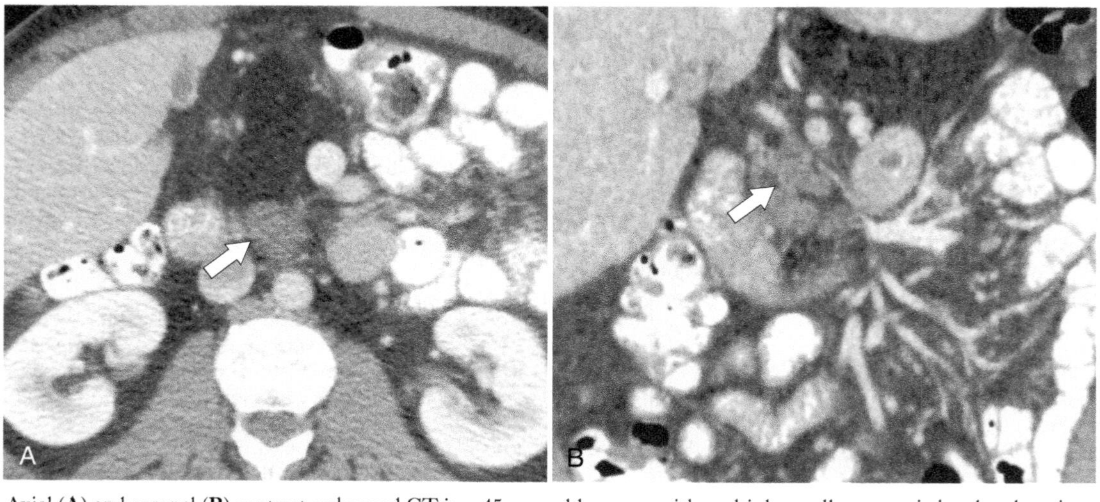

FIGURE 9-77. Axial (**A**) and coronal (**B**) contrast-enhanced CT in a 45-year-old woman with multiple small pancreatic head and uncinate cysts (*arrows*) caused by pancreatic cystosis in cystic fibrosis. Note that the remaining pancreas has been fatty replaced.

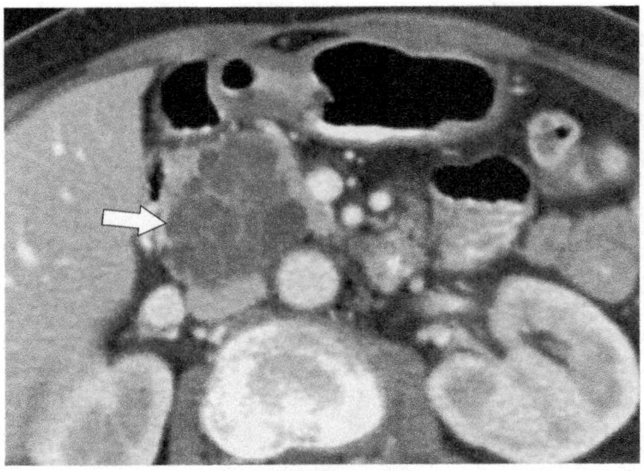

FIGURE 9-78. Axial contrast-enhanced CT in a 44-year-old woman with a 6-cm multicystic mass in the head of the pancreas (*arrow*). The numerous small cysts are consistent with a serous cystadenoma.

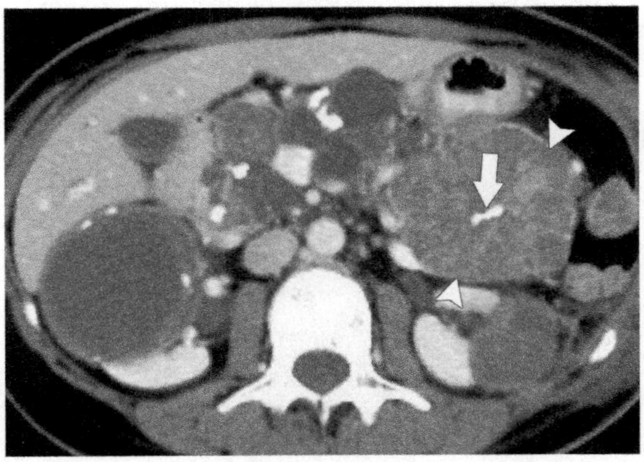

FIGURE 9-79. Axial contrast-enhanced CT in a 48-year-old woman with an 8-cm pancreatic tail mass (*arrowheads*) with central scar calcification (*arrow*) characteristic of serous cystadenoma. There are multiple other pancreatic cystic changes caused by chronic pancreatitis in the head.

pancreatic duct dilatation. Imaging with MRI may delineate the size and number of cysts better than CT, particularly in small lesions, because of MRI's better contrast characteristics with T2-weighted images (particularly when fat saturated) (Fig. 9-80). Cyst wall and central scar enhancement is also noted after gadolinium administration.

Once the cystic lesion is detected, usually by CT, and before a definitive diagnosis is made, the main concern is whether it is serous or mucinous. Mucinous lesions require more aggressive management because of their propensity to become malignant. Despite this conundrum, these lesions can be managed less aggressively (partly because they occur in the elderly) and are generally not removed unless they are large and produce symptoms, even if a simple-appearing mucinous tumor has not been totally excluded. The lead time for mucinous tumors to become malignant is usually sufficiently long that delaying surgical removal (a procedure not without complications) may be prudent if the lesion shows no malignant features. Definitive diagnosis may require endoscopic US (Fig. 9-81), which can often show the multiple small cystic masses to even better advantage than MRI. Percutaneous aspiration of cyst contents is then usually performed and yields negative carcinoembryonic antigen values.

Mucinous Pancreatic Neoplasms

Mucinous pancreatic neoplasms are differentiated into mucinous cystic neoplasms and intraductal pancreatic mucinous neoplasms because both produce mucin.

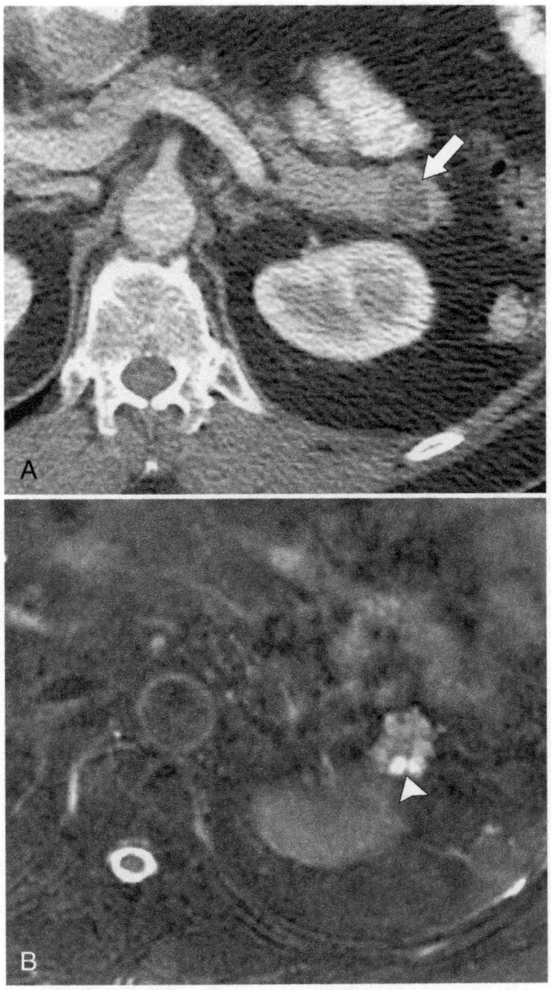

FIGURE 9-80. Axial contrast-enhanced CT (**A**) and T2-weighted MR images (**B**) in a 64-year-old woman with a 2-cm pancreatic tail serous cystadenoma (*arrow*). The multiple small septa (*arrowhead*) are better appreciated with fat-saturated T2-weighted MRI.

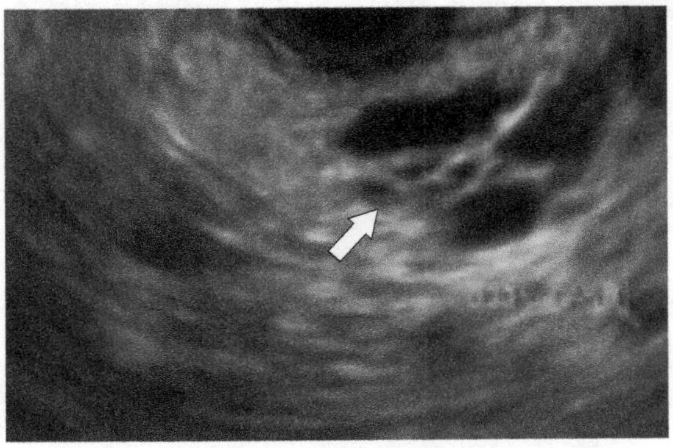

FIGURE 9-81. Endoscopic US in a 78-year-old woman with a serous cystadenoma. The mass has multiple small cystic components (*arrow*).

Mucinous Cystic Neoplasms

Mucinous cystic neoplasms result from mucinous production from tall columnar epithelium and are far more common than serous tumors. They most commonly occur in the pancreatic tail (90%) and in middle-aged women (40 to 60 years of age; 9:1). The diagnosis therefore should be considered mucinous until proven

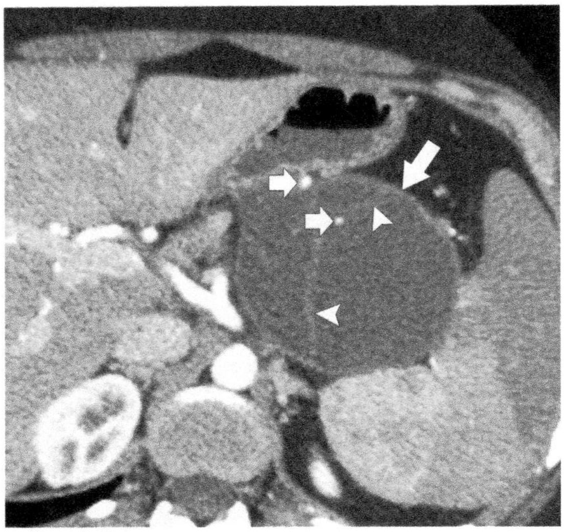

FIGURE 9-82. Axial contrast-enhanced CT in a 76-year-old man with a 10-cm macrocystic lesion (*large arrow*) in the pancreatic tail representing a mucinous cystadenoma. Septa separating larger cysts are seen (*arrowheads*), and there are two punctate areas of calcification (*small arrows*).

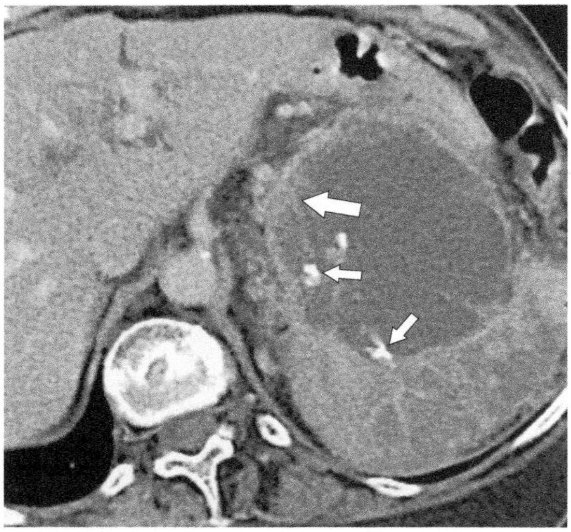

FIGURE 9-83. Axial contrast-enhanced CT in a 66-year-old woman with a 12-cm complex cystic mass in the pancreatic tail representing a malignant cystadenocarcinoma. Note scattered calcification (*small arrows*) and mural nodules (*large arrow*).

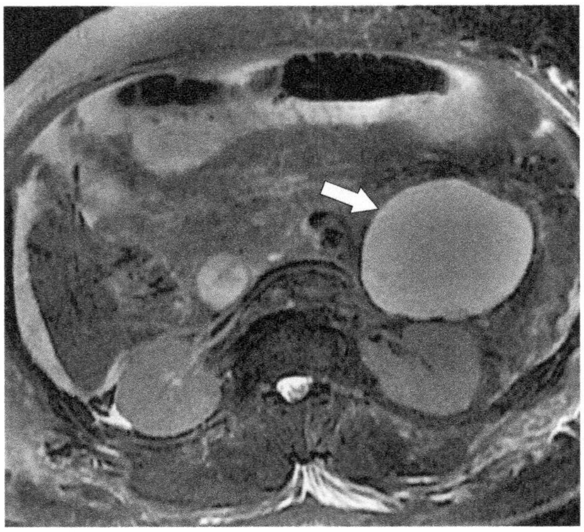

FIGURE 9-84. Axial T2-weighted fat-saturated MRI in a 75-year-old woman with a unilocular 7-cm mucinous cystadenoma in the pancreatic tail (*arrow*).

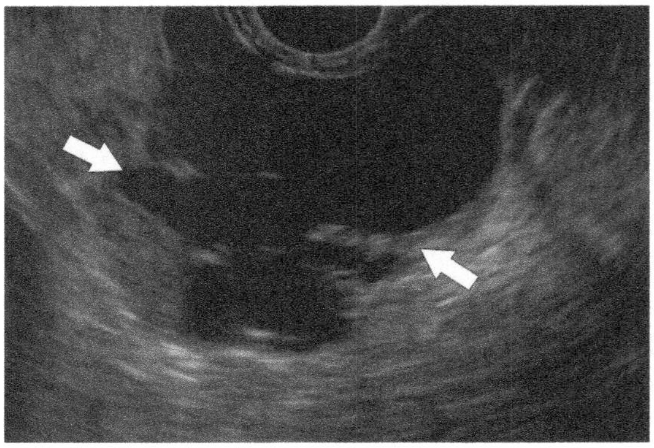

FIGURE 9-85. Endoscopic US of a 57-year-old woman with a 4-cm macrocystic neoplasm of the pancreas. The cysts are few in number and relatively larger than microcystic disease (*arrows*).

otherwise in a middle-aged woman with a cystic tail pancreatic lesion. However, when small, these neoplasms may be very difficult to differentiate from other cystic neoplasms. Given this, and their 10% chance of malignant transformation, the threshold for needle aspiration (endoscopic US) is relatively low. The neoplasms are then usually surgically removed if mucinous. Sometimes, benign-appearing lesions are periodically followed with imaging (6 months to 1 year) if the patient is elderly because the chance of malignancy is still low and surgical removal is not without risks.

At imaging, several features distinguish mucinous cystic neoplasms from other cystic pancreatic neoplasms (Table 9-7). Cysts are generally fewer (<6) and may sometimes even be unilocular. The cysts are usually larger (>2 cm) than those seen in serous cystic pancreatic neoplasms. Enhancement can be seen in the cyst walls, including any internal septa. Wall or septal calcification is observed in approximately 15% of lesions (Fig. 9-82). Cyst walls may contain mural nodules, which markedly increase the likelihood of malignancy, particularly if they enhance (Fig. 9-83). The mass more commonly causes proximal pancreatic duct dilatation than do serous neoplasms. On MRI with T1-weighted imaging, the cyst contents can be of mixed signal if contents are proteinaceous or hemorrhagic, but they are generally hyperintense on T2-weighted imaging (Fig. 9-84). Endoscopic US is often performed to evaluate cyst features and to aspirate fluid contents. Elevated carcinoembryonic antigen 19-9 levels are commonly observed and are specific for mucinous cystic neoplasms (Fig. 9-85).

Intraductal Papillary Mucinous Neoplasms

Intraductal papillary mucinous neoplasms (IPMNs) are also known as intraductal papillary mucinous tumors (IPMTs). These are not as rare as once thought and are relatively frequently detected with high-resolution cross-sectional imaging. They are ductal epithelial in origin, arising either from the side (30%) or combined main and side (70%) pancreatic ducts and producing excessive thick mucin (hence, mucinous-producing tumor), which almost always obstructs the immediate duct or main duct with resulting ductal dilatation.

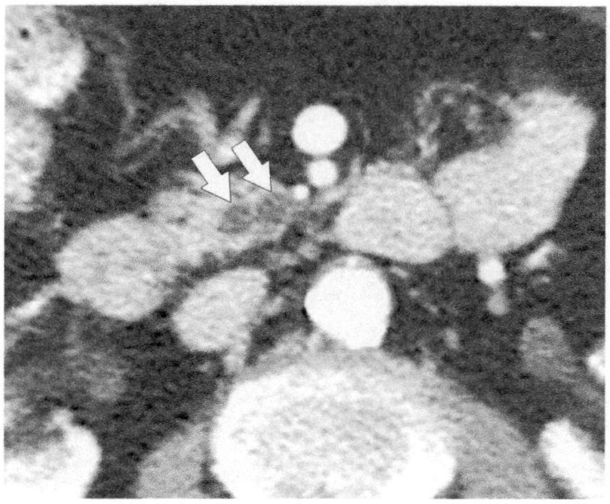

FIGURE 9-86. Axial contrast-enhanced CT in a 79-year-old man with two 8-mm cystic lesions in the uncinate (*arrows*) consistent with side branch IPMNs.

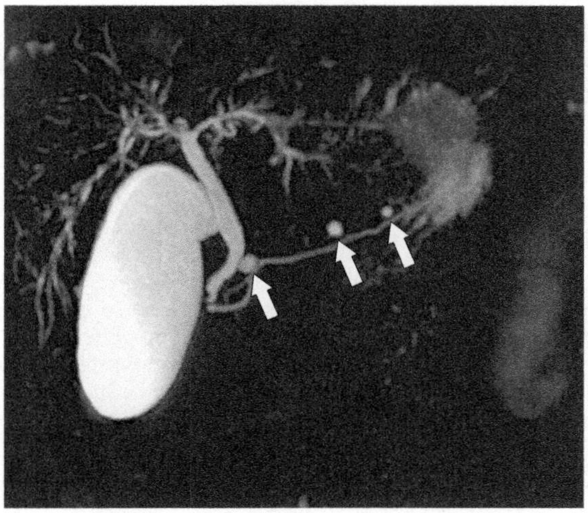

FIGURE 9-87. MRCP in a 74-year-old man demonstrating three small side branch IPMNs (*arrows*).

Most IPMNs are asymptomatic, occurring in elderly men in the head and uncinate of the pancreas (Fig. 9-86) (approximately 55%), with a minority (10%) in the tail. The remainder (35%) are multiple and diffusely located throughout the pancreas (Fig. 9-87). Most are small and cyst like, but main duct variants simply cause duct dilatation owing to excessive mucin production. Main duct IPMNs can involve either the entire duct or a segment (Fig. 9-88). They are more frequently detected by MRCP because of the high T2 mucin signal characteristics (Fig. 9-88), and side branch lesions can often be observed to communicate with the main pancreatic duct (Figs. 9-86 and 9-87).

The lesions are premalignant, with up to 25% showing hyperplastic features, 50% showing dysplastic features, and 25% showing frank adenocarcinoma. Malignant degeneration is more common in main duct tumors than in side branch lesions, and features include presence or development of a solid mass, pancreatic duct dilatation greater than 10 mm, mucin calcification, and polypoid main duct lesions (Fig. 9-89). Therefore annual follow-up is recommended for incidentally detected IPMNs, especially if the patient is younger. Follow-up should ideally be performed with MRCP rather than CT because of better contrast characteristics and avoidance of ionizing radiation. The management of small IPMNs, particularly the more common side branch lesions, in the elderly is more challenging given that they are relatively common and the risk of malignant degeneration may be small. Less frequent monitoring is therefore sometimes practiced.

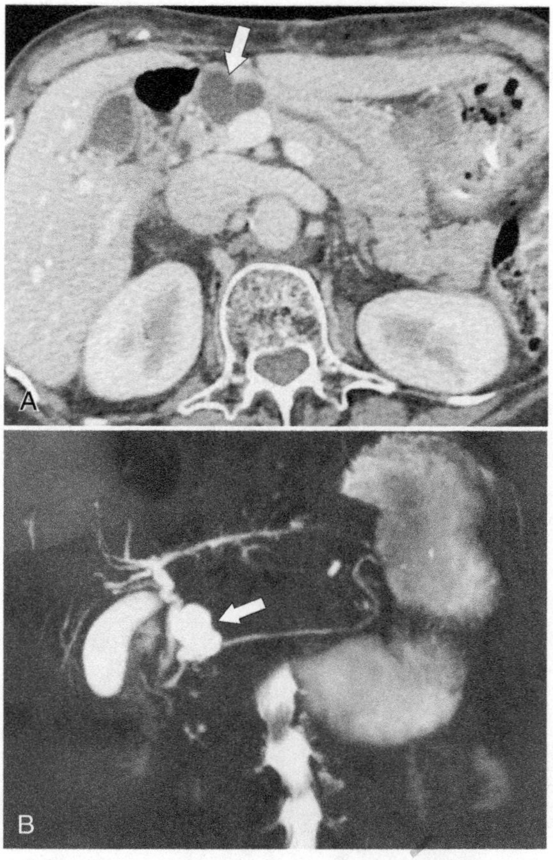

FIGURE 9-88. Axial contrast-enhanced CT (**A**) and MRCP (**B**) in an 80-year-old woman with a main duct IPMN and dilatation of a segment of the main pancreatic duct in the head (*arrows*).

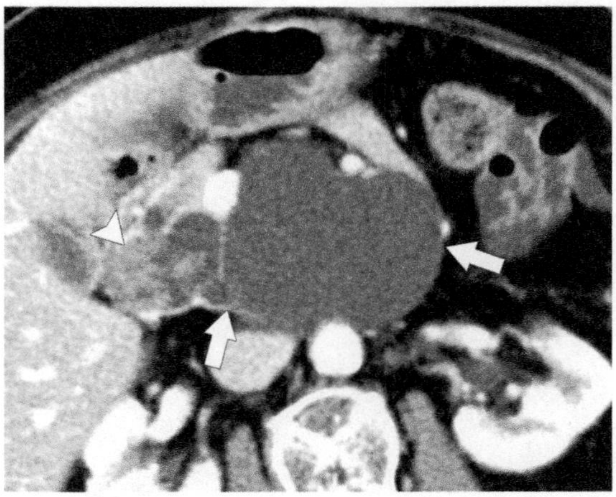

FIGURE 9-89. Axial contrast-enhanced CT in a 78-year-old man with a malignant IPMN demonstrates a multicystic complex mass (*arrows*) and a soft tissue mass projecting into the duodenum (*arrowhead*).

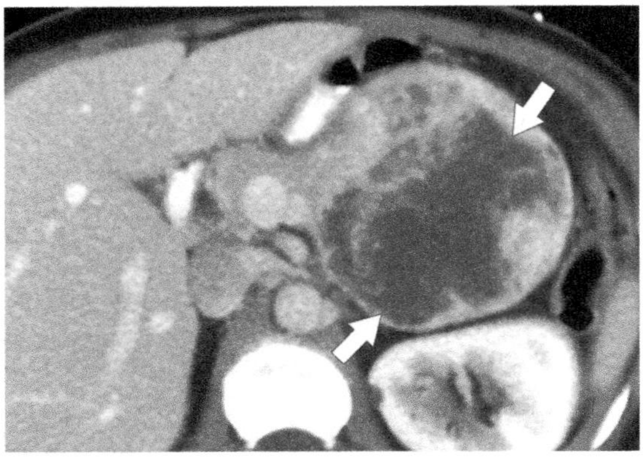

FIGURE 9-90. Axial contrast-enhanced CT in a 57-year-old man with a 9-cm complex predominantly low-density necrotic mass (*arrows*) representing a nonfunctioning pancreatic neuroendocrine tumor.

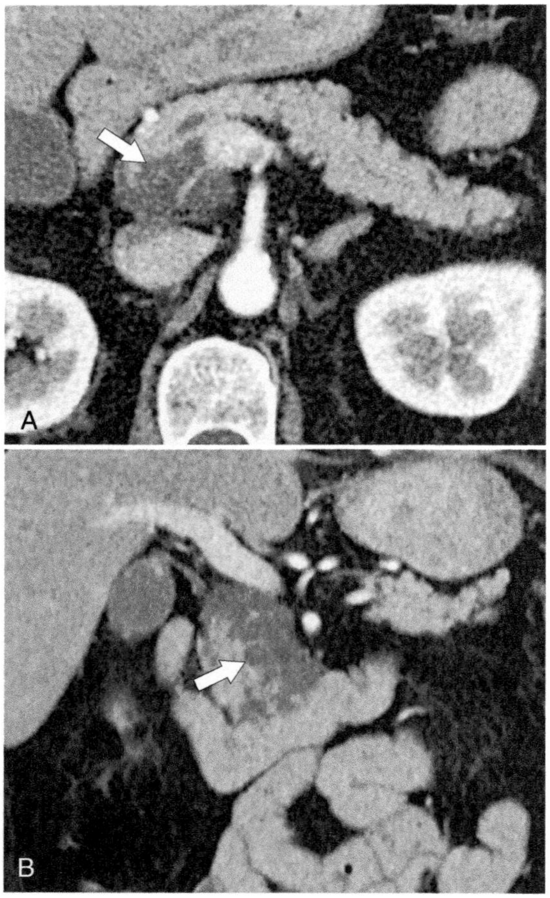

FIGURE 9-91. Axial (**A**) and coronal (**B**) contrast-enhanced CT in a 65-year-old man with a 4-cm complex cystic mass in the head of the pancreas (*arrows*) owing to acinar cell carcinoma.

Cystic Pancreatic Neuroendocrine Tumors

Some PNETs are predominantly cystic (Figs. 9-60 and 9-62), whether functioning or nonfunctioning. Larger nonfunctioning PNETs may undergo central necrosis and appear cystic at presentation (Fig. 9-90).

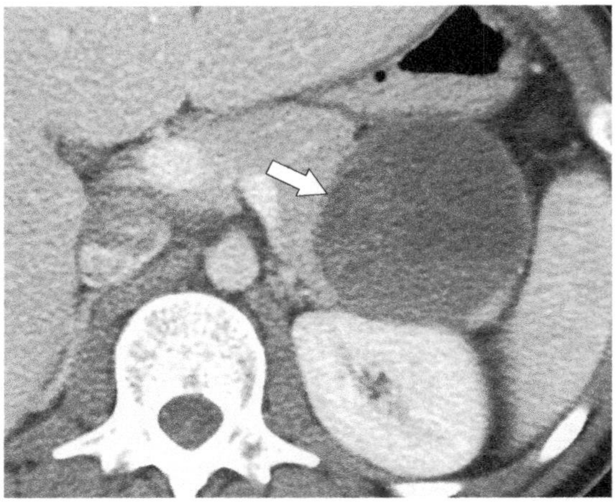

FIGURE 9-92. Axial contrast-enhanced CT in a 17-year-old woman with an 8-cm complex cystic mass (*arrow*) representing a solid and papillary epithelial neoplasm of the pancreas, not dissimilar to mucinous pancreatic neoplasms.

Acinar Cell Tumor

Acinar cell tumors are usually heterogeneous, but some are predominantly cystic and can be confused with other pancreatic cystic neoplasms (Fig. 9-91). These tumors are, however, extremely rare, and the diagnosis may be made only after biopsy or surgery.

Cystic Teratoma of the Pancreas

Cystic teratomas of the pancreas are extremely rare. They usually present late and large and are discovered because of their mass effect on adjacent organs. They tend to be homogeneous and uniform with a rounded, smooth-walled mass, sometimes with rim calcification, but like teratomas elsewhere, they can present with fat, soft tissue, and coarse calcification.

Pancreatic Lymphangioma

Pancreatic lymphangioma, a very rare presentation of lymphangioma, is usually identified in the neck or axilla, retroperitoneum, or mesentery. Similar to lymphangiomas elsewhere, pancreatic lymphangiomas are multicystic with thin septa and uniformly hypodense cyst contents.

Solid and Papillary Epithelial Neoplasm

Solid and papillary epithelial neoplasms (SPENs), also known as solid and pseudopapillary neoplasms, papillary cystic carcinoma tumors, papillary epithelial neoplasms, and Frantz* tumors, are composed of epithelial tissue. These tumors are rare, more common in younger women (90%; often non-Caucasians), and usually large at initial imaging presentation because of their indolent growth pattern. At imaging they are usually located in the pancreatic body and tail. They show complex solid and cystic masses (with or without calcification) and a well-defined capsule, which often avidly enhances. They can therefore appear similar to other cystic pancreatic neoplasms, particularly mucinous tumors (Fig. 9-92). Internal hemorrhage is common because they are highly vascular masses, which can be observed after administration of IV contrast medium, helping to differentiate the lesion from mucinous tumors (Fig. 9-93). Despite these rather alarming imaging features, only 10% are malignant.

*Virginia Kneeland Frantz (1896-1967), American surgical pathologist.

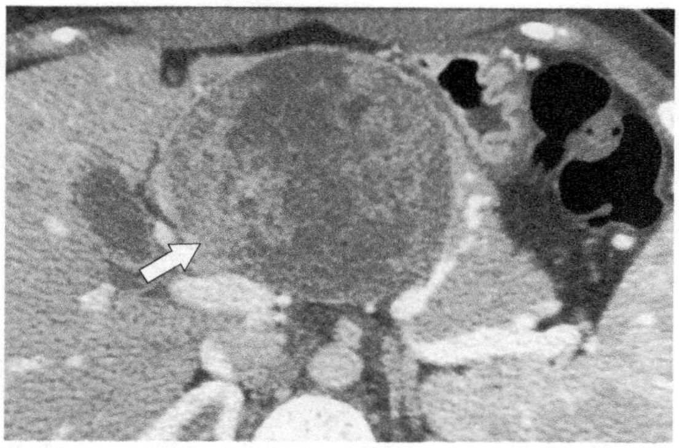

FIGURE 9-93. Axial contrast-enhanced CT in a 24-year-old woman with a 10-cm complex solid and cystic pancreatic head mass (*arrow*) caused by a solid and papillary epithelial neoplasm.

Box 9-4. Pancreatic Calcification

CHRONIC PANCREATITIS
Pancreatic cystic neoplasm (mucinous > serous)
Cystic fibrosis
Ductal stones

PANCREATIC PSEUDOCYST
Hyperparathyroidism/hypercalcemia
Kwashiokor
Hereditary pancreatitis

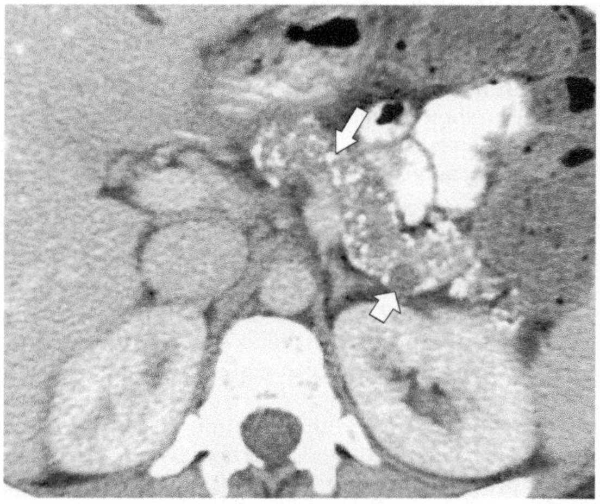

FIGURE 9-94. Axial contrast-enhanced CT in a 27-year-old woman with diffuse pancreatic calcification secondary to cystic fibrosis (*large arrow*). There is also pancreatic cystosis (*small arrow*).

Most are removed for formal diagnosis because of their complex imaging features.

PANCREATIC CALCIFICATION (BOX 9-4)

The most common cause of pancreatic calcification is chronic pancreatitis, usually presenting with multiple variably sized coarse calcifications, which lie within the distorted ducts (Figs. 9-10 and 9-30 through 9-32). The walls of chronic pseudocysts can calcify and are typically thicker and more circumferential than those observed in pancreatic cystic mucinous neoplasms (15% of cases). Calcification is also curvilinear, or sometimes possibly septal (Fig. 9-83), but is not usually circumferential. Calcification in serous tumors is more stellate with a calcification of the central scar (Fig. 9-79).

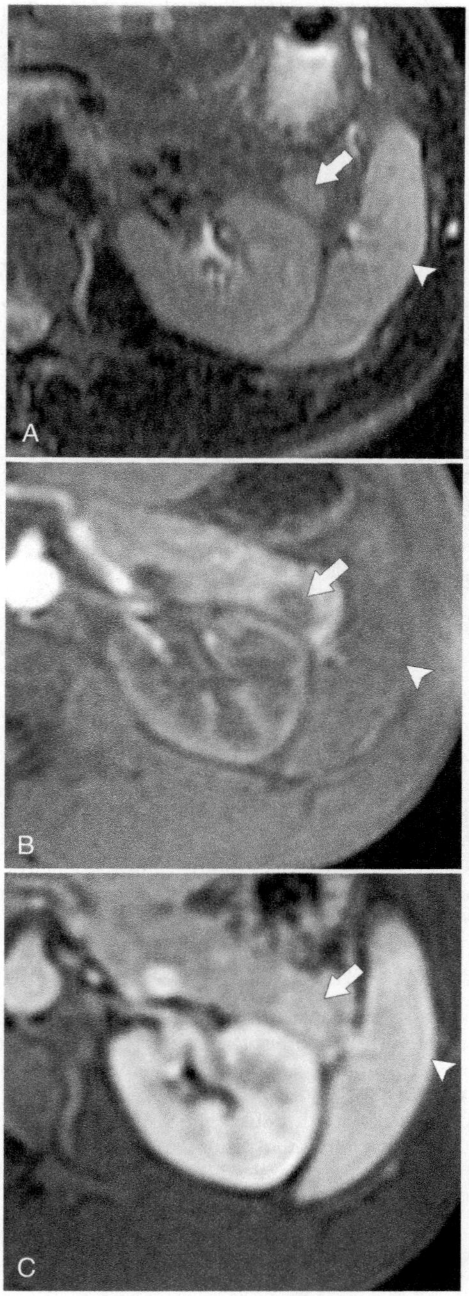

FIGURE 9-95. Axial T2-weighted fat-saturated (**A**) and T1-weighted fat-saturated arterial- (**B**) and portal venous–phase (**C**) postcontrast images in a 29-year-old man with a 1.5-cm pancreatic tail lesion (*arrows*) with similar signal characteristics to the spleen (*arrowheads*) on all pulse sequences, which proved to be an intrapancreatic accessory spleen.

Congenital calcification from cystic fibrosis and hereditary pancreatitis tends to lie within pancreatic ducts. Cystic fibrosis affects the pancreas by developing thick inspissated mucous plugs that "plug" the pancreatic ducts with consequent calcification (Fig. 9-94). Over the longer term the pancreas becomes atrophic and fatty replaced (Figs. 9-12 and 9-15), and patients usually develop diabetes mellitus. Hereditary pancreatitis is a rare autosomal-dominant disease characterized by recurrent bouts of pancreatitis. The resulting chronic pancreatitis and development of ductal pancreatic calcification are typically larger than those seen in other, more common forms of chronic pancreatitis.

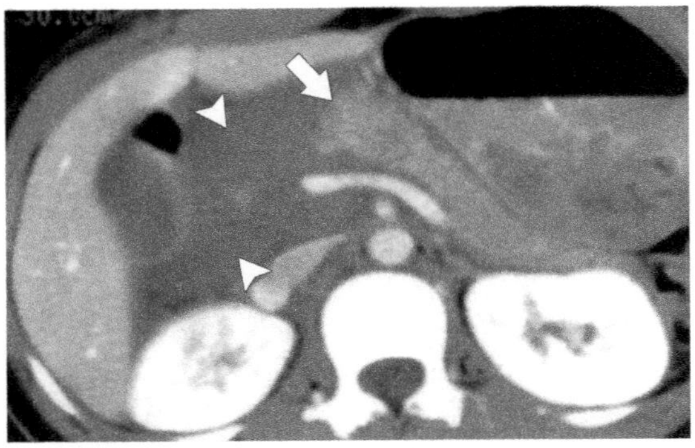

FIGURE 9-96. Axial contrast-enhanced CT in a 38-year-old man with a pancreatic fracture (*arrow*) and diffuse hemorrhage (*arrowheads*).

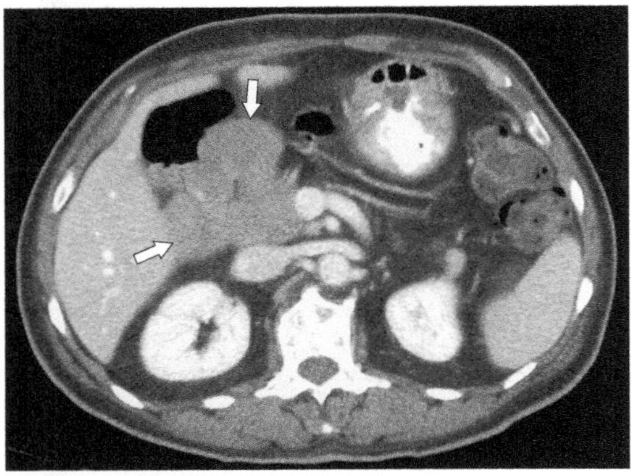

FIGURE 9-97. Axial contrast-enhanced CT in a 56-year-old man with a right upper quadrant mass (*arrows*) caused by a normal afferent loop after a Whipple procedure.

INTRAPANCREATIC ACCESSORY SPLEEN

An accessory spleen (splenules or splenunculi) is relatively common, usually in the region of the splenic hilum, but occasionally is present in the pancreas, particularly the pancreatic tail (Fig. 9-95). Accessory spleens are usually small and enhance similarly to the spleen and may therefore be confused with hypervascular pancreatic tumors, particularly neuroendocrine tumors. Diagnosis may require ^{99m}Tc sulfur colloid imaging to identify the mass as splenic tissue (see Chapter 7).

PANCREATIC TRAUMA

Pancreatic trauma is either penetrating (e.g., stab or gunshot) or blunt (e.g., motor vehicle accident). Contrast-enhanced CT is the investigation of choice, and depending on the severity of the trauma, the pancreas can be enlarged and inflamed because of contusion, although more severe injuries lead to laceration and even transection (Fig. 9-96). With more severe trauma, there may be areas of nonvascularization with the consequent lack of enhancement. Patients with laceration or transection should be evaluated intraoperatively with contrast pancreatography to determine the integrity of the pancreatic duct. Longer term complications include pancreatitis, pancreatic fluid collections, fistula, and abscess formation.

POSTSURGICAL PANCREAS

The Whipple* procedure, the standard surgical maneuver to remove pancreatic head tumors, involves resection of the pancreatic head, duodenum, gastric antrum, and usually gallbladder. A pylorus-sparing Whipple procedure is often performed, which preserves the stomach and pylorus to normalize gastric emptying. With either procedure, a loop of jejunum is used to connect to the bile ducts (choledochojejunal anastomosis) and the remaining pancreas (pancreaticojejunal anastomosis), which usually is referred to as the afferent loop. At follow-up imaging, the radiologist should recognize normal postoperative findings. The normal afferent loop is often partially fluid filled but can appear mass like and should not be mistaken for local recurrence (Fig. 9-97).

Complications of the Whipple procedure include delayed gastric emptying (common to other anastomotic gastric procedures), pancreatic fistula (usually resolves spontaneously), pancreatitis (Fig. 9-98), hemorrhage (Fig. 9-99), abscess, and biliary strictures (common to all biliary-enteric procedures). The afferent loop can become obstructed because of edema, tumor, or adhesions (Fig. 9-100).

Other pancreatic procedures include the Puestow* procedure, performed to facilitate pancreatic duct drainage (usually from chronic pancreatitis) by filleting the pancreas along its length and oversewing a loop of small bowel onto it (pancreaticojejunostomy). The imaging appearances are similar to those of a Whipple procedure, except the pancreatic head is preserved.

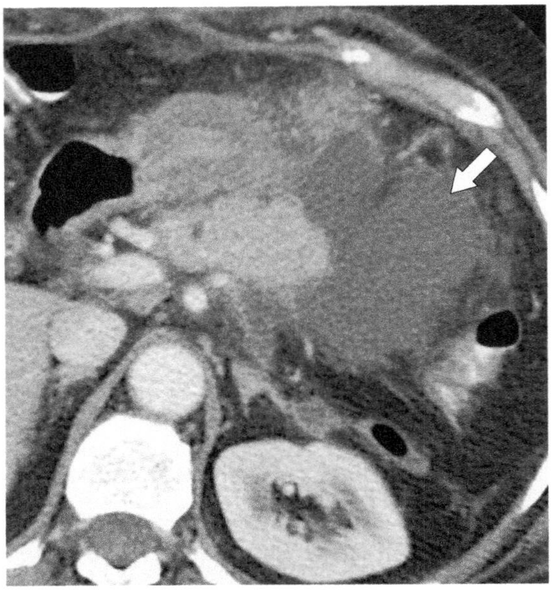

FIGURE 9-98. Axial contrast-enhanced CT in a 66-year woman after pancreatic tail resection for adenocarcinoma. A large postoperative fluid collection (*arrow*) in the operative bed is due to a combination of pancreatitis and a pancreatic duct transection.

PANCREATIC TRANSPLANT

Pancreatic transplant is an innovative procedure that is performed primarily for patients with type 1 diabetes mellitus. The pancreas is transplanted alone or more commonly with simultaneous renal transplantation. With older surgical transplants the pancreatic duct drainage occurred into the bladder via a duodenal interposition with the vascular supply to the pancreas delivered from the iliac arteries. More recently, the procedure has enabled drainage directly into a loop of small bowel with pancreatic vascularization from the iliac vessels. Pancreatic transplantation usually occurs on the right side, and renal transplantation occurs on the left.

*Allen Whipple (1881-1963), American surgeon.

*C.B. Puestow (1902-1973), American surgeon.

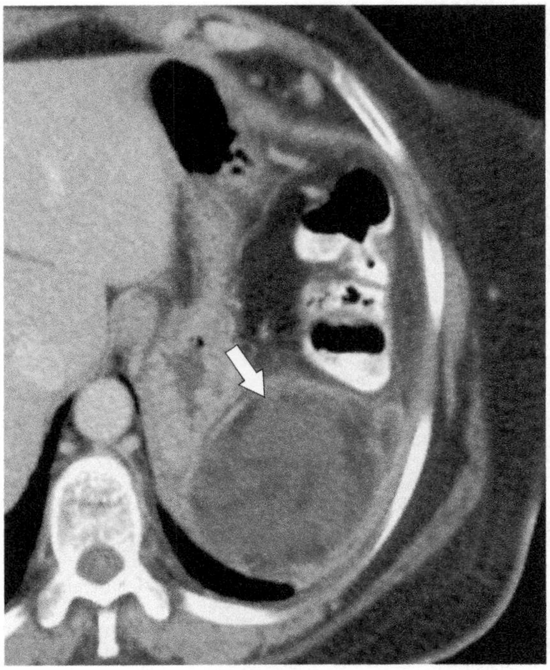

FIGURE 9-99. Axial contrast-enhanced CT in a 50-year-old man with distal pancreatic resection and splenectomy and a hematoma in the operative bed (*arrow*).

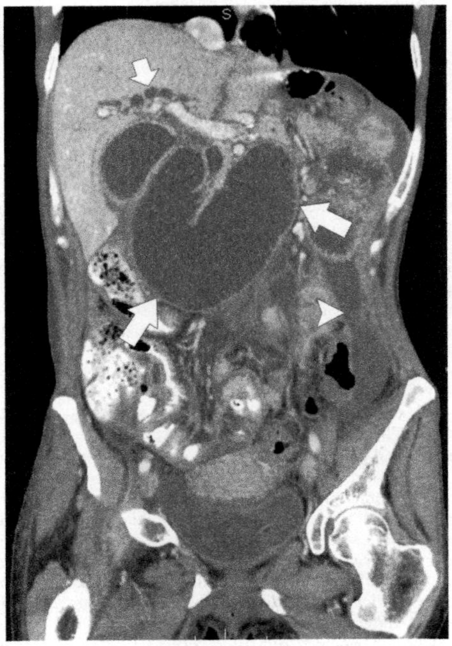

FIGURE 9-100. Coronal contrast-enhanced CT in a 71-year-old man with an obstructed afferent loop (*arrows*) after a Whipple procedure. There is also intrahepatic duct dilatation caused by the obstructed loop (*small arrow*) and intraabdominal ascites (*arrowheads*).

The follow-up imaging of the transplant is preferentially performed with US or MRI because of potential renal complications from iodinated contrast material, although with normal posttransplant function, smaller doses of iodinated contrast are not contraindicated. Complications include pancreatitis (Fig. 9-101), thrombosis, hemorrhage, infection, and rejection. For patients who have undergone this procedure, the 5-year allograft survival rate approaches 70%.

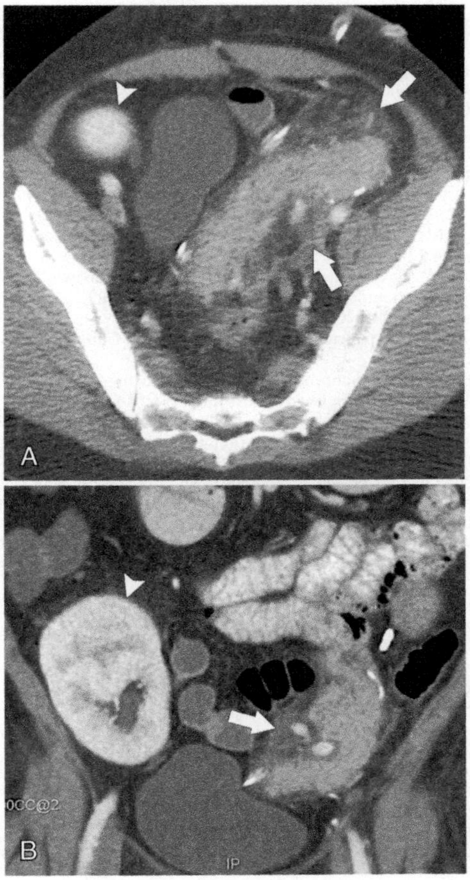

FIGURE 9-101. Axial and coronal contrast-enhanced CT in a 43-year-old woman with a combined renal (*arrowheads*) and pancreas transplant with pancreatic swelling and peripancreatic inflammation (stranding) (*arrows*) caused by transplant pancreatitis.

SUGGESTED READINGS

Anderson SW et al: Pancreatic duct evaluation: accuracy of portal venous phase 64 MDCT. Abdom Imaging 34(1):55-63, 2009.

Axon ATR: Endoscopic retrograde cholangiopancreatography in chronic pancreatitis: Cambridge classification. Radiol Clin North Am 27:39-50, 1989.

Balthazar E: CT diagnosis and staging of acute pancreatitis. Radiol Clin North Am 27:19-37, 1989.

Balthazar EJ: Acute pancreatitis: assessment of severity with clinical and CT evaluation. Radiology 223(3):603-613, 2002.

Balthazar EJ et al: Acute pancreatitis: value of CT in establishing prognosis. Radiology 174:331-336, 1990.

Baudin G et al: CT-guided percutaneous catheter drainage of acute infectious necrotizing pancreatitis: assessment of effectiveness and safety. AJR 199:192-199, 2012; doi:10.2214/AJR.11.6984.

Blasbalg R et al: MRI features of groove pancreatitis. AJR 189(1):73-80, 2007.

Bodily KD et al: Autoimmune pancreatitis: pancreatic and extrapancreatic imaging findings. AJR 192:431-437, 200910.2214/AJR.07.295.

Bollen TL et al: Comparative evaluation of the modified CT severity index and CT severity index in assessing severity of acute pancreatitis. AJR 197:386-392, 2011; doi:10.2214/AJR.09.4025.

Brennan DDD et al: Comprehensive preoperative assessment of pancreatic adenocarcinoma with 64-section volumetric CT. Radiographics 27(6):1653-1666, 2007; doi:10.1148/rg.276075034.

Bret PM et al: Pancreas divisum: evaluation with MR cholangiopancreatography. Radiology 199:99, 1996.

Bronstein YL et al: Detection of small pancreatic tumors with multiphasic helical CT. AJR 182:619-623, 2004.

Buccimazza I et al: Isolated main pancreatic duct injuries spectrum and management. Am J Surg 191(4):448-452, 2006.

Buetow PC et al: Islet cell tumors of the pancreas: clinical, radiologic, and pathologic correlation in diagnosis and localization. Radiographics 17:453-472, 1997.

Buetow PC et al: Solid and papillary epithelial neoplasm of the pancreas: imaging-pathologic correlation on 56 cases. Radiology 199(3):707-711, 1996.

Choi BI et al: Solid and papillary epithelial neoplasms of the pancreas: CT findings. Radiology 166(2):413-416, 1988.

Choi JY et al: Typical and atypical manifestations of serous cystadenoma of the pancreas: imaging findings with pathologic correlation. AJR 193(1):136-142, 2009.
Chung EM et al: From the archives of the AFIP: pancreatic tumors in children: radiologic-pathologic correlation. Radiographics 26(4):1211-1238, 200610.1148/rg.264065012.
Coakley FV et al: Pancreatic imaging mimics: part 1, imaging mimics of pancreatic adenocarcinoma. AJR 199:301-308, 2012; doi:10.2214/AJR.11.7907.
Cohen-Scali F et al: Discrimination of unilocular macrocystic serous cystadenoma from pancreatic pseudocyst and mucinous cystadenoma with CT: initial observations. Radiology 228(3):727-733, 2003.
Dodds WJ et al: MEN I syndrome and islet cell tumors of the pancreas. Semin Roentgenol 20:17-63, 1985.
Fletcher JG et al: Pancreatic malignancy: value of arterial, pancreatic, and hepatic phase imaging with multi-detector row CT. Radiology 229(1):81-90, 2003; doi:10.1148/radiol.2291020582.
Friedman AC et al: Rare pancreatic malignancies. Radiol Clin North Am 27:177-190, 1989.
Fugazzola C et al: Cystic tumors of the pancreas: evaluation by ultrasonography and computed tomography. Gastrointest Radiol 16:53-61, 1991.
Fukukura Y et al: Pancreatic duct: morphologic evaluation with MR cholangiopancreatography after secretin stimulation. Radiology 222(3):674-680, 2002. published online January 18, 2002; doi: 10.1148/radiol.2223010684.
Fukukura Y et al: Pancreatic adenocarcinoma: variability of diffusion-weighted MR imaging findings. Radiology 263(3):732-740, 2012; doi:10.1148/radiol.12111222. published online April 24, 2012.
Graf O et al: Arterial versus portal venous helical CT for revealing pancreatic adenocarcinoma: conspicuity of tumor and critical vascular anatomy. AJR 169:119-123, 1997.
Gupta R et al: Pancreatic intraductal papillary mucinous neoplasms: role of CT in predicting pathologic subtypes. AJR 191(5):1458-1464, 2008. Erratum in AJR 191(6):1876, 2008.
Hagspiel KD et al: Evaluation of vascular complications of pancreas transplantation with high-spatial-resolution contrast-enhanced MR angiography. Radiology 242(2):590-599, 2007.
Horton KM et al: Multi-detector row CT of pancreatic islet cell tumors. Radiographics 26(2):53-464, 2006; doi:10.1148/rg.262055056.
Ichikawa T et al: Atypical exocrine and endocrine pancreatic tumors (anaplastic, small cell, and giant cell types): CT and pathologic features in 14 patients. Abdom Imaging 25(4):409-419, 2000.
Ichikawa T et al: MDCT of pancreatic adenocarcinoma: optimal imaging phases and multiplanar reformatted imaging. AJR 187:1513-1520, 2006; doi:10.2214/AJR.05.1031.
Kalb B et al: MR imaging of cystic lesions of the pancreas. Radiographics 29(6):1749-1765, 2009; doi:10.1148/rg.296095506.
Kawamoto S et al: Lymphoplasmacytic sclerosing pancreatitis (autoimmune pancreatitis): evaluation with multidetector CT. Radiographics 28(1):157-170, 2008; doi:10.1148/rg.281065188.
Kettritz U et al: Contrast-enhanced MR imaging of the pancreas. MRI Clin North Am 4:87, 1996.
Khrana B et al: Macrocystic serous adenoma of the pancreas: radiologic-pathologic correlation. AJR 181:119-123, 2003.
Kim JH et al: Metallic stent placement in the palliative treatment of malignant gastric outlet obstructions: primary gastric carcinoma versus pancreatic carcinoma. AJR 193(1):241-247, 2009.
Kim JH et al: Visually isoattenuating pancreatic adenocarcinoma at dynamic-enhanced CT: frequency, clinical and pathologic characteristics, and diagnosis at imaging examinations. Radiology 257(1):87-96, 2010; published online August 9, 2010; doi: 10.1148/radiol.10100015.
Kim SY et al: Macrocystic neoplasms of the pancreas: CT differentiation of serous oligocystic adenoma from mucinous cystadenoma and intraductal papillary mucinous tumor. AJR 187(5):1192-1198, 2006.
Kim YH et al: Imaging diagnosis of cystic pancreatic lesions: pseudocyst versus nonpseudocyst. Radiographics 25(3):671-685, 2005; doi: 10.1148/rg.253045104.
Lane MJ et al: Diagnosis of pancreatic injury after blunt abdominal trauma. Semin Ultrasound CT MR 17:177, 1996.
Lenhart DK et al: MDCT of acute mild (nonnecrotizing) pancreatitis: abdominal complications and fate of fluid collections. AJR 190:643-649, 2008; doi:10.2214/AJR.07.2761.
Lewis RB et al: Pancreatic endocrine tumors: radiologic-clinicopathologic correlation. Radiographics 30(6):1445-1464, 2012; doi:10.1148/rg.306105523.
Linsenmaier U et al: Diagnosis and classification of pancreatic and duodenal injuries in emergency radiology. Radiographics 28(6):1591-1602, 2008; doi:10.1148/rg.286085524.
Macari M et al: Differentiating pancreatic cystic neoplasms from pancreatic pseudocysts at MR imaging: value of perceived internal debris. Radiology 251(1):77-84, 2009; doi:10.1148/radiol.2511081286.
Manfredi R et al: Autoimmune pancreatitis: pancreatic and extrapancreatic MR imaging–MR cholangiopancreatography findings at diagnosis, after steroid therapy, and at recurrence. Radiology 260(2):428-436, 2011. published online May 25, 2011; doi: 10.1148/radiol.11101729.
Manfredi R et al: Idiopathic chronic pancreatitis in children: MR cholangiopancreatography after secretin administration. Radiology 224(3):675-682, 2002.
Manfredi R et al: Main pancreatic duct intraductal papillary mucinous neoplasms: accuracy of MR imaging in differentiation between benign and malignant tumors compared with histopathologic analysis. Radiology 253(1):106-115, 2009. published online July 31, 2009; doi: 10.1148/radiol.2531080604.
Mathiu D et al: Pancreatic cystic neoplasms. Radiol Clin North Am 27:163-176, 1989.
Matos C et al: MR imaging of the pancreas: a pictorial tour. Radiographics 22:1, 2002. e2.
McNulty NJ et al: Multi-detector row helical CT of the pancreas: effect of contrast-enhanced multiphasic imaging on enhancement of the pancreas, peripancreatic vasculature, and pancreatic adenocarcinoma. Radiology 220:97-102, 2001.
Mergo PJ et al: Pancreatic neoplasms: MR imaging and pathologic correlation. Radiographics 17:281-301, 1997.
Merkle EM et al: Imaging findings in pancreatic lymphoma: differential aspects. AJR 174(3):671-675, 2000.
Mitchell DG: MR imaging of the pancreas. MRI Clin North Am 3:51, 1995.
Morgan DE et al: Resectability of pancreatic adenocarcinoma in patients with locally advanced disease downstaged by preoperative therapy: a challenge for MDCT. AJR 194:668-674, 2010; doi:10.2214/AJR.09.3285.
Mortelé KJ et al: CT-guided percutaneous catheter drainage of acute necrotizing pancreatitis: clinical experience and observations in patients with sterile and infected necrosis. AJR 192:110-116, 2009; doi:10.2214/AJR.08.1116.
Nijs E et al: Disorders of the pediatric pancreas: imaging features, Pediatr Radiol 35(4):358-373, 2005. quiz 457.
Oshikawa O et al: Dynamic sonography of pancreatic tumors: comparison with dynamic CT. AJR 178(5):1133-1137, 2002.
Reinhold C et al: MR cholangiopancreatography: potential clinical applications. Radiographics 16:309-320, 1996.
Rizzo RJ et al: Congenital abnormalities of the pancreas and biliary tree in adults. Radiographics 15:49-68, 1995.
Roche CJ et al: CT and pathologic assessment of prospective nodal staging in patients with ductal adenocarcinoma of the head of the pancreas. AJR 180(2): 475-480, 2003.
Ros P et al: Cystic masses of the pancreas. Radiographics 12:673-686, 1992.
Sahani DV et al: Autoimmune pancreatitis: disease evolution, staging, response assessment, and CT features that predict response to corticosteroid therapy. Radiology 250(1):118-129, 2009. published online November 18, 2008; doi: 10.1148/radiol.2493080279.
Sahani DV et al: Autoimmune pancreatitis: imaging features. Radiology 233(2):345-352, 2004. published online September 30, 2004; doi: 10.1148/radiol.2332031436.
Sahani DV et al: Cystic pancreatic lesions: a simple imaging-based classification system for guiding management. Radiographics 25(6):1471-1484, 2005; doi:10.1148/rg.256045161.
Sahani DV et al: Pancreatic cysts 3 cm or smaller: how aggressive should treatment be? Radiology 238(3):912-919, 2006. published online January 26, 2006; doi: 10.1148/radiol.2382041806.
Sahani DV et al: State-of-the-art PET/CT of the pancreas: current role and emerging indications. Radiographics 32(4):1133-1158, 2012; doi:10.1148/rg.324115143.
Sandrasegaran K et al: Disconnection of the pancreatic duct: an important but overlooked complication of severe acute pancreatitis. Radiographics 27(5): 1389-1400, 2007.
Scatarige JC et al: Pancreatic parenchymal metastases: observations on helical CT. AJR 176(3):695-699, 2001.
Shanbhogue AKP et al: A clinical and radiologic review of uncommon types and causes of pancreatitis. Radiographics 29(4):1003-1026, 2009; doi:10.1148/rg.294085748.
Soto JA et al: Pancreas divisum: depiction with multidetector row CT. Radiology 235(2):503-508, 2005.
Sun MRM et al: Intraoperative ultrasonography of the pancreas. Radiographics 30(7):1935-1953, 2010; doi:10.1148/rg.307105051.
Takahashi N et al: Dual-phase CT of autoimmune pancreatitis: a multireader study. AJR 190:280-286, 2008; doi:10.2214/AJR.07.2309.
Takahashi N et al: Autoimmune pancreatitis: differentiation from pancreatic carcinoma and normal pancreas on the basis of enhancement characteristics at dual-phase CT. AJR 193:479-484, 2009; doi:10.2214/AJR.08.1883.
Takeshita K et al: Differential diagnosis of benign or malignant intraductal papillary mucinous neoplasm of the pancreas by multidetector row helical computed tomography: evaluation of predictive factors by logistic regression analysis. J Comput Assist Tomogr 32(2):191-197, 2008.
Tamura R et al: Chronic pancreatitis: MRCP versus ERCP for quantitative caliber measurement and qualitative evaluation. Radiology 238(3):920-928, 2006.
Taylor AJ et al: Filling defects in the pancreatic duct on endoscopic retrograde pancreatography. AJR 159:1203-1208, 1992.
Thoeni RF et al: The revised Atlanta classification of acute pancreatitis: its importance for the radiologist and its effect on treatment. Radiology 262(3):751-764, 2012; doi:10.1148/radiol.11110947.
To'o KJ et al: Pancreatic and peripancreatic diseases mimicking primary pancreatic neoplasia. Radiographics 25(4):949-965, 2005; doi:10.1148/rg.254045167.
Triantopoulou C et al: Groove pancreatitis: a diagnostic challenge. Eur Radiol 19(7):1736-1743, 2009.
Vandermeer FQ et al: Imaging of whole-organ pancreas transplants. Radiographics 32(2):411-435, 2012; doi:10.1148/rg.322115144.
Vlachou PA et al: IgG4-related sclerosing disease: autoimmune pancreatitis and extrapancreatic manifestations. Radiographics 31(5):1379-1402, 2011; doi:10.1148/rg.315105735.

Yamada Y et al: Intraductal papillary mucinous neoplasms of the pancreas: correlation of helical CT and dynamic MR imaging features with pathologic findings. Abdom Imaging 33(4):474-481, 2008.
Yamauchi FI et al: Multidetector CT evaluation of the postoperative pancreas. Radiographics 32(3):743-764, 2012; doi:10.1148/rg.323105121.
Yoon SH et al: Small (≤20 mm) pancreatic adenocarcinomas: analysis of enhancement patterns and secondary signs with multiphasic multidetector CT. Radiology 259(2):442-452, 2011. published online March 15, 2011; doi: 10.1148/radiol.11101133.
Yu J et al: Normal anatomy and disease process of the pancreatic duodenal groove: imaging features. AJR 183:839-846, 2004.
Zamboni GA et al: Pancreatic adenocarcinoma: value of multidetector CT angiography in preoperative evaluation. Radiology 245(3):770-778, 2007. published online October 19, 2007; doi: 10.1148/radiol.2453061795.

CHAPTER 10

Peritoneum, Retroperitoneum, and Mesentery

ANATOMY

The abdominal cavity is divided into both intraperitoneal and retroperitoneal spaces. The peritoneal cavity is lined by visceral and parietal peritoneum (a thin mesothelial membrane) and lies within the abdominal cavity, with two potential spaces, the greater and lesser sacs. The lesser sac communicates with the greater sac via the epiploic* foramen. The mesentery represents a double layer of visceral peritoneum that encloses the small bowel, transverse, and sigmoid colon. These mesenteries are fixed to the posterior abdominal wall, with small bowel mesentery extending from the lower right abdomen to the upper left and the sigmoid mesentery also passing obliquely within the pelvis. The remaining ascending and descending colon are covered by peritoneum only on their anterior surface and are predominantly retroperitoneum, as is most of the duodenum. The greater curvature of the stomach, another double-layered peritoneum, gives rise to the greater omentum, which drapes over the transverse colon before turning back on itself to enfold the transverse colon and attach to the posterior abdominal wall. The lesser omentum passes from the lesser curvature of the stomach to cover the proximal duodenum and attaches to the inferior hepatic margin. The peritoneum contains a number of recesses formed by the folds of peritoneum and peritoneal ligaments.

The retroperitoneum lies behind the peritoneum within the abdominal cavity and is covered by parietal peritoneum and bordered posteriorly by the abdominal wall. Various organs and anatomical structures lie within this space, including the kidneys, ureters, bladder, adrenal glands, aorta, inferior vena cava, lower esophagus, duodenum (except for first part), pancreas, ascending and descending colon, and rectum.

HERNIAS (see Chapters 1 to 5)

Abdominal hernias are defined as internal or external. Internal hernias are secondary to defects within the peritoneal mesentery, either congenital or acquired (usually after surgery). External hernias occur far more frequently, the most common being inguinal hernia followed by femoral hernia. There are, however, numerous other external abdominal hernias (see Chapter 4).

The significance of both internal and external hernias is that small, and to a lesser extent large, bowel can pass through the hernia, which may lead to bowel obstruction, particularly if the afferent and efferent loops of bowel pass through a narrow or tight hiatus. Usually, when the hiatus is wide mouthed, the bowel is free to "slide" in and out of the hernial orifice, but as this orifice becomes narrower, the bowel may become fixed, at which point it is known as being incarcerated. The proximal (or afferent) loop may or may not become obstructed by external compression at this stage. As bowel contents pass into the herniated loop, however, the herniated bowel becomes distended, further constricting the afferent loop at its entry point, and proximal bowel dilatation develops. Small (or large) bowel obstruction can then present with distention of the proximal bowel and collapse of the distal bowel (Fig. 10-1). The bowel is now at risk of ischemia at the hiatal margin as the tight orifice further constricts the arterial and venous blood supply. Ultimately, if hernias are left untreated, bowel infarction (see Chapter 4) and sometimes death occur. All external hernias are at risk of this dynamic.

*From epipluo (Greek root) "to float upon" as in the omentum that floats upon abdominal contents (omentum in Latin).

Diaphragmatic Hernia

Diaphragmatic hernias can be congenital or develop as a result of trauma (blunt injury or iatrogenic).

Bochdalek Hernia

Bochdalek* hernia accounts for approximately 95% of congenital diaphragmatic hernias and is situated in a posterolateral position, mostly on the left. Sometimes the hiatus is large enough for stomach, small or large bowel, and rarely the spleen to freely enter the chest, which can cause compression of the left lung and mediastinal displacement. Many patients are asymptomatic, however, and the hernia is detected at CT performed for incidental reasons (Fig. 10-2).

Morgagni Hernia

Morgagni† hernia is uncommon, comprising approximately 2% of congenital diaphragmatic hernias. It is situated anteriorly and occurs when the colon and omentum (less commonly stomach, small bowel, and liver) herniate through the foramen of Morgagni, situated adjacent to the sternal xiphoid process. Most are asymptomatic, but the heart may be compressed by the herniated bowel (Fig. 10-3).

*Vincent Bochdalek (1801-1883), Bohemian anatomist.
†Giovanni Morgagni (1682-1771), Italian anatomist.

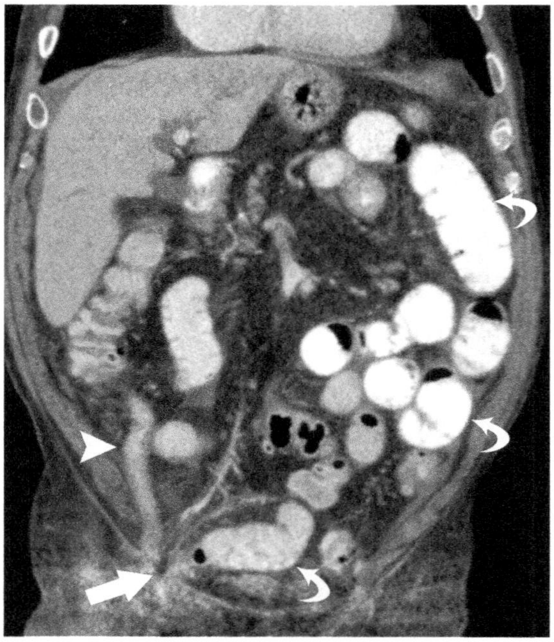

FIGURE 10-1. Coronal contrast-enhanced CT in an 85-year-old woman with an obstructed right inguinal hernia (*large arrow*), dilated proximal bowel (*curved arrows*), and collapsed distal small bowel (*arrowhead*).

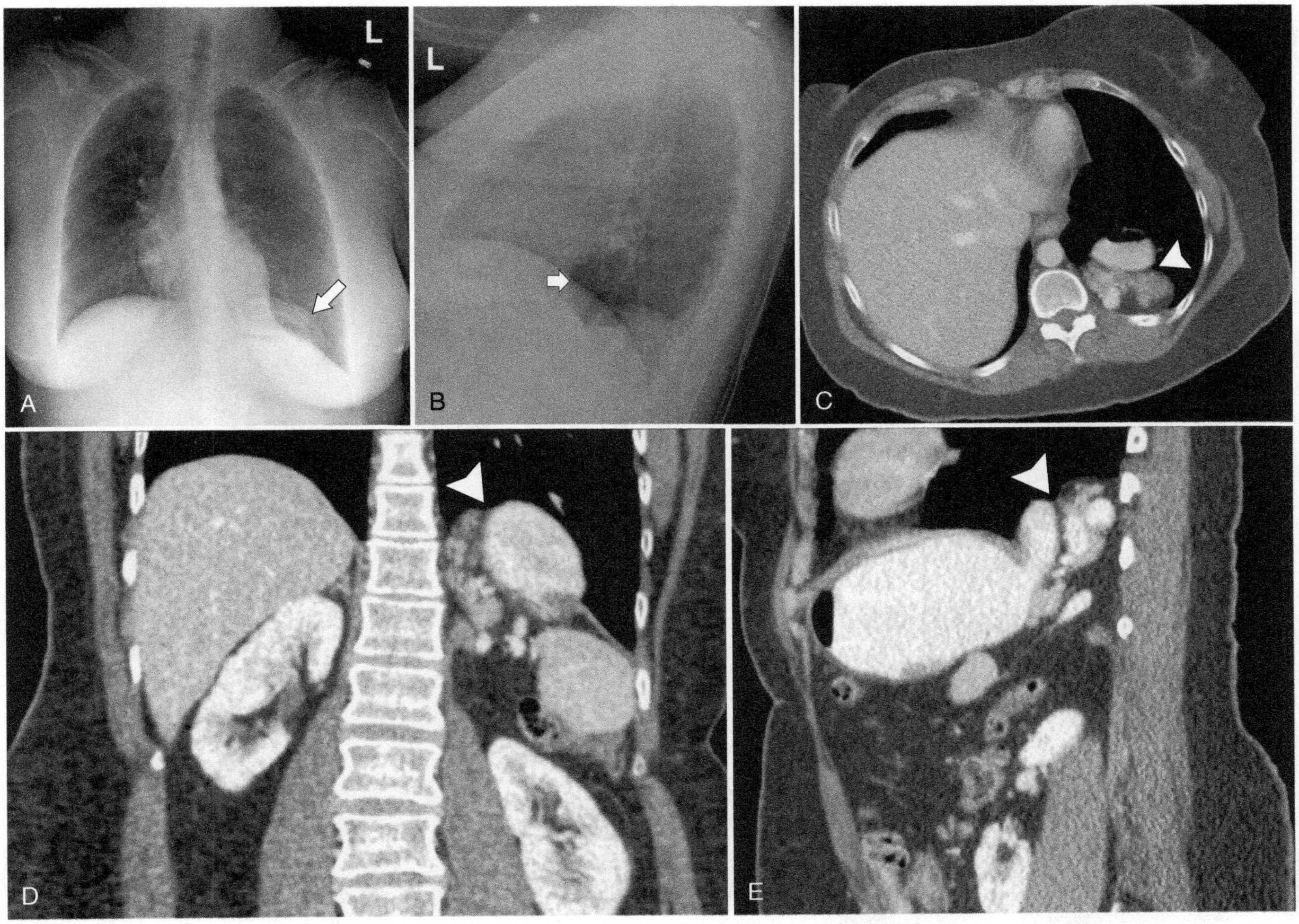

FIGURE 10-2. Posteroanterior (A) and lateral plain chest radiograph (B) and axial (C), coronal (D), and sagittal (E) contrast-enhanced CT in a 39-year-old woman with a Bochdalek hernia. A posterior soft tissue supradiaphragmatic density (*large arrow*) and gas lucency (*small arrow*) are identifiable on chest radiograph, and represent stomach and pancreas, identified on axial, coronal, and sagittal CT images (*arrowheads*).

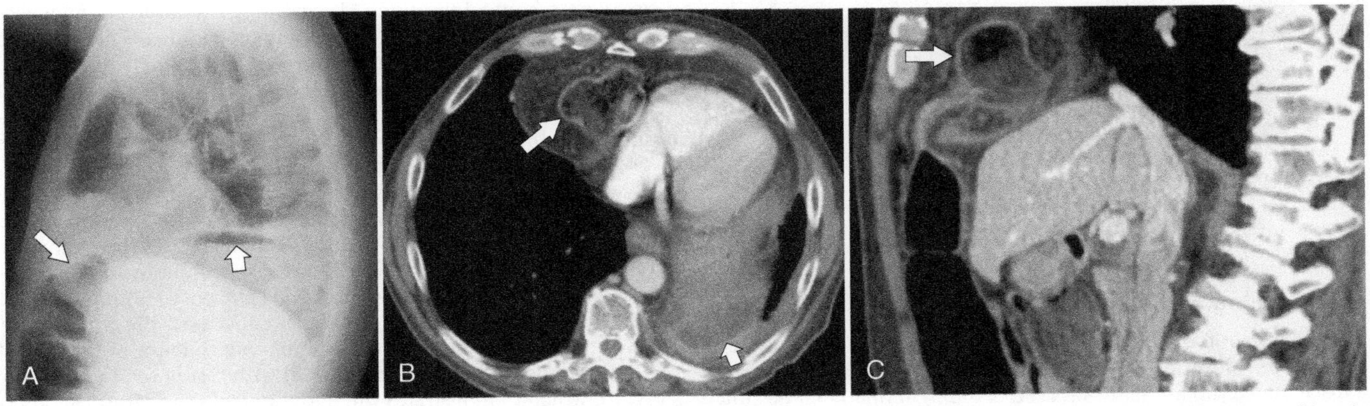

FIGURE 10-3. Lateral plain radiograph of the chest (A) and axial (B) and sagittal (C) contrast-enhanced CT in a 77-year-old man with a Morgagni hernia and the hepatic colonic flexure passing into the chest anteriorly (*large arrows*). There is also a small left subphrenic collection (*small arrows*).

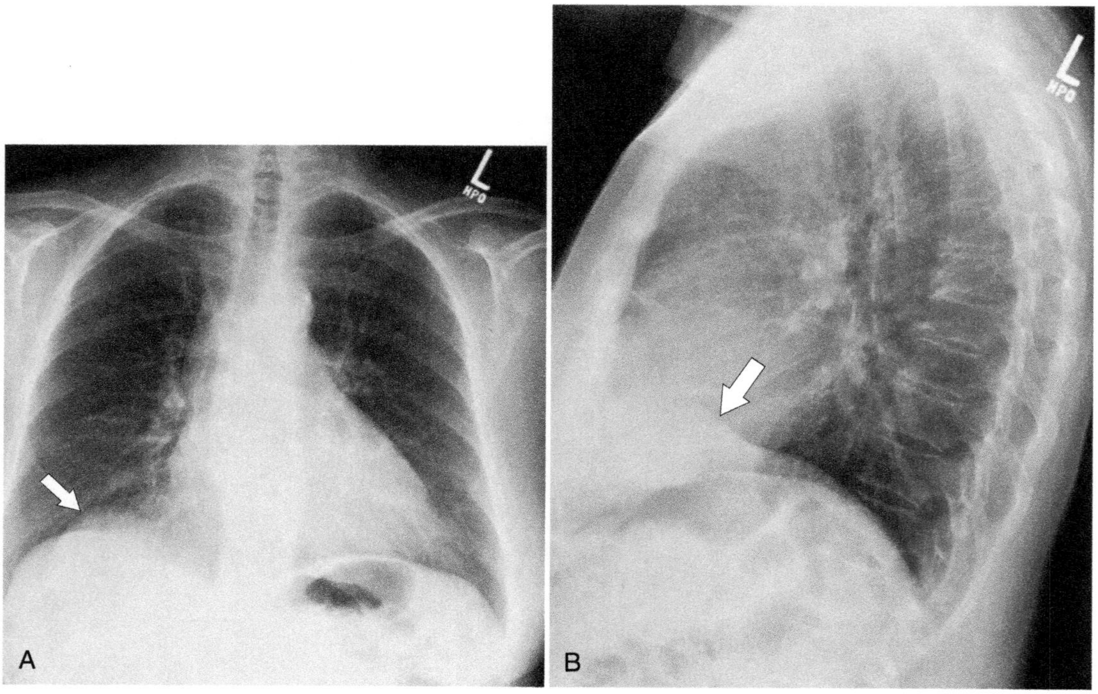

Figure 10-4. Plain posteroanterior (**A**) and lateral chest radiograph (**B**) in a 66-year-old woman with right hemidiaphragmatic elevation caused by slight eventration (*arrows*).

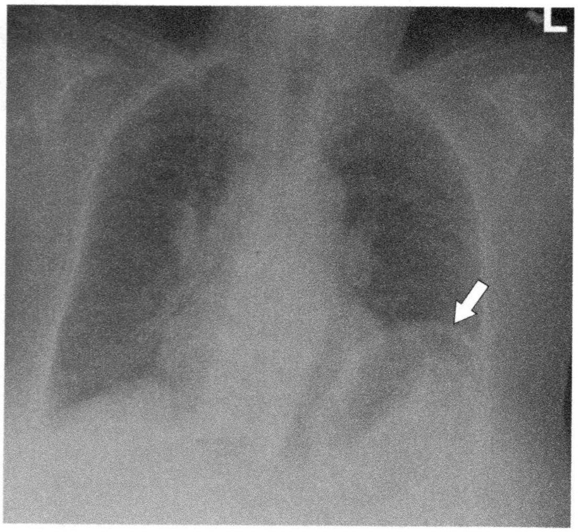

Figure 10-5. Posteroanterior chest radiograph in an 83-year-old woman with a large left diaphragmatic eventration with elevation of the splenic flexure (*arrow*), which remains in the abdomen.

Diaphragmatic Eventration

Diaphragmatic eventration is not actually a hernia, but rather a congenital elevation of one side of an intact diaphragm, creating a space above the normally situated diaphragm that becomes filled by the bowel. It is quite common, usually small (Fig. 10-4) but occasionally large (Fig. 10-5), and asymptomatic in most cases. In the newborn, however, it can cause respiratory distress.

Diaphragmatic Rupture

Diaphragmatic rupture is a tear of the diaphragm and is usually traumatic. Given that abdominal pressure is higher than chest pressure, the bowel often herniates through the diaphragmatic rent, which may sometimes be sufficient to cause symptomatic compression of the lungs or heart. The diagnosis is usually made by multiplanar CT or MRI (Figs. 10-6 and 10-7), although oral contrast material injected through a nasogastric tube should demonstrate herniated bowel contents in the chest. Most traumatic diaphragmatic hernias require surgical repair.

PNEUMOPERITONEUM

Although pneumoperitoneum is sometimes referred to as "free air," the gas is generally not "air," but rather carbon dioxide inserted from laparoscopic procedures or bowel gas that is present in an extraluminal location. The gas may resemble air, however, for a short while after open laparotomy procedures. The presence of pneumoperitoneum may therefore be a benign postsurgical finding or may represent more sinister causes secondary to bowel ischemia or perforation (Box 10-1). The detection of pneumoperitoneum is important and sometimes critical because it may be the only imaging sign of bowel perforation. Its detection, however, can be challenging (especially on plain radiograph) but is more likely when the x-ray beam is tangential to the location of the gas, which rises to the most nondependent part of the abdomen. Therefore, on an upright view the gas is most likely to be identified under the diaphragm (Fig. 10-8), but on an anteroposterior view the gas may not be appreciated because the x-ray beam does not pass tangential to it. Pneumoperitoneum in the lateral or sagittal plane is better appreciated with computed tomography (CT), which demonstrates the extraluminal gas against the anterior abdominal wall (Fig. 10-9). Smaller volumes of pneumoperitoneum can be quite subtle to detect on plain radiograph (Fig. 10-10), and a lateral chest view may be required before small volumes of gas are identified (Fig. 10-11). The most sensitive plain radiograph procedure is the left decubitus (right side up) view of the right upper quadrant, where as little as 1 mL of extraluminal gas can be detected between the liver margin and diaphragm. This procedure is rarely performed, primarily because CT is a far

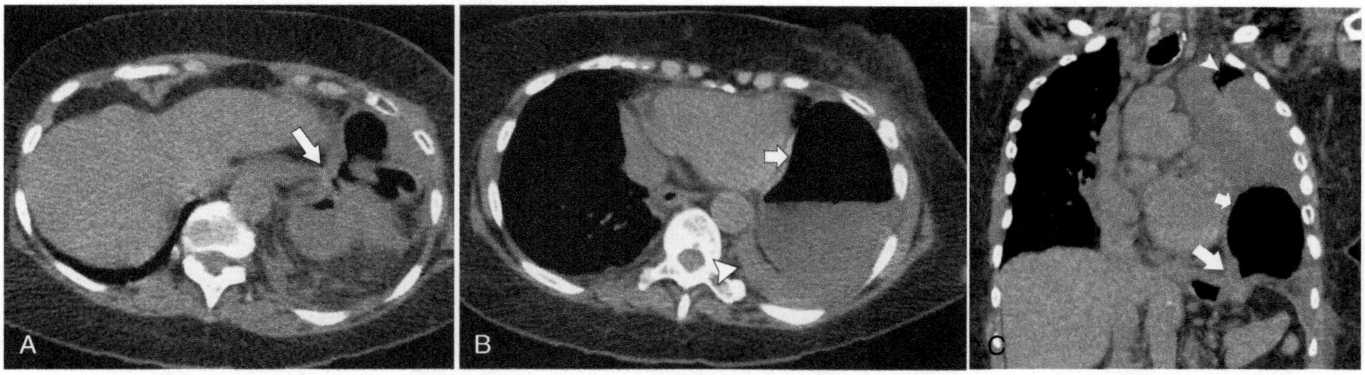

FIGURE 10-6. Axial (**A** and **B**) and coronal (**C**) noncontrast CT in a 78-year-old woman who was recently involved in a motor vehicle accident. She has left diaphragmatic rupture (*large arrows*) and herniation of the splenic flexure (*small arrows*) into the chest, causing lung compression (*arrowheads*).

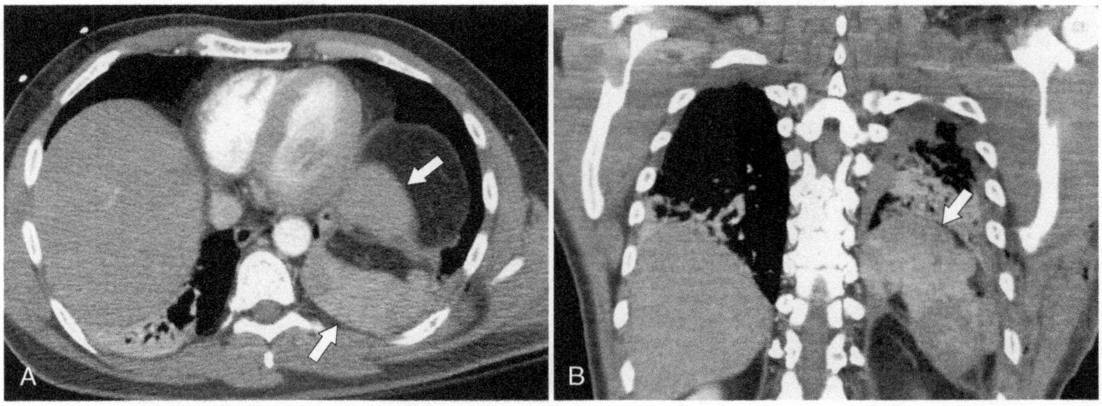

FIGURE 10-7. Axial (**A**) and coronal (**B**) contrast-enhanced CT in a 29-year-old man who was recently involved in a motor vehicle accident and has left diaphragmatic rupture and splenic herniation into the chest (*arrows*).

Box 10-1. Causes of Pneumoperitoneum

IATROGENIC
Postsurgery
Postlaparoscopy
Endoscopy
Peritoneal hemodialysis
Barium enema

PERFORATED VISCUS
Bowel obstruction (e.g., volvulus)
Ischemia (e.g., obstructed hernia)
Peptic ulcer disease
Diverticulitis
Appendicitis
Colitis (e.g., Crohn, infectious)
Malignancy
Steroids

PNEUMATOSIS

INTRATHORACIC
Pneumomediastinum
Pneumothorax

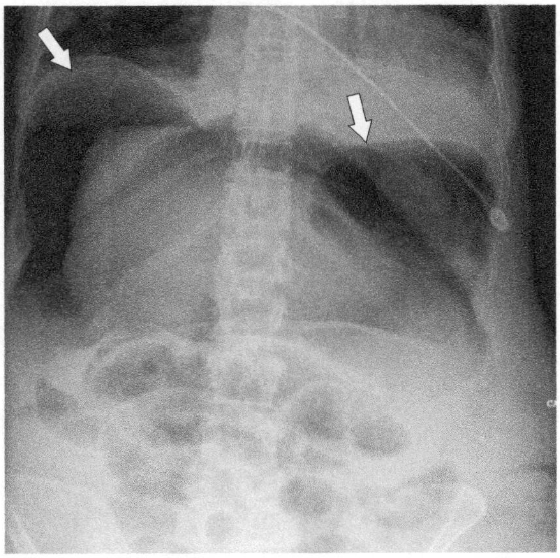

FIGURE 10-8. Upright plain abdominal radiograph in a 51-year-old woman who recently underwent abdominal surgery. A large pneumoperitoneum is best appreciated in the most nondependent part under the diaphragms (*arrows*).

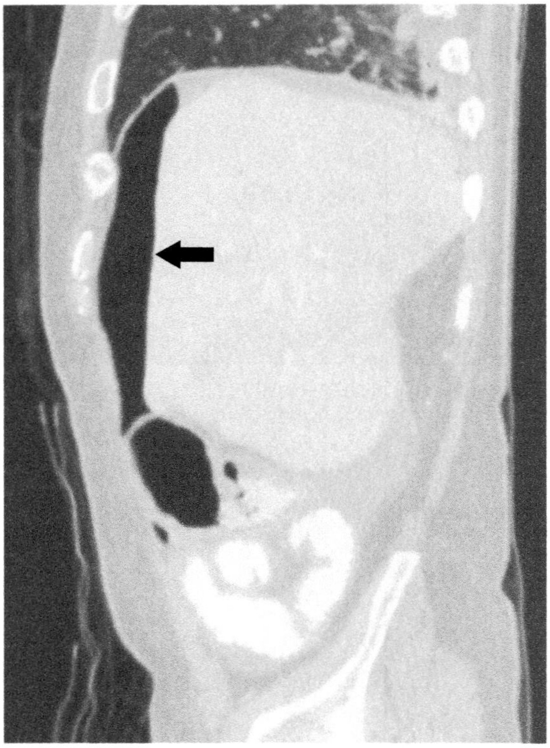

FIGURE 10-9. Sagittal reconstruction CT on lung window settings in a 41-year-old man with extraluminal gas against the anterior abdominal wall (*arrow*).

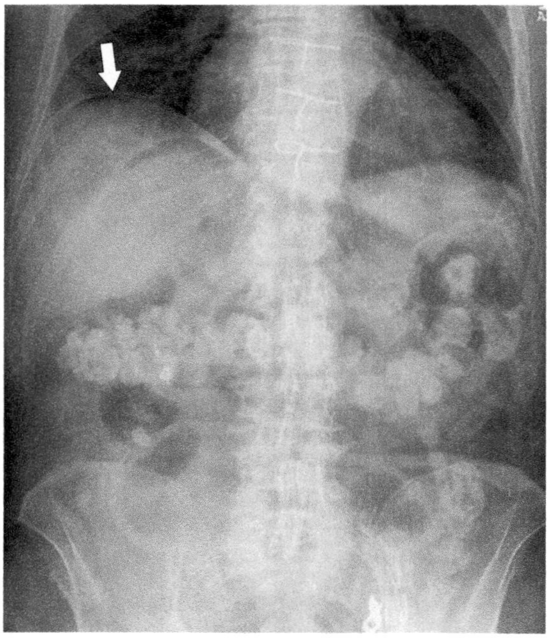

FIGURE 10-10. Upright abdominal radiograph in an 83-year-old man who recently underwent abdominal and chest surgery. A "sliver" of gas (*arrow*) under the right hemidiaphragm represents pneumoperitoneum.

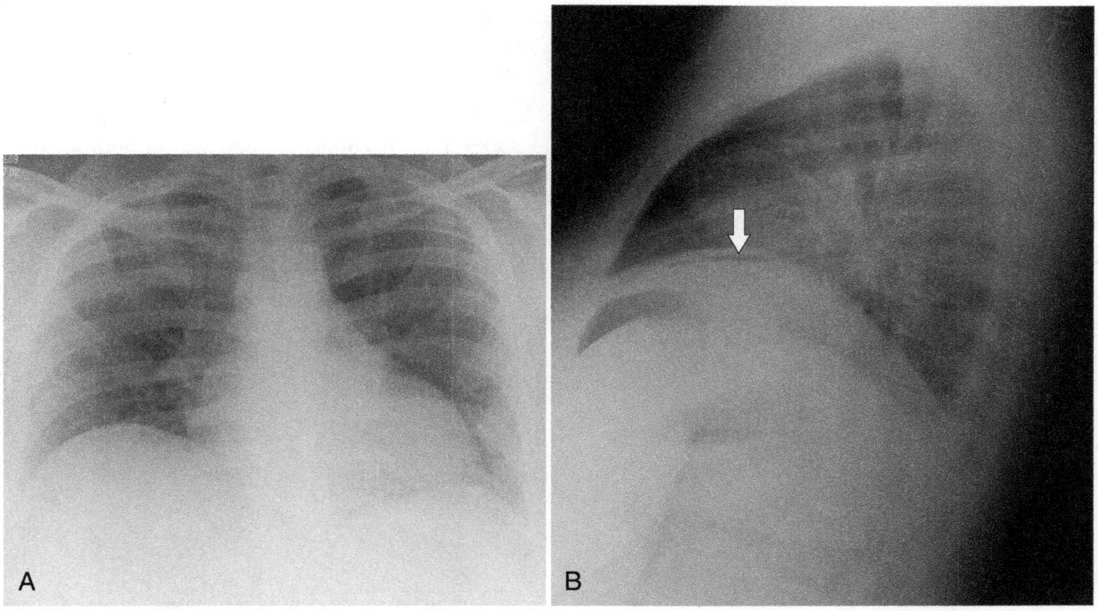

FIGURE 10-11. Posteroanterior (**A**) and lateral chest radiograph (**B**) in a 40-year-old woman who recently underwent abdominal surgery. Subtle pneumoperitoneum is detected only on the lateral view (*arrow*).

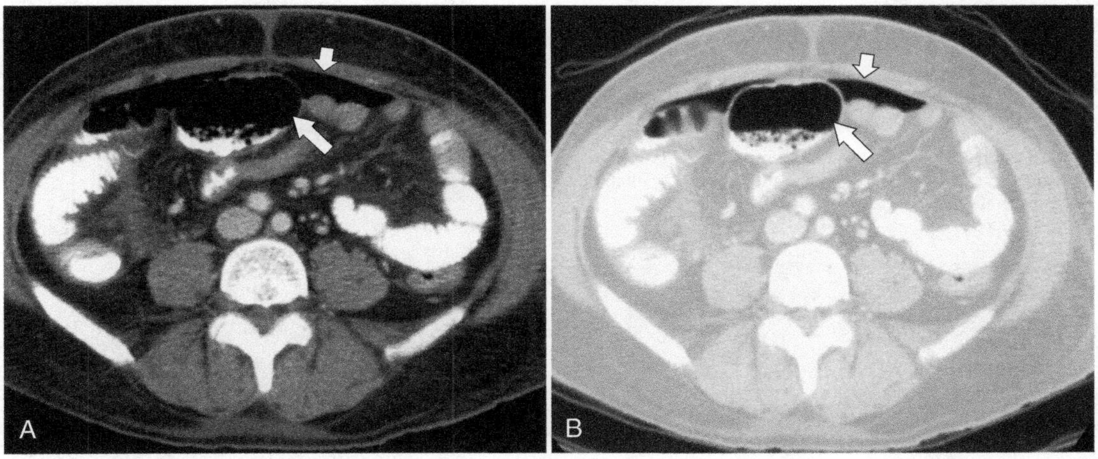

FIGURE 10-12. Axial contrast-enhanced CT on soft tissue (**A**) and lung window (**B**) contrast settings in a 51-year-old man. The differentiation of intraluminal (*large arrows*) from extraluminal (*small arrows*) gas is far better appreciated on lung window settings.

more sensitive tool for the detection of pneumoperitoneum, especially for small volumes of gas. However, even larger volumes of extraluminal gas may be missed unless viewed using lung window contrast settings, since the gas might otherwise be confused with intraluminal gas (Fig. 10-12). Other plain radiograph findings can be demonstrated with larger volumes of gas. These include the visualization of the falciform ligament (Fig. 10-13), which is also better visualized by CT (Fig. 10-14) or recognized as a "football" sign, representing a large ovoid lucency in the center of the abdomen on supine radiographs. Gas can also sometimes be visualized in the Morison* pouch or may outline the lateral umbilical ligaments, but more often both sides of the bowel wall are outlined, usually referred to as the Rigler† sign (less commonly, double-wall sign). This sign is generally identified on the supine view, and large volumes of extraluminal gas are usually present (Fig. 10-15). The sign may be quite subtle or obvious (Fig. 10-16).

PERITONEAL DISEASE

As a potential space, the peritoneal cavity can fill with fluid (ascites) and is susceptible to a number of inflammatory conditions. There are also a number of rare primary neoplastic lesions involving the mesentery, although metastatic deposits from intraabdominal malignancies are more common, particularly given its larger surface area.

Peritonitis

Peritonitis is an inflammatory process within the peritoneum, either infectious or otherwise but usually bacterial, which can be spontaneous or caused by rupture of an intraabdominal viscus (traumatic, inflammatory, neoplastic, or iatrogenic). Patients

*James Rutherford Morison (1853-1939), British surgeon.
†Leo George Rigler (1896-1979), American radiologist.

on peritoneal hemodialysis are particularly susceptible because they are often immunosuppressed. Tuberculosis is a common cause worldwide and is usually hematogenous in origin. Common symptoms of peritonitis are abdominal pain, fever, and sometimes distention, particularly because ileus is often associated with inflammatory disease. Most causes of peritonitis are associated with the development of ascites. Indeed, the absence of ascites normally excludes the diagnosis of peritonitis. Early in the process there may be simple ascites, which is difficult to differentiate from other causes of ascites (see later in the chapter). As the peritonitis worsens, however, the mesenteric fat becomes infiltrated and edematous (fat stranding) and the peritoneal linings become thickened and may show enhancement after the administration of IV contrast medium at CT. Peritoneal loculations, in which ascitic fluid becomes trapped within peritoneal folds and is not free to move throughout the abdomen, then develop as an inflammatory response. These can further develop into secondary loculated abscesses.

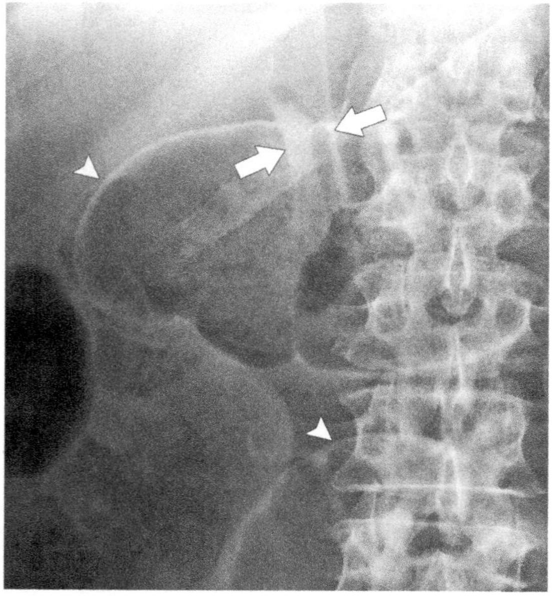

FIGURE 10-13. Magnified view of supine abdominal radiograph in a patient with pneumoperitoneum that outlines the falciform ligament (*arrows*) and a Rigler sign (*arrowheads*).

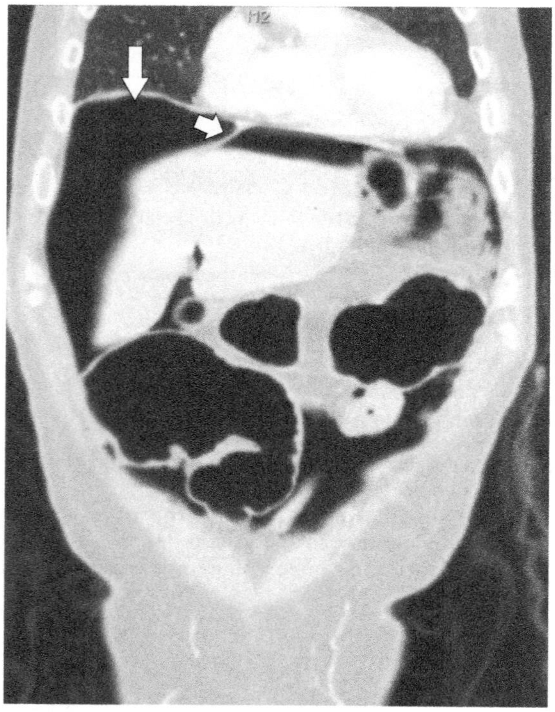

FIGURE 10-14. Coronal contrast-enhanced CT on lung windows in a 53-year-old man with pneumoperitoneum (*arrow*) with the falciform ligament outlined (*small arrow*).

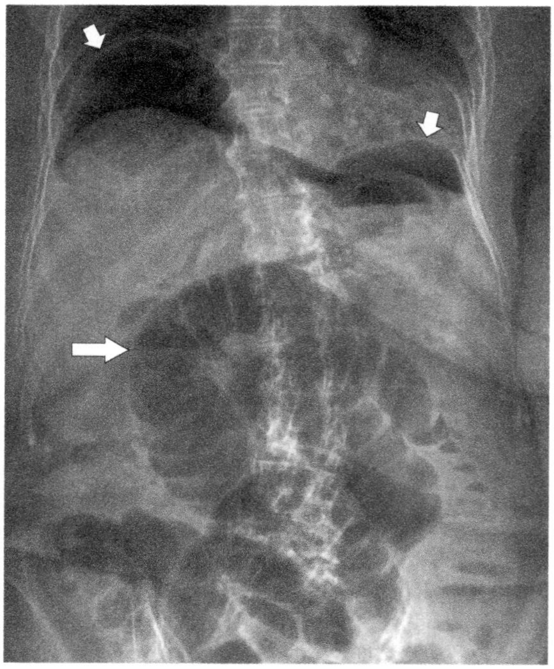

FIGURE 10-15. Upright abdominal radiograph in a 78-year-old woman with Rigler sign (*arrow*) and gas under both diaphragms (*small arrows*).

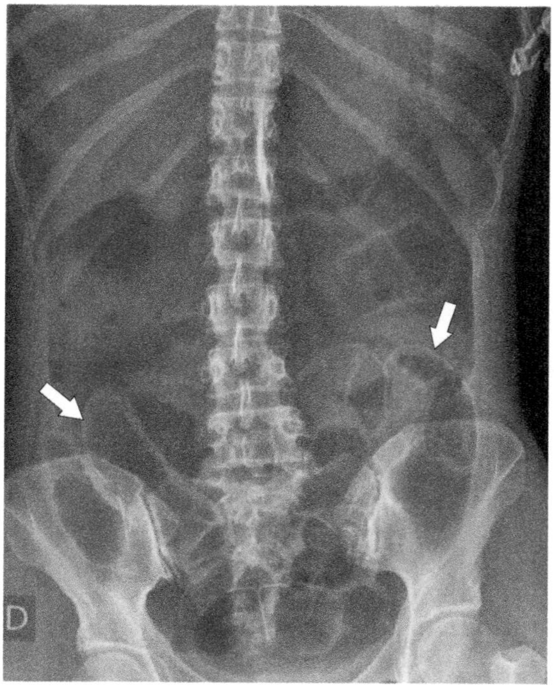

FIGURE 10-16. Supine plain abdominal radiograph in a 63-year-old woman with obvious Rigler sign (*arrows*) caused by pneumoperitoneum.

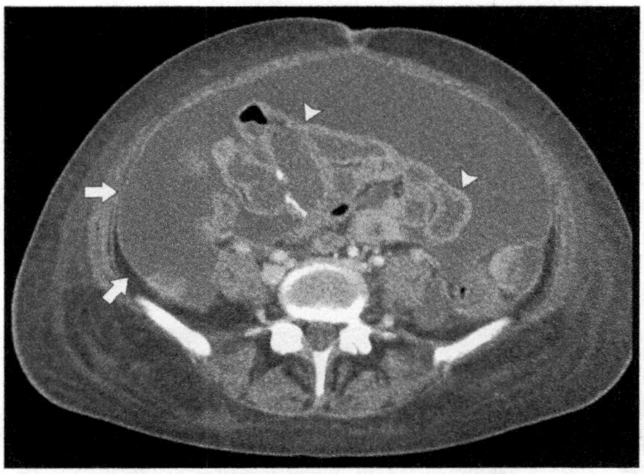

FIGURE 10-17. Axial contrast-enhanced CT in a 35-year-old man with tuberculous peritonitis and enhancing peritoneal lining (*arrows*) and a cocoon-like appearance to the small bowel (*arrowheads*).

At imaging, the presence of ascites, loculated or otherwise (Fig. 10-17), can be confirmed by ultrasound (US) or contrast-enhanced CT. The features are generally nonspecific, and the diagnosis is based on clinical symptoms and signs (e.g., history of recent endoscopic procedure). Chronic peritonitis (which is sometimes recognized in patients undergoing peritoneal hemodialysis) may heal by peritoneal calcification that envelops the intraabdominal organs (Fig. 10-18). Tuberculous peritonitis often demonstrates regional adenopathy, terminal ileitis, diffuse ascites, and omental thickening (Fig. 10-19). Sometimes there is a characteristic "cocoon" appearance as the fibrotic mesenteric process encapsulates the small bowel (also known as sclerosing encapsulating peritonitis) (Fig. 10-20).

Peritoneal Abscess

Peritoneal abscess represents a peritoneal collection of pus. The abscesses may be single or multiple and are usually secondary to infection of intraabdominal organs (appendicitis,

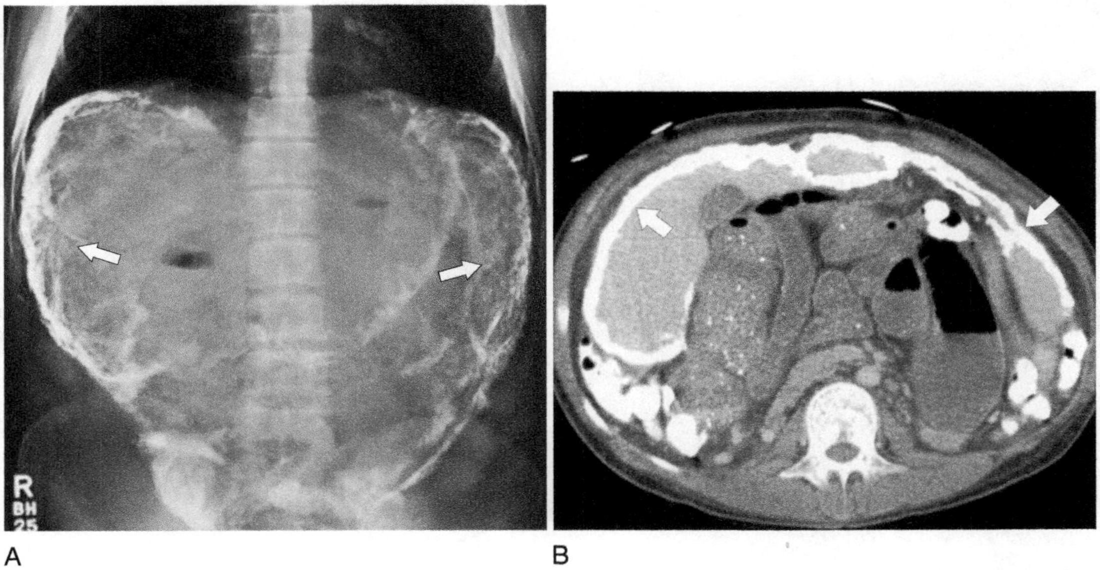

FIGURE 10-18. Plain abdominal radiograph (**A**) and axial contrast-enhanced CT (**B**) in a 25-year-old woman with diffuse peritoneal calcification (*arrows*) from multiple prior episodes of peritonitis resulting from hemodialysis.

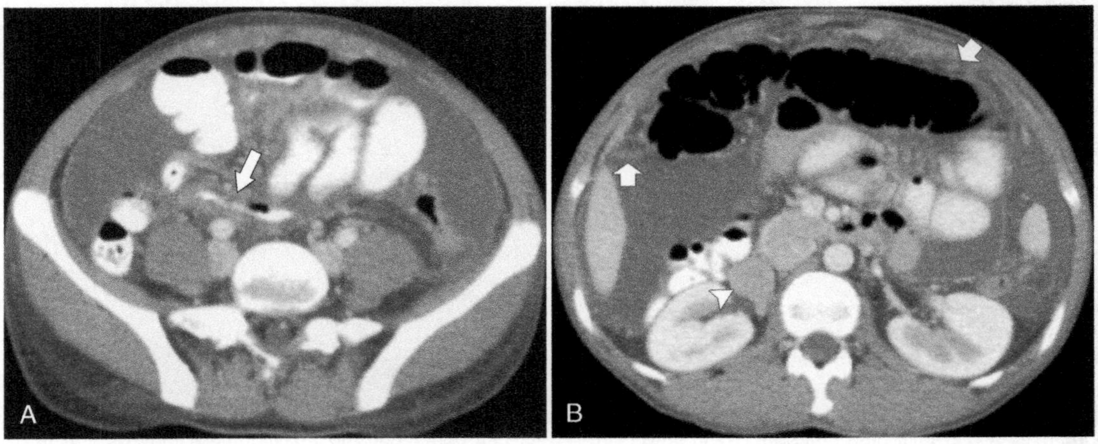

FIGURE 10-19. Axial contrast-enhanced CT in a 20-year-old woman with tuberculous peritonitis and diffuse ascites, terminal ileal thickening (**A**; *arrow*), and omental thickening (**B**; *small arrows*). There are also retroperitoneal nodes (*arrowhead*).

diverticulitis) or localized perforation from inflammatory bowel disease. They may result from peritonitis and often reside within peritoneal spaces (subhepatic, subdiaphragmatic, Morison pouch, or the cul-de-sac). Patients usually have abdominal pain and fever and demonstrate a peripheral leukocytosis. Imaging demonstrates a well-circumscribed, low-density collection, but definitive confirmation of abscess may require percutaneous aspiration and microbiological evaluation because infected and noninfected intraabdominal fluid can appear identical in the early stages. As the abscess develops, however, gas may form, which may be evidenced as multiple gas bubbles (Fig. 10-21) or show a fluid level (Fig. 10-22), and the lining to the abscess may enhance after administration of IV contrast material at CT (Fig. 10-23). Tumor necrosis can have similar features (Fig. 10-24).

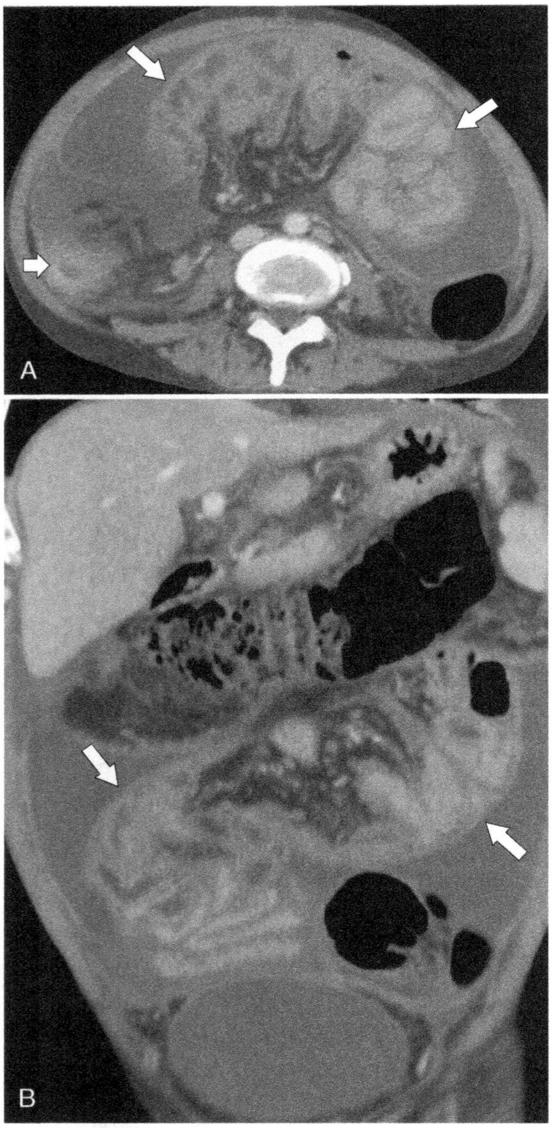

FIGURE 10-20. Axial (**A**) and coronal (**B**) contrast-enhanced CT in a 29-year-old man with diffuse tuberculous peritonitis with peritoneal fibrosis and confinement of the small bowel mesentery and bowel centrally (*arrows*) in a cocoon-like appearance. There is also colonic tuberculous disease (*small arrow*).

Mesenteritis

Mesenteritis is a benign process of unknown cause and is also known as fibrosing mesenteritis, sclerosing mesenteritis, retractile mesenteritis, or mesenteric panniculitis. It represents inflammation of the mesenteric fat that is identified at CT as a "hazy" mesentery produced by inflammatory change (Fig. 10-25). It often heals by fibrosis as a simple mesenteric mass (with or without associated calcification) (Fig. 10-26) or

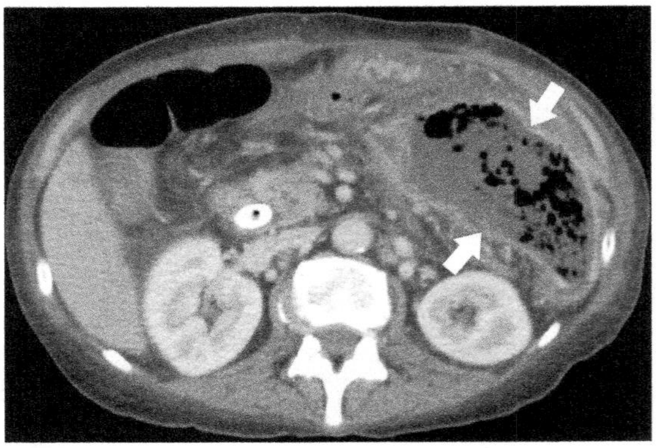

FIGURE 10-21. Axial contrast-enhanced CT in a 67-year-old man with intraabdominal abscess (*arrows*) and multiple small gas bubbles.

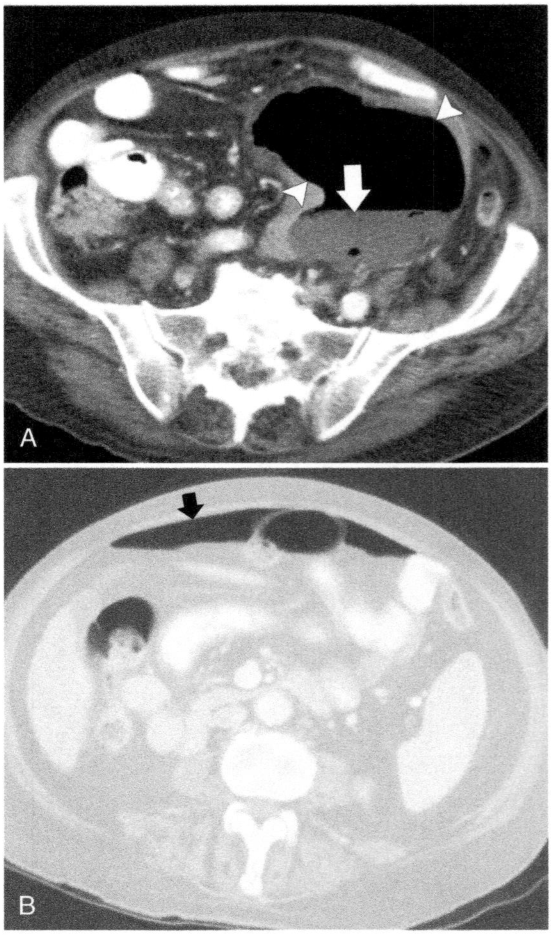

FIGURE 10-22. Axial contrast-enhanced CT in a 75-year-old man with colonic perforation and intraabdominal abscess (**A**; *arrowheads*) with a gas-pus fluid level (**A**; *arrow*) and anterior extraluminal gas (**B**; *arrow*) as seen on lung window settings.

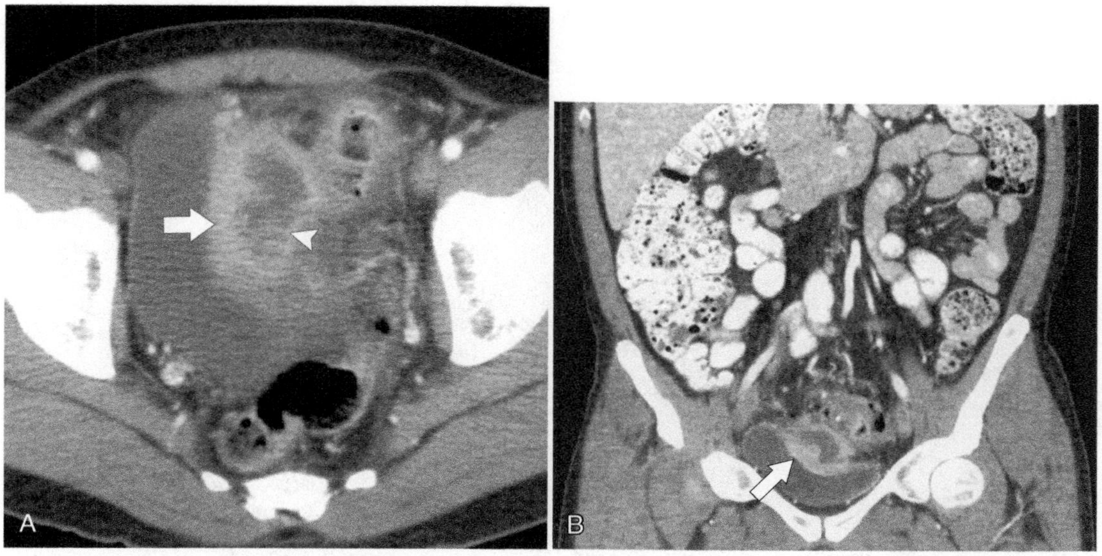

FIGURE 10-23. Axial (A) and coronal (B) contrast-enhanced CT in a 59-year-old man with a sigmoid diverticular abscess (*arrowhead*) and an enhancing wall (*arrows*).

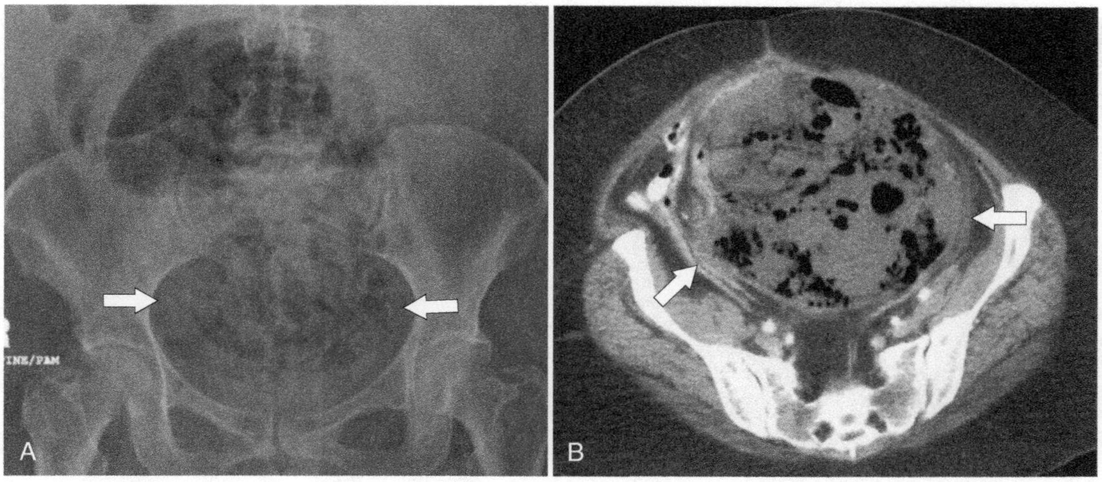

FIGURE 10-24. Plain abdominal radiograph (A) and axial contrast-enhanced CT (B) in a 59-year-old woman with a large necrotic pelvic sarcoma (*arrows*).

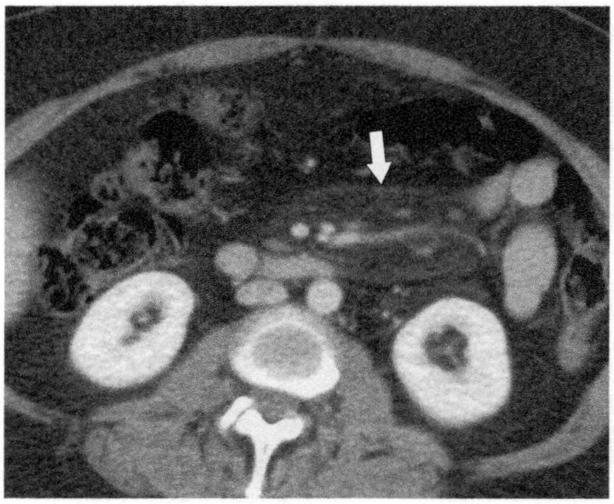

FIGURE 10-25. Axial contrast-enhanced CT in a 58-year-old woman with "hazy" mesentery (*arrow*) resulting from mesenteritis.

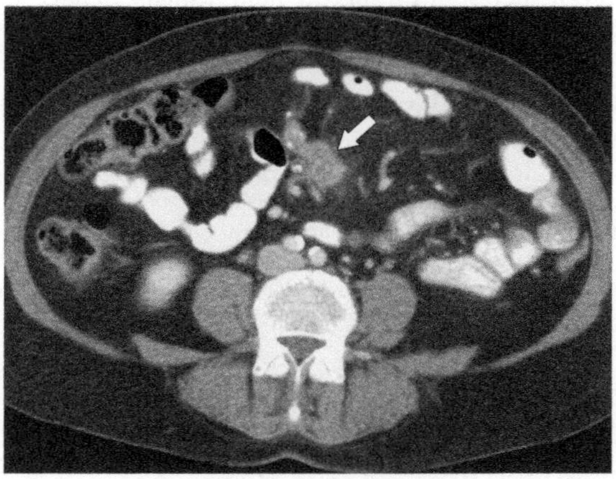

FIGURE 10-26. Axial contrast-enhanced CT in a 56-year-old woman with an irregular calcified mesenteric mass (*arrow*) caused by prior mesenteritis.

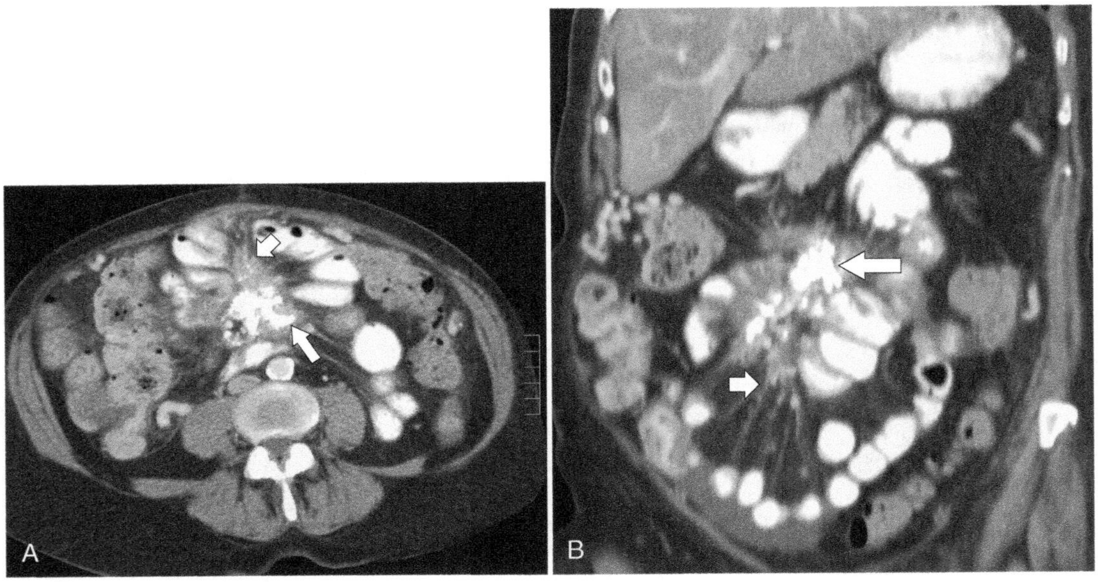

FIGURE 10-27. Axial (**A**) and coronal (**B**) contrast-enhanced CT in a 73-year-old woman with a calcified mesenteric mass (*large arrows*) with mesenteric retraction (*small arrow*) caused by retractile mesenteritis.

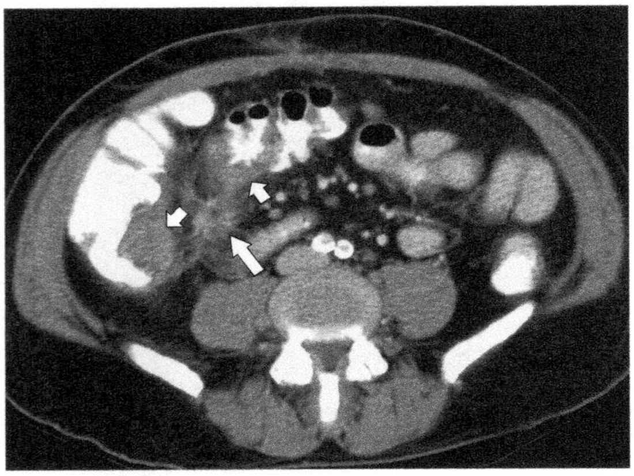

FIGURE 10-28. Axial contrast-enhanced CT with a right lower quadrant mass representing carcinoid (*large arrow*) and a mesenteric desmoplastic reaction and associated colonic thickening (*small arrows*).

with constriction or retraction of the mesentery, often with calcification (Fig. 10-27). It should be differentiated from mesenteric metastases from carcinoid, which can have similar appearances (Fig. 10-28).

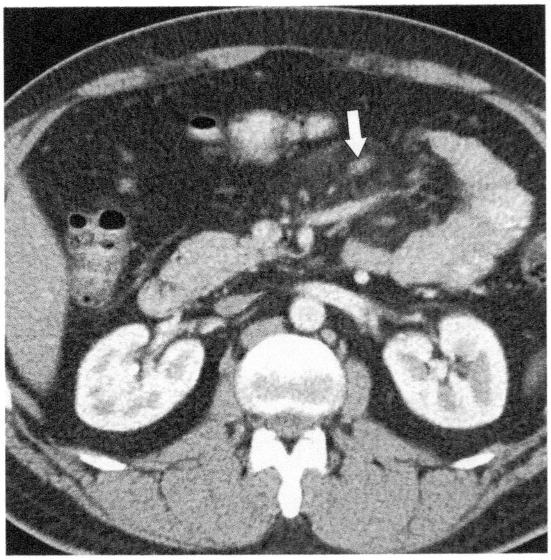

FIGURE 10-29. Axial contrast-enhanced CT in a 56-year-old man with several slightly enlarged mesenteric nodes (*large arrow*) and inflammatory fat changes resulting from mesenteric adenitis.

Mesenteric Adenitis

Inflammation of the mesenteric nodes is not uncommon. It is usually nonspecific and recognized on CT as a number of slightly enlarged mesenteric lymph nodes associated with inflammatory fat changes (fat stranding) (Fig. 10-29). It is most often idiopathic but can be bacterial (Fig. 10-30) or tuberculous (Fig. 10-31). Reactive adenitis can also occur with small or large bowel infections or inflammatory bowel disease (see Chapter 4).

Mesenteric Fat Necrosis

Mesenteric fat necrosis is often referred to as an omental infarct and simply represents arterial disruption of a small area of mesentery, leading to infarction. It is most commonly identified in obese elderly patients and in those who have had recent abdominal surgery. Patients present with acute abdominal pain, which

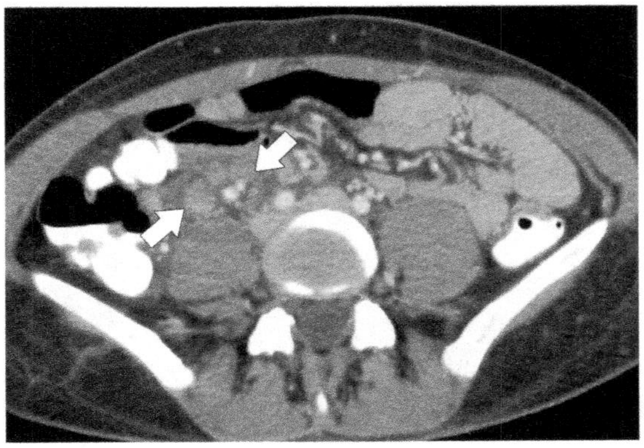

FIGURE 10-30. Axial contrast-enhanced CT in a 61-year-old man with a number of enlarged right lower quadrant mesenteric nodes (*arrows*) due to bacterial mesenteric adenitis.

can be mistaken for appendicitis, diverticulitis, or epiploic appendagitis. CT findings, which can be quite subtle, are a focal area of omentum or peritoneal fat with heterogeneous edematous change (Fig. 10-32). Larger areas of fat necrosis may show gas within the infarction (Fig. 10-33, *A*) and even fat/fluid levels (Fig. 10-33, *B*).

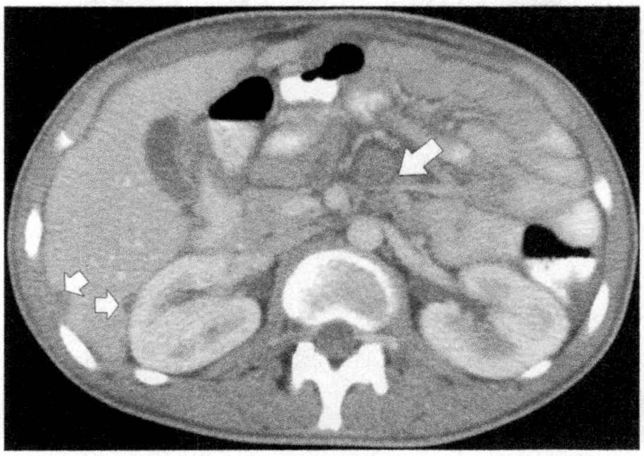

FIGURE 10-31. Axial contrast-enhanced CT in a 29-year-old woman with intraabdominal tuberculosis and multiple mesenteric nodes (*arrow*). There are also tuberculous deposits on the liver capsule (*small arrows*).

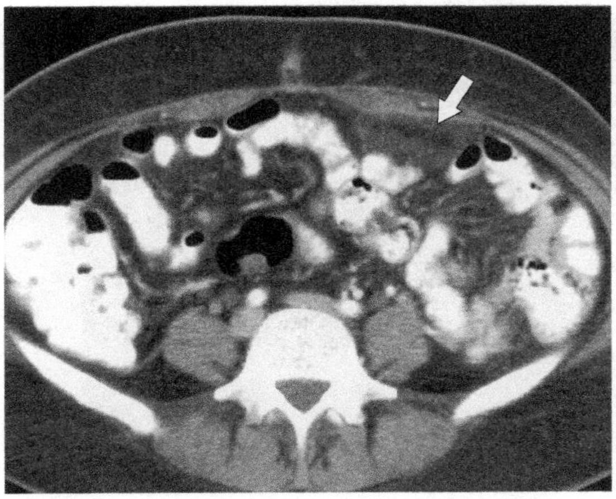

FIGURE 10-32. Axial contrast-enhanced CT in a 39-year-old woman with omental fat necrosis (*arrow*).

Necrotizing Fasciitis

Necrotizing fasciitis is a rare, often fatal, infection of the skin and subcutaneous tissue that is caused by gram-positive and -negative bacteria, most commonly in patients with immunosuppression, diabetes mellitus, malignancy, or alcoholism. The infection is usually secondary to trauma (surgical or nonsurgical) and develops rapidly, along with widespread fat necrosis (Fig. 10-34).

Injection Fat Necrosis and Granuloma

Injection fat necrosis and granuloma are commonly identified in patients who are hospitalized and have received multiple subcutaneous injections. Their features are characteristic at CT and include rounded, soft tissue changes in the subcutaneous fat because of localized fat necrosis (Fig. 10-35, *A*). Sometimes they show increased fluorodeoxyglucose (FDG) activity on positron emission tomography (PET) (Fig. 10-35, *B*). They often heal by dystrophic calcification (Fig. 10-36).

Benign Peritoneal Masses

Peritoneal Inclusion Cyst

Peritoneal inclusion cysts represent loculated simple fluid within the abdomen, usually resulting from adhesions, and are identified primarily in an adnexal location. Therefore they must be differentiated from ovarian cysts. They are seen in women, mostly those of reproductive age, who have had prior pelvic inflammatory diseases or surgery. At imaging the cysts are usually complex with fluid and thin septa but do not typically contain solid elements (Fig. 10-37). They can become large, filling almost the entire pelvis (Fig. 10-38).

Lymphangioma (Mesenteric Cyst)

Lymphangiomas (mesenteric cysts) are cystic lesions arising within the abdomen and are usually caused by obstructed lymphatics. They are to be differentiated from mesenteric duplication cysts, which are also cystic. They are usually identified incidentally at CT as simple irregular cystic structures (Fig. 10-39) that may show punctate calcification in the cyst wall. These cysts can also occur in a retroperitoneal location (Fig. 10-40).

Seroma

Seroma refers to a well-circumscribed, low-density mass representing a pocket of serous fluid that most commonly has collected as leakage from surgically damaged regional vasculature. Seromas less commonly result from trauma. Their appearances at CT are

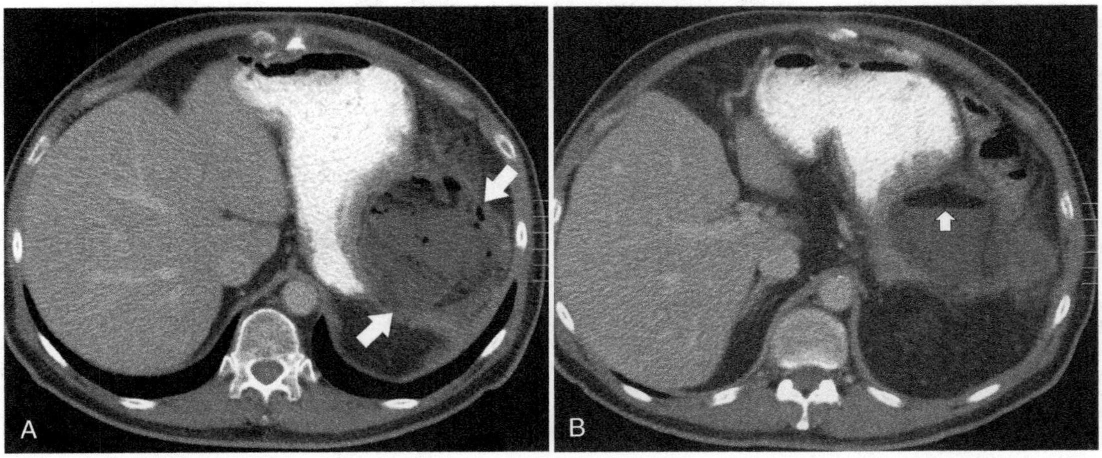

FIGURE 10-33. Axial contrast-enhanced CT in a 54-year-old man with left upper quadrant fat necrosis and gas formation (**A**; *arrows*). Slightly cephalad, there is a fat/fluid level (**B**; *arrow*).

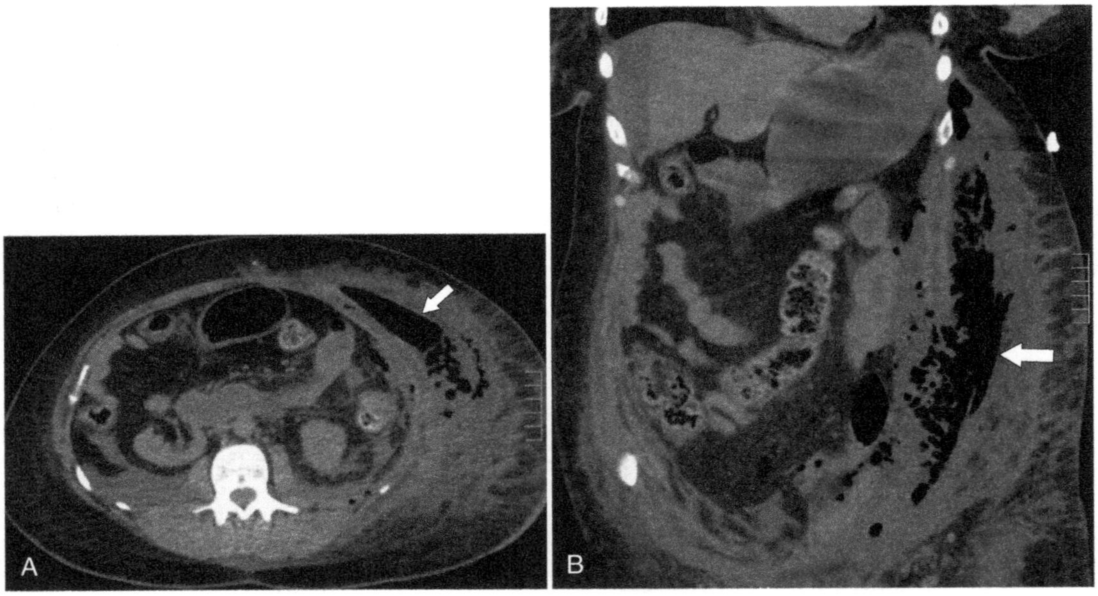

FIGURE 10-34. Axial (**A**) and coronal (**B**) noncontrast CT in a 44-year-old woman with necrotizing fasciitis. There is diffuse fat necrosis and gas formation in the abdominal wall (*arrows*).

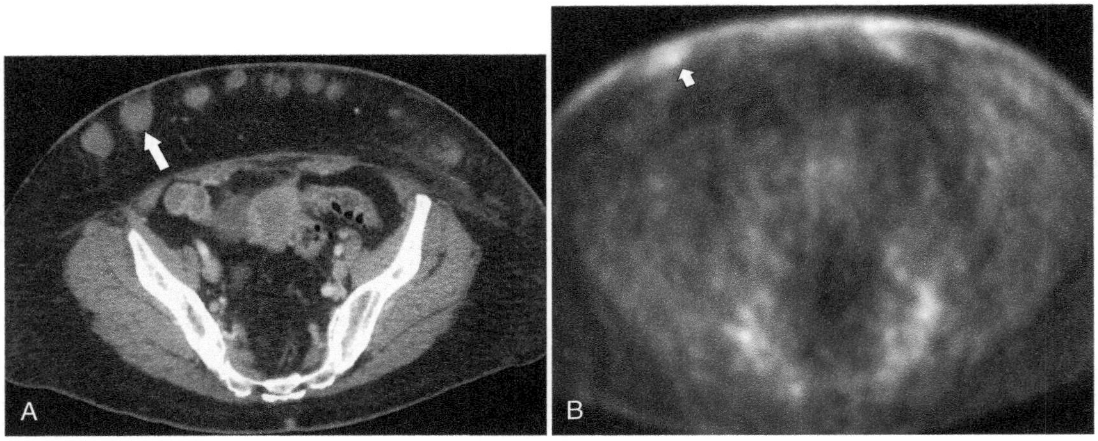

FIGURE 10-35. **A**, Axial contrast-enhanced CT in a 71-year-old woman with multiple subcutaneous soft tissue masses (*large arrow*) in the anterior abdominal wall caused by fat necrosis from subcutaneous injections. **B**, These can demonstrate mild fluorodeoxyglucose uptake at PET (*small arrow*) because of the inflammatory nature of the fat necrosis.

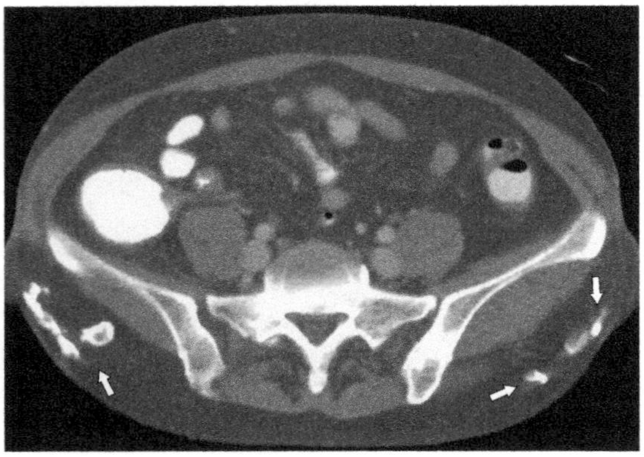

FIGURE 10-36. Axial contrast-enhanced CT in a 73-year-old woman with multiple calcified buttock injection granulomata (*arrows*).

characteristic, with a well-defined smooth mass (Fig. 10-41) of uniform fluid density. The diagnosis is likely in patients with the appropriate surgical history.

Lymphangiectasia

Lymphangiectasia is a benign, usually congenital disease that is caused by dilated peritoneal lymphatics, usually idiopathic in nature but sometimes resulting from the lymphatic obstructive effects of granulomatous disease or malignancies. The lymphatic obstruction can lead to diarrhea, hypoproteinemia, and small bowel mucosal thickening (see Chapter 4). The disease is usually identified at CT as cystic structures (sometimes similar to lymphangioma) along the route of the mesentery (Fig. 10-42).

Desmoid Tumor

Desmoid tumors are of unknown origin (although often identified in patients with prior abdominal surgery and commonly

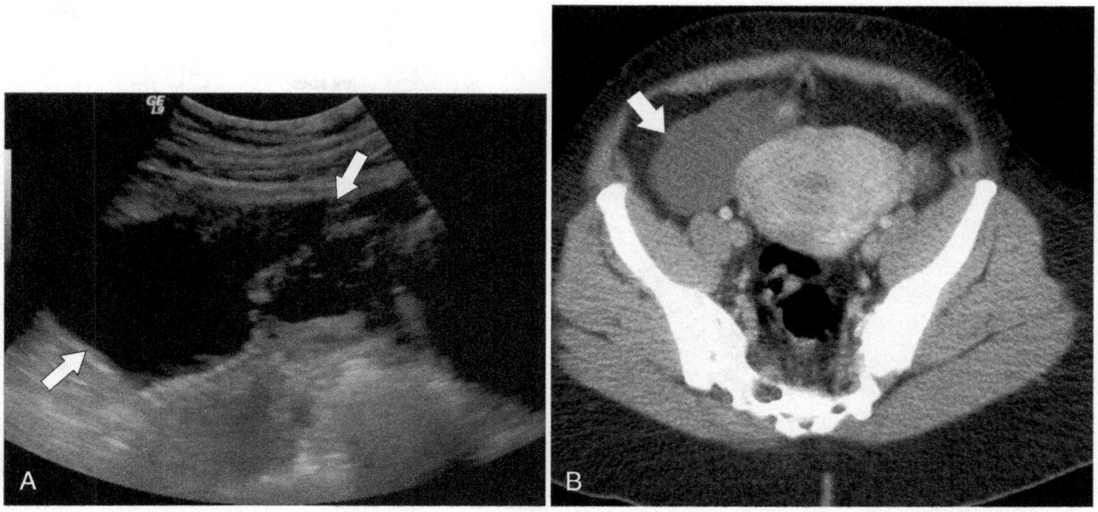

FIGURE 10-37. Transvaginal US (**A**) and axial contrast-enhanced CT (**B**) in a 39-year-old woman with a complex cystic lesion representing a peritoneal inclusion cyst (*arrows*).

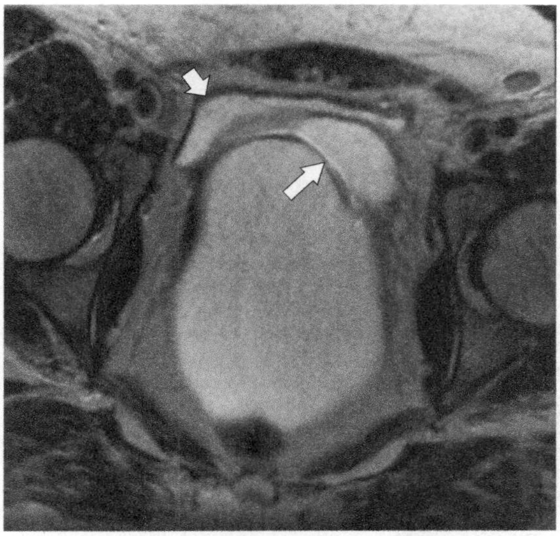

FIGURE 10-38. Axial T2-weighted MRI in a 37-year-old woman with a large peritoneal inclusion cyst (*large arrow*), distinct from the bladder (*small arrow*).

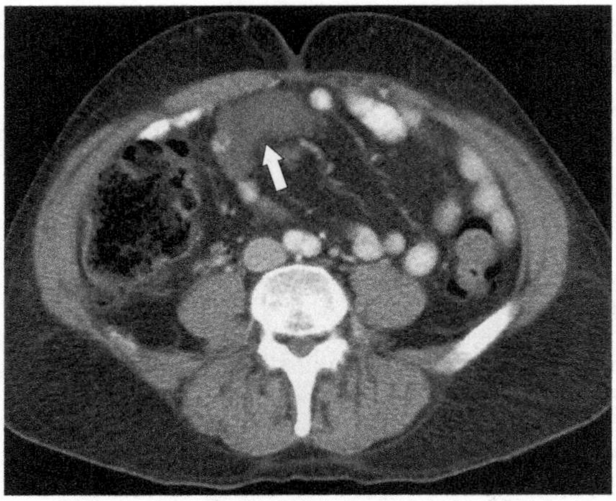

FIGURE 10-39. Axial contrast-enhanced CT in a 53-year-old man with a lower abdominal cystic mesenteric lesion (*arrow*) representing lymphangioma.

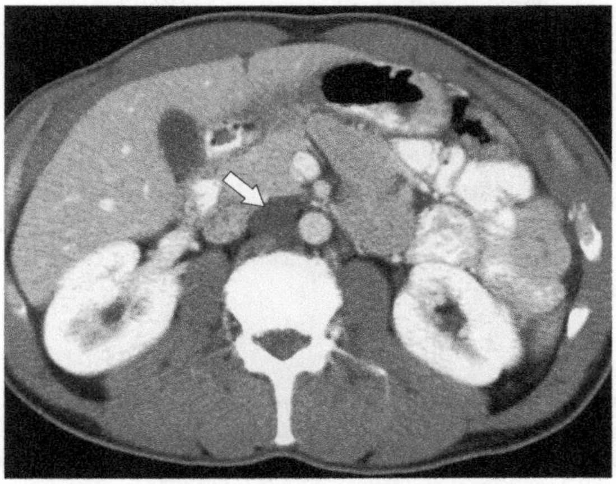

FIGURE 10-40. Axial contrast-enhanced CT in a 39-year-old woman with a 3-cm retroperitoneal cystic structure (*arrow*) representing lymphangioma.

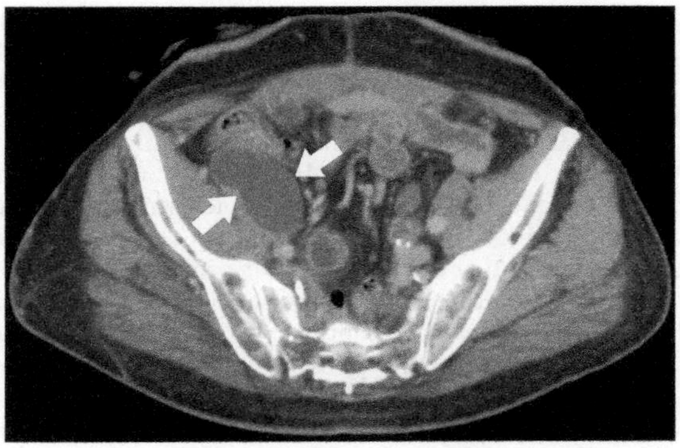

FIGURE 10-41. Axial contrast-enhanced CT in a 67-year-old man with a postoperative seroma (*arrows*).

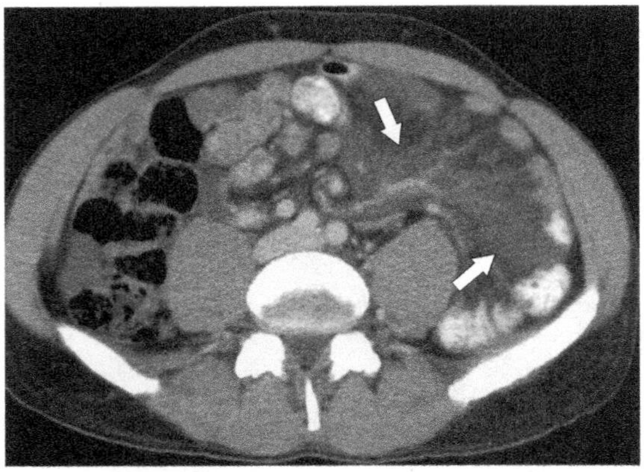

FIGURE 10-42. Axial contrast-enhanced CT in a 49-year-old woman with congenital lymphangiectasia (*arrows*).

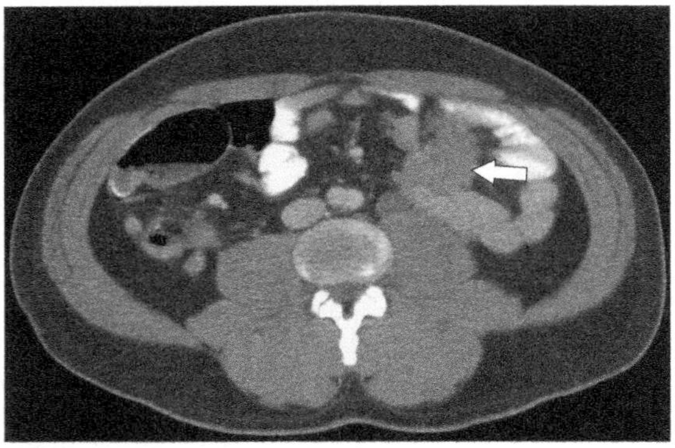

FIGURE 10-43. Axial contrast-enhanced CT in a 41-year-old man with a solitary soft tissue mass in the central mesentery (*arrow*) that represents a desmoid tumor.

associated with Gardner syndrome, particularly when multiple), can be single or multiple, and are also known as fibromatosis. Although benign, these tumors can recur after resection and locally invade surrounding bowel. Therefore they are difficult to remove completely. They are usually located within the mesentery but can reside in the retroperitoneum or abdominal wall. Desmoid tumors are most commonly identified incidentally at CT, typically as single (sometimes multiple), nonspecific, rounded soft tissue masses within the mesentery (Fig. 10-43). They can cause displacement or retraction of bowel loops.

Dermoid Tumor

Dermoid tumors are most commonly present in the pelvis, but larger lesions can extend into the abdomen and are ovarian in origin. They are also known as dermoid cysts or cystic teratomas and represent a primitive tumor that contains multiple tissue elements, including fat, teeth, hair, and cartilage, among other tissues. Almost all of these tumors are benign, although a malignant teratoma is recognized. They are readily identifiable at CT by their fat content (Fig. 10-44) (and sometimes other soft tissue or calcified features) and at US by diffuse hyperechogenicity resulting from the fat content. Rarely, multiple well-circumscribed fatty dermoid masses can be identified throughout the abdomen after traumatic rupture of the pelvic neoplasm, which disseminates throughout the peritoneum. At ultrasound, dermoid tumors are thought to appear similar to falling snow or a snowstorm (Fig. 10-45), but they might also be identified by other calcified or soft tissue elements.

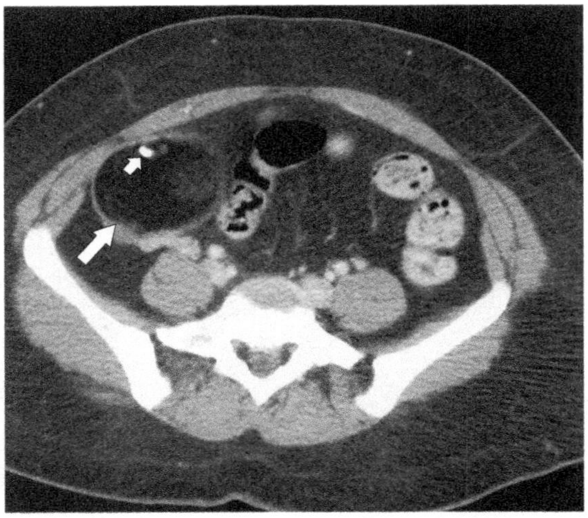

FIGURE 10-44. Axial contrast-enhanced CT in a 41-year-old woman with a predominantly fatty mass due to a dermoid tumor (*large arrow*). There is also dense internal calcification (*small arrow*).

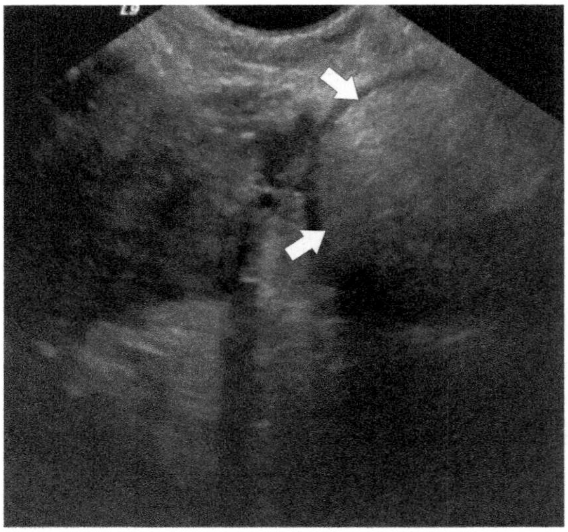

FIGURE 10-45. Transvaginal US in a 33-year-old woman with a left adnexal dermoid tumor (*arrows*) and a diffuse hyperechogenicity caused by its fat content.

Malignant Peritoneal Masses

Metastases

Metastatic deposits are by far the most common malignant peritoneal mesenteric masses or retroperitoneal deposits. They arise by direct invasion or ascitic spread (Figs. 10-46 and 10-47) or via hematogenous or lymphatic routes. The deposits can be either single and focal (Fig. 10-48) or diffuse. Diffuse involvement can invade the omentum, causing it to be studded with tumor deposits (known as omental "caking"), an appearance that can be subtle (Fig. 10-49) or obvious (Fig. 10-50). This should be differentiated from the omental caking resulting from diffuse tuberculous abdominal disease (Fig. 10-51).

Abdominal Mesothelioma

Abdominal mesothelioma is a rare primary malignancy of the peritoneum and is a similar tumor to the more common pleural mesothelioma. It is associated with prior asbestos exposure. In fact, up to 50% of patients show calcified pleural plaques. The

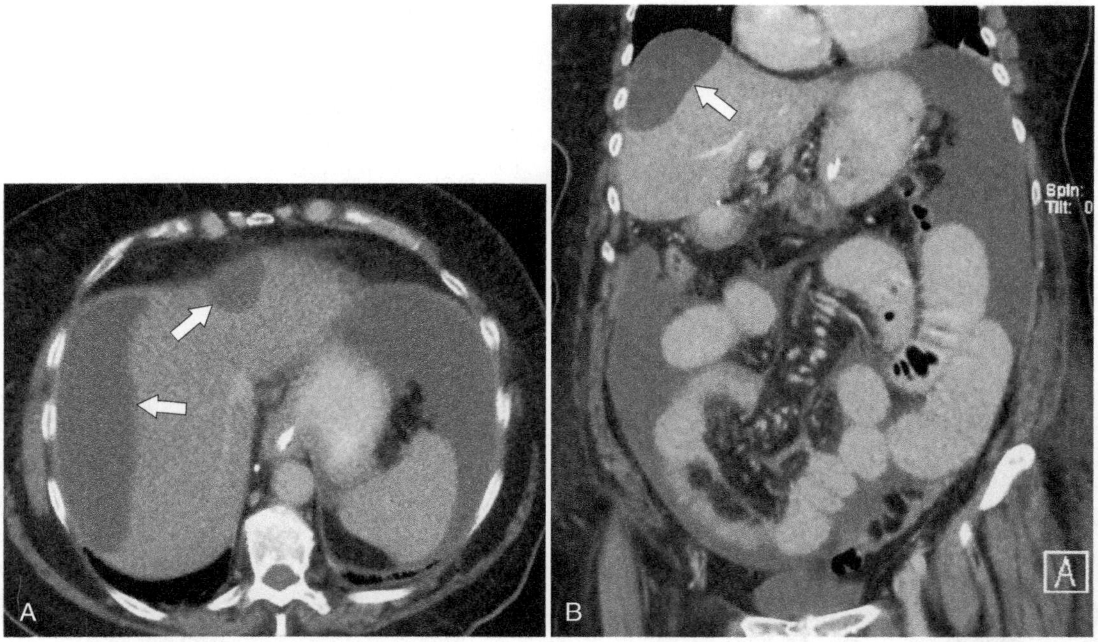

FIGURE 10-46. Axial (**A**) and coronal (**B**) contrast-enhanced CT in a 61-year-old woman with metastatic ovarian cancer that characteristically "scallops" the liver capsule (*arrows*). There is widespread malignant ascites.

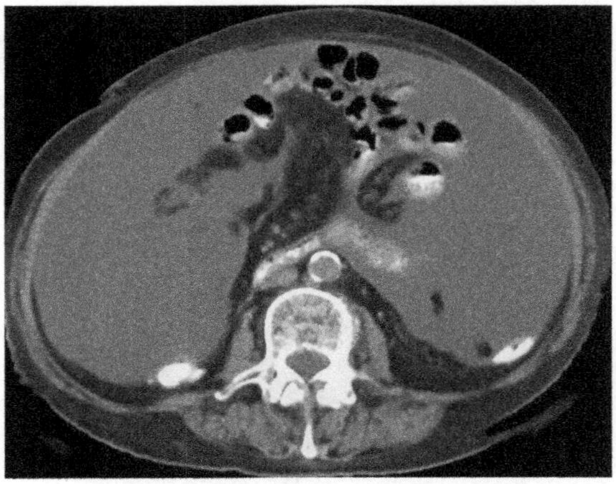

FIGURE 10-47. Axial contrast-enhanced CT in an 83-year-old woman with diffuse peritoneal ascites and crowding of small bowel caused by metastatic ovarian cancer.

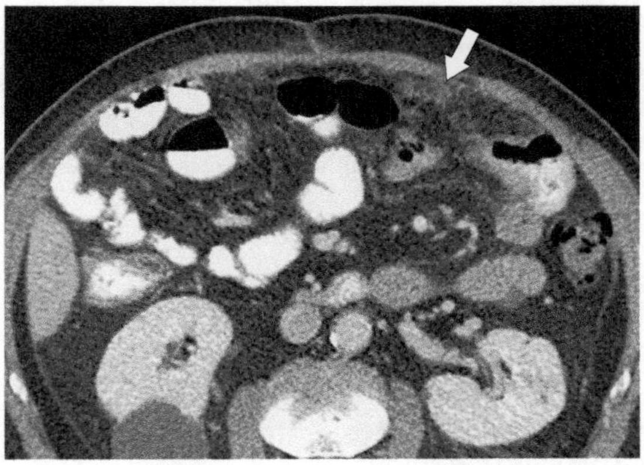

FIGURE 10-49. Axial contrast-enhanced CT in a 56-year-old man with several omental nodules (*arrow*) representing gastric cancer metastases.

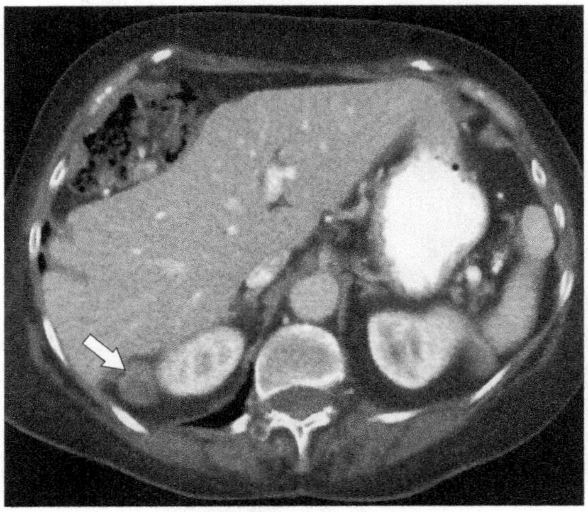

FIGURE 10-48. Axial contrast-enhanced CT in a 64-year-old woman with a soft tissue metastatic deposit (*arrow*) in Morison pouch from ovarian cancer.

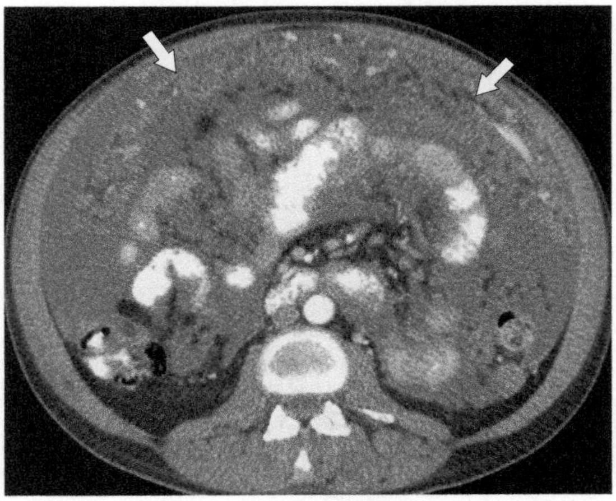

FIGURE 10-50. Axial contrast-enhanced CT in a 48-year-old woman with diffuse omental "caking" (*arrows*) and ascites caused by metastatic gastric cancer.

diagnosis is therefore suggested in patients with peritoneal or omental thickening and calcified pleural plaques. The findings at CT vary, from ascites and fine reticular-like peritoneal changes (Fig. 10-52) to more mass-like deposits (Fig. 10-53).

Pseudomyxoma Peritonei

Pseudomyxoma peritonei is caused by the widespread peritoneal deposition of mucinous material usually from a ruptured appendix. Other mucin-producing tumors, including those of the colon and rectum among others, can also metastasize to produce pseudomyxoma. It produces multiple low-density globular masses throughout the abdomen and can envelop the small bowel, causing multiple areas of stricturing. It surrounds the liver capsule and, like ovarian metastatic disease, causes a scalloped appearance of the liver capsule (Fig. 10-54). Pseudomyxoma peritonei is difficult to treat because it is usually impossible to remove all the intraabdominal mucinous material, which therefore frequently recurs. Most patients ultimately die of the relentless mucinous process.

Liposarcoma

Liposarcoma is a malignant tumor of adipose tissue in the retroperitoneum or peritoneum (it can also occur elsewhere, such as the thigh). These are usually large bulky tumors with mass

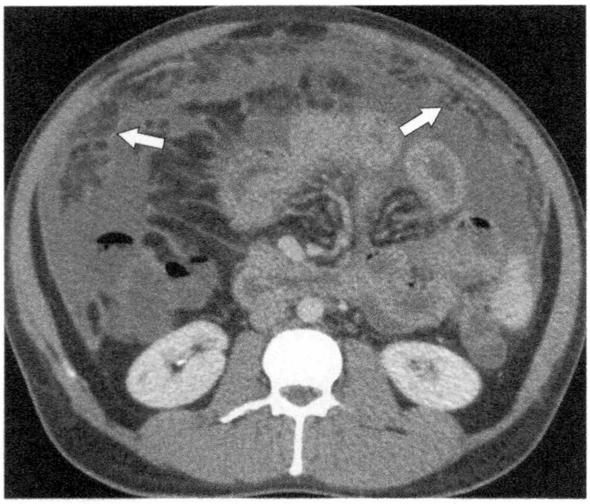

FIGURE 10-51. Axial contrast-enhanced CT in a 33-year-old woman with omental thickening (*arrows*) and ascites caused by abdominal tuberculosis.

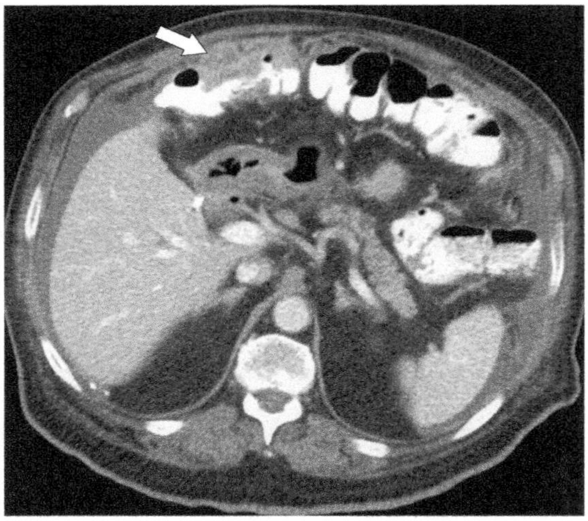

FIGURE 10-53. Axial contrast-enhanced CT in a 65-year-old man with ascites and omental mass (*arrow*) caused by abdominal mesothelioma.

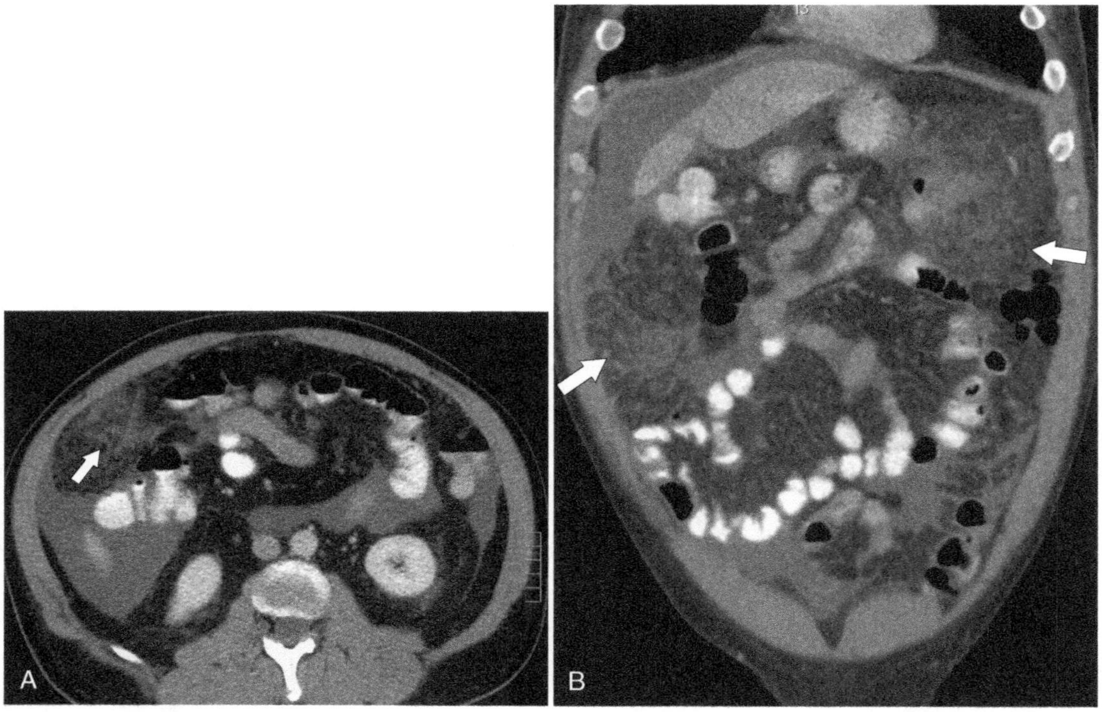

FIGURE 10-52. Axial (**A**) and coronal (**B**) contrast-enhanced CT in a 50-year-old man with ascites and mesenteric and omental reticular thickening (*arrows*) caused by abdominal mesothelioma.

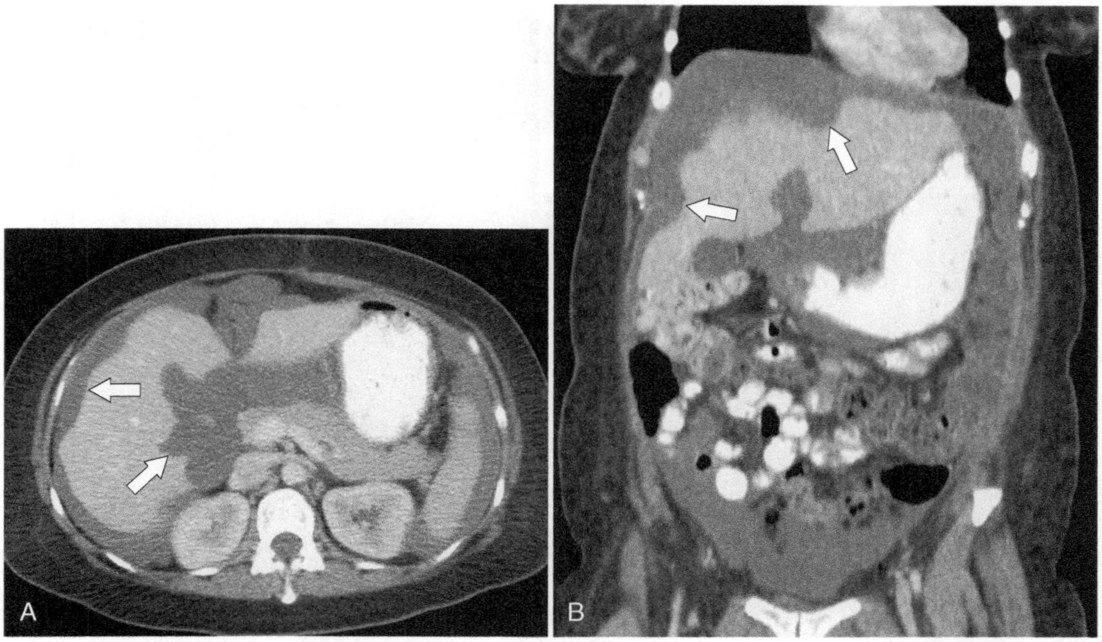

FIGURE 10-54. Axial (**A**) and coronal (**B**) contrast-enhanced CT in a 38-year-old woman with pseudomyxoma peritonei, scalloping of the liver margin (*arrows*), and diffuse intraabdominal mucinous deposits.

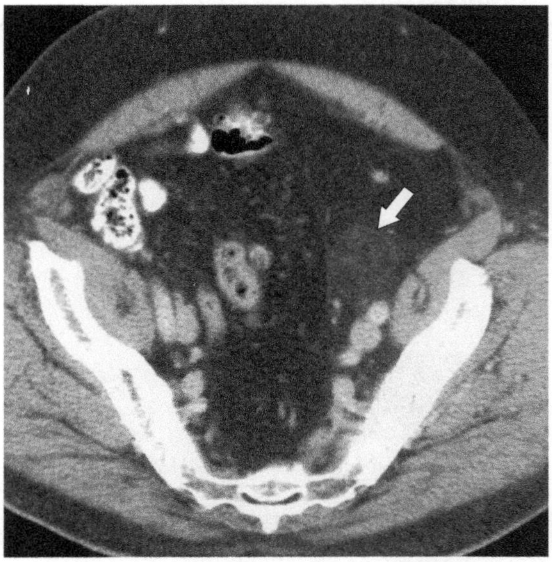

FIGURE 10-55. Axial contrast-enhanced CT in a 53-year-old man with a subtle fatty mass (*arrow*) in the left pelvis resulting from liposarcoma. Fat necrosis could have similar appearances.

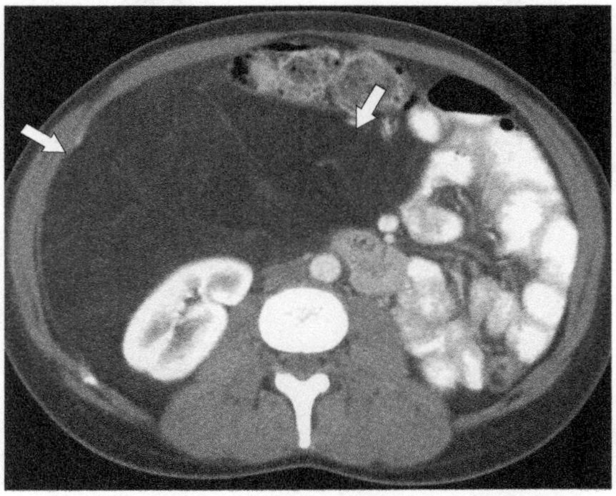

FIGURE 10-56. Axial contrast-enhanced CT in a 49-year-old man with a right retroperitoneal fatty mass (*arrows*) that has mass effect on the colon and small bowel and is caused by a liposarcoma.

effect. On CT they can be quite subtle (Fig. 10-55) or may be recognized only by their mass effect (Fig. 10-56). Most masses are more obvious and multilobulated and predominantly fatty with few soft tissue elements (Fig. 10-57), although occasionally there is a larger soft tissue component (Fig. 10-58). These tumors require differentiation from uterine lipoleiomyoma, a benign fatty fibroid identified rarely in postmenopausal women (Fig. 10-59).

Lymphoma (see Chapters 2 and 4)

Multiple enlarged mesenteric lymph nodes are most likely caused by intraabdominal lymphoma, especially if associated with retroperitoneal adenopathy. There are numerous subtypes of lymphoma, discussed in greater detail in Chapter 2. The disease is usually evaluated by CT, which readily demonstrates intraabdominal lymphadenopathy as discrete nodes (Fig. 10-60) or a conglomerate mesenteric or retroperitoneal mass (Fig. 10-61). After chemotherapy there is often a dramatic response with almost complete resolution of the lymphoid masses, but subtle residual disease that resembles mesenteric panniculitis frequently remains (Fig. 10-60). However, there is usually no residual tumor within the mass. The disease is frequently monitored with PET/CT and may show response to chemotherapy earlier on the PET than the CT study (Figs. 10-61 and 10-62).

Retroperitoneal Lymphadenopathy

Small (<1 cm in short axis) lymph nodes are often present in the retroperitoneum and mesentery. Although usually clinically insignificant, they are also a common site for neoplastic and

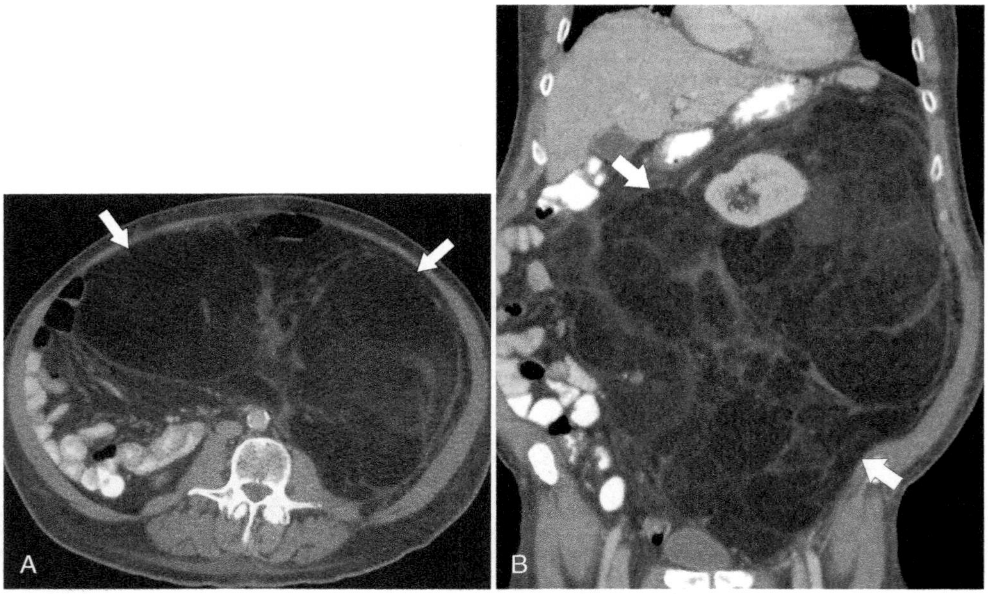

Figure 10-57. Axial (**A**) and coronal (**B**) contrast-enhanced CT in an 83-year-old man with a large multilobulated peritoneal fatty mass (*arrows*) with minor soft tissue components, caused by liposarcoma.

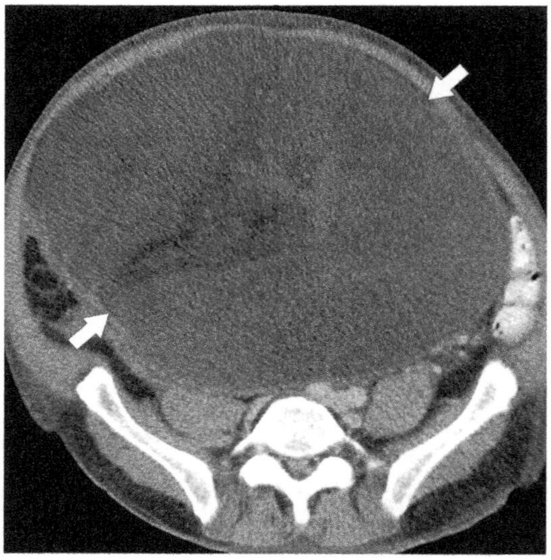

Figure 10-58. Axial contrast-enhanced CT in a 75-year-old woman with a large mixed fatty/soft tissue abdominal mass caused by liposarcoma (*arrows*).

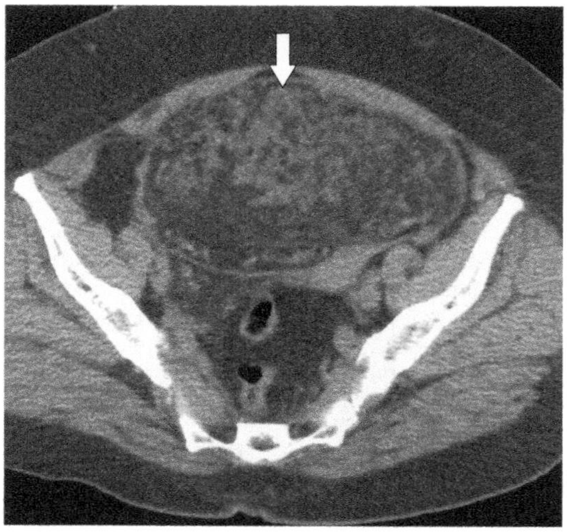

Figure 10-59. Axial noncontrast CT in a 57-year-old woman with lipoleiomyoma of the uterus (*arrow*).

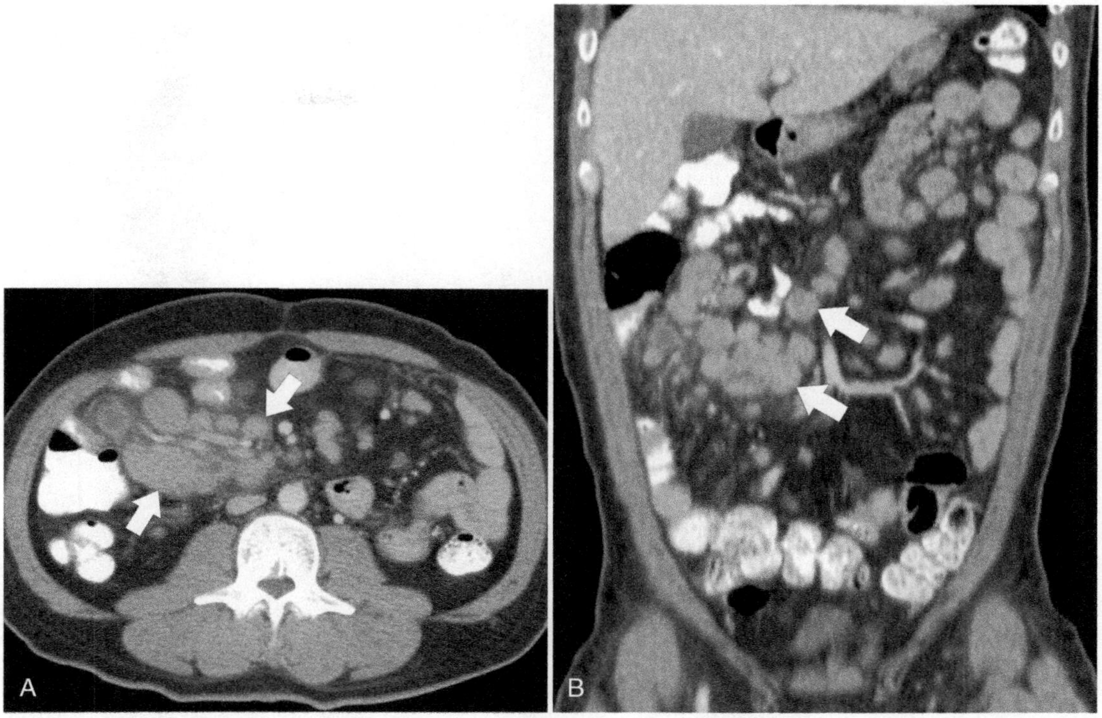

FIGURE 10-60. Axial (**A**) and coronal (**B**) contrast-enhanced CT in a 40-year-old man with intraabdominal lymphadenopathy (*arrows*) caused by lymphoma.

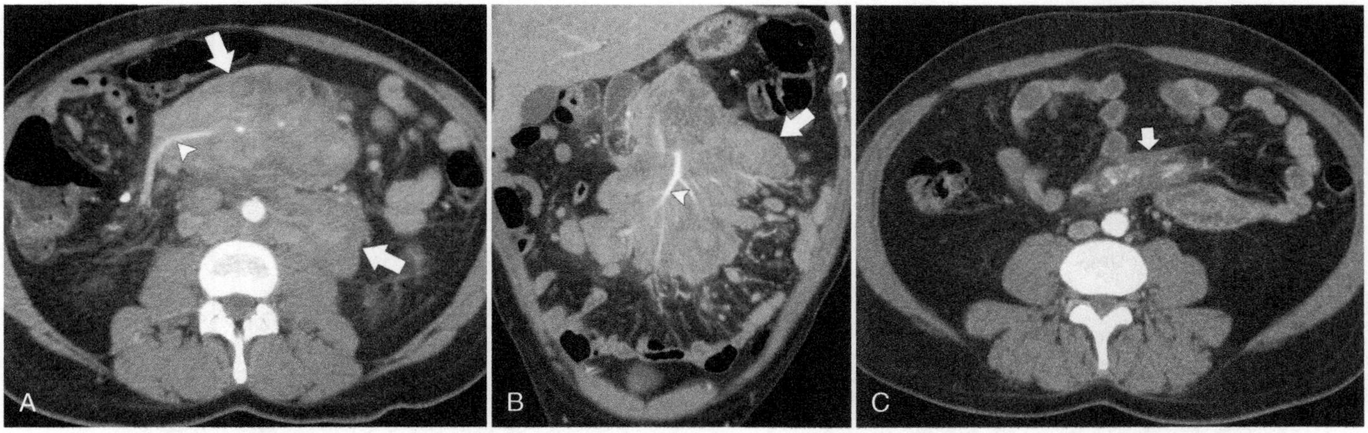

FIGURE 10-61. Axial (**A**) and coronal (**B**) contrast-enhanced CT in a 52-year-old man with bulky abdominal lymphadenopathy (*large arrows*) caused by lymphoma. After chemotherapy, on contrast-enhanced CT (**C**) there is almost complete disappearance of the disease, with residual hazy fat changes (*small arrow*). This is most likely a metabolic response with no active residual tumor. Note that vascular integrity is preserved as is characteristic with lymphoma (*arrowheads*).

nonneoplastic disease. Neoplastic disease is often secondary to lymphoma, but many intraabdominal and extraabdominal malignancies metastasize to the retroperitoneum, either as discrete, sometimes single nodes (Fig. 10-63) or as multiple and sometimes less-defined nodes (Fig. 10-64). Many infectious (e.g., tuberculosis, appendicitis, cholecystitis), autoimmune (rheumatoid arthritis), and systemic (e.g., sarcoidosis, systemic lupus erythematosus, amyloidosis, mastocytosis) diseases can also cause retroperitoneal lymphadenopathy, but these are often part of a wider spectrum of lymphadenopathy elsewhere. Lymphadenopathy caused by tuberculosis or *Mycobacterium avium-intracellulare* infection (often seen in acquired immune deficiency syndrome) is characteristically hypodense (Fig. 10-65).

Retroperitoneal Fibrosis

Retroperitoneal fibrosis is a fibrotic disease of the retroperitoneum, usually the lower retroperitoneum. The cause is most commonly idiopathic but can also be autoimmune disease (ankylosing spondylitis, systemic lupus erythematosus, scleroderma), inflammatory periaortitis (secondary to aortic aneurysms), some malignancies (lymphoma, sarcoma, carcinoma), and drug therapy (beta-blockers, methyldopa). Depending on the cause, patients respond well to immunosuppressive therapy. Patients present with nonspecific back pain or peripheral edema caused by venous compressive effects; deep venous thrombosis is therefore a complication. On imaging, a soft tissue mass envelops the lower aorta and inferior vena cava (Fig. 10-66) and may also involve the

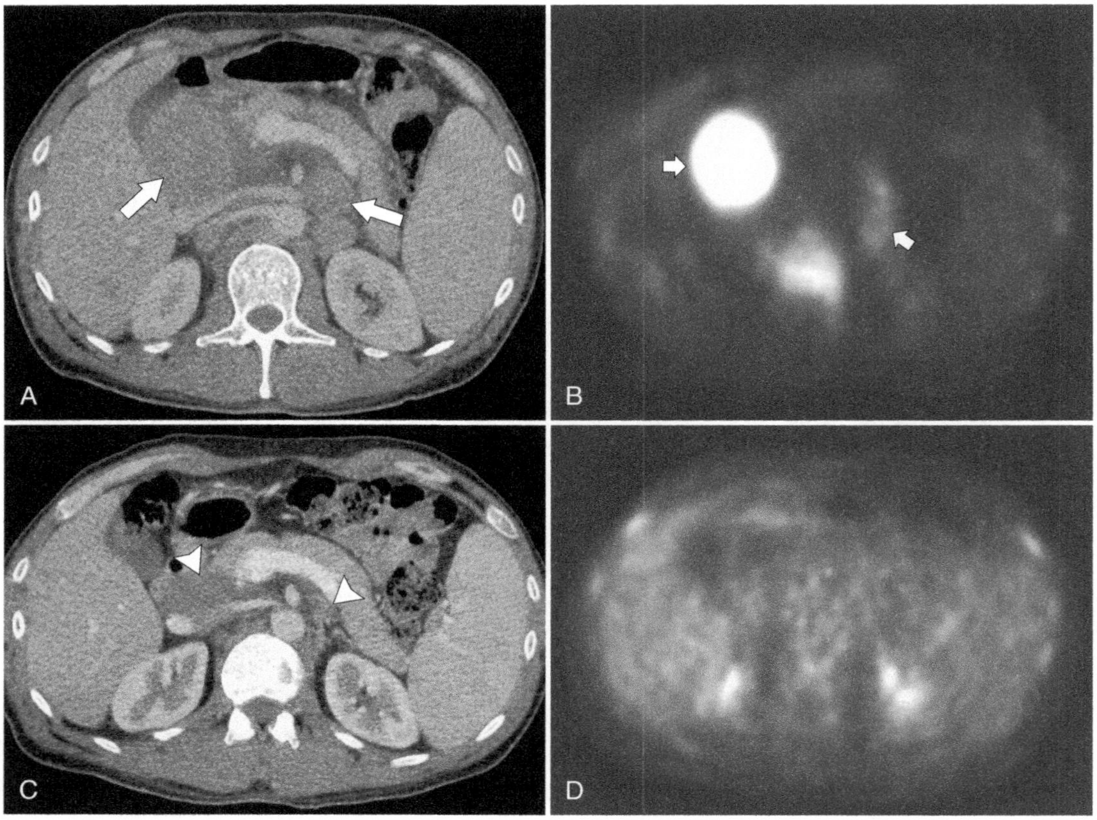

FIGURE 10-62. Axial contrast-enhanced PET/CT in a 40-year-old man with follicular lymphoma with abdominal lymphadenopathy (**A**; *arrows*), which are fluorodeoxyglucose avid (**B**; *small arrows*). After chemotherapy, there is still residual, but less, disease seen on CT (**C**; *arrowheads*) but complete response seen on PET (**D**).

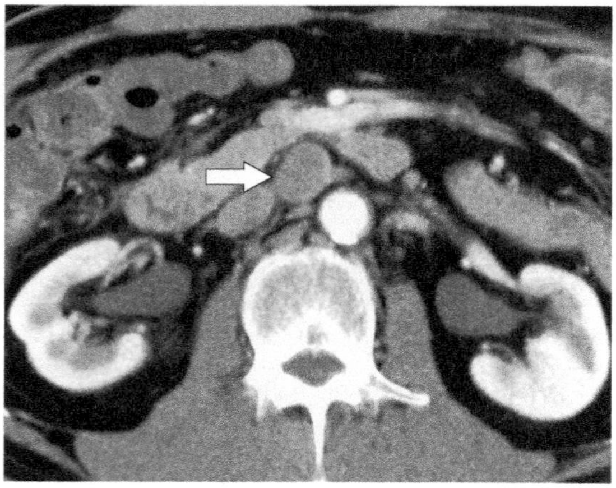

FIGURE 10-63. Axial contrast-enhanced CT in a 56-year-old woman with colon cancer and a single discrete retroperitoneal 2.3-cm lymph node (*arrow*).

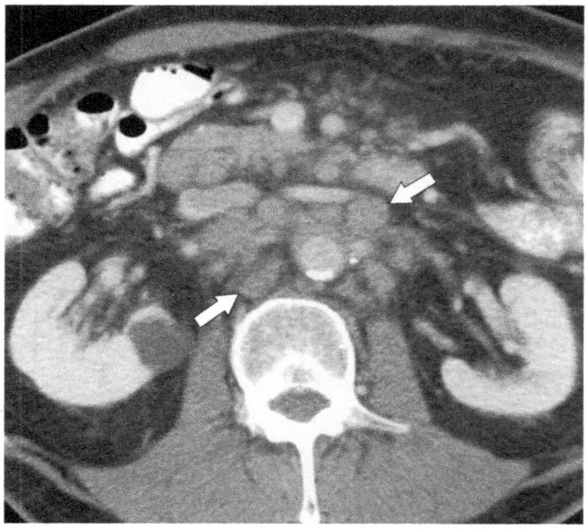

FIGURE 10-64. Axial contrast-enhanced CT in a 66-year-old woman with colon cancer and multiple ill-defined retroperitoneal nodes (*arrows*).

ureters, resulting in hydronephrosis. Because of its inflammatory nature, retroperitoneal fibrosis in the acute phase may demonstrate intense uptake at FDG-PET (Fig. 10-66). Diffuse retroperitoneal lymphadenopathy from lymphoma can appear similar and may also demonstrate increased uptake on PET imaging, but the retroperitoneum is often not the only site of disease and therefore it can be differentiated from retroperitoneal fibrosis (Fig. 10-67).

Extramedullary Hematopoiesis

Extramedullary hematopoiesis refers to ectopic hematopoiesis outside the bony medulla. It is therefore associated with conditions causing bone marrow displacement, particularly myelofibrosis but also congenital hemolytic anemias and thalassemia. Patients are usually asymptomatic, but mediastinal, retroperitoneal, or pelvic sites of hematopoiesis can develop and can be mistaken for lymphadenopathy or other malignant masses (Fig. 10-68).

Abdominal Wall Hemorrhage

Hemorrhage in the abdominal wall musculature is a relatively common event in patients receiving anticoagulant therapy. However, it may be traumatic (blunt injury or surgery) or caused by excessive coughing or sometimes pregnancy. At imaging, the diagnosis is usually straightforward with a hyperdense mass in the affected musculature (Fig. 10-69), which may demonstrate a hematocrit level (Fig. 10-70).

Propylene (Prolene) Plug

Propylene (Prolene) plug is a nonabsorbable material that is used to "fill" the hernial orifice and thus prevent hernial recurrence. Its appearance at CT imaging should be recognized (Fig. 10-71) and not confused with other, more sinister soft tissue masses. It is usually identified based on the appropriate history and expected location of the plug.

AlloDerm Spacers

AlloDerm spacers are a patented human tissue matrix (acellular human dermis) increasingly used in patients undergoing radiation or proton beam therapy. The cadaveric human tissue separates vital normal anatomical strictures from the radiation portal. AlloDerm has also been used for graft repair, breast reconstructive surgery, and hernia repairs. Its appearances are characteristic at CT with a multilayered, sometimes whorled appearance of the dermal collagen matrix (Fig. 10-72). The spacer involutes after a period of time and can be mistaken for a soft tissue mass and

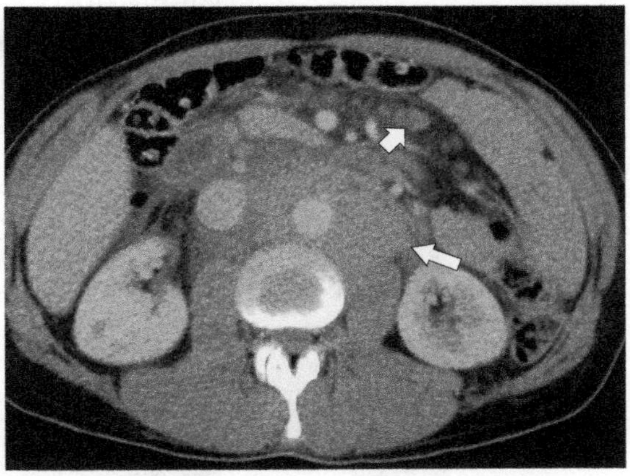

FIGURE 10-67. Axial contrast-enhanced CT in a 44-year-old woman with retroperitoneal lymphoma (*large arrow*) with appearances similar to retroperitoneal fibrosis. There are, however, smaller nodes in the mesentery (*small arrow*).

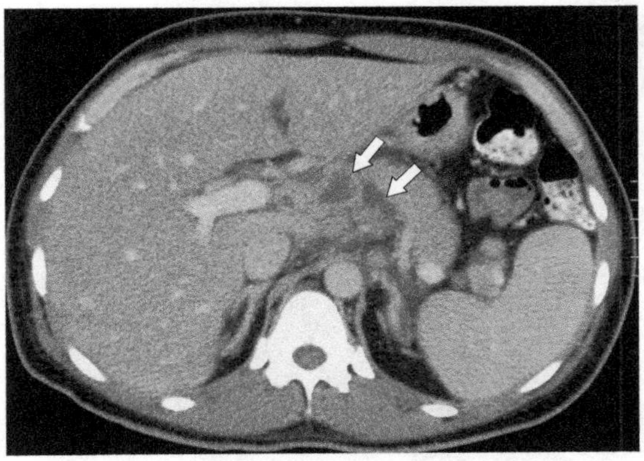

FIGURE 10-65. Axial contrast-enhanced CT in a 23-year-old woman with tuberculosis and multiple hypodense retroperitoneal lymph nodes (*arrows*).

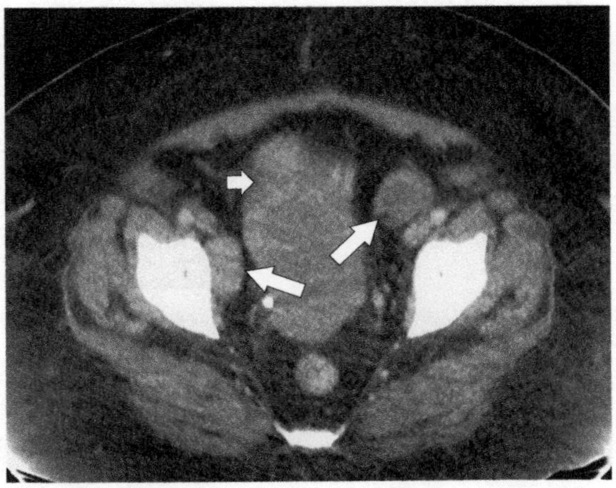

FIGURE 10-68. Axial contrast-enhanced CT in a 48-year-old woman with extramedullary hematopoiesis in the pelvis (*large arrows*). There is a fibroid uterus (*small arrow*).

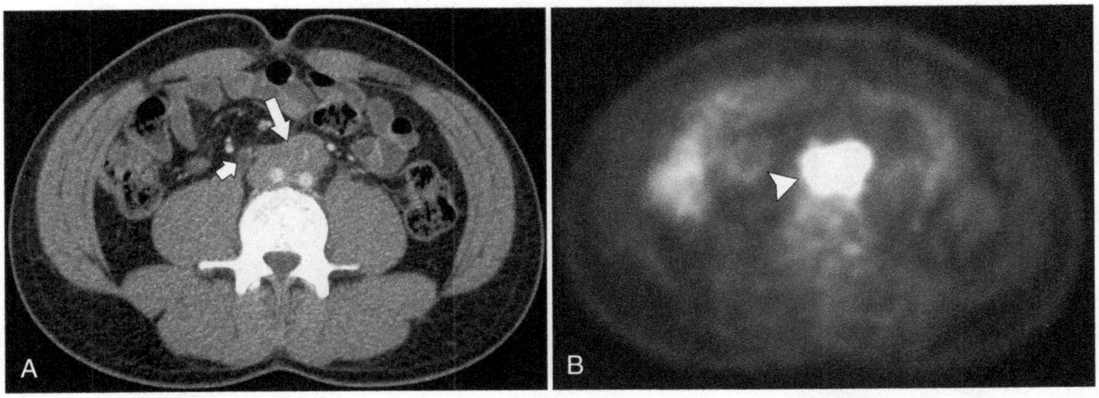

FIGURE 10-66. A, Axial contrast-enhanced CT in a 44-year-old woman with idiopathic retroperitoneal fibrosis and a soft tissue mass that envelops the aortic bifurcation and inferior vena cava (*large arrow*). There is right ureter dilatation (*small arrow*) caused by inflammatory involvement more caudally. **B,** The disease is fluorodeoxyglucose avid at PET (*arrowhead*).

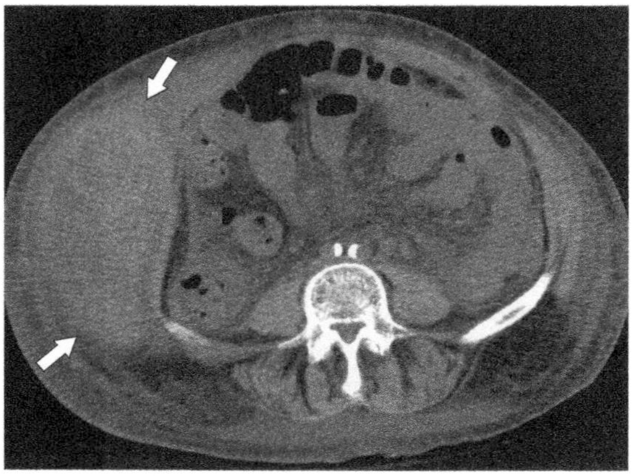

FIGURE 10-69. Axial noncontrast CT in a 71-year-old woman with a right-sided hyperdense mass representing an external oblique muscle hematoma (*arrows*).

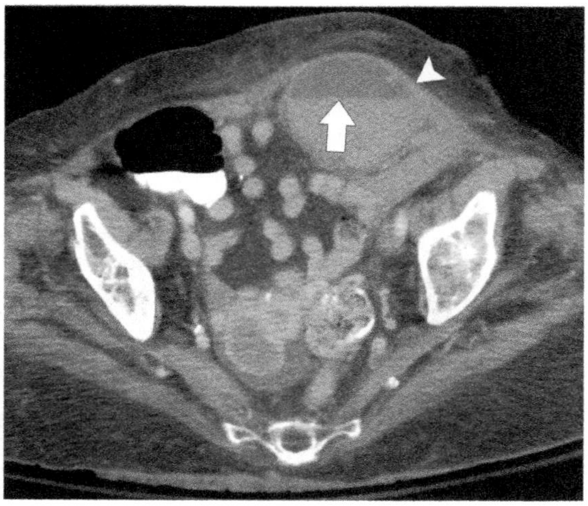

FIGURE 10-70. Axial contrast-enhanced CT in a 68-year-old woman with a left-sided rectus sheath hematoma (*arrowhead*) that demonstrates a hematocrit level (*arrow*).

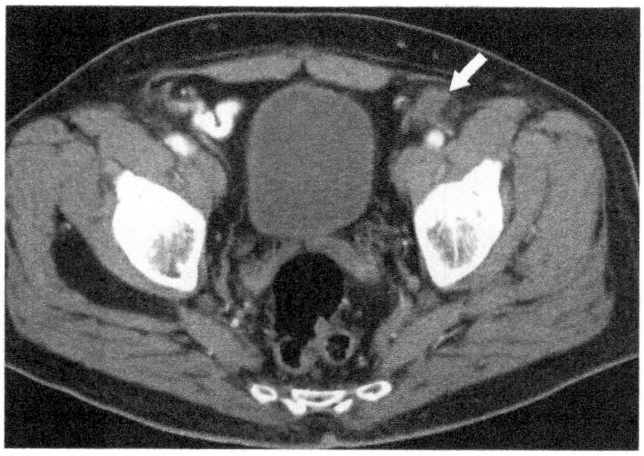

FIGURE 10-71. Axial contrast-enhanced CT in a 51-year-old man with a left-sided propylene (Prolene) plug (*arrow*) used in prior left hernia repair.

possible metastatic deposit, particularly because many patients are being treated for an underlying malignancy (Fig. 10-72).

Gossypiboma

Gossypiboma refers to retained intraabdominal surgical material that is accidently left within the abdominal cavity. The name gossypiboma is derived from the Latin word for cotton (gossypium) and usually refers to retained surgical sponge material. Gossypibomas are thought to occur in only approximately 1 in 5000 surgeries. Patients usually present with a sign and symptom of abscess formation (Fig. 10-73). If uninfected, patients present with adhesions and a foreign body granuloma.

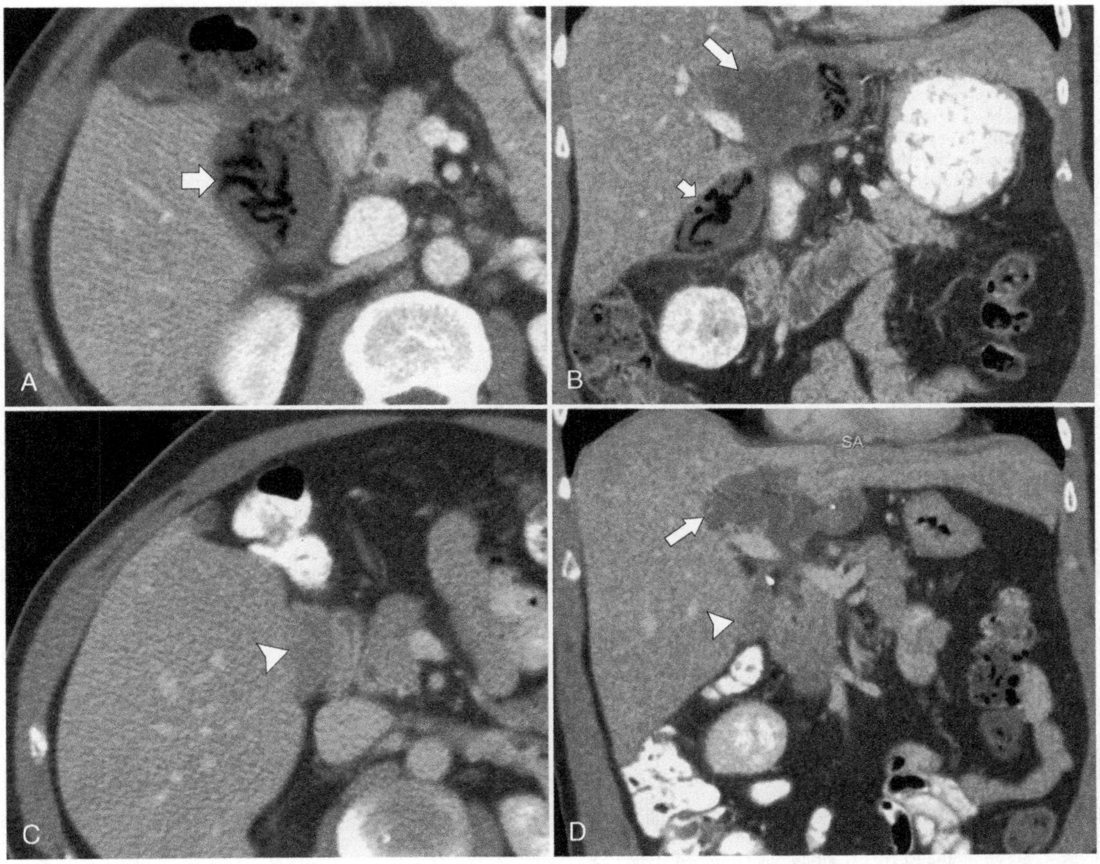

FIGURE 10-72. Axial (**A** and **C**) and coronal (**B** and **D**) contrast-enhanced CT in a 53-year-old man with cholangiocarcinoma (*large arrows*) and AlloDerm spacers (*small arrows*). Recent placement demonstrates serpiginous formation but later appears as a soft tissue density, mimicking a mass and recurrent disease (*arrowheads*).

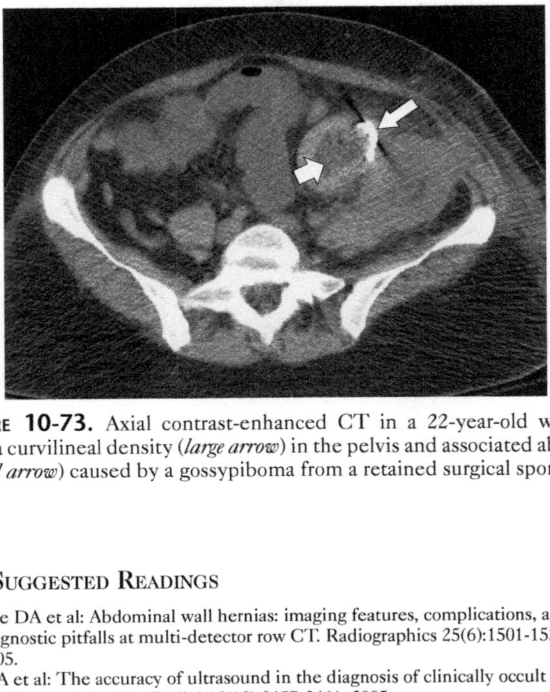

FIGURE 10-73. Axial contrast-enhanced CT in a 22-year-old woman with a curvilineal density (*large arrow*) in the pelvis and associated abscess (*small arrow*) caused by a gossypiboma from a retained surgical sponge.

SUGGESTED READINGS

Aguirre DA et al: Abdominal wall hernias: imaging features, complications, and diagnostic pitfalls at multi-detector row CT. Radiographics 25(6):1501-1520, 2005.

Alam A et al: The accuracy of ultrasound in the diagnosis of clinically occult groin hernias in adults. Eur Radiol 15(12):2457-2461, 2005.

Atr M et al: Surgically important bowel and/or mesenteric injury in blunt trauma: accuracy of multidetector CT for evaluation. Radiology 249(2):524-533, 2008.

Burkhardt JH et al: Diagnosis of inguinal region hernias with axial CT: the lateral crescent sign and other key findings. Radiographics 31(2):E1-E12, 2011.

Carucci LR et al: Internal hernia following Roux-en-Y gastric bypass surgery for morbid obesity: evaluation of radiographic findings at small-bowel examination. Radiology 251(3):762-770, 2009.

Catalano OA et al: Internal hernia with volvulus and intussusception: case report. Abdom Imaging 29(2):164-165, 2004.

Chavhan GB et al: Multimodality imaging of the pediatric diaphragm: anatomy and pathologic conditions. Radiographics 30(7):1797-1817, 2010.

Cherian PT et al: Radiologic anatomy of the inguinofermal region: insights from MDCT. AJR 189(4):W177-W183, 2007.

Cherian PT et al: The diagnosis and classification of inguinal and femoral hernia on multisection spiral CT. Clin Radiol 63(2):184-192, 2008.

Cioppa T et al: Cytoreduction and hyperthermic intraperitoneal chemotherapy in the treatment of peritoneal carcinomatosis from pseudomyxoma peritonei. World J Gastroenterol 14(44):6817-6823, 2008.

Cronin CG et al: Retroperitoneal fibrosis: a review of clinical features and imaging findings. AJR 191(2):423-431, 2008.

Cronin CG et al: Pictorial essay: multitechnique imaging findings of prolene plug hernia repair. AJR 195:701-706, 2010.

Demir MK et al: Case 108: sclerosing encapsulating peritonitis. Radiology 242(3):937-939, 2007.

Desir A, Ghaye B: CT of blunt diaphragmatic rupture. Radiographics 32(2): 477-498, 2012.

Dinauer PA et al: Pathologic and MR imaging features of benign fibrous soft-tissue tumors in adults. Radiographics 27(1):173-187, 2007.

Fuks D et al: CT can help the surgeon consider conversion from laparoscopic to open cholecystectomy. Radiology 263(1):128-138, 2012.

Fukukura Y et al: Autoimmune pancreatitis associated with idiopathic retroperitoneal fibrosis. AJR 181(4):993-995, 2003.

Garg PK et al: Subcutaneous and breast metastasis from asymptomatic gallbladder carcinoma. Hepatobiliary Pancreat Dis Int 8(2):209-211, 2009.

Gayer G et al: Foreign objects encountered in the abdominal cavity at CT. Radiographics 31(2):409-428, 2011.

George C et al: Computed tomography appearances of sclerosing encapsulating peritonitis. Clin Radiol 62(8):732-737, 2007.

Hanbidge AE et al: US of the peritoneum. Radiographics 23(3):663-684, 2003. discussion 684-685.

Harshen R et al: Pseudomyxoma peritonei. Clin Oncol (R Coll Radiol) 15(2):73-77, 2004.

Horton KM et al: CT findings in sclerosing mesenteritis (panniculitis): spectrum of disease. Radiographics 23(6):1561-1567, 2003.

Iannuccilli JD et al: Sensitivity and specificity of eight CT signs in the preoperative diagnosis of internal mesenteric hernia following Roux-en-Y gastric bypass surgery. Clin Radiol 64(4):373-380, 2009.

Jacquemin G et al: Pseudomyxoma peritonei: review on a cluster of peritoneal mucinous diseases. Acta Chir Belg 105(2):127-133, 2005.

Jaffe TA et al: Practice patterns in percutaneous image-guided intraabdominal abscess drainage: survey of academic and private practice centers. Radiology 233(3):750-756, 2004.

Jayne DG: The molecular biology of peritoneal carcinomatosis from gastrointestinal cancer. Ann Acad Med Singapore 32(2):219-225, 2003.

Johnson PT et al: The elephant trunk procedure for aortic aneurysm repair: an illustrated guide to surgical technique with CT correlation. AJR 197: W1052-W1059, 2011.

Kamaya A et al: Imaging manifestations of abdominal fat necrosis and its mimics. Radiographics 31(7):2021-2034, 2011.

Kandpal H et al: Combined transmesocolic and left paraduodenal hernia: barium, CT and MRI features. Abdom Imaging 32(2):224-227, 2007.

Kim SH et al: Esophageal varices in patients with cirrhosis: multidetector CT esophagography—comparison with endoscopy. Radiology 242(3):759-768, 2007.

Kreuzberg B et al: Diagnostic problems of abdominal desmoids tumors in various locations. Eur J Radiol 62(2):180-185, 2007.

Larici AR et al: Helical CT with sagittal and coronal reconstructions: accuracy for detection of diaphragmatic injury. AJR 179(2):451-457, 2002.

Lee JC et al: Aggressive fibromatosis: MRI features with pathologic correlation. AJR 186(1):247-254, 2006.

Lee WK et al: Infected (mycotic) aneurysms: spectrum of imaging appearances and management. Radiographics 28(7):1853-1868, 2008.

Levy AD et al: From the archives of the AFIP: benign fibrous tumors and tumorlike lesions of the mesentery: radiologic-pathologic correlation. Radiographics 26(1):245-264, 2006.

Lockhart ME et al: Internal hernia after gastric bypass: sensitivity and specificity of seven CT signs with surgical correlation and controls. AJR 188:745-750, 2007.

Low RN: Diffusion-weighted MR imaging for the whole body metastatic disease and lymphadenopathy. Magn Reson Imaging Clin N Am 17(2):245-261, 2009.

Ly JQ: The Rigler sign. Radiology 228(3):706-707, 2003.

Martin LC et al: Review of internal hernias: radiographic and clinical findings. AJR 186(3):703-717, 2006.

McCarville MB et al: MRI and biologic behavior of desmoids tumors in children. AJR 189(3):633-640, 2007.

McDonald ES et al: Best cases from the AFIP: extraabdominal desmoids-type fibromatosis. Radiographics 28(3):901-906, 2008.

Morikawa T et al: Recurrent prostatic stromal sarcoma with massive high-grade prostatic intraepithelial neoplasia. J Clin Pathol 60(3):330-332, 2007.

Nason LK et al: Imaging of the diaphragm: anatomy and function. Radiographics 32(2):E51-E70, 2012.

Nishie A et al: Fitz-Hugh-Curtis syndrome: radiologic manifestation. J Comput Assist Tomogr 27(5):786-791, 2003.

Nishino M et al: Primary retroperitoneal neoplasms: CT and MR findings with anatomic and pathologic diagnostic clues. Radiographics 23(1):45-57, 2003.

Osadchy A et al: Small bowel obstruction related to left side paraduodenal hernia: CT findings. Abdom Imaging 30(1):53-55, 2005.

Park CM et al: Recurrent ovarian malignancy: patterns and spectrum of imaging findings. Abdom Imaging 28(3):404-415, 2003.

Power N et al: CT assessment of anastomotic bowel leak. Clin Radiol 62(1):37-42, 2007.

Purysko AS et al: Beyond appendicitis: common and uncommon gastrointestinal causes of right lower quadrant abdominal pain at multidetector CT. Radiographics 31(4):927-947, 2011.

Raptopoulos V et al: Peritoneal carcinomatosis. Eur Radiol 11(11):2195-2206, 2001.

Reddy SA et al: Clinical observations: diagnosis of transmesocolic internal hernia as a complication of retrocolic gastric bypass: CT imaging criteria. AJR 189:52-55, 2007.

Rees O et al: Multidetector-row CT of right hemidiaphragmatic rupture caused by blunt trauma: a review of 12 cases. Clin Radiol 60(12):1280-1289, 2005.

Robinson P et al: Inguinofemoral hernia: accuracy of sonography in patients with indeterminate clinical features. AJR 187(5):1168-1178, 2006.

Sai VF et al: Colonoscopy after CT diagnosis of diverticulitis to exclude colon. Radiology 263:383-390, 2012.

Schwartz SA et al: CT findings of rupture, impending rupture, and contained rupture of abdominal aortic aneurysms. AJR 188(1):W57-W62, 2007.

Shadbolt CL et al: Imaging of groin masses: inguinal anatomy and pathologic conditions revisited. Radiographics 21(Spec. No):S261-S271, 2001.

Shinagare AB et al: Pictorial essay: A to Z of desmoid tumors. Am J Roentgenol 197(6):W1008-W1014, 2011.

Singh AK et al: Neoplastic iliopsoas masses in oncology patients: CT findings. Abdom Imaging 33(4):493-497, 2008.

Singh AK et al: Omental infarct: CT imaging features. Abdom Imaging 31:549-554, 2006.

Sunnapwar A et al: Taxonomy and imaging spectrum of small bowel obstruction after Roux-en-Y gastric bypass surgery. AJR 194:120-128, 2010.

Tamsma JT et al: Pathogenesis of malignant ascites: Starling's law of capillary hemodynamics revisited. Ann Oncol 12(10):1353-1357, 2001.

Tateishi U et al: Nodal status of malignant lymphoma in pelvic and retroperitoneal lymphatic pathways: PET/CT. Abdom Imaging 35(2):232-240, 2010.

Thornton E et al: Pattern of the month: patterns of fat stranding. AJR 197: W1-W14, 2011.

Ti JP et al: Pictorial essay: imaging features of encapsulating peritoneal sclerosis in continuous ambulatory peritoneal dialysis patients. AJR 195:W50-W54, 2010.

Tirkes T et al: Peritoneal and retroperitoneal anatomy and its relevance for cross-sectional imaging. Radiographics 32(2):437-451, 2012.

Tombak MC et al: Clinical perspective: an unusual cause of intestinal obstruction: abdominal cocoon. AJR 194:W176-W178, 2010.

Wong WL et al: Best cases from the AFIP: multicystic mesothelioma. Radiographics 24(1):247-250, 2004.

Zarvan NP et al: Abdominal hernias: CT findings. AJR 164:1391-1395, 1995.

Index

Page numbers followed by *f* indicate figures; *t*, tables; *b*, boxes.

T